AF511992

Clinical Obstetrics and Gynecology

History Taking, Case Discussion, Practical Viva Voce Topics, and OSCE

Second Edition

As per the Competency-Based Medical Curriculum

Clinical Obstetrics and Gynecology

History Taking, Case Discussion, Practical Viva Voce Topics, and OSCE

Second Edition

As per the Competency-Based Medical Curriculum

Sharmila Arun Babu

MBBS, MS ObsGyn (JIPMER), Dip. RM, FMAS, MBA (HM)
Additional Professor and Head
Department of Obstetrics and Gynecology
All India Institute of Medical Sciences (AIIMS)
Mangalagiri, Andhra Pradesh, India

Wolters Kluwer

Sr. *Publishing Manager:* P Sangeetha
Development Editor: Dr Richa Sharma
Production Editor: Pooja Chauhan
Assistant Manager-Manufacturing: Sumit Johry

Copyright © 2023 by Wolters Kluwer (India) Pvt. Ltd.

3rd Floor, Tower B, Building No. 10, Phase – II, DLF Cyber City
Gurgaon, Haryana - 122002

All rights reserved. This product, consisting of the printed book, is protected by copyright. No part of this book may be reproduced in any form or by any means, including photocopying, or utilized by any information storage and retrieval system without written permission from the copyright owner.

The publisher is not responsible (as a matter of product liability, negligence, or otherwise) for any injury resulting from any material contained herein. This publication contains information relating to obstetrics and gynecology that should not be construed as specific instructions for individual patients. Manufacturers' product information and package inserts should be reviewed for current information, including contraindications, dosages, and precautions. All products/brands/names/processes cited in this book are the properties of their respective owners. Reference herein to any specific commercial products, processes, or services by trade name, trademark, manufacturer, or otherwise is purely for academic purposes and does not constitute or imply endorsement, recommendation, or favoring by the publisher. The views and opinions of authors expressed herein do not necessarily state or reflect those of the publisher, and shall not be used for advertising or product endorsement purposes.

Care has been taken to confirm the accuracy of the information presented and to describe generally accepted practices. However, the authors, editors, and publishers are not responsible for errors or omissions or for any consequences from application of the information in this book and make no warranty, expressed or implied, with respect to the currency, completeness, or accuracy of the contents of the publication. Application of this information in a particular situation remains the professional responsibility of the practitioner. Readers are urged to confirm that the information, especially with regard to drug dose/usage, complies with current legislation and standards of practice.

Please consult full prescribing information before issuing prescription for any product mentioned in the publication.

The publishers have made every effort to trace copyright holders for borrowed material. If they have inadvertently overlooked any, they will be pleased to make the necessary arrangements at the first opportunity.

First Edition, 2019
Second Edition,2022
Sixth Impression, 2025
ISBN: 978-93-93553-35-5

Published by Wolters Kluwer (India) Pvt. Ltd., Gurgaon
Compositor: B2K - Bytes 2 Knowledge
Printed and bound at *SDR Printers, Trans Delhi Signature City, Ghaziabad (U.P.)*

For product enquiry, please contact– Marketing Department (marketing@wolterskluwerindia.co.in) or log on to our website www.wolterskluwerindia.co.in.

Dedicated to

My parents, for their unconditional support and blessings
My teachers, for teaching me the ABCs of Medicine
My husband, Dr Arun Babu, for believing in my abilities and motivating me to write this book
My kids, Akshaya and Akash, for sacrificing their share of time with me

Preface to the Second Edition

We are extremely pleased and excited in bringing out the second edition of *Clinical Obstetrics and Gynecology* following the resounding success and popularity of the first edition. The driving force for this edition has been the positive feedback and appreciation from students and faculty across the country. The first edition, which primarily aimed at the complete coverage of clinical aspects in obstetrics and gynecology, has given students the confidence to face the practical examination. While retaining the essence of the first edition, the content has been thoroughly revised and updated to include the latest clinical recommendations and guidelines.

The current emphasis in medical education is on integration of knowledge with skills, attitude, and communication. Competency-based medical education (CBME) has been introduced to make medical education learner centric as well as to help students become competency-based learners thereby enabling them to serve the patients and community better. To be in line with the new curriculum, the content has been meticulously updated focusing on the practical aspects.

Chapters in Parts 1 and 2 that include obstetric and gynecology clinical cases presented in a systematic format have been revised as per the recent guidelines; practical viva voce topics in Part 3 that serve as a ready reckoner during preparation for clinical exams have been updated with new color images, illustrations, and surgical procedures. This edition features a new Part 4 on Objective structured Clinical examination (OSCE) which has been introduced as per the requirement of the new CBME. This section gives a detailed step-by-step description of the clinical procedures, examination, counseling sessions, and informed consent that can appear in OSCE practical exam.

The special features of the first edition such as *High-yield points, Viva corner, Note, Extra edge, Frequently asked viva questions* and practical viva voce topics—largely responsible for the success of the book—have been retained with updated and revised content. Bulleted points, simple illustrations, and tables which were the other highlights of the first edition have been retained in this edition as well. All these will serve to make reading, understanding, and retention easier and effective.

This book covers all the practical aspects of the new CBME curriculum making it a "one-stop solution" for students. Extreme care has been taken to include accurate information and most recent evidence-based guidelines in each chapter. The content has been thoroughly peer-reviewed by subject experts of national repute.

I sincerely hope that this thoroughly updated second edition will be of immense value to the medical students and practicing clinicians. For updates about the book, please visit Facebook page http://www.facebook.com/sharmila.author. Feedback regarding the book will be appreciated.

Sharmila Arun Babu
sharu_jipmer@yahoo.co.in

Preface to the First Edition

It gives me great pleasure in bringing out this book which is primarily aimed at complete coverage of clinical aspects in obstetrics and gynecology.

Case presentation and case discussion are an integral part of teaching in medicine. During clinical exams, a medical student is expected to demonstrate knowledge and skills in history taking, clinical examination, case presentation, and case discussion which includes arriving at a diagnosis and planning management strategies. As a medical teacher and examiner in obstetrics and gynecology, I have observed that medical students often struggle to understand basic clinical concepts and they face difficulty in demonstrating clinical skills. I have always felt the need for a single comprehensive book which will help students acquire all the necessary knowledge and skills to deal with the clinical aspects in obstetrics and gynecology. This motivated me to come up with this book which deals with all the aspects that a medical student needs to know while preparing for clinical exams.

This book covers clinical cases and practical viva voce topics, making it a "one-stop solution" for the students and practicing clinicians. I have incorporated a systematic approach while discussing the clinical cases which can be appreciated while reading this book. Bulleted points, simple illustrations, tables, and colored images are the highlights of this book that will make reading, understanding, and retention easier and effective. *High-yield points, Viva corner, Note,* and *Extra edge* are special segments included in each chapter to create interest in the reader and to avoid monotony. This book also includes an elaborate part on practical viva voce topics in the subject that will serve as a ready reckoner during preparation for clinical exams. Extreme care has been taken to include accurate information and most recent evidence-based guidelines in each topic. The content has been thoroughly peer-reviewed independently by experts in the field.

I would like to thank Mrs Sangeetha Parthasarathy, Sr. Publishing Manager, for being a huge pillar of support to this project. I would also like to extend my sincere appreciation and thanks to Dr Vallika Devi Katragadda and the entire production team of Wolters Kluwer (India) for bringing out this book. Last but not the least, I thank my husband, Dr Arun Babu, for being a great source of inspiration and motivating me to edit this book.

I sincerely hope that this book will be of immense value to the medical students and practicing clinicians. Any feedback regarding the book will be appreciated. Write to the author at sharu_jipmer@yahoo.co.in.

For updates about the book, please visit Facebook page, Clinical Obstetrics and Gynecology by Dr Sharmila Arun Babu (http://www.facebook.com/sharmila.author)

Sharmila Arun Babu

Acknowledgments

I would like to thank my teachers and mentors at my alma mater, JIPMER, for imparting the knowledge and skills that are helping me in my career everyday and have enabled me to edit this book.

I would like to express my everlasting gratitude to the elders in my family—Mr. Vijayan and Mrs. Sagoundala (my parents) and Mr. Thirunavukkarasu and Mrs. Sampurnam (my in-laws) for their wishes and blessings.

I thank my husband Dr. Arun Babu for being a huge pillar of strength, a great source of inspiration, and for encouraging me to push my boundaries, and my children Akshaya and Akash for sacrificing their share of time with me.

I want to sincerely thank the faculty and resident reviewers for reviewing the chapters despite their busy schedule. I am grateful to all the students and faculty members who have always supported and encouraged me since the time of release of the first edition.

I would also like to extend my heartfelt gratitude to Prof. (Dr.) Mukesh Tripathi, Director and CEO, AIIMS, Mangalagiri, for all his support and wishes.

My sincere gratitude and thanks to the team at Wolters Kluwer (India): Ms. Sheenam Aggarwal, Associate Director-Content Management & Publishing, for encouraging me to go forward with this edition; Ms. Sangeetha Parthasarathy, Sr. Publishing Manager, for being a huge pillar of support to this project right from the first edition; Dr. Richa Sharma, Development Editor, for her excellent and diligent editing work and the entire production team for bringing out this book.

Last but not the least, I would like to thank God Almighty for giving me the strength, knowledge, and opportunity to work on this book.

Sharmila Arun Babu

Acknowledgments

Reviewers

Faculty Reviewers

Anitha Yadav
Associate Professor
Department of OBG
AIIMS, Nagpur

Anshuja Singla
Professor
Department of OBG
UCMS & GTB Hospital, New Delhi

Banishree Pati
Associate Professor
Department of OBG
HIMS, Jollygrant, Uttarakhand

Bupathy A
Senior Professor
Department of OBG
SMVMC & RI, Puducherry

Chitra T
Additional Professor
Department of OBG
JIPMER, Puducherry

Dilip Kumar Maurya
Professor
Department of OBG
JIPMER, Puducherry

Habeebullah Syed
Senior Professor
Department of OBG
MGMCRI, Puducherry

Hemali Heidi Sinha
Professor and Head
Department of OBG
AIIMS, Patna

Ipshita Mohapatra
Associate Professor
Department of OBG
AIIMS, Kalyani

Jasmina Begum
Assistant Professor
Department of OBG
AIIMS, Bhubaneshwar

Kanika Chopra
Assistant Professor
Department of OBG
LHMC, New Delhi

Kavitha Garikapati
Assistant Professor
Department of OBG
AIIMS, Mangalagiri

Latha Chaturvedula
Senior Professor
Department of OBG
JIPMER, Puducherry

Medha Davikle
Assistant Professor
Department of OBG
AIIMS, Nagpur

Mukta Agarwal
Additional Professor
Department of OBG
AIIMS, Patna

Murali S
Additional Professor
Department of OBG
JIPMER, Puducherry

Nabnita Patnaik
Additional Professor and Head
Department of OBG
AIIMS, Bibinagar

Naina Kumar
Associate Professor
Department of OBG
AIIMS, Bibinagar

Natasha Gupta
Assistant Professor
Department of OBG
AIIMS, Jammu

Neha Gangane
Assistant Professor
Department of OBG
AIIMS, Nagpur

Papa Dasari
Senior Professor
Department of OBG
JIPMER, Puducherry

Pushpalatha K
Additional Professor and Head
Department of OBG
AIIMS, Bhopal

Pragati Trigunait
Assistant Professor
Department of OBG
AIIMS, Mangalagiri

Pratibha Singh
Professor and Head
Department of OBG
AIIMS, Jodhpur

Priyanka Garg
Associate Professor
Department of OBG
AIIMS, Bathinda

Priyanka Kathuria
Associate Professor
Department of OBG
AIIMS, Jodhpur

Priyanka Rai
Associate Professor
Department of OBG
AIIMS, Deoghar

Priyanka Yoga
Assistant Professor
Department of OBG
AIIMS, Mangalagiri

Rajlaxmi Mundhra
Associate Professor
Department of OBG
AIIMS, Rishikesh

Reddy Rani
Senior Professor (Retd.)
Department of OBG
JIPMER, Puducherry

Renu Sharma
Associate Professor
Department of OBG
AIIMS, Jammu

Rupa Vani K
Associate Professor
Department of OBG
IGMC & RI, Puducherry

Sairem Mangolnganbi Chanu
Associate Professor
Department of OBG
AIIMS, Mangalagiri

Sarita Agrawal
Professor and Head
Department of OBG
AIIMS, Raipur

Sasirekha R
Professor
Department of OBG
JIPMER, Puducherry

Saubhagya Kumar Jena
Professor and Head
Department of OBG
AIIMS, Bhubaneshwar

Suchita Mundle
Professor and Head
Department of OBG
AIIMS, Nagpur

Sushruti Kaushal
Assistant Professor
Department of OBG
AIIMS, Bilaspur

Thirunavukkarasu Arun Babu
Additional Professor and Head
Department of Pediatrics
AIIMS, Mangalagiri

Veena P
Professor
Department of OBG
JIPMER, Puducherry

Resident Reviewers

- **Deepti Yedla**, Senior Resident, Department of OBG, AIIMS, Mangalagiri.
- **Gaurang Narayan**, MBBS Graduate, Diplomate in Medical Law and Ethics National Law School of Indian University, Bengaluru.
- **Padmapriya**, Resident, Department of Pathology, Andhra Medical College, Andhra Pradesh.
- **Shalini Singh**, Senior Resident, Department of OBG, AIIMS, Mangalagiri.

Student Reviewers

- **Chandrasekar**, MBBS Student AIIMS, Mangalagiri.
- **Liya Aji**, MBBS Student AIIMS, Mangalagiri.
- **Soumika Kesani**, MBBS Student AIIMS, Mangalagiri.

Faculty Reviewers (Previous edition)

- **Gowri Dorairajan**, Professor and Head, Department of OBG, JIPMER, Puducherry.
- **Hima Bindu**, Professor, Department of OBG, IGMC & RI, Puducherry.
- **Jayalakshmi**, Professor, Department of OBG, JIPMER, Puducherry.
- **Minakshi Vivek Shukla**, Assistant Professor, Department of OBG, Dr DY Patil Med College, Navi Mumbai.
- **Sabita Saichandan**, Professor and Head, Department of OBG, IGMCRI, Puducherry.
- **Seetesh Ghose**, Professor, Department of OBG, MGMCRI, Puducherry.
- **Sindhuja Sekar**, Assistant Professor, Department of OBG, SVMCRI, Puducherry.
- **Shyjus P**, Consultant, ARMC IVF Fertility Centre, Kannur, Kerala.
- **Swaramya C**, Consultant, Department of OBG, East Coast Hospitals, Puducherry.
- **Usha Rani**, Professor, Department of OBG, SRMC, Porur, Chennai.

Publisher's Acknowledgments

The Publisher would like to thank the following for their reviews and recommendations of the first edition.

Faculty

Aparajita Sophia D'Souza, Professor and Head, Department of Obstetrics and Gynecology, ESIC Medical College, Hyderabad, Telangana.

K Chitra, Professor and Head, Department of Obstetrics and Gynecology, Velammal Hospital and Medical College, Madurai, Tamil Nadu.

M G Dhanalakshmi, Professor, Department of Obstetrics and Gynecology, Sri Ramachandra Institute of Higher Education and Research, Chennai, Tamil Nadu.

K Durga, Associate Professor, Department of Obstetrics and Gynecology, Sri Lakshmi Narayana Institute of Medical, Sciences (SLIMS), Puducherry.

P B Hiremath, Professor and Head, Department of Obstetrics and Gynecology, Sri Venkateswaraa Medical College Hospital & Research Institute (SVMC&RI), Puducherry.

M Jayalakshmi, Professor and Head, Department of Obstetrics and Gynecology, Maharaja Institute of Medical Sciences, Vizianagaram, Andhra Pradesh.

R Jayanthi, Professor and Head, Department of Obstetrics and Gynecology, Meenakshi Medical College Hospital and Research Institute, Kancheepuram, Tamil Nadu.

Mahati Sudhakar, Assistant Professor, Department of Obstetrics and Gynecology, NRI Medical College, Visakhapatnam, Andhra Pradesh.

R Manomani, Professor and Head, Department of Obstetrics and Gynecology, Coimbatore Medical College, Coimbatore, Tamil Nadu.

Parvathy Deth, Associate Professor, Department of Obstetrics and Gynecology, Government Medical College, Ernakulam, Kerala.

Pradeep Patil, Assistant Professor, Department of Obstetrics and Gynecology, Ashwini Rural Medical College, Solapur, Maharashtra.

Pradeep S, Professor, Department of Obstetrics and Gynecology, PES Medical College, Kuppam, Andhra Pradesh.

T Punithavathi, Associate Professor, Department of Obstetrics and Gynecology, Government Medical College and ESIC Hospital, Coimbatore, Tamil Nadu.

B Rajeshwari, Professor and Head, Department of Obstetrics and Gynecology, Osmania Medical College, Hyderabad, Telangana.

Rajkumar Patange, Professor and Head, Department of Obstetrics and Gynecology, Krishna Institute of Medical Science, Karad, Maharashtra.

Ramalingam K, Professor, Department of Obstetrics and Gynecology, N R I Academy of Sciences, Guntur District, Andhra Pradesh.

N Rekha, Professor and Head, Department of Obstetrics and Gynecology, BGS Global Institute of Medical Sciences, Bengaluru, Karnataka.

Rohini N S, Professor and Head, Department of Obstetrics and Gynecology, Akash Institute of Medical Sciences and Research Centre, Bengaluru, Karnataka.

B M Rupakala, Professor and Unit Chief, Department of Obstetrics and Gynecology, RajaRajeswari Medical College and Hospital, Bengaluru, Karnataka.

M P A Sailakshmi, Professor and Head, Department of Obstetrics and Gynecology, RajaRajeswari Medical College and Hospital, Bengaluru, Karnataka.

Sangeetha Shah, Professor and Head, Department of Obstetrics and Gynecology, Gandhi Medical College, Hyderabad, Telangana.

K A Sarumathy, Assistant Professor, Department of Obstetrics and Gynecology, Aarupadai Veedu Medical College, Puducherry.

Sathiya, Professor, Department of Obstetrics and Gynecology, Melmaruvathur Adiparasakthi Institute of Medical Sciences and Research, Melmaruvathur, Tamil Nadu.

Seetha Panicker, Professor and Head, Department of Obstetrics and Gynecology, PSG Institute of Medical Sciences and Research, Coimbatore, Tamil Nadu.

Shashikala Karanth, Professor, Department of Obstetrics and Gynecology, St. Johns Medical College and Hospital, Bengaluru, Karnataka.

Shilpa Kshirsagar, Associate Professor, Department of Obstetrics and Gynecology, Dr D Y Patil Medical College, Pune, Maharashtra.

Shilpa Naik, Assistant Professor, Department of Obstetrics and Gynecology, B J Govt Medical College, Pune, Maharashtra.

Shiny Varghese, Ex-Professor OBG CMC Ludhiana, *Presently,* Senior Consultant and Head, Department of Obstetrics and Gynecology, Bangalore Baptist Hospital, Bengaluru, Karnataka.

Shreedhar Venkatesh, Principal cum Professor, Department of Obstetrics and Gynecology, Vydehi Institute of Medical Sciences and Research Centre, Bengaluru, Karnataka.

Smitha M V, Associate Professor, AIIMS College of Nursing, Bhubaneswar, Odisha.

Suparna Grover, Professor, Department of Obstetrics and Gynecology, Government Medical College, Amritsar, Punjab.

Sushma Sharma, Professor and Head, Department of Obstetrics and Gynecology, Maharashtra Institute of Medical Education and Research, Pune, Maharashtra.

V Usha Rani, Professor and Head, Department of Obstetrics and Gynecology, Mahaveer Medical College, Vikarabad, Telangana.

Vidya Gaikwad, Professor, Department of Obstetrics and Gynecology, Dr D Y Patil Medical College, Pune, Maharashtra.

G Vijayalakshmi, Professor and Head, Department of Obstetrics and Gynecology, Bhaskar Medical College, Hyderabad, Telangana.

Students

Aisiri Deepak, MBBS Third Year, BGS Global Institute of Medical Sciences, Bengaluru, Karnataka.

Ajinkya Shende, MBBS Final Year, Lokmanya Tilak Municipal Medical College, Mumbai, Maharashtra.

Ananya G Gupta, MBBS Third Year, Pramukh Swami Medical College, Karamsad, Gujarat.

Avinash, MBBS Intern, Andhra Medical College, Visakhapatnam, Andhra Pradesh.

Bhumika C, MBBS Third Year, BGS Global Institute of Medical Sciences, Bengaluru, Karnataka.

Charan V, MBBS Intern, Andhra Medical College, Visakhapatnam, Andhra Pradesh.

Dev Pandhi, MBBS Final Year, Smt. NHL Municipal Medical College, Ahmedabad, Gujarat.

Diteshna, MBBS Third Year, NRI Medical College, Visakhapatnam, Andhra Pradesh.

Deena Mariyam, Vice President, South Indian Medical Student's Association, Kempegowda Institute of Medical Science, Bengaluru, Karnataka.

Divyanshi, MBBS Final Year, Ramaiah Medical College, Bengaluru, Karnataka.

Joshita Veeramachineni, MBBS Intern, Andhra Medical College, Visakhapatnam, Andhra Pradesh.

Kavya, MBBS Final Year, Dr D Y Patil Medical College, Pune, Maharashtra.

Kiran Krishna A S, MBBS Intern, Mount Zion Medical College, Adoor, Kerala.

Kishan G Adodariya, MBBS Final year, B J Medical College, Ahmedabad, Gujarat.

Kriti Barui, MSc (Nursing) II Year, Obstetrics and Gynaecological Nursing, AIIMS College of Nursing, Bhubaneswar, Odisha.

Krutarth Thacker, MBBS Final Year, B J Medical College, Ahmedabad, Gujarat.

Krutik P Modi, MBBS Third Year, B J Medical College, Ahmedabad, Gujarat.

Niharika Naresh, MBBS Intern, Bengaluru Medical College and Research Institute, Bengaluru, Karnataka.

Prasham Shah, MBBS Final Year, Pramukh Swami Medical College, Karamsad, Gujarat.

Prem Shah, MBBS Final Year, Pramukh Swami Medical College, Karamsad, Gujarat.

Prudhvi Kalyan, MBBS Third Year, Government Medical College, Suryapet, Telangana.

Radhika Agarwal, MBBS Final Year, Government Medical College, Gondia, Maharashtra.

Sajith KM, MBBS Intern, Sri Ramachandra Institute of Higher Education and Research, Chennai, Tamil Nadu.

Sanil Karanth, MBBS Final Year, St. Johns Medical College and Hospital, Bengaluru, Karnataka.

Saurabh Sangam, MBBS Third Year, Sri Siddhartha Institute of Medical Sciences and Research Center, Bangalore, Karnataka.

Sindhu S, MBBS Final Year, MVJ Medical College and Research Hospital, Hoskote, Karnataka, Bengaluru, Karnataka.

Sharanu Rajole, MBBS Final Year, Joint Secretary, BMCRI Students' Association, Bangalore Medical College and Research Institute, Bengaluru, Karnataka.

Shimoni Jain, MBBS Final Year, General Secretary, BMCRI Students' Association, Bangalore Medical College and Research Institute, Bengaluru, Karnataka.

Shobith M A, MBBS Final Year, Cultural Secretary, BMCRI Students' Association, Bangalore Medical College and Research Institute, Bengaluru, Karnataka.

Sreelal, MBBS Intern, ESIC Medical College, Hyderabad, Telangana.

A Sri Amrutha Sai, MS (OG) Third Year, Obstetrics and Gynaecology, Stanley Medical College, Chennai, Tamil Nadu.

Sushrut Agarwal, MBBS Final Year, Maulana Azad Medical College, Delhi.

Shushrutha K, MBBS Final Year, MVJ Medical College and Research Hospital, Hoskote, Karnataka.

Suvarna Sharma, MBBS Third Year, Sri Siddhartha Institute of Medical Sciences and Research Center, Bengaluru, Karnataka.

Swarnim Deshwal, MBBS Final Year, Lady Hardinge Medical College, Delhi.

Tanvi Deshpande, MBBS Final Year, St. Johns Medical College and Hospital, Bengaluru, Karnataka.

Tanya Avis Cherian, MBBS Final Year, Kempegowda Institute of Medical Sciences, Hoskote, Karnataka.

Umme Shifa, MBBS Final Year, Kempegowda Institute of Medical Sciences, Bengaluru, Karnataka.

Vaishali Goswami, MBBS Final Year, Dr. BSA Medical College, Delhi.

Veerapaneni Kiran, MBBS Intern, ACS Medical College and Hospital, Chennai, Tamil Nadu.

Contents

CBME Topics*

The following competencies are covered in the scope of Clinical Obstetrics and Gynecology.

Competency No.	Competency Description	Chapter No.
Part 1 – Obstetrics		
OG8.1	Enumerate, describe and discuss the objectives of antenatal care, assessment of period of gestation; screening for high-risk factors.	1
OG8.2	Elicit document and present an obstetric history including menstrual history, last menstrual period, previous obstetric history, comorbid conditions, past medical history and surgical history	1
OG8.3	Describe, demonstrate, document and perform an obstetrical examination including a general and abdominal examination and clinical monitoring of maternal and fetal well-being	1
OG8.7	Enumerate the indications for and types of vaccination in pregnancy	1
OG8.8	Enumerate the indications and describe the investigations including the use of ultrasound in the initial assessment and monitoring in pregnancy	1
OG9.1	Classify, define and discuss the aetiology and management of abortions including threatened, incomplete, inevitable, missed and septic	1
OG35.1	Obtain a logical sequence of history, and perform a humane and thorough clinical examination, excluding internal examinations (per-rectal and per-vaginal)	1
OG35.2	Arrive at a logical provisional diagnosis after examination.	1
OG12.2	Define, classify and describe the etiology, pathophysiology, diagnosis, investigations, adverse effects on the mother and foetus and the management during pregnancy and labor, and complications of anemia in pregnancy	2
OG12.3	Define, classify and describe the etiology, pathophysiology, diagnosis, investigations, criteria, adverse effects on the mother and foetus and the management during pregnancy and labor, and complications of diabetes in pregnancy	3
OG12.1	Define, classify and describe the etiology and pathophysiology, early detection, investigations; principles of management of hypertensive disorders of pregnancy and eclampsia, complications of eclampsia	4
OG12.4	Define, classify and describe the etiology, pathophysiology, diagnosis, investigations, criteria, adverse effects on the mother and foetus and the management during pregnancy and labor, and complications of heart diseases in pregnancy	5
OG14.3	Describe and discuss rupture uterus, causes, diagnosis and management	6
OG13.2	Define, describe the causes, pathophysiology, diagnosis, investigations and management of preterm labor, PROM and postdated pregnancy	7

Reference: National Medical Commission. Competency Based Undergraduate Curriculum for the Indian Medical Graduate, Vol. 3 (2018), pages 100 to 129. Available at https://www.nmc.org.in/wp-content/uploads/2020/01/UG-Curriculum-Vol-III.pdf

Competency No.	Competency Description	Chapter No.
OG11.1	Describe the etiopathology, clinical features; diagnosis and investigations, complications, principles of management of multiple pregnancies	8
OG14.2	Discuss the mechanism of normal labor, Define and describe obstructed labor, its clinical features; prevention; and management	9
OG12.8	Describe the mechanism, prophylaxis, fetal complications, diagnosis and management of isoimmunization in pregnancy	10
OG16.3	Describe and discuss causes, clinical features, diagnosis, investigations; monitoring of fetal well-being, including ultrasound and fetal Doppler; principles of management; prevention and counselling in intrauterine growth retardation	11
OG13.2	Define, describe the causes, pathophysiology, diagnosis, investigations and management of preterm labor, PROM and postdated pregnancy	13
OG10.1	Define, classify and describe the aetiology, pathogenesis, clinical features, ultrasonography, differential diagnosis and management of antepartum haemorrhage in pregnancy	15
OG10.2	Enumerate the indications and describe the appropriate use of blood and blood products, their complications and management.	15
OG8.5	Describe and demonstrate pelvic assessment in a model	16
OG5.2	Determine maternal high risk factors and verify immunization status	17.I
OG13.1	Enumerate and discuss the physiology of normal labor, mechanism of labor in occipito-anterior presentation; monitoring of labor including partogram; conduct of labor, pain relief; principles of induction and acceleration of labor; management of third stage of labor.	17.II
OG13.3	Observe/assist in the performance of an artificial rupture of membranes	17.II
OG16.1	Enumerate and discuss causes, prevention, diagnosis, management, appropriate use of blood and blood products in postpartum haemorrhage	17.III
OG35.16	Diagnose and provide emergency management of antepartum and postpartum hemorrhage in a simulated/guided environment	17.III
OG19.1	Describe and discuss the physiology of puerperium, its complications, diagnosis and management; counselling for contraception, puerperal sterilization	17.IV
Part 2 – Gynecology		
OG35.1	Obtain a logical sequence of history, and perform a humane and thorough clinical examination, excluding internal examinations (perrectal and per-vaginal)	18
OG35.2	Arrive at a logical provisional diagnosis after examination.	18
OG24.1	Define, classify and discuss abnormal uterine bleeding, its aetiology, clinical features, investigations, diagnosis and management	19
OG29.1	Describe and discuss the etiology; pathology; clinical features; differential diagnosis; investigations; principles of management, complications of fibroid uterus	20
OG34.2	Describe and discuss the etiology, pathology, classification, staging of ovarian cancer, clinical features, differential diagnosis, investigations, principal of management including staging laparotomy	21
OG33.1	Classify, describe and discuss the etiology, pathology, clinical features, differential diagnosis, investigations and staging of cervical cancer	22

Competency No.	Competency Description	Chapter No.
OG33.2	Describe the principles of management including surgery and radiotherapy of Benign, Pre-malignant (CIN) and Malignant Lesions of the Cervix	22
OG33.3	Describe and demonstrate the screening for cervical cancer in a simulated environment	22
OG33.4	Enumerate the methods to prevent cancer of cervix including visual inspection with acetic acid (VIA), visual inspection of cervix with Lugol's iodine (VILI), pap smear and colposcopy	22
OG32.2	Enumerate the causes of postmenopausal bleeding and describe its management	23
OG34.1	Describe and discuss aetiology, pathology, staging clinical features, differential diagnosis, investigations, staging laparotomy and principles of management of endometrial cancer	23
OG31.1	Describe and discuss the etiology, classification, clinical features, diagnosis, investigations, principles of management and preventive aspects of prolapse of uterus	24
OG28.1	Describe and discuss the common causes, pathogenesis, clinical features, differential diagnosis; investigations; principles of management of infertility – methods of tubal patency, ovulation induction, assisted reproductive techniques	25
OG28.2	Enumerate the assessment and restoration of tubal latency	25
OG28.3	Describe the principles of ovulation induction	25
OG28.4	Enumerate the various Assisted Reproduction Techniques	25
OG25.1	Describe and discuss the causes of primary and secondary amenorrhea, its investigation and the principles of management.	26
OG30.1	Describe and discuss the etiopathogenesis; clinical features; differential diagnosis; investigations; management, complications of PCOS	26
OG22.1	Describe the clinical characteristics of physiological vaginal discharge.	27
OG22.2	Describe and discuss the etiology (with special emphasis on Candida, T. vaginalis, bacterial vaginosis), characteristics, clinical diagnosis, investigations, genital hygiene, management of common causes and the syndromic management	27
Part 3 – Practical Viva Voce Topics		
OG21.1	Describe and discuss the temporary and permanent methods of contraception, indications, technique and complications; selection of patients, side effects and failure rate including Ocs, male contraception, emergency contraception and IUCD	31
OG21.2	Describe & discuss PPIUCD programme	31
OG8.5	Describe and demonstrate pelvic assessment in a model	32
OG14.1	Enumerate and discuss the diameters of maternal pelvis and types	32
OG13.1	Enumerate and discuss the physiology of normal labor, mechanism of labor in occipito-anterior presentation; monitoring of labor including partogram; conduct of labor, pain relief; principles of induction and acceleration of labor; management of third stage of labor.	33
OG13.3	Observe/assist in the performance of an artificial rupture of membranes	33
OG13.5	Observe and assist the conduct of a normal vaginal delivery	33

Competency No.	Competency Description	Chapter No.
OG14.2	Discuss the mechanism of normal labor, Define and describe obstructed labor, its clinical features; prevention; and management	33
OG14.4	Describe and discuss the classification; diagnosis; management of abnormal labor	34
OG13.1	Enumerate and discuss the physiology of normal labor, mechanism of labor in occipito-anterior presentation; monitoring of labor including partogram; conduct of labor, pain relief; principles of induction and acceleration of labor; management of third stage of labor.	35
OG8.4	Describe and demonstrate clinical monitoring of maternal and fetal well-being	36
OG9.2	Describe the steps and observe/assist in the performance of an MTP evacuation	37
OG15.1	Enumerate and describe the indications and steps of common obstetric procedures, technique and complications: Episiotomy, vacuum extraction; low forceps; Caesarean section, assisted breech delivery; external cephalic version; cervical cerclage	37
OG19.3	Observe/assist in the performance of tubal ligation	37
OG20.1	Enumerate the indications and describe and discuss the legal aspects, indications, methods for first and second trimester MTP; complications and management of complications of Medical Termination of Pregnancy	37
OG37.1	Observe and assist in the performance of a Caesarean section	37
OG37.6	Observe and assist in the performance of outlet forceps application of vacuum and breech delivery	37
OG37.7	Observe and assist in the performance of MTP in the first trimester and evacuation in incomplete abortion	37
OG34.4	Operative Gynaecology: Understand and describe the technique and complications: Dilatation & Curettage (D&C); EA-ECC; cervical biopsy; abdominal hysterectomy; myomectomy; surgery for ovarian tumours; staging laparotomy; vaginal hysterectomy including pelvic floor repair; Fothergill's operation, Laparoscopy; hysteroscopy; management of postoperative complications	38
OG36.3	Demonstrate the correct technique of biopsy of uterus in a simulated/supervised environment	38
OG37.2	Observe and assist in the performance of Laparotomy	38
OG37.3	Observe and assist in the performance of Hysterectomy – abdominal/vaginal	38
OG37.4	Observe and assist in the performance of Dilatation & Curettage (D&C)	38
OG37.5	Observe and assist in the performance of Endometrial aspiration - endocervical curettage (EA-ECC)	38
OG38.1	Laparoscopy	38
OG38.2	Hysteroscopy	38
Part 4 – Objective Structured Clinical Examination (OSCE)		
OG18.2	Demonstrate the steps of neonatal resuscitation in a simulated environment	39
OG19.4	Enumerate the indications for, describe the steps in and insert and remove an intrauterine device in a simulated environment	39
OG35.5	Determine gestational age, EDD and obstetric formula	39

Competency No.	Competency Description	Chapter No.
OG35.6	Demonstrate ethical behavior in all aspects of medical practice.	39
OG35.12	Obtain a PAP smear in a stimulated environment	39
OG35.13	Demonstrate the correct technique to perform artificial rupture of membranes in a simulated/supervised environment	39
OG35.14	Demonstrate the correct technique to perform and suture episiotomies in a simulated/supervised environment	39
OG35.15	Demonstrate the correct technique to insert and remove an IUD in a simulated/supervised environment	39
OG35.17	Demonstrate the correct technique of urinary catheterisation in a simulated/ supervised environment	39
OG36.3	Demonstrate the correct technique of punch biopsy of uterus in a simulated/ supervised environment	39
OG8.6	Assess and counsel a patient in a simulated environment regarding appropriate nutrition in pregnancy	40
OG13.4	Demonstrate the stages of normal labor in a simulated environment/ mannequin and counsel on methods of safe abortion.	40
OG19.2	Counsel in a simulated environment, contraception and puerperal sterilisation	40
OG35.4	Demonstrate interpersonal and communication skills befitting a physician in order to discuss illness and its outcome with patient and family	40
OG35.7	Obtain informed consent for any examination/procedure	40
OG20.2	In a simulated environment administer informed consent to a person wishing to undergo Medical Termination of Pregnancy	41

Part 1

Obstetrics

1 History Taking and Examination

Introduction

History in medicine refers to recording of the medical events that have already taken place in the patient. Physical examination is determination of the clinical state of the patient at the time of examination of the patient. Every disease has a behavior pattern; a well-recorded history and physical examination combined with a sound knowledge of the subject will help the doctor in identifying the likely cause of the patient's problem in majority of the cases. Therefore, history taking and physical examination are the fundamental tools that help the physician in making a provisional diagnosis, based on which further evaluation is done.

Clinical competency expected from the medical students in the subject of Obstetrics and Gynecology includes the ability to:

- Elicit a detailed obstetric history in a normal pregnancy and in a pregnancy with complications
- Carry out general, systemic, and obstetric examinations in a normal pregnancy and in a pregnancy with complications
- Summarize and integrate the history and examination findings and to arrive at a probable diagnosis or differential diagnosis
- Formulate a management plan for the patient that includes further investigations and treatment

BASICS IN OBSTETRICS

Terminologies

Obstetric indices

These are gravida (G), para (P), live (L), and abortion (A) (Table 1.1).

Table 1.1 Obstetric indices and their definitions

Obstetric index	Definition
Gravida	Refers to the number of pregnancies including the present pregnancy the woman has had, irrespective of the period of gestation and pregnancy outcome
Para*,†	Refers to the number of pregnancies that have crossed the period of viability, excluding the present pregnancy
Live	Refers to the number of living children at present (while taking history)
Abortion‡	Refers to the expulsion of products of conception before the period of viability

* Viability refers to the ability of the fetus to survive outside the uterus after birth. Period of viability varies in different countries:
- In developing countries such as India the period is 28 weeks.
- In developed countries such as the United States and the United Kingdom the period is 24 weeks.

† Previous H/o multiple pregnancy: Parity is determined by the number of previous viable pregnancies and not by the number of fetuses delivered. Hence, parity remains the same if previous twins or triplets were born.

‡ Previous H/o vesicular mole and ectopic pregnancy is included under abortion.

Additional terminologies

See Table 1.2

Duration of pregnancy

Pregnancy is divided into three trimesters (Table 1.3).

Term/preterm/post-term pregnancy

See Table 1.4

Table 1.2 Various terminologies used in obstetrics

Terminology	Definition
Primigravida	Woman who is pregnant for the first time
Multigravida	A woman who is or has been pregnant for at least second time
Nulliparous	Woman who has never carried a previous pregnancy up to the period of viability
Primiparous	Woman who has had one previous viable pregnancy
Multiparous	Woman who has had two or more previous viable pregnancies
Grand multipara	Woman who has had five or more previous viable pregnancies
Nulligravida	Woman who has never been pregnant so far
Parturient	Woman who is in labor
Puerperium	It refers to the period of about 42 days/6 weeks after childbirth

Table 1.3 Trimesters in pregnancy

Trimester	Time period during pregnancy
First trimester	From the time of conception up to 12 completed weeks of gestation
Second trimester	From the 13th week up to 28 completed weeks of gestation
Third trimester	From the 29th week up to delivery

Table 1.4 Definitions based on the period of gestation

Terminology	Definition
Term pregnancy	Pregnancy after 37 completed weeks of gestation and before 42 completed weeks of gestation
Preterm	Pregnancy after viability is attained but before 37 completed weeks of gestation
Postdated pregnancy	Pregnancy continuing beyond 40 weeks of gestation up to 42 weeks
Prolonged or post-term pregnancy	Pregnancy continuing beyond 42 weeks of gestation

Calculation of expected date of delivery and period of gestation

Expected date of delivery

Expected date of delivery (EDD) is calculated from the first day of last menstrual period (LMP) using the Naegele's rule.

Naegele's rule

EDD = LMP + 9 months + 7 days (for a woman with 28-day regular menstrual cycles)

- Naegele's rule can be used to calculate EDD, only if the woman had regular menstrual cycles prior to conception and there is no H/o oral contraceptive pill (OCP) intake prior to conception. In case of the latter, ovulation may not resume immediately following the withdrawal of hormonal pills and there may be a delay of 2–3 weeks in resuming ovulation. Hence, EDD may not be accurately determined with Naegele's rule.

Note *Ovulatory or fertilization age is typically 2 weeks less than the period of gestation (POG) calculated from LMP. This 2-week period is based on the calculation of the day of ovulation, which is generally 14 days prior to the date of menstruation. it is mainly used by embryologists in assisted reproductive techniques (ARTs).*

Corrected expected date of delivery

- **For cycle length >28 days:** Add up to extra 14 days to the EDD calculated from Naegele's formula.
  - *Example*: For a 35-day cycle, add extra 7 days (35 days – 28 days = 7 days) and the corrected EDD = LMP + 9 months + 7 days + 7 days.
- **For cycle length <28 days:** Deduct the number of days from the EDD calculated from Naegele's formula.
  - *Example*: For a 25-day cycle, deduct 3 days (28 days – 25 days = 3 days) and the corrected EDD = LMP + 9 months + 7 days – 3 days.
- **If cycle length is >45 days or cycles are irregular:** LMP is not reliable and hence dating ultrasound and clinical examination findings are used for determining the period of gestation (POG) and EDD.

Note *Only 4% of women will deliver on the EDD. Majority of women will deliver either 2 weeks before or 1 week after EDD.*

Part 1

Viva corner

Q1 What should be done if the patient does not remember her LMP?

If LMP is not known or the patient is not sure of LMP, the details may be collected from the following:

- History
  - Woman may be asked to relate her LMP to some important festivals or occasions that she might remember.
  - Ask when her urine pregnancy test (UPT) first became positive (UPT becomes positive 11–15 days after conception, 1–2 days after a missed period, in a woman with regular 28 days menstrual cycle).
  - Ask for date of quickening—quickening or perception of fetal movements for the first time during pregnancy is felt around 16–18 weeks in multigravida and 18–20 weeks in primigravida.
  - Details/dates of intrauterine insemination (IUI)/invitro fertilization (IVF) are known in woman treated for infertility.
- Obstetric examination
  - Check the patient's antenatal records for uterine size in early gestation and for fundal height in subsequent antenatal visits.
- Obstetric ultrasound
  - Check whether the patient has done dating ultrasound in the first trimester or any ultrasound in the second trimester.

Note

- *First documentation of fetal heart rate (FHR) by transabdominal scan is at 7 weeks, by handheld Doppler at 10 weeks, and by auscultation with stethoscope at 20 weeks.*
- *In postnatal period, pediatricians assess maturity of the newborn based on Ballard's scoring.*

Period of gestation

Add the total number of days from the first day of LMP till date and then divide it by 7 to calculate the POG in weeks.

Good, excellent, and bad dates

- **Excellent dates**
  - Women with adequate clinical information (i.e., known normal LMP, 28-day cycle, no recent use of OCPs, with uterine size in correlation with gestational age) and with one ultrasound done between 16 and 24 weeks of gestation correlating with POG as per LMP
  - Women with inadequate clinical information and with two ultrasound examinations between 16 and 24 weeks of gestation showing linear fetal growth and similar EDD
- **Good dates**
  - Women with adequate clinical examination (i.e., known normal LMP, 28-day cycle, no recent use of OCPs, with uterine size in correlation with gestational age) and with one ultrasound done after 24 weeks of gestation correlating with POG as per LMP
  - Women with inadequate clinical examination and with two or more ultrasound examinations after 24 weeks of gestation showing linear growth and similar EDD
- **Poor dates**
  - Any situation other than the above

Extra edge

Other Naegele's terminologies in obstetrics

Naegele's pelvis It is a type of asymmetrical contracted pelvis due to arrested development of one ala of the sacrum. Delivery is by cesarean section.

Naegele's obliquity It refers to anterior acynclitism or anterior parietal bone presentation during vaginal delivery.

ANTENATAL CARE AND BOOKING

Antenatal care

It refers to systematic supervision of a woman during pregnancy, to monitor the progress of fetal growth and to ascertain the well-being of the mother and the fetus.

Objective The objective is to achieve a healthy mother and a healthy baby at the end of the pregnancy.

Aims

- To screen for "high-risk" cases
- To prevent, detect, and treat any complications at the earliest
- To educate the mother about the physiology of pregnancy and labor, to alleviate fears regarding childbirth, and to promote breastfeeding following delivery

- To motivate the couple for family planning and educate them regarding the available options
- To give appropriate advice to couple seeking medical termination of pregnancy

Booking

It refers to the number of visits made by the pregnant woman to the doctor.

- Ideal number of antenatal visits: 13
  - *First trimester*: One visit
  - *Second trimester*: Once in 4 weeks
  - *Third trimester*: 28–36 weeks, once in 2 weeks; 36 weeks till term, once in a week

However, for a high proportion of mothers from lower socioeconomic group, it may not be possible to follow this schedule due to reasons such as the following:

- The antenatal clinic may be far away from home
- Going to the clinic may result in loss of wage
- Other personal/family problems preventing the mother from attending the antenatal clinic

In these cases, it is recommended that a **minimum of 4 AN visits** should be made as per the following schedule:

- **Timing of registration (first visit):** The registration or first visit of a pregnant woman for antenatal care should take place as soon as the pregnancy is suspected. Ideally, the first visit should be within 12 weeks. This visit is utilized for registration of pregnancy and first antenatal check up
- **Second visit:** In second trimester
- **Third visit:** Between 28 and 34 weeks
- **Fourth visit:** Between 36 weeks and term

Part 1

Proforma for history taking and clinical examination in antenatal cases

The following is a detailed account of various elements that should be considered during history taking and clinical examination in all antenatal cases. The case/disease-specific elements in history taking and clinical examination are discussed in respective chapters under the heading "Case presentation." Therefore, "Case presentation" in subsequent chapters will include only the salient points pertaining to the specific case being discussed in order to avoid repetition of content.

A few examples of how to present a clinical case in obstetrics during the viva voce examination taken by undergraduate medical students are presented in Appendix 1.

History taking

Consider the following relevant points during the history taking in obstetric cases.

Patient profile

She is Mrs. ________, ____ years of age, W/o Mr. _______, resides at _______, educated up to _______, and works as a _______. She belongs to _____ (mention the class) socioeconomic status. Her nearest health center is _______, which takes __ (time) to reach by ___ (means of transport).

- *She is Gravida (G) __ Para (P) __ Live (L) __ Abortion (A) __ (or) her obstetric index is "GPLA."*
- *Her last menstrual period (LMP) was on ______ (mention whether previous regular menstrual cycles and whether OCPs were taken prior to conception—e.g., "Her LMP was on _ (date), with previous regular 28-day menstrual cycles and no H/o OCPs prior to conception").*
- *Her expected date of delivery (EDD) is on ____.*
- *Period of gestation (POG) is _____ weeks and ______ days.*
- *Mention whether she is booked and immunized.*
- *Blood group of the patient is ____.*

Note *Students are advised not to use short forms such as LMP, POG, and EDD while presenting the case. Instead, use the expanded terms such as "last menstrual period, period of gestation, and expected date of delivery."*

(CONTD...)

(...CONTD)

Presenting complaints

The various presenting complaints of the patient are listed in chronological order from the time of onset.

Common presenting complaints during antenatal period are the following:

- *Excessive vomiting*
- *Swelling of feet*
- *Bleeding per vaginum*
- *Leaking per vaginum*
- *Pain abdomen*
- *Decreased fetal movements*
- *Breathlessness*
- *White discharge per vaginum*
- *Burning micturition*
- *Any other specific complaints*

If no complaints, mentioned that the patient has come for routine antenatal checkup or admitted for safe confinement.

H/o presenting complaints

- *Elaborate or describe the presenting complaints with details such as mode of onset, severity, duration, and aggravating or relieving factors.*
- *Mention current admission and treatment history if the patient is an inpatient (admitted in the ward).*

H/o present pregnancy

First trimester

- *Whether it is a spontaneous conception or following infertility treatment* (if so, the details on the type of treatment option taken should be asked)
- *The pregnancy was confirmed at __ days of amenorrhea, by ____ [urine pregnancy test (UPT) or ultrasonography (USG)], at ___ (place)*
- *H/o hyperemesis gravidarum*
- *H/o fever with rashes*
- *H/o bleeding P/V*
- *H/o exposure to radiation*
- *H/o drug intake*
- *Whether antenatal investigations and dating scan have been done and said to be normal*

Second trimester

- *Number of antenatal visits*
- *Time when quickening was felt*
- *H/o tetanus vaccination—number of doses and POG at which the injections were received*
- *H/o iron and calcium supplementation*
- *H/o bleeding P/V*
- *H/o symptoms suggestive of preeclampsia such as excessive weight gain, swelling of feet, decreased urine output, headache, blurring of vision, and epigastric pain*
- *Whether screening test for gestational diabetes mellitus was performed*
- *Whether fetal anomalies scan was done and said to be normal*

Third trimester

- *Number of antenatal visits*
- *H/o symptoms of preeclampsia such as excessive weight gain, swelling of feet, decreased urine output, headache, blurring of vision, and epigastric pain*
- *Whether perceiving normal fetal movements*
- *H/o iron and calcium supplementation*
- *H/o bleeding P/V*
- *H/o leaking P/V*
- *H/o pain abdomen*
- *H/o bowel and bladder disturbances*

Menstrual history

- *Age at menarche*
- *Menstrual cycles*
  - *Regular/irregular*
  - *Cycles once in _____ days/lasting for _______ days*
  - *Whether flow is moderate/profuse/scanty in amount*
  - *H/o associated clots/dysmenorrhea*
  - *LMP __*

Note Always end the menstrual history with LMP.

Marital history

- *Married for the past _______ years*
- *Consanguineous/nonconsanguineous marriage (if it is a consanguineous marriage, mention the degree of consanguinity—first degree/second degree/third degree)*

(CONTD...)

(...CONTD)

Past obstetric history

Note Detailed H/o all the previous pregnancies has to be elicited.

- *Pregnancy was confirmed at ____ days of amenorrhea by ____ (UPT or USG)*
- *Whether she was booked and immunized*
- *Whether antenatal period was uneventful or had any complications such as preeclampsia, gestational diabetes mellitus (GDM), and antepartum hemorrhage*
- *Name of the institute where the patient delivered*
- *Admission details*
  - *POG at which the patient was admitted*
  - *Whether admitted with labor pains/leaking P/V/bleeding P/V/or any specific complaints*
- *Delivery details*
  - *Onset of labor—spontaneous/induced labor*
  - *Whether term/preterm/postdated delivery*
  - *Whether spontaneous vaginal delivery (SVD)/instrumental delivery/cesarean section (if cesarean section was done, detailed history has to be taken as mentioned in a case of previous LSCS, Part 1, Chapter 6, Postcesarean Pregnancy)*
  - *H/o blood transfusion*
- *Baby details*
  - *Live/stillbirth*
    - *If stillbirth, whether fresh/macerated*
    - *Cause of death, if known*
  - *Sex of the baby*
  - *Birth weight*
  - *Whether cried immediately after birth/any neonatal intensive care unit (NICU) admission*
  - *Any congenital anomaly*
  - *Time of starting breastfeeding the baby—"breastfed the baby ____ hours after birth")*
  - *Time period for which exclusive breastfeeding was given*
  - *Present age of the child and whether healthy*
- *Puerperium*
  - *Mention whether uneventful or whether had complications such as fever, foul-smelling lochia, wound gaping, and H/o prolonged hospital stay for any specific reason*
- *Contraception details*
  - *H/o contraceptive usage in between pregnancies*
  - *Method of contraception used and for how long*

In case of past H/o abortion, ask the following:

- *Confirmed pregnancy by _____ (UPT or USG) at _______ days of amenorrhea*
- *Spontaneous/induced abortion*
- *If induced, reason for induced abortion*
- *POG at which she aborted*
- *Whether medical or surgical abortion*
- *Any fever/foul-smelling discharge following abortion*
- *Time when the patient resumed menstrual cycles following abortion*
- *H/o any contraception following abortion*

Past history

- *Medical history such as diabetes/hypertension/tuberculosis/jaundice/epilepsy/bronchial asthma/thyroid disorder or any other medical illness*
- *Surgical history—past H/o of any surgery*
- *H/o blood transfusion*
- *H/o sexually transmitted diseases (STDs)*

Personal history

- *Sleep and appetite*
- *H/o any addictions such as tobacco usage, alcohol, or smoking*
- *H/o drug allergies/drug intake for chronic illness*

Diet history

- *Mixed/vegetarian diet*
- *A record of the patient's daily food intake should be documented to calculate the daily calorie and protein intake*
- *It is mentioned as "Calorie intake is ___ kcal/day and protein intake is __ g/day"*
- *It is mentioned whether diet is adequate in calories and protein intake or else mentioned that diet is __% deficient in calories and ___% deficient in protein intake*

Family history

- *Diabetes mellitus*
- *Hypertension*

(CONTD...)

(...CONTD)

- *Tuberculosis*
- *Multiple pregnancy*
- *Congenital anomalies*
- *Genetic disorders*

Summary of history

A summary is made at the end of history taking, which should include the patient's name, age, obstetric index (GPLA), LMP, EDD, POG, chief complaints, significant positive and negative history, and any associated complications. Pregnancy can be identified as a low-risk or high-risk case at the completion of history taking in majority of the cases.

Clinical examination

Consider the following relevant points during examination of an antenatal case.

Gadgets required for examination of an antenatal case

See Figure 1.1

General examination

- *Whether the patient is comfortable at rest*
- *Built—medium built/well built/thin built*
- *Nourishment—adequate/poorly nourished*
- *Height*
- *Weight*
- *Body mass index (BMI)—weight (kg)/[height (m)]^2 (Prepregnancy body weight or weight in the early first trimester is taken for calculation of BMI)*
- *Check for any abnormal gait and spinal deformities such as kyphoscoliosis*

Check for pallor/icterus/cyanosis/clubbing/lymphadenopathy/pedal edema.

Note Presence or absence of pallor and pedal edema are the two general examination findings that are usually noted during each antenatal visit.

Vitals

- *Temperature—whether afebrile or febrile (if febrile, mention the temperature in degree Celsius or Fahrenheit)*
- *Pulse rate __/min. Describe the rhythm, volume, character, and whether all peripheral pulses are equally felt (e.g., pulse rate is 84/min, regular in rhythm, normal volume and character, and all peripheral pulses are equally felt)*
- *Respiratory rate __/min (generally, in pregnancy, it is abdomino-thoracic type of respiration; any audible grunt/wheeze)*
- *Blood pressure (BP) __ mmHg, measured in right upper limb in sitting/left lateral position*

Thyroid examination

Mention whether "normal" or presence of any thyroid swelling (thyroid moves with deglutition).

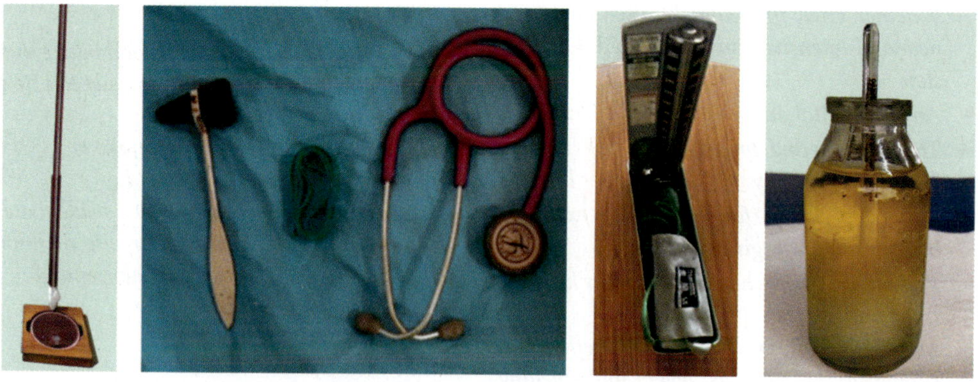

a. b. c. d.

Figure 1.1 Gadgets required for examination of an antenatal case. **a.** Weight and height measurement tool. **b.** Knee hammer, inch tape, and stethoscope. **c.** Sphygmomanometer. **d.** Thermometer.

(CONTD...)

(...CONTD)

Breast examination

Mention whether breasts are "normal" or whether there is presence of any retracted nipple/fissures/discharge from nipple/any palpable mass.

Systemic examination

Cardiovascular system (CVS) *If it is normal, mention as "clinically normal"/"S1 S2 heard and no murmurs"/"within normal limits" (CVS abnormalities are mentioned in Part 1, Chapter 5, Cardiac Disease in Pregnancy).*

Respiratory system (RS) *If it is normal, mention as "clinically normal"/"normal vesicular breath sounds are heard"/"within normal limits" or mention if any abnormal findings are detected (crepts, rhonchi, diminished breath sounds, etc.).*

Obstetric abdominal examination

Prerequisites for obstetric examination include the following:

- *Explain the procedure to the patient.*
- *Obtain her consent.*
- *Ask the patient to empty her bladder.*
- *Ensure privacy (get a screen prior to examination).*
- *Ensure adequate lighting.*
- *Stand on the right side of the patient.*
- *A male doctor should have the presence of a female attendant during examination.*
- *Ask the patient to lie down in supine position and cover the lower limbs with a blanket.*
- *Request the patient to undress the parts to be examined.*
- *Warm your fingers and examine from nontender to tender area.*

Inspection

- *Abdominal distension and contour. Note whether flanks are full or not.*
- *Umbilicus—whether normal/everted/flushed with skin surface*
- *Linea nigra and striae gravidarum looked for (Figure 1.2)*
- *Any scars/sinuses*
- *Cough impulse at hernia orifices checked (mention as cough impulse is present/absent at hernia orifices) [if any scar is present, check for cough impulse at scar sites (to rule out incisional hernia)]*

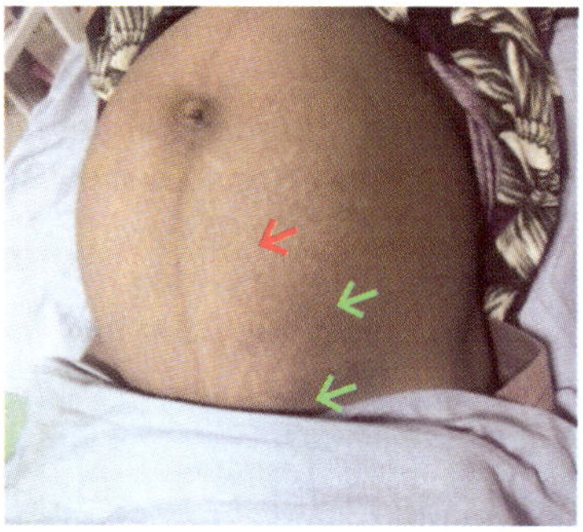

Figure 1.2 Linea nigra (red arrow) and striae gravidarum (green arrows).

Palpation

Fundal height

- *Patient position: The patient should be in dorsal position with legs flexed and slightly abducted (Figure 1.3a).*
- *Correct the dextrorotation of uterus with the right hand.*

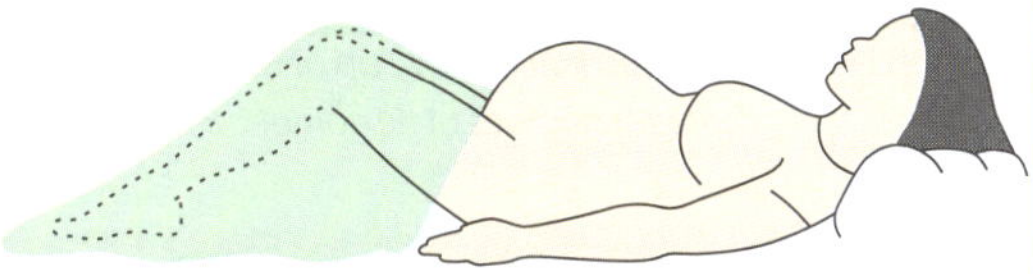

a.

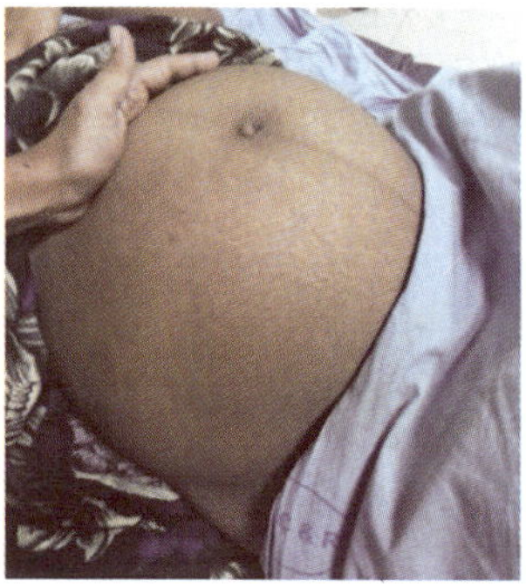

b.

Figure 1.3 Obstetric palpation. **a.** Position of the patient for obstetric palpation. **b.** Demonstration of fundal height.

(CONTD...)

(...CONTD)

- *Palpate with the ulnar border of left hand to determine the upper border of the uterus—either from below upwards till disappearance of resistance of uterus or from above downwards till fundus of uterus is felt (appearance of resistance) (Figure 1.3b).*
- *Before taking away the palpating hand, ask permission of the patient and mark the fundal height on the abdomen.*

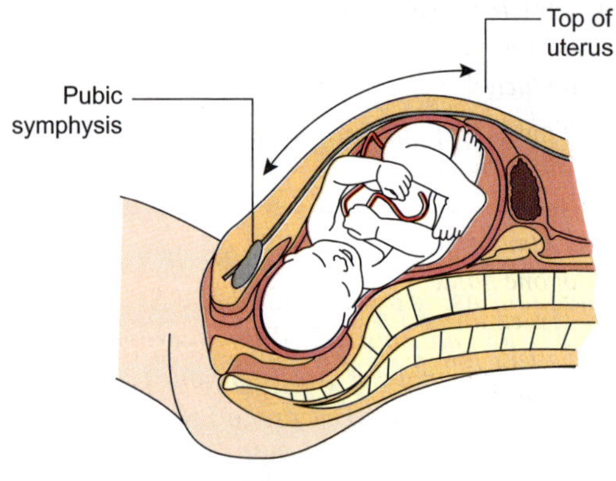

a.

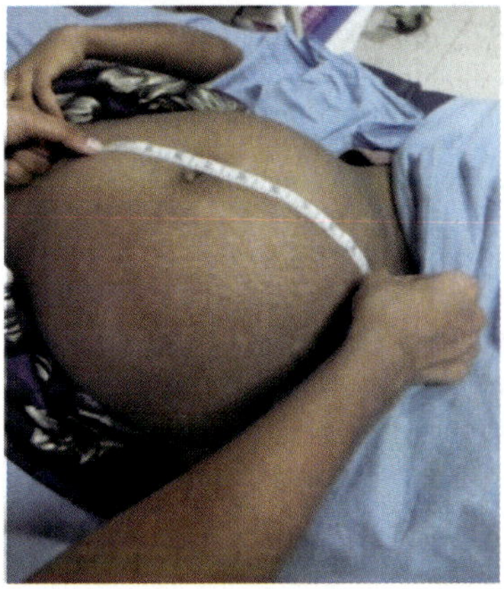

b.

Figure 1.4 Symphysiofundal height measurement. **a.** Landmarks for measuring the symphysiofundal height. **b.** Measuring the symphysiofundal height.

Symphysiofundal height (SFH; Figure 1.4)

- *Patient position: The patient should be in dorsal position with legs extended.*
- *Measure with a measuring tape with the inches side facing up (this is to avoid examiner bias for equating the SFH to POG).*
- *Place one end of measuring tape over pubic symphysis and take the tape across umbilicus up to the marking of fundal height on the abdomen.*
- *Turn the tape to check for the SFH measurement in centimeters.*

Note *SFH measurement is the only examination done with legs of the patient in extended position. With extended legs, reference point of pubic symphysis remains the same at each visit while symphysis may move up or down with different degrees of flexion of the thighs.*

Obstetric grips (Leopold's maneuvers; Figure 1.5)

Aim *Obstetric grips help in determining fetal lie and presentation. Grips are performed usually after 34 weeks of gestation as the fetal lie and presentation remain variable prior to this period.*

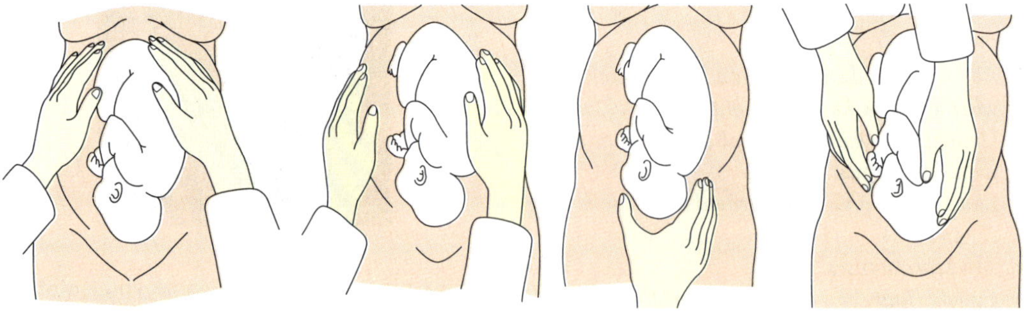

a. b. c. d.

Figure 1.5 Demonstration of obstetric grips. **a.** Fundal grip. **b.** Lateral grip. **c.** First pelvic grip. **d.** Second pelvic grip.

(CONTD...)

(...CONTD)

- *Obstetric grips are done with the patient in dorsal position with legs flexed and slightly abducted (relaxes the abdominal muscles which makes palpation easier).*
- *Obstetric grips must be performed in a relaxed uterus.*
- *Palpate gently with ventral aspect of the fingers of one hand.*
- *The examiner faces toward the head end of the patient for the first three maneuvers and faces toward her feet for the fourth maneuver.*

Fundal grip (first Leopold; Figure 1.6)

- *Palpation is done facing the head end of the patient.*
- *Palpate fundus of uterus with both the hands.*
- *Inference*

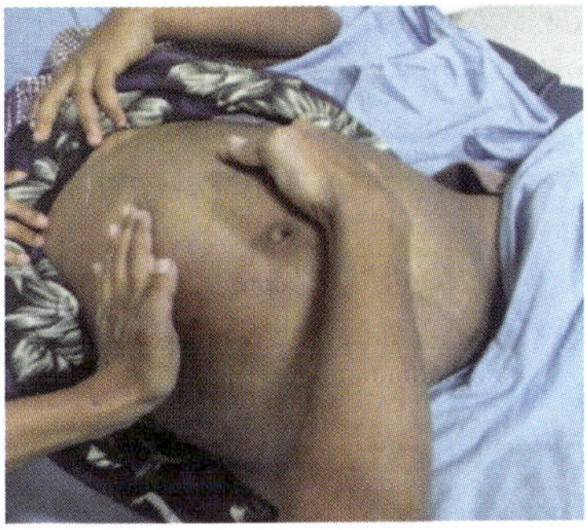

Figure 1.6 Demonstration of fundal grip.

  - *If a smooth, hard, globular, ballotable mass is felt, it is suggestive of fetal head.*
  - *If a broad, soft, irregular, nonballotable mass is felt, it is suggestive of breech.*

Lateral/umbilical grip (second Leopold; Figure 1.7)

- *Palpation is done facing the head end of the patient.*
- *Steady one side of the uterus with the palm of one hand while palpating the other side and then do vice versa.*
- *Palpate one side first and then the other side.*
- *Inference*
  - *If a smooth curved, uniform resistance is felt, it is suggestive of fetal back.*
  - *If small, knobby, irregular parts are felt, it is suggestive of fetal limb buds.*

First pelvic grip/Pawlik's grip (third Leopold; Figure 1.8)

- *Palpation is done facing the head end of the patient.*
- *The ulnar border of the right hand is placed on the upper border of pubic symphysis.*
- *Palpate the fetus between the outstretched thumb and the four fingers of right hand.*
- *Inference*

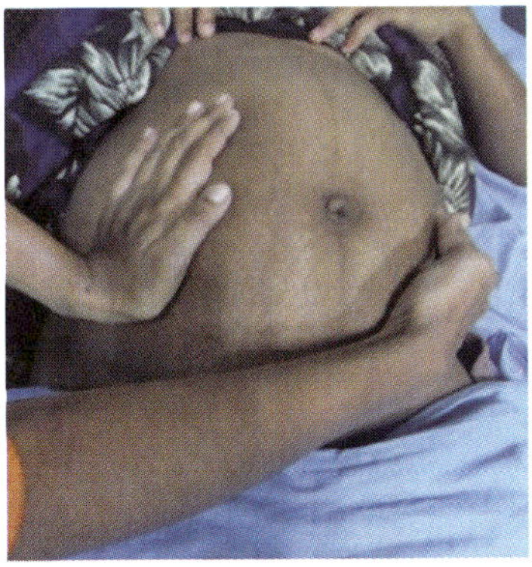

a.

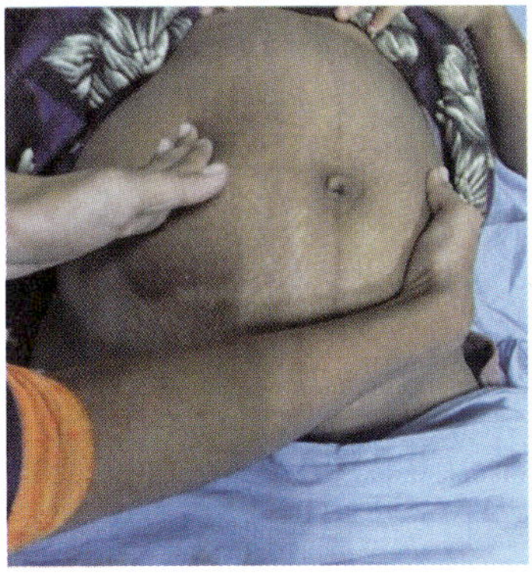

b.

Figure 1.7 Demonstration of lateral grip. a. Left hand is used for stabilizing one side of the abdomen and palpation of the other side of the abdomen is done with the right hand. b. Right hand is used for stabilizing the abdomen and palpation of the opposite side of the abdomen is done with left hand.

(CONTD...)

(...CONTD)

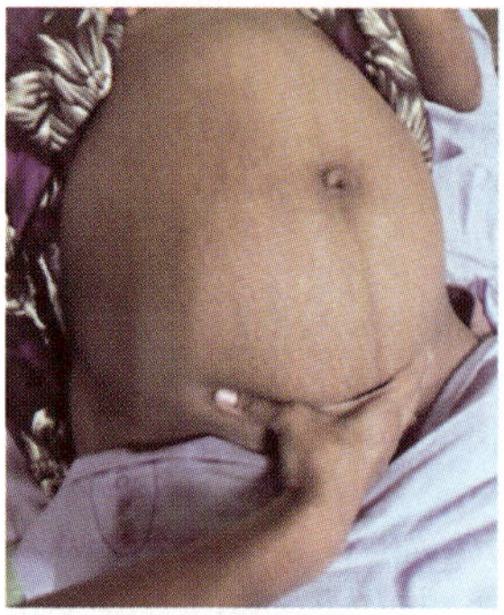

Figure 1.8 Demonstration of first pelvic grip.

- *Presentation of fetus*
  - *If a smooth, hard, globular, ballotable mass is felt, it is suggestive of fetal head.*
  - *If a broad, soft, irregular, nonballotable mass is felt, it is suggestive of breech.*
- *Whether presenting part is engaged or not*
  - *If the presenting part is freely ballotable, it is not engaged.*
  - *If the presenting part is fixed or nonballotable, it may be engaged.*

Note *In transverse lie, the first pelvic grip is empty.*

Second pelvic grip (fourth Leopold; Figure 1.9)

- *Examination is done facing the foot end of the patient (only obstetric grip that is done facing the foot end of the patient). This grip is usually done at term pregnancy to check if the presenting part is engaged or not.*

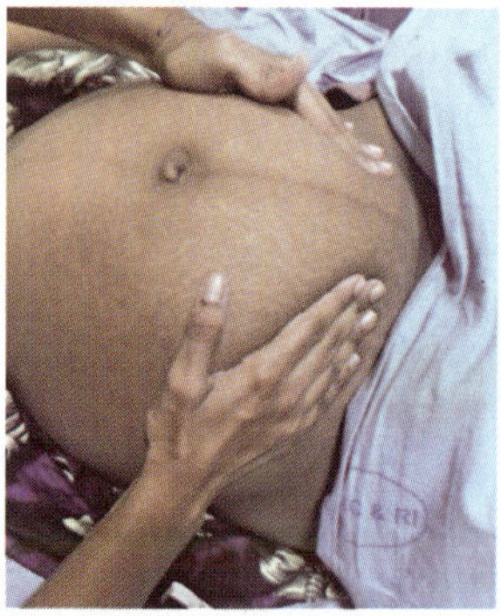

Figure 1.9 Demonstration of second pelvic grip.

- *Place both hands on either side of abdomen above and parallel to inguinal ligament.*
- *Palpate simultaneously with both hands and move medially and downwards.*
- *Inference*
  - *The second pelvic grip confirms the findings of first pelvic grip, that is, presentation of fetus and whether presenting part is engaged or not.*
  - *It gives additional information on attitude of the head in cephalic presentation (whether well flexed/deflexed/extended head).*

Following the obstetric grips, mention regarding the following:

- ***Uterine activity**: Whether uterus is relaxed/irritable/acting*
- ***Liquor content**: Whether average/excessive/re-duced in amount*
- ***Scar tenderness**: To be checked in previous cesarean pregnancy to rule out impending scar rupture. (Figure 1.10). The suprapubic region is gently palpated with palmar aspect of fingers of right hand and the patient's face is simultaneously looked at for any wincing or discomfort due to pain.*

Auscultation of fetal heart rate (Figure 1.11)

- *Check for fetal heart rate (FHR) on the side of fetal back along the spinoumbilical line.*
- *FHR is heard best with the bell of a stethoscope.*
- *Count for 1 minute; mention the rate and regularity (normal FHR: 120–160 beats/min).*

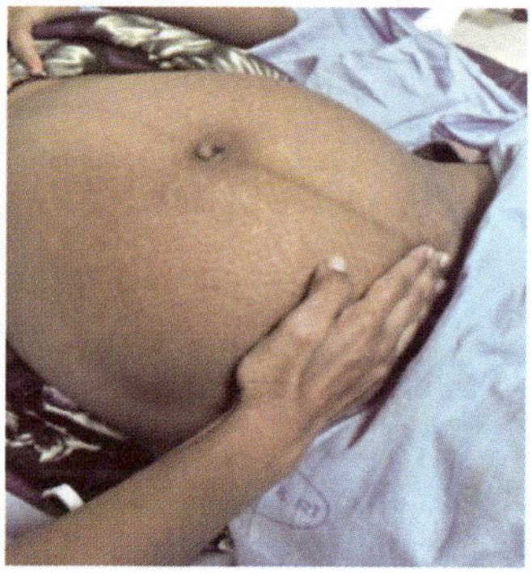

Figure 1.10 Eliciting scar tenderness.

(CONTD...)

(...CONTD)

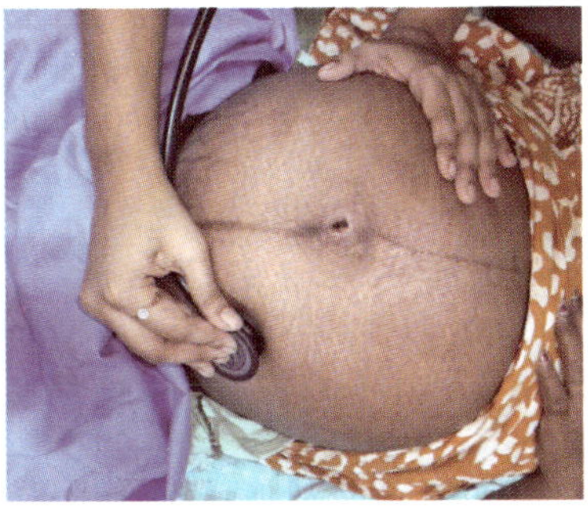

Figure 1.11 Auscultation of fetal heart rate along the spinoumbilical line.

Note *Fetal heart sounds are heard through the back of the fetus (left scapular region) in vertex and breech presentations and through the chest of the fetus in face presentation.*

Estimated fetal weight (EFW)

It is calculated using Johnson's formula:

$$EFW = (SFH - 11 \text{ or } 12) \times 155 \text{ (grams)}$$

- *Take the value as 11, if head is below the level of ischial spines.*
- *Take the value as 12, if head is at or above the level of ischial spines.*

Obstetric pelvic examination

Routine vaginal examination is not required in the antenatal period. It may be indicated in cases with complaints of vaginal discharge, and pelvic pain. A vaginal examination may be performed at or after 38 weeks' gestation and during labor to obtain information about the cervix, presenting part, membranes, and pelvis.

Note *Undergraduate medical students are expected to perform only the obstetric abdominal examination and the inspection of external genitalia. However, one should be able to answer viva questions regarding pelvic examination. Postgraduates are expected to do obstetric pelvic examination in indicated antenatal cases.*

Prerequisites for vaginal examination

- *The patient is asked to empty her bladder.*
- *Explain the procedure and get informed consent.*
- *Ensure adequate privacy and lighting.*
- *The patient should be in dorsal position with thighs flexed and slightly abducted and buttocks placed at the foot end of the table (Figure 1.12).*

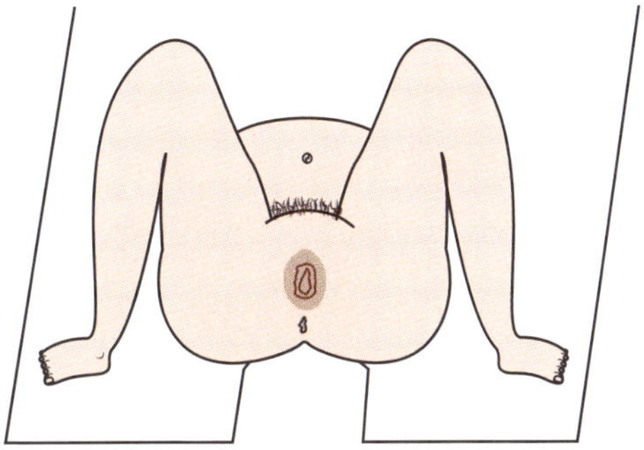

Figure 1.12 Dorsal position of the patient for speculum and vaginal examination.

- *Hands are washed with soap or antiseptic solution and sterile gloves are worn before examination.*
- *The patient's vulva and perineum are swabbed with Savlon or Betadine prior to the procedure.*

Obstetric pelvic examination procedure

Inspection of the external genitalia *Inspect them on symphysis pubis, labia majora, labia minora, perineum, and anal region for any ulcers, warts, skin lesions, varicosities, and any vulvar edema. Then the labia are separated to inspect the urethra, clitoris, and introitus.*

Speculum examination (Figure 1.13) *Speculum examination is done prior to bimanual or vaginal examination to visualize the vagina and cervix. With the help of a good light source, Sims' speculum or Cusco's bivalve speculum is inserted into the vagina under aseptic precautions.*

Look for the following:

- *Any abnormal discharge, leaking P/V, and bleeding P/V*

(CONTD...)

(...CONTD)

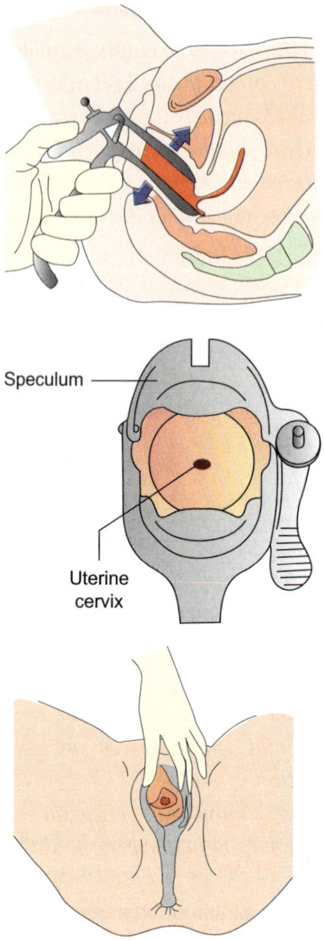

Figure 1.13 Speculum examination. **a.** Insertion of Cusco's speculum. **b.** Visualization of cervix after insertion of Cusco's speculum. **c.** Sims' speculum examination.

- *Any ulcers and lesions*
- *Cervical smear for exfoliative cytology (PAP smear) or vaginal swab for culture may be taken, if indicated.*

Bimanual examination (Figure 1.14) *This is done in early pregnancy when uterus remains a pelvic organ. The index and middle fingers of the examiner's right hand are introduced into the vagina, while the left hand is placed in the suprapubic region and the uterus is palpated between the abdominal hand and the hand in the vagina. Do a gentle and systematic examination and note the following:*

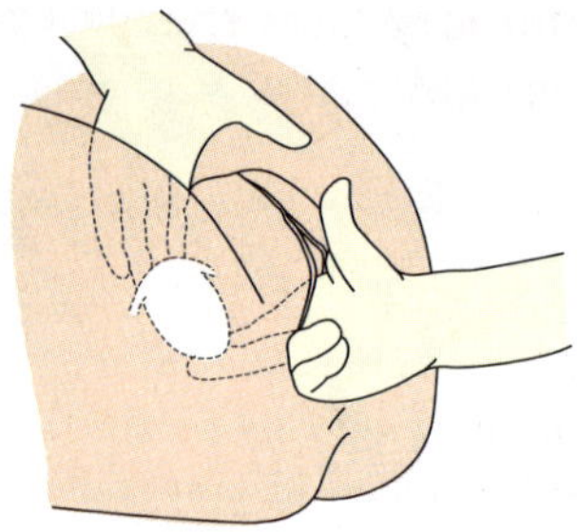

Figure 1.14 Bimanual pelvic examination.

- ***Cervix:*** *Consistency, position, and any cervical pathology*
- ***Uterus:*** *Size, shape, position, and consistency (to corroborate the size of the uterus with the period of amenorrhea in early pregnancy)*
- ***Adnexae:*** *Any mass/tenderness felt through the fornix*

Vaginal examination (Figure 1.15) *Vaginal examination is indicated usually prior to induction of labor or during labor for the following reasons:*

- *To do pelvic assessment to rule out cephalopelvic disproportion (CPD)*
- *To assess cervical ripening prior to induction of labor*
- *To assess fetal presenting part and position*
- *To do artificial rupture of membranes*
- *To note the color of liquor, if membranes have ruptured*
- *To rule out cord prolapse following rupture of membranes*
- *To assess cervical effacement and dilatation during labor*
- *To assess station of the presenting part*
- *To note progress of labor*
- *To confirm second stage of labor*

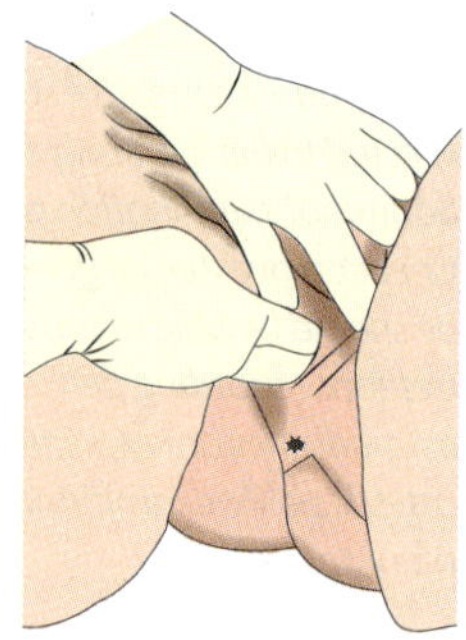

Figure 1.15 Vaginal examination.

(CONTD...)

(...CONTD)

Case summary (summary of history and examination)

A summary is made at the end of history and examination, which should include the patient's name, age, obstetric index (GPLA), LMP, EDD, POG, chief complaints, significant positive and negative history, any associated complications, and salient findings in general and obstetric examinations.

Provisional case diagnosis

A provisional diagnosis is made, which should include the patient's age, obstetric index, POG, complications (if any), and the current status of this pregnancy.

Example *___ years of age, GPLA _____, at _______ POG, with diagnosis of ___, with a singleton live fetus in cephalic presentation, not in labor.*

Booked pregnancy A pregnant woman is said to be booked if:

- She has had a minimum of three antenatal visits after her pregnancy was registered, out of which two visits should be in the third trimester.
- She has been provided with iron and calcium supplementation.
- She has been immunized with two doses of tetanus toxoid (TT).

Note *It should be emphasized that the three visits following registration of pregnancy are a minimum requirement and more visits may be required, depending on the pregnancy need.*

Proforma for history taking and examination in obstetrics followed by significance/relevance of the history taken and examination performed is described in the following subsections.

INVESTIGATIONS AND MANAGEMENT PLAN FOR THE CASE

The investigations relevant to the given case that aid in diagnosis and/or management and a brief plan of management for the given case are to be noted, following the summary and provisional diagnosis.

Note *Always be ready with the summary of the case, as examiner may ask you to present only the summary of the case and can start the discussion.*

DISCUSSION POINTS IN HISTORY TAKING AND CLINICAL EXAMINATION

The time-honored method of history taking and clinical examination can give significant information regarding diagnosis of pregnancy, identification of risk factors, and appropriate management for the patient.

Relevance of the various items in the history taken and the examination performed is described below.

Discussion points in history taking

Relevance of the history taken in patient profile

Name of the patient Documentation of the patient's name is necessary for the following:

- Identification of the patient
- Addressing the patient
- To build rapport with the patient

Husband's name To avoid confusion among patients with the same name in the ward. *(Considering that the present abortion laws have changed the term from "husband" to "partner," usage of the terms "Mrs" and "husband" may be noninclusive. The term "Ms." for salutation of the woman and the term "Partner" instead of husband may be used during case presentation.)*

Importance of age Obstetric complications are more common in teenage pregnancies and in advanced maternal age. Risks associated with teenage pregnancy (age ≤18 years) and advanced maternal age (age >35 years) are given in Tables 1.5 and 1.6, respectively.

Importance of residence

- Accessibility to health services in case of obstetric emergencies

Part 1

Table 1.5 Risks associated with teenage pregnancy

Antenatal	Intrapartum	Postpartum
• Anemia • Malnutrition • Abortion • Preterm labor • Intrauterine growth restriction • Preeclampsia	• Contracted pelvis • Cephalopelvic disproportion • Increased rate of cesarean section • Perineal injuries during delivery	• Failed lactation • Emotional upset

Table 1.6 Risks associated with advanced maternal age

Antenatal	Intrapartum	Postpartum
• Abortion • Preeclampsia • Chronic hypertension • Gestational diabetes mellitus • Overt diabetes mellitus • Fibroid complicating pregnancy • Intrauterine growth restriction • Fetal risk—chromosomal abnormalities such as trisomies (Down syndrome)	• Uterine inertia • Incoordinate uterine action • Operative interferences such as instrumental deliveries and cesarean section	• Failed lactation

- To plan admissions
  - A woman from remote area may require admission at term for safe confinement, while a woman residing close to the hospital may be asked to come for admission with onset of labor pain.
  - A patient residing close to the hospital may be managed on outpatient department (OPD) basis in case of mild preeclampsia, GDM, etc.
- Some areas endemic for certain diseases—filariasis, leprosy, iodine deficiency, etc. Further, studies have shown that built environment has a lot of impact on the perinatal outcomes.

Importance of education

- Educated women are in a better position to understand the importance of antenatal care and follow-up.
- Compliance may be more in educated women regarding diet advice, drug intake, etc.
- To decide on management plan for cases with GDM, preeclampsia, etc.—whether to treat on OPD basis or as inpatient. Educated women are more compliant for follow-up and can be managed on OPD basis.

Importance of occupation

- Women may be prone to occupational hazards such as the following:
  - *Radiology department*: Exposure to radiation
  - *IT sector*: Stress
  - *Agricultural workers*: Hookworm infestation
  - *Construction workers*: Abortion due to lifting heavy weights

Importance of socioeconomic status (SES) The complications associated with lower and higher economic status are given in Table 1.7.

- Based on SES
  - Advice on diet (in anemia—patients can be advised to take meat, liver, egg yolk, etc., if they can afford these, while those not able to afford such foods can be advised cheaper alternatives rich in iron such as green leafy vegetables, jaggery, and ragi)
  - Prescription of drugs (cheaper brand of drugs may be prescribed for patients who cannot afford to buy costly medications)

SES is one of the important determinants of health status. There is no direct measure of the social status of an individual. Several methods or scales have been proposed for classifying population by SES. The commonly used scales are given in Table 1.8. These scales are revised periodically to meet the fast-growing economy.

Table 1.7 Pregnancy complications associated with socioeconomic status (SES)

Complications associated with lower SES	Complications associated with higher SES
• Anemia and malnutrition • Rheumatic heart disease • Tuberculosis • Sexually transmitted diseases • Hookworm infestation	• Sedentary lifestyle—obesity, postdated pregnancy • Pregnancy-induced hypertension, gestational diabetes mellitus

Table 1.8 Different scales to classify population on the basis of socioeconomic status

Scale	Applicable to
Kuppuswamy's scale	Urban areas
Modified BG Prasad scale	Both urban and rural areas
Uday Pareek scale	Rural areas

- Kuppuswamy's socioeconomic status scale
  - The modified Kuppuswamy scale is based on a composite score considering the education and occupation of the head of the family, and the monthly income of the family that yields a score of 3–29 (Tables 1.9–1.12).
  - The scale classifies the study population into high, middle, and low SES.

Table 1.9 Kuppuswamy's scale—scores based on the education of the head of the family

Education of head of family	Score
Profession or honors	7
Graduate or postgraduate	6
Intermediate or post-high school diploma	5
High school certificate	4
Middle school certificate	3
Primary school certificate	2
Illiterate	1

Table 1.10 Kuppuswamy's scale—scores based on the occupation of the head of the family

Occupation of the head of the family	Score
Legislators, senior officials and managers	10
Professionals	9
Technicians and associate professionals	8
Clerks	7
Skilled workers and shop and market sales workers	6
Skilled agricultural and fishery workers	5
Craft and related trade workers	4
Plant and machine operators and assemblers	3
Elementary occupation	2
Unemployed	1

Table 1.11 Kuppuswamy's scale—scores based on the monthly income of the family

Updated monthly family income in INR (2021)	Score
>123,322	12
61,663–123,321	10
46,129–61,662	6
30,831–46,128	4
18,497–30,830	3
6,175–18,496	2
≤6,174	1

Table 1.12 Kuppuswamy's socioeconomic status scale

Socioeconomic class	Total score defined by Kuppuswamy*
I (upper)	26–29
II (upper middle)	16–25
III (lower middle)	11–15
IV (upper lower)	5–10
V (lower)	<5

* Scores based on the education and occupation of the head of the family, and monthly income of the family.

  - Education and occupation of head of the family are not changeable with time. However, the income range in the scale has to be updated regularly for socioeconomic classification of the study population.
  - The changes in the income scale are proportional to the change in the consumer price index numbers for industrial workers [CPI (IW)].
- Modified BG Prasad scale is based on per capita monthly income (Table 1.13).

Table 1.13 Modified BG Prasad scale (2019)

Socioeconomic class	Per capita monthly income (₹)
Upper class	≥7,008
Upper middle class	3,504–7,007
Middle class	2,102–3,503
Lower middle class	1,051–2,101
Lower class	<1,050

Part 1

Importance of nearest health center

- Accessibility to health services in case of emergencies
- To decide on management—whether to treat on OPD basis or as inpatient

Importance of POG and EDD It helps in many aspects of diagnosis and decision making in pregnancy.

Complications in a primigravida Increased risk of the following:

- Preeclampsia
- Preterm labor
- CPD

Complications in a grand multigravida See Table 1.14

Relevance of history of present pregnancy

Importance of various history taken in first trimester

Hyperemes is gravidarum

- **Definition:** Hyperemesis gravidarum refers to excessive vomiting in pregnancy that has got deleterious effects on the health of the mother.
- Causes
  - Molar pregnancy
  - Multiple pregnancy
  - More common in primigravida
  - Previous H/o hyperemesis
  - Strong family history
  - Nonobstetric causes for vomiting (Table 1.15)

Table 1.14 Complications in a grand multigravida

Antenatal	Intrapartum	Postnatal
• Anemia • Malpresentations due to pendulous abdomen • Multiple pregnancy • Placenta previa	• Incoordinate uterine action • Rupture uterus • Postpartum hemorrhage	• Subinvolution • Failed lactation

Table 1.15 Nonobstetric causes for vomiting

Medical causes	Surgical causes	Gynecological causes
• Urinary tract infections • Hepatitis • Diabetic ketoacidosis • Peptic ulcer	• Appendicitis • Cholecystitis	• Twisted ovarian cyst • Red degeneration of fibroid

Viva corner

Q1 What is implantation bleeding?

In some women, spotting P/V may occur approximately on the day of expected menstruation, due to implantation of fertilized ovum that may be confused with last menstrual period. This is referred to as implantation bleeding. There might be a discrepancy in the gestational age in women who have implantation bleeding. Also, women might commonly mistake it for abortions.

Q2 What are the different types of abortions?

See the table and figure given below

Table Different types of abortion, their clinical features (C/F) per abdominal (P/A), per vaginal (P/V), and ultrasonography (USG) observations

Abortion type	C/F	P/A	P/V	USG
• Threatened abortion	Pain abdomen, spotting or bleeding P/V	Fundal height (FH) corresponds to period of gestation (POG)	Spotting+, cervical os closed	Cardiac activity (CA) good
• Inevitable abortion	Pain abdomen, bleeding P/V	FH may correspond to POG	Bleeding+, os open	CA+
• Incomplete abortion	Pain abdomen, bleeding P/V	FH <POG	Bleeding+, os open	Retained products of conception+

(CONTD...)

(...CONTD)

Viva corner

Table *(CONTD...)*

Abortion type	C/F	P/A	P/V	USG
• Complete abortion	Pain subsided, minimal or no bleeding P/V	Normal uterine size	No or minimal bleeding, os closed	Uterine cavity empty
• Missed abortion	No symptoms or bleeding P/V	FH < POG	Altered blood-stained discharge, os closed	CA absent

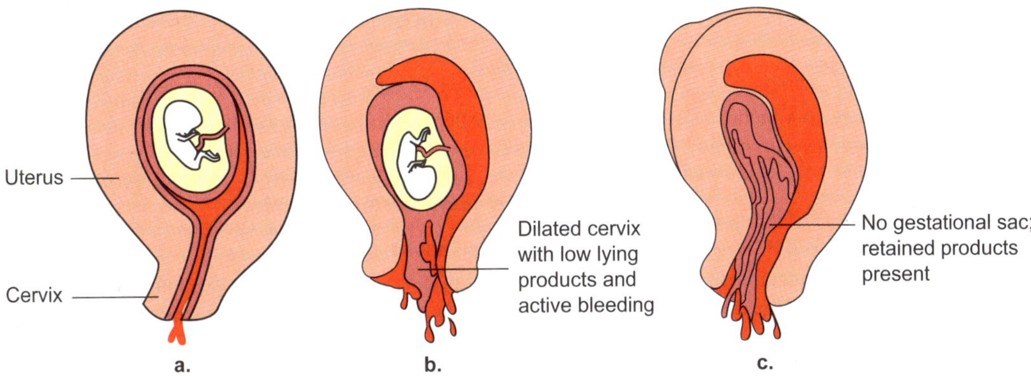

Figure Types of abortion. **a.** Threatened abortion. **b.** Inevitable abortion. **c.** Incomplete abortion.

Bleeding P/V

- Causes of bleeding P/V in first trimester
  - Implantation bleeding
  - Abortion
  - Ectopic pregnancy
  - Molar pregnancy
  - Local lesions—cervical erosion, polyp, carcinoma cervix, etc.

Fever with rashes High-grade fever can lead to abortion, intrauterine death, and preterm delivery.

- Causes of fever with rashes
  - Rubella
  - Chicken pox (varicella)
  - Measles

Exposure to radiation

- Radiation hazards
  - Teratogenic effects can occur when the cumulative dose of radiation exposure is ≥5 rad.
  - Radiation exposure in the first trimester can be associated with an increased risk of childhood malignancy.
- Common indications for radiation exposure during pregnancy
  - Maternal reasons
    - Patients with cardiac or pulmonary diseases may require chest X-rays.
    - Patients with bone fractures may require X-rays.
  - Fetal reasons for radiation exposure have become obsolete with the availability of USG, MRI, etc.

Drug intake

- Periconceptional folic acid intake (500 mcg OD oral) decreases the incidence of neural tube defects.

High-yield points

Rubella infection during pregnancy

Risks of major fetal anomalies are 50%, 25%, and 10% when infection occurs in the first, second, and third trimesters, respectively.

Congenital rubella syndrome It includes multisystem abnormalities such as the following:

- Triad of sensorineural deafness, congenital cataract, and cardiac defects (patent ductus arteriosus, septal defects)
- Hematological (anemia, thrombocytopenia)
- Hepatosplenomegaly
- Osteopenia
- Chromosomal abnormalities
- Medical termination pregnancy is advised when acute rubella infection occurs during pregnancy (IgM antibody).
- Rubella vaccine is a live vaccine given to nonimmunized, nonpregnant women.
- Rubella vaccine is not recommended during pregnancy and pregnancy should be avoided within 4 weeks of vaccination.

Varicella infection during pregnancy

Risk of congenital malformation is more when infection occurs in the first trimester.

Congenital varicella syndrome It is characterized by the following:

- Limb hypoplasia
- Limb deformity
- Chorioretinal scarring
- Microcephaly
- Cutaneous scarring
- Varicella vaccine is a live attenuated vaccine contraindicated during pregnancy.
- Varicella zoster immunoglobulin (VZIG) should be given to exposed, nonimmune patients.
- VZIG should be given to newborns in case of exposure to infection within 5 days of delivery.

Measles during pregnancy

- It is not teratogenic.
- However, any high-grade fever during pregnancy can lead to abortion, intrauterine death, and preterm delivery.

- Teratogens are chemical or physical agents that cause permanent alteration in structure or function of an organ during embryonic or fetal life, resulting in congenital malformations.
- Examples of teratogenic drugs
  - Antiepileptics—phenytoin and valproate
  - Antihypertensives—ACE inhibitors (captopril, enalapril)
  - Anticoagulants—warfarin
  - Antibiotics—tetracycline and chloramphenicol (some safe antibiotics in pregnancy are penicillins, cephalosporins, and erythromycin)
  - Chemotherapy drugs

Extra edge

Rule of 10: No woman should be exposed to radiation 10 days outside her LMP.

Radiation exposure in various investigation procedures

Procedure	Dose (rad)
Chest X-ray	<0.001
Abdominal X-ray	0.3
Pelvic X-ray	0.5–1
Abdominal CT	0.5–1

Note *USG and MRI are devoid of any ionizing radiation.*

FDA risk category for drugs during pregnancy

See Table 1.16

Importance of history taken in second trimester

Number of antenatal visits It is required to know the booking status.

Tetanus vaccination The Health Ministry of India in 2018 replaced the tetanus toxoid (TT) vaccine with tetanus-diphtheria toxoid (Td) vaccine on WHO guidance, as it would be more beneficial than using a TT vaccine alone. Tetanus and diphtheria (Td) vaccine is a

Table 1.16 Risk category [as per Food and Drug Administration (FDA)] of drugs during pregnancy

Category	Definition	Remarks
A	Safest drugs during pregnancy	No fetal risk in well-controlled studies. *Examples*: Folic acid, levothyroxine
B	No evidence of fetal risk in humans	Well-controlled studies show no fetal risk, despite risk in animal studies. *Examples*: Penicillin V, amoxicillin, erythromycin, paracetamol, metformin
C	Fetal risk cannot be ruled out. Potential benefit may outweigh the risk	Well-controlled studies in humans are lacking. *Examples*: Corticosteroids, adrenaline, thiopentone, atropine, tramadol, gabapentin, amlodipine
D	• Positive evidence of fetal risk • Potential benefit (life-threatening situations) may outweigh the risk	Studies in humans have demonstrated risk. *Examples*: Phenytoin, phenobarbitone, doxycycline, clonazepam
X	Contraindicated in pregnancy	Proven fetal risks. *Examples*: ACE inhibitors, mifepristone, danazol, isotretinoin, methotrexate, radioactive iodine, atorvastatin

combination of tetanus and diphtheria with lower concentration of diphtheria antigen (d) as recommended for older children and adults.

- The use of Td instead of TT is recommended during pregnancy to protect against maternal and neonatal tetanus and diphtheria during prenatal care.
- Vaccination during pregnancy also serves to boost immunity and increases the duration of protection in those pregnant women who had not received the full set of recommended booster doses.
- Td is safe during pregnancy and the dose is 0.5 mL given as intramuscular injection in the deltoid or upper outer quadrant of buttocks.
- The National Immunization Schedule in India recommends two doses of Td for unknown immunization status of pregnant women.
  - First dose of Td is administered early in pregnancy (in many clinics, it is administered at 16–20 weeks, when the patient comes to get anomaly scan done)
  - Second dose of Td is administered 4 weeks after the first dose or at least 4 weeks prior to EDD.

If a mother received two Td doses in the last pregnancy and the next pregnancy is within 3 years, then only one booster dose of Td is recommended.

The WHO recommends a third dose of Td to be given 6 months after the second dose, to provide protection for at least 5 years.

Viva corner

Q1 What is warfarin embryopathy?

Warfarin intake during organogenesis period can result in fetal anomalies termed warfarin embryopathy or Conradi syndrome. It includes the following:

- Skeletal and facial anomalies
- Optic atrophy
- Microcephaly
- Chondrodysplasia punctata

Note *CDC advices the use of Tdap (Tetanus toxoid, reduced diphtheria toxoid, and acellular Pertussis vaccine) during each pregnancy. Optimal timing for vaccination is 27–36 weeks of gestation to maximize the maternal antibody response and passive antibody transfer to the infant. Pertussis component has been added to prevent deaths due to pertussis among infants who are too young to be protected by the childhood pertussis vaccine series that starts at 2 months of age.*

Quickening

- **Definition:** Perception of fetal movements for the first time during pregnancy is called quickening.
  - Quickening is usually felt at:
    - 18–20 weeks in primigravida

- 16–18 weeks in multigravida (a multigravida feels earlier because she already knows how a fetal movement feels like)

- Significance of quickening
  - It assures a live fetus at that point of time.
  - Date of quickening may be helpful in calculating the POG, in case of irregular cycles or if LMP is not known.
    - In primigravida: Quickening + 20 weeks = EDD
    - In multigravida: Quickening + 22 weeks = EDD

Bleeding P/V in second trimester

- Causes
  - Abortion
  - Molar pregnancy
  - Local lesions—cervical erosion, polyps, and cervicitis

Drug intake

- Iron and calcium supplementation is started when the nausea and vomiting of pregnancy settles down, usually around 14 weeks.
- Recommended prophylaxis included 100 mg of elemental iron and 1 g of calcium daily during pregnancy (National Nutritional Anemia Control Program 2013, Govt. of India, Iron Plus Initiative).

> **High-yield points**
>
> **Immunizations that can be given during pregnancy**
>
> - Vaccines that provide active immunity
>   - TT and diphtheria toxoid
>   - Rabies (inactivated virus)
>   - Hepatitis A and B (inactivated virus)
>   - Vaccination against pneumococcal, meningococcal, and *Haemophilus* (inactivated bacterial)
> - Immunoglobulins for postexposure prophylaxis (passive immunity)
>   - Hepatitis A and B
>   - Tetanus
>   - Rabies
>   - Varicella
>   - Measles
>
> **Immunizations that are contraindicated in pregnancy**
>
> - Measles (live viral vaccine)
> - Mumps (live viral vaccine)
> - Varicella zoster (live viral vaccine)

- Current recommendation: Anemia Mukt Bharat Program (2018–2022) by the Govt. of India recommends daily intake of one iron and folic acid tablet containing 60 mg elemental iron +500 μg folic acid, starting from the second trimester and continued throughout pregnancy for a minimum 180 days followed by intake for 180 days in the postpartum period.

Symptoms of preeclampsia Excessive weight gain, swelling of feet, decreased urine output, headache, blurring of vision, and epigastric pain are the symptoms suggestive of preeclampsia (elaborated in Part 1, Chapter 4, *Hypertensive Disorders in Pregnancy).*

- Importance of excessive weight gain
  - Normal weight gain during pregnancy is 10–12 kg for an average Indian woman.
  - Weight gain is distributed as 1–2 kg in the first trimester, 5 kg in the second trimester, and 5 kg in the third trimester.
  - Weight gain should not be more than 0.5 kg in a week or more than 2 kg in a month.
- Importance of swelling of feet: The causes and characteristics of swelling of feet during pregnancy are mentioned in Table 1.17.

Note *Pedal edema is not included in diagnostic criteria for preeclampsia. Headache, blurring of vision, epigastric pain, and decreased urine output are imminent symptoms of eclampsia.*

Table 1.17 Causes and characteristics of swelling of feet in pregnancy

Physiological edema	Pathological edema
• Cause – Physiological edema of pregnancy develops due to pressure of the gravid uterus on inferior vena cava, thereby decreasing venous return	• Causes – Pregnancy-induced hypertension – Congestive cardiac failure – Anemia – Hypoproteinemia – Renal failure
• Characteristics – Usually develops in the third trimester – Relieved by rest – Dependent edema	• Characteristics – Can present in any trimester – Not relieved by rest – Can develop in non-dependent sites such as abdomen, hands, face, and vulva

Screening for GDM

Universal screening for GDM is recommended in the first antenatal visit and repeated at 24–28 weeks when glucose intolerance during pregnancy is maximum manifested

Ultrasonography in second trimester

USG to detect fetal anomalies is usually done between 16 and 24 weeks.

Importance of history taken in third trimester

Number of antenatal visits It helps to know the booking status.

Perception of fetal movements It assures that the fetus is alive.

H/o bleeding P/V in third trimester Causes of bleeding P/V in the third trimester are given in Table 1.18.

Table 1.18 Causes of bleeding P/V in third trimester

Physiological causes	Pathological causes
• "Show"—passage of blood-stained discharge P/V with the onset of labor	• Antepartum hemorrhage—placenta previa and abruption • Scar rupture in previous cesarean pregnancy • Local lesions—cervical erosion, carcinoma cervix, cervical polyp, etc.

Viva corner

Q1 How is a fetal kick count kept?

Cardiff's "count to 10" formula:

- The patient starts to count fetal movements from a particular time in the morning.
- The counting comes to end as soon as 10 movements are perceived.
- Admitted patients are usually given a thread and asked to make a knot during each fetal movement.
- Perception of <10 fetal movements over 12 hours on successive days or no fetal movement over 12 hours in a single day is considered abnormal.

Viva corner

Q1 What is antepartum hemorrhage (APH)?

APH refers to bleeding from or into the genital tract after 28 weeks of gestation but before the delivery of the baby.

- **Placenta previa:** Placenta is attached partially or completely onto the lower uterine segment. Bleeding occurs due to the shearing effect between the placenta and the uterine wall, when the lower uterine segment gets formed.
- **Abruption:** Premature separation of a normally located placenta (usually placenta separates only after the delivery of the baby).

H/o drug intake The patient is advised to take iron and calcium supplementation throughout pregnancy.

Symptoms of preeclampsia Already discussed under second trimester.

H/o pain abdomen

Causes of pain abdomen in the third trimester are given in Table 1.19.

H/o leaking P/V It implies rupture of membranes.

Premature rupture of membranes or prelabor rupture of membranes

- **Definition:** It refers to the rupture of membranes before the onset of labor.
  - *Term prelabor rupture of membranes (PROM):* When the rupture of membranes

Table 1.19 Causes of pain abdomen in third trimester

Obstetric causes	Nonobstetric causes
• Labor pain • Abruption • Scar dehiscence in previous cesarean section	• Medical: Peptic ulcer, urinary tract infection • Surgical: Appendicitis, cholecystitis • Gynecological: Red degeneration of fibroid, twisted ovarian cyst

Viva corner

Q1 How are true and false labor pains differentiated?

Table Differentiating features of true and false labor pain

True labor pain	False labor pain
• Increase in frequency, duration, and intensity of uterine contractions as time advances	• Irregular uterine contractions
• Pain in lower back radiating to front of abdomen and thighs	• Lower abdominal pain mostly
• Associated with cervical changes—cervical dilatation and effacement	• No associated cervical dilatation or effacement
• Does not subside with enema or sedation	• Subsides with enema/sedation

occurs beyond 37 completed weeks but before the onset of labor
- *Preterm PROM (PPROM):* When the rupture of membranes occurs prior to 37 completed weeks of gestation

Clinical diagnosis of rupture of membranes

- H/o leaking per vagina
- Speculum examination to look for leaking of liquor
- Valsalva maneuver (ask the patient to cough and look for escape of liquor)

Importance of menstrual history

- To know the regularity of cycles (LMP may not be reliable in women with irregular cycles)
- H/o menorrhagia in previous cycles (patient may be anemic/associated hypothyroidism may be present)

Importance of marital history

- The risk of congenital and chromosomal abnormalities is higher in consanguineous marriages.
  - Degree of consanguinity is given in Table 1.20.

Viva corner

Q1 What is the reason for increased frequency of micturition in the first and third trimesters?

- In the first trimester, congestion and compression of bladder by the pressure of the growing uterus causes increased frequency of micturition that disappears in the second trimester, as the uterus becomes an abdominal organ.
- It reappears in the third trimester as the head descends into the pelvis and exerts pressure on the bladder.

Q2 How will you differentiate liquor from urine or vaginal discharge?

Confirmation tests for liquor may be done to rule out urine or vaginal discharge.

- **Nitrazine paper test:** Nitrazine paper turns from yellow to blue due to alkalinity (pH >6) of amniotic fluid.
- **Fern test:** The pooled fluid is collected from posterior fornix and the smear prepared is examined under microscope—appearance of arborization or ferning pattern confirms liquor.
- **Nile blue sulfate test:** Presence of orange blue cells on staining with Nile blue sulfate indicates the presence of fetal fat cells in liquor.

Table 1.20 Degree of consanguinity

First degree (incest)	Brother–sister/parent–child
Second degree	Uncle–niece/aunt–nephew
Third degree	First cousins (half-uncle–niece/half-aunt–nephew)

- When was the conception after marriage?
  - *High fecundity*: Conception immediately after marriage
  - *Low fecundity*: Conception after a period of infertility

Importance of past obstetric history

- Past obstetric history is one of the important histories that determines the plan of management in the present pregnancy.

- Examples
  - *H/o previous LSCS*: Decision on repeat cesarean section or trial of labor is based on the previous obstetric history.
  - *H/o recurrent pregnancy loss*: The cause has to be identified and treated if possible. Example: Second trimester loss due to cervical incompetence → cervical encerclage has to done in the present pregnancy to prevent pregnancy loss.
  - *H/o preeclampsia, GDM, anemia, and preterm labor in previous pregnancy*: There is an increased chance of recurrence in the subsequent pregnancy.

Importance of past medical and surgical history

- The significance of past obstetric history is mainly to categorize whether the pregnancy is potentially a high-risk pregnancy based on women's previous experience of conception, pregnancy, and childbirth.
- Past medical history has clinical implication during present pregnancy—monitoring of medical conditions is required during pregnancy as:
  - Certain conditions may worsen during pregnancy—cardiac disease and DM.
  - Certain conditions may remain unchanged—bronchial asthma.
  - Certain conditions may improve during pregnancy—autoimmune disorders (pregnancy is an immunosuppressive condition).
- Difficulties are anticipated during cesarean section in cases with previous abdominal surgeries.

Importance of personal history

- **Alcohol consumption during pregnancy:** Can lead to fetal malformations and intrauterine growth restriction (IUGR)
- **Heavy smoking during pregnancy:** Can lead to abortion and IUGR

Importance of diet history

- Diet history helps in identifying dietary deficiencies and excesses of calories and proteins.
- Dietary history is particularly important in some pregnancy-related complications where dietary modifications are suggested, for example, diabetic diet in case of gestational diabetes, and iron-rich, high-protein diet in case of anemia in pregnancy.

Additional calorie and protein requirement during pregnancy is given in Table 1.21.

Table 1.21 Additional requirement of calories and proteins during pregnancy

	Pregnancy	Lactation
Calories (kcal/day)	+350	+500
Proteins (g/day)	+15	+25

Importance of family history

- Certain conditions can have familial inheritance—DM and hypertension.
- Certain disorders can run in families—autosomal dominant disorders.
- There is an increased chance of occurrence of multiple pregnancy or congenital anomalies in women with such family history.

Discussion points in examination

Relevance of performing general examination

Whether the patient is comfortable at rest The patient may be uncomfortable at rest in the following conditions:

- Cardiac diseases (New York Heart Association (NYHA) class IV) and anemia in failure
- Respiratory diseases such as lower respiratory infection, chronic obstructive pulmonary disease (COPD), and bronchial asthma (due to tachypnea, and working of accessory muscles)
- Overdistension of abdomen such as in polyhydramnios and multiple pregnancy

Built

- Built refers to the skeletal framework of a person.
- Medium built refers to one who is average in height and weight. The person is neither tall nor short, neither fat nor skinny.
- Well-built refers to one who does exercises for conditioning of the body and has a muscular built.
- Thin built refers to one who has a lean body mass.

Nourishment

- Nourishment is clinically assessed by the following:
  - Examining for features of vitamin deficiency

- Measurement of skin-fold thickness and midarm circumference
- Nourishment is expressed as "patient is averagely nourished/well nourished/poorly nourished."
- Clinical significance: A poorly nourished woman may be at an increased risk of anemia, infections, etc., during pregnancy.

Height

- Clinical significance
  - Height ≤145 cm is referred to as short stature. The incidence of contracted pelvis and CPD is more in short-statured women.
  - Height is one of the parameters used to calculate the BMI.

Weight

- Clinical significance
  - Serial maternal weight gain is monitored during pregnancy—excessive weight gain may be an initial symptom of preeclampsia.
  - Women with prepregnancy body weight of <45 kg are more prone to have low-birth-weight babies and growth-restricted babies.
  - Obese women are prone to develop complications during pregnancy such as preeclampsia, DM, big baby, and increased risk of operative interferences.
- Causes of excessive maternal weight gain: Preeclampsia, diabetes, multiple pregnancy, big baby, and polyhydramnios
- Causes of poor maternal weight gain: Malnutrition, IUGR, oligohydramnios, and intrauterine death
  - Weight is one of the parameters used to calculate the BMI.

Body mass index

- BMI = weight (kg)/[height $(m)^2$]. Classification of weight based on BMI is given in Table 1.22.

Table 1.22 WHO BMI classification for the general population and for Asian populations

	General population	Asian population
Underweight	<18.5 kg/m^2	<18.5 kg/m^2
Ideal	18.5–24.9 kg/m^2	18.5–23 kg/m^2
Overweight	25.0–29.9 kg/m^2	23–27.5 kg/m^2
Obese	≥30 kg/m^2	>27.5 kg/m^2

- Clinical significance
  - BMI is used to calculate the diet chart or meal plan for the patient (based on the BMI calculated from prepregnancy body weight).
  - Preeclampsia and GDM are more common in women with increased BMI.
  - Malnutrition and anemia are more common in underweight women.

Pallor (Figure 1.16)

- Pallor is paleness of skin due to reduced oxyhemoglobin or decreased peripheral perfusion.
- Mentioned as "pallor present or absent." Grade of anemia (mild/moderate/severe) is assessed by checking hemoglobin level.
- Anemia and pallor are not synonymous. Anemia is one of the causes for pallor.
- Indian Council of Medical Research (ICMR) classification of anemia during pregnancy is given in Table 1.23.

Pedal edema (Figure 1.17)

- Physiological edema accounts for 80% of pedal edema during pregnancy.

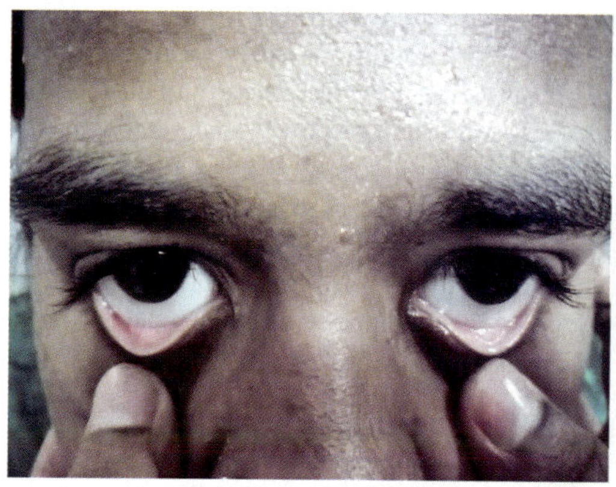

Figure 1.16 Demonstration of pallor.

Table 1.23 ICMR classification of anemia during pregnancy

Grade	Hemoglobin (g/dL)
Mild	10–11
Moderate	7–9.9
Severe	<7
Very severe	≤4

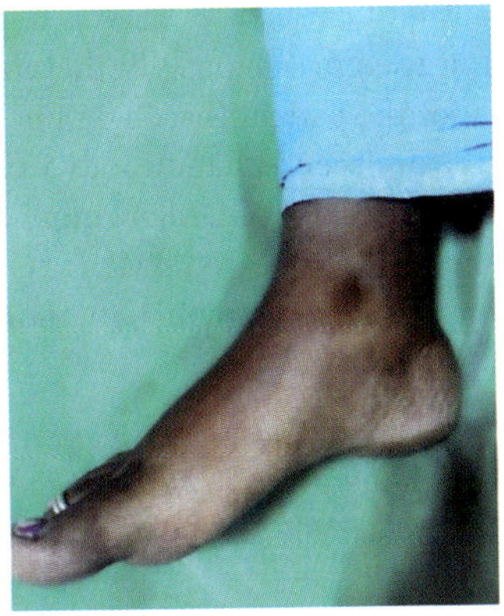

Figure 1.17 Pitting pedal edema.

Viva corner

Q1 What are the sites to look for pallor?

- Lower palpebral conjunctiva
- Dorsum of the tongue
- Soft palate
- Nail beds
- Palms and sole
- Skin

Q2 What are the causes of pallor other than anemia?

Anemia is one of the causes of pallor. Other causes are the following:

- Neurogenic shock
- Hypoglycemia and other metabolic derangements
- Pheochromocytoma

Table 1.24 Causes of bilateral and unilateral pedal edema during pregnancy

Bilateral pedal edema	Unilateral pedal edema
• Physiological edema of pregnancy • Preeclampsia • Anemia • Hypoproteinemia • Cardiac causes—congestive cardiac failure • Renal causes (glomerulonephritis, nephrotic syndrome, etc.) • Hypothyroidism (bilateral non-pitting ankle edema)	• Filariasis • Lymphangitis • Deep vein thrombosis • Cellulitis

- Features that differentiate physiological edema from pathological edema have already been mentioned in Table 1.17.
- Causes of unilateral and bilateral pedal edema are mentioned in Table 1.24.

High-yield points

Sites to look for edema

- Just above medial malleolus, elicited by pressing with the thumb for at least 15 seconds
- Dorsum of foot
- Sacrum (in bedridden patients)
- Abdomen
- Vulva
- Hands and face

Icterus

- **Definition:** Icterus or jaundice refers to yellowish discoloration of the skin and sclera of the eyes due to high bilirubin levels. When serum bilirubin exceeds 2 mg%, icterus appears (normal values: Total bilirubin 0.2–1.2 mg/dL; direct bilirubin <0.3 mg/dL).
- **Causes of jaundice during pregnancy:** See Table 1.25

Table 1.25 Causes of jaundice during pregnancy

Jaundice peculiar to pregnancy	Jaundice unrelated to pregnant state	Jaundice in cases of pregnancy superimposed on chronic liver diseases
• Intrahepatic cholestasis (obstetric hepatosis) • Severe pre-eclampsia, eclampsia, HELLP syndrome • Acute fatty liver of pregnancy • Severe hyperemesis gravidarum • Disseminated intravascular coagulation	• Viral hepatitis • Obstructive jaundice due to gallstones • Drug induced—isoniazid therapy • Hemolytic jaundice—mismatched blood transfusion, malaria, etc.	• Chronic hepatitis • Cirrhosis

High-yield points

Sites to look for icterus (examine under sunlight)

- Upper bulbar conjunctiva
- Undersurface of tongue
- Soft palate
- Sole and palm
- Skin

Cyanosis

- **Definition:** It is defined as bluish discoloration of skin and mucous membranes.

Causes of cyanosis can be central or peripheral, which are described in Table 1.26.

Clubbing

- **Definition:** It refers to selective bulbous enlargement of distal segment of digits (Figure 1.18). Mention as "Clubbing present or absent."
- **Causes of clubbing**
  - *Cardiac:* Cyanotic heart diseases
  - *Respiratory:* Bronchiectasis and interstitial lung diseases
  - *GIT:* Crohn disease and ulcerative colitis

Table 1.26 Central and peripheral cyanosis

Central cyanosis	Peripheral cyanosis
• Circulatory or ventilatory problem causing poor blood oxygenation in the lungs, leading to ≤85% fall in arterial oxygen saturation • Causes – Central nervous system—seizures, intracranial hemorrhage – Respiratory system—chronic obstructive pulmonary disease – Cardiovascular system—congenital heart diseases, cardiac failure – Methemoglobinemia	• Reduction in blood flow to extremities • Causes – All causes of central cyanosis – Reduced cardiac output—hypovolemia, cardiac failure – Local vasoconstriction—cold exposure, peripheral vascular diseases

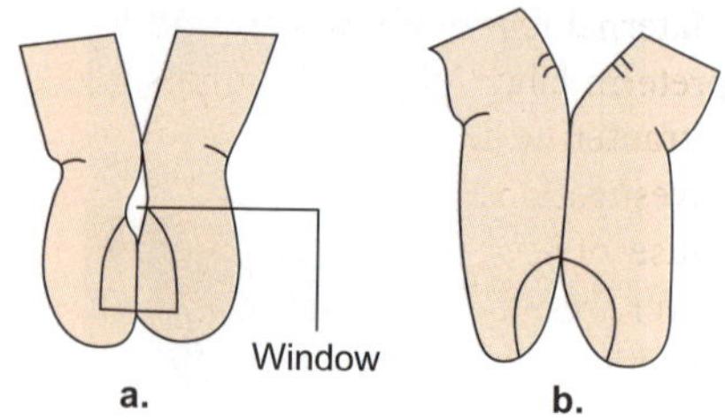

Figure 1.18 Clubbing of fingers. **a.** Normal fingers. **b.** Clubbing of fingers—obliteration of the diamond-shaped window (Schamroth sign).

Note *Look for cyanosis and clubbing especially in cases with cardiac disease complicating pregnancy*

Extra edge

Grades of clubbing

Table Grades of clubbing

Grade of clubbing	Features
I	Increased fluctuation of nail bed
II	Obliteration of Lovibond's angle (angle between nail and nail bed)
III	Increased curvature of nails leading to parrot beaking or drumstick appearance
IV	Hypertrophic osteoarthropathy (painful, tender swelling of wrist and elbows)

Lymphadenopathy

- Palpate for any enlarged lymph nodes—mention the number, site, size, mobility, and whether the nodes are tender or nontender.
- Cervical nodes may be palpable in tuberculosis and enlarged nodes may be present in any local infection.
- Mention as "lymphadenopathy present or absent."

Vitals

Temperature

- Significance of recording temperature

- Maternal febrile illness can lead to abortion, preterm labor, oligohydramnios and sudden intrauterine death.
- Investigations should be done to identify the cause of fever (upper respiratory infection, lower respiratory infection, urinary tract infection, chorioamnionitis, etc.).

Pulse Radial pulse is palpated at the wrist by pulp of three fingers with the patient's forearm in semiprone position and slight flexion of wrist.

- In cardiac disease, pulse may be abnormal in rate, rhythm, volume, and character, and radiofemoral delay may be present.
- In anemia, patient may have a high volume pulse.

Respiratory rate Physiological breathlessness during pregnancy may be present due to the following:

- Distension of uterus pushing the diaphragm up
- Decrease in the central nervous system (CNS) threshold for CO_2

High-yield points

Table Causes of maternal tachycardia and bradycardia

Causes of maternal tachycardia	Causes of maternal bradycardia
• Fever • Cardiac failure • Hyperthyroidism • Arrhythmias • Anemia • Acute hemorrhage such as APH • Scar rupture • Drugs—beta-agonists	• Heart block • Hypothyroidism • Drugs—beta-blockers

Table Causes of low and high volume pulse

Causes of low-volume pulse (hypokinetic pulse)	Causes of high-volume pulse (hyperkinetic pulse)
• Cardiac failure • Shock • Aortic and mitral stenosis	• Anemia • Mitral and aortic regurgitation

Causes of breathlessness during pregnancy

- Cardiac diseases
- Respiratory diseases: Lower respiratory infection, bronchial asthma, and COPD
- Anemia complicating pregnancy especially when in failure
- Obstetric causes: Multiple pregnancy and polyhydramnios

Viva corner

Q1 How is BP checked?

- Position of the patient in one of the following positions:
  - Sitting position
  - Semirecumbent position at an angle of 30° with horizontal
  - Left lateral position
- Position of cuff
  - Cuff is wrapped firmly but not tightly, 2–3 cm above elbow.
- Size of the cuff
  - Bladder of the cuff should go 80% around the arm.
  - Bladder width should be 40% of arm circumference.
  - Small-sized cuff for obese women may overestimate BP.
  - Large-sized cuff for any woman underestimates BP.
- Recording BP
  - Systolic BP is first recorded manually by palpating the radial pulse and then with sphygmomanometer.
  - Systolic BP is recorded when repetitive Korotkoff sounds are first heard (K1).
  - Diastolic BP is recorded at the point when the sound disappears (K5).
- Korotkoff sounds
  - *K1*: First appearance of tapping sound occurs.
  - *K2*: Sounds are like murmur or swishing quality.
  - *K3*: Sounds become crisper with increased intensity.
  - *K4*: Sounds become muffled.
  - *K5*: Sounds disappear.

Note *Respiratory rate is one of the parameters to be monitored while administering $MgSO_4$ in eclampsia.*

Blood pressure BP is recorded during each antenatal visit to watch out for preeclampsia. Preeclampsia is a multisystem disorder of unknown etiology characterized by the following:

- BP of ≥140/90 mmHg, recorded for the first time during pregnancy, after 20 weeks of gestation on at least two occasions, 4 hours apart and associated with proteinuria

Breast examination

- Retracted nipples, if detected should be treated during antenatal period to establish normal lactation and suckling by infant following delivery. Treatment is with syringing (done after 36 weeks as nipple stimulation may lead to preterm labor)
- Cracked nipples—can lead to painful lactation and mastitis; treated with local application of paraffin
- Discharge from nipples and any palpable mass should be evaluated further

High-yield points

Breast changes during pregnancy

- Pronounced pigmentation of areola and nipples
- Appearance of secondary areola and Montgomery's tubercles
- Increased vascularity

Thyroid examination

In case of obvious enlargement of the thyroid gland or if it feels nodular, the patient must be subjected to further investigations.

Effects of untreated maternal hypothyroidism

Untreated hypothyroidism increases the risk of abortion, preterm delivery, and preeclampsia, and affects the intellectual development of the child.

Effects of untreated maternal hyperthyroidism

- **Maternal effects:** Abortion, preterm delivery, preeclampsia, congestive cardiac failure (CCF), abruption, and thyroid storm
- **Fetal/neonatal effects:** Prematurity, stillbirth, fetal hyperthyroidism or hypothyroidism, and increased perinatal morbidity and mortality

Gait and spine examination

Lower limb deformities and kyphoscoliosis may be associated with CPD; difficulty encountered while giving regional anesthesia for cesarean section.

Relevance of performing systemic examination

Cardiovascular system

- Auscultation of CVS has to be done in all antenatal cases during the initial antenatal visit to detect any cardiac abnormalities.

Note *Rheumatic heart diseases may be identified for the first time during pregnancy.*

- If the patient is a known case of heart disease, detailed CVS examination has to be presented (mentioned in Part 1, Chapter 5, *Cardiac Disease in Pregnancy*).

High-yield points

Table Differentiating features that simulate heart disease during pregnancy and those specific to heart disease

Pregnancy changes that simulate organic heart disease	Features that are specific to organic heart disease
• Palpitation • Dyspnea • Pedal edema • Easy fatigue • Short systolic murmur • Third heart sound • Rotation of the axis of heart	• Progressive dyspnea • Paroxysmal nocturnal dyspnea • Chest pain • Syncope with exertion • Evidence of pulmonary congestion (hemoptysis, fine basal crepitations) • Cyanosis • Clubbing • Palpable thrill • Loud systolic murmur (grade 3/6 or more) • Diastolic murmur • Cardiomegaly • Arrhythmia

Respiratory system

Auscultation of RS is performed for normal vesicular breath sounds. RS examination may be abnormal in the following cases:
- Cardiac diseases (fine crepts in CCF)
- Lower respiratory infections (coarse crepts or rhonchi)
- Pneumonia (decreased breath sounds)
- Tuberculosis
- COPD

Relevance of performing an obstetric abdominal examination

Inspection

Shape or distension of the abdomen
- Longitudinally distended in cephalic and breech presentation
- Transversely distended in transverse lie of fetus
- Flattening of abdomen below umbilicus is present in occipitoposterior position
- Overdistended in multiple pregnancy and polyhydramnios
- Flanks full in term pregnancy

Linea nigra
- Linea nigra is a brownish black–colored line that develops in the midline of the abdomen during pregnancy.
- Cause may be due to increase in aldosterone production and melanocyte-stimulating hormone during pregnancy.
- It usually disappears following delivery.

Striae gravidarum
- Striae gravidarum are stretch marks that may develop over the skin of abdomen, breast, or thighs in the later months of pregnancy.
- Striae are caused by tears in the dermis, due to rapid stretching of the skin associated with growth of fetus or weight changes. Stretch marks may also be influenced by hormonal changes associated with pregnancy.
- They may disappear or persist following delivery.

Palpation

Fundal height Anatomical landmarks used for estimation of fundal height include symphysis pubis, umbilicus, and xiphisternum (Figure 1.19).

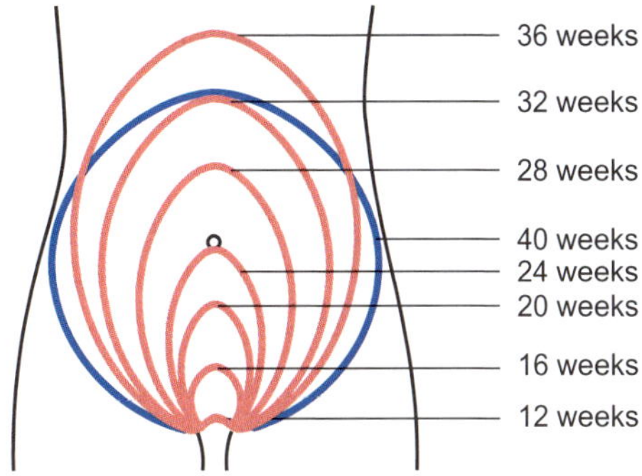

Figure 1.19 Fundal height at different weeks of gestation.

- Up to 12 weeks (first trimester), uterus remains a pelvic organ and there is primarily an increase in the anterior posterior diameter of the uterus.
- After 12 weeks of gestation, uterus becomes an abdominal organ. Uterus is palpable just above the symphysis pubis at 12 weeks.
- Fundal height at the level of umbilicus corresponds to 24 weeks of gestation.
- Fundal height at the level of xiphisternum corresponds to 36 weeks of gestation.
- The distance between the symphysis pubis and the umbilicus is divided into three equal parts by two imaginary lines corresponding to 16, 20, and 24 weeks.
- The distance between umbilicus and xiphisternum is divided into three equal parts by two imaginary lines corresponding to 28, 32, and 36 weeks.
- At 40 weeks of gestation, due to the engagement of fetal head, the fundal height reduces and corresponds to the level at 32 weeks with flank fullness.
- After determining fundal height, assess whether it corresponds to the POG calculated from LMP.
- **Significance of fundal height:** Causes of discrepancy in fundal height are mentioned in Table 1.27. Further evaluation with ultrasonography is required if the discrepancy between POG and fundal height is ±4 weeks

Symphysiofundal height
- SFH in centimeters corresponds to the POG in weeks from 18 to 32 weeks of gestation.
- Significance

Table 1.27 Causes of discrepancy in fundal height

Causes of fundal height more than POG	Causes of fundal height less than POG
• Wrong dates • Full bladder • Multiple pregnancy • Polyhydramnios • Big baby • Concealed abruption • Associated fibroid uterus or ovarian mass	• Wrong dates • Intrauterine growth restriction • Oligohydramnios • Intrauterine death • Transverse lie

POG, period of gestation.

- To assess growth of fetus
  - Variation in SFH of ±2 cm is considered as normal
  - Discrepancy in SFH by values more than ±2 cm → suspect causes that are mentioned in Table 1.27
- To calculate the clinically estimated fetal weight using Johnson's formula that uses SFH as a parameter
- For gravidogram charting (Figure 1.20)
  - Gravidogram is a graphical representation of the growth of fetus, where the SFH (Y-axis) is plotted against the POG (X-axis).
  - If the measurement falls below the 10th percentile, fetal growth restriction is suspected.

Obstetric grips or Leopold's maneuvers of abdominal palpation

Obstetric grips are performed to identify the fetal lie, presentation and attitude of the fetal head, and to know whether the head is engaged or not.

Fundal grip It helps to identify the fetal pole that occupies the fundus of uterus.

- In longitudinal lie, either breech or head occupies the fundus of the uterus.
- Description of head—"hard, globular, ballotable mass" is suggestive of head.
- Description of breech—"soft, broad, irregular, nonballotable mass" is suggestive of breech (**Hint:** *Remember "SBI"*).

Lateral grip

- It helps to identify the position of fetal back and limbs.
- Identifying the side of back helps to determine the position of fetal head.
- In longitudinal lie, back is felt on one side and fetal limbs are felt on the other side.
- In transverse lie, fetal head is felt on one of the sides.
- Description of the back: "Uniformly curved, smooth resistance felt" is suggestive of back
- Description of limbs: "Irregular, knob-like structures felt" is suggestive of limb buds

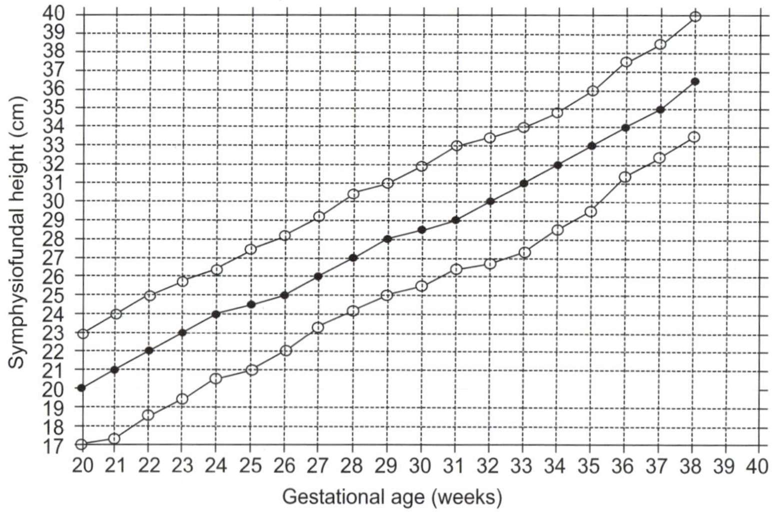

Figure 1.20 Gravidogram for plotting symphysiofundal height.

Viva corner

Q1 How is a 32-week pregnancy differentiated from a term pregnancy as the fundal height is same at both these periods of gestation?

Table Differentiating features of 32-week pregnancy and a term pregnancy

32 weeks	Term
• Fundal height is 32 weeks; abdomen is longitudinally distended • Flanks are not full • Head feels preterm on palpation • Head is free floating in cephalic presentation	• Fundal height is 32 weeks; abdomen is spherical in shape • Flanks are full • Head feels term • Head may be fixed or engaged

Q2 How should one look for fullness of flanks?

While the patient is in a sitting position, look from the posterior aspect (from the back) of the patient. Flanks are said to be full if there is any obvious bulge on the sides of the flanks, seen from the posterior aspect.

Q3 What is the reason for dextrorotation of uterus in some cases?

The uterus at term may be dextrorotated because of the presence of sigmoid colon on the left side.

First pelvic grip It helps:

- To know the presentation of the fetus: To identify the fetal pole that occupies the lower pole of uterus
  - In longitudinal lie, either head or breech occupies the lower pole of the uterus—cephalic or breech presentation, respectively.
  - In transverse lie, the first pelvic grip is empty.
- To know whether the head is engaged or not: When the head is engaged, two-fifth or less of the head palpable

Note *Fetal head may be fixed, but not necessarily engaged. An engaged or fixed head will be nonballotable.*

Second pelvic grip It helps:

- To confirm the findings of the first pelvic grip
  - Confirms presentation
  - Confirms whether the head is engaged or not
    - Engaged head: Hands will be diverging
    - Head not engaged: Hands will be converging
- To make out attitude of the fetal head (additional findings made in the second pelvic grip)
  - Determined by observing the relative position of sinciput and occiput of the fetal head
  - Occiput—the pole that lies on the side of fetal back
  - Sinciput—the pole that lies on the side of fetal limbs
- **Well-flexed head:** Sinciput at a higher level than occiput
- **Deflexed head:** Sinciput and occiput at the same level
- **Extended head:** Occiput at a higher level than sinciput

Relationship between sinciput and occiput (Figure 1.21)

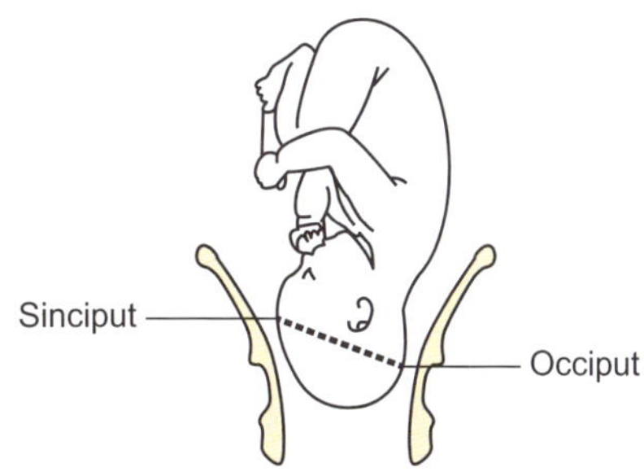

Figure 1.21 Relationship between sinciput and occiput in a well-flexed head.

Uterine activity

- **Braxton Hicks contractions:** Rhythmic, irregular, painless uterine contractions are present throughout pregnancy called Braxton Hicks contractions.
- **Effective uterine contractions:** During labor, contractions are said to be effective if three contractions are felt in 10 minutes, each lasting for up to 45 seconds. Painful uterine contractions at <37 weeks of gestation, may be suggestive of preterm labor.

Liquor amount

- **Polyhydramnios (excess liquor):** Fundal height will be >POG; fetal parts will be difficult to palpate. Difficult to auscultate fetal heart rate/heard at a distance. Causes of polyhydramnios are mentioned in Table 1.28.
- **Oligohydramnios (reduced liquor):** Fundal height will be <POG; Uterus appears full of fetus due to scanty liquor. Causes of oligohydramnios are mentioned in Table 1.29.

Table 1.28 Causes of polyhydramnios

Maternal	Fetal	Placental
• GDM • Rh iso-immunization	• Multiple pregnancy • Fetal anomalies – Esophageal and duodenal atresia – Anencephaly	• Chorio-angioma of placenta

Table 1.29 Causes of oligohydramnios

Maternal	Fetal	Placental
• PROM • Prolonged pregnancy	• Chromosomal anomalies • Renal agenesis • IUGR	• Amnion nodosum

Viva corner

Q1 What is engagement of presenting part?

- Engagement occurs when the largest transverse diameter of the presenting part crosses the pelvic brim.
- In cephalic presentation, head is said to be engaged when the biparietal diameter crosses the pelvic brim (see figure below).

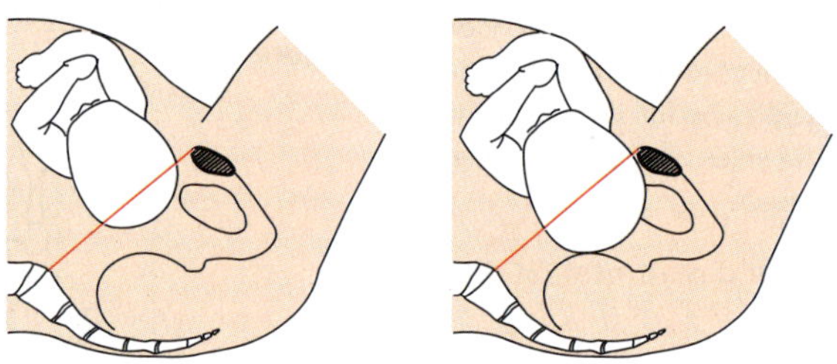

a. b.

Figure Engagement of the fetal head in vertex presentation. **a.** The biparietal diameter lies above the pelvic brim when the head is not engaged. **b.** The biparietal diameter lies below the pelvic brim when the head is engaged.

Q2 When will you say that the head is engaged from abdominal examination?

- Head cannot be moved from side to side.
- Examining fingers are divergent in the second pelvic grip (fingers cannot reach below the presenting part).
- Two-fifth or less of fetal head is palpable by abdominal fifth method (see figure below).
- Sinciput and occiput are not palpable or one pole may be palpable.

Q3 When will you say that the head is not engaged from abdominal examination?

- Head can be moved from side to side (ballotable).
- Examining fingers are convergent in the second pelvic grip.
- Three-fifth or more of fetal head is palpable by abdominal fifth method.
- Both sinciput and occiput are palpable.

(CONTD...)

(...CONTD)

Viva corner

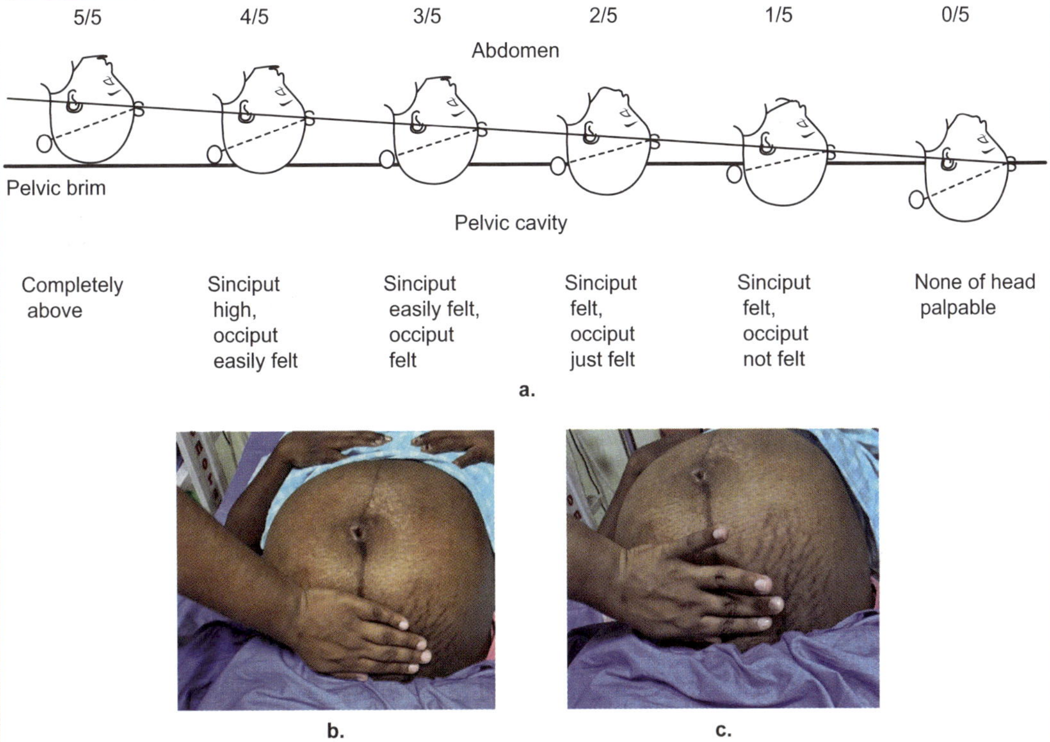

Figure Abdominal fifth method of palpation of descent of fetal head (Crichton's score). **a.** Diagrammatic representation of descent of fetal head in fifths palpable above pubic symphysis. **b.** Five-fifth palpable when the whole head is above the pelvic brim. **c.** Two-fifth palpable—head accommodates two fingers above the pubic symphysis.

Auscultation of fetal heart rate

- FHR is usually heard well on the side of the fetal back.
- Site of auscultation of FHR may vary depending on the presentation of the fetus (Table 1.30).
- Normal FHR is 110–160 bpm.
- FHR abnormalities may indicate fetal hypoxia during pregnancy and labor.
- FHR <110/min is termed fetal bradycardia. Causes of fetal bradycardia are mentioned in Table 1.31.

Table 1.30 Sites of auscultation of fetal heart rate (FHR) depending on the presentation of the fetus

Fetal presentation	Site of FHR
Cephalic presentation, occipitoanterior	Heard along or below the spinoumbilical line
Cephalic presentation, occipitoposterior	Heard laterally near the flanks
Breech presentation	Heard above the level of umbilicus
Transverse lie	Heard around the umbilicus

Table 1.31 Causes of fetal bradycardia

Maternal causes	Fetal causes
• Placental insufficiency • Abruption • Uterine hyperstimulation • Uterine scar dehiscence and rupture • Maternal drugs—beta-blockers	• Fetal conduction heart blocks • Fetal distress

Viva corner

Q1 How frequently should FHR be auscultated during labor?

Table Auscultation of FHR during labor

	Low-risk cases	High-risk cases
First stage of labor	Every 30 minutes	Every 15 minutes
Second stage of labor	Every 15 minutes	Every 5 minutes

Timing: Each auscultation should last for at least 1 minute. Auscultate during a uterine contraction and continue for at least 30 seconds after the contraction. If the FHR is not always in the normal range (i.e., 110–160 bpm), auscultation should be prolonged to cover at least three uterine contractions.

Q2 What are the instances when it is difficult to auscultate FHR?

- FHR is heard with difficulty in cases of maternal obesity, polyhydramnios, and occipitoposterior position, and is absent in intrauterine death

Q3 What are the other sounds that can be heard over the abdomen of a pregnant woman?

- Uterine souffle—soft, blowing sound, synchronous with maternal pulse due to blood flow through the dilated uterine vessels
- Umbilical cord souffle or funic souffle—sharp whistling sound, synchronous with fetal heart rate due to rush of blood through the umbilical arteries
- Fetal thuds (fetal movements)
- Maternal intestinal peristaltic sounds

- FHR >160/min is termed fetal tachycardia. Causes of fetal tachycardia are mentioned in Table 1.32.

Table 1.32 Causes of fetal tachycardia

Maternal causes	Fetal causes
• Anemia • Cardiac failure • Hyperthyroidism • Maternal fever • Drugs—CCB, beta-agonists	• Prematurity • Anemia • Arrhythmias • Fetal infections

Estimated fetal weight

- Calculated using the Johnson's formula
- Common causes of macrosomia
  - Maternal diabetes
  - Prolonged pregnancy
  - Maternal obesity

DIAGNOSIS OF PREGNANCY

Clinical symptoms and signs of pregnancy are given in Table 1.33.

Table 1.33 Clinical symptoms and signs of pregnancy

Maternal	Clinical symptoms	Clinical signs
First trimester	• Amenorrhea • Morning sickness—giddiness, vomiting, nausea, loss of appetite, pica • Increased frequency of micturition • Breast changes—engorgement, fullness	• Uterus increases in size, becomes more vascular and soft – *At 8 weeks*: Size of hen's egg – *At 10 weeks*: Size of orange – *At 12 weeks*: Size of coconut/fetal head

(CONTD...)

Table 1.33 *(CONTD...)*

Maternal	Clinical symptoms	Clinical signs
Second trimester	• Amenorrhea • Skin changes—chloasma, linea nigra, striae gravidarum • Breast changes – Appearance of secondary areola – Secretion of colostrum—12 weeks • Progressive enlargement of abdomen • Quickening felt	• Uterus becomes palpable per abdomen in the second trimester • Fetal parts and fetal movements can be felt from 20 weeks • Fetal heart sound—heard with stethoscope at 20 weeks • Braxton Hicks contractions—begin in early pregnancy and continue till term • Internal and external ballottement can be elicited
Third trimester	• Amenorrhea persists • Enlargement of the abdomen is progressive • Lightening—at about 38th week, especially in primigravidae, a sense of relief of the pressure symptoms is felt due to engagement of the presenting part • Frequency of micturition reappears at term • Fetal movements are more pronounced	• Cutaneous changes are more prominent with increased pigmentation and striae • Fundal height progressively increases • Braxton Hicks contractions are more evident • Fetal movements are easily felt • Palpation of the fetal parts and their identification become easier • Lie, presentation, and position of the fetus are determined • Fetal heart sound is heard distinctly

High-yield points

Various signs elicited during the first-trimester obstetric examination

Table Signs elicited during the first trimester

Signs	Description
Chadwick's sign/ Jacquemier's sign	Bluish discoloration of cervix and vaginal mucosa due to local vascular congestion
Osiander's sign	Increased pulsations felt through lateral fornices
Goodell's sign	Softening of cervix (feels like the lips of mouth)
Hegar's sign	During bimanually palpation at 6–10 weeks, the fingers of the examiner's abdominal and vaginal hands can be opposed at the level of isthmus due to softening of the isthmus
Palmer's sign	Rhythmic contractions of uterus on bimanual examination

Absolute signs of pregnancy

- Palpation of fetal parts
- Palpation of fetal movements
- Auscultation of FHR
- Confirmed by performing USG examination

Differential diagnosis for pregnancy

- Distended bladder
- Fibroid
- Ovarian mass
- Pyometra/hematometra
- Pseudocyesis

Warning signs of pregnancy

- Pain abdomen
- Bleeding P/V
- Leaking P/V
- Headache, blurring of vision, and epigastric pain (imminent symptoms of preeclampsia)

(CONTD...)

(...CONTD)

High-yield points

Common uses of USG in various trimesters

- **First-trimester USG**
  - To confirm intrauterine pregnancy
  - To confirm viability of fetus
  - To accurately estimate the POG. Most accurate parameter in estimating gestational age is crown–rump length (CRL)
  - Anencephaly is the only anomaly that can be detected in the first-trimester USG. It is identified by absence of fetal skull and protruding eyeballs (frog's-eye appearance).
  - Best time to diagnose multiple pregnancy
  - Screening for chromosomal abnormalities at 11–13 weeks by assessing nuchal translucency
- **Second-trimester USG**
  - To estimate gestational age (±10 days)—biparietal diameter (BPD), femur length (FL), abdominal circumference, and head circumference are assessed
  - To detect congenital anomalies (anomalies scan is done between 16 and 24 weeks)
- **Third-trimester USG**
  - To monitor fetal growth—serial USG for fetal parameters
  - To localize placenta (to rule out placenta previa)
  - To assess amniotic fluid index

ANTENATAL CARE

See Table 1.34

Table 1.34 Antenatal care to be provided during antenatal visits

During first antenatal visit (preferably before 12 weeks of gestation)	• Pregnancy is confirmed • Antenatal registration is done and antenatal card is provided to the patient • Detailed history is taken and complete examination is done • Accurate period of gestation is established by first-trimester ultrasound • Folic acid tablets are prescribed • High-risk women are identified and referred to tertiary care center for further management • Routine investigations done during the first visit for all antenatal women – Blood grouping and typing (if the patient is Rh-negative, husband's blood grouping and typing should be done) – Hemoglobin estimation – Urine—albumin, sugar, and microscopy (pus cells >5/high-power field is significant) – Screening for diabetes—oral glucose tolerance test or fasting and post prandial blood sugars tested – Serology—VDRL, HIV, HBsAg, HCV – Dating USG (accuracy of crown–rump length in estimating gestational age is ±5 days) – USG for nuchal translucency is done at 11–14 weeks in indicated cases
During subsequent antenatal visits	• Ask for any fresh complaints • Watch out for complications that may develop during pregnancy such as preeclampsia, GDM, and APH • Complete general and obstetric examinations are done • Two doses of tetanus toxoid immunization are given at interval of at least 4 weeks • Iron and calcium supplementation is started from the second trimester onwards Investigations at subsequent visits • Urine for proteins is checked at each visit • Hemoglobin level is repeated at 28 and 36 weeks • Screening for GDM at 24–28 weeks (if negative in initial test) and again at 32 weeks in high-risk cases • In women with Rh-incompatible pregnancy, indirect Coombs' test is done according to guidelines (mentioned in Part 1, Chapter 10, *Rh Isoimmunization*) • USG for nuchal translucency (NT scan) at 11–14 weeks • Targeted USG for fetal anomalies is done at 16–24 weeks • USG may be done in the third trimester to assess liquor amount, placental location, interval growth of fetus (frequency of USG depends on other medical and obstetric risk factors)

ADVICE GIVEN TO ANTENATAL WOMEN

- Emphasis on the need for regular antenatal checkup
- Advice on diet—need for additional calories and proteins
- Advice on adequate sleep of 2 hours in afternoon and 8 hours at night
- Exercises (walking and upper trunk exercises can be undertaken)
- Smoking and alcohol to be avoided
- Periconceptional folic acid supplementation
- IFA (iron and folic acid supplementation) and calcium supplementation
- Can travel safely in the second trimester (avoid long journeys and jerky movements)
- Can have coitus unless contraindicated
- Patient informed on warning symptoms

Frequently asked viva questions

1. Define gravida and para. How often should a woman be examined in antenatal clinic?
2. What investigations are commonly advised to a pregnant woman?
3. What investigations are repeated in subsequent visits?
4. What are the common causes of edema during pregnancy?
5. How will you differentiate physiological edema from pathological edema?
6. How will you measure SFH and what is its significance?
7. What information can be obtained from pelvic grips?
8. What are the methods to assess the POG?
9. What are the uses of ultrasound in pregnancy?
10. What advice will you give to a pregnant woman?

2 Anemia in Pregnancy

Introduction

Anemia is the most common medical disorder during pregnancy, resulting in increased maternal morbidity and mortality. Prevalence of anemia during pregnancy in India is almost 80% (high-prevalence country). This chapter deals with the discussion on nutritional anemias which are the major cause of anemia in pregnancy.

Definition of anemia

Anemia refers to quantitative and qualitative decrease in RBC count and/or hemoglobin concentration, in relation to age and sex, resulting in lowering of the oxygen-carrying capacity of blood.

The World Health Organization (WHO) defines anemia during pregnancy as hemoglobin (Hb) concentration of less than 11 g/dL or a hematocrit of less than 33%.

The Centers for Disease Control and Prevention (CDC) defines anemia during pregnancy as follows:

- Hb <11 g/dL in the first and third trimesters
- Hb <10.5 g/dL in the second trimester

Indian Center for Medical Research (ICMR) classification of anemia during pregnancy

See Table 2.1

Table 2.1 ICMR classification of anemia during pregnancy

Grading	Hemoglobin (g/dL)
Mild	10–10.9
Moderate	7–9.9
Severe	<7
Very severe	<4

CAUSES OF ANEMIA DURING PREGNANCY

- Physiological anemia (usually mild anemia)
- Nutritional anemia (most common)
  - Iron deficiency anemia (most common nutritional anemia)
  - Folic acid deficiency anemia
  - Vitamin B_{12} deficiency anemia
  - Dimorphic anemia
- Anemia due to blood loss (hemorrhagic anemia)
  - Antepartum hemorrhage, hookworm infestation, bleeding piles, etc.
- Hemolytic anemia
  - Thalassemia, sickle cell anemia, and hereditary spherocytosis (hereditary causes)
  - Malaria (acquired cause)
- Others include anemia caused by diseases such as the following:
  - Bone marrow insufficiency (aplastic anemia)
  - Neoplasms
  - Chronic renal disease
  - Tuberculosis

Note

- *Nutritional anemias are the most common causes of anemia in pregnancy.*
- *Iron deficiency anemia is the most common nutritional anemia in pregnancy.*

Causes of iron deficiency anemia in pregnancy

- Decreased intake of iron
  - Inadequate diet intake due to nausea and vomiting of pregnancy
  - Faulty dietary habits such as pica and diet poor in iron content

  - Inadequate antenatal care (not taking iron supplementation)
- Decreased absorption
  - Due to malabsorption syndrome and giardiasis
- Increased loss of iron
  - Hookworm infestation
  - Bleeding piles, malaria, etc.
- Increased demand during pregnancy
  - Increase in total iron requirement during pregnancy
  - Multiple pregnancy
- Inadequate storage of iron
  - Repeated and frequent childbirths

Case presentation

Salient points in history

Consider the following relevant points during history taking in cases of anemia during pregnancy.

Patient details

- *Age (anemia is common in teenage pregnancy)*
- *Occupation (e.g., agricultural workers prone to hookworm infestation resulting in anemia)*
- *Socioeconomic status (more common in low socioeconomic group)*

Presenting complaints and H/o presenting complaints

H/o symptoms of anemia *These include easy fatigability, tiredness, weakness, lethargy, breathlessness, palpitation, and swelling of feet. Elaborate with details such as onset, duration, and progression of symptoms.*

H/o possible causes for anemia

- *H/o bleeding per rectum, melena, hematuria, hematemesis, and hemoptysis*
- *H/o worms in stools*
- *H/o chronic diarrhea (malabsorption)*
- *H/o burning micturition [to rule out recurrent/chronic urinary tract infection (UTI)]*
- *H/o fever with chills and rigors (to rule out malaria)*
- *H/o gastric surgery (malabsorption)*

H/o other causes of breathlessness

- *H/o cardiac symptoms such as chest pain, palpitation, orthopnea, paroxysmal nocturnal dyspnea, and syncopal attack (to rule out cardiac causes of breathlessness)*
- *H/o bronchial asthma*

H/o other causes of swelling of feet

- *H/o symptoms of preeclampsia such as headache, blurring of vision, epigastric pain, and decreased urine output*
- *H/o cardiac symptoms (as mentioned under "H/o causes for breathlessness")*
- *H/o symptoms of renal disease such as facial puffiness*

H/o present pregnancy

- *Whether on regular antenatal visits*
- *Whether taking iron supplementation regularly (noncompliance in hematinic intake leads to anemia)*
- *H/o bleeding P/V in third trimester (to rule out antepartum hemorrhage as a cause for anemia)*

Menstrual history

H/o heavy menstrual bleeding (HMB) in previous menstrual cycles (leads to anemia)

Past obstetric history

- *Parity (repeated pregnancy is a likely cause of anemia)*
- *Spacing between pregnancies (spacing of at least 2 years is required to replenish iron stores)*
- *Whether had regular antenatal checkup*
- *H/o hematinic intake during pregnancy*
- *H/o blood transfusion*
- *H/o postpartum hemorrhage (PPH)*
- *H/o puerperal sepsis*
- *H/o low-birth-weight baby*
- *Whether taken postnatal iron supplementation*

Past medical and surgical history

- *H/o chronic medical illness (chronic illness can lead to anemia)*
- *H/o any gastric surgeries*

(CONTD...)

(...CONTD)

Nutritional/diet history

- *This carries significance in an anemia case and should be mentioned in detail along with protein and calorie intake and deficiency, if any (You may be asked sources of iron rich foods).*

Family history

Family H/o sickle cell anemia and thalassemia

Salient points in examination

Consider the following relevant points during examination in cases of anemia during pregnancy.

General examination

- *Nutrition (may be undernourished)*
- *Weight (serial weight gain may be less in malnourished women)*
- *Pallor (Figure 2.1)*
- *Pedal edema [may be due to congestive cardiac failure (CCF) and associated hypoproteinemia]*
- *Icterus (may be present in hemolytic anemia)*
- *Signs of vitamin deficiency such as dry lusterless hair, glossitis, and angular stomatitis*
- *Platonychia (flat nails), koilonychia (spoon-shaped nails), and brittle nails may be present in chronic anemia*

Vitals

- *Pulse rate (tachycardia may be present in acute cause of anemia such as hemorrhage and in CCF; high-volume pulse is present in anemia)*
- *BP (anemia is associated with increased risk of preeclampsia)*

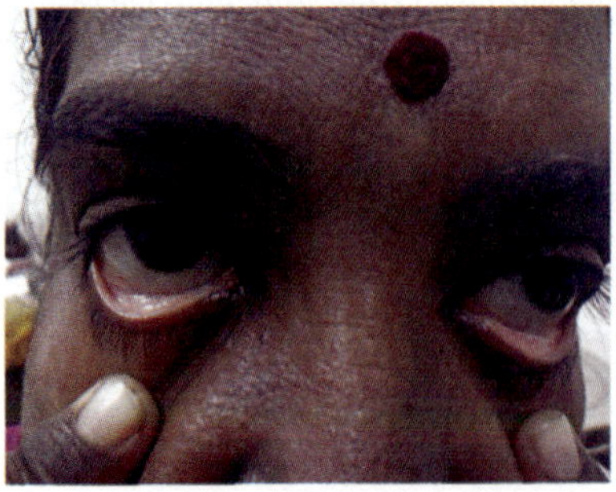

Figure 2.1 Demonstration of pallor.

Systemic examination

Cardiovascular system

The following may be present:

- *Jugular venous pressure (JVP; may be elevated in CCF)*
- *Hyperdynamic apex beat*
- *Hemic murmur (ejection systolic murmur) in pulmonary area (due to volume overload)*

Respiratory system

Basal lung crepts may be present in the case of CCF due to severe anemia.

Gastrointestinal tract

Look for hepatosplenomegaly (may be present in malaria, leukemia, lymphomas, and hemolytic anemia).

Obstetric examination

Fundal height and symphysiofundal height (SFH) may be less than period of gestation (POG) if associated intrauterine growth retardation (IUGR) is present (IUGR may be present in long standing cases of severe anemia due to chronic hypoxia).

Case summary

An example of writing diagnosis in cases of anemia in pregnancy is given below.

Example *Mrs. A, 28 years of age, G3P2L2 at 32 weeks of gestation, presents with the complaints of tiredness and easy fatigability for the past 2 months and breathlessness on exertion for the past 15 days.*

On examination, pallor is present; there is no pedal edema and the patient's BP is 120/80 mmHg. Her cardiovascular and respiratory system examination are normal. Her obstetric examination reveals fundal height up to 32 weeks with single live fetus in cephalic presentation, fetal heart rate (FHR) is 140 beats/min, regular, with adequate amount of liquor, and she is not in labor.

Case diagnosis

An example of writing diagnosis in cases of anemia in pregnancy is given below.

(CONTD...)

(...CONTD)

Example *28 years of age, G3P2L2 at 32 weeks of gestation, with anemia complicating pregnancy with a single live fetus in cephalic presentation, not in failure, not in labor, admitted for further evaluation and management*

Case discussion

Investigations to be done in a case of anemia

Investigations These are done to know the severity, type, and cause of anemia.

- Complete blood count includes the following:
  - Hemoglobin estimation which indicates the severity of anemia
  - Hematocrit and packed cell volume (PCV)
  - Red cell indices—mean corpuscular volume (MCV), mean corpuscular hemoglobin (MCH), and mean corpuscular hemoglobin concentration (MCHC)
  - Total RBC count
  - Total and differential WBC count (elevated in infections)
  - Platelet count
  - Reticulocyte count
- Peripheral smear examination
  - To study the morphology of RBCs that indicates the type of anemia
  - To look for hemoparasites such as malarial parasite
  - To look for abnormal cells such as blast cells in leukemia and burr cells in renal failure
  - To look for evidence of hemolysis
  - Platelet count
- Blood grouping and typing

Investigations to evaluate the cause

- Urine: Albumin, sugar, and microscopy for pus cells, casts, and deposits
- Urine: Culture and sensitivity (possibility of anemia due to chronic UTI)
- Stool: Ova/cyst/parasites/occult blood
- Serum total proteins (possibility of the presence of associated hypoproteinemia)
- Investigations such as ECG and cardiac ECHO are done to rule out cardiac cause for breathlessness and pedal edema, if cardiac murmur is detected on clinical examination.
- Other routine antenatal investigations that include oral glucose tolerance test (OGTT), HIV, HBsAg, and venereal disease research laboratory (VDRL) test are performed.
- Ultrasonography (USG) is done to assess fetal biometry and well-being (IUGR is a complication of anemia).

Other investigations helpful in evaluation of iron deficiency anemia (labeled as "Serum iron profile")

- Serum iron (decreased)
- Serum ferritin (decreased)
- Serum transferrin saturation (decreased)
- Total iron-binding capacity (TIBC; increased)

Note *Iron profile is done to differentiate iron deficiency anemia from other causes of microcytic hypochromic anemia.*

The various hematological parameters in iron deficiency anemia are mentioned in Table 2.2. Mean corpuscular hemoglobin concentration (MCHC) is the most sensitive of all the red cell indices.

Table 2.2 Hematological parameters in iron deficiency anemia

	Normal values in pregnancy	Iron deficiency anemia
Hb (g/dL)	12–16	<11
RBC count (million/mm^3)	4–5	<3.2
PCV (%)	32–36	<30
MCH (pg): Hb/RBC	26–31	<25
MCV (fL): PCV/RBC	75–95	<75
MCHC (%): Hb/PCV	30–35	<30
Serum iron (µg/dL)	60–120	<60
Serum ferritin (µg/L)	15–200	<15
TIBC (µg/dL)	300–400	>400
Transferrin saturation (%)	20–50	<10

Part 1

Extra edge

Blood loss in hookworm infestation

- **Ancylostoma duodenale:** 0.2 mL blood loss/worm/ day
- **Necator americanus:** 0.03 mL blood loss/worm/ day

Characteristics of hookworm egg

- Oval or elliptical
- Colorless
- Not bile stained
- Floats in saturated salt solution
- Has a thin, transparent shell membrane
- A segmented ovum with four to eight blastomeres is present in egg found in feces (see figure below).

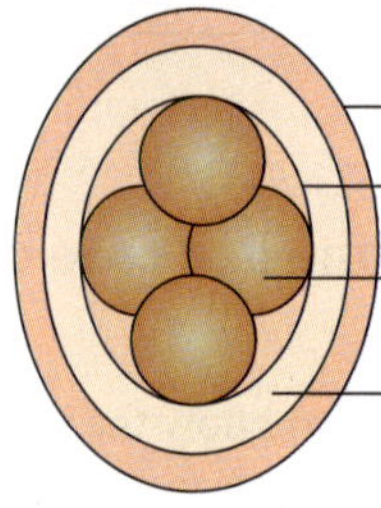

Figure Hookworm egg.

Viva corner

Q1 What are the methods of estimation of hemoglobin?

- Spectrophotometric/calorimetric method
- Acid hematin method/Sahli's method

Q2 How is a peripheral smear examination done?

- Blood smear is prepared on a glass slide and air dried.
- It is stained with Leishman's stain for 2 minutes, then washed with distilled water, dried, and then examined under microscope.

Q3 What are the causes of microcytic hypochromic anemia?

- Iron deficiency anemia
- Thalassemia
- Sideroblastic anemia
- Anemia due to chronic diseases
- Lead poisoning

Q4 What are the causes of normocytic normochromic anemia?

- Acute blood loss
- Bone marrow failure

Q5 What are the causes of macrocytic anemia?

- Vitamin B_{12} deficiency
- Folic acid deficiency
- Hereditary spherocytosis

Q6 What are the peripheral smear findings in various types of anemia?

See table below

Table **Peripheral smear findings in various types of anemia**

Type of anemia	Peripheral smear findings
Iron deficiency anemia	Microcytic hypochromic anemia (RBCs are smaller in size with central pallor). Anisocytosis (variation in size) and poikilocytosis (variation in shape) may be present (see figure below).
Folic acid and vitamin B_{12} deficiency	Macrocytic anemia, hypersegmented neutrophils (5% of neutrophils showing five lobes or more or a single neutrophil with six or more lobes)
Dimorphic anemia	All three types of erythropoiesis can usually be detected—hypochromic, megaloblastic, and normoblastic (the latter predominating)
Hemolytic anemia	Schistocytes, target cells
Leukemia	Abnormal cells such as blast cells
Renal failure	Burr cells

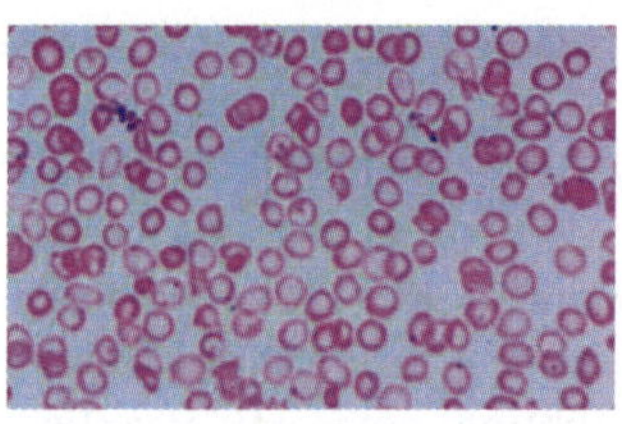

Figure Microcytic hypochromic anemia in peripheral smear picture.

Special investigations for evaluation of other types of anemia

See Table 2.3

Indications for bone marrow study in anemia

- Aplastic anemia (suspected in cases with low total count, differential count)
- Refractory anemia (nonresponders to iron therapy)
- Suspected kala-azar

Table 2.3 **Special investigations for evaluation of anemia other than iron deficiency anemia**

Type of anemia	Investigation required for diagnosis
Megaloblastic anemia	Serum folate, RBC folate, serum vitamin B_{12}
Autoimmune hemolytic anemia	Coombs' test, serum bilirubin
Hereditary spherocytosis	Serum osmotic fragility test
Sickle cell anemia	Sickle cell test, hemoglobin electrophoresis
Hemoglobinopathies (thalassemia)	Hemoglobin electrophoresis by high performance liquid chromatography (HPLC)

Complications of anemia during pregnancy

See Table 2.4

Management of iron deficiency anemia during pregnancy

The aim of treatment of anemia during pregnancy is to achieve a safe level of hemoglobin at the time of delivery to reduce the complications.

Approach to management of anemia in pregnancy

- Confirm the diagnosis and grade the severity of anemia according to hemoglobin level.
  - *Hb <7 g/dL*: Severe anemia
  - *Hb 7–10 g/dL*: Moderate anemia
  - *Hb 10–10.9 g/dL*: Mild anemia
- Determine the type of anemia by doing RBC indices (MCV, MCH, MCHC) and peripheral smear.
- Investigate for the causes of anemia and treat possible causes.

High-yield points

Stages of iron deficiency anemia (IDA)

Stage	Finding	Inference
I	Decreased serum ferritin	Depleted iron stores
II	Decreased serum iron and increased TIBC	Deficient erythropoiesis
III	Effects of decreased iron on Hb and RBCs	Iron deficiency anemia

Difference between IDA and thalassemia

Blood index	IDA	Thalassemia
Peripheral smear	Microcytic hypochromic anemia	Microcytic hypochromic anemia
MCV, MCHC, MCH	All reduced proportionate to the severity of anemia	All reduced to very low levels in relation to the severity of anemia
Serum iron	Reduced	Normal or high
Serum ferritin	Reduced	High
TIBC	High	Normal
Transferrin saturation	Reduced	Normal or high
HbF and HbA2	Normal	High
Bone marrow iron stores	Decreased hemosiderin	Increased hemosiderin

Table 2.4 Complications of anemia during pregnancy

Maternal			Fetus and neonate
Antenatal	Intrapartum	Puerperium	
• Increased risk of infections • Increased risk of preeclampsia • Preterm labor • Congestive cardiac failure	• Congestive cardiac failure • Postpartum hemorrhage and shock	• Cardiac failure • Puerperal sepsis • Subinvolution • Failed lactation • Venous thrombosis	• Prematurity • Intrauterine growth restriction • Low birth weight • Decreased iron stores in the neonate, if the mother had severe anemia during pregnancy

Viva corner

Q1 What is physiological anemia of pregnancy?

- Physiological anemia occurs in pregnancy because the increase in plasma volume (30–40%) is much more than the increase in red cell mass (10–15%) leading to apparent decrease in hematocrit.
- Hb does not fall below 11 g% in the first trimester and below 10 g% in the second and third trimesters in physiological anemia.

Q2 Why does hemodilution occur during pregnancy?

Hemodilution occurs in pregnancy for the following reasons:

- Reduces blood viscosity, thereby enhancing placental perfusion and facilitating oxygen delivery to the fetus
- Reduces work load on the heart
- Reduces postpartum loss of RBCs

- Correction of anemia is done with oral or parenteral iron therapy or blood transfusion depending on the severity of anemia and POG.

Correction of anemia

Need for admission

- Women with mild to moderate anemia without other complications can be managed on OPD basis.
- Patients with severe anemia should be hospitalized.
- There should be liberal admission and treatment of anemia near term.

Dietary advice

Iron-rich, high-protein diet is advised.

Mild anemia (10–10.9 g/dL)

- Oral iron therapy is given.
- Parenteral iron therapy can be given as an alternative to oral therapy if there is intolerance to oral iron or noncompliance or malabsorption.

Moderate anemia (7–10 g/dL)

- Oral iron therapy can be given, if there are no associated complications.
- Parenteral iron therapy can be given as an alternative to oral therapy in the following situations:
  - If there is intolerance to oral iron or noncompliance or malabsorption
  - In cases with moderate anemia in later half of pregnancy (more than 32 weeks of gestation) to ensure compliance and bioavailability
- Packed cell transfusion is given, if Hb is <8 g near term, as rapid improvement in Hb is essential when the woman is close to term (there is less time available for correction of anemia with oral or parenteral therapy).

Severe anemia at any period of gestation (<7 g/dL)

Packed cell transfusion is given.

Oral iron therapy

Indications

Mild to moderate anemia

- Therapeutic dose—180–200 mg/day of elemental iron is given in two or three divided doses (60 mg TDS or 100 mg BD).
  - Iron is best absorbed when taken on an empty stomach, with water or fruit juice,

Viva corner

Q1 What are the dietary sources of iron?

- **Rich sources of iron:** Organ meat (liver, heart, kidney), fish, egg yolk, and dry beans
- **Good sources of iron:** Green leafy vegetables, cereals, pulses, ragi, and dates
- **Poor sources of iron:** Milk

Q2 Why is routine iron supplementation required during pregnancy?

Iron supplementation is essential for all pregnant women for the following reasons:

- Developing countries like India have high prevalence (>40%) of iron deficiency anemia and low iron stores during pregnancy
- Iron requirement during pregnancy steadily increases and is as follows:
- *First trimester:* 2 mg/day
- *Second trimester:* 4–6 mg/day
- *Third trimester:* 6–8 mg/day
- Only 10% of dietary iron is absorbed. Daily diet contains 10–20 mg of elemental iron, of which only 10% is absorbed (1–2 mg)

  Hence, dietary iron intake is inadequate to meet the body's iron demand in second and third trimesters and therefore routine iron supplementation is required during pregnancy.
- Iron requirement for the entire pregnancy is approximately 1000 mg, which is distributed as shown in the table below.

Table Distribution of iron requirement during pregnancy

Factors that require iron during pregnancy	Iron requirement
Fetus and placenta	+300 mg
Maternal increase in RBC mass	+500 mg
Basal loss (loss through urine, sweat, and feces)	+200 mg
Blood loss at delivery	+300 mg
Iron saved due to amenorrhea	−300 mg (30 × 10)*
Total iron demand during pregnancy	1000 mg

* Iron saved due to 10 months of amenorrhea during pregnancy (no menstrual blood loss) (30 mg × 10) = 300 mg

about 1 hour before or 2 hours after meals. However, to lessen the possible gastrointestinal (GI) side effects, iron may be taken with food or immediately after meals.

– Hemoglobin levels start rising in 2–3 weeks and reach the normal value after 6 weeks of therapy. To replenish the iron stores, treatment should be continued for 3 months after the hemoglobin levels return to normal.

- Other drugs given along with oral iron therapy are the following:
  - Folic acid 500 µg/day
  - Vitamin C (helps in absorption)
  - Deworming with oral albendazole 400 mg stat or mebendazole 100 mg BD for 3 days

High-yield points

Factors influencing the iron absorption

Factors increasing iron absorption	Factors decreasing iron absorption
• Acidity • Ascorbic acid (vitamin C) • Absorption of heme iron is two to three times more than that of nonheme iron • Iron absorption increases during pregnancy and in iron deficiency anemia	• Phytates (cereals) • Oxalates (leafy vegetables) • Phosphates (egg yolk) • Calcium salts • Tea, coffee, antacids, and H2 receptor blockers

Oral iron preparations

Ferrous salts Ferrous salts are the most effective oral iron preparations. The various ferrous salts used for therapy are mentioned in Table 2.5.

Other oral iron preparations A number of other iron preparations are available, though not superior to ferrous salts.

- Ferric hydroxide (iron) polymaltose complex (IPC complex). It is a combination of ferric iron with polymaltose molecules and is anionic
  - Does not stain teeth
  - No metallic taste
  - No interaction with food or other drugs
  - Has less absorption than ferrous salts
  - May be tried as an alternative to those who cannot tolerate ferrous salts
- Sustained-release iron preparations
  - *Advantage*: Less GI side effects
  - *Disadvantage*: Less iron is released in the main absorptive area, that is, duodenum and upper jejunum, hence absorption is less
- Carbonyl iron—highly purified form of iron (it has high bioavailability and is less toxic)

Main disadvantage of oral iron therapy

Main disadvantage is that oral iron therapy has an unpredictable absorption rate.

Side effects of oral iron therapy

- **Upper GI tract:** Metallic taste, staining of teeth, nausea, and gastric discomfort
- **Lower GI tract:** Constipation, diarrhea, and flatulence

Prescription of oral iron (methods to increase absorption and decrease side effects)

- It is advisable to start with one iron tablet per day and gradually increase the dose every 3–5 days up to three times per day.
- Oral iron may be prescribed along with meals to reduce the side effects and to increase compliance. (Iron is better absorbed when taken before meals but the side effects are more.)
- Taking vitamin C along with the drug helps in absorption (citrus fruits).
- Avoid tea/coffee for at least 2 hours after oral iron intake as milk reduces iron absorption.
- Calcium salts and antacids reduce iron absorption and hence should not be taken along with oral iron. There should be a gap of at least 2 hours between iron and calcium supplementation.
- To ensure compliance, ask for color of feces (black discoloration of stools).

Viva corner

Q1 What should be done if the patient does not tolerate oral iron therapy?

The patient is advised to

- Take oral iron along with meals. If no response, then change the iron salt preparation. If still no response, then change to parenteral route.

Signs of improvement

Positive response to iron therapy is indicated by the following:

- A sense of well-being

Table 2.5 Ferrous salts as oral iron preparations

Ferrous salt	Characteristics
Ferrous sulfate (200 mg contain 60 mg elemental iron)	• Has high amount of elemental iron • Cheaper • Has good bioavailability but is associated with GI side effects
Ferrous fumarate (300 mg contain 100 mg elemental iron)	• Has similar efficacy and GI tolerance to ferrous sulfate • It is a commonly used salt in commercial preparation
Ferrous gluconate (300 mg contain 30 mg elemental iron)	• Well tolerated but has low iron content
Ferrous ascorbate (contain 100 mg elemental iron)	• Has high amount of elemental iron • Converts ferric to ferrous iron, thereby increases iron absorption • Inhibits the formation of insoluble iron complexes

GI, gastrointestinal.

- Increase in appetite
- Improvement in other symptoms

Laboratory parameters showing signs of improvement are as follows:

- **By 5–7 days:** Increase in reticulocyte count to up to 5% (normal 0.2–2%) (reticulocytosis is the earliest hematological response to iron therapy)
- **By 2–3 weeks:** Increase in hemoglobin level at the rate of 0.8–1 g/dL per week
- **By 6–8 weeks:** Return of hemoglobin to normal level (peripheral smear shows normocytic normochromic RBCs; serum ferritin level increases)

Causes for failure of oral iron therapy

- Noncompliance
- Intolerance
- Malabsorption
- Inaccurate diagnosis of the cause of anemia (e.g., anemia due to thalassemia does not improve with iron supplementation; dimorphic anemia)
- Ongoing blood loss—hookworm infestation, hemorrhoids, etc.
- Coexisting infections (infection impairs erythropoiesis)
- Coexisting deficiencies—folic acid deficiency, protein deficiency, etc.

Parenteral iron therapy

Indications

- Noncompliance to oral iron
- Intolerance to oral iron
- Malabsorption of oral iron—peptic ulcer, inflammatory bowel disease, etc.
- Moderate anemia in later half of pregnancy (>32 weeks)

Main advantage of parenteral iron over oral iron

- There is certainty of administration of parenteral iron as it bypasses GI absorption (it has a predictable absorption rate).
- Parenteral iron is usually preferred over oral iron for cases with moderate anemia in later half of pregnancy (>32 weeks) due to its predictable absorption rate and ensuring compliance.

Note *Parenteral iron therapy does not give faster response when compared with oral therapy. The rise in hemoglobin after parenteral therapy is 0.8–1.0 g% per week, which is same as seen with oral iron therapy. The main advantage of parenteral iron therapy is the certainty of its administration.*

Formulas for calculation of total requirement of parenteral iron

- [Hb deficit × BW (kg) × 2.2] + 1000 mg (to replenish iron stores)
- [Hb deficit × BW (kg) × 4.4] + 50% for stores
- (Hb deficit × 250) + 50% for stores
- [Hb deficit × 0.3 × BW (lb)] + 1000 mg (for stores)

Hb deficit = Target or desired Hb – Patient's Hb (target Hb usually taken as 11 g/dL in pregnancy)

BW refers to body weight. Prepregnancy body weight is used for calculation.

Parenteral iron preparations

Parenteral iron preparations are available for intramuscular and intravenous use (Table 2.6).

Note *Iron dextran is available for IM and IV use.*

Intramuscular iron preparations

- Iron dextran (Imferon) and iron sorbitol citric acid complex (Jectofer)
- Both the preparations contain 50 mg of elemental iron in 1 mL

Administration of intramuscular iron

- The total dose needed is calculated using the formula for calculation of total requirement of parenteral iron.
- Initial intramuscular (IM) test dose is given—0.5 mL (25 mg).
- IM iron is administered in the dosage of 2 mL (100 mg) on a daily or alternate-day basis.

Table 2.6 Parenteral iron preparations

Intramuscular iron preparations	Intravenous iron preparations
• Iron dextran • Iron sorbitol citrate complex	• Iron dextran • Iron sucrose • Ferric carboxymaltose

- Multiple injections are required to administer the total dose.
- The dose is administered as deep IM injection on the upper outer quadrant of buttocks by "Z" track technique to prevent staining of skin.
- The injection site should not be massaged.

Intravenous iron preparations

Iron dextran (Imferon)

The calculated total dose can be given as one large dose [total dose infusion (TDI)] or as divided multiple dose regimen on daily/alternate days.

Total dose infusion Total dose calculated is given on a single day.

- Initial intravenous (IV) test dose of 0.5 mL is given as slow IV.
- The total dose of iron dextran is given as IV infusion in 500 mL normal saline over 6–8 hours (5% dextrose can lead to phlebitis).
- If the total dose required is >1000 mg, it is given as two divided doses on alternate days.
- Currently, TDI is not given due to increased risk of anaphylactic reactions.

Multiple dose regimen

- Initial IV test dose of 0.5 mL (25 mg) is given as slow IV.
- Repeated doses of 2 mL (100 mg) is given either as IV infusion by diluting in 250 mL of saline, over 30–60 minutes, or as undiluted slow IV push at a maximum of 20 mg/min on daily/alternate-day basis.

Iron sucrose

- It is a dextran-free IV preparation, available as 5 mL ampoules containing 100 mg iron (20 mg/mL) (Figure 2.2).
- Advantages of iron sucrose over other preparations are as follows:
  - Hypersensitivity reactions are very rare and hence test dose is not recommended.
  - Iron sucrose is safer than iron dextran with rare anaphylactic reactions.
  - It has minimal side effects.

Viva corner

Q1 What is "Z" track technique?

- The main aim of "Z" track technique is to prevent staining of skin with IM iron injections (see figure below).
- Deep IM injections are given in the upper outer quadrant of buttocks with 2- or 3-in. long 20-gauge needle.
- While giving the injection, the patient should be in lateral position, with the injection site being the uppermost.
- Slide the skin covering the muscle at the chosen site with fingers of the nondominant hand.
- The needle is placed at right angles to the skin and is penetrated quickly. Needle is pushed till bone resistance is felt. Then the needle is withdrawn slightly, so that the tip of the needle is in the muscle. The plunger is then withdrawn to look for any blood (if any vessel is pierced). Injection is then given and needle is withdrawn quickly.
- The superficial tissues are then slid back into place.
- As the skin puncture site is away from the injection deposition site, skin staining is avoided.

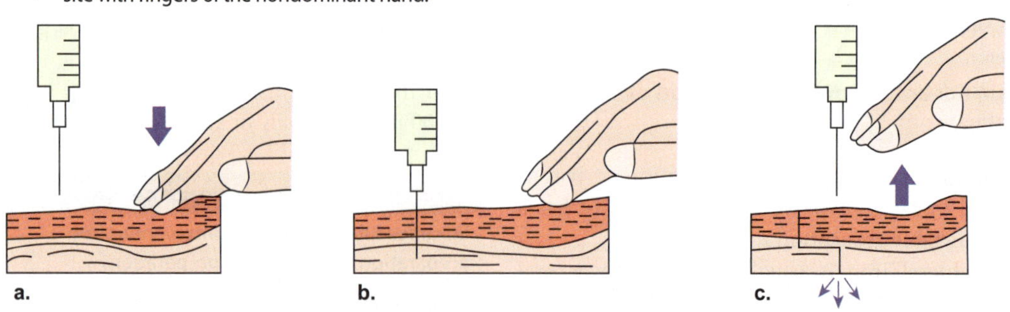

Figure Z track technique for deep intramuscular injections. **a.** The skin over the injection site retracted and held. **b.** Muscular injection given. **c.** Skin released.

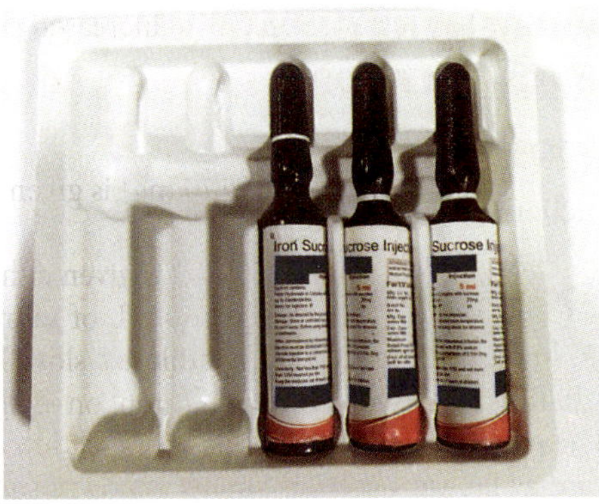

Figure 2.2 Iron sucrose ampoules.

- It can be given undiluted as slow IV push at 20 mg/min (maximum dose is 100 mg).
- Alternatively, 5 mL containing 100 mg iron is diluted in 100 mL normal saline and administered over 20 minutes. The initial 25 mL is given slowly to look for any reactions. A maximum dose of 200 mg can be given at a time.
- Infusion can be repeated on alternate days.
- The disadvantage is that multiple doses are required.

Ferric carboxymaltose (FCM)

- It is a new dextran-free iron preparation that can be given as a single-dose IV infusion.
- Large dose up to 1000 mg can be administered over 15 minutes. Available as 500 mg/10 mL and 1 g/20 mL vials.
- Advantages over other parenteral preparations are as follows:
  - Administered as single dose (avoids multiple doses) over short time period
  - Dextran free and hence risk of anaphylaxis or serious hypersensitivity reactions is very low
  - Test dose is not required
  - Good safety and efficacy profile.
- Ferric carboxymaltose is an attractive alternative to iron sucrose in terms of safety profile, efficacy, patient comfort, and resource utilization.

Note *Oral iron is withheld while giving parenteral iron to prevent toxicity.*

Advantages of parenteral iron

- There is certainty of iron administration, that is, parenteral iron has a predictable absorption rate.
- Side effects of oral iron are avoided.
- Risk of transmission of infections and incompatibility associated with blood transfusions is avoided.

Side effects of parenteral iron

- Local—pain, skin discoloration, and abscess formation with IM preparations, and thrombophlebitis with IV administration
- General—myalgia, arthralgia, fever, lymphadenopathy, and anaphylaxis
- Possibility of iron toxicity in iron overload conditions such as thalassemia

Disadvantages of intramuscular iron over intravenous iron

IM iron preparations are not preferred for the following reasons:
- It is more painful.
- It causes staining of the skin and abscess formation at the injection site.
- Its absorption is irregular.

Contraindications to parenteral iron

- H/o anaphylactic reactions to parenteral iron therapy
- Liver diseases (acute or chronic infection)
- Oral iron intake should be stopped within 24 hours prior to parenteral therapy to avoid toxic reaction.

Blood transfusion

Indications

- Severe anemia at any POG
- Moderate anemia with Hb <8 g% near term (rapid improvement in Hb is essential as woman is close to term and there is not enough time to achieve a reasonable hemoglobin level before delivery with oral or parenteral therapy)
- Anemia due to acute blood loss such as antepartum hemorrhage
- Refractory anemia not responding to oral or parenteral iron therapy
- Associated infections

Precautions to be taken during blood transfusion

- Packed cell transfusion is preferred to whole blood (to prevent volume overload).
- Check bag no. and blood group and type.
- Diuretic such as furosemide 20 mg is given IV prior to the transfusion to prevent volume overload and congestive cardiac failure.
- Blood transfusion must be administered slowly over 4–6 hours.
- Clinical parameters (pulse, respiratory rate, and intermittent chest auscultation for crepts) must be regularly monitored.

Note *Each unit of packed cells improves hemoglobin by 1 g/dL. Usually hemoglobin is corrected to at least 7 g/dL with packed cell transfusion and then parenteral or oral iron therapy is started depending on the time available before onset of labor.*

Advantages

- Blood transfusion is the fastest way to improve Hb
- Improves oxygen-carrying capacity of blood
- Stimulates erythropoiesis

Disadvantages

- Possibility of transfusion reactions
- Risk of transfusion transmitted infections such as HIV, HBsAg
- Can precipitate CCF
- Can precipitate preterm labor

Partial exchange transfusion

- It is rarely performed.
- Blood is withdrawn from the patient and centrifuged, serum is separated, and RBCs are reinfused back into the patient.
- It may be indicated in cases of severe anemia with cardiac failure to avoid circulatory overload.

Note *When there is no response to iron therapy, investigate for other types of anemia.*

MANAGEMENT OF PATIENTS WITH ANEMIA IN LABOR

Intrapartum

Induction of labor can be done in indicated cases.

I stage

- IV line is secured; blood is cross-matched and additional units are reserved.
- The patient is put in a propped-up position if in cardiac failure, otherwise in left lateral position.
- Oxygen is given by mask.
- Adequate analgesia is given for pain relief.
- To maintain hydration, oral fluids are encouraged and IV fluids are restricted to <75 mL/h (to prevent volume overload).
- Monitor for symptoms and signs of CCF (tachycardia, raised JVP, fine crepitations in base of lungs).
- Strict aseptic precautions are followed.
- Restrict the number of vaginal examination (monitor descent of fetal head by abdominal palpation of fetal poles).
- Prophylactic antibiotics are given (anemic patients are at an increased risk of infection).
- Partogram is maintained to monitor maternal and fetal well-being and progress of labor.
- Monitor FHR by continuous electronic fetal monitoring, if facilities are available. Otherwise, intermittent auscultation with stethoscope is done for every 15 minutes in the first stage and every 5 minutes in the second stage.
- Oxytocin can be given for augmentation of labor
- Cesarean section is done only for obstetric indications. Regional anesthesia is preferred over general anesthesia.

Note
- *In case of preterm labor, beta-agonists and steroids must be administered with caution in anemic patients to prevent pulmonary edema.*

II stage

- Prolonged second stage should be avoided. Forceps or vacuum can be applied to reduce maternal straining especially in women with CCF.
- Injection Frusemide is administered in severely anemic women to prevent heart failure.

III stage

- Active management of the third stage of labor (AMTSL) is performed to prevent PPH.
- Oxytocin is the drug of choice for AMTSL and should be given in concentrated form.
- Methergin 0.2 mg IV/IM is not contraindicated except in cases with severe anemia in failure (can lead to volume overload).
- Restrict IV fluids.
- PPH has to be managed aggressively, as even a small amount of blood loss can lead to decompensation.

Postpartum

- Intensive monitoring is done for the initial 24 hours following delivery as there is a risk of CCF.
- Antibiotics are given to prevent infections.
- Correction of anemia is continued in postpartum period.
- Patient is advised iron therapy for at least 3–6 months following delivery to replenish iron stores.
- Contraception counseling is given. Postpartum sterilization is offered if the patient has completed her family.
- Spacing of at least 2 years is advised in between pregnancies.

PREVENTION OF IRON DEFICIENCY ANEMIA DURING PREGNANCY

Measures to prevent iron deficiency anemia during pregnancy include the following:

- Provision of iron prophylaxis to all preschool children and adolescent girls (WHO, Government of India)
- Deworming with anthelmintic agents such as Albendazole or Mebendazole should be done every 6 months for children and adults. The national guidelines for deworming in pregnancy by the MoHFW, Government of India, recommend a single dose of 400 mg of albendazole tablet after the I trimester, preferably in the II trimester
- Health education—to avoid frequent childbirths (educate on methods of contraception)
- Early detection of anemia during pregnancy—hemoglobin estimation at the first antenatal visit and repeated at 28 and 36 weeks
- Iron and folic acid prophylaxis during pregnancy
- Detection and treatment of any underlying cause for anemia such as infections (management of endemic infections such as malaria and hookworm infestation)
- Advice on diet rich in iron
- Fortification of food with iron (iron-fortified foods available in market are the following: wheat flour, sugar, salt, and cereal-based food)

National Nutritional Anemia Control Program

Ministry of Health and Family Welfare, Government of India (2013) recommended prophylaxis with 100 mg elemental iron (in the form of ferrous sulfate) and folic acid 500 µg for at least 100 days during pregnancy starting from 14– to 16 weeks of gestation. This should be followed by the same dose for 100 days in the postpartum period.

The beneficiaries of NNACP included children aged 6–59 months, 5–10 years, adolescents aged 10–19 years, pregnant and lactating women, and women in reproductive age group under the National Iron Plus Initiative (NIPI).

Note *The dose recommendation has currently been changed in the Anemia Mukt Bharat Program 2018 as detailed in the text below.*

A 12 by 12 initiative was launched in 2007, jointly undertaken by MOHFW, WHO, and UNICEF, to ensure that every child would have hemoglobin levels of 12 g/dL by the age of 12 years.

Anemia Mukt Bharat Initiative

- The Ministry of Health and Family Welfare (MoHFW) launched the Anemia Mukt Bharat Program in 2018. This program was designed to achieve the WHO target of 50% reduction of anemia in women of reproductive age by 2025 and the Poshan Abhiyaan (2018–2022) to reduce the prevalence of anemia among young children, adolescents, and women of reproductive age group by 3% per year.
- Aim: To strengthen the existing mechanisms and promote newer strategies for tackling anemia.

- It focusses on six target beneficiary groups through six interventions and six institutional mechanisms to achieve the envisaged targets under the POSHAN Abhiyaan.
- Six Beneficiaries: Children (6–60 months); adolescent girls (15–19 years); adolescent boys (15–19 years); women of reproductive age group; pregnant women; lactating women.
- Anemia Mukt Bharat strategy recommends daily intake of one iron and folic acid tablet containing 60 mg elemental iron + 500 µg folic acid, starting from the second trimester and continued throughout pregnancy for a minimum 180 days followed by intake for 180 days in the postpartum period.

Interventions

The Anemia Mukt Bharat strategy will focus on the following interventions:

1. Prophylactic iron and folic acid supplementation
2. Deworming
3. Intensified year-round behavior change communication campaign (Solid Body, Smart Mind) focusing on four key behaviors:
    a. Increase in the intake of iron-rich food through diet diversity/quantity/frequency and/or fortified foods
    b. Improving compliance to iron folic acid supplementation and deworming
    c. Ensuring delayed cord clamping after delivery
    d. Appropriate infant and child feeding practices
4. Testing and treatment of anemia with special focus on pregnant women and school-going adolescents
5. Provision of iron and folic acid fortified foods in government-funded public health programs
6. Intensifying awareness, screening, and treatment of non-nutritional causes of anemia in endemic areas, with special focus on malaria and hemoglobinopathies

Poshan Abhiyaan or National Nutrition Mission

- Government of India launched the Poshan Abhiyaan Program in 2018 to improve nutritional outcomes for children, pregnant women, and lactating mothers.
- The focus of Abhiyaan is to lay emphasis on nutritional status of adolescent girls, pregnant women, lactating mothers, and children from 0 to 6 years of age.

WHO recommendation for iron prophylaxis during pregnancy

The WHO recommends 60 mg elemental iron and 400 µg of folic acid for 6 months during pregnancy in countries with prevalence of anemia less than 40%, and additional 3 months during postpartum in countries with prevalence of anemia greater than 40%.

Extra edge

- Iron is a trace element required for erythropoiesis.
- Dietary iron is found in two forms:
    - *Heme iron*: Found in meat and meat products (5–10% of dietary iron; it is the most bioavailable source of iron)
    - *Nonheme iron*: Found in cereals, pulses, and vegetables (90–95% of dietary iron)

Iron metabolism (see figure below)

- Iron is absorbed in duodenum and upper jejunum. Only 10% of ingested iron is absorbed.
- Ingested iron contains mostly ferric iron (Fe^{3+}) that is converted to ferrous form by ferrireductase in stomach.
- Iron is absorbed in ferrous form (Fe^{2+}) in the duodenum and jejunum and is released into the plasma in ferrous form.
- In the plasma, it is oxidized again to ferric form (Fe^{3+}) that binds to transferrin, which is the transport protein.
- Iron circulates in the plasma bound to transferrin and binds to transferrin receptors on the surface of marrow erythroid cells. Once transferrin binds with its receptor, the transferrin–receptor complex is internalized via clathrin-coated pits. The iron is then made available for heme synthesis while the transferrin receptor complex is recycled back into circulation.
- The excess ferrous iron in the GI mucosal cell binds to the storage protein, apoferritin, to form ferritin, which is the storage form of iron. When apoferritin gets saturated, absorption of iron is inhibited. This is called mucosal block theory or ferritin curtain. Ferritin stored in mucosal cells is lost when the cells are shed after a life span of 2–4 days.

(CONTD...)

(...CONTD)

Extra edge

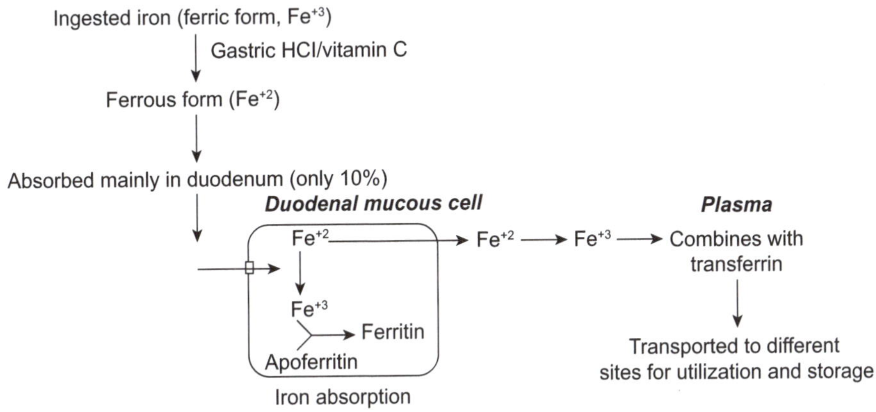

Figure Iron metabolism.

OTHER NUTRITIONAL ANEMIAS

Megaloblastic anemia

Megaloblastic anemia is characterized by macrocytic blood picture and megaloblastic bone marrow which is seen in folic acid and vitamin B_{12} deficiency.

- Folic acid and vitamin B_{12} are coenzymes required for red cell DNA synthesis. Lack of vitamin B_{12} and/or folic acid leads to impaired DNA synthesis. The DNA synthesis is impaired while the cytoplasmic maturation is normal, leading to formation of megaloblasts or macrocytosis.

Diagnosis of megaloblastic anemia

See Table 2.7

Confirmatory tests for folate and vitamin B_{12} deficiency

The diagnostic tests to confirm folate and vitamin B_{12} deficiency are not available easily and are costly. If facilities are available, serum B_{12} levels and

Table 2.7 Various investigations in diagnosis of megaloblastic anemia

Parameter	Value
Hemoglobin	<10 g/dL
Hematocrit	<33%
MCV	>96 fL
MCH	>33 pg
MCHC	Within normal range
Peripheral smear	• Presence of macrocytes and megaloblasts (characteristic finding) • Hypersegmented neutrophils: 5% of neutrophils with five or more lobes or even a single neutrophil with six or more lobes • Presence of nucleated RBCs • Howell–Jolly bodies in RBC
Unconjugated bilirubin and serum LDH	As there is ineffective erythropoiesis, hemolysis can occur due to which serum unconjugated bilirubin and LDH can be elevated

LDH, lactate dehydrogenase; *MCH*, mean corpuscular hemoglobin; *MCHC*, mean corpuscular hemoglobin concentration; *MCV*, mean corpuscular volume.

Table 2.8 Vitamin B_{12} and folate deficiencies

Deficiency	Serum levels
Vitamin B_{12} deficiency	• Serum B_{12} level <100 pg/mL
Folate deficiency	• Serum folate level <2 ng/mL • Fasting serum folate level <6 μg/L • RBC folate <165 μg/L Fasting folate and RBC folate levels are more specific, as there is no interference by food

serum folate levels can be measured (Table 2.8). If the complete blood count and peripheral smear picture is suggestive of megaloblastic anemia, empirical treatment with folate and vitamin B_{12} is usually started.

Viva corner

Q1 Which deficiency is more common—vitamin B_{12} or folate deficiency?

Folate deficiency is more common than vitamin B_{12} deficiency because:

- Folate stores last only for 2–4 months, whereas vitamin B12 stores are sufficient for 2–3 years.
- Folate gets destroyed by prolonged cooking.
- Dietary deficiency of vitamin B_{12} occurs only in pure vegetarians.

Folic acid deficiency

- Megaloblastic anemia in pregnancy is almost always secondary to folate deficiency.
- Folic acid is absorbed in jejunum.
- Folate stores last only for 2–4 months and deficiency occurs in 6 months with reduced intake.
- Dietary sources of folic acid include yeast, liver, green leafy vegetables, and fruits.
- Treatment: Folic acid 5 mg is given orally daily during pregnancy that is continued till 3 months postpartum.

Vitamin B_{12} deficiency

- Intrinsic factor secreted by mucosal cells of stomach is required for B_{12} absorption. Vitamin B_{12} deficiency is most often caused due to malabsorption; therefore, it is usually administered in parental form.
- Vitamin B_{12} has a high quantity of storage in the body and hence deficiency is manifested only after a prolonged period of reduced intake of 3–4 years.
- Dietary sources of B_{12} include meat, poultry, fish, and dairy products (animal sources mainly). Hence, deficiency is common in strict vegetarians.
- Treatment: Vitamin B_{12} (hydroxycobalamin 1000 μg) 1000 μg is given as IM injection on alternate days for 2 weeks followed by 1000 μg IM once a month for 6 months.

Note

- *Along with folate or B_{12} therapy, iron preparations are also given, as demand for iron increases with increase in erythropoiesis.*
- *Dimorphic anemia is due to deficiency of both iron and folic acid/vitamin B_{12} (macrocytic/normocytic with hypochromic/normochromic blood picture).*

Frequently asked viva questions

1. Summarize the case.
2. What is the diagnosis of the case?
3. What are the investigations you want to do for the case?
4. How will you treat the patient?
5. How will you prescribe oral iron therapy? What advice will you give the patient?
6. What are the various parenteral iron preparations?
7. What are the advantages of parenteral iron therapy?
8. Can you list some sources of iron-rich food?
9. What are the complications of anemia in pregnancy?
10. How will you manage the patient during labor?
11. What advice will you give the patient during postnatal period?
12. How can you prevent anemia during pregnancy?

3 Diabetes in Pregnancy

Introduction

Diabetes is a common medical problem complicating pregnancy that is associated with adverse maternal and perinatal outcomes. Pregnancy may be complicated by diabetes mellitus (DM) either due to preexisting overt DM or due to glucose intolerance that develops during pregnancy. This chapter deals with the case discussion on DM complicating pregnancy.

Definition of GDM

Until recently, GDM has been defined as "any degree of glucose intolerance with the onset or first recognition during pregnancy." This definition included women with pre-existing diabetes, not identified prior to pregnancy. However, it blurs the line between morbidities associated with diabetes in pregnancy and GDM (risk of maternal and fetal complications are high in DM antedating pregnancy).

Hence, there is continuous effort to improve the definition and classification of hyperglycemia during pregnancy.

FIGO 2016 statement Hyperglycemia first detected at any time during pregnancy should be classified either as DM in pregnancy (DIP) or GDM. Refer Figure 3.1 for classification of hyperglycemia in pregnancy.

- FIGO adopts the WHO (2013) criteria for diagnosis of DIP
- FIGO adopts the WHO (2013) and IADPSG (2010) criteria for diagnosis of GDM
- However, FIGO suggests various options for diagnosis of GDM based on the resource settings

DM in pregnancy (DIP)

Definition

The diagnosis of diabetes in pregnancy as defined by the WHO criteria is based on one or more of the following results, recorded by routine testing at any time during the course of pregnancy:

1. Fasting plasma glucose ≥126 mg/dL; and/or
2. 2-hour plasma glucose (≥200 mg/dL following a 75-g oral glucose load; or
3. Random plasma glucose ≥200 mg/dL in the presence of diabetes symptoms.

Concerns

- In DIP, the risk of complications is high because of the following:
  - The degree of hyperglycemia
  - The uncertainty as to whether the onset of hyperglycemia was prior to pregnancy or developed during early pregnancy.
- DIP might be type 1 or type 2, but a diagnosis of type 2 is more likely.
- Compared with GDM, DIP is more likely to be detected as early as in first trimester.

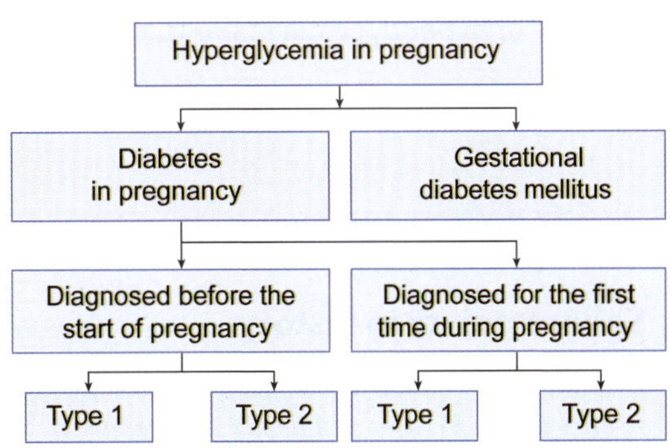

Figure 3.1 DIP classification.

Note *Pregestational DM, overt DM have all been replaced by single terminology of DIP. However, these terminologies are still being used widely.*

Gestational diabetes mellitus (GDM)

Definition

When hyperglycemia detected during routine testing in pregnancy (generally between 24 and 28 weeks) does not meet the criteria of DIP it is termed as GDM.

The diagnosis of GDM as defined by IADPSG (2010) and WHO (2013) is based on a single-step 75-g OGTT when one or more of the following results are recorded during routine testing specifically between weeks 24 and 28 of pregnancy or at any other time during the course of pregnancy:

1. Fasting plasma glucose 92–125 mg/dL
2. 1-hour post 75-g oral glucose load 180 mg/dL
3. 2-hour post 75-g oral glucose load 153–199 mg/dL

Concerns

- GDM implies a relatively milder form of hyperglycemia compared to DIP due to its usual diagnosis and appearance later in pregnancy and less severe hyperglycemia
- Associated with increased risk of poor pregnancy outcome if not managed appropriately
- Associated with future risk of diabetes and cardiovascular disease

Note
- *Definition applies regardless of the use of insulin for treatment.*
- *Refer Figure 3. 2 for differences between DIP and GDM.*

Incidence of hyperglycemia in pregnancy

It is 5–15% of which GDM accounts for 90% of the cases.

Diabetes in pregnancy	Gestational diabetes mellitus
Pregnancy in previously known diabetes	Hyperglycemia during pregnancy that is not diabetes
Or Hyperglycemia diagnosed for the first time during pregnancy that meets WHO criterion for diabetes mellitus in the nonpregnant state	Hyperglycemia diagnosed for the first time during pregnancy
May occur anytime during pregnancy including the first trimester	May occur anytime during pregnancy but most likely after 24 weeks

Figure 3.2 Differences between diabetes in pregnancy and gestational diabetes mellitus.

High-risk factors for GDM

See Table 3.1

Table 3.1 High-risk factors for GDM

Present pregnancy	Past obstetric history
• Elderly gravida • Obesity • K/C/O polycystic ovarian disease • Recurrent urinary tract infection, vulvovaginal candidiasis—to screen for DM in such cases • Persistent glycosuria • Polyhydramnios • Fetal macrosomia • Family history—H/o GDM in first-degree relative	• H/o GDM in previous pregnancy • H/o intrauterine death • H/o stillbirth • H/o unexplained neonatal deaths • H/o macrosomic baby • H/o congenital anomalies • H/o shoulder dystocia • H/o nerve injuries (Erb's palsy) • H/o birth trauma • H/o early onset preeclampsia • H/o recurrent pregnancy loss

Case presentation

Salient points in history

Consider the following relevant points during history taking in cases of diabetes in pregnancy.

Age of the patient

Overt DM and GDM are more common with advancing maternal age.

(CONTD...)

(...CONTD)

Present pregnancy

- *If the patient is a diagnosed case of GDM:*
  - *When was she diagnosed, that is, at what period of gestation (POG)?*
  - *How was she diagnosed, that is, by what method—oral glucose tolerance test (OGTT), random blood sugar (RBS) sample, or fasting and postprandial blood sugar (PPBS)?*
  - *How is she managed following diagnosis?*
    - *Is she on diabetic diet or insulin therapy?*
    - *If she is on insulin therapy, ask the following:*
      - *Is she aware of the dosage?*
      - *Who gives the insulin injection (self-administration or by any other person such as family member or staff nurse)?*
      - *Does she perform self-monitoring of blood glucose (SMBG)?*
  - *Are blood sugars regularly monitored?*
  - *Are blood sugars under control at present?*
  - *What were the last blood sugar values, if known?*
- *If the patient is a known case of overt DM prior to pregnancy:*
  - *Was she on insulin or oral hypoglycemic drugs before pregnancy?*
  - *Were blood sugars under control at the time of conception (increased risk of abortion and fetal anomalies, with uncontrolled sugars during conception and organogenesis)?*
- *Whether fetal anomaly scan was done and told to be normal (increased risk of congenital anomalies in overt DM)*
- *H/o recurrent urinary tract infection (UTI) and recurrent vaginal infections*
- *H/o increased weight gain and symptoms of preeclampsia (10–25% risk of preeclampsia in GDM patients)*

Past obstetric history

- *Ask for H/o GDM in previous pregnancy; if present:*
  - *POG at diagnosis*
  - *Whether on diet or insulin therapy*
  - *Any other antepartum complications such as preeclampsia, polyhydramnios, and antepartum hemorrhage*
- *Delivery details—induced or spontaneous labor (patients with GDM on insulin are usually induced at 38 completed weeks), mode of delivery, and baby details*
- *H/o intrauterine death, big baby, birth trauma, difficult delivery, stillbirth, perinatal death, and congenital anomalies*
- *Whether OGTT was repeated after 6 weeks following delivery*

Family history

H/o DM in first-degree relatives

Diet history

Whether patient is taking a diabetic diet

Salient points in examination

Consider the following relevant points during examination in cases of diabetes in pregnancy.

General examination

- *Height, weight, and BMI*
- *Pallor*
- *Pedal edema*
- *BP (preeclampsia is common in patients with GDM)*
- *Features of polycystic ovarian disease (PCOD) such as acne, hirsutism, and acanthosis nigricans are looked for.*

Obstetric examination

- *Fundal height and symphysiofundal height (SFH) (may be >POG if macrosomia or polyhydramnios is present)*
- *Amount of liquor (polyhydramnios may be present)*
- *Estimated fetal weight (macrosomia may be present)*

Case summary

An example of writing summary in cases of diabetes in pregnancy is given below.

Example *Mrs. T, 26 years of age, primigravida at 34 weeks of gestation, a diagnosed case of GDM on insulin since 28 weeks of gestation, has been*

(CONTD...)

Part 1

(...CONTD)

admitted for blood sugar profile. She has no specific complaints. She is perceiving normal fetal movements. There is no H/o bleeding P/V, leaking P/V, or labor pains. Both of her parents are diabetic. Her obstetric examination reveals a singleton live fetus in cephalic presentation. Uterus is relaxed and liquor appears average in amount. Fetal heart rate (FHR) is 144 beats/min, regular, heard on the left spinoumbilical line.

Case diagnosis

An example of writing diagnosis in cases of diabetes in pregnancy is given below.

Example *26 years of age, primigravida at 34 weeks of gestation, with GDM on insulin, with a singleton live fetus in cephalic presentation, not in labor.*

Case discussion

Screening for GDM

- It is important to screen, diagnose, and treat hyperglycemia in pregnancy to prevent adverse maternal and perinatal outcomes.
- There is no international consensus regarding the timing of screening, method of screening, and diagnostic criteria for GDM. Hence, a simplified version of all the available recommendations on GDM screening and diagnosis are described in this section.

Whom to screen?

Universal versus selective screening

- **Universal screening:** Screening for GDM is done for all pregnant women.
- **Selective screening:** Screening is based on risk stratification. Risk is assessed at the first antenatal visit. Refer to Table 3.2 for risk stratification as per recommendations at the Fifth International Workshop for Gestational Diabetes, 2005.

Disadvantage of selective screening Ninety percent of pregnant women have some risk factor that necessitates screening and there is a chance of missing cases with risk-based or selective screening. Hence, selective screening is not cost-effective and time-effective.

Current guidelines for screening of pregnant women for GDM

Universal screening of all pregnant women is widely accepted (Table 3.3).

Table 3.2 Risk stratification to screen for GDM in pregnancy

Risk category	Members who belong to the risk category	Screening for GDM
Low risk	All the following factors should be fulfilled: • Age <25 years • Normal prepregnancy body weight • No H/o diabetes in first-degree relatives • No H/o abnormal glucose metabolism • No H/o poor obstetric outcome	No screening required
Average risk	Members of ethnic group belonging to Hispanic, African Americans, Southeast Asians, Native Americans	Done at 24–28 weeks using two-step or one-step procedure.
High risk	• Age >30 years • Obesity • Family H/o type 2 DM in first-degree relative • Previous H/o GDM • Past H/o bad obstetric outcome • Persistent glycosuria	Done as soon as feasible and repeated at 24–28 weeks

Table 3.3 Current guidelines for screening of pregnant women for GDM

Guidelines	Recommendation
ADA 2016 guidelines	• Test women with high-risk factors at the first antenatal visit (women diagnosed in the first trimester are treated as overt DM) • Test women without prior diabetes at 24–28 weeks
ACOG 2017 guidelines (has adopted ADA guidelines)	• Test women with high-risk factors at the first antenatal visit (women diagnosed in the first trimester are treated as overt DM) • Test women without prior diabetes at 24–28 weeks
IADPSG guidelines	Screening of all women during the first antenatal visit. If screening is negative, the test should be repeated at 24–28 weeks

ADA, American Diabetes Association; *ACOG*, American College of Obstetricians and Gynecologists; *IADPSG*, International Association of Diabetes in Pregnancy Study Group.

Note *Universal screening is recommended for women belonging to Southeast Asians countries (includes India), as they belong to an ethnic group that is at high risk for developing type 2 DM.*

When to screen?

- Screening in the first trimester helps to identify cases of overt DM that are diagnosed for the first time during pregnancy.
- Screening for GDM at 24–28 weeks of gestation is recommended because placental hormone-mediated insulin resistance increases during the second trimester and glucose levels rise in women who cannot cope up with this insulin resistance. The glucose intolerance is unrevealed during 24–28 weeks.
- Screening in the third trimester limits the time period during which metabolic interventions could be done.

Current guidelines on time of screening for GDM

See Table 3.4. Recommendations of ADA and ACOG are already mentioned in Table 3.3.

Note *It is recommended to screen pregnant women at first antenatal visit and if the test is negative, screening should be repeated at 24–28 weeks.*

How to screen for GDM?

Screening may be done by two-step or one-step procedures.

Table 3.4 Current guidelines on time of screening of pregnant women for GDM

Guidelines	Recommendation
IADPSG (2010)	FBS or HbA1c or RBS is done for all women on the first antenatal visit. If results are not diagnostic of overt DM, 75 g OGTT is done at 24–28 weeks
DIPSI (2006)	Test is done at the first visit and if negative, repeat at 24–28 weeks and again at 32–34 weeks

DIPSI, Diabetes in Pregnancy Study Group in India; *FBS*, fasting blood sugar; *IADPSG*, International Association of Diabetes in Pregnancy Study Groups; *OGTT*, oral glucose challenge test; *RBS*, random blood sugar.

Two-step procedure for diagnosis of GDM

It includes screening with 50 g oral glucose challenge test (OGCT) followed by diagnostic OGTT for those meeting the threshold value in OGCT.

OGCT (50 g) screening test

- **Patient preparation**: It is not necessary to be in the fasting state before the test. Test is done irrespective of time of the day and time of last meal.
- **Procedure:** The patient is asked to take 50 g of oral glucose load. Venous plasma glucose is measured 1 hour later.
- **Cutoff values**
  - OGCT value of ≥140 mg/dL is taken as the cutoff value for doing an OGTT (80% sensitivity, false-positive rate 15%).

- OGCT cutoff value of ≥130 mg/dL increases sensitivity to 90% but the false-positive rate increases to 25%.
- *If glucose level is between 120 and 140 mg/dL:* Repeat the test after a week.
- *OGCT value >200 mg/dL:* The patient is more likely to be a case of overt diabetes.

OGTT diagnostic test

- The patients who meet the threshold value in OGCT are subjected to a 100 g, 3-hour OGTT or 75 g, 2-hour OGTT for diagnosis of GDM (the procedures are described below).
- Disadvantages of the two-step procedure: Two visits are required for diagnosis of GDM and the patient is subjected to several needle pricks.

One-step procedure for diagnosis of GDM

Diagnostic 100 g or 75 g OGTT is performed without doing a screening test.

Note *With simplification of diagnostic tests for GDM, the two-step procedure is not commonly used at present.*

Various diagnostic tests for GDM

100 g OGTT diagnostic test

- **Patient preparation**: The test is done following 3 days of carbohydrate-unrestricted diet (>150 g/day). The test is performed in the morning following an overnight fasting of 8 hours but not more than 14 hours.
- **Procedure**: Fasting blood glucose is estimated. This is followed by intake of 100 g glucose load and blood glucose is estimated at the first, second, and third hours following glucose load.
- **Diagnostic criteria of GDM:** Criteria for interpretation of the 100-g diagnostic OGTT are mentioned in Table 3.5.

Note *Glucose oxidase method of estimation of plasma glucose with Carpenter and Coustan cutoff values is commonly practiced.*

- **Interpretation:**
  - *Two or more values are abnormal:* Diagnose as GDM.
  - *One value is abnormal:* Repeat the test after 1–2 weeks.
    - Abnormal fasting glucose: Increased risk of macrosomia and sudden intrauterine death
    - Abnormal first-, second-, or third-hour value: Increased risk of polyhydramnios
  - *GCT is abnormal but OGTT is normal:* There is an increased risk of macrosomia. The patient is kept under surveillance. Repeat the OGTT test at 24–28 weeks and at 32 weeks.
- American College of Obstetricians and Gynecologists (ACOG) recommends the two step 100 g, 3-hour OGTT for diagnosis of GDM.

Table 3.5 Diagnostic criteria (O'Sullivan and Mahan, 1964; NDDG, 1979; and Carpenter and Coustan, 1982) of GDM by 100 g OGTT and the cutoff values

	O'Sullivan and Mahan criteria (not done these days)	NDDG criteria	Carpenter and Coustan criteria*
Blood sample	Whole blood glucose estimation (whole blood values are 15% less than plasma values)	Plasma glucose estimation	Plasma glucose estimation
Method of estimation of glucose	Somogyi–Nelson method (detects other saccharides in addition to glucose)	Somogyi–Nelson method	Glucose oxidase method (more specific for glucose and values are 5% less than those in Somogyi–Nelson method)
Blood sugar cutoff values (mg %)			
Fasting	≥90	≥105	≥95
First hour	≥165	≥190	≥180
Second hour	≥145	≥165	≥155
Third hour	≥125	≥145	≥140

*These cutoff values are commonly used for diagnosis of GDM by 100 g OGTT.
NDDG, National Diabetes Data Group.

75 g OGTT diagnostic test

- International Association of the Diabetes and Pregnancy Study Groups (IADPSG) recommends the 75 g, 2-hour OGTT for diagnosis of GDM.
- IADPSG criteria for GDM is based on the Hyperglycemia and Adverse Pregnancy Outcome (HAPO) Study.
- **Procedure:** Fasting blood glucose is estimated. This is followed by intake of 75 g glucose load and blood glucose is estimated at the first and second hour following glucose load.
- **Diagnostic criteria of GDM:** IADPSG criteria for interpretation of the 75 g diagnostic OGTT are mentioned in Table 3.6.
- **Interpretation:** GDM is diagnosed if one or more value is abnormal.

American Diabetes Association criteria for GDM

American Diabetes Association (ADA) recommends either 75 g OGTT with IADPSG cutoff values or 100 g OGTT with Carpenter and Coustan/National Diabetes Data Group (NDDG) cutoff values for diagnosis of GDM (Table 3.7).

WHO diagnostic criteria for GDM

- WHO (2013) recommends the 75 g OGTT with IADPSG cutoff values for diagnosis of GDM.

Table 3.6 75 g OGTT diagnostic criteria by IADPSG (2010)

Blood sample	Blood sugar cutoff values (mg/dL)
Fasting	≥92
First hour	≥180
Second hour	≥153

IADPSG, International Association of the Diabetes and Pregnancy Study Groups.

American College of Obstetricians and Gynecologists 2017 recommendations

- American College of Obstetricians and Gynecologists (ACOG) still recommends the two-step approach (50 g GCT followed by 100 g OGTT) with use of either Carpenter and Coustan or NDDG cutoff values for diagnosis of GDM.

Disadvantage of all of the above-mentioned OGTT criteria Overnight fasting is required, so the patient should have another visit to the hospital in fasting state to get the test done. This disadvantage is overcome by Diabetes in Pregnancy Study Group in India (DIPSI) 75 g OGTT.

The Diabetes in Pregnancy Study Group in India (DIPSI) test

Experience from India setting:

- Asian Indians are considered to be at the highest risk of gestational diabetes. Based on studies from India—rising prevalence of diabetes, resource constraints within the health system, and high rate of deliveries—the Diabetes in Pregnancy Study Group in India (DIPSI) developed the following guideline for diagnosis of GDM in the community.
- DIPSI guideline has been endorsed by the Ministry of Health, Government of India; the Federation of Obstetrics and Gynecological Societies of India (FOGSI); and the Association of Physicians of India (API).

Whom to test?

All pregnant women in the community should be tested for hyperglycemia during pregnancy, i.e., there should be universal testing.

Table 3.7 ADA (2016) diagnostic criteria for GDM based on 75 or 100 g OGTT

Blood samples	Blood glucose cutoff values (mg/dL)		
	75 g OGTT	100 g OGTT—Carpenter and Coustan values	100 g OGTT—NDDG values
Fasting	≥92	≥95	≥105
First hour	≥180	≥180	≥190
Second hour	≥153	≥155	≥165
Third hour		≥140	≥145

ADA, American Diabetic Association; *NDDG*, National Diabetes Data Group.

Part 1

When to test?

- Testing for GDM is recommended twice during pregnancy.
- The first testing should be done during first antenatal visit as early as possible in pregnancy. The second testing should be done ideally during 24–28 weeks of pregnancy if the first test is negative.
- If women present beyond 28 weeks of pregnancy, test is to be done at the first point of contact.

How to test?

- Test for diagnosis should be simple, economical, and feasible both within the resource challenged public health system as well as the equally overburdened private practice.
- A Single Step Test measures plasma glucose 2 hours after ingestion of 75 g glucose dissolved in approximately 300 mL water irrespective of the last meal (fasting or non-fasting).
- A glucose level of ≥140 mg/dL is taken as the cut-off for diagnosis of GDM (Table 3.8).

Advantages of the DIPSI test

- Single test: Serves as both screening and diagnostic procedure (universal testing is possible).
- Convenient and feasible: Most women do not come in fasting state for the antenatal visit. When asked to come back again in the fasting state for the test, the dropout rate is high owing to travel time and cost; even if women come, their fasting gets unduly prolonged because of clinic schedules and high patient volume, causing discomfort and inconvenience to them.

Table 3.8 DIPSI (2006) recommendations on OGTT cutoff values

Second-hour venous plasma glucose (mg/dL)	Interpretation
>200	DM
140–200	GDM
120–140	DGGT—may increase the risk of polyhydramnios

DGGT, decreased gestational glucose tolerance; *DIPSI*, Diabetes in Pregnancy Study Group in India.

The nonfasting test increases convenience as well as implementation feasibility.

- In the absence of available laboratory facilities, a plasma standardized glucometer may be used to evaluate blood glucose. Using the glucometer provides an opportunity to communicate results instantly and initiate counseling, avoiding the need for the patient to return for test result.
- Economical [DIPSI is more cost-effective than a single 100 g OGTT (four blood samples drawn for a single test) or 75 g GTT of IADPSG (3 blood samples drawn].

Why the DIPSI diagnostic cutoff point of 2 hour 75 g is ≥ 140 mg/dL?

- DIPSI guidelines were initiated before the WHO endorsed the IADPSG guideline and have been ratified by the Ministry of Health and other professional bodies. The DIPSI guidelines follow the old WHO 2-hour cutoff value.
- Given the positive relationship of poor pregnancy outcomes with increasing maternal plasma glucose values in Asian Indian women, a 2-hour cutoff value of 140 mg/dL of the earlier WHO (1999) criteria is considered more appropriate to identify those at risk for macrosomia-related birth complications.
- Treatment of women with GDM identified with nonfasting 2-hour post-75 g glucose cutoff values (140 mg/dL) is associated with reduced adverse pregnancy outcomes.

Extra edge

- IADPSG criteria is the only outcome-based criteria. IADPSG 75 g, 2-hour OGTT cutoff values for GDM are based on blood glucose values that resulted in adverse pregnancy outcomes, while 100 g OGTT diagnostic criteria cutoff values are based on blood glucose values associated with the development of subsequent type 2 DM.
- DIPSI cutoff value has not been put to test to find the correlation with adverse perinatal outcome.

Summary of all the diagnostic criteria for GDM as per different organizations

See Table 3.9.

Table 3.9 Diagnostic criteria for GDM as per different organizations

Recommendation by	Glucose load	Criteria	Venous plasma glucose cutoff values (mg%)			
			Fasting	1st hour	2nd hour	3rd hour
ADA (2016)	100 g (two steps) 100 g (two steps) 75 g	Carpenter and Coustan NDDG IADPSG	≥95 105 ≥92	≥180 ≥190 ≥180	≥155 ≥165 ≥153	≥140 ≥145 NR
IADPSG (2010)	75 g	Based on HAPO study results	≥92	≥180	≥153	NR
ACOG (2017)	100 g (two steps)	Carpenter and Coustan NDDG	≥95 105	≥180 ≥190	≥155 ≥165	≥140 ≥145
WHO (2013)	75 g	IADPSG	≥92	≥180	≥153	NR
DIPSI (2006)	75 g	DIPSI	NR	NR	≥140	NR

ADA, American Diabetes Association; *ACOG,* American College of Obstetricians and Gynecologists; *DIPSI,* Diabetes in Pregnancy Study Group in India; *HAPO,* hyperglycemia and adverse pregnancy outcome; *IADPSG,* International Association of the Diabetes and Pregnancy Study Groups; *NDDG,* National Diabetes Data Group; *NR,* not recorded.

Extra edge

DIPSI testing is done irrespective of the last meal—justification:

- Fasting test is done mainly for the convenience of patients. If Fasting test has to be done, there will be two visits.
- GDM is a state of insulin resistance due to diabetogenic hormones of pregnancy (cortisol, estrogen, progesterone, human placental lactogen). In normal women with adequate pancreatic reserve, insulin secretion increases to overcome the insulin resistance in pregnancy. Patients with GDM are not able to cope up with the insulin demand to meet the peripheral insulin resistance that occurs during pregnancy.
- Glucose challenge irrespective of last meals results in adequate and brisk insulin response in normal women to maintain euglycemic state, while women with GDM have impaired insulin secretion resulting in an increase in glucose levels.

DIPSI recommends 75 g OGTT to be done in the first antenatal visit—justification:

- It helps to identify cases of overt DM.
- Fetal pancreas starts developing by 9 weeks of gestation. If hyperglycemia is present at this time, pancreatic memory of this hyperglycemic insult may result in the development of DM in the offspring later in life.

Other methods of screening for GDM

- **Fasting blood sugar (FBS):** It is not useful as pregnancy is a state of fasting hypoglycemia and postprandial hyperglycemia.
- **Random blood sugar (RBS):** It is not recommended for diagnosis of DM.
- **Glycosylated hemoglobin (HbA1c):** It reflects glycemic control over the past 2 months (half-life of RBC is 60 days) and is not affected by recent or transient increase in blood glucose levels.
  - For nondiabetic patients, the normal range of HbA1c is 4–5.6%.
  - Incidence of congenital anomalies increases with higher values of HbA1c (HbA1c >10%—incidence of congenital anomalies is 14%).
- **Fructosamine assay:** It reflects glycemic control over the past 1–3 weeks.
- **Glucose polymer challenge test:** Glucose polymer saccharide can be used instead of glucose for OGTT.
  - *Advantage*: Lesser gastrointestinal symptoms
- **Intravenous (IV) glucose tolerance test (GTT):**
  - Indications
    - Intolerance to oral glucose such as vomiting
    - Altered gastrointestinal absorption
- **Urine glucose:** It is not specific as renal glycosuria can be present during pregnancy in 5–50% of cases. Renal threshold decreases during pregnancy due to the following:
  - Increased glomerular filtration rate
  - Impaired tubular reabsorption of glucose

- **Capillary blood glucose estimation (using glucometer):** It is not recommended for diagnosis of GDM due to lack of standard threshold values. However, glucometer is widely being used to follow-up patients with GDM, following diagnosis by standard method.

Diagnostic criteria for DIP (previously termed overt DM in pregnancy)

- FBS ≥126 mg/dL
- RBS ≥200 mg/dL
- HbA1c ≥6.5

Complications of diabetes in pregnancy

Effects of pregnancy on DM

Pregnancy worsens pregestational or overt DM.

- Those on diabetic diet may require insulin therapy.
- Those on oral hypoglycemic drugs have to be changed to insulin.
- Those on insulin may require higher doses of insulin.
- Pregnancy worsens diabetic vasculopathy such as nephropathy, retinopathy, and microangiopathy.
- There is an increased risk of diabetic ketoacidosis.

Effect of DM on pregnancy

Maternal complications

- Poor glycemic control is the most important cause for maternal complications.
- Pregestational diabetes is associated with a higher rate of maternal complications than GDM (Table 3.10).

Viva corner

Q1 Why does insulin requirement increase with advancing pregnancy?

Insulin requirement increases with advancing pregnancy because of increase in diabetogenic hormones of pregnancy.

Diabetogenic hormones of pregnancy

- Human placental lactogen (HPL)
- Increased estrogen
- Increased progesterone
- Increased cortisol
- Placental insulinase

Fetal and neonatal complications

Maternal hyperglycemia is the most important cause of fetal and neonatal complications (see Tables 3.11 and 3.12).

Table 3.11 Fetal and neonatal complications due to DM

Fetal complications	Neonatal complications
• Abortions (in DIP) • Congenital malformations (in DIP) • Macrosomia (Figure 3.3) • Prematurity • Sudden intrauterine deaths • Birth injuries during delivery	• Respiratory distress syndrome • Hypoglycemia • Hypothermia • Hypocalcemia • Hyperbilirubinemia • Polycythemia • Myocardial hypertrophy (overt DM) • Future risk of DM and obesity

DIP, diabetes mellitus in pregnancy; *DM*, diabetes mellitus.

Table 3.10 Maternal complications due to DM

Antenatal	Intrapartum	Postpartum
• Infections—recurrent urinary tract infection, pyelonephritis, vulvovaginal candidiasis • Preeclampsia—25% incidence • Polyhydramnios • Preterm labor	• Prolonged labor • Increase in instrumental delivery and lower-segment cesarean section • Perineal trauma • Postpartum hemorrhage *(Intrapartum complications are mainly due to macrosomia and shoulder dystocia)*	• Infections • Puerperal sepsis

Table 3.12 Reasons for various pregnancy complications in DM

Complications	Reasons
Congenital malformations	• Hyperglycemia can lead to abnormal embryogenesis • Microangiopathy-induced tissue hypoxia • Increased free radicals • Hyperketonemia • Decreased arachidonic acid and myoinositol
Polyhydramnios	• Hyperglycemia in fetus leading to increased fetal urine excretion • Irritation of fetal membranes by glucose in amniotic fluid leads to increased transudation across fetal membranes • Associated central nervous system anomalies such as neural tube defects result in absent fetal swallowing reflux and hence decreased swallowing of amniotic fluid
Preterm labor	• Infections • Polyhydramnios • Premature rupture of membranes (due to polyhydramnios and infections) • Iatrogenic (induction of labor)
Sudden IUD	• Chronic aberration in oxygen transport in poorly controlled DM → chronic hypoxia → leads to reduced oxygen delivery to tissues → sudden IUD • Villous edema due to hyperglycemia can impair oxygen transport • Associated vasculopathy can lead to intrauterine growth restriction (IUGR) and fetal death
Postpartum hemorrhage	• Uterine overdistension (polyhydramnios and big baby) • Associated preeclampsia • Operative interferences
Macrosomia in GDM (birth weight ≥4 kg)	• Explained by Pederson's hypothesis: Maternal hyperglycemia → fetal hyperglycemia → stimulates fetal pancreas to secrete insulin → fetal hyperinsulinemia → increased glycogen synthesis, lipogenesis, protein synthesis → deposition of fat in fetus → macrosomia
RDS in newborn	• Due to delayed fetal lung maturity: Maternal hyperglycemia → fetal hyperglycemia → fetal hyperinsulinemia → high insulin inhibits cortisol action on pulmonary fibroblasts → decreased surfactant synthesis → RDS
Neonatal hypoglycemia	• Maternal hyperglycemia → fetal hyperglycemia → fetal hyperinsulinemia. Following delivery, glucose load from the mother is cut off and existing hyperinsulinemia in the newborn leads to hypoglycemia
Neonatal hypothermia	• Large surface area of the newborn • Less of thermogenic brown fat and more of yellow fat
Neonatal polycythemia	• Chronic intrauterine hypoxia → stimulates erythropoietin synthesis → increased red cell production and polycythemia
Neonatal hyperbilirubinemia	• Polycythemia and increased viscosity • Prematurity
Neonatal hypocalcemia	• Prematurity • Relative neonatal hypoparathyroidism

DM, diabetes mellitus; *GDM*, gestational diabetes mellitus; *IUD*, intrauterine death; *RDS*, respiratory distress syndrome.

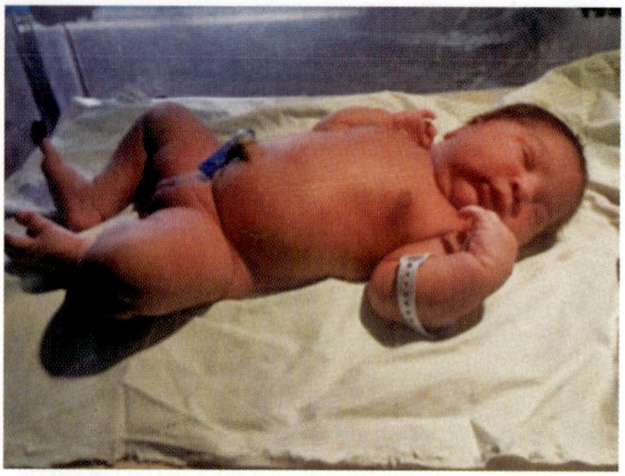

Figure 3.3 A macrosomic baby born to a gestational diabetes mellitus mother.

Extra edge

Cutoff values for detection of important neonatal complications

Terminology	Cutoff value
Neonatal hypoglycemia	Blood glucose <45 mg/dL
Neonatal hypocalcemia	Serum calcium <7 mg/dL
Neonatal polycythemia	Hematocrit >65%

Management of DM complicating pregnancy

- Diagnosis and treatment of DM in pregnancy reduces maternal and fetal complications.
- Women with DM complicating pregnancy are managed with a team of specialists that include an obstetrician, a physician, a dietician, and a pediatrician.
- Management includes the following:
  - Medical management to control blood sugars
  - Obstetric management to monitor the mother and fetus for early detection of complications

Management goals

- To achieve glycemic control
- To reduce maternal and fetal complications
- To plan the time and mode of delivery
- To provide neonatal care

Medical management—achieving glycemic control

- Glycemic control is achieved by diet, exercise, and oral antidiabetic drugs +/– insulin therapy. Maintaining euglycemia throughout pregnancy is essential to prevent complications.

High-yield points

Usually GDM is associated with fetal macrosomia. However, it may be associated with intrauterine growth restriction (IUGR) in the following conditions:

- Pregestational DM associated with vasculopathy such as nephropathy and microangiopathy (due to uteroplacental insufficiency)
- GDM associated with preeclampsia

Fetal complications specific to DIP (pregestational or overt DM)

- Increased risk of abortions and congenital anomalies are specific to overt DM (in true GDM, hyperglycemia usually occurs in the second trimester and hence associated with late fetal complications such as macrosomia and polyhydramnios).
- Neonatal complications are similar in both true GDM and pregestational DM.

Congenital malformations in DM

These occur in overt DM when blood glucose levels are uncontrolled during organogenesis.

Incidence

- It is 6–10% in DM (in normal population—3%). HbA1c >10 is associated with 14% risk of congenital malformations.

Common congenital anomalies in fetuses of diabetic mothers are as follows:

- Cardiac anomalies (most common anomalies)—transposition of great vessels, ventricular septal defect, atrial septal defect, patent ductus arteriosus, and coarctation of aorta
- Neural tube defects—anencephaly and microcephaly
- Renal and gastrointestinal tract anomalies
- Most specific defect—caudal regression syndrome (very rare)

- Patients diagnosed with GDM should be started on medical nutrition therapy (MNT) for 2 weeks (MNT is described later in this chapter).
- After 2 weeks of MNT, a 2 hours postprandial blood sugar (PPBS) level is checked.
  - If PPBS is <120 mg/dL, repeat test every 2 weeks in second trimester and every week in third trimester.
  - If PPBS is ≥120 mg/dL, oral antidiabetic agents (OAD)/insulin therapy should be started as per the guidelines.
- Goals of blood sugar control (current therapeutic targets recommended by ADA and ACOG) are given in Table 3.13.
- GDM is most often diagnosed in midtrimester. Target glucose levels can be achieved and maintained by diet alone or diet plus OAD +/– insulin.
- When dietary therapy is insufficient to maintain euglycemia in women with GDM, use of OADs (metformin or glyburide) has been considered as the first option for drug treatment in many settings and recommended by several organizations (NICE guidelines). However, ACOG still considers insulin as gold standard for GDM.
- Patients with preexisting overt DM and GDM diagnosed in first trimester (more likely to be a case of overt DM) often require insulin therapy to achieve euglycemia. Insulin requirement increases in the second half of pregnancy and should be adequately adjusted.

Obstetric management

Antenatal management of GDM

- The patient is advised on frequent antenatal visits once in every 2 weeks till 32 weeks and then every week.
- Maternal and fetal surveillance are done.

Table 3.13 Goals of blood sugar control in patients with GDM

Blood sample	Cutoff value (mg/dL)
Fasting	≤95
Premeal	≤100
1 hour postprandial	≤140
2 hours postprandial	≤120
Fasting 2–4 am	60–90
During labor and delivery	72–126

Maternal surveillance

- Screen for infections
  - P/S examination done to rule out vaginal infections
  - Urine routine and microscopy—to check for proteinuria, glycosuria, and pus cells
  - Urine culture sensitivity
- Close watch on BP (patients with GDM are at a high risk of developing preeclampsia)

Fetal surveillance

- Fetal anomalies scan is done between 16 and 24 weeks.
- The patient is advised to keep a daily fetal kick count (DFMC).
- Fundal height and SFH are measured during antenatal visits.
- Serial ultrasonography (USG) for fetal growth, fetal weight, and amniotic fluid index (AFI) is done every 2 weeks (abdominal circumference (AC) is an important predictor of macrosomia).
- From 32 weeks onward, nonstress test (NST) is done twice a week and fetal biophysical profile (BPP) is done every week.

Note *If GDM is diagnosed in the first trimester, the patient is more likely to be a case of overt DM—management is similar to that in overt DM.*

Periconceptional management of overt DM

- Provide patient education and counseling on the need for strict blood sugar control and the complications of DM.
- Advise on a diabetic diet.
- Optimize blood sugar control prior to conception.
  - FBS <95 mg/dL
  - HbA1c <7.5 (to prevent congenital malformations)
- Periconceptional folic acid 500 µg/day is given (decreases the incidence of neural tube defect).
- Evaluate diabetic status and complications.
  - HbA1c
  - Urine—albumin, sugar, and ketones
  - 24-Hour urine protein
  - Renal function test

- Fundus examination for hypertensive retinopathy changes
- ECG
- ECHO cardiogram

- If the patient is on oral hypoglycemic drugs, change to insulin therapy.

> **Extra edge**
>
> - **Microalbuminuria:** Urine albumin excretion of 30–300 mg/day
> - **Overt albuminuria:** Urine albumin excretion of >300 mg/day

Antenatal management of overt DM

- Maternal and perinatal complications are higher in pregestational diabetes.
- The patient is advised on frequent antenatal visits once in every 2 weeks till 32 weeks and then every week.
- Maternal and fetal surveillance are done.

Maternal surveillance

- Screen for vasculopathy
  - Urine for proteinuria every visit
  - 24-Hour urine protein every trimester
  - Renal function test every trimester
  - Fundus examination for diabetic retinopathy every trimester
  - ECG and ECHO cardiogram
- Screen for infections
  - P/S examination to look for vaginal infections
  - Urine routine and microscopy (to check for proteinuria, glycosuria, and pus cells)
  - Urine culture sensitivity to rule out asymptomatic bacteriuria
- Close watch on BP (high risk for developing preeclampsia)

Fetal surveillance

First trimester

- HbA1c (HbA1c levels >10 → associated with 25% risk of congenital anomalies)
- USG for dating pregnancy and confirming viability
- USG between 11 and 13 weeks for nuchal translucency, to rule out anencephaly

Second trimester

- Maternal serum alpha-fetoprotein (MSAFP) at 15–18 weeks
- Level II anomalies scan at 16–24 weeks
- Fetal ECHO cardiogram at 24–26 weeks

Third trimester

- Antepartum fetal surveillance (APFS) is started from 28 weeks due to risk of macrosomia, polyhydramnios, and intrauterine death (IUD) in the third trimester.
- The patient is advised to keep a DFMC.
- Fundal height and SFH are measured during antenatal visits.
- Serial USG for fetal growth, fetal weight, and AFI is done every 2 weeks.
- NST to assess fetal well-being is done twice a week from 32 weeks onwards.
- Biophysical profile is done every week.

> **Viva corner**
>
> **Q1 Which component of biophysical profile can be misleading in GDM cases?**
>
> Amniotic fluid index can be misleading as polyhydramnios may be present in GDM cases.

Time of delivery in pregnancy with DM

- **GDM on diet (GDM A1):** With antepartum fetal surveillance, we can wait up to 40 weeks for spontaneous onset of labor; however, the pregnancy is not allowed to cross the EDD.
- **GDM on insulin (GDM A2):** Elective induction is done at 38 completed weeks as there is a risk of sudden unexplained IUDs in the last few weeks of pregnancy. Elective induction, in addition, reduces risk of shoulder dystocia.
- **Overt DM:** Pregnancy is terminated at 38 completed weeks.
- **DM associated with complications such as preeclampsia, vascular disease, uncontrolled sugars, and IUGR:** Early termination at <38 weeks may be considered.

Mode of delivery

- Elective induction of labor can be done if macrosomia and cephalopelvic disproportion (CPD) are ruled out.

- Elective cesarean section is indicated for the following reasons:
  - Big baby (4.5 kg/5 kg in diabetic/nondiabetic (ACOG);—increased incidence of shoulder dystocia)
  - Obstetric indications such as placenta previa, malpresentations, CPD, severe IUGR, and bad obstetric history

Viva corner

Q1 Why are GDM cases not induced at 37 completed weeks as in preeclampsia?

In GDM, there is delayed fetal lung maturity as hyperinsulinemia delays surfactant production. Hence, to reduce the risk of respiratory distress syndrome, we wait for 1 more week after reaching term (37 weeks) for termination of pregnancy.

Intrapartum management

- Elective induction of labor is done.
- Night dose of insulin is given and morning dose withheld. Induction is planned in the morning.
- If cervix is unfavorable, cervical ripening with Foley's catheter/PGE2 is done prior to induction.
- Induction of labor is done with PGE2/oxytocin depending on the Bishop's score.
- Blood glucose is monitored every 2 hours.
- Aim is to maintain intrapartum blood glucose at <140 mg/dL.
- Buffered dextrose (glucose infusion with insulin) is started and titrated according to capillary blood glucose values.
- Urine ketones are checked every 4 hours, and serum electrolytes every 12 hours.

Titration of insulin according to sliding scale

Five units of plain insulin in 500 mL of 5% dextrose is started at a rate of 100 mL/h.

- If blood sugar >140 mg/dL, plain insulin is titrated accordingly (Table 3.14).
- If blood sugar <80 mg/dL, infuse 5% dextrose at rate of 100 mL/h.

Table 3.14 Titration of insulin—sliding scale

Blood sugar (mg/dL)	Plain insulin given subcutaneously (units)
140–180	4
181–250	8
251–400	12
>400	16

Alternative method of titration of insulin in buffered dextrose infusion

- This method of insulin titration is used in many Indian labor room settings (Table 3.15).

Table 3.15 Alternative method of titration of insulin in buffered dextrose infusion

Blood sugar (mg/dL)	Buffered dextrose at 100 mL/h
<60	25% dextrose
61–100	5% dextrose
101–150	5 units plain insulin in 5% D + 10 mEq KCl in each pint
151–200	10 units plain insulin in 5% D + 10 mEq KCl in each pint
201–250	15 units plain insulin in 5% D + 10 mEq KCl in each pint
≥250	20 units plain insulin in normal saline + 10 mEq KCl in each pint

Management during labor

I stage

- A partogram is plotted to monitor the progress of labor and maternal and fetal well-being.
- Monitor FHR with continuous electronic monitoring if facilities are available; otherwise, intermittent auscultation with a stethoscope (every 15 minutes in the first stage and 5 minutes in the second stage) is done.
- Give adequate labor analgesia and hydration. Epidural analgesia is preferred, if facilities are available (if LSCS is indicated during labor, anesthesia can be administered through the same epidural catheter)
- Strict asepsis is followed as there is an increased risk of infections.
- Restrict the number of P/V examinations.

- Augmentation of labor is done with artificial rupture of membranes (ARM) + oxytocin. Controlled ARM is done in case of polyhydramnios to prevent cord prolapse.
- Prophylactic antibiotics are given following rupture of membranes or ARM.

II stage
- Anticipate shoulder dystocia.
- Anticipate perineal trauma due to big baby.

III stage
- Active management of third stage of labor is done
- Anticipate postpartum hemorrhage (PPH) (atonic PPH—overdistended uterus due to big baby or polyhydramnios, traumatic PPH due to perineal injuries)

Preparation for elective cesarean section

- Night dose of insulin is given. Withhold the morning dose of insulin.
- FBS and serum electrolytes are estimated.
- Regional anesthesia (epidural) is preferred.
- Postoperative blood sugars are checked every 2 hours for initial 12 hours, and then 4 hourly. Insulin in buffered dextrose infusion is administered in women with overt DM.
- Urine albumin, sugar, and ketone charting is done.

Postpartum management

- Early breastfeeding is started to avoid hypoglycemia in the baby.
- Continue prophylactic antibiotics.
- Insulin requirement falls immediately after delivery. Blood sugar levels should be tested 24–48 hours after delivery.
- Most women with true GDM will not require insulin in the postnatal period and are advised a normal diet.
- Patients should be followed up with a 75 g OGTT at or after 6 weeks following delivery to detect impaired glucose tolerance or overt DM. The test is repeated every year, since women with GDM are at a high risk for developing type 2 diabetes.
- In patients with overt DM, the dose of insulin should be adjusted accordingly or may be changed to oral hypoglycemic drugs.

Contraception

- If the patient has completed family, advise on permanent methods of contraception.
- For spacing between pregnancies
  - Barrier methods can be advised (failure rate is high).
  - Progesterones (pills, implants, intrauterine devices) can be given during lactation.
  - Oral contraceptives pills should be avoided in the initial 6 months during lactation. It is contraindicated in women with complications or risk factors for vascular diseases.
  - IUCDs can be inserted.

Long-term follow-up of patients with GDM

- There is a 50% chance of developing GDM in the next pregnancy.
- There is a 50% chance of developing overt DM later in life.

Viva corner

Q1 What is controlled artificial rupture of membranes (ARM)?

In cases with polyhydramnios, ARM can result in cord prolapse. Hence, the presenting part is fixed onto the pelvis by the assistant and ARM is done with a Kocher's forceps or a needle to allow slow escape of liquor.

Following the procedure:

- Rule out cord prolapse.
- Auscultate fetal heart sound to rule out FHR abnormalities due to cord compression or occult cord prolapse.

Role of diet, physical activity, and pharmacotherapy in patients with GDM (FIGO recommendations)

Role of diet therapy (medical nutrition therapy)

- Dietary counseling in GDM is referred to as medical nutritional therapy (MNT).
- Medical nutritional therapy in pregnancy can be described as "a carbohydrate-controlled meal plan that promotes adequate nutrition with

appropriate weight gain, normoglycemia, and the absence of ketosis."

- It is the first-line therapy in all women diagnosed with GDM. However, there is paucity of data to provide evidence-based recommendations for most of the nutrition interventions.
- Goals of medical nutrition therapy:
  - To provide adequate nutrition to the mother
  - To maintain glycemic control.
- To prevent starvation ketosis, blood sugar targets for MNT are FBG value <95 mg/dL and 2-hour PP value <120 mg/dL.
- Effects of diet on blood sugar values are apparent after 2 weeks of starting diet therapy.

Calories

- Modest caloric restriction (1600–1800 calories/day, 33% reduction) does not lead to ketosis.
- Daily energy intake of almost 2050 calories in all BMI categories in women with GDM was reported to reduce weight gain, maintain euglycemia, avoid ketonuria, and achieve average birth weights.
- For dietary requirements during pregnancy, see Table 3.16.

Carbohydrates

- Focusing on total amount, quality, and distribution of carbohydrate intake helps attain metabolic control in all patients with diabetes.
- The total amount of carbohydrates, distribution of carbohydrates in various meals and snacks, type of carbohydrates, and the glycemic index (GI) of foods can be modified without affecting the total caloric intake.
- Carbohydrates should be distributed throughout the day in three small-to-moderate-sized meals and three snacks to reduce postprandial glucose fluctuations (Table 3.17).
- Carbohydrate intake should be limited to 35–45% of total calories, with a minimum of 175 g carbohydrates/day.
- Determining the carbohydrate intake in meals and snacks is termed carbohydrate counting.
- Carbohydrate counting estimates carbohydrate amount in each meal by determining carbohydrate serving. Each 15 g of carbohydrate is equivalent to one carbohydrate serving. 1 g of carbohydrate produces 4 kcal of energy.

Table 3.16 Dietary requirements of patients with GDM

Weight	Recommended calorie intake (kcal/kg/day)
Underweight women	35–40
Normal weight women	30–35
Overweight women	25–30

Table 3.17 Breakup of calorie intake among meals and snacks in patients with GDM

Meal	Calories (% of daily intake)
Breakfast	10–15
Snack	5–10
Lunch	20–30
Snack	5–10
Dinner	20–30
Snack	5–10

- The glycemic index (GI) of foods (ranges between 50 and 100) is also an important factor, as food with a low GI may reduce postmeal glycemic levels and flatten the glucose curve while foods with a high GI (>70) may show higher postprandial values.

Dietary Fibers

- Restriction of saturated fats (<10%) and increase in intake of dietary fibers are advised.
- Fiber intake, particularly soluble fiber, is beneficial in lowering serum lipid levels, reducing glucose excursions and reducing constipation.
- Low GI foods often have higher fiber content.
- Up to 28 g fiber intake per day is recommended for pregnant women.

The following principles should be adhered while advising MNT for all pregnant women with diabetes:

- Design an appropriate diet with respect to prepregnancy BMI, desired body weight, physical activity, habits, personal and cultural preferences.
- Provide routine follow-up and diet adjustments throughout pregnancy to achieve and maintain treatment goals.

- Offer education, support, and follow-up by a qualified dietician experienced in care of women with diabetes. Topics for discussion include weight control, food records, carbohydrate counting, prevention of hypoglycemia, healthy foods, and physical activity.

Role of physical activity

Recommendations for physical activity in women with GDM:

- Exercise increases insulin sensitivity and cardiorespiratory reserve. Exercise in conjunction with diet therapy improves blood glucose control and may reduce the need for insulin.
- ACOG recommends at least 30 min/day of moderate-intensity exercise for 5 days in a week or a minimum of 150 minutes per week. Simple exercise such as walking for 10–15 minutes after each meal can lead to improved glycemic control and is recommended.
- Effect of exercise on blood sugar values is apparent after 4 weeks of training.
- Exercises advised during pregnancy are as follows:
  - Exercises involving upper trunk do not provoke uterine contractions. Brisk walking is safe during pregnancy.
  - Cycling, swimming, and low-impact aerobics can be done during pregnancy.

Part 1

Pharmacotherapy during pregnancy

Pharmacological therapy is usually added to MNT, if FBS levels ≥95 mg/dL, 1-hour levels consistently ≥140 mg/dL, or 2-hour levels consistently ≥120 mg/dL.

Role of oral hypoglycemic agents during pregnancy

- Glyburide and metformin are the oral hypoglycemic drugs studied to be relatively safe during pregnancy.
- Metformin and glyburide (OADs) are safe and effective therapies for GDM during the second and third trimesters and may be initiated as first-line treatment after failing to achieve glucose control with lifestyle modification.
- Among OADs, metformin may be a better choice than glyburide.
- Women should be counseled regarding:
  - The lack of superiority of OADs when compared with insulin
  - No long-term evidence on the safety of OADs.

Role of insulin therapy

- When blood glucose targets cannot be reached by diet and/or OADs, insulin is required.
- Insulin should be considered as the first-line treatment in women with GDM who are at high

High-yield points

Types of insulin

Table **Types of insulin and their action**

Type of insulin	Onset of action	Peak time of action	Duration of action
• Ultrashort acting – Insulin aspart – Lispro	5–15 minutes	1–2 hours	4–6 hours
• Short acting – Regular insulin	0.5–1 hour	2–4 hours	6–8 hours
• Intermediate acting – NPH (isophane) – Human lente	1–2 hours	4–6 hours	12 hours
• Long acting – Ultralente – Glargine – Detemir	1–1.5 hours	No peak time	12–24 hours

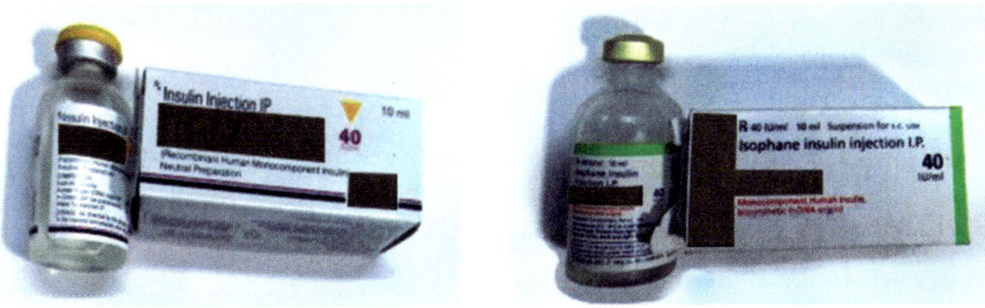

a. b.

Figure 3.4 Insulin vials. **a.** Regular (short acting) insulin. **b.** Isophane (intermediate acting) insulin.

risk of failing on OAD therapy, including the following factors:
- Diagnosis of diabetes <20 weeks of gestation
- Need for pharmacologic therapy >30 weeks
- Fasting plasma glucose levels >110 mg/dL
- 1-hour postprandial glucose >140 mg/dL
- Pregnancy weight gain >12 kg

- Insulin does not cross the placenta and can achieve tight metabolic control.
- Insulin requirement in pregnancy: Insulin requirement increases during pregnancy. Insulin requirements in various trimesters are as follows:
  - *First trimester*: 0.7 unit/kg
  - *Second trimester*: 0.8 unit/kg
  - *Third trimester*: 0.9 unit/kg
- There is no evidence supporting the advantages of any one type of insulin or regimen of insulin over another. Thus, insulin type and regimens should be individualized.
- Two-third of insulin dose is given before breakfast [70 intermediate (NPH)/30 regular insulin]. One-third of insulin dose is given before dinner (50 intermediate/50 regular insulin).
- It is beneficial to pair rapid-acting with intermediate or long-acting insulin, in order to simulate the physiologic insulin secretion throughout the day. Usually short-acting insulin in three divided doses and one or two doses of long-or intermediate-acting insulin are prescribed (Figure 3.4).
- However, if there are only isolated abnormal values at a specific time of day, focusing the insulin regimen to correct the specific hyperglycemia is preferred.
- NPH insulin (intermediate-acting) and regular insulin (short-acting) are the mainstay of insulin therapy in hyperglycemia in pregnancy. However, more recently, insulins such as insulin lispro and aspart (short-acting) and detemir (long-acting) can be safely used in pregnancy. There is paucity of data on the use of insulin glargine during pregnancy.
- Insulin lispro and aspart have a more rapid onset of action, enabling the patient to administer her insulin right at the time of a meal rather than 10–15 minutes before an anticipated meal. This provides better glycemic control and helps avoid hypoglycemic episodes from errors in timing.
- Target plasma glucose levels with insulin therapy
  - *FBS:* <95 mg/dL
  - *One hour PPBS:* <140 mg/dL
  - *Two hours PPBS:* <120 mg/dL

High-yield points

Dawn phenomenon

- High fasting blood sugar levels in the absence of nocturnal hypoglycemia (plasma blood glucose at 2 am is high; fasting blood glucose is high)
- Treatment: Dose of intermediate acting insulin given at bedtime is increased

Somogyi phenomenon

- Nocturnal hypoglycemia leads to counterregulatory response resulting in high fasting blood sugars (plasma blood glucose at 2 am is low; fasting blood glucose is high).
- Treatment: Dose of intermediate acting insulin given at bedtime is decreased.

- Educate to recognize and treat signs of hypoglycemia: To ingest 15 g of simple carbohydrate (sugar, rapidly absorbed tablets, sweetened liquids). Glucagon injection should be made available in hospitals settings.

Shoulder dystocia

Shoulder dystocia is one of the anticipated complications during delivery in women with DM complicating pregnancy. It is an obstetric emergency that occurs without warning and can lead to serious neonatal and maternal morbidity (Figure 3.5).

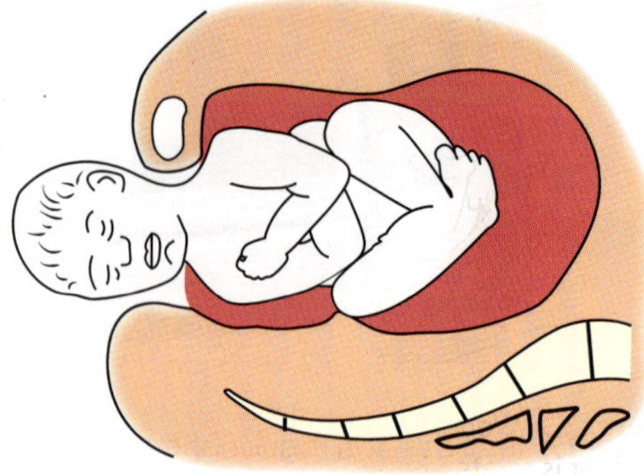

Figure 3.5 Shoulder dystocia.

Definition It refers to difficulty in delivery of fetal shoulders that requires additional maneuvers, other than the gentle downward traction of fetal head.

Risk factors (Hint: *Remember the pneumonic "DOPE")*
- Diabetes
- Obesity
- Past dates and prior big baby
- Excessive weight gain in pregnancy

Complications See Table 3.18

Table 3.18 Fetal and maternal complications due to shoulder dystocia

Fetal complications	Maternal complications
• Brachial plexus injury • Fractures • Birth asphyxia • Fetal death	• Operative interferences • Postpartum hemorrhage • Perineal trauma • Diastasis of pubic symphysis • Femoral neuropathy

Management ACOG criteria for management of shoulder dystocia include the following:
- Call for help.
- Drain the bladder.
- Give liberal episiotomy.
- McRoberts maneuver: Perform hyperflexion and abduction of both hips and provide suprapubic pressure with downward traction on the fetal head (Figure 3.6).

If the above-mentioned measures fail, then try other maneuvers such as the following:
- **Wood's screw maneuver:** Posterior shoulder that is below the pelvic brim is rotated anteriorly

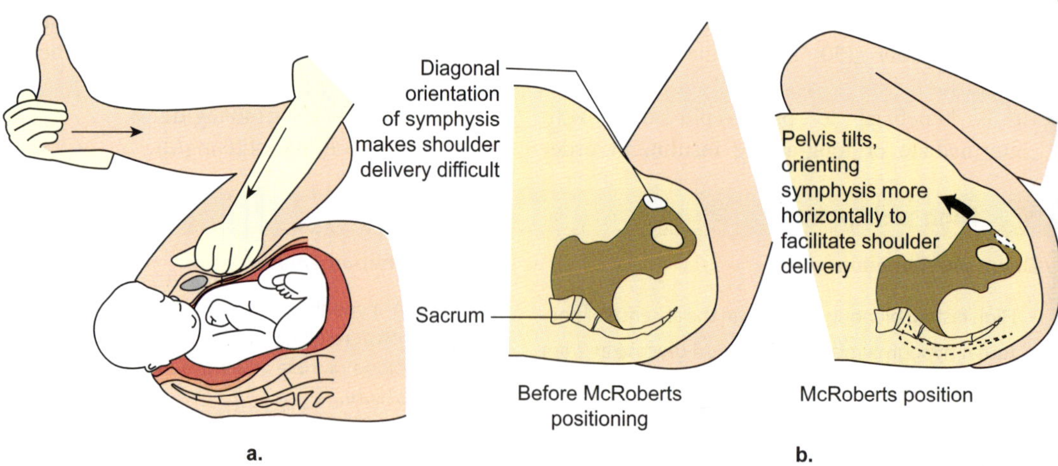

Figure 3.6 McRoberts maneuver. **a.** Mother's legs are hyperflexed onto the abdomen along with suprapubic pressure. **b.** The sacrum straightens and the pubic symphysis tilts anteriorly, reducing the angle of inclination.

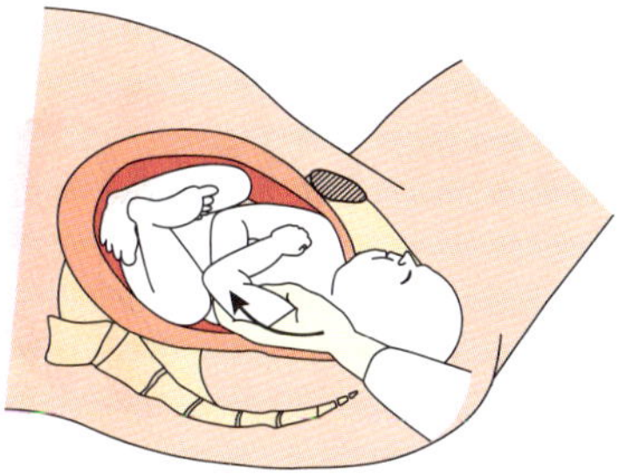

Figure 3.7 Wood's screw maneuver. The posterior shoulder is rotated by 180° to bring it under the pubic symphysis.

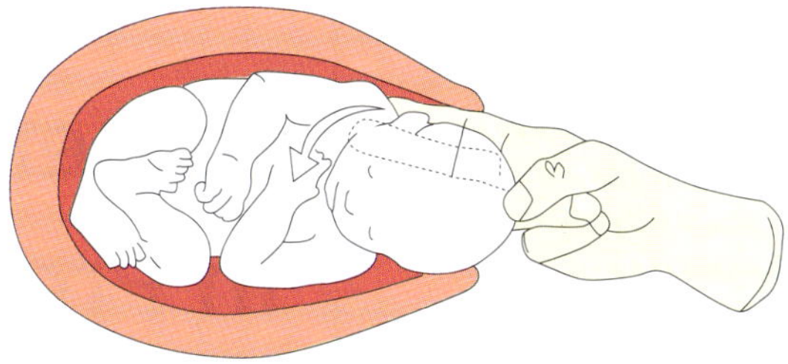

Figure 3.8 Rubin's maneuver. Fetal shoulder is pushed toward the chest to produce adduction of shoulders resulting in decrease in bisacromial diameter and delivery of the shoulders.

by 180° to get it below pubic symphysis and delivered. The opposite shoulder is now below the pelvic brim that can be hooked out after another 180° rotation (Figure 3.7).

- **Rubin's maneuver:** Hand is inserted into vagina and fetal shoulder is pushed toward the chest to produce adduction of shoulders resulting in decrease in bisacromial diameter and delivery of the shoulders (Figure 3.8).
- **Gaskin's maneuver:** The patient is placed on all four limbs to dislodge the shoulder from behind pubic symphysis.
- **Intentional fracture of clavicle:** It reduces the bisacromial diameter.
- **Zavanelli maneuver:** It includes pushing the head back into vagina and performing cesarean section.

Frequently asked viva questions

1. Summarize the case.
2. What is the diagnosis of the case?
3. What is the plan of management for the case?
4. What investigations do you want to do?
5. When do you want to terminate pregnancy?
6. What are the indications for elective LSCS in GDM?
7. What are the maternal and fetal complications of DM in pregnancy?
8. How will you induce labor?
9. How will you monitor the patient during labor?
10. What should be the treatment following delivery?
11. What contraception will you advise the patient?
12. What is the chance of recurrence of GDM in subsequent pregnancies?

4 Hypertensive Disorders in Pregnancy

Introduction

Hypertension is a common medical problem complicating pregnancy that contributes significantly to maternal and perinatal morbidity and mortality. Hypertension is a sign of some underlying pathology and it may preexist a pregnancy or appear for the first time during pregnancy. Preeclampsia (PE), a pregnancy-specific hypertension, is a standard clinical case for exams and is dealt in this chapter.

Definition of hypertensive disorders in pregnancy

Blood pressure (BP) of more than or equal to 140/90 mmHg recorded on at least two occasions 4 hours apart during pregnancy is termed hypertension during pregnancy.

> **High-yield points**
>
> **Criteria (other than BP ≥140/90 mmHg) for defining hypertension in pregnancy**
>
> - Mean arterial pressure (MAP) ≥105 mmHg
> - Rise in systolic BP (SBP) of ≥30 mmHg or diastolic BP (DBP) of ≥15 mmHg above baseline
> - Rise in MAP by 20 mmHg over baseline
>
> MAP = (SBP + 2DBP)/3 or DBP + (1/3) pulse pressure (PP)
>
> where PP = SBP − DBP. These criteria are nonspecific, but warrant close observation.

Classification of hypertensive disorders in pregnancy (Table 4.1)

This is done as per the National High BP Education Program Classification (NHBPEP, 2000) and recommended by American College of Obstetricians and Gynecologists (ACOG, 2013).

Table 4.1 Classification of hypertensive disorders in pregnancy

Type of hypertension	Characteristics
Gestational hypertension	Defined as BP of ≥140/90 mmHg during pregnancy, not associated with proteinuria, and returns to normal within 12 weeks postpartum
Preeclampsia	Characterized by the following: • BP of ≥140/90 mmHg • On at least two occasions 4 hours apart • Recorded for the first time during pregnancy after 20 weeks of gestation • Associated with proteinuria
Eclampsia	Convulsions or coma occurring in a woman with preeclampsia, not attributed to other causes, is termed eclampsia
Chronic hypertension	Preexisting hypertension before pregnancy or hypertension detected before 20 weeks
Superimposed preeclampsia	Preeclampsia superimposed on chronic hypertension. Superimposed preeclampsia complicates 25% of pregnancies in women with chronic hypertension

Note

- *Gestational hypertension (GHT) is de novo hypertension after 20 weeks' gestation in the absence of proteinuria and without biochemical or hematological abnormalities or fetal growth restriction.*
- *Outcomes in pregnancies complicated by GHT are normally good, but about 25% of women with GHT (particularly those who present at <34 weeks) will progress to preeclampsia and may have poorer outcomes.*
- *BP returns to normal within 12 weeks postpartum in patients with gestational hypertension and preeclampsia.*

Terminologies

Pregnancy-induced hypertension (PIH) It is a term used to describe any new-onset pregnancy-related hypertension. It includes gestational hypertension, preeclampsia, and eclampsia (this is an old but widely used terminology; it lacks precision and hence not preferred currently).

Proteinuria It is defined by the presence of one of the following:

- 24-Hour urine protein excretion of greater than or equal to 300 mg/day
- Spot urine protein/creatinine ratio (PCR) of greater than or equal to 0.3 (24-hour urine protein measurement has widely been replaced with a spot urine PCR, as this method eliminates the inherent difficulties in undertaking 24-hour urine collection and speeds up the process of decision making)
- Dipstick urine protein of 2+ or more (false positives and false negatives are high and should be performed only when other quantitative methods are not available or rapid decisions are required)

Early onset preeclampsia Preeclampsia usually develops in the second half of the third trimester. However, in some women, it may develop before 34 weeks of gestation, termed early onset preeclampsia, which is associated with high maternal and perinatal morbidity and mortality.

Imminent eclampsia It is the occurrence of symptoms and signs in a woman with preeclampsia which indicate that eclampsia is impending or imminent.

Eclampsia often is preceded by premonitory signs of cerebral irritation such as severe and persistent occipital or frontal headaches, visual disturbances, photophobia, right hypochondriac pain, hyperreflexia, and altered mental status. However, eclampsia can occur in the absence of warning signs or symptoms.

Currently, these symptoms and signs are classified as severe preeclampsia and the term "imminent eclampsia" is not used.

Note

Although hypertension and proteinuria are considered as classical criteria to diagnose preeclampsia, other criteria are also important. Women with gestational hypertension in the absence of proteinuria, presenting with any of the following severe features are managed in same lines as severe preeclampsia:

- *High BP (SBP ≥160 mm Hg or DBP ≥110 mm Hg)*
- *Thrombocytopenia (platelet count less than 100,000/mm^3)*
- *Impaired liver function (abnormally elevated liver enzymes to twice the upper limit of normal)*
- *Renal insufficiency (serum creatinine ≥1.1 mg/dL or a doubling of the serum creatinine in the absence of other renal disease)*
- *New-onset headache unresponsive to medication, visual disturbances, severe persistent right upper quadrant or epigastric pain, and pulmonary edema.*

Therefore, preeclampsia can be diagnosed if there is presence of new onset hypertension after 20 weeks of gestation associated with proteinuria and/or presence of maternal renal dysfunction, liver dysfunction, neurological clinical features, thrombocytopenia, or fetal growth restriction.

Pedal edema during pregnancy

Pedal edema is present in 85% of cases of preeclampsia. However, it is also present in 50% of normal pregnancies. Hence, it is not included in the diagnostic criteria for preeclampsia.

Causes of pedal edema during pregnancy

Bilateral pedal edema

Physiological edema It is seen in 50% of normal pregnancies.

Viva corner

Q1 What are the conditions in which preeclampsia can develop before 20 weeks of gestation?

- Molar pregnancy
- Multiple pregnancy
- Hydrops fetalis

Q2 Why does physiological edema occur during pregnancy?

- The increase in femoral venous pressure due to pressure on the inferior vena cava by gravid uterus leads to pedal edema.
- Decrease in albumin levels during pregnancy by 30% leads to reduction in colloid oncotic pressure and can result in edema.

Q3 How is physiological pedal edema differentiated from pathological pedal edema?

See table below

Table Clinical differences between physiological and pathological pedal edema

Physiological edema	Pathological edema
Usually develops in the third trimester	Can develop anytime during pregnancy
Dependent edema—only in the legs	Can be nondependent edema—face, hands, abdomen, vulva, etc.
Subsides after rest for 12 hours	Does not subside after rest
Not associated with increased BP recordings	May be associated with raised BP recordings in preeclampsia

Pathological edema

- Preeclampsia
- Anemia
- Hypoproteinemia
- Renal causes (renal failure, glomerulonephritis, etc.)
- Cardiac causes—congestive cardiac failure
- Hypothyroidism (causes bilateral non pitting pedal edema)

Unilateral pedal edema

- Cellulitis
- Filariasis
- Deep vein thrombosis

Proteinuria in pregnancy

- Preeclampsia is hypertension in pregnancy associated with proteinuria while gestational hypertension is hypertension in pregnancy without associated proteinuria.
- Causes of proteinuria during pregnancy
  - Preeclampsia
  - Urinary tract infection (UTI)
  - Pyelonephritis
  - Renal diseases
  - Diabetic nephropathy
  - Contamination of urine
- Gestational proteinuria

PREECLAMPSIA

Incidence

It is 5–10%.

Risk factors for preeclampsia

- Primigravida (incidence is 10% in primigravida, 5% in multigravida)
- Maternal age of <20 and >35 years
- Obesity (Prepregnancy BMI >30)
- Maternal medical diseases
  - Preexisting chronic hypertension
  - Preexisting renal or vascular diseases
  - Gestational diabetes
- Antiphospholipid antibodies (APLA) syndrome, systemic lupus erythematosus
- Thrombophilias—protein C and S deficiency, and factor V Leiden deficiency
- Obstetric problems
  - Molar pregnancy
  - Multiple pregnancy
  - Rh incompatibility (hydrops fetalis)
- Assisted reproductive technology
- H/o preeclampsia in previous pregnancy
- Family history of hypertension
- Genetic and immunological factors

Clinical features

Preeclampsia is a syndrome of more signs than symptoms.

Symptoms

- Excessive weight gain
- Swelling of feet, not relieved by rest
- Nondependent edema such as swelling of hands, abdominal wall, face, and vulva
- Headache (frontal headache not relieved by analgesics)

- Visual disturbances such as blurring of vision, dimness, flashing of lights, and sudden loss of vision in both eyes
- Epigastric or right upper quadrant pain
- Decreased urine output

Signs

- BP recording of ≥140/90 mmHg on at least two occasions 4 hours apart
- Sudden or excessive weight gain (weight gain of more than 0.5 kg in a week or 2 kg in a month)
- Edema—pedal edema (Figure 4.1) and nondependent edema of abdomen, face, hands, vulva, etc.
- Tenderness in right upper quadrant of the abdomen
- Maternal ascites may be present in cases with severe preeclampsia
- Brisk deep tendon reflexes; knee jerks are usually checked for (Figure 4.2)
- Possibility of fundal height being less than period of gestation (POG) [preeclampsia is associated with an increased risk of intrauterine growth restriction (IUGR) and oligohydramnios]

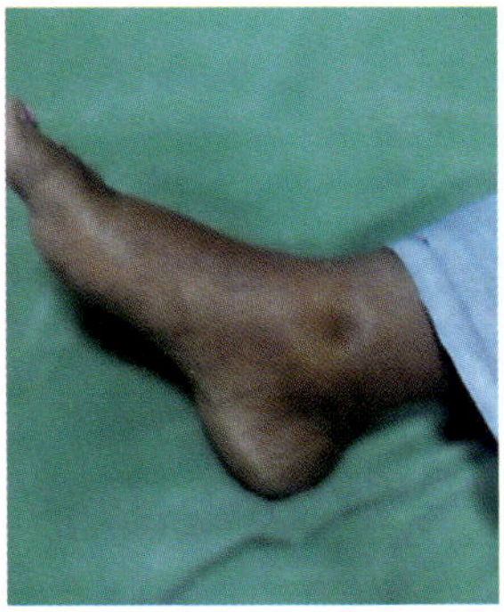

Figure 4.1 Pitting pedal edema.

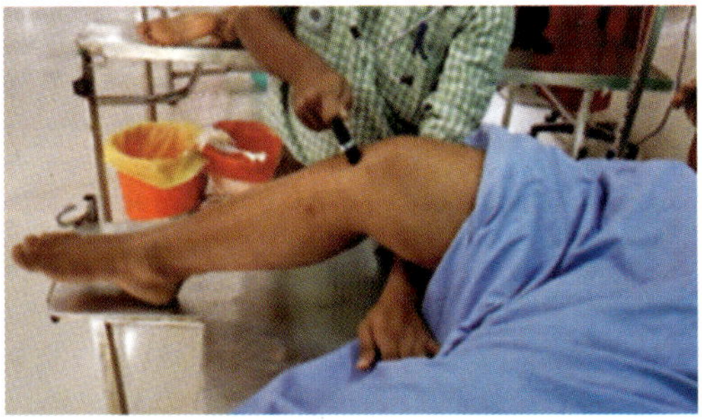

Figure 4.2 Demonstration of knee jerk.

High-yield points

Pathogenesis in preeclampsia

The main cause for preeclampsia is defective second wave of trophoblastic invasion of myometrial spiral arterioles that normally occurs between 16 and 18 weeks of gestation (see figure below).

Defective trophoblastic invasion → increase in resistance to placental blood flow → placental ischemia and hypoxia resulting in release of inflammatory mediators and cytokines from placenta → endothelial damage and generalized vasospasm.

Vasospasm leads to hypertension and endothelial damage leads to leakage of fluid into third space, platelet aggregation, and activation of coagulation system. Thus, the pathophysiology and organ damage in preeclampsia mainly involve vasospasm and endothelial dysfunction (see tables below).

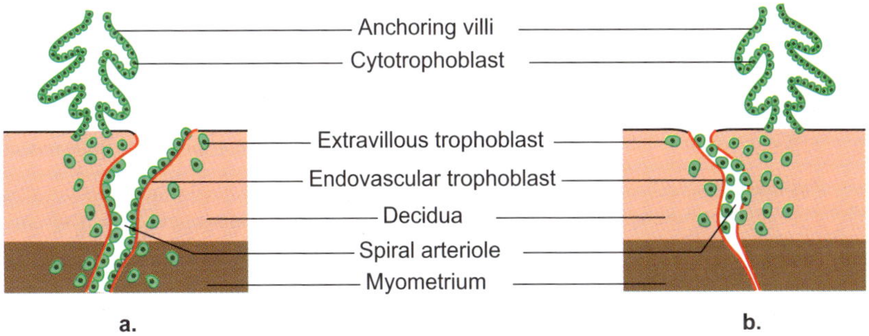

Figure Defective second wave of trophoblastic invasion—main pathogenesis in preeclampsia. **a.** Trophoblastic invasion of myometrial spiral arterioles in normal pregnancy. **b.** Defective trophoblastic invasion of myometrial spiral arterioles in preeclampsia.

(CONTD...)

(...CONTD)

High-yield points

Table Pathophysiology of various symptoms and signs in preeclampsia

Symptoms/signs	Pathophysiology (cause)
Hypertension	Generalized vasospasm
Proteinuria	Renal endothelial damage
Edema	Capillary endothelial damage → capillary leak → edema
Right upper quadrant pain	Subcapsular hemorrhage causing stretching of Glisson's capsule of liver
Pulmonary edema	Capillary leak in lungs
Headache, convulsions	Cerebral edema
Blurring of vision (reversible blindness)	Occipital lobe edema, retinal edema, and retinal artery spasm
Thrombocytopenia	Endothelial damage results in excess thrombin activity and increased consumption of platelets (platelet aggregation and activation)
Intrauterine growth restriction	Increased resistance in uteroplacental circulation

Table Specific organ damage in preeclampsia

Organ	Damage caused due to preeclampsia
Blood vessels	Vasospasm
Kidney	Glomerular endotheliosis
Liver	Periportal hemorrhagic necrosis, subcapsular hemorrhage
Lungs	Pulmonary edema
Heart	Subendothelial hemorrhages and focal necrosis
Brain	Cerebral hemorrhage, edema
Hematology	Hemoconcentration, thrombocytopenia, disseminated intravascular coagulation

Classification of preeclampsia

Preeclampsia is classified as "preeclampsia without severe features" and "severe preeclampsia based on the risk of morbidity and mortality." The term "mild" preeclampsia which was used earlier has been replaced by "preeclampsia without severe features" in current practice (Table 4.2).

Table 4.2 Features of nonsevere and severe preeclampsia

	"Preeclampsia without severe features" (previously termed as "mild preeclampsia")	Severe preeclampsia
BP	≥140/90 mmHg but <160/110 mmHg	SBP ≥160 and/or DBP ≥110 mmHg
Platelet count	Normal	Thrombocytopenia (platelet count ≤100,000/mm^3)
Liver function tests	Normal	Impaired liver function (elevated blood liver enzymes AST and ALT to more than twice the upper limit of normal concentrations)
Renal function test	Normal	Renal insufficiency (serum creatinine ≥1.1 mg/dL or a doubling of the serum creatinine)
Symptoms suggestive of severe eclampsia	Absent	• New-onset headache unresponsive to medication • Visual disturbances • Pulmonary edema • Severe persistent right upper quadrant or epigastric pain unresponsive to medications

ALT, alanine aminotransferase; *AST*, aspartate aminotransferase; *IUGR*, intrauterine growth restriction; *SBP*, systolic blood pressure.

Changes made by ACOG (2013) in preeclampsia classification

According to ACOG (2013), the following changes have been made in the classification of preeclampsia:

- The term "mild preeclampsia" is now replaced by the term "nonsevere preeclampsia" or "preeclampsia without severe features" (as the usage of the term "mild" can be misleading, as morbidity and mortality can be increased even in the absence of severe features of preeclampsia).
- Proteinuria of >5 g/24 hours (>2 + on dipstick) has been excluded now in the classification. Following the initial documentation of proteinuria and the establishment of the diagnosis of preeclampsia, additional quantifications of proteinuria are no longer necessary. Although the amount of proteinuria is expected to increase over time with expectant management, this change is not predictive of perinatal outcome and should not influence the management of preeclampsia.
- Serum creatinine of ≥1.1 mg/dL or a doubling of serum creatinine, in the absence of preexisting renal disease, is used as a sign of renal involvement, instead of oliguria that was used earlier.
- Fetal growth restriction has been excluded in the classification, since management of growth restriction does not depend on the severity of preeclampsia.

Case presentation

Salient points in history

Consider the following relevant points during history taking in cases of hypertensive disorders in pregnancy.

Patient details

- ***Age:*** *Preeclampsia is more common in teenage pregnancy and advanced maternal age.*
- ***Parity:*** *Primigravida are at an increased risk for preeclampsia.*

Presenting complaints

- *Swelling of feet*
  - *Onset*
  - *Duration*
  - *Whether relieved by rest or not*
- *Swelling of other nondependent parts such as face, abdominal wall, vulva, or whole body (anasarca)*
- *H/o headache, visual disturbances such as blurring of vision, epigastric pain (imminent symptoms), and decreased urine output*
- *If the patient is already diagnosed to have new-onset hypertension during pregnancy, ask the following:*
  - *What was the POG at which the new-onset hypertension was detected [whether hypertension was detected before or after 20 weeks is crucial in differentiating chronic hypertension from preeclampsia/gestational hypertension (GHT)]?*
  - *Is the patient on any antihypertensive drug?*
  - *Has she been admitted earlier?*
- *Is the patient perceiving normal fetal movements (decreased fetal movements may indicate fetal hypoxia due to uteroplacental insufficiency)?*
- *If swelling of feet is the only complaint, history suggestive of other causes of swelling of feet such as anemia and cardiac disease should be asked.*

H/o present pregnancy

- *Whether it is a spontaneous conception (preeclampsia is more common in IVF pregnancies using donor sperm or ovum)*
- *H/o increased BP recording during previous antenatal visits*
- *History suggestive of preeclampsia such as excessive weight gain, swelling of feet, headache, blurring of vision, epigastric pain, or reduced urine output in the second and third trimesters*
- *Whether ultrasonography (USG) has been done and said to be normal (multiple pregnancy can be associated with preeclampsia; IUGR is a complication of preeclampsia)*

Past obstetric history (in a multigravida)

- *Whether the patient was booked and immunized*

(CONTD...)

(...CONTD)

- *Antenatal period—any significant history such as preeclampsia, gestational diabetes mellitus (GDM), antepartum hemorrhage (APH), or any other complications*

If the patient has H/o hypertension in previous pregnancy, ask the following:

- *At what POG was the hypertension diagnosed?*
- *Was the patient on antihypertensive drugs?*
- *Was labor induced? If so, at what POG?*
- *Was there any H/o convulsions (eclampsia)? If yes, ask details of the following:*
  - *Number of episodes of convulsions*
  - *How long each episode of convulsion lasted*
  - *H/o regaining consciousness in between convulsions*
  - *Time period between last convulsion and delivery*
- *Was there any H/o complications such as APH, coagulopathy, and renal failure?*

Labor details

- *H/o induction of labor [if yes, POG at induction (mild preeclampsia, induction is done at 37 completed weeks; severe preeclampsia, induction is done at 34 completed weeks)]*
- *Duration of labor*
- *Any intrapartum complications such as eclampsia*
- *Mode of delivery*
  - *Spontaneous vaginal delivery*
  - *Forceps/vacuum (indication)*
  - *Cesarean section (CS)—elective/emergency and indication (ask all other details as mentioned in a case of previous CS pregnancy in Part 1, Chapter 6, Postcesarean Pregnancy)*
- *H/o postpartum hemorrhage (PPH) and blood transfusion (patients with preeclampsia have intravascular volume depletion and hence cannot tolerate blood loss)*
- *Birth weight of baby (IUGR is one of the fetal complications of preeclampsia)*
- *Whether the baby cried immediately after birth, and any need for NICU admission*
- *When was breastfeeding initiated following delivery?*
- *Duration of stay in hospital (patients with preeclampsia are discharged following control of BP)*

Puerperium

- *How long was the BP elevated? How long was the patient on antihypertensive therapy? (BP returns to normal within 12 weeks postpartum in patients with gestational hypertension and preeclampsia.)*
- *Ask about H/o contraception in between pregnancies.*

Significant past history

H/o chronic hypertension, DM, and renal disease (patient may be a case of chronic hypertension or superimposed preeclampsia)

Significant family history

- *F/H/o hypertension (hypertension may run in families)*
- *H/o preeclampsia in mother or siblings (risk is 20–25%)*

Salient points in examination

Consider the following relevant points during examination in cases of hypertensive disorders in pregnancy.

General examination

- *Built and nourishment*
- *Height, weight, and BMI*
  - *Significance of weight charting in preeclampsia—obese women are at an increased risk of preeclampsia than those with normal BMI; excessive weight gain indicated by weight gain of >0.5/week or >2 kg in a month is one of the premonitory signs of preeclampsia*
- *Pallor*
- *Icterus*
- *Pedal edema, edema of hands, orbit and face*

Vitals

- *Temperature*
- *Pulse rate*
- *BP ___ mmHg measured in right upper limb in sitting position/left lateral position*
- *Respiratory rate*

(CONTD...)

Part 1

(...CONTD)

Note *BP should be recorded after a period of rest of 10 minutes, no caffiene intake in past half an hour, with back support in sitting position, foot support and arm resting on a table.*

Cardiovascular and respiratory system examination *Pulmonary edema is one of the complications of preeclampsia.*

Central nervous system *Deep tendon reflexes may be exaggerated in imminent eclampsia (knee jerks are checked).*

Grading of deep tendon reflexes *See Table 4.3*

Table 4.3 Grading of deep tendon reflexes

Grade	Interpretation
0	Absent
1+	Diminished/low normal
2+	Average/normal
3+	Brisker than average
4+	Very brisk/hyperactive with clonus

Brisk deep tendon reflex results from central nervous system irritability.

Abdomen *Look for abdominal wall edema and ascites.*

Obstetric examination *Check if the fundal height corresponds to the POG. Fundal height more than POG may suggest conditions such as twins, hydramnios, or molar pregnancy that can be associated with hypertension in pregnancy. Fundal height less than POG is suggestive of IUGR or oligohydramnios that may develop as a complication of hypertension in pregnancy.*

External genitalia *Look for vulvar edema.*

Case summary

An example of writing summary in cases of hypertensive disorders in pregnancy is given below.

Example *Mrs. V, 24 years of age, a primigravida at 34 weeks of gestation, admitted with complaints of swelling of feet for the past 2 weeks, not relieved with rest. She is perceiving normal fetal movements. There is no H/o imminent symptoms. On general physical examination, there is no pallor and B/L pitting pedal edema is present. Her BP is 140/100 mmHg. Her cardiovascular and respiratory systems are normal. Obstetric examination reveals uterus corresponding to 32 weeks of gestation with a singleton live fetus in cephalic presentation. Liquor appears average and uterus is relaxed. On auscultation, FHR is 140 beats/min, regular, and heard on the left spinoumbilical line.*

Case diagnosis

An example of writing the diagnosis in cases of hypertensive disorders in pregnancy is given below.

Example *24 years of age, primigravida at 34 weeks of gestation with new-onset hypertension complicating pregnancy, with a singleton live fetus in cephalic presentation and not in labor, admitted for further evaluation and management (the diagnosis in this case can be either gestational hypertension or preeclampsia that can be confirmed only by checking for urine proteins)*

Case discussion

Diagnosis of hypertensive disorders in pregnancy

- Hypertensive disorders in pregnancy are clinical diagnosis that are made by recording of elevated BP of ≥140/90 mmHg, confirmed by repeat examination of BP after 4 hours. However, if BP recordings are ≥160/100 mmHg, it has to be rechecked in 15 minutes, to avoid undue delay in initiating treatment.
- Once hypertension in pregnancy is detected, the next step is to determine if it is gestational hypertension or preeclampsia. Urinalysis for proteinuria is the first step in evaluation.
  - If proteinuria is absent, it is gestational hypertension.
  - If proteinuria is present, it is preeclampsia.

The next step is to assess the severity of the disease.

Investigations

Investigations are done:

- To assess the severity of the disease in the mother
- To assess fetal condition

Maternal evaluation

In addition to routine antenatal investigations, investigations specific for preeclampsia are the following:

- Hb%
- Packed cell volume (PCV) and hematocrit
- Platelet count
- Peripheral smear for schistocytes
- Urine analysis—proteins, sugar, and microscopy
  - Proteins—preeclampsia is confirmed if elevated BP is associated with proteinuria
  - Microscopy—for granular casts/RBC casts—suggestive of underlying renal disease
- 24-Hour urinary proteins or spot urine protein/creatinine ratio (PCR)
- Blood urea and serum creatinine
- Serum uric acid
- Liver enzymes [alanine aminotransferase (ALT), aspartate aminotransferase (AST), lactate dehydrogenase (LDH)] and serum bilirubin
- Serum total proteins and serum albumin (may be decreased due to proteinuria)
- Fundus examination—to look for hypertensive retinopathy changes
- Bleeding time and clotting time
- Prothrombin time and activated partial thromboplastin time (aPTT)
- Serum fibrinogen and fibrin degradation products (FDPs)—in suspected disseminated intravascular coagulation (DIC) such as in abruption and intrauterine death (IUD)

Significance of the various investigations is mentioned in Table 4.4.

Table 4.4 Significance of various investigations in preeclampsia

Investigation	Significance
Packed cell volume and hematocrit	• Hematocrit is increased in preeclampsia due to hemoconcentration
Peripheral smear	• Microangiopathic hemolytic anemia may be present in preeclampsia • Schistocytes may be seen in peripheral smear due to hemolysis • To assess the number of platelets (<4 platelets/high-power field in peripheral smear indicates thrombocytopenia)
Platelet count	• Thrombocytopenia may be present in preeclampsia due to vasospasm-induced microangiopathic hemolysis. Endothelial damage leads to excess thrombin activity and increased intravascular consumption of platelets • Thrombocytopenia—platelet count of <1.5 lakh/mm^3 • Thrombocytopenia is a component of HELLP syndrome
Urine examination	• Urine proteins: To diagnose preeclampsia *(Proteinuria in preeclampsia is nonselective, as a result of increased tubular permeability to most large molecular-weight proteins (albumin, globulin, transferrin)* • Urine microscopy: To evaluate for renal diseases
Liver function test	• Elevated liver enzymes indicate ischemic injury to hepatocytes • AST is the dominant transaminase released into the peripheral circulation in liver dysfunction due to preeclampsia and is related to periportal necrosis • Elevated LDH indicates hepatic dysfunction (LDH derived from ischemic or necrotic tissues) and hemolysis (LDH from red blood cell destruction) • Elevated bilirubin indicates excessive hemolysis (in advanced stages) • Hemolysis and elevated liver enzymes are seen in HELLP syndrome • Alterations in hepatic synthetic function, as reflected by abnormalities of PT, aPTT, and fibrinogen, usually develop in advanced preeclampsia. Evaluation of these coagulation parameters is required when the platelet count is <150,000/mm^3, or in the presence of significant liver dysfunction, or in suspected placental abruption
Uric acid estimation	• Uric acid may be elevated in preeclampsia due to vasospasm-induced renal tubular dysfunction and decreased clearance • Placental ischemia may lead to increased trophoblastic turnover and production of purines • Rising levels of serum uric acid correlate directly with fetal morbidity

(CONTD...)

Table 4.4 *(CONTD...)*

Investigation	Significance
Fundus examination	• Fundus changes seen in preeclampsia are as follows: – Retinal artery spasm – Generalized narrowing of vessels – Altered arteriovenous ratio (A:V) from 2:3 to 1:2 • Retinal hemorrhage, exudates, and extensive arteriolar changes are seen in chronic hypertension • Papilledema is a rare feature in preeclampsia

HELLP, hemolysis, elevated liver enzymes, low platelet count; *LDH*, lactate dehydrogenase.

Fetal evaluation

Obstetric USG

- To assess fetal growth (to look for IUGR)
- To assess fetal weight
- To assess amount of liquor

Nonstress test (NST) and biophysical profile (BPP) These are done to assess fetal well-being.

Doppler studies Doppler studies of the umbilical artery, middle cerebral artery, cerebro placental ratio (CPR), and venous Doppler are done in suspected IUGR cases.

Frequency of repeating the investigations

Investigations that need to be repeated to assess the progression of disease are the following:

- PCV, platelets, peripheral smear, RFT, and liver function test (LFT)—repeated every week or every fortnight depending on the severity of the disease
- USG for fetal growth and liquor every 2 weeks
- BPP and NST weekly or twice weekly depending on the fetal condition

Extra edge

Methods for urine protein estimation

Semiquantitative method for urine protein estimation

Dipstick urine protein test (see figure below)

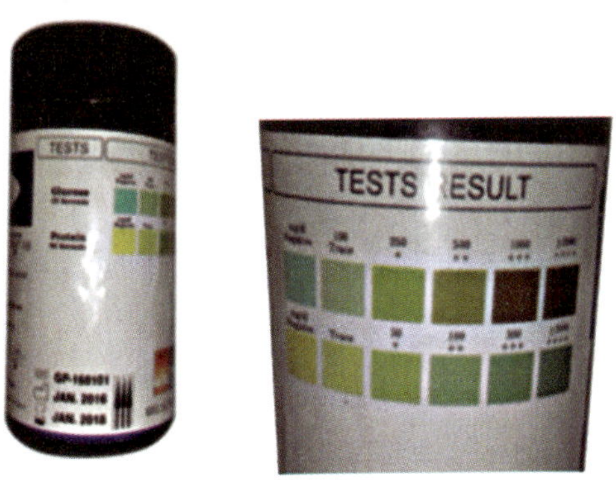

a. b.

Figure Dipstick for urine proteins. **a.** Urine protein dipstick container. **b.** Color coding marked on the container indicating the amount of proteins in urine.

- Dipstick has a stiff absorbent cellulose impregnated with tetrabromophenol blue indicator and salicylate buffer at one end.
- If urine protein is present, color changes from light yellow to blue.
- Reports are read with color coding comparator provided.
- Reports are interpreted as given in the table below.

Table Interpretation of dipstick for urine proteins

Dipstick interpretation	Urine proteins (g/L)
Trace	0.1
1+	0.3
2+	1
3+	3
4+	10

(CONTD...)

(...CONTD)

Extra edge

Note *Dipstick test is used as a screening test for initial evaluation. If dipstick urine protein is ≥ 1+, a spot urine protein/creatinine ratio or 24-hour urinary protein may be performed.*

Advantages

- Cheap and quick method to estimate urine proteins

Disadvantages

- Variations in protein excretion may be missed
- False-positive and false-negative results are high
- There is a high observer-dependent variation

Heat and acetic acid test

- Take 5–10 mL of urine in a test tube and heat the upper portion over a flame (see figure below).

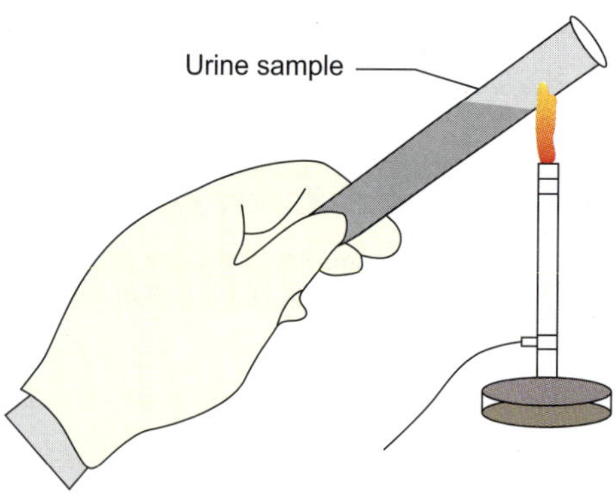

Figure Heat coagulation test.

- If turbidity develops, add one to two drops of 3% glacial acetic acid.
  - If acetic acid clears up the turbidity, then turbidity is due to phosphates or carbonates.
  - If turbidity does not disappear, then turbidity is due to proteins.

Turbidity is graded against a dark background and interpreted as given in the table below.

Table **Grading of turbidity in heat and acetic acid test**

Grading	Turbidity
Negative	No cloudiness
Trace	Barely visible cloudiness
1+	Dense cloudiness
2+	Cloudiness with granules and definite flocculation
3+	Cloudiness with flocculation
4+	Cloudiness with precipitation

The turbidity can be interpreted easily when placed against a background containing letters in black like a newspaper (see figure below).

Quantitative tests for urine protein estimation

24-Hour urine protein estimation

- It is done on 24-hour urine collection to detect the exact amount of protein excretion using the Esbach's method.
- There is no need for frequent quantification of proteinuria as it will not alter the management.

Disadvantages

- Patient inconvenience (urine voided over 24 hours has to be collected)
- Cumbersome procedure
- Expensive

Spot urine protein/creatinine ratio

This ratio cancels the time factor in expression of protein and creatinine excretion and allows for 24-hour urine protein estimation.

Advantages

- More reliable than spot urine protein
- Easier than 24-hour urine protein estimation

(CONTD...)

(...CONTD)

Extra edge

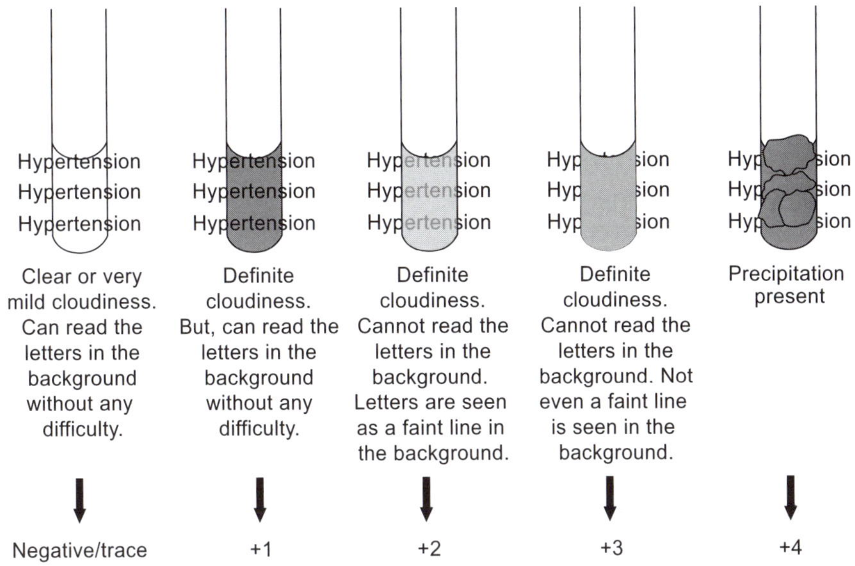

Figure Interpretation of heat coagulation test for urine proteins. A heat coagulation test is performed and then the test tube is placed in front of a background that contains letters in black such as a newspaper. Compare what you see with the given figure.

Complications of preeclampsia

Complications are minimal with GHT; preeclampsia is associated with increased maternal and perinatal morbidity and mortality (Table 4.5).

Table 4.5 Maternal and fetal complications in preeclampsia

Maternal complications			Fetal complications
Antenatal (Hint: *Remember complications in CNS, eyes, lungs, heart, liver, kidneys, uterus, hematology)*	**Intrapartum**	**Postpartum**	
• Eclampsia • Cerebral hemorrhage • Eye—cortical blindness • Pulmonary edema • Left ventricular failure • Rupture of liver due to hematoma • HELLP syndrome • Acute renal failure • Antepartum hemorrhage (abruption) • Disseminated intravascular coagulation • Preterm labor (mostly iatrogenic) • Posterior reversible encephalopathy syndrome (PRES syndrome)	• Eclampsia • Postpartum hemorrhage	• Eclampsia • Shock • Late complications – Recurrent preeclampsia in subsequent pregnancies (25%) – Chronic hypertension in future—40% risk, especially in women with familial or personal predisposition	• Intrauterine growth restriction • Intrauterine death • Prematurity • Birth asphyxia

HELLP, hemolysis, elevated liver enzymes, low platelet count.

Viva corner

Q1 What is the cause for hemoconcentration and its significance in preeclampsia?

Reasons for hemoconcentration in preeclampsia are as follows:

- Blood volume expansion that occurs during normal pregnancy is less in preeclampsia.
- Endothelial damage leads to increased capillary permeability that results in leakage of fluid from intravascular compartment to extravascular compartment (interstitial or third space compartment leak).
- Preeclampsia is thus a state of volume contraction with intravascular volume depletion.

Significance of hemoconcentration

Patients with preeclampsia have intravascular volume depletion and hence cannot tolerate blood loss and are at a risk of hemorrhagic shock. At the same time, the patient cannot be overloaded with intravenous (IV) fluids as it can lead to pulmonary edema and congestive cardiac failure due to extravasation of fluid into interstitial space.

Management of preeclampsia

Objectives in management of preeclampsia

- Prevention of eclampsia
- Early identification of worsening of the disease by close monitoring
- Appropriate timing and mode of delivery with least possible adverse effects of the disease on the mother and fetus
- Restoration of the health of the mother following delivery

Antenatal management

- The patient is admitted to assess the severity of the disease.
- All investigations for preeclampsia (as mentioned earlier) are done.
- BP charting is done every 4 hours except during night (10 pm to 6 am).
- High-protein diet is advised.
- Restriction of physical activity and rest in left lateral position are advised (increases placental and renal perfusion).
- Watch for imminent symptoms such as headache, visual disturbances, epigastric pain, and decreased urine output.
- Iron and calcium supplementation should be continued.
- Antihypertensives are usually started if diastolic BP (DBP) is ≥100 mmHg and/or systolic BP is >150 mmHg on two or more occasions. However, sudden or drastic fall in BP should be avoided, as it can affect the already compromised uteroplacental circulation.
- Daily urine output charting is maintained.
- Weekly maternal weight gain charting is maintained.
- Fetal well-being is assessed by:
  - Daily fetal movement count (DFMC)
  - Daily clinical examination—fundal height and FHR
  - USG for assessment of fetal growth and liquor done every 2 weeks
  - BPP and Doppler studies done once a week

Definitive treatment of preeclampsia is termination of pregnancy. Hence, further management depends on the following:

- Severity of preeclampsia
- POG
- Maternal and fetal condition

Management of nonsevere (earlier termed "mild") preeclampsia

Gestational hypertension Delivery can be delayed until 39+6 weeks provided BP can be controlled, fetal monitoring is reassuring, and preeclampsia has not developed *(ACOG recommends delivery at 37 completed weeks in both GHT and preeclampsia without severe features).*

Preeclampsia without severe features at or after 37 weeks Delivery rather than expectant management is recommended. Pregnancy is terminated by induction of labor after confirming the dates.

Preeclampsia without severe features at POG <37 weeks Following admission and initial evaluation, the patient can be discharged and managed on OPD basis if:

- BP is under control (DBP <100 mmHg) and investigations are normal.
- The patient understands the seriousness of the problem and is compliant for regular follow-up.
- The patient has facility for daily blood pressure measurement.
- The patient can reach the hospital quickly in case of emergency.

Advice on management at home (management on OPD basis)

- The patient is advised adequate bed rest of at least 2 hours in afternoon and 8 hours in night.
- Advise on a high-protein diet.
- There is no need of salt restriction in preeclampsia unlike chronic hypertension.
- Antihypertensives are not required if DBP is <100 mmHg.
- BP is recorded daily at home or in a local hospital and the patient should report immediately if DBP is ≥100 mmHg.
- The patient is advised to keep a DFMC.
- Warn the patient of ominous signs such as imminent symptoms, decreased urine output, and bleeding P/V, pain abdomen, reduced fetal movements, and to report immediately to the hospital.
- The patient is advised to attend antenatal clinic every week. The following are assessed: review of home BP charting, urine protein estimation, maternal weight, BP, and fetal movement count and fetal growth charting (fundal height, SFH).
- Monitor for disease progression and fetal wellbeing by doing periodic investigations.
- Pregnancy is terminated at 37 completed weeks.

Viva corner

Q1 Why is pregnancy terminated at 37 completed weeks in mild preeclampsia?

In preeclampsia, maternal and perinatal morbidity increases as pregnancy advances. There is no maternal or fetal benefit in continuing the pregnancy beyond term, as preeclampsia is a progressive disease that gets cured only with termination of pregnancy.

Management of severe preeclampsia

If the patient is diagnosed to have severe preeclampsia at the initial assessment or mild preeclampsia progresses to severe preeclampsia, then the following measures are taken:

- Patient is admitted
- **Evaluation of maternal and fetal condition is done:** This consists of investigations to look for multiorgan involvement in the mother (urine proteins, peripheral smear for schistocytes, liver enzymes AST, ALT, LDH, platelet count, and serum creatinine) and evaluation of fetal status by doing an USG and NST.
- **Immediate management:** It includes antihypertensives, seizure prophylaxis, and steroids for fetal lung maturity.
  - *Antihypertensives:* Antihypertensives are started to reduce the SBP to 140–150 mmHg and DBP to 90–100 mmHg. Antihypertensives of choice are nifedipine and labetalol.
  - *Seizure prophylaxis:* Magnesium sulfate regimen is administered for prevention of convulsions.
  - *Corticosteroids:* Betamethasone or Dexamethasone is administered to accelerate fetal lung maturity if gestational age is <34 weeks.
  - Magnesium sulphate for neuroprotection of fetus can be given, if pregnancy is likely to be terminated prior to 32 weeks of gestation.
- **Subsequent management:** Further management depends on the following:
  - POG
  - Maternal and fetal evaluation

POG ≥34 weeks Delivery is recommended when preeclampsia with severe features is diagnosed at or beyond 34 weeks of gestation, after maternal stabilization (The clinical course of preeclampsia with severe features is characterized by progressive deterioration of maternal and fetal condition. At POG ≥ 34 weeks, prognosis for fetal survival is good and further waiting will jeopardize the mother and fetal condition. Hence, immediate delivery is recommended).

Note *In developed countries, the POG cutoff for viability is 24 weeks. In developing countries, perinatal survival is poor at <28 weeks; hence, the institutional cutoff of 28 weeks may be used as a limit of viability.*

POG 24–34 weeks

- Maternal and fetal conditions are evaluated.
- If features of preeclampsia are under control (i.e., BP is under control, investigations are normal, and fetal condition is stable):
  - Continue the pregnancy up to 34 weeks.
  - Maternal and fetal statuses are assessed periodically.
  - Give steroids for fetal lung maturity.
  - Terminate pregnancy at 34 completed weeks of gestation.

Part 1

- If BP is not under control despite antihypertensive therapy or if features of severe preeclampsia aggravate, terminate the pregnancy irrespective of gestational age. Consent for termination of pregnancy to save maternal life has to be taken in written from the patient and responsible attender.

POG <24 weeks (lower limit of 28 weeks may be considered in developing countries) Both maternal and perinatal outcomes are poor in previable severe preeclampsia and waiting will jeopardize the maternal condition. Hence, severe preeclampsia is best managed by termination of pregnancy after counseling the couple.

High-yield points

Expectant management in preeclampsia

- Aim: To prolong pregnancy and improve fetal survival, thereby avoiding prematurity and its complications.
- Expectant management is not beneficial to the mother as the disease is a progressive condition that stops only on termination of pregnancy.
- Indications: Expectant management can be given in gestational hypertension and preeclampsia without severe features up to 37 weeks and in severe preeclampsia up to 34 completed weeks, after which the pregnancy is terminated.
- Expectant management includes the following:
  - Management in a tertiary care center
  - Close monitoring of maternal and fetal conditions for severity and progression of the disease
  - Use of antihypertensives
  - Corticosteroids for fetal lung maturity
- Indications for termination of pregnancy during expectant management are
  - At 37 completed weeks in mild preeclampsia
  - At 34 completed weeks in severe preeclampsia
  - Worsening of maternal or fetal conditions or development of maternal complications is an indication for immediate delivery

Indications for admission in preeclampsia irrespective of gestational age

- DBP ≥100 mmHg
- Presence of imminent symptoms
- Features of severe preeclampsia/eclampsia
- Fetal compromise

Indications for termination of pregnancy in preeclampsia

- At 37 completed weeks in nonsevere preeclampsia
- At 34 completed weeks in severe preeclampsia.
- In severe preeclampsia at <24 weeks
- Uncontrolled hypertension (if BP is not under control with ≥2 classes of antihypertensives in appropriate doses)
- Imminent eclampsia
- Eclampsia
- Increasing organ dysfunction such as thrombocytopenia, abnormal LFT, and serum creatinine >1.1 mg/dL

Viva corner

Q1 How does bed rest help a woman with preeclampsia?

- Bed rest improves glomerular filtration rate (GFR) and urine output.
- It improves venous return and decreases edema.
- It increases uteroplacental blood flow.
- It decreases BP.

Q2 Why is a high-protein diet advised?

Proteins are lost in urine and into the interstitial space due to endothelial damage leading to hypoproteinemia in preeclampsia. Hence, a high-protein diet is advised.

Q3 Why is a sudden drastic fall in BP avoided?

Sudden fall in BP can compromise the uteroplacental blood flow, which is already in a compromised state and hence can lead to intrauterine death. Hence, the purpose of antihypertensives is to reduce the BP to a level that will reduce maternal complications such as severe hypertension, abruption, and multiorgan involvement without reducing placental perfusion.

Q4 When are antihypertensives started in preeclampsia?

- Patients with persistent DBP ≥100 mmHg are started on antihypertensives. Rise in DBP above 100 mmHg increases the risk of eclampsia. A drastic fall in BP can compromise uteroplacental blood flow.
- Antihypertensives will not alter the course of disease. The main purpose of antihypertensives is to prevent complications such as severe hypertension, multiorgan dysfunction, abruption, and IUD.

- If the patient develops complications of preeclampsia such as pulmonary edema, hemolysis, elevated liver enzymes, low platelet count (HELLP) syndrome, abruption, and DIC
- Nonreassuring fetal heart tracing in NST/abnormal BPP/abnormal Doppler studies
- Severe IUGR

Mode of termination

Induction of labor is done based on the Bishop's score:

- Oxytocin and/or artificial rupture of membranes (ARM), if cervix is favorable
- PGE2, if cervix is unfavorable

Indications for elective lower-segment cesarean section (LSCS) in preeclampsia Elective LSCS is done only for obstetric indications such as contracted pelvis, cephalopelvic disproportion (CPD), major degree placenta previa, malpresentations, bad obstetric history (BOH), and severe IUGR.

Note *Preeclampsia as such is not an indication for LSCS.*

Management during labor

I stage

- No ambulation is allowed; the patient is shifted to labor room for monitoring.
- Intravenous (IV) line is secured, and blood sent for crossmatching and reservation.
- Maintain hydration with oral fluids. Restrict IV fluids as there is risk of fluid overload and pulmonary edema (restricted to ≤75 mL/h).
- Provide adequate analgesia.
- Maintain partogram to monitor maternal and fetal conditions and progress of labor.
- Antihypertensives are given when DBP is ≥100 mmHg. Tab. nifedipine 10 mg stat dose can be given orally if DBP ≥110 mmHg.
- Prophylactic magnesium sulfate therapy for prevention of eclampsia is administered in imminent and severe preeclampsia cases.
- Intense monitoring of maternal condition is required (worsening of hypertension, convulsions, and pulmonary edema can occur during labor)
  - Pulse, BP, and urine output charting
  - BP recorded every hourly
  - Respiratory system (RS) auscultation to rule out pulmonary edema
  - Imminent symptoms watched for
- Monitor FHR by continuous electronic monitoring, if facilities are available, or by intermittent auscultation every 15 minutes in the first stage and every 5 minutes in the second stage.
- Augmentation of labor is done by oxytocin and/or ARM.

II stage Do not allow undue prolongation of the second stage. Prophylactic cut short of the second stage is done with forceps or vacuum in severe/imminent eclampsia and in eclampsia cases.

III stage

- Anticipate PPH (patients with preeclampsia are intravascular volume depleted and hence cannot tolerate blood loss).
- Active management of the third stage of labor is followed—10 units oxytocin IV/IM is given following delivery of baby, delayed cord clamping, delivery of placenta by controlled cord traction, and palpation of uterine tone (patients with preeclampsia cannot tolerate blood loss).
- Methergin is contraindicated (as it can lead to sudden increase in BP).
- Following delivery, the patient is monitored in labor room—monitor BP and watch for excessive bleeding P/V.
- Aggressive fluid therapy should be avoided as it can lead to pulmonary edema.
- Magnesium sulfate regimen is continued for 24 hours following delivery or last convulsions, whichever is later.

Postpartum management

- Monitor BP and close monitoring is required for 48–72 hours as the risk is high because of mobilization of fluid.
- The patient is discharged when BP is under control and advised on regular follow-up to monitor BP and taper the dose of antihypertensives.
- BP usually returns to normal by 12 weeks postpartum.
- If BP does not return to normal by 12 weeks postpartum, the patient is labeled as a case of chronic hypertension.

High-yield points

Antihypertensives in preeclampsia

See table below

Table Antihypertensives used in preeclampsia

Drug name	Mechanism of action	Dose	Side effects
Labetalol: First line drug of choice; safe in pregnancy	Alpha-adrenergic + beta-adrenergic blocker	• 100 mg BD oral initial dose, maximum up to 1200 mg/day • Can be used for rapid reduction of BP in hypertensive crisis: 20 mg IV bolus → 40 mg IV → 80 mg IV → 80 mg IV → 80 mg IV (response to IV bolus is checked every 10 minutes, maximum dose—300 mg)	• Maternal: Flushing, hypotension, bradycardia • Fetal: Safe; IV Labetalol can lead to fetal heart rate irregularities
Nifedipine: First line drug of choice; safe in pregnancy	Calcium channel blocker causing direct arteriolar vasodilation	• 5 mg BD up to 80 mg/day oral in divided doses • Can be used for rapid lowering of BP in hypertensive crisis: Oral nifedipine 10 mg → 20 mg, can be repeated up to a maximum dose of 90 mg, every 10–20 minutes	• Maternal: Flushing, headache, tachycardia, palpitation, hypotension
Methyldopa: Effective and safe for mother and fetus	Central and peripheral antiadrenergic action	250 mg BD oral up to 2000 mg/day, effect appears after 48 hours (hence, it is not useful in severe preeclampsia for rapid lowering of BP)	• Maternal: Postural hypotension, drowsiness, hemolytic anemia, positive Coombs' test • Fetal: Safe
Hydralazine	Peripheral arterial vasodilator, used in hypertensive emergencies	In hypertensive crisis: 5–10 mg IV every 15 minutes till desired BP is achieved (maximum dose per episode—30 mg)	• Maternal: Flushing, headache, tachycardia, palpitation, hypotension, lupus-like syndrome • Fetal: Safe, can cause fetal thrombocytopenia
Sodium nitroprusside	Direct arterial and venous vasodilation	Used in CCU for hypertensive emergencies	• Maternal: Hypotension, vomiting • Fetal: Toxicity due to cyanide and thiocyanate
Nitroglycerine	Mainly venous relaxation	Used in hypertensive crisis for short period only	• Maternal: Headache, methemoglobinemia • Nitroglycerine is contraindicated in hypertensive encephalopathy as it increases cerebral blood flow and intracranial pressure

Role of antihypertensives

Benefits

Antihypertensives reduce the risk of the following:

- Cerebrovascular accidents
- Cardiac failure
- Pulmonary edema

(CONTD...)

(...CONTD)

High-yield points

- Abruption
- Commonly used antihypertensives: Methyldopa, labetalol, and nifedipine
- First-choice antihypertensive for mild to moderate elevation in BP in pregnancy: Labetalol, Nifedipine, and alpha-methyldopa
- Hypertensive emergencies: Labetalol, hydralazine, nifedipine, sodium nitroprusside, and nitroglycerine
- Hypertensives for postpartum use
  - Calcium channel blockers such as nifedipine and amlodipine
  - Beta-blockers such as atenolol
  - Alpha- + beta-adrenergic receptor blockers such as labetalol
  - Methyldopa usually not given as it can cause depression

Target blood pressure

Target BP in severe preeclampsia is 140–150 mmHg SBP and 90–100 mmHg DBP. Lowering of BP beyond this threshold level can decrease placental perfusion and result in fetal growth restriction.

Antihypertensives contraindicated in pregnancy

- Diuretics
- Angiotensin-converting enzyme (ACE) inhibitors
- Angiotensin receptor blockers

ACE inhibitors and angiotensin receptor blockers are associated with fetal complications such as oligohydramnios, renal agenesis, pulmonary atresia, and IUGR.

Contraception

Women who have completed family are counseled for sterilization. Intrauterine contraceptive devices (IUCDs), progesterone-only pills, and injectable progesterones are safe in women with hypertensive disorders. Combined oral contraceptive pills are not prescribed during lactation and when the BP is high.

Eclampsia

- **Definition:** Convulsion occurring in a woman with preeclampsia is called eclampsia.
- **Incidence**
  - *Antepartum*: 50% (more common in the third trimester)
  - *Intrapartum*: 30%
  - *Postpartum*: 20% (usually within 48 hours after delivery)
- Convulsions occurring beyond 7 days of delivery are unlikely due to eclampsia.

Note *Eclampsia can occur even without any prior documentation of either hypertension or proteinuria. Thus, the notion that preeclampsia has a natural linear progression from preeclampsia without severe features to preeclampsia with severe features and eventually to eclamptic convulsions is inaccurate.*

Status eclampticus It refers to occurrence of convulsions continuously without any seizure-free interval. Interval time is usually considered as 30 minutes. It can result in prolonged coma and death.

Intercurrent eclampsia When pregnancy is continued for at least 2 days to 2 weeks following eclampsia, it is termed intercurrent eclampsia. This is controversial as pregnancy is usually terminated within the next 24–48 hours in eclampsia due to high maternal and perinatal morbidity and mortality.

Description of convulsions in eclampsia—grand mal convulsions Typical convulsion in eclampsia last for 3–4 minutes and has four stages (Table 4.6).

Extra edge

Indications for invasive hemodynamic monitoring in preeclampsia

- Oliguria not responding to IV fluids
- Renal failure
- Pulmonary edema
- Hypertensive crisis

Table 4.6 Description of convulsions in eclampsia

Stage	Duration	Clinical features
Premonitory stage	30 seconds	Rolling up of eyeballs, twitching of limbs and face
Tonic stage	15–20 seconds	Generalized tonic contraction of entire body, opisthotonus, cessation of respiration, clenching of hands, protrusion of tongue
Clonic stage	1 minute	Muscles of the body contract and relax, tongue bite occurs, secretions from mouth
Postconvulsion stage	Few minutes	Patient is in a drowsy or confused state

Complications of eclampsia

- Cerebrovascular accident
- Aspiration pneumonia
- Cardiopulmonary arrest
- Renal failure
- Abruption and DIC
- Injuries—tongue bite, etc.
- Fetal hypoxia and death

Management of eclampsia

Management of a patient with eclampsia includes the following:

- Stabilization of the patient
- Anticonvulsants to control convulsions and prevent further convulsions
- Antihypertensives to control BP
- Immediate delivery

General measures

- Admit and shift the patient to eclampsia room (dim light with minimal noise).
- Call for help.
- The patient is put on a railed cot to prevent fall during convulsions.

During a convulsion episode

- Maintain airway, breathing, and circulation.
- Foot end elevation with head turned to one side to prevent aspiration.
- Place a mouth gag to prevent tongue from falling back and obstructing airway.
- Do suctioning to remove secretions from mouth, to clear the air passage.
- Give humidified oxygen inhalation as there is hypoxia during convulsion.
- Secure IV line, send investigations that are done for preeclampsia, and start IV drip with 10% dextrose.
- Simultaneously, take a quick history from a reliable relative regarding details of convulsions—number of convulsions, when was the first convulsion, whether the patient regained consciousness in between convulsions, etc.
- Review the patient's antenatal records and do a quick general physical and obstetric examination.

Specific management

Anticonvulsant therapy

Magnesium sulfate ($MgSO_4$) is the drug of choice (proved by collaborative eclampsia trial that compared $MgSO_4$ and phenytoin).

- Pritchard regimen is commonly used. Zuspan and Sibai are the other regimens used (Table 4.7).

Table 4.7 Magnesium sulfate regimens used in the management of eclampsia

Regimen	Loading dose	Maintenance dose
IM regimen (Pritchard regimen)—most commonly used regimen	4 g IV as 20% solution is given over 3–5 minutes, followed by 10 g as 50% solution given as deep IM injection (5 g in each buttock)	5 g IM injections—4 hourly in alternate buttock after checking respiratory rate, knee jerks, urine output
IV regimen (Zuspan regimen)	4 g in 100 mL 5% D is given IV over 15–20 minutes	1 g/h IV infusion
IV regimen (Sibai regimen)	6 g in 100 mL 5% D is given IV over 15–20 minutes	2 g/h IV infusion

- Recurrent convulsion—if the patient develops recurrent convulsion while on $MgSO_4$, further dose of 2 g of 20% $MgSO_4$ slow IV can be given.
- Duration of treatment—$MgSO_4$ is given for 24 hours following delivery or last convulsion, whichever is later.
- Therapeutic levels of magnesium sulfate are 4.8–8.4 mg/dL (4–7 mEq/L).
- Parameters monitored during magnesium sulfate therapy include urine output, knee jerks, and respiratory rate.
- Maintenance doses of $MgSO_4$ are given only if:
  - Urine output exceeds 30 mL/h or is at least 100 mL/4 hours.
  - Knee jerks are present.
  - Respiratory rate is >14/min.

Magnesium toxicity can lead to depressed deep tendon reflexes and can finally lead to respiratory depression.

- Deep tendon reflexes (Patellar reflexes/knee jerk) are lost at levels 9.5–12 mg/dL (>7 mEq/L)
- Respiratory depression occurs at levels 12–18 mg/dL (>10 mEq/L)
- Cardiac arrest occurs at levels 24–30 mg/dL (>25 mEq/L)
- $MgSO_4$ is excreted in urine and hence urine output should be adequate to avoid toxic levels in circulation.

Note *Plasma monitoring of Mg is usually not necessary. Toxic levels are monitored clinically with knee jerks, urine output, respiratory rate.*
Magnesium sulfate is more effective than phenytoin and diazepam in eclampsia and should be considered the drug of choice.
Benzodiazepines (diazepam) and phenytoin are justified only when magnesium sulfate is contraindicated or unavailable.

Management of Mg toxicity

- Withhold $MgSO_4$ IM dose or IV infusion.
- If respiratory depression is suspected, the patient is connected to pulse oxymeter, oxygen is given, and serum Mg levels are estimated.
- Calcium gluconate is the antidote for magnesium. 1 g in 10 mL of 10% calcium gluconate is given as slow IV.
- If respiratory or cardiac arrest occurs, the patient is intubated and mechanical ventilation is given.

Contraindications for $MgSO_4$

- Myasthenia gravis, moderate-to-severe renal failure, cardiac ischemia, heart block, or myocarditis

Antihypertensive therapy

BP must be controlled immediately with antihypertensives such as Tab. Nifedipine oral, Inj. labetalol IV, and Inj. hydralazine IV. The SBP should be maintained at 140–150 mmHg and DBP at 90–100 mmHg.

Other measures in a patient with eclampsia

- The patient is kept nil oral to prevent aspiration in case of further convulsions.
- Monitor blood pressure, pulse, respiratory rate, oxygen saturation, cardiovascular system and respiratory system.
- IV fluids are given with caution (restrict to 75 mL/h) to avoid volume overload and pulmonary edema.
- Prophylactic antibiotics are given as there is a risk of aspiration pneumonia.
- An indwelling Foley's catheter is inserted to monitor the patient's urine output and maintain input/output charting.
- $MgSO_4$ should be continued for 24 hours following delivery or last convulsions, whichever is later.
- Antihypertensives are given for control of BP if BP is ≥150/100 mmHg.
- USG and NST are done to assess fetal well-being.
- Steroids are given for lung maturity in case of preterm fetus.

Definitive obstetric management is by termination of pregnancy

Induction of labor is done based on Bishop's score. LSCS is done only for obstetric indications and in conditions such as status eclampticus, recurrent pulmonary edema, acute renal failure, retinal detachment, papilloedema, cerebrovascular accident, worsening hematological parameters in HELLP.

Acute fulminant preeclampsia

- Intense features of preeclampsia occurring within a short time span with rapid deterioration of the patient's condition is termed acute fulminant preeclampsia.
- There is a constant threat of convulsions or coma.

Viva corner

Q1 What is the differential diagnosis for convulsions occurring in pregnancy?

Differential diagnosis for convulsions in pregnancy includes the following:

- Eclampsia
- Epilepsy
- Meningitis
- Encephalitis
- Cortical venous thrombosis
- Metabolic abnormalities—hypoglycemia and electrolyte imbalance
- Hypertensive encephalopathy
- Intracranial tumors
- Neurocysticercosis

Note *Convulsions occurring during pregnancy and within 48 hours of delivery are assumed to be eclampsia until proved otherwise.*

Q2 What are the other therapies for control of convulsions in eclampsia?

- Phenytoin
- Lytic cocktail regimen—combination of pethidine, promethazine, and chlorpromazine

Q3 What are the drugs used in the treatment of status eclampticus?

- Lorazepam
- Phenytoin
- Thiopentone sodium

Resistant cases require intubation and mechanical ventilation.

Q4 What is prophylactic $MgSO_4$ therapy?

When $MgSO_4$ is given for prevention of convulsions in severe and imminent preeclampsia, it is termed prophylactic $MgSO_4$ therapy (MAGPIE trial—$MgSO_4$ for prevention of eclampsia).

Prophylactic $MgSO_4$ regimen is the same as in eclampsia (both IV and IM loading doses and maintenance doses are given).

Q5 What is Dhaka regimen for $MgSO_4$ administration?

According to this regimen, the loading dose of magnesium sulfate is 10 g (4 g IV + 6 g IM). Maintenance dose of $MgSO_4$ (2.5 g) is given intramuscularly every 4 hours, for 24 hours after administration of loading dose.

Inference

Half of the standard dose of magnesium sulfate appeared to be sufficient to control convulsions effectively and serum levels of magnesium remained lower than the levels that produce toxicity.

- Treatment: It involves hospitalization, administration of magnesium sulfate, antihypertensives, and immediate delivery.

HELLP syndrome

It includes hemolysis, elevated liver enzymes, and low platelets.

Complete HELLP It has all the three components.

Partial HELLP It has one or two components.

Incidence It is 20% in severe preeclampsia cases.

Pathogenesis Generalized vasospasm and endothelial damage leads to activation of coagulation system, platelet aggregation, and end-organ damage.

Criteria for diagnosis of HELLP syndrome See Table 4.8

Table 4.8 Criteria for diagnosis of HELLP syndrome

Hemolysis	Elevated liver enzymes	Low platelets
• Abnormal peripheral smear—presence of schistocytes, Burr cells • Total bilirubin >1.2 mg/dL • Low serum haptoglobin (<25 mg/dL) • Lactate dehydrogenase >600 IU/L	• Serum aspartate aminotransferase (AST) and alanine aminotransferase (ALT) >70 IU/L (more than twice the normal) • Lactate dehydrogenase >600 IU/L (nonspecific)	• Platelet count <1,00,000/mm^3

Mississippi classification of HELLP syndrome See Table 4.9

Table 4.9 Mississippi classification of HELLP syndrome

HELLP classification	Platelets
Class I	<50,000/mm^3
Class II	50,000–1,00,000/mm^3
Class III	1,00,000–2,00,000/mm^3

Tennessee diagnostic criteria for HELLP Hemolysis with increased LDH (> 600 U/L), AST (≥ 70 U/L), and platelets < 1,00,000 mm^3.

Management—immediate termination of pregnancy

- Transfuse blood components—platelet transfusion is given if counts are less than 50,000/mm^3.
- Give antihypertensives.
- Give $MgSO_4$ prophylaxis.
- Terminate the pregnancy.
  - Platelet count <20,000/mm^3—risk of spontaneous bleeding is more.
  - Platelet count >50,000/mm^3 is recommended for any procedure including vaginal delivery and to reduce PPH.
  - Platelet count >80,000/mm^3 is recommended for regional analgesia/anesthesia and CS.
  - CS is done only for obstetric indications.
  - General anesthesia is preferred to regional anesthesia, if platelets are low.
- Dexamethasone 10 mg IV q 12 hourly can be given.
  - It causes transient improvement in platelet count, urine output, LDH, and aspartate aminotransferase (AST) levels.
  - It reduces the need for blood transfusion.
  - It reduces the duration of stay in hospital.

Note *Intramuscular injections, pudendal block, and spinal/epidural anesthesia must be avoided in patients with HELLP syndrome because of risk of bleeding.*

Posterior reversible encephalopathy syndrome (PRES)

- PRES, one of the complications of preeclampsia, is a distinctive clinical and imaging syndrome, characterized by acute headaches, visual impairment, seizures, and altered sensorium.
- Neuroimaging (MRI) is characterized by cerebral edema predominantly affecting the parietal and occipital lobes.
- In addition to preeclampsia/eclampsia, PRES has been associated with other systemic conditions such as severe hypertension and renal failure.
- Risk of PRES is more in the settings of eclampsia and preeclampsia with headache, altered consciousness, or visual abnormalities.

Management of PRES

- Prompt recognition and early treatment often lead to complete reversal of the condition. However, disability or death may result from delaying the therapy.
- The principles of therapy include control of blood pressure, treatment of seizures, and prompt delivery.
- Correction of electrolyte imbalance, dehydration, and adequate oxygenation should be ensured.

Chronic hypertension in pregnancy

Definition Chronic hypertension refers to preexisting hypertension or hypertension diagnosed before 20 weeks, not attributed to trophoblastic diseases.

Common causes of chronic hypertension

- Essential hypertension (most common)
- Renal diseases
- Connective tissue disorders—systemic lupus erythematosus (SLE)
- Endocrine causes—pheochromocytoma

Complications of chronic hypertension See Table 4.10

Table 4.10 Complications of chronic hypertension

Maternal complications	Fetal complications
• Superimposed preeclampsia (25%) • Severe hypertension • Abruption	• Fetal growth restriction • Preterm delivery • Fetal anomalies (if angiotensin-converting enzyme inhibitors are taken during pregnancy)

Part 1

Additional evaluation in chronic hypertension during pregnancy

- ECG
- ECHO cardiogram
- 24-Hour urine protein estimation
- Renal function test
- USG for maternal kidneys, renal artery Doppler
- Fundus for hypertensive changes
- GDM screening

Management

- Advise on salt restriction.
- Continue antihypertensives during pregnancy. If the patient is on angiotensin-converting enzyme (ACE) inhibitors or angiotensin receptor antagonists, change to other safer antihypertensives in pregnancy.
- Low-dose aspirin can be started at 12 weeks as prophylaxis against superimposed preeclampsia.

Viva corner

Q1 Can you predict preeclampsia?

There are no screening tests that can accurately predict preeclampsia. However, the tests given in the table below may be used especially in high-risk women (see table below).

Table Screening tests for prediction of preeclampsia

Screening test	Prediction for preeclampsia
Uterine artery Doppler	Persistence of diastolic notch in uterine artery Doppler after 24 weeks predicts preeclampsia (see figure below)
Mean arterial pressure (MAP)	MAP of >90 mmHg in the second trimester predicts preeclampsia
Angiotensin sensitivity test	<8 ng/kg/min of angiotensin required to increase DBP by 20 mmHg is considered as a positive test
Rollover test	Increase in DBP by 20 mmHg when the patient changes from left lateral position (LLP) to supine position between 28 and 32 weeks predicts preeclampsia
Isometric handgrip test	Rise in DBP of >20 mmHg after isometric handgrip exercise at 28–32 weeks is a predictive test

(**Hint:** *Remember the acronym "MARI" for screening tests for preeclampsia)*

Recent advances

The use of uterine artery Doppler waveform analysis in the first trimester for prediction of preeclampsia has been studied in recent years.

Novel Predictors of Preeclampsia: Angiogenic factors implicated in the pathophysiology of preeclampsia may have the potential of identifying women earlier in their disease course. A role for angiogenic biomarkers in the diagnosis of preeclampsia is emerging.

Angiogenic factors with positive prediction of preeclampsia under evaluation include:

- Increase in the level of antiangiogenic factors such as sFlt-1, s-endoglin, and thromboxane A2
- Decrease in the levels of proangiogenic factors such as VEGF, PIGF, NO, PAPP-A, sFlt-1/PIGF ratio >38 (sFlt-1-soluble fms-like tyrosine kinase 1; PIGF-placental growth factor)
- PIGF value of >100 pg/mL

Q2 Can you prevent preeclampsia?

- Preeclampsia cannot be completely prevented. Several interventions for prevention have been studied.

Low-dose aspirin: Imbalance in prostacyclin and thromboxane A2 metabolism involved in the pathogenesis of preeclampsia led to the studies of aspirin for preeclampsia prevention because of its preferential inhibition of thromboxane A2 at lower doses (CLASP trial—collaborative low-dose aspirin trial).

- ACOG recommends low-dose (75–81 mg/day) aspirin for preeclampsia prophylaxis initiated between 12 weeks and 28 weeks of gestation (optimally before 16 weeks of gestation) and continuing until delivery for the followingcases:
  - Women with any of the high-risk factors for preeclampsia (previous pregnancy with preeclampsia, renal diseases, autoimmune diseases such as APLA and SLE, type 1 or type 2 DM, and chronic hypertension).
  - Women with more than one of the moderate-risk factors (first pregnancy, multiple pregnancy, maternal age of ≥35 years,

(CONTD...)

(...CONTD)

Viva corner

BMI >30, F/H/o preeclampsia, and inter pregnancy interval of >10 years).

- It is not recommended in low-risk cases.

Calcium supplementation: Significant reduction in preeclampsia has been noted with 2 g/day of calcium supplementation during pregnancy, with the greatest effect among women with low-baseline calcium intake.

Other nutritional agents: Evidence is insufficient to demonstrate effectiveness for vitamins C, D, and E, folic acid, fish oil, garlic supplementation, sodium restriction, and bed rest for reducing the risk of preeclampsia.

Investigational agents: Metformin, sildenafil, and statins for the prevention of preeclampsia remain investigational.

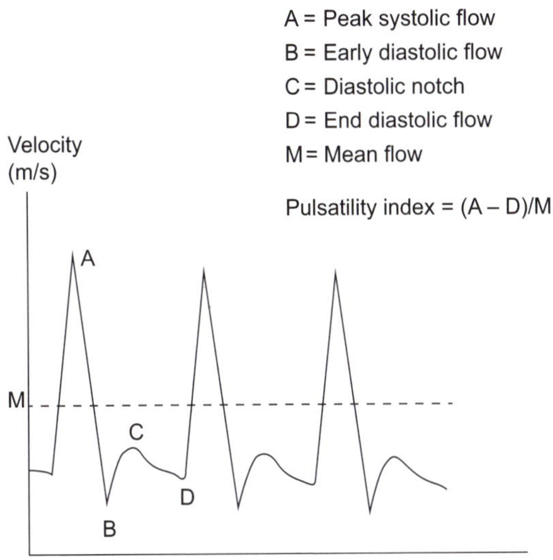

Figure Persistent diastolic notch in uterine artery Doppler (persistence of diastolic notch after 24 weeks predicts preeclampsia).

Extra edge

Grading of hypertensive retinopathy (Keith and Wegner classification) seen in chronic hypertension

See table below

Table Grading of hypertensive retinopathy

Grade	Features
I	Attenuated tortuous retinal vessels
II	Changes in arteriovenous crossing such as kinking, deflection of veins at points of crossing with arteries
III	Copper and silver wiring of vessels; retinal exudates and hemorrhage
IV	Papilledema

- Regular antenatal care is required for close monitoring of BP and proteinuria, and for monitoring of fetal growth.
- Watch for superimposed preeclampsia.
- Termination of pregnancy at 40 weeks—pregnancy is not allowed to become postdated.

Frequently asked viva questions

1. Summarize the case.
2. What is the diagnosis of the case?
3. What are the maternal and perinatal complications in preeclampsia?
4. What are the investigations you want to do for a patient with preeclampsia?

5. What are the features of severe preeclampsia?
6. What is the role of urine examination in preeclampsia?
7. How will you manage a case of mild preeclampsia?
8. When will you start antihypertensives? What are the commonly used antihypertensives in preeclampsia?
9. How will you manage a case of severe preeclampsia?
10. When will you terminate pregnancy in preeclampsia?
11. What is the mode of delivery in preeclampsia?
12. What is the role of LSCS in preeclampsia?
13. How will you monitor the patient in labor?
14. How will you manage a case of eclampsia?
15. How will you give magnesium sulfate therapy?
16. How will you monitor the patient on magnesium sulfate therapy?
17. What is the role of aspirin in the prevention of preeclampsia?

5 Cardiac Disease in Pregnancy

Introduction

Cardiac diseases in pregnancy account for significant maternal morbidity and mortality and are a leading cause of obstetrical intensive care unit admissions. Physiological changes in cardiovascular system (CVS) during pregnancy can have a profound effect on women with underlying cardiac diseases and can lead to cardiac failure in pregnancy. This chapter deals with the case discussion on cardiac disease complicating pregnancy.

Physiological changes in cardiovascular system during pregnancy

The important changes in cardiovascular system during pregnancy such as increase in cardiac output, blood volume, and heart rate and decrease in peripheral resistance may compromise cardiac function in women with heart disease (Table 5.1; Figures 5.1 and 5.2).

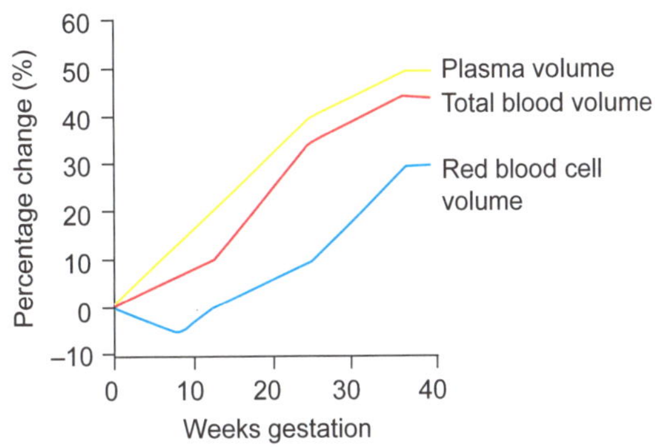

Figure 5.1 Maternal intravascular volume changes during pregnancy.

Table 5.1 Physiological changes in cardiovascular system during pregnancy

Physiological function	Change during pregnancy
Plasma volume	• Increases by 50% • Increase begins by 6 weeks, peaks at 30 weeks, and plateaus till term
Blood volume	• Increases by 40–50% • Increase begins by 6 weeks, peaks at 32–34 weeks, and plateaus till term
RBC mass	• Increases by 30%
Heart rate (HR)	• Increases by 10–15 beats/min
Stroke volume (SV)	• Increases by 30%
Cardiac output (CO = SV × HR)	• Increases by 50% • Increase starts by 6 weeks, peaks around 28–30 weeks, and plateaus till term • Additional 50% increase during labor • Increases during immediate postpartum following delivery • Cardiac output returns to nonpregnant level by 2 weeks postpartum
Blood pressure	• Midtrimester fall in diastolic BP by 10–15 mmHg due to decrease in systemic vascular resistance
Systemic vascular resistance	• Decreases by 20%

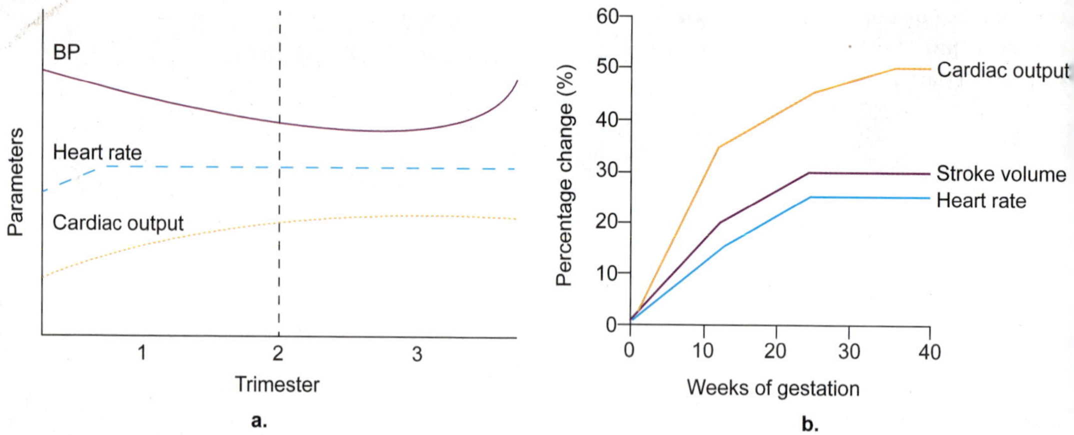

Figure 5.2 Cardiovascular changes during pregnancy. **a.** Changes in the blood pressure, heart rate, and cardiac output during pregnancy. **b.** Changes in the cardiac output, stroke volume, and heart rate during pregnancy.

High-yield points

Causes for increase in cardiac output during pregnancy

Cardiac output (CO)	Cause(s) for increase
Antepartum (CO increases by 50%)	• Increase in heart rate • Increase in stroke volume (due to increase in blood volume) • Decrease in peripheral vascular resistance
Intrapartum	
• Additional 15% increase in CO during the first stage of labor	• Uterine contractions cause return of 300–500 mL of blood into systemic circulation
• Additional 50% increase in CO during the second stage of labor	• Sympathetic response to pain and anxiety causes increase in heart rate and BP, and in turn increases cardiac output
• Additional 75% increase in CO during the third stage of labor that returns to prelabor values by 1 hour after delivery	• Approximately 500 mL of blood is returned to systemic circulation following delivery due to uterine retraction (shunting of blood from uterus) and reduction of pressure on inferior vena cava • Transfer of fluid from extracellular space into systemic circulation (mobilization of extravascular fluid) increases the venous return and stroke volume

HEART DISEASE IN PREGNANCY

Incidence of heart disease in pregnancy varies from 0.5% to 3%.

Classification of heart disease during pregnancy

- Rheumatic heart disease (RHD)
  - Mitral stenosis (MS)
  - Mitral regurgitation
  - Aortic stenosis
  - Aortic regurgitation
- Congenital heart disease
  - Atrial septal defect (ASD), ventricular septal defect (VSD), and patent ductus arteriosus (PDA)
  - Tetralogy of Fallot (TOF)
  - Eisenmenger syndrome
  - Coarctation of aorta

- Pregnancy in women with prosthetic valves
- Peripartum cardiomyopathy
- Coronary artery disease

Note

- *In India, RHD is the most common cause of heart disease during pregnancy.*
- *In India, the ratio of RHD to congenital heart disease is 3:1, while in Western countries, this ratio is equal or reverse due to the following:*
  - *Better control of rheumatic fever in childhood*
  - *Better survival rate of patients with congenital heart disease because of availability of better medical treatment*
- *The most common valve involved in RHD is mitral valve (85%), followed by aortic valve (10%).*

Changes during pregnancy that can mimic organic heart disease

See Table 5.2

Table 5.2 Symptoms and signs of cardiovascular changes during pregnancy that can mimic organic heart disease

Symptoms	Signs
• Swelling of feet • Breathlessness • Palpitation • Easy fatigability	• Pedal edema • Increased pulse rate, bounding pulse • Shift in apex beat • Short systolic murmur • Third heart sound (S3)

Clinical features of organic heart disease in pregnancy

See Table 5.3

Table 5.3 Symptoms and signs of organic heart disease in pregnancy

Symptoms	Signs
• Progressive dyspnea • Paroxysmal nocturnal dyspnea • Orthopnea • Chest pain • Syncopal attacks • Hemoptysis	• Cyanosis • Clubbing • Persistent distension of neck veins • Palpable thrill • Parasternal heave • Loud systolic murmur (grade 3/6 or more) • Diastolic murmur • Fine basal crepts • Cardiomegaly • Arrhythmias • Pulmonary hypertension

New York Heart Association (NYHA) functional classification of symptoms of heart disease

This is a functional classification based on the symptoms of fatigue, palpitation, dyspnea, and anginal pain. Women with NYHA class I and class II often have an uneventful pregnancy and women in class III and class IV are prone to complications (Table 5.4).

Table 5.4 New York Heart Association (NYHA) functional classification of symptoms of heart disease

Class	Functional capacity	Symptoms
Class I	Patients with cardiac disease with no limitation of physical activity	Ordinary physical activity does not cause fatigue, palpitations, dyspnea, or anginal pain
Class II	Patients with cardiac disease with slight limitation of physical activity	Ordinary physical activity results in fatigue, palpitations, dyspnea, or anginal pain
Class III	Patients with cardiac disease with marked limitation of physical activity	Less than ordinary physical activity results in fatigue, palpitations, dyspnea, or anginal pain
Class IV	Patients with cardiac disease with inability to carry on any physical activity without discomfort	Symptoms of cardiac insufficiency may be present even at rest, that is, symptomatic at rest. If any physical activity is undertaken, discomfort is increased

Case presentation

Salient points in history

Consider the following relevant points during history taking in cases of cardiac disease in pregnancy:

- *Age*
- *Education—to judge the patient's understanding of the disease and explain her about the treatment*
- *Occupation*
- *Socioeconomic status (SES)—RHD is more common among lower SES); to anticipate and treat complications associated with low SES such as anemia and infections (can precipitate heart failure)*

Present pregnancy

- *H/o breathlessness on exertion (NYHA class)*
- *H/o chest pain, palpitations, syncope, orthopnea, paroxysmal nocturnal dyspnea, and cough with hemoptysis*
- *Whether the patient is a known case of cardiac disease; if yes:*
  - *Age at diagnosis of the cardiac problem*
  - *Treatment details—H/o intake of cardiac drugs such as digoxin, diuretics, injection penicillin (once in every 3 weeks), and syrup potassium chloride, warfarin therapy (teratogenic)*
  - *H/o previous cardiac surgery*
  - *H/o previous admissions for cardiac complaints*
  - *H/o recurrent lower respiratory infections, urinary infections, and periodontal infections*
  - *H/o rheumatic fever in childhood*
  - *Ask for H/o cyanotic spells relieved on squatting etc., if the patient is a known case of congenital heart disease*
- *H/o fever, cough with expectoration, and burning micturition (infections can predispose to infective endocarditis)*

Obstetric history

- *Any history related to cardiac problem in previous pregnancy, and in postpartum period*
- *H/o any obstetric complications such as preeclampsia, gestational diabetes mellitus (GDM), and antepartum hemorrhage (APH)*
- *H/o contraception in between pregnancies*

Past history

- *H/o DM, hypertension, thromboembolism, tuberculosis, blood transfusion, and drug allergy*
- *H/o rheumatic fever, previous cardiac surgery, cardiac complications*
- *H/o stroke, transient ischemic attacks, and arrhythmias*

Personal history

- *History of smoking, alcohol, and drug abuse*
- *Bowel and bladder habits*
- *Sleep and appetite*

Diet history

- *Total caloric and protein intake*
- *Dietary advice given to restrict sodium (salt) and to take adequate proteins (80–90 g/day)*

Family history

- *H/o DM, hypertension, tuberculosis, and congenital anomalies*
- *H/o congenital heart disease*

Salient points in examination

Consider the following relevant points during examination in cases of cardiac disease in pregnancy.

General physical examination

- *Built*
- *Nutrition*
- *Height*
- *Weight*
- *BMI*
- *Pallor*
- *Icterus*
- *Cyanosis*
- *Clubbing*
- *Lymphadenopathy*
- *Pedal edema, dependent edema in admitted patients*
- *Oral cavity examined—tongue, teeth, gums, and tonsils—for any evidence of infection*

Vitals

- *Temperature*
- *Pulse—rate, rhythm (regular or irregular), volume, character, whether all peripheral pulses*

(CONTD...)

(...CONTD)

are equally felt, and any radiofemoral delay (to rule out coarctation of aorta)
- Blood pressure
- Respiratory rate

Cardiovascular system examination

A detailed CVS examination has to be performed.

Inspection

- Raised jugular venous pressure (JVP) is looked for
  - Procedure to check for JVP (Figure 5.3)
    - Right internal jugular vein (IJV) is used for measurement.
    - Patient position is maintained at 45° reclining position, neck turned slightly to left.
    - Vertical distance between the sternal angle and the highest point of oscillating venous column over right IJV is measured (i.e., height of the venous pressure above sternal angle).
    - Sternal angle is 5 cm from right atrium regardless of patient position, hence used as reference point.
    - JVP (cm H_2O) = height of venous column above sternal angle + 5 cm.
    - JVP provides an indirect measure of central venous pressure.
    - Normal JVP pressure does not exceed 3–4 cm above sternal angle.
    - Elevated JVP >4 cm above sternal angle is seen in right-sided heart failure.

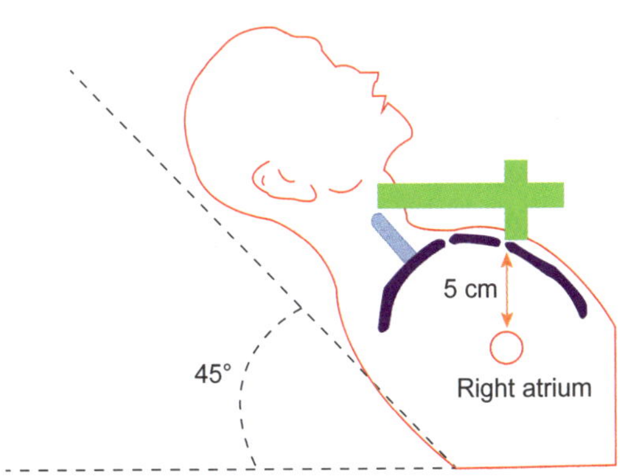

Figure 5.3 Jugular venous pressure measurement.

- Location of apex beat
  - Apex beat is the lowermost and outermost point of definitive cardiac pulsation. It is normally located in the left fifth intercostal space (ICS), 1 cm medial to midclavicular line (MCL).
  - Apex beat is shifted above and lateral, to the fourth ICS, outside the MCL during pregnancy.
- Any dilated veins
- Any precordial bulge
- Any abnormal pulsations (left parasternal pulsation indicates enlarged right ventricle)
- Any scars of previous cardiac surgery

Palpation

- Apex beat—note the character of the apex beat by palpation. Character of apex beat in various cardiac lesions is mentioned in Table 5.5.
- Any palpable thrill
- Parasternal heave

Auscultation

The sites for cardiac auscultation are depicted in Figure 5.4.

- **Mitral area:** Left fifth ICS, 1 cm medial to midclavicular line
- **Aortic area:** Right second ICS, along the sternal border
- **Pulmonary area:** Left second ICS, along the sternal border
- **Tricuspid area:** Left fourth ICS, along the sternal border

If any murmur is heard, mention the type and grade of murmur and the area over the chest where the murmur is best heard.

Table 5.5 Character of apex beat in various cardiac lesions

Character of apex beat	Condition
Hyperdynamic apex	Aortic and mitral regurgitation
Heaving apex beat (increased amplitude)	Aortic stenosis
Tapping apex beat (increased amplitude and duration)	Mitral stenosis

(CONTD...)

(...CONTD)

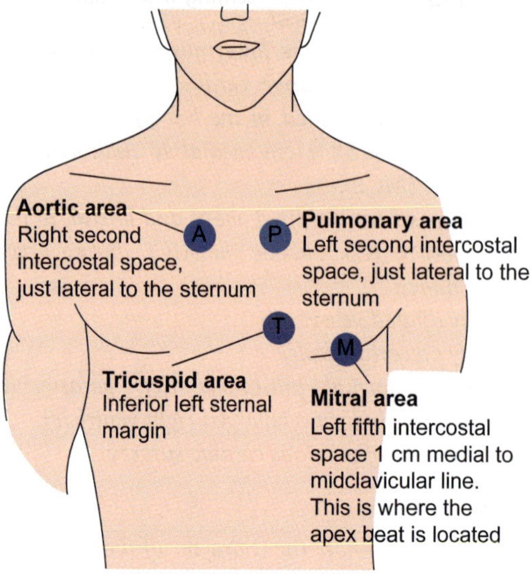

Figure 5.4 Sites for cardiac auscultation.

Various abnormal cardiac auscultation findings include:

- *Mammary souffle: It is a high-pitched sound heard in the second or third intercostal space, due to increased blood flow through mammary vessels (it is physiological and often misdiagnosed for organic heart disease).*
- *Typical auscultation finding in mitral stenosis: It is the opening snap, mid-diastolic murmur with presystolic accentuation.*
- *Murmurs heard in various cardiac lesions are mentioned in Table 5.6.*

Note *Low-grade ejection systolic murmurs are present in about 80% of pregnant women and are not clinically significant; however, diastolic murmurs are abnormal.*

Table 5.6 Murmurs heard in various cardiac lesions

Murmur	Condition
Mid-diastolic murmur	Mitral and tricuspid stenosis
Ejection systolic murmur	• Pregnancy, severe anemia • Aortic and pulmonary stenosis
Pansystolic murmur	Mitral and tricuspid regurgitation

Respiratory system examination

- *Whether air entry is equal on both sides*
- *Any abnormal breath sounds (fine basal crepts indicate left ventricular failure)*

Per abdomen

Palpate for hepatomegaly/splenomegaly.

Obstetric examination

- *Fundal height and symphysiofundal height (SFH) (look for any discrepancy in fundal height and SFH which may be suggestive of intrauterine growth restriction)*
- *Obstetric grips are performed as usual*
- *Amount of liquor, uterine activity, and fetal heart rate (FHR)*

Case summary

An example of writing summary in cases of cardiac disease in pregnancy is given below.

Example *Mrs. N, 28 years of age, primigravida at 30 weeks of gestation, a known case of RHD with mitral stenosis for the past 8 years on regular medications, is now admitted with chief complaints of dyspnea NYHA class III and palpitations for 1 week. There is no pallor or pedal edema. Her pulse rate is 100/min, regular, and BP is 124/70 mmHg. CVS examination reveals that JVP is not raised, and a mid-diastolic murmur is heard in mitral area with opening snap. Respiratory system examination is normal with no added breath sounds. Obstetric examination reveals fundal height of 28 weeks with a singleton live fetus in cephalic presentation; uterus is relaxed and FHR is 132 beats/min.*

Case diagnosis

An example of writing the diagnosis in cases of cardiac disease in pregnancy is given below.

Example *28 years of age, primigravida at 30 weeks of gestation with RHD, mitral stenosis, NYHA class III symptoms, not in failure, with a singleton live fetus in cephalic presentation, not in labor*

Case discussion

Cardiac disease is one of the differential diagnosis for breathlessness and pedal edema during pregnancy. There may be other causes for these symptoms which have to be ruled out from history, clinical examination, and investigations.

DIFFERENTIAL DIAGNOSIS FOR BREATHLESSNESS DURING PREGNANCY

- Normal pregnancy changes: Progesterone causes decrease in threshold for CO_2, resulting in slight hyperventilation that is manifested as breathlessness during pregnancy.
- Anemia
  - Patient may present with H/o palpitations, breathlessness on exertion, swelling of feet, tiredness, and easy fatigability.
  - Ask for H/o iron supplementation, H/o chronic illness such as urinary tract infection, worm infestation, bleeding piles, menorrhagia, and H/o blood transfusion (as mentioned in Part 1, Chapter 2, *Anemia in Pregnancy*).
  - On examination—look for pallor, edema, koilonychia, and signs of vitamin deficiency such as angular stomatitis.
  - In anemia cases, pulse is regular; soft systolic murmur can be heard, and JVP is not raised (except in failure).
- Respiratory illness
  - Ask for H/o fever with chills and rigors, cough with sputum expectoration, pleuritic chest pain, and hemoptysis.
  - On examination—look for any raised temperature, tachycardia, and conducted sounds on respiratory system (RS) examination.

DIFFERENTIAL DIAGNOSIS FOR PITTING PEDAL EDEMA DURING PREGNANCY

- Physiological edema
- Preeclampsia
- Anemia and hypoproteinemia
- Cardiac disease
- Renal disease

Note *In a patient presenting with pedal edema or breathlessness, the differential diagnosis should be kept in mind and relevant history should be taken and examination performed to rule out other causes.*

Diagnosis of cardiac disease

- All pregnant women should have a cardiac examination in the first antenatal visit. In case of suspicious signs and symptoms, further investigations should be performed.
- Investigations to confirm the diagnosis are the following:
  - ECG
  - ECHO cardiogram (most useful investigation–gives accurate diagnosis of cardiac disease)
  - Chest X-ray (may be done with abdominal shielding, if indicated in the first trimester)

Effects of heart disease on pregnancy

- Maternal and fetal complications associated with heart disease in pregnancy are mentioned in Table 5.7.
- Complications are higher in women with NYHA class III and IV.

Effects of pregnancy on heart disease

- Increase in cardiac output (CO) during pregnancy can lead to pulmonary edema and congestive cardiac failure (CCF).
- There is an increase in requirement of anticoagulants in women with prosthetic valves.

Factors that can precipitate cardiac failure and pulmonary edema

- There is a high risk for CCF at 28–30 weeks, labor, immediate postpartum, and during puerperium
- Anemia
- Arrhythmias
- Infections
- Infective endocarditis
- Multiple pregnancy
- Preeclampsia
- Hyperthyroidism

Table 5.7 Maternal and fetal complications of heart disease in pregnancy

Maternal	Fetal
Maternal mortality and morbidity are increased due to the following: • Congestive cardiac failure (can occur at any POG, but maximum incidence is at 30–32 weeks, when blood volume and cardiac output peaks) • Pulmonary edema • Arrhythmias – Atrial fibrillation is the most common • Infective endocarditis • Pulmonary embolism	• Spontaneous abortions • Intrauterine growth restriction • Prematurity • Congenital heart disease in the offspring – High risk of inherited congenital heart disease in the child, if the mother has congenital heart disease (3% in TOF, 10% in ASD, coarctation of aorta, and aortic stenosis) – Marfan syndrome is an autosomal dominant condition, 50% risk in offspring – A fetal ECHO is indicated if the mother has a congenital heart disease

ASD, atrial septal defect; *POG*, period of gestation; *TOF*, tetralogy of Fallot.

Management of cardiac disease during pregnancy

Prepregnancy counseling in a patient with diagnosed heart disease

Preconceptional counseling is important to achieve optimal outcome of pregnancy in women with cardiac disease. Patients with cardiac disease require a combined consultation of a cardiologist and an obstetrician. Preconceptional management in cardiac disease includes the following:

- Assessment of the nature of lesion
- Assessment of the functional status
- Assessment of the risk of maternal morbidity and mortality
- Counsel on the following:
  - Effects of cardiac disease on pregnancy
  - Fetal complications
  - Need for prolonged hospital stay
  - Need for change in medications (warfarin to heparin)
  - Advise on surgical correction in indicated cases such as severe MS

High-yield points

CARPREG (CArdiac Disease in PREGnancy Study) II Risk Score

Developed from the prospective Cardiac Disease in Pregnancy Study in women with pre-existing cardiac disease. The scoring includes 10 predictors of a cardiac event as follows:

Predictor	Points
Prior cardiac events or arrhythmias	3
Baseline NYHA III-IV or cyanosis	3
Mechanical valve	3
Ventricular dysfunction	2
High-risk left-sided valve disease/left ventricular outflow tract obstruction	2
Pulmonary hypertension	2
Coronary artery disease	2
High-risk aortopathy	2
No prior cardiac intervention	1
Late pregnancy assessment	1

Score	Predicted risk of primary cardiac event
0 to 1 points	5%
2 points	10%
3 points	15%
4 points	22%
>4 points	41%

Maternal mortality in heart diseases

Maternal mortality in cardiac disease varies with the type of cardiac lesion. Risk categorization helps in management during pregnancy (see table below).

(CONTD...)

(...CONTD)

High-yield points

Table Modified World Health Organization (WHO) classification of maternal cardiovascular risk

Risk category	Description	Conditions
I	• No detectable increased risk in maternal mortality and no/ mild increase in morbidity	• Uncomplicated, small or mild PS, PDA, or mitral valve prolapse • Successfully repaired simple lesions (ASD, VSD, anomalous pulmonary venous drainage) • Atrial or ventricular ectopic beats, isolated
II	• Small, increased risk of maternal mortality and moderate increase in morbidity	• Unoperated ASD or VSD • Repaired TOF • Most arrhythmias
II/III	• Risk as indicated in Class II (above) or Class III (below)	• Mild left ventricular impairment • HCM • Native or tissue valvular heart disease not considered WHO class I or IV • Marfan's syndrome without aortic dilatation • Aortic dilatation <45 mm in aortic disease associated with BAoV • Repaired CoA
III	• Significantly increased risk of maternal mortality or severe morbidity • Expert counseling required • If pregnancy is decided upon, intensive specialist, cardiac and obstetric monitoring needed throughout pregnancy, childbirth, and puerperium	• Mechanical valve • Systemic right ventricle • Fontan circulation • Cyanotic heart disease (unrepaired) • Other complex congenital heart disease • Aortic dilatation 40–45 mm in Marfan's syndrome • Aortic dilatation 45–50 mm in aortic disease associated with BAoV
IV	• Extremely high risk of maternal mortality or severe morbidity; pregnancy contraindicated • If pregnancy occurs, termination should be discussed • If pregnancy continues, care as for class III	• Pulmonary arterial hypertension of any cause • Severe systemic ventricular dysfunction (LVEF <30%, NYHA class III–IV) • Previous PPCM with any residual impairment of left ventricular function • Severe MS, severe symptomatic AS • Marfan's syndrome with aorta dilation >45 mm • Aortic dilatation >50 mm in aortic disease associated with BAoV • Native severe CoA

AS = aortic valve stenosis; ASD = atrial septal defect; BAoV = bicuspid aortic valve; CoA = coarctation of the aorta; HCM = hypertrophic cardiomyopathy; LVEF = left ventricular ejection fraction; MS = mitral stenosis; NYHA = New York Heart Association; PPCM = peripartum cardiomyopathy; PS = pulmonary stenosis; PDA = patent ductus arteriosus; TOF = tetralogy of Fallot; VSD = ventricular septal defect.

Antenatal management

- Patient with cardiac disease should be managed by a team of cardiologist, obstetrician, anesthetist, and neonatologist in a tertiary care center.
- Detailed history is taken and clinical examination is performed at the first visit to detect any cardiac disease (if previously not known).
- Cardiac workup—ECG and ECHO heart are done to confirm nature of lesion, and assess functional status.
- Classify the patient according to NYHA functional class.
- Advise on the following:
  - Adequate rest and restriction of physical activities

- Salt restriction to less than 2 g/day
- Rheumatic prophylaxis is continued throughout pregnancy in patients with RHD
- Patients with signs and symptoms of heart failure may require treatment with antifailure drugs that include diuretics (Frusemide) and Digoxin.
- Iron and calcium supplementation are given

- Keep a close watch on maternal hemoglobin and BP. Anemia and hypertension can precipitate CCF and should be managed appropriately.
- Detect and treat factors that can precipitate CCF such as infections and arrhythmias.
- Advise on frequent antenatal visits.
  - Cardiac risk assessment should be ongoing at each antenatal visit.
  - Antenatal visits should be scheduled once in 2 weeks up to 28 weeks and then every week thereafter.
  - Advise the patient to return earlier if there is deterioration in cardiac status, fever, or any other obstetric complaints.
- Fetal growth should be monitored by clinical examination and by periodic USG examination. Antepartum fetal surveillance is started from 32 weeks by nonstress test (NST).

Indications for admission

In NYHA classes I and II

- The patient may be admitted at the initial visit for complete cardiac workup and then followed up on OPD basis.
- The patient is admitted 2 weeks before the expected date of delivery.
- Indications for emergency admission
  - Deterioration of functional status
  - Appearance of signs and symptoms of cardiac failure
  - Complications that can precipitate cardiac failure such as anemia and infections
  - Obstetric complications such as preeclampsia

In NYHA classes III and IV

- Patients are hospitalized till delivery.
- An NYHA class III patient whose condition is stable may take short breaks from hospitalization.

Intrapartum management

- Await spontaneous onset of labor (most women with cardiac disease have spontaneous onset of labor at or near term).
- Role of induction: Induction is better avoided. Induction of labor can increase the risk of infection, failed induction, and cesarean section (CS) rates. However, if there is any obstetric indication, then there is no contraindication for induction. Prostaglandins may be used for cervical ripening. Oxytocin should be given by an infusion pump to avoid fluid overload.
- Vaginal delivery is preferred as it is associated with less morbidity and mortality. CS is performed only for obstetric indications.

First stage

- Avoid ambulation. The patient is put in propped-up position (avoid lithotomy position, as it increases venous return and thereby increases CO and can precipitate CCF).
- Oxygen is administered by mask.
- Patients with CCF require continued therapy with antifailure drugs.
- Hydration is maintained by oral fluids, as far as possible to avoid fluid overload. Restrict intravenous (IV) fluids to 75 mL/h (exception—aortic stenosis where IV fluids are given at 125 mL/h).
- Adequate analgesia for pain relief should be given. Morphine 0.3 mg/kg BW can be given IM every 4–6 hours (avoid pethidine as it causes maternal tachycardia). Continuous epidural analgesia is preferred, if facilities are available.
- Monitoring of pulse rate, BP, respiratory rate, and chest auscultation (lung bases for crepts) are done every 30 minutes.
- ECG and pulse oximetry monitoring are done, especially in NYHA class III/IV.
- Maintain strict input/output charting.
- Partogram is maintained to monitor the progress of labor.
- Oxytocin for augmentation of labor is given by infusion pump (to prevent fluid overload).
- Continuous electronic FHR monitoring is done, if facilities are available. Otherwise, intermittent auscultation with stethoscope is done every 15 minutes in the first stage and every 5 minutes in the second stage.

- Restrict the number of per vaginal examinations.
- Maintain strict asepsis during P/V examination and while conducting delivery.
- IE prophylaxis is not recommended for vaginal delivery in the absence of pelvic infection. However, in clinical practice, routine IE prophylaxis is given for vaginal delivery in all structural heart diseases, as the cost is low and it is not possible to predict whether the vaginal delivery is going to be complicated or not.

Second stage

- Lateral decubitus position is preferred. Lithotomy position should be avoided.
- Oxygen by mask, vitals charting, and intermittent chest auscultation are continued.
- Prophylactic cut short of the second stage is done with forceps or vacuum to avoid bearing-down efforts and additional strain on the heart. Vacuum is preferred over forceps, as it can be applied without placing the patient in lithotomy position.

Third stage

- Methergin is contraindicated (it results in forceful uterine contraction and returns blood rapidly from uterus into systemic circulation that can increase cardiac load and precipitate CCF; it can also cause an acute rise in blood pressure).
- A slow IV infusion of oxytocin (2 U of oxytocin given over 10 minutes immediately after birth, followed by 12 mU/min infusion for 4 h) reduces the risk of PPH and has a minimal impact on cardiovascular parameters (this regimen is recommended by European Society of Cardiology in 2018).
- Oxytocin and misoprostol can be used for PPH treatment; however, ergometrine and prostaglandin F2 analogues should be avoided.
- Injection furosemide 40 mg IV is administered after delivery of the placenta to reduce preload and the risk of pulmonary edema.

Part 1

Postpartum management

- Careful observation and monitoring is required in the initial 24–72 hours following delivery as cardiac decompensation can occur during this period. Significant hemodynamic changes and fluid shifts after delivery may precipitate heart failure. There is abrupt increase in venous return during this period because of the following:
  - Autotransfusion from uterus
  - Release of vena caval compression following delivery

Viva corner

Q1 What are the advantages of analgesia in cardiac disease?

Pain relief is mandatory in a patient with cardiac disease in labor because stress and pain during labor will cause tachycardia and increase the cardiac demand, precipitating CCF. Analgesia decreases tachycardia and thereby reduces risk of CCF.

Q2 What are the advantages of morphine for pain relief in cardiac patients?

Morphine for pain relief in cardiac patient has the following advantages:

- Relieves pain and anxiety
- Does not cause tachycardia (unlike pethidine)
- Reduces venous congestion and decreases pulmonary edema

Q3 What are the contraindications for epidural analgesia in cardiac patients?

Epidural analgesia can be given in most of the cardiac diseases except the following:

- Severe aortic stenosis
- Women on anticoagulants
- Cyanotic heart disease

Epidural narcotics such as pentazocine or fentanyl are preferred than lignocaine or bupivacaine (risk of hypotension is less).

Q4 What are the tocolytics that can be used in cardiac disease?

- Magnesium sulfate and atosiban can be used.
- Beta-agonists and calcium channel blockers are contraindicated.

- Mobilization of extravascular fluid into circulation
- Complications that are anticipated include postpartum hemorrhage (PPH), CCF, pulmonary edema, infective endocarditis and thromboembolism.
- The patient is put in propped-up position and oxygen is administered.
- Vitals monitoring, I/O charting, and chest auscultation are continued.
- Continue antifailure medications in patients with heart failure.
- Advise on adequate bed rest with gentle leg exercises and breathing exercises to prevent thromboembolism.
- Breastfeeding is allowed except in patients with cardiac failure.
- Hospitalization is required for at least 1 week for stabilization of the patient's general condition in our setup.

Advice on contraception

- Limit the family size to one or two children.
- Spacing methods
  - Barrier methods are safe but failure rates are high.
  - Oral contraceptive pills (OCPs) are contraindicated due to risk of thromboembolism.
  - Progesterone only pills, implants or injections are safe.
  - Intrauterine contraceptive devices are the safest and most effective contraceptives and should be inserted in a hospital setting under strict aseptic precautions with meticulous care. Ensure that the threads are cut short to reduce the risk of infection.
- Permanent methods
  - Vasectomy in males is the preferred and safe option than female sterilization in cardiac disease.
  - Female sterilization can be done under regional or local anesthesia by minilap technique(in women with class I and II disease—puerperal sterilization can be performed; in women with class III and IV disease—interval sterilization is advised after 6 weeks postpartum, when the cardiac status has improved).

Indications for termination of pregnancy in cardiac disease

Absolute indications (maternal mortality is >25%)

- Eisenmenger syndrome
- Primary pulmonary hypertension
- Marfan syndrome with aortic valve involvement
- Coarctation of aorta with aortic valve involvement
- Dilated cardiomyopathy

Relative contraindications

- NYHA class III or IV, refractory to medical management
- Severe aortic stenosis
- Congenital cyanotic heart disease
- H/o CCF in previous pregnancy or in early pregnancy

Indications for cesarean section in cardiac disease

- In pregnancy with heart disease, CS is done only for obstetric indications. Certain cardiac conditions are exception to this rule.
- Cardiac indications for CS
  - Marfan syndrome with aortic involvement

High-yield points

Congestive cardiac failure in pregnancy

Symptoms Progressive dyspnea, orthopnea, edema, cough with pink, frothy expectoration, and hemoptysis

Signs Elevated JVP, tachycardia, pedal edema, basal lung crepitations, and tender hepatomegaly

Treatment of congestive heart failure

- Rest in propped-up position
- Oxygen by mask
- Morphine 15 mg IM every 8 hours (to reduce pain and anxiety)
- Digoxin 0.5 mg OD per oral (it has a positive inotropic action on the heart)
- Diuretics—Frusemide 40 mg IV OD with potassium chloride (KCl) syrup (loop diuretics cause hypokalemia and hence potassium supplementation is necessary)
- Precipitating factors should be treated
- Underlying cardiac lesion treated by surgery in refractory cases

- Coarctation of aorta with valvular involvement
- Severe aortic stenosis
- Severe pulmonary hypertension
- Eisenmenger syndrome
- Uncorrected TOF

Indications for anticoagulation in cardiac disease

- Mechanical valves
- Mitral stenosis with atrial fibrillation
- Primary pulmonary hypertension
- Eisenmenger syndrome
- Cardiomyopathy

Recommended protocol for anticoagulation in pregnancy

See Table 5.8 for the recommended anticoagulant regimen during pregnancy.

- In patients on heparin therapy, activated partial thromboplastin time (aPTT) maintained at two times the control
- In patients on warfarin therapy, PT INR maintained between 2.5 and 3.5

Warfarin

It is an oral anticoagulant monitored with prothrombin time (PT INR).

Advantages

- Patient compliance is better.
- Warfarin is more effective than heparin in preventing thromboembolic complications.

Disadvantages

- Warfarin crosses placenta and when administered in the first trimester can lead to warfarin embryopathy (nasal hypoplasia, microcephaly, optic atrophy, mental retardation, frontal bossing, stippling of epiphysis).
- There is an increased risk of abortion, stillbirth, and fetal bleeding.
- If warfarin is administered prior to onset of labor or during labor, the anticoagulant effect is difficult to reverse and risk of maternal and fetal hemorrhage is high.
- Warfarin overdosage is treated by vitamin K injection and fresh frozen plasma.
- Breastfeeding is not contraindicated in patients on warfarin as negligible amount is secreted in breast milk.

Table 5.8 Recommended protocol for anticoagulation in pregnancy

Period of gestation	Anticoagulant
Conception to 12 weeks	Switch over from warfarin to heparin/LMWH
12–36 weeks	Warfarin can be restarted and continued up to 36 weeks For patients who prefer to avoid warfarin during pregnancy, heparin/LMWH can be continued
36 weeks onwards	Switch patients on warfarin to heparin/LMWH 36 hours prior to induction or cesarean delivery, all patients should be switched to heparin
At onset of labor/ 6 hours prior to planned delivery	Heparin should be stopped
6 hours following vaginal delivery and 12 hours following cesarean section	Restart heparin Once safe to start long-term anticoagulation, bridge heparin to warfarin with careful INR monitoring till desired INR is achieved, then heparin is stopped and continued with warfarin

Unfractionated heparin

- Unfractionated heparin (UFH) is given as a subcutaneous or IV injection, 5000–10,000 units every 12 hours.
- UFH is monitored with aPTT and should be given in a dose that maintains aPTT two times the control.

Advantages

- It does not cross the placenta; hence it is safe in pregnancy.
- Heparin is the drug of choice before labor and delivery as the anticoagulant effect can be quickly reversed with protamine sulfate.

Disadvantages

- It can result in osteoporosis, thrombocytopenia, and bleeding manifestation in the mother.
- Risk of thromboembolism is higher with UFH compared with that with warfarin.
- Hemorrhagic complications due to heparin are treated with protamine sulfate and blood transfusion.

Extra edge

Recommendations for infective endocarditis (IE) prophylaxis (American Heart Association—2007)

IE prophylaxis for dental procedures is recommended in the high-risk group (see the tables below).

IE prophylaxis is not recommended for either vaginal or cesarean delivery in the absence of pelvic infection.

Table High- and low-risk cardiac group for IE

High-risk group for IE	Low-risk group for IE
• Prosthetic valves • Previous H/o infective endocarditis • Unrepaired congenital heart disease • Repaired congenital heart disease with residual defects at the site • Cardiac transplantation recipients who develop cardiac valvulopathy	• Surgically corrected ASD, VSD, PDA • Mitral valve prolapse without regurgitation • Physiological or functional murmurs • Previous rheumatic fever without valve dysfunction • Previous Kawasaki disease without valve involvement • Previous coronary artery bypass graft • Cardiac pacemakers

Table Antibiotic regimens used for prophylaxis against IE

Patient group	Antibiotic	Dose (single dose, 30–60 minutes before procedure)
Able to take oral medication	Amoxycillin	2 g
Unable to take oral medication	Ampicillin	2 g IM or IV
Allergic to penicillin and able to take oral medication	• Cephalexin • Clindamycin • Azithromycin or clarithromycin	• 2 g • 600 mg • 500 mg
Allergic to penicillin and unable to take oral medication	• Cefazolin or ceftriaxone • Clindamycin	• 1 g IM or IV • 600 mg IM or IV

Low-molecular-weight heparin

- Can be used instead of UFH—enoxaparin 1 mg/kg body weight OD subcutaneously
- Low-molecular-weight heparin (LMWH) is monitored with anti Xa factor level

Advantages of low-molecular-weight heparin

- Less thrombocytopenia
- Longer half-life, which permits once-daily dosing
- Lesser incidence of osteoporosis
- Lower risk of bleeding and the need for monitoring

Disadvantage

- Protamine sulfate reverses the anticoagulant action only partially; therefore, it is preferable to switch to heparin before labor and delivery.

Salient points on various heart lesions

Rheumatic heart disease

RHD is the commonest cardiac lesion complicating pregnancy in developing countries including India. The most common rheumatic valvular lesion is MS.

Mitral stenosis

- It accounts for 80% of cases of RHD in pregnancy.
- Normal mitral valve orifice is 4–6 cm^2.
- Symptoms appear when mitral valve orifice (MVO) is <2.5 cm^2.
- MVO <1 cm^2 is called critical MS.
- MS → left atrial outflow obstruction → increase in resting pressure gradient across the mitral valve → increase in left atrial pressure → increase in pulmonary venous and capillary pressure leading to pulmonary congestion, pulmonary edema, and CCF.
- Dyspnea is due to reduced pulmonary compliance and hemoptysis is due to pulmonary congestion.
- Left atrial dilatation increases the risk of arrhythmias and atrial fibrillation.
- Stagnation of blood and atrial fibrillation increases the risk of thromboembolic complications.

Indications for surgery in mitral stenosis during pregnancy

- Critical MS
- Pulmonary edema not responding to medical therapy
- Profuse and uncontrollable hemoptysis
- Progressive pulmonary hypertension

Mitral regurgitation

- It is commonly rheumatic in origin or associated with mitral valve prolapse.
- It is generally well tolerated during pregnancy and cardiac failure is rare.
- Prognosis is usually decided by the associated mitral stenosis.

Aortic stenosis

- It can be congenital or rheumatic in origin.
- Normal valve orifice is 3–4 cm^2.
- Aortic valve orifice <1 cm^2 is termed critical stenosis.
- Pregnancy is poorly tolerated with high maternal mortality.
- Stenotic aortic valve leads to fixed CO (CO = stroke volume × heart rate). Hence, increase in CO during pregnancy can be met only by an increase in heart rate, which in turn shortens cardiac diastole, thus decreasing coronary blood flow.
- Advice
  - There should be strict limitation of physical activity.
- Avoid hypotension and hypovolemia.
  - IV fluids during labor are given at 125 mL/h (wet-side fluid management to maintain CO and to prevent hypotension and collapse).
  - Diuretics, vasodilators, and epidural anesthesia, which cause hypotension, are avoided.

Aortic regurgitation

- Regurgitant lesions are well tolerated during pregnancy because the decrease in systemic vascular resistance will increase the forward flow.
- It is commonly associated with MS.

Pulmonary and tricuspid valve diseases are usually well tolerated during pregnancy.

Congenital heart diseases

Acyanotic heart diseases (left to right shunts)

These include ASD, VSD, and PDA.

- ASD is the most common left to right shunt.
- L to R shunts are usually well tolerated during pregnancy.
- Size of the defect is the main determinant factor for complications.
- Pulmonary hypertension, right ventricular failure, and arrhythmias can occur.

Cyanotic heart diseases (right to left shunts)

Tetralogy of Fallot

Tetralogy of Fallot is the most common cyanotic heart disease. It comprises the following:

- Pulmonary stenosis
- Right ventricular hypertrophy
- Large VSD
- Overriding of aorta

Women with corrected TOF tolerate pregnancy well. In uncorrected TOF, pregnancy is poorly tolerated with frequent cyanosis, dyspnea, syncopal attacks, and increased maternal mortality.

Eisenmenger syndrome

- It is characterized by pulmonary hypertension secondary to right to left or bidirectional shunt.
- Medical termination of pregnancy (MTP) is advised, as it is associated with high maternal and perinatal mortality (due to severe maternal hypoxemia and polycythemia).

Other congenital heart diseases

Coarctation of aorta

- It is frequently associated with bicuspid aortic valve and cerebral artery aneurysms.
- There is an increased risk of aortic dissection, infective endocarditis, and cerebral hemorrhage.

Marfan syndrome

- It is an autosomal dominant connective tissue disorder.
- Aortic root dilatation can lead to aortic dissection and rupture during pregnancy.

Idiopathic hypertrophic subaortic stenosis

- There is marked hypertrophy of ventricular septum leading to outflow obstruction.
- Hypovolemia should be avoided as in aortic stenosis.

Primary pulmonary hypertension

- There is thickening of the media of pulmonary arteries resulting in pulmonary hypertension.
- Maternal mortality is high; hence, MTP is indicated.

Pregnancy with prosthetic valves

Women with prosthetic mitral or aortic valves following valve replacement surgery can have two types of valves as follows:

- Bioprosthetic valve
  - Patients with bioprosthetic valve do not require anticoagulation; hence, pregnancy is relatively safer.
  - Bioprosthetic valves have a short life of 8–12 years because of tissue degeneration.
  - Degeneration of bioprosthetic valve during pregnancy can lead to heart failure.
- Mechanical prosthetic valve
  - Requires lifelong anticoagulation
  - Associated with increased maternal morbidity and mortality—hemorrhage, thromboembolism, endocarditis, and heart failure

Peripartum cardiomyopathy

Definition Peripartum cardiomyopathy (PPCM) is defined as an idiopathic cardiomyopathy with the following characteristics *(European Society of Cardiology (ESC) working group 2010):*

- Development of heart failure toward the end of pregnancy or within 5 months following delivery.
- Absence of another identifiable cause for the heart failure.
- Left ventricular (LV) systolic dysfunction with LV ejection fraction (LVEF) of <45%.
  - Confirmed by echocardiography features—Diagnostic echocardiographic criteria for PPCM include left ventricular ejection fraction <0.45 or M-mode fractional shortening <30% (or both) and end-diastolic dimension >2.7 cm/m^2

Extra edge

Clinical findings in rheumatic fever Joint arthritis, subcutaneous nodules, erythema marginatum (rashes)

Clinical findings in infective endocarditis Splinter hemorrhages, osler's nodules

Features of left and right heart failure

Features of left heart failure Dyspnea on exertion, fine crepitations at lung bases, pulmonary edema, tachypnea, gallop rhythm, and extra heart sounds

Features of right heart failure Hepatosplenomegaly, ascitis, dependent pedal edema, distended neck veins, parasternal heave, and extra heart sounds

Cardiogenic and noncardiogenic causes of pulmonary edema

Cardiogenic causes of pulmonary edema	Noncardiogenic (occurs due to changes in capillary permeability)
• Heart failure • Coronary artery disease with left ventricular failure • Cardiac arrhythmias • Fluid overload • Cardiomyopathy • Obstructive valvular lesions • Myocarditis and infective endocarditis	• Sepsis • Hypovolemic shock • Disseminated intravascular coagulation • High altitude pulmonary edema • Near drowning

- Associated with a high risk of maternal mortality: 25–50%
- Treatment of heart failure as per usual guidelines
  - Salt restriction
  - Bed rest
  - Angiotensin-converting-enzyme (ACE) inhibitors
  - Beta-blockers
  - Diuretics
  - Digoxin
- High risk of recurrence in future pregnancies

Cardiac surgery during pregnancy

Cardiac surgery may be required during pregnancy in women with life-threatening complications such as failure to respond to medical treatment, recurrent CCF, uncontrolled hemoptysis, critical mitral stenosis (MVO< 1 sqcm), and pulmonary edema. The most commonly performed procedure is balloon mitral valvotomy.

- **Closed mitral valvotomy**: Can be performed for MS in indicated cases (mentioned under "*mitral stenosis*"). The procedure is usually performed in the second trimester, but if pulmonary edema is intractable, the procedure can be undertaken at any POG
- **Percutaneous balloon mitral valvuloplasty**: Can be performed for MS, but the radiation exposure to fetus should be minimized by decreasing the fluoroscopy time
- **Open heart surgery and valve replacement**: Has the same risks as in a nonpregnant patient, but fetal loss is high

Frequently asked viva questions

1. Summarize the case.
2. What is the diagnosis of the case?
3. What are the normal cardiac auscultation findings in pregnant women?
4. What are the physiological signs and symptoms during pregnancy that can mimic heart disease?
5. How will you manage the case?
6. How will you manage the patient in labor?
7. How will you manage the patient in postnatal period?
8. What are the family planning advices given after delivery?
9. What are the indications for MTP in heart disease?
10. What are the heart diseases with maximum mortality during pregnancy?
11. What are the precipitating factors for cardiac failure during pregnancy?
12. How will you manage a patient with cardiac failure during pregnancy?
13. How will you manage a patient who is on anticoagulants during pregnancy?

6 Postcesarean Pregnancy

Introduction

The incidence of cesarean section (CS) is on an increase across the world and with the rise in the number of primary cesarean deliveries, postcesarean pregnancies have become common in current practice. The most important aspect of management of a postcesarean pregnancy is the decision making on the mode of delivery—whether to allow for vaginal birth after cesarean (VBAC)/trial of labor after cesarean (TOLAC) or to perform an elective repeat cesarean section/delivery (ERCS/ERCD). This chapter deals with the clinical aspects of a case of postcesarean pregnancy which includes the following:

- Antenatal management of a postcesarean pregnancy
- Decision on the mode of delivery—VBAC/TOLAC or ERCS
- Management of VBAC/TOLAC
- Management of ERCS

Definition of CS

It is an operative procedure to deliver the fetus after the period of viability, through incisions on the abdominal wall and the uterus.

Note
- *Removal of the fetus from the peritoneal cavity following uterine rupture or in case of abdominal pregnancy is termed laparotomy and is not included in CS.*
- *Removal of abortus from the uterus (i.e., before the period of viability) through an incision on the uterus is termed hysterotomy.*

INDICATIONS FOR CS

See Table 6.1

Table 6.1 Indications for CS

Nonrecurrent indications (more common)	Recurrent indications
• Maternal – Cephalopelvic disproportion – Failed induction – Nonprogress of labor – Antepartum hemorrhage ▪ Major degree placenta previa ▪ Abruptio placentae with unfavorable cervix or fetal distress • Fetal – Fetal distress – Malpresentations—breech, brow, mentoposterior face – Multiple pregnancy—first twin nonvertex presentation – Cord prolapse/cord presentation – Macrosomia – Vasa previa	• Contracted pelvis • Previous classical scar • Previous two or more CS • Previous uterine rupture • Previous hysterotomy • Previous vesicovaginal fistula repair • Cervical or vaginal stenosis • Previous myomectomy where cavity has been entered

Common indications of CS

- Fetal distress
- Failed induction
- Non progress of labor
- Previous lower-segment cesarean section (LSCS)
- Cephalopelvic disproportion (CPD)
- Breech presentation

Reasons for increasing trend in performing CS

The various reasons for the increasing trend in performing CS are as follows:

- Probable overdiagnosis of fetal distress and increased rate of CS due to continuous cardiotocography (CTG) monitoring of fetal heart rate (FHR) during labor
- Increased rate of CS for breech presentation (obstetricians nowadays are afraid of the increasing number of litigations in this field)
- Decreased skill and experience in conducting vaginal instrumental deliveries (obstetricians nowadays prefer CS to difficult vaginal delivery)
- Increased rate of induction of labor (CS rate increases due to failed induction)
- Low threshold for performing CS in precious pregnancies such as in elderly primigravida, bad obstetric history, and pregnancy following infertility treatment
- Fear of medicolegal litigation for alleged neglect in vaginal delivery (lowers the threshold for performing CS during labor)
- Increased rate of repeat CS in women with previous cesarean deliveries due to fear of scar rupture

TYPES OF CS

CS may be classified based on the timing of CS, number of CS, and the type of uterine incision (Table 6.2).

PREGNANCY WITH PREVIOUS CS

Note

- *The most important risk in pregnancy with previous CS is the risk of uterine scar rupture.*
- *The most important concern in pregnancy with previous CS is the decision regarding the mode of delivery—whether VBAC or PRCS.*
- *The terms scar dehiscence and scar rupture while discussing a case of postcesarean pregnancy refer to the uterine scar.*

Part 1

Table 6.2 Types of CS

According to timing of performing CS	Elective CS: CS done at prearranged time to ensure best surgical conditions	Emergency CS: CS done due to unforeseen complications arising during pregnancy or labor
According to number of CS	Primary CS: CS done for the first time	Repeat CS: CS done in a woman with previous CS
According to type of uterine incision (Figure 6.1)	Classical or upper-segment CS	• Lower-segment cesarean section – Lower-segment transverse incision (Kerr's incision): It is the most common type of incision for CS – Lower-segment vertical incision (Kronig's incision): It may be rarely performed in preterm cases where the lower segment is not well formed

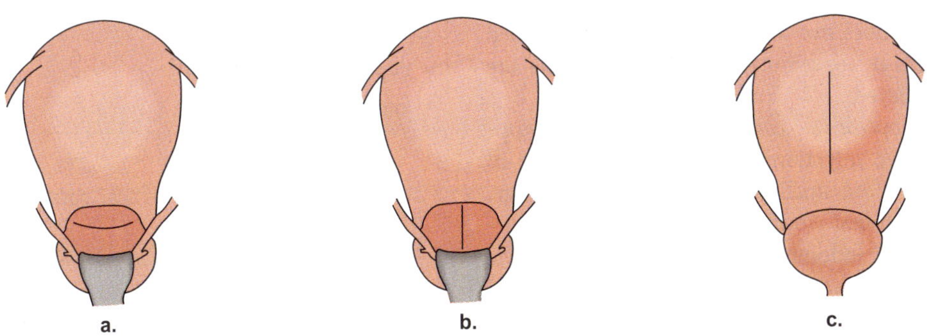

Figure 6.1 Types of uterine incision. **a.** Lower-segment transverse incision. **b.** Lower-segment vertical incision. **c.** Upper segment incision or classical cesarean section.

Factors that determine the mode of delivery in a woman with previous cesarean pregnancy

- **Type of previous CS:** Whether the previous CS was a classical CS or a LSCS (a previous classical CS is an absolute indication for performing an elective CS)
- **Integrity of the lower-segment scar:** Integrity of scar refers to how efficient a scar is to withstand the burden of the present pregnancy with regards to scar rupture. Integrity of the scar depends on the following factors:
  - *Whether previous LSCS was an elective CS/emergency CS*: Elective cesarean scar is expected to be more sound (risk of infection tends to be more in an emergency CS and can lead to a weak scar).
  - *Indication for CS*: Scar tends to be weak in previous CS done for indications such as prolonged labor, obstructed labor, second-stage CPD, and placenta previa; success rate of VBAC is more in previous CS done for indications such as fetal distress and breech presentation.
  - *Operative skill of the surgeon*: The integrity of the scar may depend on the operative skill of the surgeon.
  - *Extension of uterine incision*: Scar may be weak in cases of inverted T- and J-shaped uterine incisions (Figure 6.2) and in case of angle extension of the lower segment incision, involving the uterine vessels.
  - *Technique of uterine closure*: Traditionally, uterine incision is closed in two layers. Some data suggest that single layer closure is associated with a greater risk of rupture. Other studies suggests that single/double-layer closure does not affect scar integrity provided perfect approximation and hemostasis are achieved.
  - *Postoperative complications*: H/o postoperative infections indicated by presence of fever, foul-smelling lochia, wound discharge, abdominal wound gaping, secondary suturing of abdominal wound , etc., makes the uterine scar weak.
  - *Interpregnancy interval of <18 months*: It is said that, if the interpregnancy interval is <18 months, scar tends to be weak, increasing the chance of scar rupture in current pregnancy.
  - *Anterior placenta previa in current pregnancy*: It makes the scar weak due to implantation of the placenta at the site of previous uterine scar.
  - *Macrosomia and polyhydramnios in current pregnancy*: VBAC success rate decreases

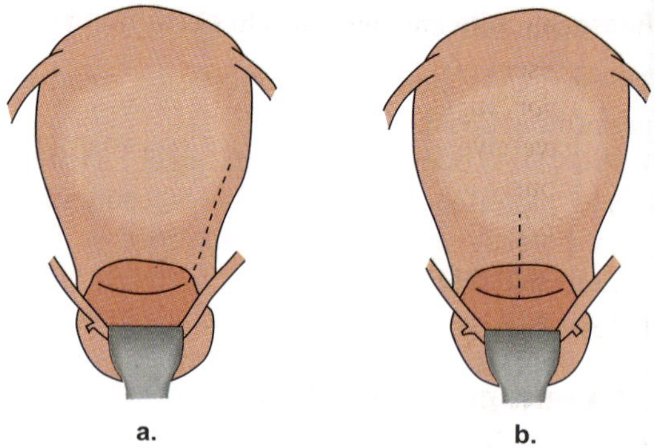

Figure 6.2 Extension of transverse uterine incision. **a.** J-shaped incision extending upward along one of the lateral edges of uterus. **b.** T-shaped incision extending into the upper segment of uterus.

Extra edge

Healing of uterine scar

- **With good approximation and perfect hemostasis:** Uterine scar heals by regeneration of smooth muscles. Scar healing and restoration of myometrium takes at least 6 months.
- **In case of inadequate approximation, incomplete hemostasis, or infection:** Uterine scar heals by formation of fibrous tissue with few regenerated smooth muscles leading to formation of a weak scar.

Factors that affect scar healing

Systemic factors

- Advancing age
- Poor nutrition
- Anemia
- Diabetes
- Infection
- Immunosuppression

Operative technique

- Imperfect approximation
- Imperfect hemostasis

with estimated fetal weight (EFW) >4 kg in present pregnancy.
- *Prior vaginal delivery*: Those women who have given birth vaginally at least once previously are more likely to have a successful VBAC.
- *Prior VBAC*: It is the single best predictor for successful VBAC and is associated with 90% VBAC success rate.
- *Maternal obesity*: As the maternal weight increases (body mass index >30), VBAC success rate decreases.

Case presentation

Salient points in history

Consider the following relevant points during history taking in cases of previous cesarean pregnancy.

Presenting complaints

- *Patient may not have any presenting complaints and may give the impression that she is admitted in view of previous CS*
- *H/o pain abdomen/bleeding P/V/leaking P/V*
- *Whether perceiving normal fetal movements*

H/o present pregnancy

Enquire history in each trimester

Past obstetric history

Note Past obstetric history is very important in cases with previous cesarean pregnancy and can be asked in detail.

Antenatal period

- *Whether she was booked and immunized?*
- *H/o any antenatal complications such as preeclampsia, gestational diabetes mellitus, and antepartum hemorrhage*
- *H/o blood transfusion (severe anemia can predispose to infection and anemia-induced hypoxia can affect scar healing)*
- *Name of the institution where the patient delivered (gives an idea about the techniques practiced during CS)*
- *The period of gestation when the patient was admitted to the hospital, and the reason if she was admitted prior to expected date of delivery*

Labor details

- *Was it spontaneous or induced labor?*
- *Was oxytocin used for labor augmentation?*
- *How long was the patient in labor?*
- *Ask for H/o prolonged rupture of membranes, H/o prolonged duration of labor (increased chance of ascending infection and intrapartum sepsis).*
- *Was the decision for LSCS taken in early labor or in the second stage of labor. Ask whether the patient was asked to bear down which indicates second stage (if LSCS is done for second-stage CPD, scar tends to be weak; VBAC is not allowed).*

Lower-segment cesarean section details

- *Elective or emergency CS (elective scar tends to be more sound than emergency scar)*
- *Indication for LSCS*
  - *Find out whether CS was done for a recurrent or a nonrecurrent indication (Integrity of scar is good in LSCS done for indications such as fetal distress and malpresentations; scar tends to be weak in LSCS done for indications such as obstructed labor and second-stage CPD)*

Procedure

- *What type of anesthesia was given—regional or general anesthesia (GA)? Usually CS is done under regional anesthesia; GA is given only for acute emergencies such as cord prolapse and rupture uterus.*
- *Type of uterine incision (check operative notes in discharge summary)*
  - *LSCS (most common type of CS—all CS are assumed to be LSCS unless specifically mentioned)*
  - *Classical CS (rarely performed nowadays, no role for trial of labor in prior classical scar)*

Check for the following details in previous discharge summary:

- *Intraoperative findings—any findings suggestive of obstructed labor such as edematous and drawn-up bladder and Bandl's ring*

(CONTD...)

(...CONTD)

- *Extension of uterine incision*
- *Technique of uterine closure—single layer/double-layer uterine closure (traditionally the uterus is closed in two layers; data on uterine incision repair and subsequent uterine rupture are unclear.)*
- *Baby details*
  - *Birth weight of baby—average/large size/small size*
  - *Whether cried immediately after birth*
  - *Time when breastfeeding was started*
  - *Whether the child is alive at present/healthy/________ years of age*
  - *If dead, cause of death (obstetric or nonobstetric cause)*

Postoperative period

- *Determine postoperative complications— H/o fever, pus discharge from wound site, and foul-smelling lochia (in cases with puerperal sepsis, the scar may be weak).*
- *Ask for H/o blood transfusion [indicates intraoperative hemorrhage/postpartum hemorrhage (PPH)].*
- *When was urinary catheter removed? (It is usually removed after 12–24 hours. Prolonged catheterization may be required in obstructed labor, bladder injury, etc.)*
- *When was skin suture removal done? (It is usually removed on the 6th–8th postoperative day.)*
- *Is there any history suggestive of wound gaping and secondary suturing? (When there is wound infection, there may be subclinical infection at underlying uterine incision, which can delay wound healing.)*
- *Determine the duration of stay of the patient in the hospital. When was she discharged?*
- *When did she resume her routine activities?*
- *Ask for H/o contraception following child birth. What was the method of contraception? How long was it used?*
- *Determine the duration of interpregnancy interval.*
- *Determine if there is any normal vaginal delivery before or after the CS. If yes, was it full term or preterm? (Prior H/o vaginal delivery increases the success rate of VBAC)*

Past history

- *H/o any medical illnesses (for anesthetic fitness and to look for complications during present pregnancy)*
- *Need to enquire about previous H/o any other uterine surgery like myomectomy (myomectomy with entry into uterine cavity increases the risk of scar rupture, hence VBAC is not allowed in such cases)*

Salient points in general examination

Consider the following relevant points during examination in cases of previous cesarean pregnancy:

- *Built and nutrition*
- *Height (height ≤145 cm is termed short stature—20% incidence of contracted pelvis; height <140 cm—40% incidence of contracted pelvis)*
- *Weight*
- *Pallor (anemia delays wound healing)*
- *Pedal edema*

Vitals

- *Pulse rate (maternal tachycardia is a sign of scar dehiscence)*
- *BP (patients with previous LSCS with associated obstetric complications such as preeclampsia—advisable to do repeat LSCS than allowing VBAC)*

Systemic examination

CVS and RS examination (for anesthetic fitness)

Obstetric examination

Inspection

- *In addition to the usual inspection findings, description of the previous cesarean scar has to be mentioned.*
- *Scar*
  - *Type of scar—midline vertical/paramedian/Pfannenstiel*
  - *Length of scar*
  - *Whether scar is healthy (healed by primary intention) or presence of any scar-related problems such as puckering/hypertrophy/keloid formation*
  - *Cough impulse at scar site is looked for (to rule out incisional hernia)*

(CONTD...)

(...CONTD)

Obstetric palpation

- *Fundal height and symphysiofundal height*
- *Fetal lie and presentation*
- *Check for scar tenderness (Figure 6.3).*
  - *Scar tenderness is checked for to assess the integrity of the lower segment uterine scar.*
  - *Scar tenderness is elicited by pressing below and behind the pubic symphysis while engaging the woman in conversation and noting for a visible wince.*
  - *If the patient is in labor, then scar tenderness is elicited in between contractions, when the uterus is relaxed.*
- *Amount of liquor*
- *Whether uterus is relaxed or acting*
- *Estimated fetal weight*

Auscultation

FHR (FHR abnormalities is one of the early signs of scar dehiscence)

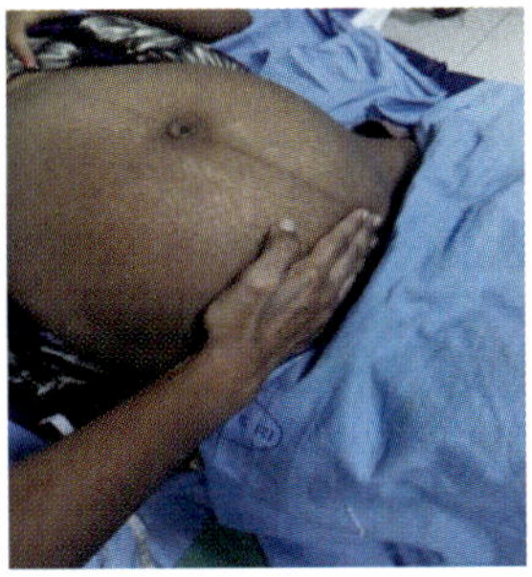

Figure 6.3 Checking for scar tenderness.

Pelvic examination

If VBAC is planned, pelvic assessment is done at or after 37 weeks:

- *To assess pelvis and to rule out CPD*
- *To assess cervix—dilatation, effacement, position, consistency, and station of the presenting part*

Note *Obstetric pelvic examination findings is expected only from postgraduates, if the patient is at term and is planned for VBAC.*

Case summary

An example of writing summary in cases of pregnancy with previous CS is given below.

Example *Mrs. S, 25 years of age, G2P1L1 at 38 + 4 weeks of gestation, is admitted for the past 2 days in view of postcesarean pregnancy. She was delivered by LSCS in previous pregnancy, indication being fetal distress with no history suggestive of any intra-op or post-op complications. She has no specific complaints. There is no history suggestive of labor pains or leaking P/V or bleeding P/V and she perceives normal fetal movements. On examination, there is no pallor or pedal edema. Her PR is 84/min and BP 120/70 mmHg. Obstetric examination reveals a term-size uterus with a singleton live fetus in cephalic presentation; head is not engaged. There is no scar tenderness. Liquor appears average and uterus is relaxed, FHR is 142 beats/min and regular.*

Case diagnosis

An example of writing diagnosis in cases of pregnancy with previous CS is given below.

Example *25 years of age, G21PL1, at 38 + 4 weeks of gestation, with postcesarean pregnancy, with a singleton live fetus in cephalic presentation, not in labor*

Case discussion

Note
- *Discussion in a case with previous cesarean pregnancy is mainly regarding risk of scar rupture and the mode of delivery in the current pregnancy—VBAC or PRCS.*
- *Chance of successful planned VBAC is 60–80%.*

Management of previous cesarean pregnancy

Antenatal management

- Pregnancy with previous LSCS is a high-risk pregnancy and the patient should be managed in a tertiary care institute.

Part 1

- Perform routine antenatal investigations.
- Accurate estimation of gestational age should be done from history, clinical examination, and ultrasonography (USG).
- Rule out associated obstetric complications such as preeclampsia and placenta previa.
- Advise on frequent antenatal visits after midpregnancy (once in 2 weeks).
- Ask for H/o pain abdomen and bleeding P/V, and check for scar tenderness during antenatal visits in the third trimester.
- Patient is usually admitted at 38 weeks of gestation or earlier if she has any complaints (e.g., pain abdomen, vaginal bleeding) or if she lives far away from the hospital. High-risk patients may be admitted near term for monitoring and timely decision.
- Perform an USG at term
  - To assess fetal growth and well-being
  - To estimate fetal weight
  - For placental localization
  - To assess uterine scar
    - Scar thickness
    - Any thinning of lower uterine segment/ wedge defect or "gutter sign" with collection of blood in the line of scar/loss of continuity of lower uterine segment
- Determine the mode of delivery—VBAC or elective repeat CS (integrity of the scar is the main factor in decision making. If there is any doubt regarding the integrity of the scar or there is a suspicion that scar might give way during labor, then it is prudent to do repeat CS).
- Explain the pros and cons (risks and benefits) of VBAC versus PRCS and discuss the decision objectively with the patient.

Extra edge

Prediction of chance of scar rupture based on the assessment of scar thickness on USG:

- Scar thickness >4.5 mm: Unlikely to rupture
- Scar thickness <2.5 mm: Scar dehiscence and rupture more likely

Disadvantages in assessing scar thickness:

- High inter observer variation
- Even a thick scar can rupture with onset of strong uterine contractions

- Final decision on the mode of delivery should be acceptable by the woman and the obstetrician, and should be taken prior to the expected date of delivery and should be documented. Written informed consent should be obtained for TOLAC.

Trial of labor after cesarean/vaginal birth after cesarean

Selection of candidates for VBAC—American College of Obstetricians and Gynecologists (ACOG) guidelines

- Not more than one previous LSCS
- No other uterine scars or previous uterine rupture
- Clinically adequate pelvis
- Obstetrician available throughout labor to monitor the labor and perform an emergency CS when indicated
- Availability of anesthesia and personnel for performing emergency CS

Criteria for selection of candidates for VBAC—elaborated

- **Factors to be considered from past obstetric history**
  - It should be a previous LSCS (previous classical scar, previous uterine rupture, hysterotomy scar, and inverted T incision are contraindications for VBAC)
  - Not more than previous one LSCS (previous two or more LSCS is an indication for repeat LSCS)
  - Good scar integrity: Integrity of scar depends on the following (discussed in detail earlier in this chapter):
    - Type of CS—LSCS/upper-segment CS
    - Elective/emergency CS
    - Indication for CS
    - Operative skill of the surgeon
    - Extension of uterine incision
    - Technique of uterine closure
    - Postoperative complications—fever, wound discharge, wound gaping, secondary suturing, etc.
    - Interpregnancy interval
    - Prior vaginal deliveries
- **Factors to be considered from current pregnancy**
  - No obstetric complications such as preeclampsia and placenta previa in current pregnancy

- Vertex presentation (no malpresentation, multiple pregnancy)
- Average estimated weight of the baby (macrosomia is a relative contraindication for VBAC)
- Adequate pelvis
- **Prerequisites for allowing VBAC**
  - VBAC should be allowed only in a tertiary care center with the following facilities—facilities for performing emergency CS, continuous monitoring during labor, blood transfusion, maternal intensive care unit and NICU facilities
  - Availability of expert obstetrician during labor to monitor the progress of labor and to perform emergency CS if necessary
  - Availability of anesthetist and anesthetic facilities for emergency CS
  - Informed consent of the patient

Note

- ***Criteria for selection of candidates for VBAC are summarized as follows:*** *"A patient with previous LSCS performed for nonrecurrent indication, wherein the integrity of scar is good, with no associated complications in the current pregnancy, with average size baby in cephalic presentation and adequate pelvis, may be allowed a vaginal delivery in a place where obstetrician is available to monitor labor, and anesthetist and facilities for emergency CS are available after taking informed consent."*
- ***Emergency CS:*** *Less than 30 minutes from the time of decision for CS to the time of start of surgery.*

Contraindications for VBAC

- Previous classical scar
- Previous T/J-shaped uterine incision
- Previous uterine rupture/hysterotomy
- Previous CS done for recurrent indications—contracted pelvis and vaginal/cervical stenosis
- Integrity of the scar is doubtful
- Medical/obstetric complications in present pregnancy (CPD, placenta previa, severe preeclampsia, bad obstetric history)
- Fetal macrosomic baby
- Inability to perform emergency CS due to nonavailability of facilities (obstetric, anesthetic, pediatric, blood bank facilities and personnel)
- Patient not consenting for VBAC

Benefits and risks of VBAC

These are given in Table 6.3.

Table 6.3 Benefits and risks of vaginal birth after cesarean (VBAC)

Benefits of VBAC	Risks or complications of VBAC
• Less hemorrhagic complications • Less pain • Early ambulation • Rapid recovery in postnatal period • Short hospital stay • Infectious morbidity is less • Complications related to CS procedure are avoided • Economical • Subsequent vaginal delivery becomes possible	• 1% risk of scar rupture • Complications associated with scar rupture—need for emergency laparotomy and/or hysterectomy due to hemorrhage, and need for blood transfusion • Increased perinatal morbidity and mortality associated with scar rupture

Success rates for VBAC About 50–60% patients with previous cesarean pregnancy are found eligible for VBAC after screening and 60–80% of them have a successful VBAC.

Scar rupture

Scar rupture is the main issue of concern during monitoring of a patient allowed for VBAC and has been elaborated prior to discussion on labor management of VBAC.

Definition

Scar rupture refers to giving way of the previous uterine scar.

Types (Figure 6.4)

- **Complete scar rupture:** It refers to disruption of the entire length of the scar including the visceral peritoneum. Fetus may lie in the peritoneal cavity and varying amount of internal hemorrhage is present.
- **Incomplete rupture or scar dehiscence**: It refers to disruption of the uterine scar but visceral peritoneum and fetal membranes are intact. Bleeding is minimal and small hematoma along the scar line may be present.

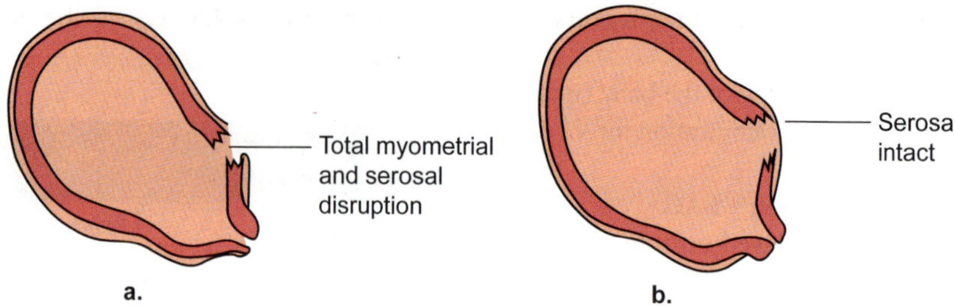

Figure 6.4 Types of scar rupture. **a.** Complete scar rupture. **b.** Incomplete rupture or scar dehiscence.

Symptoms and signs of scar dehiscence and scar rupture (Table 6.4)

Table 6.4 Symptoms and signs of scar dehiscence and scar rupture

	Scar dehiscence	Scar rupture
Symptoms	• Continuous abdominal pain persisting in between contractions • Suprapubic pain • Bladder tenesmus • Slight vaginal bleeding	• Severe pain followed by sensation of something giving way and sudden cessation of pain abdomen and uterine contractions • Probable fainting/collapse immediately following cessation of pain • Excessive vaginal bleeding • Gross hematuria • Possibility of presence of shoulder pain due to hemoperitoneum
Signs	• Unexplained maternal tachycardia (considered as the earliest sign of scar dehiscence) • Scar tenderness • FHR abnormalities (deceleration of FHR on CTG is a specific sign of uterine rupture) • Nonprogress of labor • Vaginal bleeding *Note:* • Suprapubic tenderness can also be due to cystitis and dense adhesions • We can also have silent scar dehiscence	• Signs of shock—thready and rapid pulse, hypotension, sweating, and restlessness Per abdominal findings: • Tenderness all over the abdomen • Superficially felt fetal parts • Loss of uterine contour—two hard globular structures are palpable (one is the contracted uterus and the other is the fetal head) • Free fluid in peritoneal cavity • Absent fetal heart sounds Per vaginal findings: • Excessive vaginal bleeding • Receding of presenting part and loss of station • Collapse of cervix due to receding of the presenting part

CTG, cardiotocography; *FHR*, fetal heart rate.

High-yield points

Scar rupture with various uterine incisions

Uterine incision	Scar rupture rate (%)
Classical scar	4–9
Inverted T incision	4–9
Low vertical	1–7
Low transverse	0.2–1.5

Scar rupture during labor

Labor	Rupture rate (%)
Spontaneous labor	0.4
Augmented labor	1
Induced labor	2.3
Induction with PGE2	1.3
Misoprostol	5.6

Management of labor in a patient allowed for VBAC

- Await spontaneous onset of labor, as spontaneous labor has a high success for vaginal delivery.
- Role of induction of labor: Induction of labor with prostaglandins and oxytocin is not practiced, as the risk of scar rupture increases with induction. Misoprostol is contraindicated as it induces strong uterine contractions and can lead to uterine rupture. However, sweeping of membranes and cervical ripening with Foley's catheter can be advocated for induction of labor in indicated cases.
- Oxytocin can be used for augmentation of labor with careful maternal and fetal monitoring.

I stage

- Following onset of labor, the patient is put on labor board.
- IV line is secured and blood sample is sent for cross-match and reservation.
- Patient is kept nil oral and IV fluids are given to maintain hydration (as patient may be taken up for emergency CS anytime during labor)
- Adequate analgesia is given—epidural analgesia can be given (advantage is that anesthesia can be given through the same epidural catheter, if patient is taken up for emergency CS. However, there is an opinion that epidural analgesia given during VBAC may mask the pain and one may miss signs of scar rupture/dehiscence)
- The anesthetist, OT staff, and pediatrician are kept informed about the case, in order to be prepared for emergency LSCS at any time during labor.
- Partogram is maintained to monitor maternal and fetal condition and the progress of labor.
- If facilities are available, continuous electronic FHR monitoring is done with CTG. Otherwise, perform intermittent auscultation of FHR with a stethoscope, every 15 minutes in the first stage and every 5 minutes in the second stage.
- Maternal monitoring: Monitor half-hourly pulse rate, hourly BP, and check for scar tenderness.
- Watch for symptoms and signs of scar dehiscence and scar rupture (newly occurring scar tenderness intrapartum is an important sign of scar dehiscence).
- Good uterine contraction, early engagement of head, progressive dilatation, and effacement of cervix with descent of fetal head are favorable factors indicating successful vaginal delivery.
- Perform emergency CS if the following are present:
  - Symptoms and signs of scar dehiscence or rupture
  - Failure of progress of labor
  - Fetal distress

> **High-yield points**
>
> **Epidural analgesia**
>
> Advantages
> - Patient can be taken up for emergency LSCS during labor with the epidural catheter
> - Instrumental deliveries can be easily performed
>
> Disadvantages
> - Can mask pain resulting from uterine scar rupture (however, the fear that it would mask the signs and symptoms of uterine rupture has not been substantiated)
> - Increased rate of instrumental deliveries

II stage

- FHR is monitored every 5 minutes.
- Watch for signs and symptoms of scar dehiscence and scar rupture.
- Prolonged second stage should not be allowed. If the patient does not deliver within 1 hour in second stage, cut short with prophylactic forceps or vacuum, provided all criteria for operative vaginal delivery are fulfilled—shortening the second stage reduces the strain on the uterine scar.

III stage

- Active management of third stage of labor (AMTSL) is practiced—IV/IM oxytocin following delivery of the baby, uterine massage, and delivery of placenta by controlled cord traction.
- Watch for any excessive bleeding.
- Usually, routine digital exploration of scar is not done if, on clinical examination, the placenta is complete and uterus is well retracted without any significant vaginal bleeding.
- The patient is kept under observation for 4 hours in labor room and then shifted to postnatal ward.
  - If the patient has excessive vaginal bleeding in the absence of uterine atony or if the patient's condition becomes unstable (rising pulse rate, falling BP, worsening pallor), then resuscitate

the patient, inform the senior consultant on call and simultaneously prepare for exploration of lower uterine segment under anesthesia in OT.

- In case of scar rupture, emergency laparotomy is performed.

Management of uterine scar rupture

- Resuscitation of the patient and shifting the patient for emergency laparotomy are carried out simultaneously.
- Two large-bore IV lines are secured and blood is arranged for transfusion.
- Informed written consent for emergency laparotomy and rent repair or hysterectomy (in case of uncontrolled hemorrhage or irreparable rent) is taken. Consent for sterilization is taken in multiparous women.
- Bladder is catheterized.
- Antacids, antiemetics, and antibiotics are given.
- Procedure should be performed by an experienced obstetrician.
- Under GA, abdomen is opened in layers.
- Baby in peritoneal cavity is quickly extracted out along with the placenta (if scar rupture has occurred during labor).
- If the scar rupture is linear without extension, then rent repair is done. Procedure can be combined with concurrent tubal sterilization in consenting women.
- If the edges are ragged with extension into major vessels or if bleeding is intractable, hysterectomy is performed to save the patient's life.
- Hemostasis is secured and abdomen is closed in layers.
- Anemia due to blood loss should be corrected with blood transfusion.
- Continue antibiotics in the postoperative period.

Extra edge

Pregnancy following previous uterine rupture

Previous uterine rupture	Risk of future uterine rupture
Lower-segment rupture	6%
Upper-segment rupture	32%

The risk of scar rupture in women with uterine anomalies is 8%.

Planned repeat CS or elective repeat CS

Indications

When VBAC is contraindicated due to any of the reasons discussed earlier, elective repeat CS is done.

Planned repeat CS—when to perform?

- It is usually performed at or after 39 completed weeks of gestation, after confirming the dates. Iatrogenic prematurity can be avoided and lower segment will be well formed when elective CS is performed close to EDD.
- In case the patient goes into labor prior to the waiting period, CS is performed at onset of labor.

Extra edge

Routine scar exploration

Routine scar exploration after successful vaginal delivery is controversial. We generally do not explore the uterine scar as a routine. Justification for and against routine scar exploration is given in the table below.

Table Justification for and against routine scar exploration

Justification for doing routine scar exploration	Justification for not doing routine scar exploration
• Some may advocate this to document scar integrity. The argument for routine scar exploration is: in a busy labor room when you do not have adequate manpower to monitor the patient postnatally, it is better to gently explore the scar prior to placental delivery when the os is still open • It is done by inserting two fingers into the uterine cavity and the lower-segment scar is gently palpated to check for its integrity	• It is considered as unnecessary and dangerous, as digital exploration might increase the silent defect and cause bleeding. Some recommend scar exploration only if abnormal bleeding or signs of shock are present • Most of the asymptomatic scar dehiscence heals well

High-yield points

Criteria for establishing POG of more than or equal to 39 weeks before doing elective CS:

- Crown-rump length (CRL) measured by USG at 6–11 weeks supports current period of gestation (POG) of ≥39 weeks.
- Clinical examination and USG performed at 16–24 weeks supports current POG of ≥39 weeks.
- It has been 20 weeks since FHR has been documented by stethoscope or 30 weeks since FHR has been documented by Doppler.
- It has been 36 weeks since a positive serum or urine beta-hCG has been performed.
- If facilities are available, amniocentesis can be performed to assess fetal lung maturity before an elective CS [estimation of lecithin/sphingomyelin ratio (L:S) and phosphatidylglycerol].

Difficulties encountered while performing a repeat CS

- Hypertrophied scars or keloids may require skin excision.
- Difficult entry: Adhesions between various layers of abdominal wall makes the entry into the abdominal cavity and approach to lower segment difficult.
- There is risk of bowel and bladder injury while opening parietal peritoneum.
- Lower uterine segment may be inaccessible due to dense adhesions.
- Bladder may be drawn up due to adhesions. Bladder should be pushed down carefully before uterine incision to prevent bladder injury.
- Angle extension is more likely to occur in a repeat CS due to the previous scarring.
- Placenta previa and adherent placenta are more common in previous CS.
- PPH is more common during a repeat CS. This may be due to uterine atonicity, injury to uterine vessels, or morbidly adherent placenta.

Hence, repeat CS should preferably be performed by an experienced surgeon to tackle the difficulties and complications encountered.

Repeat CS is performed as an elective procedure. If the patient goes into labor during the waiting period or if the LMP is not reliable and dates are not confirmed, then CS is performed at the onset of labor. Advantages and disadvantages of performing elective repeat CS and CS at onset of labor are given in Tables 6.5 and 6.6.

Table 6.5 Advantages and disadvantages of performing an elective repeat CS

Advantages	Disadvantages
• Patient is well prepared for the surgery— kept nil oral for 8 hours before surgery (lessens the risk of Mendelson syndrome or aspiration, if general anesthesia is given) • Done during working hours, when senior consultants are available to tackle any complications • Risk of infection is less	• It can result in iatrogenic prematurity, if dates are not confirmed • Lower segment may not be well formed—risk of angle extension • Risk of atonic postpartum hemorrhage is more • Can lead to transient tachypnea of newborn

Table 6.6 Advantages and disadvantages of performing repeat CS at onset of labor

Advantages	Disadvantages
• Less chance of iatrogenic prematurity • Lower segment well formed • Risk of atonic postpartum hemorrhage is less	• Patient may be full stomach—may lead to aspiration, if general anesthesia is given • Risk of infection is more

Principle steps of LSCS

Please refer to Part 3, Chapter 37, *Common Obstetric Surgical Procedures* for preoperative preparation, principle steps, and postoperative care in CS

Types of skin incision

See Table 6.7 and Figure 6.5

Table 6.7 Types of skin incision

Pfannenstiel skin incision	• Transverse curvilinear incision above pubic hair line • Deepened through subcutaneous tissue up to rectus sheath • Rectus sheath divided transversely • The two recti muscles are laterally retracted
Joel-Cohen incision	• A modified transverse incision placed 3 cm below the line joining anterior superior iliac spines • The incision is placed higher than Pfannenstiel incision and is not curved
Maylard's skin incision	• It is an option when more exposure is needed in transverse incision • Rectus muscle is divided
Midline vertical incision	• Midline incision from a point just below umbilicus to a point above pubic symphysis

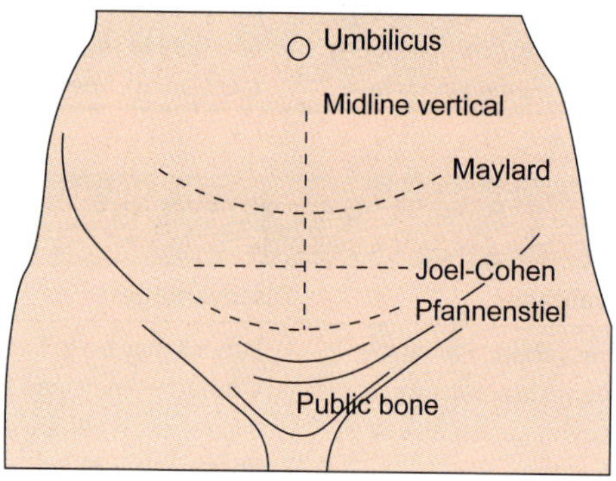

Figure 6.5 Types of skin incision for cesarean section.

Complications of CS

See Table 6.8

High-yield points

Advantages and disadvantages of midline and Pfannenstiel skin incisions are given in tables below.

Table Midline skin incision

Advantages	Disadvantages
• Entry into abdomen is quicker • Blood loss is less, as midline is less vascular	• More postoperative pain • More risk of burst abdomen
• Incision can be extended if required • Suitable for classical CS and rupture uterus	• More risk of incisional hernia • Less cosmetic

Table Pfannenstiel skin incision (see figure below)

Advantages	Disadvantages
• More postoperative comfort • Less chance of wound dehiscence • Less chance of incisional hernia • Cosmetically better	• Blood loss is slightly more when compared with that in midline incision • Incision cannot be extended unlike midline incision

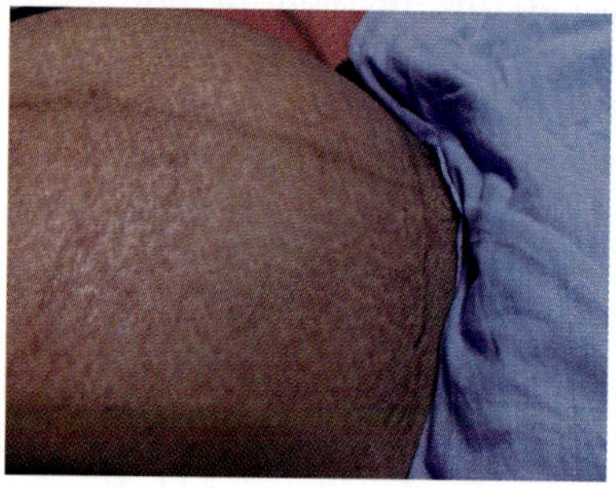

Figure Pfannenstiel scar in a woman with previous cesarean pregnancy.

Table 6.8 Complications of CS

Intraoperative	Postoperative	Delayed postoperative

• Anesthesia-related complications
  – Hypotension
  – Mendelson syndrome
• Hemorrhage
• Visceral injury—bladder, bowel
	• Paralytic ileus
	• Deep vein thrombosis
	• Infections—urinary tract infection, respiratory infections
		• Incisional hernia
		• Future obstetric complications such as scar rupture

Viva corner

Q1 Why is scar rupture more in a classical scar?

Wound healing is better in a lower-segment scar compared to a classical scar. Hence, risk of rupture is more in a classical scar. The table below shows the difference between lower-segment scar and upper-segment (classical) scar.

Table Lower-segment scar versus classical scar

Lower-segment scar	Upper-segment (classical) scar
• Perfect apposition of margins is possible	• Thick margins lead to poor approximation of edges
• Hematoma formation is less	• Hematoma formation is more due to imperfect apposition
• Healing is better as the wound is quiescent during healing process	• Healing is poor as the upper segment is contracting and retracting in postnatal period
• In future pregnancy, stretching is along the line of scar	• Stretching is at right angles to the scar
• Chance of scar being weakened by placental implantation is less	• Chance of scar being weakened by placental implantation on the scar is more
• Chance of scar rupture 0.2–1.5%	• Chance of scar rupture 4–9%

Frequently asked viva questions

1. Summarize the case.
2. What is the diagnosis?
3. What is the plan of management for the case?
4. What is the mode of delivery for the patient? Justify your answer.
5. What are the advantages of VBAC?
6. How will you monitor the patient allowed for VBAC during labor?
7. How will you elicit scar tenderness?
8. What are the symptoms and signs of scar rupture?
9. What are the indications for repeat CS?
10. What are the difficulties encountered while performing a repeat CS?
11. What are the common indications for performing a CS?
12. What are the complications of CS?

7 Post-Term Pregnancy

Introduction

A pregnancy that continues beyond 42 completed weeks of gestation is termed post-term pregnancy and it is associated with significant perinatal morbidity and mortality. Estimation of accurate period of gestation (POG) helps in the correct diagnosis and appropriate management of these cases. Confirmation of POG, fetal surveillance, and induction of labor are the main aspects of clinical discussion in a case of post-term pregnancy and has been dealt in this chapter.

Definitions

- **Prolonged pregnancy/post-term pregnancy:** It refers to pregnancy continuing beyond 42 weeks of gestation or >294 days from the day of last menstrual period, assuming that the dates are correct (FIGO, WHO). The incidence is 10%.
- **Postdated pregnancy:** It refers to pregnancy continuing beyond 40 weeks of gestation, that is, continuing after the expected date of delivery (EDD).
- **Postmaturity syndrome:** It refers to characteristic features seen in 10–20% of neonates born in cases of prolonged pregnancy. It is a postnatal diagnosis of the newborn.

Note
- *Twenty percent of post-term babies show features of postmaturity syndrome.*
- *Twenty percent of post-term babies are macrosomic.*

Causes for post-term pregnancy

Post-term pregnancy is considered to be associated with the factors mentioned in Table 7.1. However, in many instances, no cause can be attributed for pregnancy going post-term.

Table 7.1 Causes attributed to post-term pregnancy

Maternal	Fetal	Placental
• Wrong dates (most common cause) • Primigravida—more common in primigravida • Elderly gravida • Sedentary lifestyle • Previous history of post-term pregnancy • Family history	• Fetal anomalies such as anencephaly, adrenal hypoplasia	• Placental sulfatase deficiency

Note
- *POG is the most important parameter to be assessed in cases of postdated and post-term pregnancy, as the diagnosis and management are based on the calculated POG. Hence, menstrual history is very important.*
- *Wrong date is the most common cause of postdated and post-term pregnancy. If the dates are not reliable or if the patient is not sure of her last menstrual period (LMP), correct POG has to be assessed from clinical examination and ultrasound.*
- *Twenty percent of women do not remember their exact LMP.*
- *Only 5% of women deliver on the exact EDD. Others deliver either 2 weeks earlier or 1 week later.*

Last menstrual period (LMP) is reliable in the calculation of the POG if the following are fulfilled:
- The patient remembers her LMP accurately.
- The patient had normal, regular menstrual cycles prior to conception.

- There is no history of oral contraceptive pill intake for 3 months prior to conception.
- The patient is not lactating and there is no H/o recent abortion.

Case presentation

Salient points in history

Consider the following relevant points during history taking in cases of postdated pregnancy:

- *LMP*
- *Regularity of the menstrual cycles before conception (last three cycles)*
- *H/o oral contraceptive pill use prior to conception (ovulation may be slightly delayed following stoppage of the pills)*
- *Whether conceived during lactation or following a recent abortion*

Presenting complaints

- *The patient may not have any specific complaints. She may say that she has been admitted as her pregnancy has crossed the expected date of delivery.*
- *Ask for H/o labor pains, leaking P/V or bleeding P/V.*
- *Whether she is perceiving normal fetal movements*

History of present pregnancy

- *Whether dating scan was done in the first trimester*
- *Date of quickening*
- *Whether anomaly scan was done in the second trimester and told to be normal*
- *H/o any high-risk factors such as preeclampsia, gestational diabetes mellitus, and antepartum hemorrhage (APH) which precludes expectant management*

Past obstetric history

- *H/o pregnancy crossing EDD in previous pregnancies*
- *Whether had spontaneous onset of labor or induced labor*
- *H/o any abortion prior to conception*

Salient points in general examination

Consider the following relevant points during examination in cases of postdated pregnancy.

Obstetric examination

- *Fundal height—term-size uterus*
- *Symphysiofundal height (SFH)*
- *Assessment of fetal lie and presentation*
- *Whether the presenting part is engaged or not*
- *Whether liquor appears normal or reduced (if oligohydramnios is present, uterus will feel full of fetus with crowding of fetal parts)*
- *Feel of the head—whether head feels term or preterm*
- *Clinically estimated fetal weight*

Vaginal examination (expected from postgraduate students)

- *Feel of the head in vertex presentation (hard skull bones may be felt through the cervix or vaginal fornix, indicating fetal maturity)*
- *Cervical assessment—Bishop's score (for induction of labor)*
- *Pelvic assessment to rule out cephalopelvic disproportion (CPD)*

Case summary

An example of writing summary in cases of postdated pregnancy is given below.

Example *Mrs. G, 28 years of age, primigravida at 40 + 5 weeks of gestation, has been admitted for safe confinement. She has no significant complaints. She is perceiving normal fetal movements and there is no H/o leaking P/V, bleeding P/V, or labor pains. On examination, there is no pallor or pedal edema. Her vitals are normal. Obstetric examination reveals a singleton live fetus in cephalic presentation. Uterus is relaxed, liquor appears average, and fetal heart rate (FHR) is 148 beats/min, regular.*

(CONTD...)

(...CONTD)

Case diagnosis

An example of writing diagnosis in cases of postdated pregnancy is given below.

Example *28 years of age, primigravida at 40 + 5 weeks of gestation, with postdated pregnancy with a singleton live fetus in cephalic presentation, not in labor*

Case discussion

Significance of post-term pregnancy

- There is significant rise in perinatal mortality when the pregnancy crosses 42 weeks of gestation. Perinatal mortality increases sixfold after 42 weeks when compared with that of 37–41 weeks.
- Placental aging results in placental dysfunction and insufficiency that leads to increased perinatal mortality and morbidity in post-term pregnancy.
- In some cases, the placenta continues to function and the fetus continues to grow, resulting in macrosomia.

Complications of post-term pregnancy

Maternal complications

Post-term pregnancy as such is not a risk for the mother.

- Increased morbidity may be due to increased operative interferences.

Fetal complications

Fetal complications are mentioned in Table 7.2.

Postmaturity/dysmaturity syndrome

It refers to the characteristic features seen in 20% of neonates born post-term. The features include the following:

- Dry skin with wrinkling and desquamation of epidermis (peeling of skin)
- Meconium staining of skin and umbilical cord
- Absence of vernix and lanugo hair
- Loss of subcutaneous fat and muscle mass
- Long thin limbs
- Overgrown nails and hair
- Scaphoid abdomen
- Attentive apprehensive look

Management of postdated pregnancy

Obstetric management in a postdated pregnancy is based on the following:

- Determination of accurate POG
- Fetal surveillance (assessment of fetal well-being)

Table 7.2 Fetal complications in post-term pregnancy

Antepartum	Intrapartum	Neonatal
• Fetal hypoxia and intrauterine death can occur due to – Oligohydramnios – Placental insufficiency resulting from placental aging and infarcts	• Fetal hypoxia and intrapartum death can occur due to – Placental insufficiency – Cord compression resulting from ▪ Oligohydramnios ▪ Decrease in Wharton's jelly – Meconium aspiration • Prolonged labor can occur due to – Hard skull bones – Macrosomia (20% of cases) – Shoulder dystocia • Birth trauma can occur due to – Shoulder dystocia in macrosomic babies – Increased operative interferences	• Meconium aspiration syndrome can lead to chemical pneumonitis, atelectasis, pulmonary hypertension, and respiratory failure • Hypothermia • Hypoglycemia (due to poor glycogen reserve) • Polycythemia • Increased neonatal intensive care unit admissions

Note
- *High-risk pregnancies must not be allowed to become postdated. In these cases, delivery is preferred around 39–40 weeks of gestation.*
- *Pregnancy is not allowed to continue post-term, as the rate of antepartum stillbirths increases significantly after 42 weeks. Patients are delivered before reaching 42 weeks and hence the management involves mainly the postdated pregnancy, that is, beyond 40 weeks and up to 42 weeks of gestation.*

Determination of accurate period of gestation

- Accurate estimation of POG is the first step in the management of postdated pregnancy (often a pregnancy is incorrectly classified as post-term because of wrong dates).
- POG is determined from history (LMP), clinical examination, and ultrasonography (USG) assessment as described in the following sections.

Assessment of gestational age from history

- Date of LMP—check whether the patient's LMP is reliable (it should be a known normal LMP, with regular 28-day cycle, no recent use of OCPs prior to conception, not conceived during lactation or following recent abortion)

If the patient does not remember her LMP or is not sure of LMP, other points in history that can help in calculating the POG are as follows:

- Date of first positive urine pregnancy test (UPT)—UPT becomes positive at 4–5 weeks following LMP (not a reliable method if LMP is not known/irregular)
- Date of quickening—quickening is felt at 18–20 weeks in primigravida, and 16–18 weeks in multigravida (patient may not remember date of quickening)
- Patient who has conceived following infertility treatment—date of hCG injection, if conceived on ovulation induction, or date of embryo transfer in in vitro fertilization (IVF) pregnancy is documented and known
- Date of single fruitful coitus (+266 days)— may be used in rape victims

Assessment of gestational age from clinical examination

- Bimanual examination in early weeks of gestation for uterine size (replaced by USG for dating of pregnancy these days)
- Abdominal examination—fundal height and SFH (whether correlating with POG calculated from LMP); fetal parts are palpable by 20 weeks
- FHR—auscultation can be performed with stethoscope from 20 weeks onward

Part 1

Viva corner

Q1 What are excellent, good, and bad dates?

Excellent dates

- In women with adequate clinical information:
  - Women with adequate clinical information (known normal LMP, 28-day cycle, no recent use of OCPs, with fundal height correlating with gestational age) and with one USG done between 16 and 24 weeks of gestation correlating with clinically estimated gestational age
- In women with inadequate clinical information:
  - Women with inadequate clinical information and with two USG examinations done between 16 and 24 weeks of gestation showing linear fetal growth and similar EDD

Good dates

- In women with adequate clinical information:
  - Women with adequate clinical examination (known normal LMP, 28-day cycle, no recent use of OCPs, with uterine size in correlation with gestational age) and with one USG obtained after 24 weeks of gestation correlating with clinical estimated gestational age
- In women with inadequate clinical examination:
  - Women with inadequate clinical examination and with two or more USG examinations done after 24 weeks of gestation showing linear growth and similar EDD

Poor dates

- Any situation other than those mentioned above

Assessment of gestational age from ultrasound

Accuracy of ultrasound in estimating POG is mentioned in Table 7.3.

Table 7.3 Accuracy of ultrasound in estimating period of gestation (POG)

Timing of ultrasound	Parameters assessed	Accuracy in estimating POG
First trimester	CRL	±1 week (most accurate in calculating POG)
Second trimester	BPD/FL	±2 weeks
Third trimester	BPD, HC, AC, FL • Distal femoral epiphysis appears by 36–37 weeks • Proximal tibial epiphysis appears by 38–40 weeks	±3 weeks

AC, abdominal circumference; *BPD*, biparietal diameter; *CRL*, crown-rump length; *FL*, femoral length; *HC*, head circumference.

Note *When there is a discrepancy between LMP-based and USG-based EDD by more than 1 week in the first trimester or by more than 2 weeks in the second trimester, USG parameters are considered for determination of POG and EDD.*

Assessment of gestational age from biochemical tests

Biochemical tests on amniotic fluid collected from amniocentesis indicate only the fetal maturity and not the exact POG. Hence, these tests are not done for the purpose of estimating POG.

Assessment of fetal well-being

There is an increased risk of oligohydramnios and fetal hypoxia in post-term pregnancy, and hence it is advisable to start fetal surveillance from 40 weeks. Assessment of fetal well-being is outlined in the following sections (a detailed description of antepartum and intrapartum fetal surveillance is provided in Part 3, Chapter 36, *Antepartum and Intrapartum Fetal Surveillance Tests*).

Assessment of fetal well-being from history

- Daily fetal movement chart (DFMC): Ask th patient to maintain a fetal kick count chart.
  - Cardiff's count to 10: Ask the patient to star counting fetal movements from a particula time of the day and to stop counting when 1 movements are perceived. Ten fetal movement over a 12-hour period ensure fetal well-being.
  - Sadowsky's count: Ask the patient to coun the fetal movements for 1 hour followin each meal, three times a day. The total coun multiplied by four gives the total fetal move ments in 12 hours. When the patient perceive no movements or less than 10 movements i 12 hours, she must report to her doctor.
  - Fetal movements considerably decreas 24–48 hours before fetal demise.

Assessment of fetal well-being from clinical examination

- Palpation of fetal movements during examinatior
- Auscultation of FHR

Assessment of fetal well-being from biophysical studies

- **Nonstress test (NST):** It is based on the principl that there is acceleration of FHR with feta movements in a normal non-asphyxiated fetus.
  - *Reactive NST*: There should be at least 2 feta heart rate accelerations, by 15 beats abov baseline, lasting for at least 15 seconds, ove a period of 20 minutes (Figures 7.1 and 7.2).
- **Biophysical profile (BPP) or Manning's score** Based on USG and NST (Table 7.4).
  - Total score is 10.
  - Disadvantage of BPP: It is time consuming.

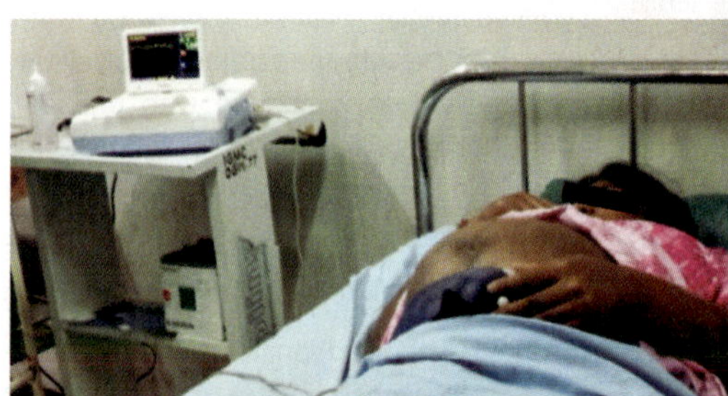

Figure 7.1 Nonstress test procedure being done o a patient.

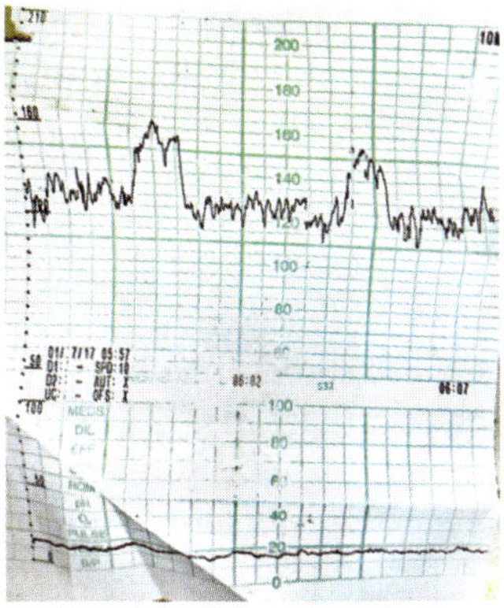

Figure 7.2 A reactive nonstress test.

Table 7.4 Biophysical profile

Component	Normal	Score
Fetal body movement	3/30 min	2
Fetal breathing movement	1/30 min	2
Fetal tone	1/30 min	2
Amniotic fluid volume [single deepest pocket (SDP)]	>2	2
Nonstress test	Reactive	2

- **Modified biophysical profile (AFI + NST)**
  - *Advantage:* Done in a short time period when compared with BPP
  - Most common method used to assess fetal well-being

Doppler waveform studies

Absent/reversed diastolic flow in fetal umbilical vessels indicates fetal jeopardy.

Viva corner

Q1 What are the uses of USG in postdated pregnancy?

In a postdated pregnancy, USG is used to assess the following:

- Fetal growth
- Amount of liquor
- Placental grading
- Estimated fetal weight
- Fetal well-being: BPP and Doppler studies

Extra edge

Pathophysiology of post-term pregnancy

- Placental function starts declining after 36 weeks of pregnancy. Structural changes in placenta such as infarcts, calcification, and decreased thickness develop beyond term resulting in utero placental insufficiency.

Amniotic fluid volume

- Amniotic fluid index is a marker of fetal well-being. Reduced amniotic fluid indicates chronic hypoxia.
- Oligohydramnios in post-term is due to uteroplacental insufficiency which leads to reduced fetal renal blood flow and fetal urine output.
- Amniotic fluid volume is maximum at 36–38 weeks, following which it starts to diminish gradually.
- Volume of amniotic fluid:
  - 36–38 weeks: 1 L (maximum)
  - 40 weeks: 800 mL
  - 42 weeks: <500 mL
  - 43 weeks: 200 mL

Protocol for management of postdated pregnancy

- Confirm the POG from LMP and early trimester scans. This step is done even in women who are sure of their LMP (20% of women do not remember their exact LMP).
- Rule out associated complications such as diabetes, preeclampsia, APH, Rh incompatibility, bad obstetric history (BOH), and intrauterine growth restriction. Postdatism is not allowed in high-risk pregnancies.
- Assess fetal well-being: Modified BPP (AFI + NST) is usually done for fetal surveillance.
- Assess pelvis for adequacy.
- If the dates are confirmed and if there are no maternal or fetal indications for termination of pregnancy, pregnancy can be continued up to 41 weeks with fetal surveillance [daily fetal movement count and twice-weekly modified BPP (AFI + NST) are usually done for fetal surveillance].
- Stripping or sweeping of membranes at 40 weeks may be helpful in spontaneous onset of labor within the next few days and reduces the number of pregnancies going post-term.

Part 1

- With this expectant management, most of the patients will go into spontaneous labor by 41 weeks.
- If the patient does not go into spontaneous labor by 41 weeks, induction of labor is done at 41 weeks.
- Induction of labor is done at 41 weeks for the following reasons:
  - Reduces perinatal mortality by 80% compared with expectant management (risk of perinatal morbidity and mortality is high after 42 weeks of gestation and hence we aim for delivery before 42 weeks of gestation, i.e., between 41 and 42 weeks)
  - Improves maternal satisfaction
  - Is cost-effective
- Cesarean section is done only for obstetric indications such as CPD, previous LSCS, malpresentations, fetal distress, failed induction, and nonprogress of labor.

Induction of labor

- Method of induction depends on the cervical assessment (Bishop's score) (induction of labor has been elaborated in Part 1, Chapter 17, *Supplementary Topics*).
  - *Bishop's score* ≥6: Indicates favorable cervix → oxytocin and/or artificial rupture of membranes (ARM) → vaginal delivery
  - *Bishop's score* <6: Indicates unfavorable cervix → cervix is ripened with Foley's catheter/PGE2 → favorable cervix → oxytocin and/or ARM → vaginal delivery

Note *Induction of labor can be asked in detail during case discussion on postdated pregnancy.*

Intrapartum management

I stage

- IV line is secured, and blood is sent for cross-matching and reservation.
- Admission cardiotocography (CTG) is done to assess fetal well-being.
- The patient is put in left lateral position.
- Maintain adequate analgesia and hydration.
- Partogram is maintained to monitor maternal and fetal condition and progress of labor.
- Continuous electronic FHR monitoring is advisable. If facilities are not available, then intermittent auscultation is done with stethoscope every 15 minutes in the first stage and every 5 minutes in the second stage (anticipate intrapartum asphyxia).
- Early ARM is usually preferred. However, the role of doing an early ARM is controversial.
  - Advantages of early ARM
    - Early detection of meconium
    - Hastens the progress of labor
    - Can insert scalp electrode or intrauterine pressure catheter for better monitoring
    - Can perform scalp pH monitoring
  - Disadvantage of early ARM
    - ARM can further reduce the amount of amniotic fluid and can lead to cord compression.
- Amnioinfusion: Infusion of 500–1000 mL of isotonic fluid such as warm normal saline through intrauterine catheter is beneficial in cases with repetitive variable deceleration by reducing/relieving cord compression.

II stage

- FHR is monitored every 5 minutes in the second stage of labor.
- Instrumental delivery may be required for prolonged second stage.
- Anticipate shoulder dystocia in cases with suspected macrosomic baby.
- Following delivery of fetal head, suctioning of oropharynx is done to prevent meconium aspiration.
- Neonatologist should be present at the time of delivery for resuscitation in cases with meconium- stained liquor.

III stage

Active management of third stage of labor is done.

Postpartum management

Contraception counseling is given

MECONIUM ASPIRATION SYNDROME

Meconium refers to the first intestinal discharge from the newborns. It is a viscous, dark green substance composed of intestinal epithelial cells, lanugo, mucus, and intestinal secretions.

- Meconium is sterile, which differentiates it from stools.

Viva corner

Q1 How can post-term pregnancy be reduced?

- Dating USG in the first trimester helps to accurately estimate the gestational age.
- Sweeping of membranes from 38 weeks onward may help in spontaneous onset of labor.

Q2 What is the role of amnioinfusion in meconium-stained liquor?

- Intrauterine infusion of warm saline 500–1000 mL (amnioinfusion) has been found to be useful to reduce cord compression in cases with repetitive variable decelerations

Advantages of amnioinfusion

- Reduces variable deceleration due to cord compression

Disadvantages of amnioinfusion

Amnioinfusion can result in:

- Cord prolapse
- Uterine scar rupture
- Intrauterine infection
- Abruption
- Amniotic fluid embolism

ACOG (2006) committee opinion on amnioinfusion

"Large proportion of women with meconium-stained amniotic fluid have infants who have taken in meconium within the trachea or bronchioles before meconium passage has been noted, and before amnioinfusion can be performed; meconium passage may predate labor. Based on current literature, routine prophylactic amnioinfusion for the dilution of meconium-stained amniotic fluid is not recommended. However, amnioinfusion remains a reasonable approach in the treatment of repetitive variable decelerations, regardless of amniotic fluid meconium status."

Types of meconium-stained liquor

- Thin meconium-stained liquor
  - It is yellow or light green and watery in consistency.
  - Vaginal delivery can be allowed with CTG monitoring.
- Thick meconium-stained liquor
  - It is dark brown and pasty in consistency (due to decreased liquor).
  - Emergency LSCS is done if the cervix is unfavorable.

Meconium aspiration syndrome (MAS) refers to the respiratory distress in the newborn, resulting from aspiration of meconium-stained amniotic fluid, which can occur before, during, or immediately following delivery.

- Fetal distress resulting from placental insufficiency, oligohydramnios, infection, and acidosis promotes the passage of meconium in utero.
- Fetal hypoxic stress causes vagal stimulation that leads to intestinal peristalsis and relaxation of the anal sphincter, resulting in passage of meconium in utero.
- Meconium is rarely found in the amniotic fluid prior to 34 weeks' gestation and therefore MAS affects only neonates born at term or post-term.

Incidence Twenty percent of fetuses have meconium- stained liquor at delivery, out of which 10% have risk of MAS.

Extra edge

Causes for respiratory distress in meconium aspiration syndrome

- Mechanical obstruction of airways due to meconium particles
- Chemical pneumonitis—inflammatory response due to release of inflammatory mediators such as cytokines and leukotrienes
- Inhibition of endogenous surfactant function by meconium, which leads to reduced lung compliance and hypoventilation

Diagnosis

- There is yellowish meconium staining of the skin, nail, and the umbilical cord of the newborn.
- Newborn may have tachypnea, cyanosis, bradycardia, or low Apgar scores.
- Meconium may be visible below the vocal cords on performing a laryngoscopy.
- These infants usually progress to develop respiratory distress syndrome within few hours after birth.

Part 1

- Investigations to confirm the diagnosis:
  - *Chest x-ray*: Shows lung hyperinflation, diaphragmatic flattening, cardiomegaly, patchy atelectasis, and consolidation
  - *Arterial blood gas (ABG) analysis*: Shows decreased oxygen levels

Management

- Ventilatory support often required for newborns with MAS
- Inhaled nitrous oxide (iNO)
- Surfactant therapy
- Extracorporeal membrane oxygenation (ECMO) - final rescue therapy

Complications of meconium aspiration syndrome in the newborn

- Pneumothorax
- Persistent pulmonary hypertension of the newborn
- Associated with high morbidity and mortality

Extra edge

ACOG updated recommendations on delivery of a newborn with Meconium-Stained liquor (MSL)

- *Routine prophylactic amnioinfusion for the dilution of MSL is not recommended.* This is because a large proportion of women with MSL have infants who have taken in meconium within the trachea or bronchioles before meconium passage has been noted and before amnioinfusion can be performed and the meconium passage may predate labor. However, amnioinfusion remains a reasonable approach in the treatment of repetitive variable decelerations, regardless of amniotic fluid meconium status.
- Infants with MSL, regardless of whether they are vigorous or not, should no longer routinely receive intrapartum suctioning. However, MSL is a condition that requires the notification and availability of Neonatology team with full resuscitation skills, including endotracheal intubation.
- Resuscitation should follow the same principles for infants with MSL as for those with clear fluid.
- Routine intubation and tracheal suctioning are no longer recommended for infants born through MSL.
  - Infant is vigorous with good respiratory effort and muscle tone:
    - Gentle clearing of meconium from the mouth and nose with a bulb syringe may be done.
  - Infant born through MSL has poor muscle tone and inadequate breathing efforts:
    - The initial steps of resuscitation should be completed under the radiant warmer.
    - Appropriate intervention to support ventilation and oxygenation should be initiated as indicated for each neonate and, if the airway is obstructed, this may include intubation and suction.
    - This new recommendation to no longer routinely suction nonvigorous neonate is to emphasis on prevention of harm (i.e., delay in providing bag-mask ventilation and potential consequences of unnecessary interventions) instead of the unknown benefit of routine tracheal intubation and suctioning.

Frequently asked viva questions

1. Summarize the case.
2. What is the diagnosis of the case?
3. What is your next step of management?
4. How will you confirm the patient's POG?
5. How will you assess fetal well-being?
6. What is the next step of management if the patient does not go into spontaneous labor?
7. When will you induce labor?
8. What are the risks of post-term pregnancy?
9. How will you monitor the patient in labor?
10. What is the role of amnioinfusion?

8 Multiple Pregnancy

Introduction

Pregnancy carrying more than one fetus is described as multiple pregnancy. Of late, advances in the management of infertility such as usage of ovulation induction drugs and assisted reproductive techniques have led to an increase in the incidence of multiple pregnancies. Case discussion of multiple pregnancy usually involves the following aspects that are dealt in this chapter:

- Types of multiple pregnancy
- Complications during pregnancy and labor
- Twin specific complications
- Antenatal and intrapartum management

Twin pregnancy is the most common multiple pregnancy; hence, discussion is mainly regarding twin pregnancy.

Definition

When more than one fetus develop simultaneously inside the uterus, it is termed multiple pregnancy. It is named twins, triplets, quadruplets, etc., depending on the number of fetuses that develop:

- **Two fetuses:** Twin pregnancy (most common)
- **Three fetuses:** Triplets
- **Four fetuses:** Quadruplets

Note *Pregnancies with three or more fetuses are referred to as higher order pregnancies or births.*

Types of twin pregnancy

Twin pregnancies can be monozygotic (MZ) or dizygotic (DZ) (see Tables 8.1 and 8.2; Figures 8.1 and 8.2).

Table 8.1 Types of twin pregnancy

Dizygotic twins	Monozygotic twins
• Fertilization of two ova released in the same cycle by two sperms	• Fertilization of one ova by a single sperm and the zygote thus formed divides at variable period following fertilization
• Accounts for two-third of cases of multiple pregnancy	• Accounts for one-third of cases
• Other names: Fraternal or nonidentical or binovular twins	• Other names: Identical or uniovular twins
• Incidence varies (depends on maternal age, parity, use of ovulation induction drugs, IVF conception, OCPs intake before conception, F/H/O twinning, etc.)	• Incidence is constant—1:250
• Always diamniotic dichorionic (DADC)	• Depending on the time of division after fertilization, monozygotic twins are further subclassified as follows: – Diamniotic dichorionic (DADC) – Diamniotic monochorionic (DAMC) – Monoamniotic monochorionic (MAMC) – Conjoint twins

Table 8.2 Classification of monozygotic twins based on the time of division following fertilization

Time of division following fertilization	Developmental stage	Type of placentation
0–3 days (within 72 hours)	Before the eight cell stage	Diamniotic dichorionic (DADC)—it may be two separate placentas or single fused placenta
4–8 days	Inner cell mass already formed but amniotic cavity not yet formed. So single chorion, two amnions	Diamniotic monochorionic (DAMC)—accounts for two-third of all monozygotic twins
9–13 days	Amniotic cavity is also formed. So single amnion	Monoamniotic monochorionic (MAMC)
Division after 13 days	Primitive streak formed. So incomplete splitting of germinal disc	Conjoint twins

(**Hint:** *Remember it as DAD, DAM, MAM)*

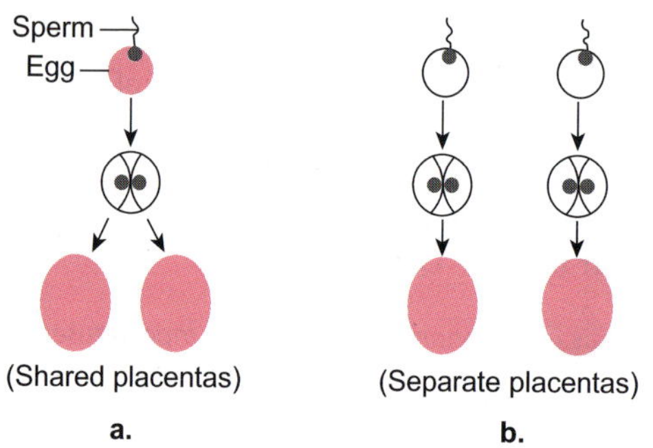

Figure 8.1 Types of twin pregnancy. **a.** Monozygotic (identical) twins. **b.** Dizygotic (fraternal) twins.

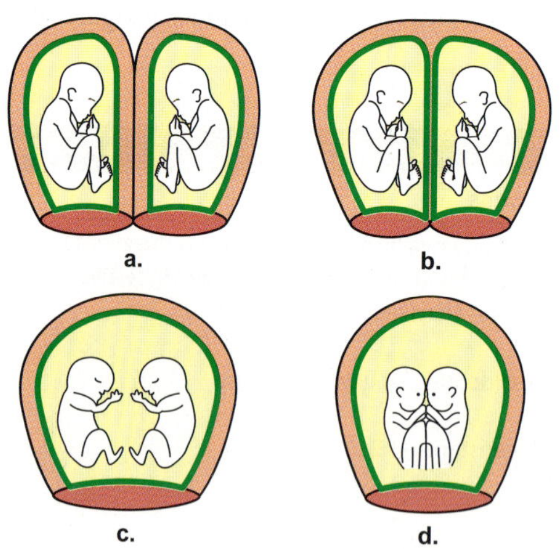

Figure 8.2 Types of placentation in monozygotic twins. Four types of monozygotic pregnancies can occur depending on the time of cleavage. **a.** Diamniotic dichorionic (separate placentas). **b.** Diamniotic monochorionic. **c.** Monoamniotic monochorionic. **d.** Monoamniotic monochorionic with conjoint twins.

Etiology of multiple pregnancy

- Ethnicity—highest among Africans
- Increased maternal age (maximum at 30–35 years due to higher FSH)
- Increased parity
- Conception following ovulation induction:
  - GnRH analogues (20–40% chance of multiple pregnancy)
  - Clomiphene citrate (5–15% chance of multiple pregnancy)
- Conception after in vitro fertilization (IVF) treatment
- Oral contraceptive pill (OCP) usage prior to conception
- Previous H/o multiple pregnancy
- Family H/o multiple pregnancy—hereditary predisposition more likely to be transmitted from the maternal side

Note *The etiologies are for dizygotic twins only. The incidence of monozygotic twins remains constant throughout the world.*

Viva corner

Q1 How does the usage of OCPs prior to conception increase the incidence of multiple pregnancy?

There is a sudden increase in the release of pituitary gonadotropins in the first spontaneous menstrual cycle, after stopping OCPs. Multiple ova may get released and hence higher rates of multiple pregnancy.

Case presentation

Salient points in history

Consider the following relevant points during history taking in cases of multiple pregnancy.

Patient profile

- *Age (incidence increases with advanced maternal age)*
- *Parity (incidence increases with increase in parity)*

Presenting complaints

- *H/o hyperemesis gravidarum (due to increased hCG secretion)*
- *H/o breathlessness (due to overdistension of abdomen, associated anemia)*
- *H/o difficulty in walking and backache (due to overdistension of abdomen)*
- *H/o symptoms of anemia (nutritional anemia is common due to increased demand)*
- *H/o symptoms of preeclampsia (increased incidence of early onset preeclampsia)*
- *Pressure symptoms—pedal edema, varicosities, and hemorrhoids (due to inferior vena cava compression)*
- *H/o bleeding P/V [increased incidence of antepartum hemorrhage (APH)]*
- *H/o labor pains (preterm labor is common)*

H/o present pregnancy

- *H/o conception following treatment for infertility such as ovulation induction drugs and IVF conception*
- *H/o OCP usage prior to conception*

Obstetric history

Previous H/o twin pregnancy

Family history

H/o twin pregnancy in the family

Salient points in examination

Consider the following relevant points during examination in cases of multiple pregnancy.

General examination

- *Whether patient is comfortable at rest. Respiratory discomfort may be present due to overdistension of abdomen*
- *Weight (multiple pregnancy is associated with excessive weight gain; excessive weight gain is a premonitory sign of preeclampsia)*
- *Pallor*
- *Pedal edema*
- *BP*

Obstetric examination

Inspection

Abdomen appears overdistended

Obstetric palpation

- *Fundal height and symphysiofundal height (SFH) are greater than period of gestation (POG).*
- *Abdominal girth at level of umbilicus is increased.*
- *Multiple fetal parts are felt.*
- *Presence of two distinct fetal heads or three fetal poles confirms the diagnosis of twin pregnancy.*
- *Liquor may be increased (polyhydramnios may be associated with twin pregnancy).*

Auscultation

Two distinct fetal heart rate (FHR), at two different sites (10 cm apart), with a difference of at least 10 beats/min, and heard by two observers simultaneously is suggestive of twins.

*(**Hint:** Two sites, two observers, 10 cm apart, 10 beats difference)*

Case summary

An example of writing summary in cases of multiple pregnancy is given below.

Example *Mrs. P, 30 years of age, G3P2L2 at 34 weeks of gestation, has been admitted with c/o pedal edema for the past 2 weeks. Clinical examination revealed no pallor; pedal edema was present and BP was 130/84 mmHg. Cardiovascular and respiratory system examinations were normal.*

(CONTD...)

(...CONTD)

Obstetric examination revealed an overdistended abdomen with SFH of 38 cm. Multiple fetal poles could be palpated. On auscultation, two FHS could be heard at two different sites, one over the right spinoumbilical line at 130 bpm and the other over the left spinoumbilical line at a higher level at 144 bpm.

Clinical diagnosis

An example of writing diagnosis in cases of multiple pregnancy is given below.

Example *30 years of age, G3P2L2 at 34 weeks of gestation with twin pregnancy, not in labor*

Case discussion

Differential diagnosis for overdistended uterus

In an antenatal case with overdistended uterus, differential diagnosis includes all the causes of fundal height greater than POG (Table 8.3).

Diagnosis of twin pregnancy

The diagnosis of twin pregnancy is based on high index of clinical suspicion and is confirmed by ultrasonography (USG).

- Two distinct gestational sacs can be appreciated as early as 6–7 weeks of gestation.
- In later months, USG visualization of two fetal heads in two perpendicular planes confirms diagnosis (in order to prevent mistaking abdominal cross-section for fetal head).

Table 8.3 Causes of fundal height greater/less than period of gestation (POG)

Causes of fundal height more than POG	Causes of fundal height less than POG
• Wrong dates • Full bladder • Multiple pregnancy • Polyhydramnios • Big baby • Fibroid uterus • Molar pregnancy	• Wrong dates • Intrauterine growth restriction • Intrauterine death • Oligohydramnios • Transverse lie

Uses of USG in multiple pregnancy

See Table 8.4

Determination of chorionicity

See Table 8.5

During antenatal period

Ultrasound is used to determine the chorionicity and is most reliable in the late first trimester or early second trimester.

In early gestation

- **DADC:** Two gestational sacs with two separate fetuses separated by thick chorion
- **DAMC:** One gestational sac with two fetuses separated by thin membrane (amnion)
- **MAMC:** One gestational sac with two fetuses and no dividing membranes

Placenta

- **Two separate placental masses**: Dichorionic (DC) twin
- **Single placental mass:** Can be a DC twin with single fused placenta or a monochorionic (MC) twin

Table 8.4 Uses of ultrasonography in multiple pregnancy

First trimester	Second trimester	Third trimester
• Confirms diagnosis • Confirms fetal viability • Confirms dates • Determines chorionicity • Nuchal translucency • Therapeutic fetal reduction can be done in higher order pregnancies	• Fetal anomalies can be ruled out • Determines chorionicity • Fetal biometry • Placental localization	• Fetal biometry • Identifies complications such as fetal growth restriction (FGR) and twin-to-twin transfusion syndrome • Amniotic fluid index • Placental localization • Fetal presentation • Doppler and biophysical profile

Table 8.5 Determination of chorionicity

Criteria for diagnosis of diamniotic dichorionic twins	Criteria for diagnosis of diamniotic monochorionic twins	Criteria for diagnosis of monoamniotic monochorionic twins
Ultrasonography • Two gestational sacs with two separate fetuses, separated by thick chorion • Two separate placenta • Intertwin membrane thickness ≥2 mm • Twin peak sign is seen • May be same or opposite fetal gender Placenta • Three or four layers are present in the intervening membranes (two amnions, two chorions)	Ultrasonography • One gestational sac with two fetuses, separated by a thin membrane • Single placenta • Intertwin membrane thickness <2 mm • Twin peak sign is absent • Always same fetal gender Placenta • Only two layers in intervening membranes (two amnions)	Ultrasonography • One gestational sac with two fetuses and no dividing membrane • Single placenta • Absent intertwin membrane • Same fetal gender • Conjoint twins may be present Placenta • Single placenta with no intervening membranes

Part 1

Viva corner

Q1 What is the difference between zygosity and chorionicity?

- **Zygosity:** Refers to the type of conception
- **Chorionicity:** Refers to the type of placenta

Zygosity (type of conception)

- It refers to whether it is a dizygotic or monozygotic twins.

Chorionicity (type of placentation)

- Dizygotic twins are always DADC.
- Monozygotic twins can be DADC, DAMC, or MAMC depending on the time of division.
- Monochorionic twins are at increased perinatal risk due to placental sharing or anastomosis between the fetal circulations.

It is very important to know the chorionicity because:

- It determines the degree of perinatal risk in twin pregnancy.
- Management protocols, complication rates, and outcome of twin pregnancies depend on chorionicity.

Intervening membranes

- **DC twin:** "Lambda sign" or "twin peak sign" seen [triangular projection of chorionic tissue extending from placental surface into the intertwin membrane (Figure 8.3)]
  - Intervening membrane thickness is ≥2 mm
  - Best appreciated between 9 and 13 weeks
- **MC twin:** "T sign" seen (no extension of chorionic tissue from placenta into intertwin membrane)
  - Intervening membrane thickness is <2 mm

Fetal sex

- **Different sex:** DC
- **Same sex:** Can be MC/DC

Following delivery

Determination of chorionicity following delivery is done by examination of the placenta.

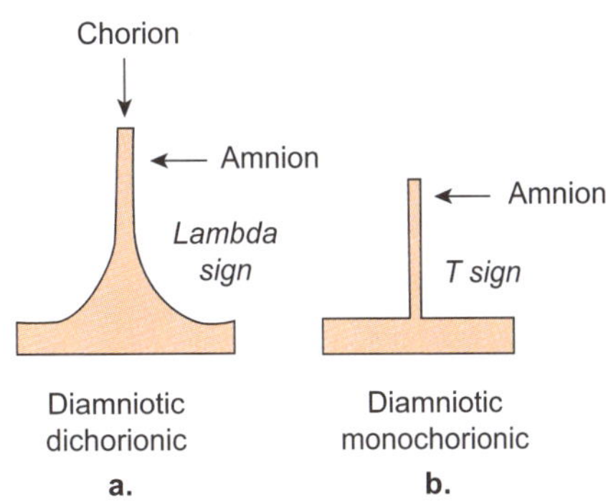

Figure 8.3 Ultrasonography findings on the intertwin membrane. **a.** "Twin peak" or "lambda sign"—triangular projection of chorionic tissue extending from placental surface into the intertwin membrane seen in dichorionic twin. **b.** "T sign"—no extension of chorionic tissue from placenta into intertwin membrane in monochorionic twin.

- **Two placenta:** DC
- **Single placenta with intervening membrane**
  - Intervening membrane has two amnions, two chorions: DC (single fused placenta)
  - Intervening membrane has two amnions only and no chorion in between the amnion: MC
- **Single placenta with no intervening membranes:** MC

Note *Prediction of chorionicity based on membrane thickness is more reliable before the 26th week, as there is thinning of membranes as pregnancy advances.*

COMPLICATIONS OF TWIN PREGNANCY

Maternal complications

Complications seen in singleton pregnancy occur more frequently in twin pregnancy (Table 8.6).

Fetal complications

Fetal complications occur at a higher rate in twin pregnancy, resulting in increased perinatal mortality and morbidity. Complications occur in both

Table 8.6 Maternal complications in twin pregnancy

Antepartum complications	Intrapartum complications	Postpartum complications
• All the symptoms of pregnancy exaggerated • Hyperemesis gravidarum (due to increased hCG) • Anemia (due to increased demand and increased blood volume expansion) • Gestational diabetes mellitus (due to increased anti-insulin hormones from placenta) • Preeclampsia—25% risk, may have early onset preeclampsia • Polyhydramnios • Preterm premature rupture of membranes (PPROM)—due to uterine overdistension and associated malpresentations • Preterm labor—mean gestational age of delivery decreases with increasing birth order (it is around 36 weeks for twins and 32 weeks for triplets) • Pressure changes—varicose veins and hemorrhoids (**Hint**: *Remember 5 P's*) • Antepartum hemorrhage—risk of placenta previa and abruption	• Increased operative interferences—due to malpresentations • Dysfunctional labor or incordinate uterine action • Postpartum hemorrhage	• Infection—due to increased operative interferences • Subinvolution • Failed lactation • Thromboembolism

Viva corner

Q1 What are the causes for preterm labor in multiple pregnancy?

- Uterine overdistension
- Polyhydramnios
- Preterm premature rupture of membranes (PPROM)

Q2 What are the causes of APH in multiple pregnancy?

- **Placenta previa**: Large placenta may encroach on the lower uterine segment.
- **Abruption:** Associated complications such as preeclampsia, polyhydramnios, and PROM can lead to abruption.
  - Abruption is more common in the second twin, following delivery of the first twin.

Q3 Why is postpartum hemorrhage (PPH) common in multiple pregnancy?

- Uterine overdistension leading to atonic PPH
- Large placenta—may take time to separate and opens up multiple sinuses
- Placenta previa—no retraction of lower uterine segment
- Abruption—causes APH and PPH
- Preexistent anemia and preeclampsia — increased risk of PPH
- Operative interferences and manipulations—lead to traumatic PPH

DC and MC twins, but there are specific complications that are unique to MC twins.

Fetal complications common to dichorionic and monochorionic twins

See Table 8.7

Malpresentations in twin pregnancy (Figure 8.4)

- More common in the second twin
- Vertex–vertex: 40% (most common type of twin presentation)
- Vertex–breech: 25%
- Breech–breech, breech–vertex, vertex–transverse lie, breech–transverse lie, and both transverse are the other presentations

Specific fetal complications of monochorionic twins

Perinatal mortality is higher in MC twins compared with that in DC twins. Complications that are specific to MC twins are as follows:

- Discordant growth (more common in MC twins)
- Death of one twin (more common in MC twins)
- Twin-to-twin transfusion syndrome (TTTS) (unique complication of MC twins)
- Twin reverse arterial perfusion (TRAP) (unique complication of MC twins)

Table 8.7 Fetal complications in twin pregnancy

Antepartum	Intrapartum	Postpartum
• Spontaneous abortion • Congenital malformations (doubled than in singleton pregnancy) • Prematurity • IUGR • Low birth weight—due to increased incidence of prematurity and IUGR • Discordant twins • Intrauterine death—due to congenital malformations • Malpresentations	• Cord prolapse—due to malpresentations • Birth asphyxia	• Increased neonatal intensive care unit admissions • Increased perinatal mortality

IUGR, intrauterine growth restriction.

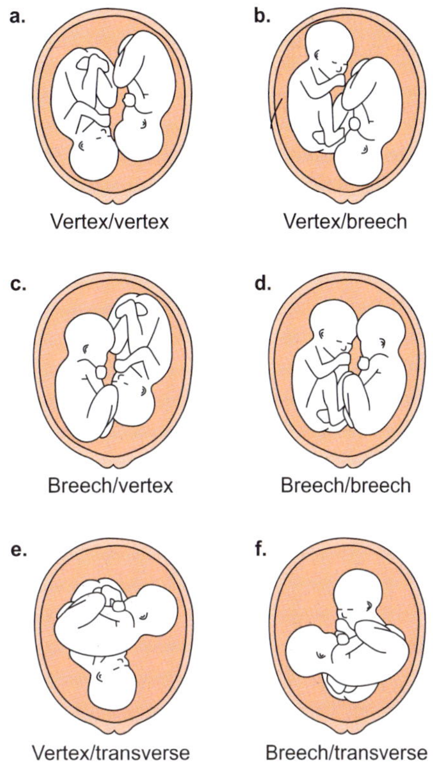

Figure 8.4 Twins Presentation. **a–f.** Various types of presentation in twin pregnancy. Vertex-vertex is the most common type of twin presentation.

- Cord entanglement (unique complication of monoamniotic twins)
- Conjoint twins (unique complication of monoamniotic twins)

(**Hint:** *Remember it as* $D^2\ T^2\ C^2$)

Discordant growth

Definition

It is defined as the difference in estimated fetal weight (EFW) of >20% between the two fetuses, expressed as percentage of weight of the larger twin. It can occur in DC and MC twins, but it is more common in MC twins.

Criteria for discordance

- Difference in EFW ≥20% (most accepted criterion)
- Difference in biparietal diameter of ≥5 mm
- Difference in abdominal circumference of ≥20 mm

- Difference in head circumference of ≥5%
- Difference in Hb ≥5 g%

Grades of discordance

- **Grade I:** Difference in EFW of 15–25%
- **Grade II:** Difference in EFW of >25%

Causes of discordant growth

- In DC twins, it can be due to:
  - Difference in genetic makeup of both the twins
  - Unequal placental masses
- In MC twins, it is due to:
  - TTTS

Death of one twin

It can occur in DC and MC twins, but it is more common in MC twins.

First trimester

Death of one twin at <14 weeks results in "vanishing twin." The dead fetus gets absorbed and pregnancy continues as singleton pregnancy.

Second trimester

Death of one twin in the second trimester results in fetus compresses or fetus papyraceous. The dead fetus gets compressed between the uterine wall and the sac of living twin, identified by USG or at the time of delivery of the normal twin.

Third trimester

Death of one twin in the third trimester increases the risk of disseminated intravascular coagulation (DIC), neurological damage, and multiple organ damage in the surviving twin and risk of DIC in the mother—due to release of thromboplastin from the dead twin. Complications are more in death of one twin in MC twins than DC twins.

Twin-to-twin transfusion syndrome (Figure 8.5)

- Unique complication of MC twins
- Cause for TTTS—due to deep arteriovenous anastomosis in placenta circulation
- Pathogenesis—unidirectional blood flow from one twin into the other results in hemodynamic imbalance, causing discordance in fetal growth and discrepancy in liquor volume

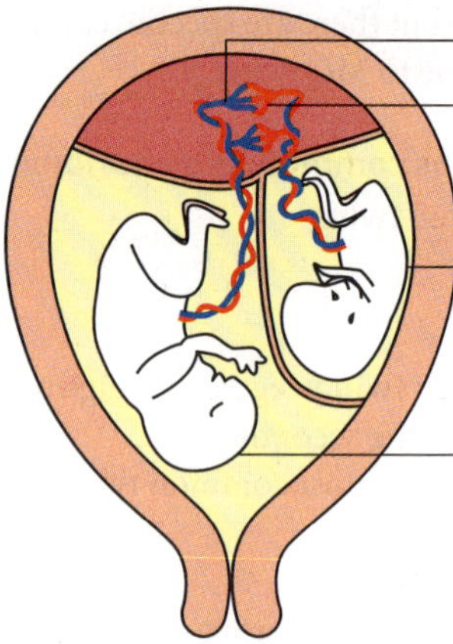

Figure 8.5 Twin-to-twin transfusion syndrome. Anastomosis between the arteries of the donor twin and veins of the recipient twin.

  - *Donor twin or "stuck twin" will be*: Hypovolemic, oligohydramniotic, anemic, and growth restricted
  - *Recipient twin will be*: Hypervolemic, polyhydramniotic, plethoric, and larger in size
- The prognosis depends on gestational age and severity of the syndrome. Survival is better in the donor twin (recipient twin usually dies in utero due to high-output cardiac failure)
- Treatment options
  - Amnioreduction of polyhydramniotic sac
  - Laser coagulation of anastomotic vessels
  - Septostomy

Twin reverse arterial perfusion (Figure 8.6)

- Unique complication of MC twins.
- Cause for TRAP: It occurs due to deep arterioarterial or vein-to-vein anastomosis in the placenta.
- Pathogenesis: It is characterized by an "acardiac twin" having blood supply from a normal co-twin via large arterioarterial or vein-to-vein anastomosis. Recipient twin has no cardiac structure and is parasitic on the other twin that provides blood supply to the acardiac twin, preferentially to the lower part of the body (iliac vessels). Desaturated blood flows to upper torso and hence there is lack of development of upper torso and head that may be absent or amorphous.

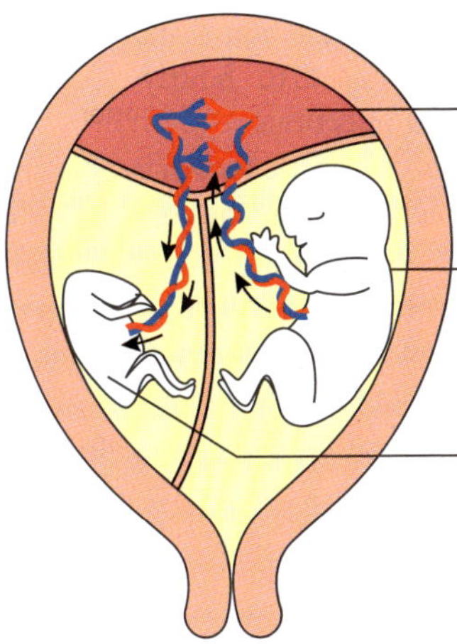

Figure 8.6 Twin reverse arterial perfusion. The donor twin pumps deoxygenated blood into the umbilical vessels of the second twin and supplies mainly to the lower half of the body. The upper half of the second twin does not develop, giving rise to acardiac twin.

- Survival: There is risk of death of both the twins. Donor twin eventually dies due to high-output cardiac failure.
- Treatment: Laser photocoagulation of the vascular anastomosis in placenta has been tried.

Cord entanglement (Figure 8.7)

- It is specific to MAMC twins.
- Cord entanglement can occur due to absence of intervening membranes and can lead to sudden intrauterine death of both the twins due to interruption in blood supply.

Conjoint twins (Figure 8.8)

- It is specific to MAMC twins due to late division of zygote after 13 days of fertilization.

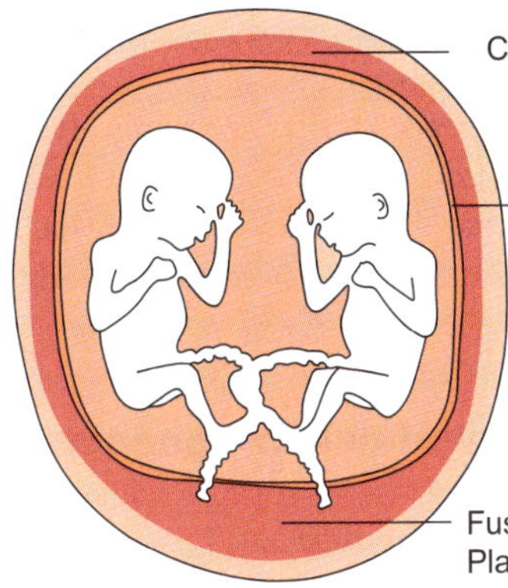

Figure 8.7 Cord entanglement—a specific complication of monoamniotic twins.

- Types of conjoint twins are as follows:
  - *Thoracophagus*: United at chest (commonest)
  - *Omphalophagus*: Fused at abdomen
  - *Pygophagus*: Fused at buttocks
  - *Ischiophagus*: Fused at ischium
  - *Craniophagus*: Fused at back of the head
  - *Cephalophagus*: Fused at head

  (**Hint**: *Remember as "TOPIC"*)
- Diagnosis: Suspect conjoint twins in USG if the following features are present:
  - Inseparable or fused body parts
  - No change in relative position of both the fetuses
  - Both heads at the same level and plane
  - Twins facing each other (thoracophagus, omphalophagus)
  - Thorax in close approximation (thoracophagus)
- Termination of pregnancy is offered when the shared organs are vital and single, such as heart and brain.

Part 1

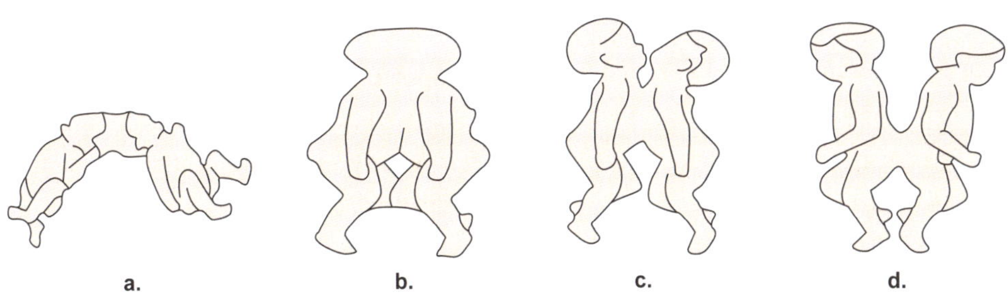

Figure 8.8 Conjoint twins. **a.** Craniophagus. **b.** Cephalophagus. **c.** Thoracophagus. **d.** Pygophagus.

- Conjoint twins are delivered by cesarean section as it can lead to obstructed labor.
- Feasibility of separation of the twins after birth should be discussed with specialists. Surgical separation may be possible in conjoint twins with no major malformations, such as only bone fusion.

Management of twin pregnancy

Antepartum management

Early diagnosis of twins and associated complications reduces perinatal morbidity and mortality.

- All women with multifetal gestations, regardless of age, should undergo routine aneuploidy screening.
- Frequent antenatal visits are advised to detect associated complications.
- Hemoglobin estimation is done at the initial visit and repeated at 28 and 36 weeks to detect anemia.
- Watch out for the development of preeclampsia and gestational diabetes mellitus (GDM)—urine for proteins during every antenatal visit and oral glucose tolerance test at the initial visit; repeated at 24–28 weeks and at 32 weeks.
- Bed rest in left lateral position for at least 2 hours in afternoon and 8 hours in night improves uteroplacental perfusion.
- Dietary advice: Advise on adequate nutrition.
  - There is increase in requirement of iron, folic acid, calories, proteins, vitamins, and minerals
  - Calorie requirement—increases by 300 kcal/day more than singleton pregnancy
  - Iron supplementation—100 mg/day
  - Folic acid—1 mg/day
- Antepartum fetal surveillance
  - Serial USG starting from second trimester helps in early detection of complications such as discordant growth, TTTS, and timely intervention can be provided.
  - Nonstress test and Doppler are done from 32 weeks onward to assess fetal well-being.
- Prevention of preterm labor
  - Limitation of physical activity
  - Steroids for lung maturity administered after 28 weeks of gestation in women at risk of delivery within 7 days—Betamethasone 12 mg two doses 24 hours apart or Dexamethasone 6 mg 12th hourly four doses intramuscular injections
  - No role for prophylactic tocolysis, although it is widely practiced (it can be given in preterm labor)
  - No role for prophylactic encerclage, prophylactic pessary, routine hospitalization, and bed rest.
  - Progesterone treatment is not recommended as it does not reduce the incidence of spontaneous preterm birth in unselected women with twin gestations
  - Magnesium sulfate reduces the severity and risk of cerebral palsy in the newborns if administered when birth is anticipated before 32 weeks of gestation (ACOG)
- Admission: The patient is admitted in case of any complications or near term.
- Hospital delivery is mandatory.
- Mode of delivery: The most important factor in deciding the mode of delivery (cesarean section or vaginal delivery) is presentation of the first twin. Vaginal delivery can be allowed when the first twin is in vertex presentation.
- Timing of delivery: Most patients have spontaneous onset of labor before expected date of delivery. Indications for induction of labor are similar to those for singleton pregnancy, such as preeclampsia and GDM.

Mode of delivery in twin pregnancy

The mode of delivery is determined by the presentation of fetuses, especially the first twin (Table 8.8; refer to Flowchart at the end of chapter).

Indications for cesarean section in twin pregnancy

See Table 8.9

Intrapartum management

Vaginal delivery can be allowed when the first twin is in vertex presentation. Anticipate complications during labor.

I stage

- Secure IV line and send blood for cross-match and reservation.

Part 1

Table 8.8 Mode of delivery in twin pregnancy

Type of presentation of twins	Mode of delivery
Both cephalic	Vaginal delivery
First twin cephalic and second twin noncephalic	Patient can be allowed for vaginal delivery (provided the obstetrician is skilled in performing intrauterine manipulations and conducting assisted breech delivery/breech extraction of the second twin)
First twin noncephalic and second twin cephalic	Cesarean section
Both twins noncephalic	Cesarean section

Table 8.9 Obstetric and fetal indications for cesarean section in twin pregnancy

Obstetric indications	Fetal indications
Twins with associated complications such as: • Previous lower-segment cesarean section • Severe preeclampsia • Placenta previa • Contracted pelvis • Bad obstetric history • *Note: Women with one previous LSCS, who are otherwise appropriate candidates for twin vaginal delivery, may be considered for trial of labor after cesarean delivery (ACOG)*	• First twin in nonvertex presentation • Conjoint twins • Monoamniotic twins (as cord entanglement can occur) • Triplets or higher-order births • Discordant twins • Twin-to-twin transfusion syndrome • Fetal head collision—heads of both twins in vertex presentation trying to enter the pelvis leading to nonengagement of either head • Cord prolapse in the first stage of labor

- Anesthetist and pediatrician are kept informed.
- There should be no ambulation. The patient is put on labor board to avoid early rupture of membranes.
- Maintain adequate hydration. Clear oral liquids can be allowed.
- Adequate analgesia should be given—preferably epidural anesthesia.
- Partogram is done to monitor maternal and fetal conditions and progress of labor.
- Abdominal and vaginal examinations are done at regular intervals to assess progress of labor and to detect complications.
- P/V should be done following rupture of membranes to exclude cord prolapse.

II stage

- Two obstetricians including one experienced obstetrician should be present at the time of delivery.
- Anesthetist should be informed about need for any emergency intervention.
- Two pediatricians and two nurses should be present to resuscitate both the babies.

Delivery of the first twin Conduct delivery as in singleton vertex presentation, with emphasis on special points such as:

- Liberal episiotomy is done to prevent intracranial hemorrhage in preterm fetus (due to sudden compression followed by decompression of head).
- Bolus oxytocin/methergin is withheld after delivery of the first twin.
- Umbilical cord is kept long enough for any further therapy such as intraumbilical transfusion.
- The baby is labeled as no. 1 and handed over to pediatrician.

Delivery of the second twin

- Management of the second twin depends on its lie and presentation.
- Obstetric abdominal and vaginal examinations are done to assess the lie and presentation of the second twin. USG can be done in doubtful cases.
  - Abdominal examination is done first to assess the lie, presentation, EFW, and fetal heart rate (FHR) of the second twin.
  - Vaginal examination is done to assess the membrane status, presenting part, and station of the presenting part.

- If the second twin is in longitudinal lie (vertex or breech):
  - Augment uterine contractions by oxytocin and/or artificial rupture of membranes (ARM)
  - Exclude cord prolapse.
  - Monitor FHR.
  - In vertex presentation, conduct it as normal vaginal delivery.
  - In breech presentation, conduct it as assisted breech delivery (ABD).
  - The second baby has good outcome, irrespective of time interval between delivery of the first and the second twin, provided there is no fetal compromise.
  - In case of fetal distress, speedy delivery is achieved by:
    - Forceps/vacuum delivery—in vertex
    - Breech extraction—in breech presentation
    - However, if the cervix is collapsed or station is high up, the second twin is delivered by lower-segment cesarean section (LSCS)
- If the second twin is in transverse lie:
  - Lie of the second twin is corrected to longitudinal lie by external version to vertex or breech presentation and delivered by spontaneous vaginal delivery (SVD) or ABD, respectively.
  - If external version fails, internal podalic version (IPV) followed by breech extraction can be done (Figure 8.9).

Note *The second twin in transverse lie is the only indication for IPV in modern obstetrics.*

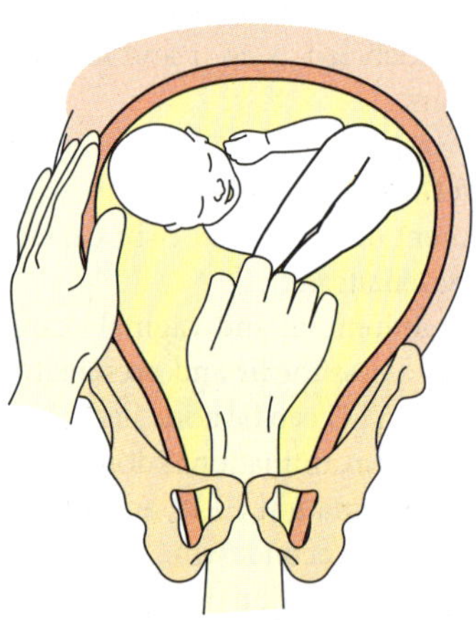

Figure 8.9 Internal podalic version and breech extraction.

High-yield points

Complications anticipated in second stage of labor

- Cord prolapse
- Abruption
- Fetal distress

All of the second-stage complications are more common in the second twin.

If methergin has been given inadvertently following delivery of the first twin, then:

- Hasten the delivery of the second twin.
- If cervical os has closed, cesarean section is done to deliver the second twin.

Time interval between delivery of the twins

According to the American College of Obstetricians and Gynecologists (ACOG), the interval between the delivery of both the twins is not critical in determining the outcome of twins. However, an urgent delivery of the second twin may be required in the following conditions:

- Excessive bleeding P/V
- Fetal distress in the second twin
- Cord prolapse of the second twin
- Inadvertent use of bolus oxytocin/methergin following delivery of the first twin
- If the first twin was delivered under general anesthesia

Indications for performing cesarean section of the second twin only

- Abruption following delivery of the first twin
- Cord prolapse
- Fetal distress with collapsed cervix
- The second twin being disproportionately larger [cephalopelvic disproportion (CPD)]
- Failure of version in transverse lie
- Failure of cervix to dilate (nonprogress of labor)
- Bolus oxytocin/methergin administered inadvertently, following delivery of the first twin

III stage

- Strict vigilance is necessary in the third stage as there is increased risk of PPH.
- Active management of the third stage of labor (AMTSL) is followed. IV oxytocin is given

Extra edge

Interlocking of twins—one fetus impedes the descent and delivery of other twin

- Body parts of the twins get interlocked causing difficulty in vaginal delivery.
- Interlocking of after-coming head of the first twin (breech) with fore-coming head of the second twin (vertex) is the commonest type of interlocking (see figure below).
- The first twin is usually dead by the time of diagnosis of this complication and cesarean section is done to salvage the second twin.

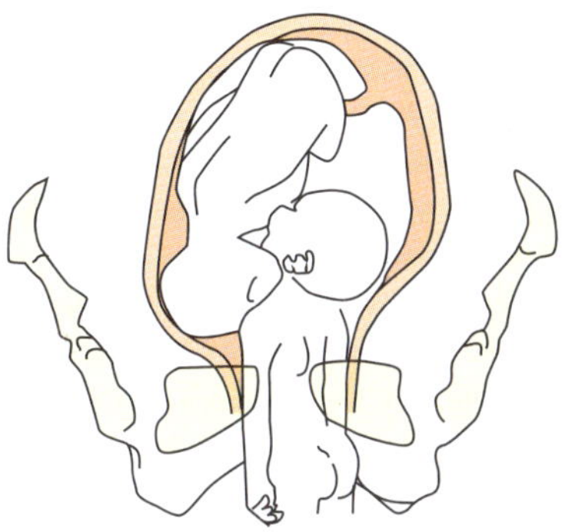

Figure Interlocking of after-coming head of the first twin (breech) with fore-coming head of the second twin (vertex).

Locked heads or collision of heads

The heads of both twins in vertex presentation collide with each other, preventing engagement of either heads (collision)

Superfetation

Fertilization of two ova released in two different cycles

Superfecundation

Fertilization of two ova released in the same cycle by two spermatozoa liberated in different acts of coitus within short interval

Selective reduction

- USG-guided reduction of fetuses, at 9–12 weeks of gestation
- Done in higher-order multiple pregnancy
- Selective feticide done by injecting potassium chloride (KCl) into fetal heart

Selective termination

- USG-guided destruction of selective fetuses in the second trimester
- Done in anomalous twin and higher-order multiple pregnancy
- Selective feticide done by injecting KCl into fetal heart

following delivery of the second twin and continued for at least 1 hour following delivery.

- Placenta is delivered by controlled cord traction and is checked for its intactness and chorionicity.
- The patient is observed for at least 2 hours in labor room.

Postpartum management

- The patient requires guidance and support to manage two babies simultaneously.
- Encourage breastfeeding of both the babies (milk secretion is usually adequate for both the babies).
- Contraception counseling should be given.

Frequently asked viva questions

1. Summarize the case.
2. What is the diagnosis of the case?
3. What is the plan of management for the case?
4. How will you confirm the diagnosis?
5. How is USG helpful in twin pregnancy?
6. What are the maternal and fetal complications of twin pregnancy?
7. How will you establish chorionicity in twin pregnancy?
8. What is the significance of chorionicity?
9. What are the complications specific to MC twins?
10. How will you manage twin pregnancy during antenatal period?
11. How will you plan the mode of delivery?
12. What are the indications for LSCS in twin pregnancy?
13. Which cases of twins can be allowed for vaginal delivery?
14. If allowed for vaginal delivery, how will you monitor the patient during labor?
15. What are the indications for LSCS of the second twin after the first twin has delivered vaginally?

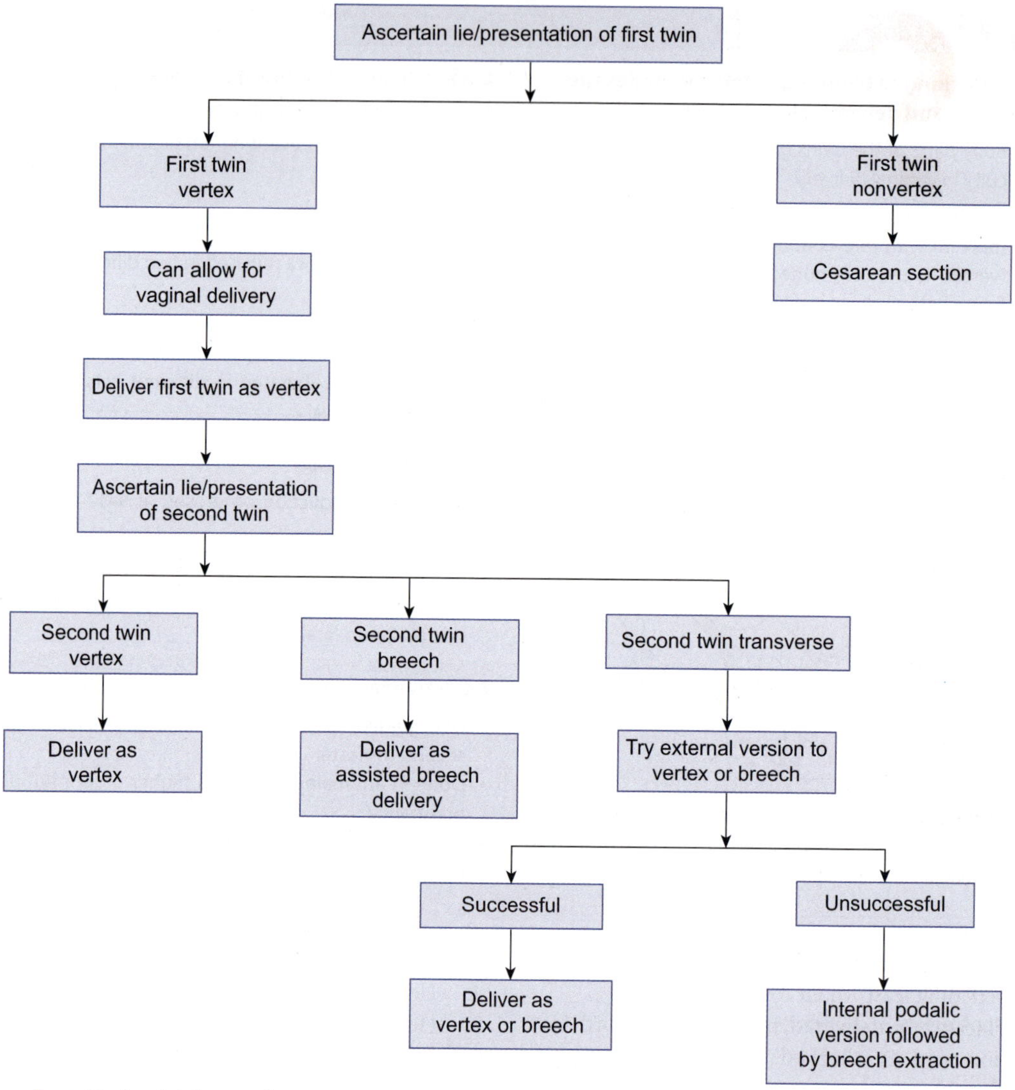

Flowchart Mode of delivery of twins.

9 Breech Presentation

Introduction

Breech presentation is the most common malpresentation seen during pregnancy and labor. Clinical case discussion of breech presentation involves the following aspects that are dealt in this chapter:

- Etiology and types of breech presentation
- Diagnosis
- Antenatal management—role of external cephalic version (ECV)
- Mode of delivery—assisted breech delivery (ABD) versus cesarean section (CS)
- ABD and complications

Definition

In breech presentation, fetus is in longitudinal lie with the podalic pole occupying the lower pole of uterus with the fetal buttocks and/or feet presenting at the maternal pelvic inlet.

Incidence

- **At 28 weeks:** 25%
- **At 32 weeks:** 8%
- **At term:** 4%

Etiology of breech presentation

The causes of breech presentation are mentioned in Table 9.1. Prematurity is the most common cause of breech presentation.

> **Extra edge**
>
> **Recurrent or habitual breech presentation**
>
> It refers to the recurrence of breech presentation in three or more consecutive pregnancies.
>
> **Causes of recurrent breech**
>
> - Congenital uterine malformations—septate, bicornuate uterus
> - Repeated cornual-fundal attachment of placenta

Types of breech presentation

Breech presentation can be of various types based on the attitude of the fetus (Table 9.2 and Figure 9.1).

Table 9.1 Causative factors for breech presentation

Maternal abdomen	• Multiparous with lax abdomen
Uterus	• Congenital malformations (septate, bicornuate) • Fibroid
Liquor	• Polyhydramnios (fetus keeps moving in excess liquor) • Oligohydramnios (less liquor preventing spontaneous version near term)
Fetus	• Prematurity (most common cause) • Multiple pregnancy • Congenital anomalies (anencephaly, hydrocephalus)
Placenta	• Placenta previa • Cornual-fundal attachment of placenta
Umbilical cord	• Short cord (prevents version)
Pelvis	• Contracted pelvis

Table 9.2 Types of breech presentation

Type of breech	Attitude	Presenting part
Complete breech (flexed breech)	Lower limbs are flexed at both hip and knee joints	Feet, buttock, external genitalia
Incomplete breech		
Frank breech (extended breech)	Breech with flexion at hip and extended legs	Buttock, external genitalia
Footling breech	Both thighs and legs are partially extended	Feet
Knee presentation	Extension at hip joint and flexion at knee joint	Knee

Note

- *Frank breech: Most common type, more common in primigravida*
- *Flexed breech: More common in multiparous women*

Viva corner

Q1 How is a flexed breech differentiated from an extended breech?

See table below

Table Differentiating features of a flexed breech from an extended breech

Flexed breech	Extended or frank breech
Head is felt in hypochondrium and is easily ballotable	Head is felt in the midline and is less ballotable due to splinting action of the legs
Breech is broad and bulky and hence engagement is usually delayed	Breech is more compact and may engage earlier
P/V—feet may be felt alongside buttocks in flexed breech	P/V—only buttocks will be felt

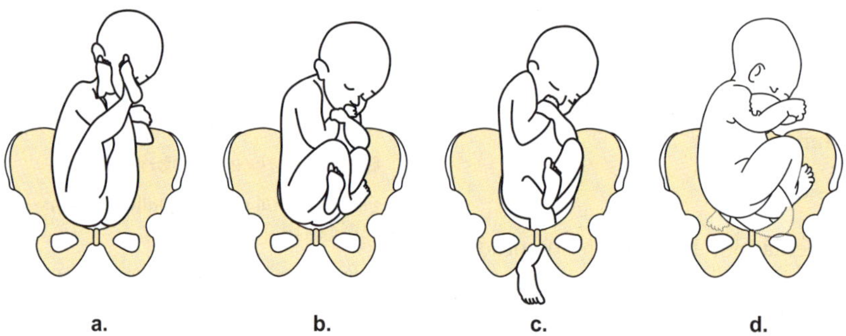

Figure 9.1 Types of breech presentation. **a.** Frank breech. **b.** Complete breech. **c.** Footling breech. **d.** Knee presentation.

Case presentation

Salient points in history

Consider the following relevant points during history taking in cases of breech presentation.

Parity—*increased incidence in multiparous women with pendulous abdomen*

Presenting complaints

The patient may say that she has been admitted as her fetus is in sitting position (probably breech presentation).

H/o present pregnancy

- *Whether anomaly scan was done and told to be normal (increased incidence of congenital anomalies)*
- *H/o antepartum hemorrhage (APH)—placenta previa is associated with fetal malpresentations*

Past obstetric history

H/o breech presentation in previous pregnancy

(CONTD...)

(...CONTD)

Salient points in examination

Consider the following relevant points during examination in cases of breech presentation.

Obstetric examination

See Table 9.3

Table 9.3 Obstetric examination findings in breech presentation

Obstetric palpation	Findings suggestive of breech presentation
Fundal grip	Hard, globular, ballotable mass—suggestive of head
Lateral grip	• Smooth, curved, uniform resistance is felt on one side—suggestive of fetal back • Irregular, knobby structures are felt on the other side—suggestive of fetal limbs
First pelvic grip	Broad, soft, irregular, nonballotable mass is felt—suggestive of breech
Second pelvic grip	Confirms findings of the first pelvic grip
Fetal heart rate	Heard above the level of umbilicus on the side of fetal back

P/V examination

The following findings in vaginal examination are suggestive of breech presentation.

During pregnancy

When os is closed, breech can be felt through fornices as a soft mass.

During labor

- *Breech is diagnosed by palpating three bony landmarks, that is, two ischial tuberosities and sacrum.*
- *In complete breech, feet are felt besides the buttocks.*
- *Anal sphincter can be felt and fresh meconium may be found on examining fingers.*
- *Male external genitalia can be palpated.*

Case summary

An example of writing summary in cases of breech presentation is given below.

Example *Mrs. F, 28 years of age, primigravida, at 38 weeks of gestation, diagnosed to have breech presentation, has presented for regular antenatal checkup. On examination, there are no significant general examination findings; her vitals are stable and obstetric examination reveals a singleton live fetus in breech presentation, not in labor.*

Case diagnosis

An example of writing diagnosis in cases of breech presentation is given below.

Example *28 years of age, a primigravida at 38 weeks of gestation with a singleton live fetus in breech presentation, not in labor.*

Case discussion

Diagnosis

In a case where clinical examination findings are suggestive of breech presentation, the diagnosis is confirmed by ultrasonography (USG) examination.

- **Role of USG in breech presentation**—information obtained are the following:
  - Confirms presentation
  - Type of breech
  - Attitude of fetal head (to rule out hyperextension of head)
  - Any congenital anomalies
  - Maturity of fetus
  - Amount of liquor
  - Estimated fetal weight (EFW)
  - Placental localization (placenta previa may be associated with breech)
  - Any uterine anomalies and fibroids

Note *The presentation of fetus is variable before 34 weeks' of gestation and most of the cases convert spontaneously to cephalic presentation near term. If the fetus persists as breech at or after 34 weeks, the patient should be reviewed after 2 weeks to confirm the presentation.*

Viva corner

Q1 How is a breech differentiated from face in P/V examination?

See table below

Table Differentiating features of a breech from face in P/V examination (see figure below)

Breech	Face
Anal sphincter and two ischial tuberosities are in one line	Mouth and two malar prominences make a triangle
Sphincteric action of anus can be felt on insertion of a finger	No such sphincteric action. Sucking of the finger inserted into the mouth can be felt
Sacrum is felt as a hard, rough surface	Hard alveolar margins and gums can be felt
Meconium staining of examining fingers	No meconium staining of examined fingers
External genitalia in male fetus can be palpated	Chin, nose, and eyes can be identified

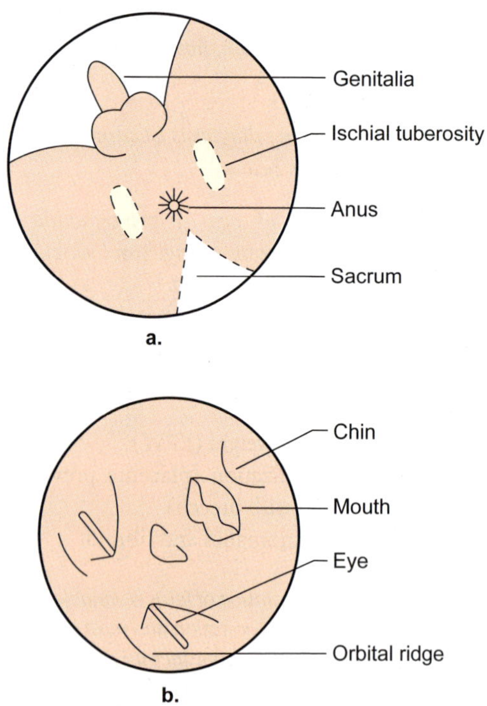

Figure Findings in breech and face presentation in P/V examination. **a.** Breech **b.** Face.

Q2 How is a foot differentiated from hand in P/V examination

See table below

Table Differentiating features of a foot from hand in P/V examination (see figure below)

Foot	Hand
Toes are of near equal length	Fingers are of unequal length
Toes are shorter	Fingers longer than toes
Great toe has lesser mobility	Thumb moves in all directions
Firm, round, knob-like heel felt	No such part felt in hand

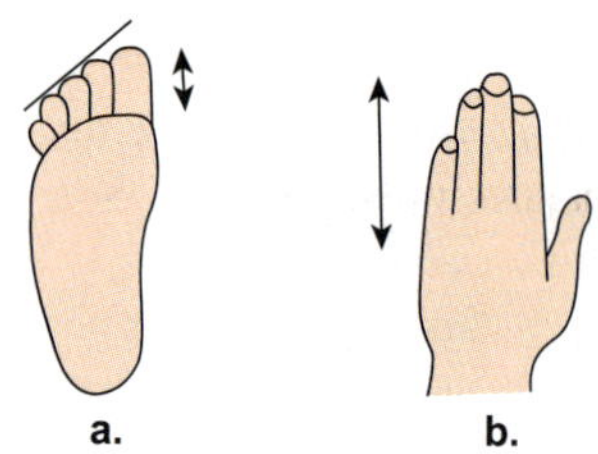

Figure Foot and hand in P/V examination. **a.** Foot. **b.** Hand. This differentiation is especially useful during internal podalic version of the second twin.

Q3 What is star-gazing fetus or flying fetus?

Breech with a hyperextended head in USG examination is termed as a star-gazing fetus (see figure below).

Significance If allowed for vaginal delivery, difficulty is encountered in the delivery of after-coming head of breech, resulting in spinal cord injury to the fetus. Hence, lower-segment cesarean section (LSCS) is indicated in breech with a hyperextended head.

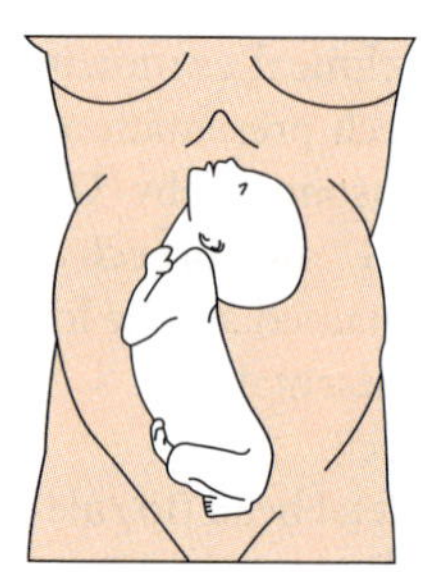

Figure Star-gazing fetus—hyperextended head.

Complications associated with breech presentation

Maternal complications

Increased morbidity due to increased incidence of lower-segment cesarean section (LSCS) and difficult vaginal breech delivery.

Fetal complications

- Risk of perinatal mortality is three to five times higher than in vertex presentation. Fetal complications may be due to:
  - Problems in the fetus such as prematurity, congenital anomalies
  - Complications of vaginal breech delivery (described below)

Complications of vaginal breech delivery

- Birth asphyxia
- Intracranial hemorrhage (ICH)
- Birth injuries

Causes of birth asphyxia

- Cord prolapse
- Cord compression
- Aspiration of amniotic fluid as a result of premature attempts at respiration while the head is still inside
- Difficulty in delivery of after-coming head (trauma to medulla oblongata by odontoid process results in hanging-like death of fetus)

Causes of intracranial hemorrhage

- Sudden compression followed by decompression of head during delivery of unmolded after-coming head of breech results in tearing of tentorium cerebelli and falx cerebri, especially in preterm breech delivery.
- Birth asphyxia can result in ICH.

Birth injuries

Various birth trauma can occur during vaginal breech delivery:

- Disruption of knee joint
- Fracture femur—during manipulation
- Dislocation of hip joint—due to traction
- Visceral injuries—liver, spleen, etc., due to faulty handling of the trunk
- Fracture humerus
- Dislocation of shoulder joint
- Fracture clavicle
- Trauma to sternocleidomastoid
- Erb's palsy due to damage to upper trunk of brachial plexus
- Klumpke's palsy due to damage to lower trunk of brachial plexus
- Fracture of cervical vertebra
- Spinal cord injury
- Dislocation of jaw
- Fracture mandible
- ICH due to sudden compression and decompression of head

(**Hint:** *Think of the fetal parts delivered in succession in vaginal breech delivery and mention the injuries accordingly from below upwards*)

High-yield points

Complicated breech

Breech presentation associated with other obstetric complications that can influence the prognosis such as contracted pelvis, placenta previa, and preeclampsia is termed complicated breech (other than inherent complications of breech such as prematurity).

Complicated breech delivery

Difficulties encountered during vaginal breech delivery such as extended arms, nuchal arm, and extended legs are termed complicated breech delivery.

Incidence of cord prolapse in various types of breech presentation

See table below

Table Incidence of cord prolapse in breech presentation

Breech type	Incidence of cord prolapse
Frank breech	0.5% (similar to vertex presentation—0.4%)
Flexed breech	5%
Footling breech	15%

Management of breech presentation

No intervention is required in cases of breech presentation prior to 34 weeks of gestation, as most of the cases convert to cephalic presentation spontaneously. If it persists as breech after 34 weeks, the patient is reviewed after 2 weeks and then the management is done as given below.

Antenatal management

- USG is done to confirm diagnosis, to rule out fetal anomalies, to locate placenta and to assess EFW.
- Identify any complicating factors such as preeclampsia and APH.
- The management options for breech presentation at near term include the following:
  - ECV to convert breech presentation into cephalic presentation
  - Delivery by CS
  - Vaginal breech delivery at term
- Spontaneous version is awaited up to 36 weeks. If it persists as breech presentation, ECV can be offered after ruling out contraindications for ECV.
- When ECV fails or is contraindicated, management is either to deliver by elective LSCS or to allow assisted vaginal breech delivery.
  - Elective CS is preferred in view of complications associated with vaginal breech delivery.
  - However, vaginal breech delivery can be offered in some cases, when required criteria are fulfilled, after patient counseling and informed consent.

External cephalic version

Definition

ECV is a procedure to convert the fetus from breech to cephalic presentation by external manipulation on the maternal abdomen.

Advantages of external cephalic version

- Decreases vaginal breech delivery and its associated perinatal morbidity and mortality
- Decreases rate of CS for breech

When to do external cephalic version?

- The procedure is done at around 36 weeks (35–37 weeks) for the following reasons:
  - Success rate is high if done at this period of gestation (POG).
  - Fetus is more likely to remain as breech after this POG (less chance of spontaneous version after this period).
- ECV is not done at <35 weeks because:
  - There is still a chance of spontaneous version.
  - There is possibility of reversion back to breech if ECV is done too early.
  - If any complications such as fetal distress, abruption occur during ECV, emergency LSCS can be done without the fear of prematurity.
- If ECV is attempted after 37 weeks, chances of failure of ECV procedure are high.

Contraindications for external cephalic version

See Table 9.4

Table 9.4 Contraindications for external cephalic version

Maternal factors	Fetal factors
• If elective LSCS is indicated like in placenta previa, contracted pelvis • Previous LSCS • PROM • Oligohydramnios • Severe preeclampsia • Precious pregnancy such as elderly gravida, bad obstetric history, and conception after infertility treatment	• Multiple pregnancy • Congenital anomalies • Intrauterine death • Intrauterine growth restriction • Abnormal cardiotocography

LSCS, lower-segment cesarean section; *PROM*, premature rupture of membranes

Unfavorable factors for external cephalic version

See Table 9.5

Table 9.5 Factors that are unfavorable for external cephalic version

Maternal factors	Fetal factors
• Obesity • Uterus is acting or irritable • Undiagnosed uterine anomalies • Oligohydramnios	• Breech with extended legs (splinting action of the spine in a frank breech prevents easy movement of the fetus) • Engaged breech • Big baby • Short cord • Anterior placenta

Procedure of external cephalic version

- It is done as an OPD procedure
- Performed in a well-equipped center with facilities for emergency CS

Extra edge

External version score (Newman Peacock Scoring System)

External version score helps in predicting the success rate of ECV. Five factors (parity, placental location, cervical dilatation, station, and EFW) are used for calculating this score. Maximum score is 10.

Version score (≥4) is associated with an increased rate of successful ECV (see table below).

Table External version score

Parameter	Score 0	Score 1	Score 2
Parity	0	1	≥2
Dilatation (cm)	≥3	1–2	0
Estimated fetal weight (g)	<2500	2500–3500	>3500
Placenta	Anterior	Posterior	Fundal
Station	≥–1	–2	–3 and above

Prior to procedure

- USG is done to confirm type of breech, amniotic fluid index (AFI), placental localization, EFW, obvious fetal anomaly, and fetal spine orientation.
- Contraindications should be ruled out.
- The patient is counseled regarding the procedure, possible complications, advantages, etc., and informed consent is obtained.
- Nonstress test (NST) is done to ensure fetal well-being.
- The patient is asked to empty the bladder.

Procedure (forward roll; Figure 9.2)

- The patient lies down in supine position with thighs and legs semiflexed.
- A pillow may be placed under the buttocks or slight Trendelenburg position (head low) is given to disengage the breech.
- Abdomen is exposed and dusting powder may be sprinkled over the abdomen to facilitate hand movements.
- Standing on the right side of the abdomen, the abdomen is palpated to confirm the presentation and state of uterus (whether relaxed or acting), and fetal heart rate (FHR) is auscultated.
- The breech is grasped by the first pelvic grip and pushed to iliac fossa toward the side of fetal back.
- The left hand presses the head down in opposite direction and the right hand pushes the breech up. Ideally fetal flexion should be maintained throughout the procedure.
- When the fetal lie becomes transverse, the hands are interchanged.
- The gentle pressure is continued till the head is brought to the lower pole of uterus.
- Auscultate FHR at the end of procedure. Transient bradycardia may be present that usually disappears in 1–2 minutes.
- If bradycardia persists for more than 10 minutes, there is a likely chance of cord entanglement and hence emergency CS is performed.

Postprocedure

- Postprocedure USG and NST are done to ensure fetal well-being.
- The patient is observed for an hour, for any vaginal bleeding, leaking P/V, or labor pains.
- Anti-D injection should be administered in case of Rh-negative pregnancy.

Indications to discontinue the procedure

- Fetal distress

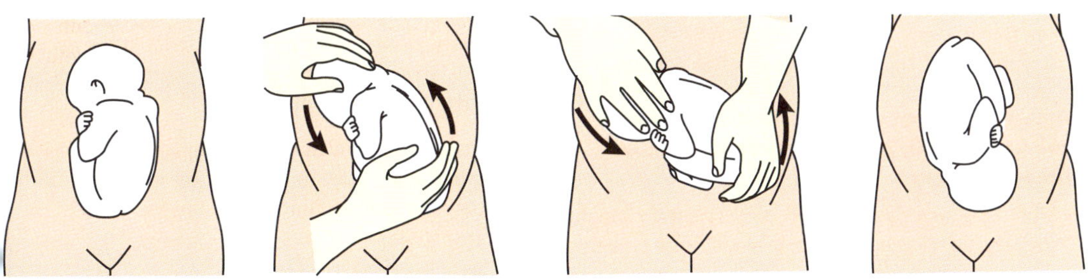

a. b. c. d.

Figure 9.2 External cephalic version. **a-d.** The fetus in breech presentation is turned in the direction in which the fetus faces and converted into cephalic presentation.

- Onset of uterine contractions
- Attempt not successful after trying for a maximum of 15 minutes

If ECV fails, the procedure may be repeated after 24 hours, after giving tocolysis. If it fails again, decision for vaginal breech delivery or LSCS is taken.

Indications for tocolysis before ECV procedure

- Primigravida (optional)
- When the first attempt fails
- Uterus irritable or mildly acting

Tocolytic drug usually given is terbutaline 250 μg subcutaneously.

Complications of external cephalic version

- Preterm labor
- Premature rupture of membranes (PROM)
- Abruption
- Cord prolapse
- Cord entanglement
- Fetal distress
- Fetomaternal hemorrhage
- Uterine rupture (rarely)

Follow-up

- If ECV is successful, the patient is examined on a weekly basis to confirm cephalic presentation and to assess fetal well-being. The patient can wait for spontaneous onset of labor and is delivered as in a normal vaginal delivery.
- When ECV has failed or is contraindicated, management is either to deliver by elective LSCS or to allow assisted vaginal breech delivery.

Mode of delivery of breech at term

- There are two choices regarding the mode of delivery in breech presentation at term: vaginal breech delivery or elective CS.
- Potential risks and benefits of vaginal breech delivery and CS should be explained to the patient.
- Current recommendation is to perform elective CS for a breech presentation at term, as vaginal breech delivery is associated with increased perinatal risks. "*Unless a patient is seen in labor where delivery is imminent, a primigravida at term with breech presentation should preferably be delivered by LSCS.*"

Indications for cesarean section in breech

- Contracted pelvis
- Fetopelvic disproportion
- EFW of >3.5 kg/EFW<1.5 kg
- Footling presentation (risk of cord prolapse)
- Hyperextended head (star gazing fetus)
- Prematurity

Extra edge

Hannah's term breech trial (Hannah et al, 2000)

- It is a multinational study done by Hannah and colleagues.
- A total of 1041 and 1042 women with singleton breech at term were randomized to planned CS and planned vaginal delivery, respectively.
- Results: Planned CS group had lower perinatal mortality and lower neonatal mortality when compared with planned vaginal delivery group.

American College of Obstetricians and Gynecologists (ACOG, 2006) recommendations on breech delivery

- The decision regarding the mode of delivery should depend on the experience of the healthcare provider.
- Cesarean delivery will be the preferred mode of delivery for most physicians because of the diminishing expertise in vaginal breech delivery.
- Obstetricians should offer and perform ECV whenever possible.
- Planned vaginal delivery of a term singleton breech fetus may be reasonable under hospital-specific protocol guidelines for both eligibility and labor management.
- Before embarking on a plan for a vaginal breech delivery, women should be informed that the risk of perinatal or neonatal mortality or morbidity may be higher than if a CS is planned.
- In instances in which breech vaginal deliveries are pursued, great caution should be exercised, and a detailed patient informed consent should be documented.
- There are no recent data to support the recommendation of CS to patients with second twin in a nonvertex presentation.

- Obstetric complications such as intrauterine growth restriction, severe preeclampsia, placenta previa, and oligohydramnios (complicated breech)
- Precious pregnancy such as bad obstetric history, infertility, and elderly gravida

Cases that can be considered for vaginal breech delivery (must fulfill all the criteria)

- Multiparous woman
- Term or near term
- Weight 2–3.5 kg
- Frank or complete breech
- Well-flexed head
- Adequate liquor
- No obstetric complications
- Adequate pelvis

Note ***Summary of the criteria for considering vaginal breech delivery:*** *Multiparous women with complete or frank breech at term, with an average-sized fetus, with well-flexed head and adequate amount of liquor, with adequate pelvis, and with no other obstetric complications can be considered for vaginal breech delivery.*

Vaginal breech delivery

Three types of vaginal breech deliveries have been described.

Viva corner

Q1 Of flexed and frank breech, which is more suitable for vaginal delivery?

Extended or frank breech is more suitable for vaginal delivery because the presenting part is more compact. Hence:

- It fits well in the pelvis and engagement occurs early.
- It causes better cervical dilatation.
- The chances of PROM and cord prolapse are less.

Spontaneous breech delivery

- There is no traction or manipulation of the baby by the obstetrician.
- The fetus delivers spontaneously on its own without any assistance.
- This occurs predominantly in extremely preterm deliveries and dead fetus.

Assisted breech delivery

- This is the most common mode of vaginal breech delivery.
- In this method, an initial "no-touch technique" is adopted, in which the baby delivers spontaneously up to umbilicus and then active assistance is provided by the obstetrician in delivering the rest of the baby.

Breech extraction

- The fetal feet are grasped and the fetus is completely extracted by the obstetrician.

Extra edge

Q1 What is Zatuchni–Andros breech scoring system?

- Zatuchni–Andros breech scoring system can be used in breech presentation to decide whether to allow a vaginal breech delivery or to perform CS (see table below).
- Total score ranges from 0–11. If the woman has a score of ≤3, she should be delivered by a CS.
- Higher scores do not guarantee a safe vaginal delivery; however, vaginal delivery can be considered with close monitoring.

Table Zatuchni–Andros breech scoring system

Parameter	0 Point	1 Point	2 Points
Parity	Primigravida	Multigravida	–
Gestational age	39 weeks or more	38 weeks	37 weeks
Estimated fetal weight	>3.5 kg	3–3.5 kg	<3 kg
Previous breech	None	One	Two or more
Cervical dilatation	2 cm or less	3 cm	4 cm or more
Station	3 or higher	–2	–1 or lower

Part 1

- Indications for breech extraction:
  - Delivery of the second twin after internal podalic version
  - In CS, fetus in breech presentation is delivered by breech extraction

Note *Total breech extraction should not be done for singleton fetuses, because the cervix may not be adequately dilated to allow passage of the fetal head.*

Assisted breech delivery

Prerequisites

- The institution should have facilities to perform emergency CS.
- Experienced obstetrician trained to conduct vaginal breech delivery should be available.
- Anesthetist and neonatologist should be available.
- Counseling should be given regarding potential risks and benefits of vaginal breech delivery and informed consent for vaginal breech delivery should be obtained.

Intrapartum management

Role of induction in breech presentation

- Role of induction or augmentation in women with breech presentation is controversial.
- CS is preferred to induction or augmentation of labor.

I stage

- Secure IV line; blood is sent for cross-match and reservation.
- Ambulation is not allowed. The patient is kept on labor board to avoid early rupture of membranes and cord prolapse.
- The patient is kept nil oral and hydration is maintained with IV fluids (as there is increased rate of CS during labor).
- Adequate analgesia is given. Epidural analgesia is preferred if facilities are available.
  - Advantages of epidural analgesia
    - Helps in pain relief
    - Helps in vaginal manipulative procedures
    - If emergency LSCS is performed, anesthesia may be administered through the same epidural catheter
- Perform continuous electronic FHR monitoring if facilities are available; otherwise, perform intermittent auscultation with stethoscope every 15 minutes in the first stage and 5 minutes in the second stage.
- Partogram is maintained to monitor the progress of labor.
- Artificial rupture of membranes (ARM) should not be done. If membranes rupture spontaneously, vaginal examination is done to exclude cord prolapse.
- Premature bearing down should be avoided in order to prevent breech delivery through incompletely dilated cervix.
- Use of oxytocin for augmentation of labor is controversial (dysfunctional labor may be an ominous sign of fetopelvic disproportion).
- Emergency LSCS is done if there is abnormal progress of labor, early rupture of membranes, cord prolapse, or fetal distress.

Viva corner

Q1 Why should ARM not be done while allowing for vaginal breech delivery?

ARM can result in:

- Cord prolapse
- Occult cord prolapse
- Difficulty in performing vaginal manipulative procedures when liquor is less
  - An intact bag of membranes is a better dilator of cervix than the irregular contour of breech

II stage (assisted breech delivery)

- Continuous monitoring of FHR is done with cardiotocography (CTG) or every 5 minutes by intermittent auscultation.
- Things to be kept ready:
  - Delivery set with a warm dry towel (breech towel)
  - Piper's forceps
  - Neonatal resuscitation equipment
- When buttocks are seen distending the perineum, the patient is brought to the edge of the delivery table and placed in dorsal position with thighs flexed.
- Antiseptic painting and sterile draping of perineum are done.
- Bladder is emptied.
- P/V examination is done to confirm the second stage and to exclude cord prolapse.

- Pudendal block or perineal infiltration with 2% lignocaine is given (if epidural analgesia has not been given).
- Mother is encouraged to bear down with contractions.
- Liberal mediolateral episiotomy is given. Advantages of liberal episiotomy are as follows:
  - It helps in vaginal manipulation.
  - It facilitates easy delivery.
  - It helps to decrease the extent of sudden compression followed by decompression of the unmolded head during delivery of after-coming head (ACH) of breech, thereby reducing the risk of intracranial hemorrhage (ICH).
- Principles to be followed while conducting a vaginal breech delivery:
  - "No pull technique"—never pull from below as it can lead to deflexion of the head and arrest of ACH.
  - Keep the back anterior.
  - Avoid undue haste particularly in delivery of ACH.
- The baby is held by femoropelvic grip and is allowed to deliver spontaneously up to umbilicus ("wait and watch policy" or "noninterference" up to umbilicus—permits full dilatation of cervix). Then, active assistance from the obstetrician starts.
- Assistant exerts suprapubic pressure to maintain flexion of fetal head.
- The trunk and limbs of the baby are wrapped in a dry, warm towel. Advantages are the following:
  - Prevents slipping while manipulation
  - Avoids external stimulus
  - Keeps the baby warm
- Umbilical cord is pulled down and placed laterally in the sacral bay to prevent its compression and traction during delivery.
- Delivery of legs and buttocks: In flexed breech, ankle is grasped and legs can be gently pulled out. In frank breech, the extended legs can be delivered by giving gentle pressure on the popliteal fossa that causes flexion and abduction of the thighs. The feet drop down that can be pulled out.
- Keep the back anterior and gentle traction may be given during contraction. When the inferior angle of scapula is visible, the flexed arms in front of the chest are delivered one after the other by hooking out at the elbow.
- Delivery of ACH: It is the most crucial stage. The baby is allowed to hang down with support, until suboccipital hair line is visible under the pubic symphysis.
  - Delay in delivery of ACH can lead in birth asphyxia, whereas hasty delivery can lead to ICH.

Viva corner

Q1 What are the conditions where written consent is required for conducting a vaginal delivery?

- Vaginal breech delivery
- Trial of labor after cesarean section (VBAC)
- HIV-positive women

Q2 What are the fetal presentations in which head delivers by flexion?

- After-coming head of breech
- Mentoanterior face presentation
- Face to pubis delivery in occipitoposterior position where wider occiput sweeps over the perineum (head is delivered by initial flexion followed by extension)

Methods for delivery of ACH

Burns-Marshall technique (Figure 9.3)

- Baby is allowed to hang by its own weight. Assistant should give suprapubic pressure in downward and backward direction to maintain flexion of the head. When the nape of neck is visible, the baby is grasped at the ankles with the right hand.

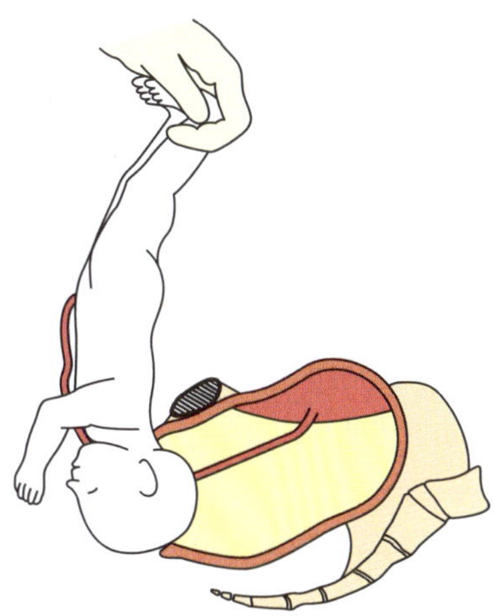

Figure 9.3 Burns-Marshall technique—the fetus is held by its feet with thumb and ring finger on either side and index and middle finger between the legs and swung in an arc over the maternal abdomen.

Steady traction is given, so that the trunk is swung in a downward, forward, and upward direction to form a wide arc of a circle over the maternal abdomen, to deliver the head. The left hand guards the perineum, slipping the perineum off successively the face and brow.

Disadvantage Full flexion of the head is not maintained in this method.

Mauriceau–Smellie–Veit technique (MSV technique) (Figure 9.4)

This includes malar flexion and shoulder traction.

- Baby's trunk rests on the operator's left supinated forearm with limbs hanging on either side.
- The obstetrician's left index and middle fingers are kept on malar prominences to maintain flexion of head. Right index and ring fingers are kept on the baby's right and left shoulders and middle finger over the suboccipit to maintain flexion.
- Having secured a firm grip, traction is given first in downward and then in forward and upward directions.
- Assistant should simultaneously give suprapubic pressure.

Advantage Flexion of the head is maintained.

Forceps delivery of the head (Figure 9.5)

- It is the best method for delivery of ACH.
- Piper's forceps or low forceps can be used.
- Forceps are applied from below after the trunk is raised by assistant.

Advantages

- Traction is directly on the head and not on the neck.
- The procedure maintains flexion of head.
- It acts as a protective cage to the head and prevents sudden compression followed by decompression.

III stage

- It includes active management of the third stage of labor to prevent postpartum hemorrhage.
- Perineum, vagina, and cervix are explored for any lacerations.

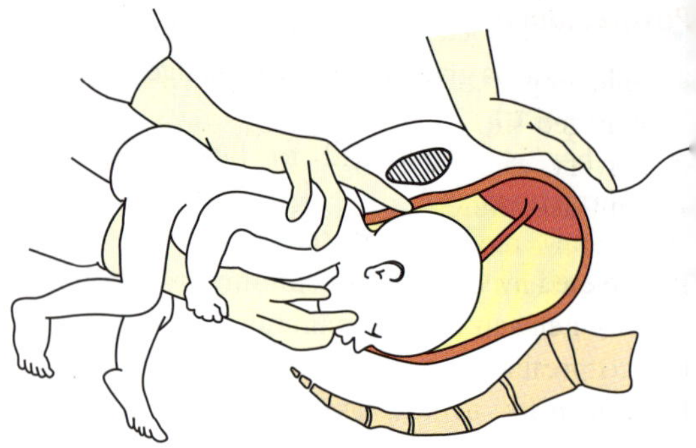

Figure 9.4 Mariceau–Smellie–Viet technique for delivery of the after-coming head.

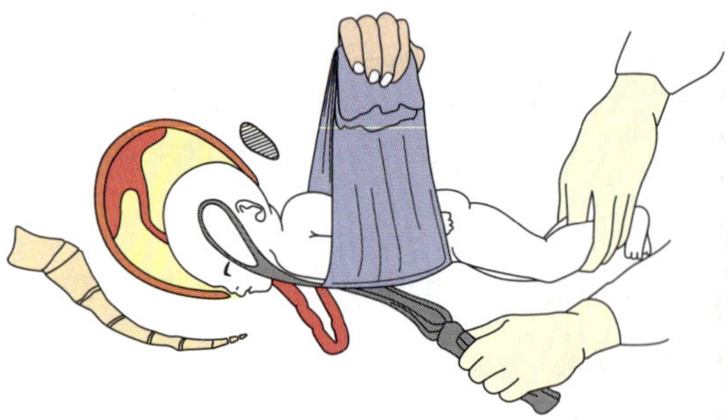

Figure 9.5 Delivery of the after-coming head by forceps—the fetus is held up and forceps applied from below.

Viva corner

Q1 What are the features of Piper's forceps?

Piper's forceps are commonly used to aid in the delivery of after-coming fetal head in ABD. The forceps has least or no pelvic curve (see figure below).

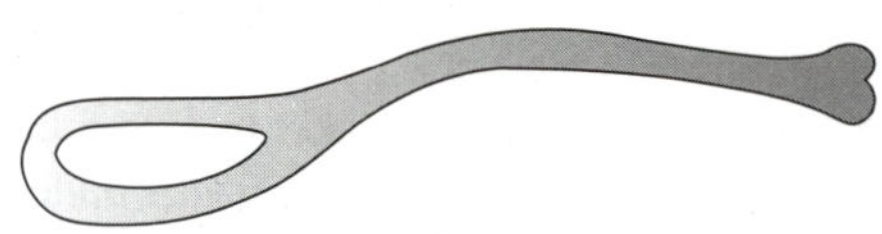

a.

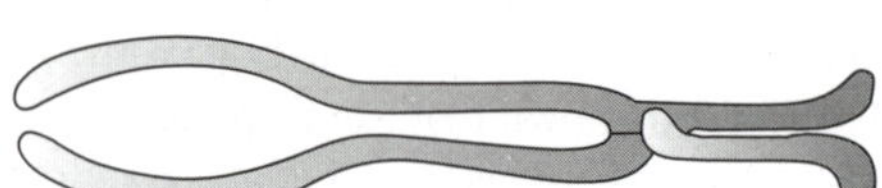

b.

Figure Piper's forceps. **a.** Single blade. **b.** Blades in locked position.

Postpartum management

- Following vaginal breech delivery, patients are managed similar to following a normal vaginal delivery
- Contraception counseling is given

If delivered by CS, look for intraoperative findings such as uterine anomalies that can lead to recurrent breech presentation. Concurrent sterilization can be done in a multiparous woman.

MANEUVERS IN VAGINAL BREECH DELIVERY

Complicated breech delivery refers to difficulties encountered during ABD such as extended legs, extended arms, posterior rotation of back, and entrapment of ACH that may be managed by certain maneuvers.

Pinard's maneuver—for delivery of extended legs (Figure 9.6)

It is done by intrauterine manipulation to convert frank breech into footling. The hand is passed along the thigh to the popliteal fossa, gentle pressure is given on the popliteal fossa to flex and abduct the thigh, following which the leg drops down, that can be pulled easily by holding at the ankle.

Lovset's maneuver—for delivery of extended arms (Figure 9.7)

Principle Sacral promontory is at a higher level than pubic symphysis because of the obliquity of the pelvis. Hence, when the anterior shoulder is above the pubic symphysis, the posterior shoulder lies below sacral promontory.

- The baby is rotated through 180° keeping the back anterior, which brings the posterior shoulder under pubic symphysis and can be easily hooked out.
- The shoulder that is now posterior can be delivered from posterior aspect or by rotating again and bringing it anterior under pubic symphysis.

Prague's maneuver (Figure 9.8)

- It is the method for delivery of ACH when back is posterior.

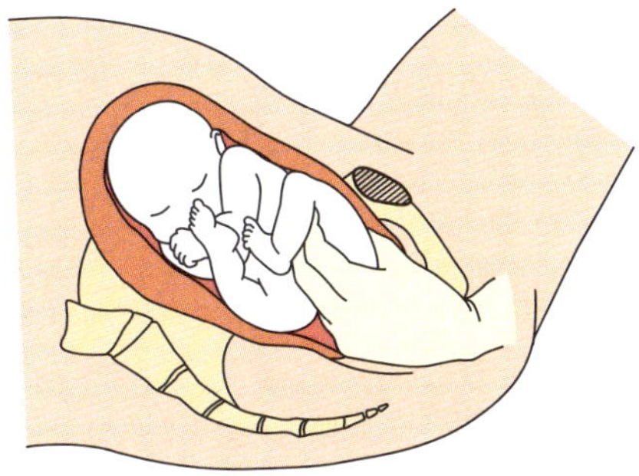

Figure 9.6 Pinard's maneuver for delivery of the extended legs. The hand is passed along the thigh to the popliteal fossa, the knee is flexed and the leg is brought down.

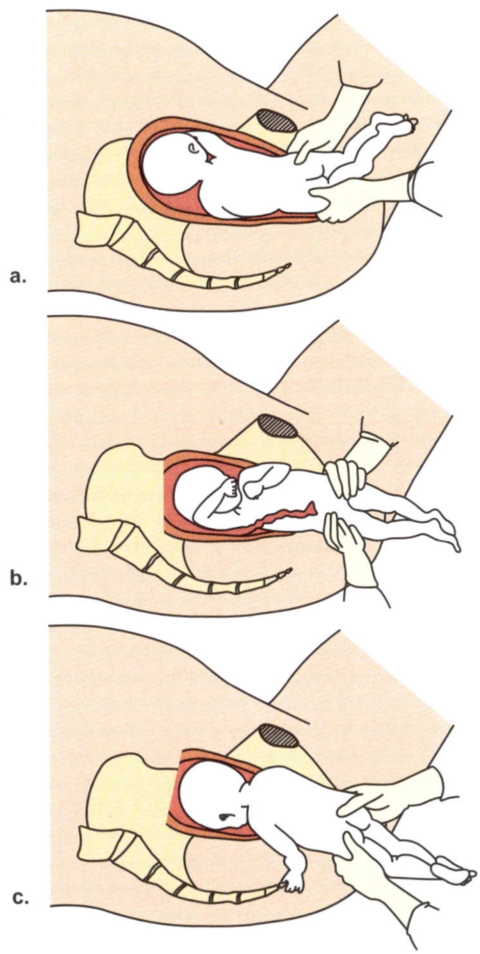

Figure 9.7 Lovset's maneuver for delivery of extended arms. **a-c.** The fetus is rotated through 180° in one direction and then in the other direction to bring the arms down.

Part 1

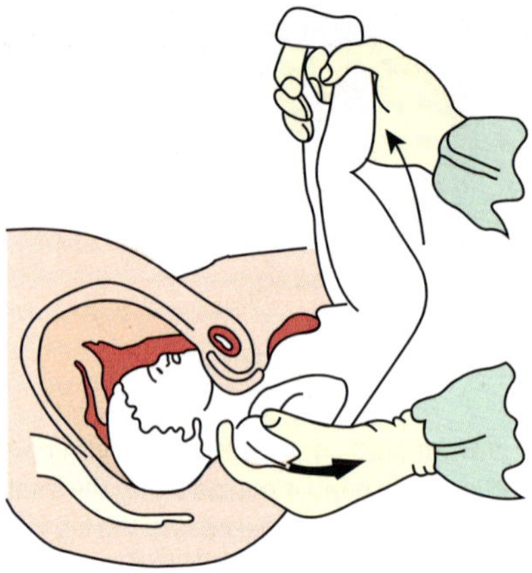

Figure 9.8 Prague's maneuver for delivery of after-coming head of breech when back is posterior.

- Rotation of back to anterior may be tried by using strong traction on fetal legs or bony pelvis.
- If back still remains posterior, fetus may be delivered by Prague's maneuver—two fingers of one hand grasp the shoulders from below while the other hand draws the feet up over the maternal abdomen.

Disadvantages This procedure may result in overstretching and injury to fetal neck.

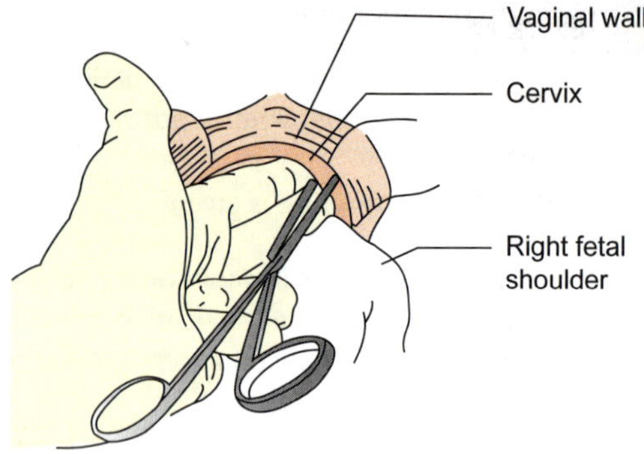

Figure 9.9 Duhrssen's incision on the cervix in case of entrapment of after-coming head by an incompletely dilated cervix.

Duhrssen's incision (Figure 9.9)

- If the head is trapped by an incompletely dilated cervix, incision is given on the cervix at 2 and 10 o'clock positions to aid in delivery of the head. This incision on cervix is termed Duhrssen's incision.
- Entrapment of ACH by incompletely dilated cervix is common in preterm breech delivery where the head is larger than the body and in cases with premature bearing-down efforts.

Viva corner

Q1 What are the major differences between vaginal delivery in cephalic and breech presentations?

Cephalic presentation	Breech presentation
• The head, which is the largest and least compressible structure of the fetus, is delivered first followed by the rest of the body. Once the head has delivered, the rest of the body follows without much difficulty	• The buttocks and trunk, which are compressible structures, are delivered first followed by the head, which is the least compressible structure. This can result in the entrapment of fetal head. It is common in footling presentation when the fetal legs deliver through partially dilated cervix followed by entrapment of fetal head
	• Breech is an irregular-fitting fetal part and a slow dilator of cervix, which increases the risk of PROM and cord prolapse
• Head delivers gradually after molding	• The head delivers suddenly without undergoing molding. As a result of this sudden compression and decompression, there is a high risk of tentorial tears and intracranial hemorrhage

There is an increased rate of performing an emergency CS, during the course of vaginal breech delivery. Thus, the vaginal breech delivery should be attempted only in a hospital with facilities for emergency CS.

Extra edge

Management of cord prolapse

Definitive management of cord prolapse is immediate delivery. If the patient is in the second stage and vaginal delivery is possible:

- **In cephalic presentation:** Instrumental delivery can be done.
- **In breech presentation:** Breech extraction can be done.

If immediate vaginal delivery is not possible, emergency CS is done.

Steps to be taken while shifting the patient for CS

- In order to prevent vasospasm of umbilical vessels, the loops of cord lying outside the vagina should be minimally handled.
- To prevent cord compression, the presenting part can be elevated either manually or by filling the urinary bladder with normal saline.
- Cord compression can be reduced by giving a head-down tilt.

Frequently asked viva questions

1. Summarize the case.
2. What is the diagnosis of the case?
3. How will you confirm the diagnosis?
4. What information will you look for in ultrasound?
5. What is the plan of management for the case?
6. Can ECV be attempted in the case?
7. What is the mode of delivery for the patient?
8. What are the causes of perinatal mortality in the case?
9. Why vaginal breech delivery is more hazardous compared to vaginal delivery in cephalic presentation?
10. What are the indications for elective LSCS?
11. What are the principles to be followed during assisted vaginal breech delivery?
12. What are the methods to deliver the after-coming head in breech?
13. What do you mean by complicated breech delivery?

10 Rh Isoimmunization

Introduction

Incompatibility of the rhesus (Rh) blood group factor between the mother and the fetus can lead to fetal hemolytic disease, termed as hemolytic disease of the fetus and newborn (HDFN) or red cell isoimmunization, that can result in increased perinatal morbidity and mortality. However, the mortality has considerably reduced with the availability of anti-D immunoglobulin for prevention of isoimmunization and tests for detection of isoimmunization and fetal hemolysis. This chapter deals with the case discussion of Rh-incompatible pregnancy.

Blood group systems

The two most important blood group systems are the following:

- ABO group (Table 10.1)
- Rhesus group (Table 10.2)

Table 10.1 ABO blood group system

Blood group	A antigen	B antigen	Anti-A antibody	Anti-B antibody
A	+	–	–	+
B	–	+	+	–
AB	+	+	–	–
O	–	–	+	+

Table 10.2 Rhesus system

Rhesus type	Rh antigen	Rh antibody
Rhesus positive (DD or Dd)	+	–
Rhesus negative (dd)	–	–

Definition of isoimmunization

Isoimmunization refers to production of antibodies in an individual, in response to an antigen derived from another individual of the same species, provided the first one lacks the antigen.

MECHANISM OF ANTIBODY FORMATION AND FETAL AFFECTION IN *Rh* ISOIMMUNIZATION

- The Rh antigen present on the RBC membrane of Rh-positive individuals has the ability to stimulate an immune antibody response when presented to an individual who lacks the antigen (Rh-negative individuals). This phenomenon of development of antibodies is termed isoimmunization (Figure 10.1).
- An Rh-negative woman gets sensitized with Rh-positive blood during the following events:
  - Pregnancy with an Rh-positive fetus (fetomaternal hemorrhage can result in mixing of fetal blood with maternal blood)
  - Mismatched blood transfusion (mismatched transfusion of Rh-positive blood to Rh-negative woman—very rare)
- About 75% of pregnant women have fetal RBCs in their circulation sometime during pregnancy and delivery. If the fetal RBCs that enter the maternal circulation are Rh positive, they stimulate a maternal immune response against the Rh antigen by formation of antibodies.
- A primary exposure leads to production of antigen-specific IgM antibodies and this response takes minimal of 12–16 weeks to occur.
- The IgM antibodies are high-molecular-weight antibodies that do not cross the placenta and

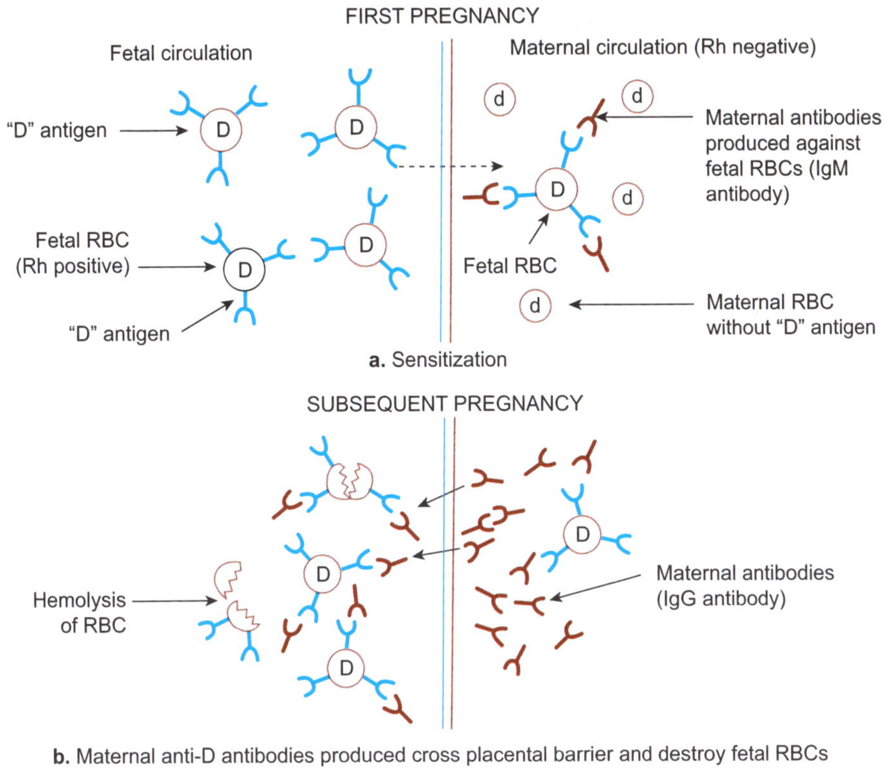

Figure 10.1 Mechanism of antibody formation and fetal affection in Rh isoimmunization. **a.** Events in first pregnancy. **b.** Events in subsequent pregnancy.

hence there is no harm to the fetus in the first pregnancy (primary sensitizing pregnancy). The first sensitizing pregnancy is usually unaffected.

- A subsequent exposure of the mother to the antigen in her second pregnancy produces an amnestic response and rapid production of large amounts of IgG antibodies from the previously primed B cells. IgG antibodies can cross the placenta and bind to Rh antigen on the fetal RBCs, causing sequestration and destruction of fetal RBCs. Affected RBCs are rapidly removed from the circulation by the reticuloendothelial system.
- Depending on the degree of RBC destruction, various manifestations of the disease occur, leading to a spectrum of hemolytic disease of the fetus and neonate.

Situations when fetomaternal hemorrhage can occur

Leakage of fetal blood into maternal circulation is termed as fetomaternal hemorrhage (FMH) and it occurs in about 75% of women during delivery. The frequency and volume of spontaneous FMH increase with advancing period of gestation (POG) and is highest during delivery. FMH that occurs in a Rh-negative mother who carries a Rh-positive fetus can result in sensitization of the mother and subsequent isoimmunization. The conditions that can result in FMH are listed in Table 10.3.

Types of antibodies

Types of maternal antibodies formed against the Rh antigen are mentioned in Table 10.4.

Table 10.3 Situations for fetomaternal hemorrhage

• Abortion • Ectopic pregnancy • Chorionic villous sampling • Amniocentesis • Cordocentesis	• Antepartum hemorrhage • Abdominal trauma • External cephalic version • During delivery • Manual removal of placenta

Table 10.4 Types of maternal antibodies formed against the Rh antigen

IgM antibody	IgG antibody
• First antibody to appear • Large molecule, hence cannot cross the placenta • Not harmful to fetus • Agglutinates RBCs when suspended in saline	• Appears after few months • Small molecule, hence crosses the placental barrier • Harmful to the fetus—causes hemolytic disease of fetus and newborn • Agglutinates RBCs when suspended in albumin

Case presentation

Salient points in history

Consider the following relevant points during history taking in cases of Rh isoimmunization.

Presenting complaints

The patient may say that her blood group is Rh negative and has been admitted close to her expected date of delivery or admitted in view of bad obstetric history.

- *Ask the blood group of the woman and her husband.*

Present pregnancy

- *H/o bleeding P/V (risk of FMH)*
- *H/o trauma (risk of FMH)*
- *H/o any invasive procedure undergone such as chorionic villous sampling and amniocentesis*
- *H/o whether indirect Coombs test (ICT) was done (patient may give H/o certain test that is repeated periodically during antenatal period)*
- *H/o anti-D immunoglobulin injection during midpregnancy*
- *H/o symptoms suggestive of preeclampsia*

Past obstetric history

There may be a bad obstetric history (elicit a detailed obstetric history):

- *H/o abortions*
- *H/o polyhydramnios or preeclampsia*
- *H/o neonatal jaundice within 24 hours of birth*
- *H/o stillbirths or intrauterine death (IUD)*
- *Blood group and Rh typing of previous babies*
- *H/o receiving anti-D immunoglobulin injection following abortions and delivery*

Past history

H/o blood transfusion

Salient points in examination

Consider the following relevant points during examination in cases of Rh isoimmunization.

General examination

Nothing specific to this case

Vitals

BP (preeclampsia may be present in Rh-isoimmunized pregnancy due to hyperplacentosis)

Obstetric examination

Look for the presence of excess liquor.

Case summary

An example of writing summary in cases of Rh isoimmunization is given below.

Example *Mrs. Y, 30 years of age, G2P1L1 at 39 + 5 weeks of gestation, with A negative blood group, has been admitted 1 day back for safe confinement. She has no specific complaints. She is perceiving normal fetal movements and there is no H/o labor pains or leaking P/V. Her previous pregnancy was uneventful, delivered vaginally at term, and she gives a history of receiving an IM injection related to her negative blood group (probably anti-D immunoglobulin) on the second day of delivery. On examination, there is no pallor or pedal edema. Her BP is 120/70 mmHg. Obstetric examination*

(CONTD...)

(...CONTD)

reveals a singleton live fetus in cephalic presentation; liquor appears average, uterus is relaxed, and FHR is 132 beats/min heard in right spinoumbilical line.

Case diagnosis

An example of writing diagnosis in cases of Rh isoimmunization is given below.

Example *30 years of age, G2P1L1 at 39 + 5 weeks of gestation with Rh-incompatible pregnancy, with a singleton live fetus in cephalic presentation, not in labor*

Note *While writing diagnosis, if sensitization has not occurred (ICT is negative) mention as Rh-incompatible pregnancy. If sensitization has occurred (ICT is positive) or if there is H/o previous affected babies then mention as Rh-isoimmunized pregnancy.*

Case discussion

Investigations—screening for isoimmunization

- Routine antenatal investigations including ABO blood grouping and Rh typing is done in all women during the first antenatal visit.
- If the mother is Rh-negative, then the partner's blood grouping and typing should be tested.
- If the partner is Rh negative, no further investigations are required.
- If the partner is Rh positive, the woman should be screened for the presence of Rh antibodies (anti-D antibodies) by doing an ICT. Further management depends on the result of ICT test for maternal anti-D antibodies screening, which is discussed under *"antenatal management of Rh-incompatible pregnancy."*

Note *All Rh-negative pregnant women with Rh-positive partner should be screened for anti-D antibodies by doing ICT, including those who have received postpartum anti-D prophylaxis in their previous pregnancy (as anti-D prophylaxis does not guarantee 100% prevention of Rh isoimmunization).*

Viva corner

Q1 Can the partner's genotype help to predict chance of affection in fetus?

Yes. The chance of affection in the fetuses of an Rh-negative mother depends on the Rh status of the father (see table and figure below).

- A homozygous Rh-positive father will have 100% Rh-positive babies with an Rh-negative mother.
- A heterozygous Rh-positive father will have 50% Rh-positive babies with an Rh-negative mother. The other 50% will be Rh negative.
- An Rh-negative father will have 100% Rh-negative babies with an Rh-negative mother.

Table Inheritance of Rh factor and chance of affection in the fetuses

Blood group of the partner of an Rh-negative female (dd)	Blood group of fetuses	Chance of affection (see figure below)
Rh-positive homozygous (DD) male	All the fetuses are Rh positive	All the fetuses are likely to be affected in an isoimmunized mother
Rh-positive heterozygous (Dd) male	50% of fetuses are Rh positive	50% of fetuses are likely to be affected in an isoimmunized mother
Rh-negative male (dd)	All fetuses will be Rh negative	None of the fetuses will be affected (isoimmunization does not occur)

(CONTD...)

(...CONTD)

Viva corner

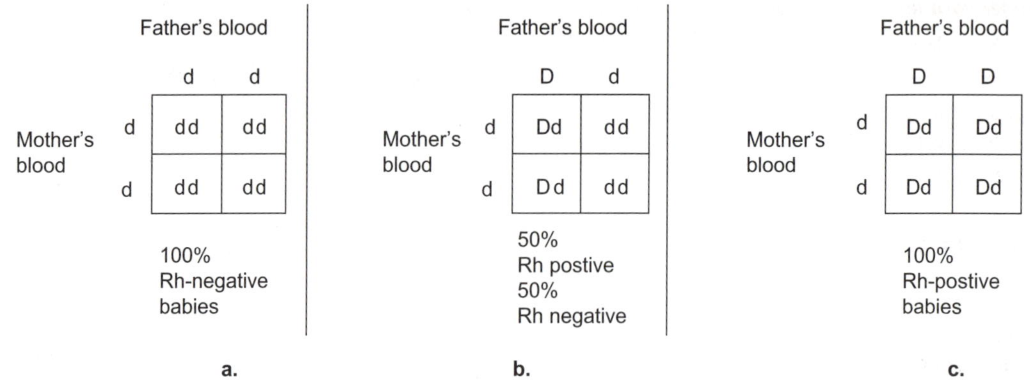

Figure Inheritance of Rh factor. **a.** An Rh-negative father will have 100% Rh-negative babies with an Rh-negative mother. **b.** A heterozygous Rh-positive father will have 50% Rh-positive babies with an Rh-negative mother. The other 50% will be Rh negative. **c.** A homozygous Rh-positive father will have 100% Rh-positive babies with an Rh-negative mother.

Q2 How can you determine the blood group of the fetus while in utero?

Determination of fetal Rh group Amniocentesis is performed under ultrasound guidance and the amniocytes obtained are cultured and amplified by polymerized chain reaction (PCR) to identify the Rh gene locus on chromosome 1.

Recent advances Free fetal DNA from fetal red cells in maternal plasma is now being used as a noninvasive method for the detection of fetal Rh gene sequence using PCR.

Complications of Rh isoimmunization

The various complications that can develop due to Rh isoimmunization are described below, prior to the discussion on management of Rh-incompatible pregnancy.

Maternal complications

The fetus is primarily affected, but the isoimmunized mother is at an increased risk of the following:

- Preeclampsia (due to hyperplacentosis)
- Polyhydramnios
- Postpartum hemorrhage (PPH) due to big-size placenta and uterine overdistension
- Probable increase in morbidity in an isoimmunized mother due to the intrauterine fetal interventions required

Fetal complications

Depending on the degree of fetal RBC destruction, various manifestations of the disease can occur, termed erythroblastosis fetalis or HDFN.

Hydrops fetalis

It is the most severe form with severe anemia due to RBC destruction.

- Severe anemia and hypoxia lead to damage to various organs.
  - Heart—high-output congestive cardiac failure
  - Liver dysfunction due to fetal anoxemia and acidosis → decreased protein synthesis → hypoproteinemia → edema at various sites → edema of scalp, skin edema, pericardial and pleural effusion, and ascites
  - Placental hyperplasia (hyperplacentosis) occurs to increase the oxygen transport to fetus
  - Ultimately fetal death due to congestive cardiac failure (CCF)

Icterus gravis neonatorum

It is a less severe form of hemolytic disease.

- Baby develops jaundice within 24 hours of birth.
- When bilirubin exceeds 20 mg/dL, it crosses blood–brain barrier to get deposited in the basal

nuclei leading to kernicterus and death. Baby may need exchange transfusion.

Congenital anemia of newborn

It is the mildest form of disease.

- Destruction of RBC continues up to 6 weeks postnatal period.
- Baby develops anemia over the first few weeks of life, but jaundice is not evident.

Antenatal management of Rh-incompatible pregnancy

- **If blood group of partner is Rh negative**: No further evaluation is required and the patient is cared for as in normal pregnancy.
- **If blood group of partner is Rh positive**: ICT is done at the first antenatal visit to screen for the presence of maternal anti-D antibodies.

Extra edge

Pathogenesis in hydrops fetalis

Hydrops fetalis is a condition characterized by abnormal accumulation of fluid in the fetal extravascular compartments and serous body cavities.

- Rh isoimmunization is the major cause of immune hydrops.
- Sequestration of fetal RBCs by maternal IgG antibodies results in severe hemolysis and fetal anemia.
- There is marked erythroid hyperplasia and extramedullary hematopoiesis in the liver and spleen leading to hepatosplenomegaly and hepatic dysfunction.
- Normal hepatic protein synthesis is impaired and portal venous pressure is increased leading to fetal ascites.
- Umbilical venous hypertension develops and the placenta shows hydropic changes and enlargement to increase the oxygen transport to fetus.
- Decrease in colloid oncotic pressure and accumulation of fluid in the extravascular spaces leads to generalized subcutaneous edema of the fetal skin, placental enlargement, pericardial and pleural effusion, and ascites. Fetal pleural effusion and diaphragmatic elevation due to ascites and hepatosplenomegaly may compress the fetal lungs with consequent lung hypoplasia.
- The hydropic fetus may die in utero due to cardiac failure resulting from severe anemia.

Diagnosis of hydrops

Ultrasound features suggestive of hydrops

- Hepatosplenomegaly.
- Increase in diameter of umbilical vein and intrahepatic portal vein due to increased blood flow in umbilical vein.
- Presence of fluid in serous cavities.
  - The first site of fluid collection is the pericardial space.
  - The earliest sign of fetal ascites is a clear delineation of small bowel due to fluid in between the loops.
  - Pleural effusion
  - Skin and scalp edema is characterized by skin thickness of >5 mm. The ideal site of measurement is the forehead.
- Cardiomegaly is diagnosed when the cardiac to thoracic circumference ratio is >50%.

X-ray

Scalp edema leads to "Buddha position sign."

Cardiotocography

Severe anemia and impending death produces a sinusoidal FHR pattern on cardiotocography (CTG; see figure below)

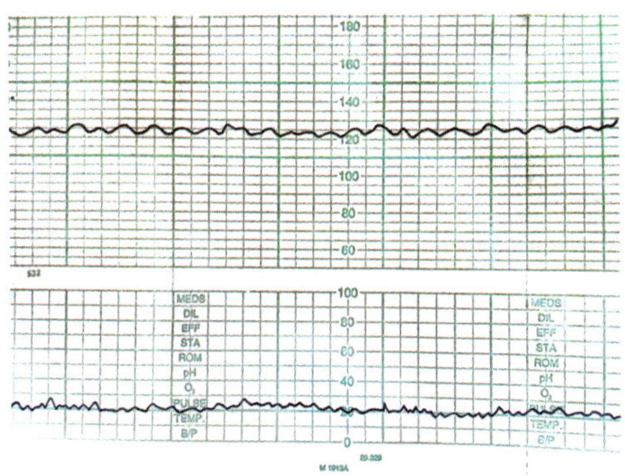

Figure Sinusoidal pattern in cardiotocography.

At birth

- Baby is pale and edematous with enlarged abdomen due to ascites and hepatosplenomegaly.
- Placenta appears pale, edematous, and enlarged, and histopathology shows villous edema.

- The presence of anti-D antibodies in the maternal serum is diagnostic of maternal Rh isoimmunization.
- **If ICT is negative**: Manage as an Rh nonimmunized pregnancy.
- **If ICT is positive**: Manage as an Rh isoimmunized pregnancy.

Hence, in the antenatal period, the women can be divided into two groups: Rh-negative nonimmunized women and Rh-negative isoimmunized women.

- In the Rh nonimmunized women, the objective of the antenatal management is prevention of Rh isoimmunization.
- In women who are already Rh isoimmunized, the objective of management is early detection and treatment of anemia in the fetus.

Management of both these cases is discussed in the subsequent sections.

Extra edge

Indirect Coombs test

- It is a test done in the mother to detect Rh (IgG) antibodies in maternal circulation (see figure below).
- It is the most sensitive and reliable method to determine the degree of isoimmunization.
- Maternal serum is incubated with Rh-positive RBCs. Agglutination of RBCs on addition of serum containing antihuman globulin (AHG) antibody (Coombs serum) indicates the presence of IgG Rh antibody in the mother's serum.
- The concentration of anti-D antibody is determined by a titration procedure. A titer value of 1:4 indicates isoimmunization.
- Critical titer is the titer level at or below which no perinatal death has occurred due to erythroblastosis.
- Titer values vary between laboratories, so the same laboratory should be used when repeat titers are done. The critical titer varies between 8 and 32; usually it is 1:16.

Mother's serum + Rh-positive RBCs → RBCs absorb antibodies if present in maternal serum → Add antihuman globulin—if agglutination occurs → ICT positive

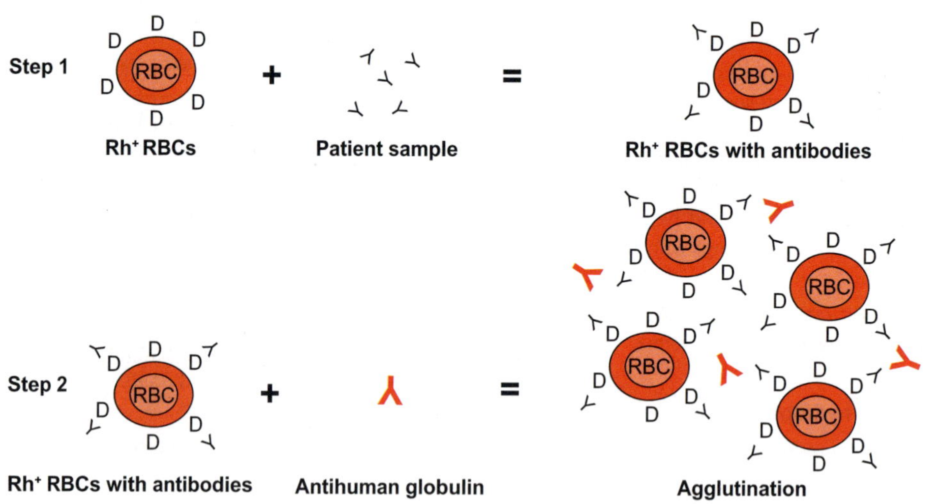

Figure Indirect Coombs test.

Example: A mother who is Rh negative can have prenatal testing to determine the presence of IgG Ab in her blood stream that will attack the fetal RBCs, if the fetus is Rh positive.

(CONTD...)

(...CONTD)

Extra edge

Direct Coombs test

- It is a test done in the baby to detect fetal RBCs that are already bound to maternal antibodies (see figure below).

Fetal RBCs + Antihuman globulin → If agglutination occurs → DCT positive

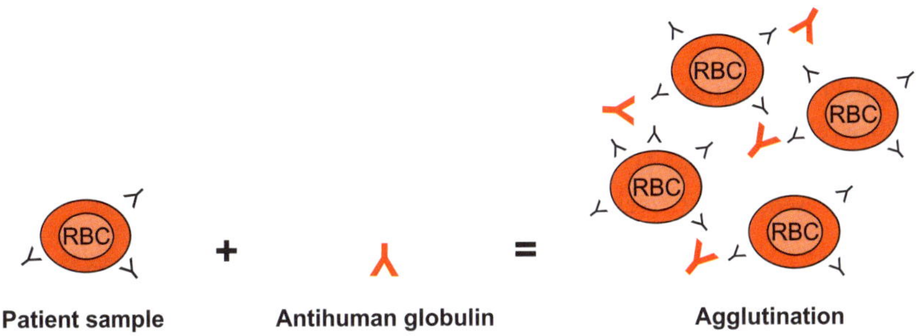

Figure Direct Coombs test.

Example: Baby's serum sample is positive for the presence of the maternal Ab on the surface of RBCs in erythroblastosis fetalis.

Management of Rh-negative non-iso immunized pregnancy (ICT negative)

The main objective in the management of an Rh-negative nonimmunized pregnant woman is prevention of isoimmmunization by passive administration of Rh immunoglobulin and minimizing the chances of FMH (refer to Flowcharts 10.1–10.3 at the end of the chapter).

Prevention of Rh isoimmunization—anti-D immunoglobulin immunoprophylaxis

Aim The aim is to prevent antibody formation in the mother.

Current recommendations for the prevention of Rh isoimmunization

- Routine antenatal anti-D prophylaxis (RAADP) given at 28 weeks along with postpartum anti-D prophylaxis within 72 hours of delivery.
- Apart from this, anti-D should also be given after potential sensitizing events during pregnancy.

Routine antenatal anti-D prophylaxis

- If ICT for Rh antibody screening is negative, the screening should be repeated every 4 weeks. Antibody screening every 4 weeks is not universally accepted as the incidence of Rh isoimmunization in the antenatal period is less (<1%), and a repeat test may be done at 28 weeks. However, screening every 4 weeks will detect the rare cases who get sensitized before delivery.
- Usual protocol is as follows:
  - *In a primigravida*: Repeat ICT at 28 weeks.
  - *In a multigravida*: Repeat ICT every 4 weeks.
- RAADP in a dose of 300 μg intramuscularly should be given to all Rh nonimmunized women at 28 weeks to prevent isoimmunization due to FMH that occurs during the antenatal period. Antenatal anti-D will provide protection for 12 weeks, that is, up to delivery.
- RAADP is not recommended before 28 weeks as sensitization is <0.1%.
- The cost-effectiveness of RAADP has been questioned, as FMH mostly occurs during delivery.

However, RAADP is still recommended, as it reduces the incidence of antenatal isoimmunization from 2% to 0.1%. The option for an informed choice of RAADP should be given to the patient, when RAADP is not necessary or cost-effective, like in the woman who has opted for sterilization after delivery.

- After RAADP, the ICT for antibody screening may show anti-D antibodies in the maternal serum but the titer values do not go beyond 1:4. A titer of >1:4 results from isoimmunization rather than anti-D administration.
- RAADP at 28 weeks should be offered even if the patient has received anti-D prophylaxis for a potentially sensitizing event early in pregnancy.

Postnatal immunoprophylaxis

- A standard postnatal dose of 300 μg IM is given within 72 hours of delivery, if the baby is Rh positive and direct Coombs test (DCT) on cord blood is negative (which detects the presence of antibodies in the fetal circulation). Postnatal prophylaxis reduces the incidence of Rh sensitization from 15% to 1–2%.
- The maximal protection occurs if anti-D is given within 72 hours, but it may be given up to 4 weeks after delivery (should not be withheld if >72 hours have passed postpartum).

Other potential sensitizing events during pregnancy that require anti-D prophylaxis

See Table 10.5

Table 10.5 Antepartum events that require anti-D prophylaxis

Event	Dose of anti-D
First-trimester spontaneous or induced abortion	50 μg
Threatened abortion in the first trimester	50 μg
Ectopic pregnancy or partial molar pregnancy	50 μg
Chorionic villus sampling	50 μg
Second-trimester spontaneous or induced abortion	300 μg
Second-trimester threatened abortion	300 μg
Amniocentesis or fetal blood sampling	300 μg
External cephalic version	300 μg
Antepartum hemorrhage	300 μg

Note *Anti-D injection is not required following evacuation of a complete mole (does not contain blood vessels, hence no chance of FMH).*

Time of delivery of Rh-nonimmunized pregnancy

- In case RAADP is not given at 28 weeks, the patient is followed up with ICT every 4 weeks till term.

High-yield points

Estimation of fetomaternal hemorrhage

- A total of 300 μg of anti-D protects the mother from 15 mL of Rh-positive fetal RBCs or 30 mL of fetal whole blood, that is, 10 μg of anti-D, protects the mother from 1 mL of FMH. However, the exact dose depends on the amount of FMH.
- FMH can be estimated by Kleihauer–Betke test, which is based on the principle of acid elution technique.
- Principle: Fetal RBCs are resistant to acid elution and remain intact as dark refractile bodies while maternal RBCs undergo elution leaving behind RBC membrane (ghost-like appearance) (see figure below)

Amount of fetal bleed is calculated by the following formula:

$$\text{Fetal bleed (mL)} = \frac{\text{No. of fetal cells}}{\text{1000 maternal cells}} \times 5000$$

The Kleihauer-Betke test

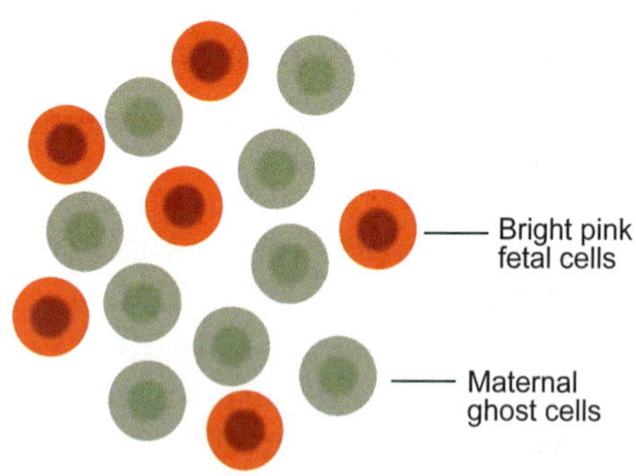

Figure Acid elution technique. Fetal RBCs are resistant to acid elution and remain intact as dark refractile bodies while maternal RBCs undergo elution leaving behind RBC membrane.

- Deliver the patient by 40 weeks (the pregnancy is not allowed to cross the expected date of delivery).

Intrapartum management

- Precautions should be taken to prevent FMH.
  - Methergin is withheld following delivery of the baby (increases FMH).
  - Manual removal of placenta should be avoided.
  - Vigorous massaging of uterus should be avoided.
  - Precautions during cesarean section
    - Avoid spillage of blood into peritoneal cavity.
    - Avoid manual removal of placenta.
    - Avoid vigorous massaging of uterus.
    - Avoid methergin.
- Keep the umbilical cord long (may require exchange transfusion).
- Collect cord blood for blood grouping and typing, Hb estimation, serum bilirubin, and DCT.

Postpartum management

Postnatal immunoprophylaxis If baby is Rh positive and DCT is negative, administer 300 μg of anti-D (IM) to the mother within 72 hours of delivery (Figure 10.2).

- **"A few women can still get sensitized despite measures to prevent sensitization."**

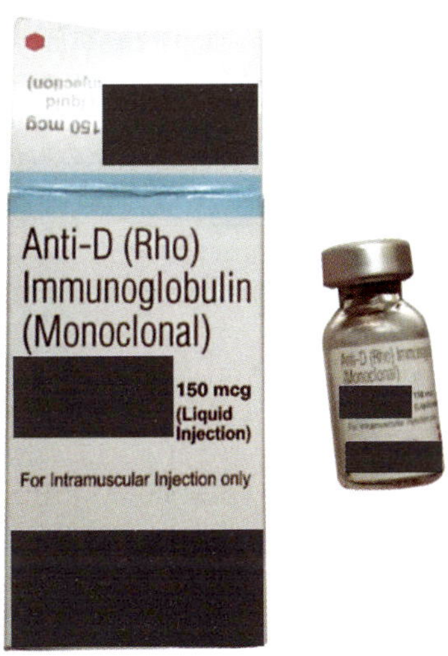

Figure 10.2 Anti-D vial.

All of the above-mentioned measures (RAADP + Postnatal prophylaxis) prevent sensitization to the extent of <1%. But a few women can still get sensitized, which may be due to the following:

- Larger volume of FMH
- Lesser potency of anti-D administered
- Delay in administration of anti-D immunoglobulin
- Sensitization of the mother has already occurred during pregnancy
- **"Not all 'at risk' Rh-negative women become sensitized"**
  - At least 0.1 mL of fetal blood should enter the maternal circulation for sensitization to occur.
  - Fetal red cells may enter the maternal circulation during pregnancy or at the time of delivery. The frequency and volume of FMH increases as pregnancy advances.
  - In the majority of cases, FMH sufficient to cause isoimmunization occurs at the time of delivery. However, an immune response is mounted only by 10–15% of the "at-risk" Rh-negative women during delivery and by <1% during pregnancy. This may be because of the following:
    - Lesser volume of FMH (size of the inoculum)—greater the number of fetal cells entering the maternal circulation, greater the possibility of maternal sensitization
    - Weak strength of Rh antigenic stimulus
    - Immunological nonresponders—30% of Rh-negative women are immunogenic nonresponders that is genetically controlled and they do not become sensitized to the Rh-positive antigen
    - Coexistent ABO incompatibility between mother and fetus reduces the risk of sensitization because of rapid clearance of ABO-incompatible fetal cells from the maternal circulation by naturally occurring antibodies in the mother, before Rh sensitization could occur. Risk of Rh isoimmunization is 2–3% in ABO-incompatible pregnancy as compared to 10–15% in ABO-compatible pregnancy (e.g., O negative group mother carrying a positive group fetus—fetal cells entering maternal circulation are destroyed by anti-A and anti-B antibodies in maternal circulation).

Viva corner

Q1 How does anti-D immunoglobulin prevent isoimmunization?

The exact mechanism by which anti-D Ig prevents isoimmunization is not known. It could be due to masking of the Rh D antigenic sites on fetal RBCs in maternal circulation, thereby preventing its expression and sensitization of maternal immune system, or may be due to downregulation of B lymphocytes.

Q2 Is postnatal anti-D prophylaxis still mandatory even if antenatal prophylaxis is given?

Postnatal prophylaxis is mandatory regardless of antenatal prophylaxis at 28 weeks because protection level lasts for only 12 weeks following administration, that is, up to delivery. Hence, postnatal anti-D prophylaxis is required to prevent Rh isoimmunization due to FMH that occurs at the time of delivery.

Q3 Why is antenatal anti-D given at 28 weeks?

FMH in the first trimester is 5%, while in the third trimester it occurs in 50% of pregnancies. Hence, maximum protection is achieved when anti-D is given during the start of the third trimester, that is, at 28 weeks, and the protection lasts for 12 weeks, that is, up to delivery.

Management of Rh-isoimmunized mother (ICT positive)

The main objective of management of an Rh-negative pregnant woman who is already sensitized is early detection and treatment of fetal anemia (refer to Flowcharts 10.1–10.3 at the end of the chapter).

Antenatal management

- If ICT is positive, do serial anti-Rh antibody titers (ICT in titers), which can determine the risk of development of fetal anemia. As long as the titer remains below the critical titer of 1:16, the risk of fetal anemia or severe erythroblastosis or perinatal death is low.

Further management is based on ICT titer levels.

- If the antibody titer remains below the critical level, repeat the titers every 4 weeks up to 28 weeks and then every 2–3 weeks thereafter.
  - The patient can be followed up with serial ultrasound till term.
  - If no other indication for early termination exists, deliver the patient at term.
  - The pediatrician should be informed during delivery so that early evaluation and treatment of the newborn is started.
  - Keep the umbilical cord long, in case exchange transfusion is required.
  - The cord blood should be collected for Rh typing, DCT, hemoglobin, and serum bilirubin.
- If at any point of time, the antibody titers exceeds the critical level or there is a significant rise in titers between two consecutive samples, further evaluation is done by Doppler velocimetry of the middle cerebral artery peak systolic velocity (MCA PSV)
- MCA Doppler has revolutionized the management of Rh-isoimmunized pregnancy by minimizing the need for invasive tests by 70%. The sensitivity of MCA PSV for the prediction of moderate to severe fetal anemia is almost 100%.

Extra edge

Principle involved in MCA changes in fetal anemia

Fetal anemia is associated with decrease in oxygen-carrying capacity and low hemoglobin and albumin levels resulting in decrease in blood viscosity. The compensatory hemodynamic changes lead to increase in cardiac output and increase in blood flow velocity. These changes are generalized and seen throughout the entire fetal circulatory system, but the middle cerebral artery depicts these changes very accurately, as it is very sensitive to hypoxemia.

Further management is based on the interpretation of MCA PSV.

- If the MCA PSV is <1.5 multiples of median (MoM), repeat the study every 2 weeks and the patient may be delivered at 37–38 weeks.
- If the MCA PSV is ≥1.5 MoM, further evaluation is required.
- If the MCA PSV is >1.5 MoM, and the patient is >34 weeks, the patient can be delivered and exchange transfusion may be given postnatally to the newborn.
- If the MCA PSV is >1.5 MoM, and the patient is <34 weeks, fetal blood sampling (FBS) is

done by cordocentesis to estimate cord blood hematocrit.
- If cord blood hematocrit is >30%, FBS is to be repeated once a week. Delivery should be planned between 34 and 36 weeks.
- If cord blood hematocrit is <30%, intrauterine transfusion (IUT) is indicated.

Viva corner

Q1 What are the advantages of MCA PSV in the detection of affected fetus?

- Noninvasive technique to detect fetal anemia
- Detects fetal anemia at an early stage
- Correlates directly with fetal anemia while spectrophotometric analysis of amniotic fluid correlates directly with fetal hyperbilirubinemia
- No worsening of fetomaternal hemorrhage
- Fetal response to in utero transfusion can be monitored

Serial amniocentesis and Liley's curve

- This method was used in the past and has now been replaced by MCA PSV (refer to Flowcharts 10.1–10.3 at the end of the chapter).
- If the mother had a critical antibody titer (≥1:16), serial amniocentesis was done to plot the Liley's curve. Fetuses affected by hemolytic disease secrete high levels of bilirubin into the amniotic fluid, and hence amniocentesis done to obtain the amniotic fluid for assessment of bilirubin levels.

Further management is based on amniotic fluid analysis.

- Principle: Spectrophotometric analysis of the amniotic fluid is done and the optical density of amniotic fluid is plotted on a semilogarithmic graph against wavelength. Bilirubin causes a shift in the optical density with a peak at a wavelength of 450 nm. The deviation or peak at 450 nm wavelength is proportionate to the amount of bilirubin in amniotic fluid. The amount of deviation at 450 nm (ΔOD 450) is used to estimate the degree of fetal hemolysis (increased fetal hemolysis leads to increased bilirubin in amniotic fluid).
- Deviation value at 450 nm (ΔOD 450) is plotted on a graph versus the gestational age from 27 to 40 weeks. This graph is divided into three zones to obtain the Liley's chart, which indicates the risk of fetal anemia (Figure 10.3).

Note *Amniocentesis is usually done after 26 weeks of gestation but not before 20 weeks. Prior to 20 weeks, fetal reticuloendothelial system is not mature enough to cause sufficient destruction of RBCs, even when they are affected by antibodies.*

Further management is based on the zones in Liley's chart.

Interpretation of Liley's graph

- **ΔOD 450 values in zone 1 (lowest zone):** Fetuses with mild anemia
- **ΔOD 450 values in zone 2:** Fetuses with moderate anemia
- **ΔOD 450 values in zone 3 (highest zone):** Severely affected fetuses (Hb <8 g%) with the possibility of developing hydrops within 7 days

Note *The boundaries of the zones slope downward with increasing gestational age because amniotic fluid (AF) bilirubin decreases with advancing gestational age.*

Extra edge

Limitations of Liley's graph

- Liley's graph begins at 27 weeks of gestation because ΔOD 450 levels in the second trimester are less reliable predictors of true fetal anemia.
- The Liley's graph was modified by Queenan et al. who developed a curve from 14 to 40 weeks. As the bilirubin levels are naturally high in amniotic fluid at midpregnancy, a large indeterminate zone is created where bilirubin levels do not accurately predict fetal Hb.
- Therefore, when severe fetal anemia or hydrops develops before 25 weeks, cordocentesis is a better method of fetal assessment than amniocentesis.

Further management depends on serial amniocentesis to determine the trend of ΔOD 450 values over time (Table 10.6).

Further management of moderate to severely affected fetus is based on cordocentesis.

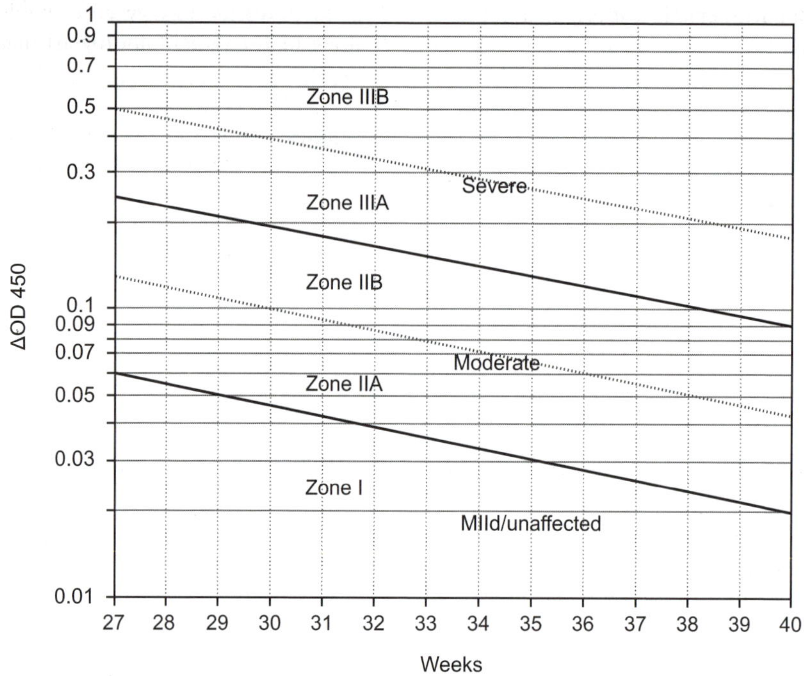

Figure 10.3 Liley's chart. The optical density (ΔOD) at 450 nm wavelength is plotted against gestation in weeks.

- Ultrasound-guided cordocentesis allows precise measurement of fetal Hb and hematocrit and the need for intrauterine blood transfusion.
- If >34 weeks, deliver and then give exchange transfusion
- If <34 weeks, do cordocentesis
  - *Hematocrit <30%:* Give intrauterine transfusion
  - *Hematocrit >30%:* Follow up with ultrasonography (USG) and cordocentesis

Table 10.6 Zones and management based on Liley's graph

Zone	Management	
Zone 1 (nonaffected or mildly affected)	• Do serial amniocentesis every 4 weeks and if it continues to remain in zone 1, deliver at term	
Zone 2 (moderately affected)	• Repeat amniocentesis after 1 week – If in zone 1 repeat at a 4-week interval – If still in zone 2, repeat the test in 1 week and do the following:	
	If the repeat value shows a horizontal trend	• **<34 weeks**: Cordocentesis for evaluation of fetal hematocrit is indicated • **>34 weeks:** Induction of labor is done
	If the repeat value shows a decreasing trend	The test may be repeated in 2–4 weeks
	If the repeat value has gone up to a higher level in zone 2 or to zone 3	Cordocentesis for evaluation of fetal hematocrit is indicated
Zone 3 (severely affected, death expected in 7–10 days if not treated)	• If **>34 weeks,** deliver and then give exchange transfusion • If **<34 weeks,** do cordocentesis – *Hematocrit <30%*: Give intrauterine transfusion – *Hematocrit >30%*: Follow-up with ultrasonography and cordocentesis	

MCA PSV is a more sensitive, specific, and noninvasive method of determining fetal anemia and has thus replaced the use of Liley's curve.

Indications for fetal cord blood sampling

- MCA PSV >1.5 MoM and amniotic fluid (AF) ΔOD 450 in upper zone 2 or zone 3
- Rising trend of AF ΔOD 450 and ultrasound features of fetal anemia
- Early onset hydrops

Indications for intrauterine transfusion as indicated by fetal blood sampling

Hematocrit below 30% at 24–34 weeks of gestation (affected fetuses with cord blood hematocrit <30% at POG >34 weeks are delivered)

Note *IUT can be started earliest at around 20 weeks.*

The objectives of intrauterine transfusion are the following:
- To correct anemia
- To reduce extramedullary hematopoiesis leading to a fall in portal venous pressure and improved hepatic function

Time of delivery in Rh-isoimmunized pregnancy

Mildly affected fetuses

They can be delivered at term.

Moderate to severely affected fetuses

The main objective is to allow pregnancy to complete 34 weeks, if necessary by intrauterine transfusion (the risk of continued invasive sampling and transfusions should be weighed against the risk of prematurity).

Determine fetal lung maturity by assessing L:S ratio or phosphatidylglycerol in amniotic fluid and then terminate the pregnancy at 34–35 weeks of gestation.

Mode of delivery in Rh-isoimmunized pregnancy

Vaginal delivery can be allowed in the following:
- Mildly affected cases
- Near-term fetuses

Induction of labor (IOL) is done based on the Bishop's score.

Favorable cervix In case of favorable cervix, IOL is done with oxytocin and/or artificial rupture of membranes (ARM)

Unfavorable cervix In case of unfavorable cervix, intracervical PGE2 is instilled for cervical ripening followed by oxytocin and/or ARM

LSCS is indicated in the following:
- Moderate to severely affected cases
- Preterm babies

Intrapartum management

I stage

Careful intrapartum monitoring is required as the fetuses are prone to intrapartum hypoxia and acidosis. Continuous electronic fetal monitoring is done, if available, or else intermittent auscultation of FHR every 15 minutes in I stage and every 5 minutes in II stage is done to detect fetal distress.

II stage

- Neonatologist should be present during delivery to evaluate the baby and to start treatment.
- Methergin is contraindicated following delivery.
- Cord is kept long enough, in case exchange transfusion is required.
- Collect cord blood for blood grouping and Rh typing, Hb, bilirubin, and DCT.

III stage

- Avoid manual removal of placenta.
- Avoid vigorous massaging of uterus.

Extra edge

Amniocentesis

Amniotic fluid is aspirated under ultrasound guidance, centrifuged, and analyzed by spectrophotometry.

Indications for amniocentesis in Rh-isoimmunized pregnancy

- When ICT titer exceeds the critical value
- Sudden increase in antibody titers
- If there is an affected baby in previous pregnancy

(CONTD...)

Part 1

(...CONTD)

Extra edge

Uses of amniotic fluid assessment in Rh-isoimmunized pregnancy

- Detection of fetal anemia
- Detection of fetal genotype
- Detection of lung maturity

Complications of amniocentesis

- Preterm labor
- Fetal distress
- Bloody tap
- Infection

Cordocentesis

- Fetal blood sampling through umbilical cord under USG guidance
- Done for estimation of fetal Hb, hematocrit, blood grouping and typing, and DCT
- Provides access for direct intrauterine transfusion

Complications of cordocentesis

- Preterm labor
- Fetal distress
- Cord hematoma and fetal death
- Risk of fetomaternal hemorrhage and infection
- Failure of the procedure

Other methods that can indicate the severity of the affected fetus in Rh isoimmunization

- **Freda's grading:** This method uses absolute net values of optical density at 450 nm to correlate with bilirubin concentration in amniotic fluid (Table 10.7).

Table 10.7 Freda's grading for estimating severity of affected fetus in Rh isoimmunization

Grade	Net OD values	Fetal status
I	0–0.2	Normal or possibly affected
II	0.2–0.3	Affected but not jeopardized
III	0.3–0.7	Distressed probably in failure
IV	>0.7	Impending fetal death

- **Estimation of antibody levels:** Estimation of antibody level is more accurate than that of antibody titers and can be used at earlier POG than Liley's chart for interpretation. Maternal antibody levels are measured serially from 16 weeks onwards:
  - *<4 IU/mL*: Mild fetal hemolysis
  - *4–10 IU/mL*: Moderate fetal hemolysis
  - *>10 IU/mL*: Severe hemolysis, warrants intervention
- **Nonstress test:** Sinusoidal pattern correlates with severe fetal anemia and impending death when done after 28 weeks of gestation.
- **Role of USG in Rh isoimmunization**
  - Diagnosis of affected pregnancy—features of polyhydramnios, fetal ascites, pleural and pericardial effusion, hepatosplenomegaly, and placentomegaly
  - Estimation of gestational age and assessment of fetal well-being
  - To perform USG-guided amniocentesis or cordocentesis
  - To perform USG-guided intrauterine transfusion

Management of the affected newborn

Objectives of management are as follows:

- Treatment of anemia
- Prevention of hyperbilirubinemia

Clinical manifestations of the affected newborn

The newborn may present with a wide spectrum of clinical manifestations:

- Newborn who develops mild jaundice (responds to conservative treatment)
- Newborn who develops severe jaundice within 24 hours of birth (requires exchange transfusion)
- Baby with hydrops fetalis
- Stillborn baby or early neonatal death in extreme cases

Investigations

- Cord blood is sent for estimation of Hb, hematocrit, blood grouping and Rh typing, DCT, and bilirubin level.
- Cord stump should be maintained, in case catheterization is required for exchange transfusion.

- In severely affected babies, serum bilirubin is done every 6–12 hours and bilirubin is plotted on charts against gestational age and need for phototherapy or exchange transfusion is decided accordingly.

Exchange transfusion in newborn

Indications

- Cord blood Hb <10 mg/dL
- Cord blood bilirubin >5 mg/dL
- Rise in bilirubin by >1 mg/dL/hour
- Total bilirubin >20 mg/dL

Aim of exchange transfusion

- To lower the serum bilirubin level and reduce the risk of brain damage (kernicterus)
- To remove the affected RBCs and circulating maternal antibodies from the newborn's circulation and thereby reduce the hemolysis of RBCs.
- To correct anemia while maintaining euvolemia to prevent any potential for heart failure

Exchange transfusion procedure

- It is done in NICU.
- Double-volume exchange transfusion with 160 mL/kg of fresh O negative blood is recommended.
- O negative RBCs less than 5 days old are used. They do not have major blood group antigens and hence they are not hemolyzed by maternal antibodies present in the newborn's circulation.
- Route is through umbilical vein in early transfusion. Femoral vein is used in late transfusion.
- For every 15 mL of blood withdrawn, 10 mL is pushed in return slowly.
- For every 100 mL of transfusion, give 1 mEq $NaHCO_3$ to correct metabolic acidosis and 1 mL of 10% calcium gluconate to prevent tetany.
- Estimate Hb% and bilirubin concentration before and after exchange transfusion.
- Antibiotics are given for 5 days.
- Repeat transfusion may be required according to bilirubin levels and Hb%.

Phototherapy (Figure 10.4)

- Given for a moderately affected baby or as an adjunct to exchange transfusion
- Principle: Decreases hyperbilirubinemia by photooxidation of bilirubin that converts unconjugated bilirubin to soluble isomers that are readily excreted
- Protect the eyes and external genitalia from UV light during phototherapy

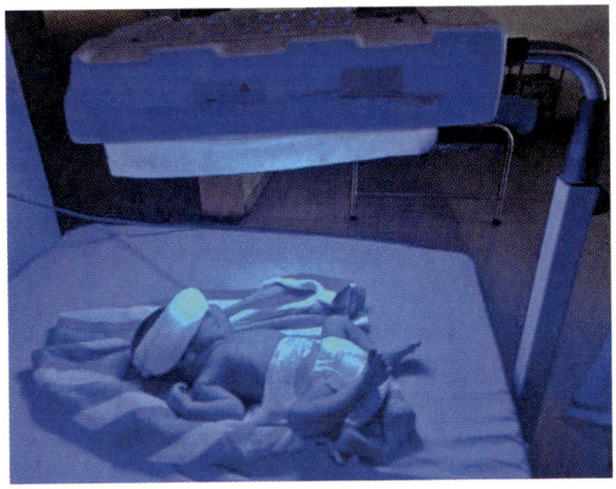

Figure 10.4 Baby receiving phototherapy.

Phenobarbitone

- The drug enhances bilirubin conjugation by increasing the activity of glucuronyl transferase (conjugated bilirubin is readily excreted)
- Dose: 2 mg/kg TDS

Complications in the affected newborn

The newborn is at risk of the following:

- Prematurity
- Anemia
- Jaundice (as bilirubin is no longer cleared across the placenta into the maternal circulation)
- DIC
- Severe thrombocytopenia
- Necrotizing enterocolitis
- Bronchopulmonary dysplasia
- Kernicterus (if unconjugated bilirubin exceeds 20 mg%)

PROGNOSIS

The prognosis of the baby in Rh-isoimmunized pregnancy depends on the following (Table 10.8):

- H/o previous babies affected with hemolytic disease
- Availability of advanced diagnostic and therapeutic facilities

Part 1

Viva corner

Q1 Why does baby not develop jaundice in utero, although RBC destruction occurs?

In utero, unconjugated bilirubin resulting from hemolysis of fetal RBCs is washed away through placenta into maternal circulation. Hence, jaundice does not develop in utero.

Following delivery, increased levels of bilirubin cannot be excreted by newborn's liver due to failure of conjugation of a large amount of bilirubin (low levels of glucuronyl transferase).

Q2 What are the causes of nonimmune hydrops fetalis?

Definition

Nonimmune hydrops fetalis is defined as accumulation of fluid in extracellular tissues and serous cavities in conditions other than Rh incompatibility.

Causes of nonimmune hydrops fetalis

Fetal causes

- **Chromosomal abnormalities:** Trisomies, Turner syndrome, triploidy, aneuploidy
- **Congenital abnormalities:** Diaphragmatic hernia, renal abnormality, cystic hygroma
- **Congenital cardiac lesions:** Congenital heart block
- **Hematological:** Beta thalassemia, glucose-6-phosphate dehydrogenase (G6PD) deficiency
- **Infections:** Parvovirus, rubella, toxoplasmosis, syphilis, cytomegalovirus

Placental and umbilical cord causes

- Twin-to-twin transfusion
- Chorioangioma
- Umbilical vein thrombosis

Maternal causes

- Uncontrolled diabetes
- Severe anemia
- Thyrotoxicosis

Idiopathic

Cause is not known in 20% cases

Table 10.8 Prognosis of the baby in Rh-isoimmunized pregnancy

Affection in previous baby	Chance of survival
H/o previous affected baby who required treatment	40%
H/o previous stillbirth due to hemolytic disease	30%
H/o death of >1 baby due to hemolytic disease	20%

Frequently asked viva questions

1. Summarize the case.
2. What is the diagnosis?
3. What do you mean by isoimmunization?
4. What investigations do you want to do for this patient?
5. How will you manage an Rh-negative mother who is ICT negative?
6. How much anti-D should be given to prevent Rh isoimmunization?
7. How will you manage an Rh-negative mother who is ICT positive?
8. Why are some mothers not sensitized even when the baby is Rh positive and anti-D was not given?
9. Why do some mothers become sensitized even when anti-D was given in time?
10. What precautions will you take to prevent fetomaternal hemorrhage?
11. What investigations are done in newborn of an Rh-negative mother?
12. How is the ideal dose of anti-D calculated?

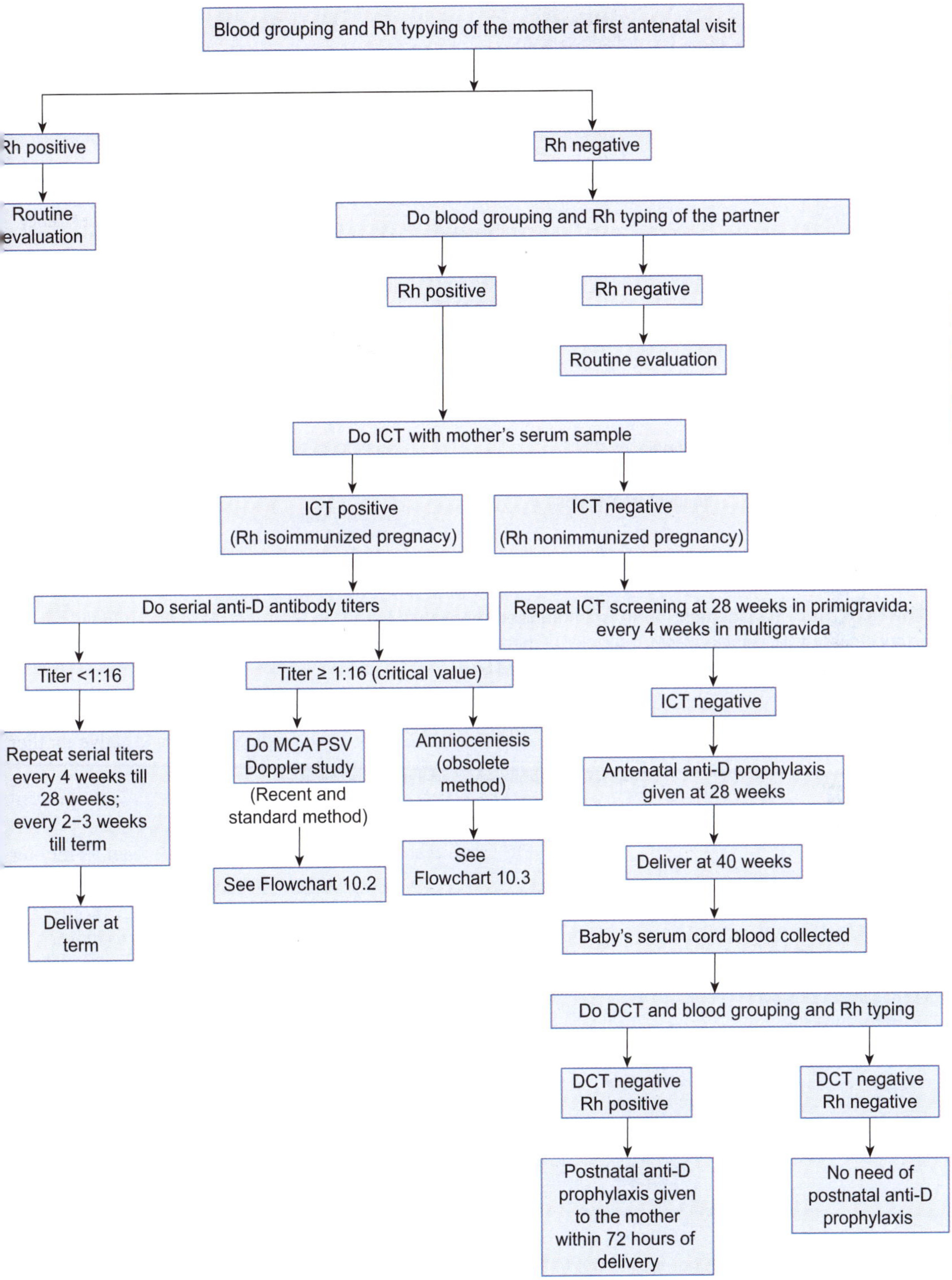

Flowchart 10.1 Mangement of Rh incompatible prenancy. *ICT*, indirect Coombs test; *MCA PSV*, middle cerebral artery peak systolic velocity; *DCT*, direct Coombs test.

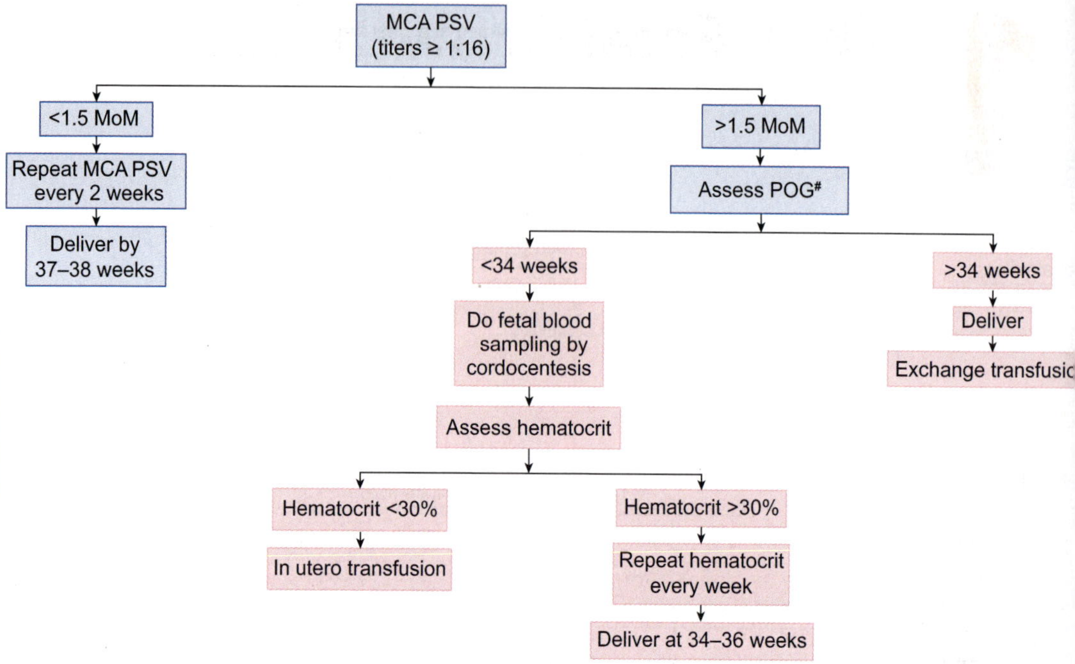

Flowchart 10.2 Management of Rh isoimmunized pregnancy based on MCA PSV. *MCA PSV*, middle cerebral artery peak systolic velocity; *MoM*, multiples of median; *POG*, period of gestation.# The rest of the Flowchart from this point is common with Flowchart 10.3 (indicated by #).

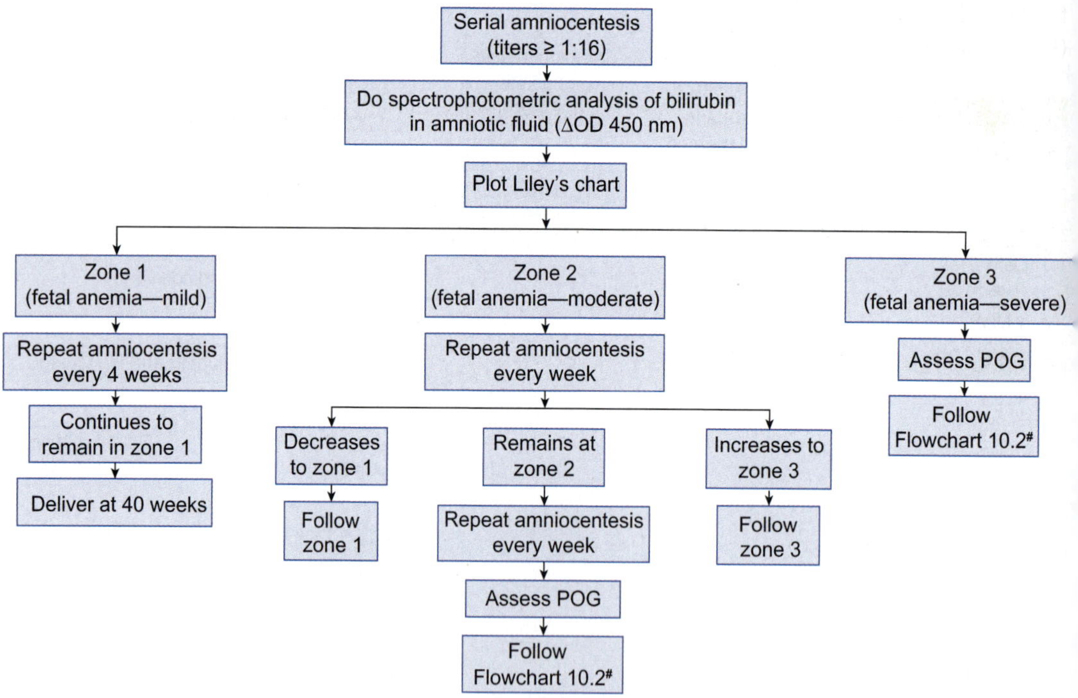

Flowchart 10.3 Management of Rh isoimmunized pregnancy based on serial amniocentesis. *POG*, period of gestation.# Part of the Flowchart 10.2 (colored in pink) to be followed from here.

11 Fetal Growth Restriction

Introduction

Fetal growth restriction (FGR) is a condition characterized by reduced fetal growth potential, leading to increased risk of perinatal morbidity and mortality. Fetal growth restriction (FGR) is the same as intrauterine growth restriction (IUGR). The term IUGR is now replaced by FGR; The etiology of FGR is not clear and hence the focus should be on early detection and appropriate management during pregnancy, labor, and neonatal period. This topic can be discussed in clinical cases with fundal height less than the period of gestation (POG) during obstetric examination.

Various terminologies with reference to the birth weight of the baby are mentioned in Table 11.1.

Definition of FGR

- Failure of fetus to grow to its genetic growth potential for that gestational age.
- FGR is defined as ultrasound estimated fetal weight (EFW) of less than the 10th percentile or abdominal circumference less than the 10th percentile for gestational age.
- Growth restricted fetuses will have a birth weight of <10th percentile for gestational age with pathological restriction in growth (Figure 11.2)

Table 11.1 Terminologies with reference to the birth weight of the baby

Terminology	Definition (Figure 11.1)	Newborns that are included under the terminology
LBW	BW less than 2.5 kg	• Preterm babies • FGR babies • Small and healthy babies
Very LBW	BW <1.5 kg	–
Extremely LBW	BW <1 kg	–
SGA	• A fetus that is unable to achieve a specific biometric or estimated weight threshold by a specific gestational age is termed SGA fetus • Infants with weight <10th percentile for their gestational age; infants with weight <2 SD of the mean weight for their gestational age.	• FGR babies • Small and healthy babies (constitutionally small babies)
FGR	BW <10th percentile for gestational age with pathological restriction in growth, i.e., failure of the fetus to reach its optimal growth potential	• Term FGR • Preterm FGR
Small and healthy babies	BW <10th percentile for gestational age, without pathological restriction in growth	• Constitutionally small babies due to constitutionally small parental size, different race, or ethnicity

BW, birth weight; *FGR*, fetal growth restriction; *LBW*, low birth weight; *SGA*, small for gestational age.

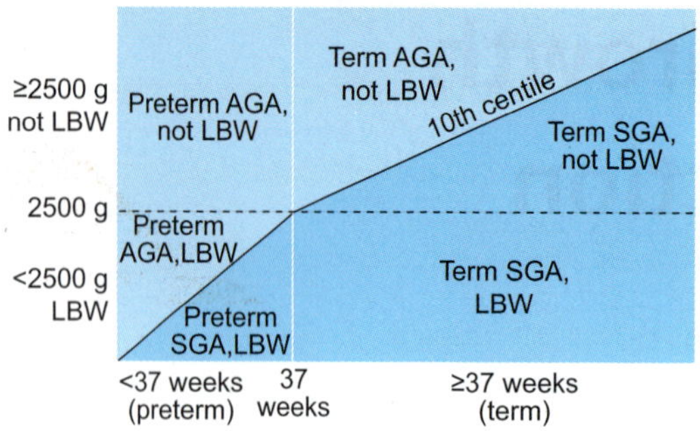

Figure 11.1 Pictorial representation of the various terms used with reference to the birth weight of the baby. *AGA,* appropriate for gestational age; *LBW,* low birth weight; *SGA,* small for gestational age.

- FGR is classified into two types based on the period of gestation when the insult to the fetus would have occurred
  - Early onset FGR
  - Late onset FGR

Early onset FGR

- Growth compromise is recognized before 28 weeks of gestation
- Occurs in 20–30% of FGR; early insult affects cell division
- Causes (intrinsic): Fetal factors such as chromosomal aberration, congenital anomaly, inborn errors of metabolism, viral infection, exposure to teratogen or idiopathic

Late-onset FGR

- Growth compromise is recognized after 28 weeks of gestation
- Occurs in 70–80% of FGR; less severe
- Causes (extrinsic): Placental insufficiency due to factors such as extremes of maternal age, low socioeconomic status, malnutrition, anemia, preeclampsia, vascular disease, heart disease, renal disease, smoking, alcohol and drug abuse

Incidence of FGR

It is 6–10%.

Etiological causes/risk factors for FGR

Maternal causes

- Maternal age <20 and >35 years
- Prepregnancy weight <45 kg
- Maternal malnutrition
- Decreased weight gain during pregnancy
- Calorie restriction during pregnancy
- Maternal diseases with vasculopathy
  - Preeclampsia
  - Chronic hypertension
  - Diabetes mellitus (DM) with vasculopathy
  - Chronic renal disease
  - Antiphospholipid antibody (APLA) syndrome
  - Thrombophilias

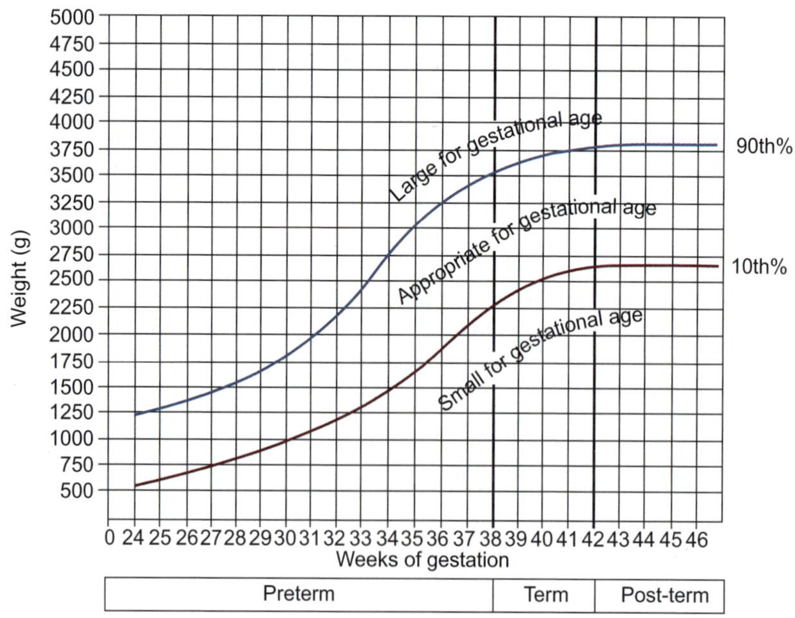

Figure 11.2 Growth profile chart.

- Chronic hypoxia—chronic obstructive pulmonary disease (COPD), bronchial asthma, cardiac disease, and living at high altitudes
- Addictions—smoking, alcohol, and cocaine abuse

Fetal causes

- Multiple pregnancy
- Congenital anomalies
- Chromosomal abnormalities
- Fetal infections—toxoplasmosis, rubella, cytomegalovirus, herpes, and syphilis (**Hint:** *Remember the acronym "TORCHeS"*)

Placental causes

- Chronic abruption
- Velamentous insertion of cord
- Placental infarcts and thrombosis
- Circumvallate placenta
- Single umbilical artery (UA)

Previous H/o FGR

There is 25% chance of recurrence in the present pregnancy, if previous H/o FGR is present.

Idiopathic

Cause for FGR is not known in 40% of cases.

Case presentation

Salient points in history

Consider the following relevant points during history taking in cases of FGR.

Present pregnancy

Remember all the etiological causes of FGR while taking history.

- *Age (FGR more common in extremes of age)*
- *Socioeconomic status (maternal malnutrition and resulting FGR)*
- *Last menstrual period (LMP)—accurate dating of pregnancy is important in diagnosing FGR. Reliability of LMP is checked for by asking the following details:*
  - *Date of LMP, whether sure of dates, and whether menstrual cycles were regular prior to conception*
  - *History of use of OCPs prior to conception*
  - *H/o recent abortions or whether conceived during lactation*
  - *Any ultrasound done in the first trimester (it will help to assess the POG most accurately)*
- *H/O present pregnancy*
  - *First trimester: H/o fever, drugs, and exposure to radiation*
  - *Second trimester: History suggestive of preeclampsia (FGR is a complication of preeclampsia)*
  - *Third trimester: H/o preeclampsia, bleeding P/V [antepartum hemorrhage (APH)], leaking P/V, whether perceiving normal fetal movements (fetal movements may be reduced)*

Menstrual history

- *Regularity of menstrual cycles (to assess reliability of LMP)*
- *LMP*

Obstetric history

- *H/o any complications such as preeclampsia*
- *H/o low birth weight in previous pregnancies (may be suggestive of FGR)*
- *H/o recurrent first trimester abortions (suggestive of APLA syndrome)*

Past history

- *Chronic hypertension*
- *DM*
- *Chronic renal disease*
- *Any other chronic medical illness*

Personal history

- *Smoking*
- *Alcoholism*
- *Drug addiction*

Dietary history

Whether dietary intake is adequate in calories and proteins

(CONTD...)

(...CONTD)

Family history

- *Hypertension*
- *DM*
- *Multiple pregnancy, chromosomal abnormalities, or congenital anomalies*

Salient points in examination

Consider the following relevant points during examination in cases of FGR:

- *Built and nourishment*
- *Height*
- *Weight*
  - *Prepregnancy weight <45 kg is a risk factor for FGR*
  - *A constitutionally small mother may have a small and healthy fetus*
  - *In FGR, decreased maternal weight gain is noted in subsequent visits*
  - *Preeclampsia patients may have excessive weight gain*
- *Pallor (chronic hypoxia in severe anemia can lead to FGR)*
- *Pedal edema—may be an indicator of anemia, hypoproteinemia, or preeclampsia*
- *BP—indicator of preeclampsia*
- *CVS/RS examination—patients with cardiac or respiratory diseases have chronic hypoxia which is a risk factor for FGR*

Obstetric examination

- *Fundal height: Fundal height is <POG in FGR. Discrepancy of 4 weeks or more in fundal height may be suggestive of FGR.*
- *Symphysiofundal height (SFH): SFH is <POG in FGR. Suspect FGR when there is discrepancy in SFH by 2 cm or more*
- *Fetal lie, presentation (it may be difficult to palpate fetal parts, if liquor is reduced)*
- *Amount of liquor (may be decreased)*
- *Auscultate fetal heart rate (FHR)*

Case summary

An example of writing summary in cases of FGR is given below.

Example *Mrs. Q, 28 years of age, a primigravida, at 36 weeks of gestation, came for routine antenatal checkup. She has no specific complaints. She is perceiving normal fetal movements and there is no H/o leaking P/V, bleeding P/V, or labor pains. On examination, mild pallor is present and her BP is 120/80 mmHg. Obstetric examination reveals fundal height corresponding to 32 weeks of gestation; SFH measures 32 cm. A single live fetus is present in cephalic presentation, uterus is relaxed and liquor volume appears reduced. On auscultation, FHR is 146 beats/min, regular heard in the left spinoumbilical line.*

Case diagnosis

An example of writing diagnosis in cases of FGR is given below.

Example *28 years of age, a primigravida at 36 weeks of gestation with suspected FGR, with clinically reduced liquor, with a singleton live fetus in cephalic presentation, not in labor*

Case discussion

Diagnosis of FGR

For diagnosis of FGR, it is important to accurately date the pregnancy from history, clinical examination, and USG.

Various methods for estimating POG are given in Table 11.2.

Note *Crown-rump length (CRL) measured in the first trimester is the most accurate method of dating a pregnancy.*

Clinical examination findings in FGR

- Inadequate maternal weight gain
- Fundal height—less than POG by 4 weeks or more
- SFH—less than POG by 2 cm or more
- Amount of liquor—may be less in FGR

Table 11.2 Accuracy in the methods for estimation of period of gestation

Method	Parameters	Accuracy
History	• LMP (excellent dates) • Conception following ovulation induction • Conception following in vitro fertilization	• ±7–14 days • ±3 days • ±1 day
Clinical examination	• P/V in the first trimester • Fundal height in the second and third trimesters	• ±2 weeks • ±4 weeks
Ultrasonography (approximate figures are given for easy remembrance)	• First trimester—CRL • Second trimester—BPD, HC, FL, AC • Third trimester—BPD, HC, FL, AC	• ±1 week • ±2 weeks • ±3 weeks

AC, abdominal circumference; *BPD*, biparietal diameter; *CRL*, crown-rump length; *FL*, femur length; HC, head circumference; *LMP*, last menstrual period.

Note *Clinical assessment has low sensitivity, high false-positive rates, and high interobserver variation. Clinical examination detects only 40% of cases of FGR. Hence, USG is required for confirmation of FGR.*

Ultrasonography findings suggestive of FGR

Obstetric USG is the mainstay in the diagnosis of FGR.

- **Biparietal diameter (BPD):** It may show a slow-growth profile or a late-flattening profile.
  - Slow-growth profile
    - BPD less than 10th percentile at all times
    - Seen in symmetrical FGR
  - Late-flattening profile
    - Normal growth curve up to 34 weeks followed by a fall in BPD growth
- **Abdominal circumference (AC)**
  - It is the most sensitive index.
  - Serial measurement of AC shows AC <10th percentile in FGR.
- **AC growth rates**
  - AC increases by 1 cm/week.
  - AC growth rate is <1 cm/week for 2 weeks → FGR.
- **Estimated fetal weight (EFW):** Serial measurement of EFW shows EFW less than 10th percentile for POG.
- **Estimated gestational age (EGA):** It refers to the discrepancy between LMP-calculated gestational age and USG-calculated gestational age (provided that the dates provided by the patient are excellent).
- **Head circumference (HC)/AC ratio:** It is the ratio between the most preserved organ (brain) to the most compromised organ (liver). Relationship between HC and AC of the fetus during pregnancy is given in Table 11.3).
  - If HC/AC is >1 after 34 weeks, it indicates asymmetric FGR.
- **Femur length (FL)/AC ratio**
  - It is a gestational age–independent parameter
  - Normal value: 22 ± 2 after 20 weeks, constant value
  - In FGR, FL/AC ratio is >24
- **Fetal ponderal index (PI)**
  - Gestational age–independent parameter
  - $PI = EFW/(FL)^3 \times 100$
  - Normal value: 8.325 ± 2.5
  - In FGR, FPI is <7
- **Fetal transverse cerebellar diameter (TCD)**
  - Gestational age–independent parameter
  - The value has been shown to correlate well with gestational age in FGR cases
  - Reduced in symmetrical FGR
- **Amniotic fluid index (AFI)**
  - Oligohydramnios is frequently associated with FGR.
  - AFI is <5 in 40% of cases of FGR.

Table 11.3 Relationship between HC and AC of the fetus during pregnancy

Up to 32 weeks	HC > AC	HC/AC > 1
32–34 weeks	HC = AC	HC/AC = 1
After 34 weeks	AC > HC	HC/AC < 1

AC, abdominal circumference; *HC*, head circumference.

Part 1

Extra edge

Reliability of various biometric parameters in the diagnosis of FGR

- AC and EFW are the most accurate parameters in predicting FGR, as these parameters have the best specificity and positive and negative predictive values, and the lowest false-positive and false-negative values. If, in addition, HC and FL are also <10th centile, then symmetric FGR should be suspected.
- Combining AC or EFW with UA Doppler studies improves the accuracy in diagnosis of FGR.
- An individual finding alone is not predictive of FGR, but a combination of abnormal findings, such as a SGA fetus with reduced liquor and/or abnormal UA Doppler, may indicate FGR.
- Serial scans every 2 weeks are superior to a single estimation of AC or EFW in the diagnosis of FGR.
- A threshold of 10th centile for AC and EFW is commonly used for the diagnosis of FGR.

- **Doppler studies in FGR**
  - In FGR fetuses, there is impaired uteroplacental blood flow resulting in abnormal umbilical artery flow pattern that can be used as a diagnostic and surveillance tool.
  - Doppler studies help to distinguish constitutionally small fetuses from FGR fetuses.
  - Doppler indices that are used include systolic/diastolic (S/D) ratio, pulsatility index (PI), and resistance index (RI) (Figure 11.3; Table 11.4).

Note *Pulsatility index can be numerically analyzed even with absent end-diastolic velocity.*

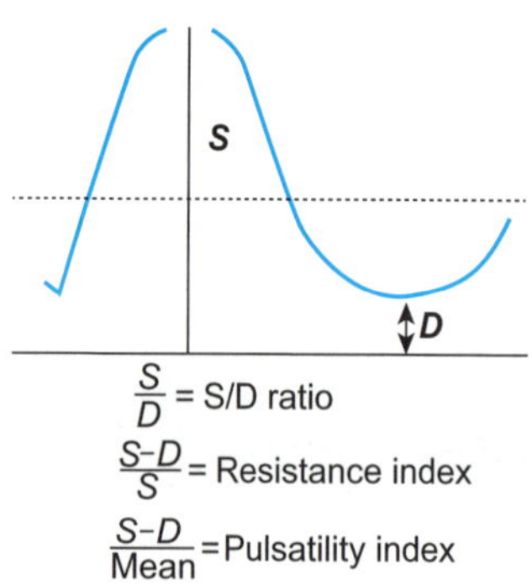

Figure 11.3 Doppler waveform analysis. *S*, peak systolic velocity; *D*, peak diastolic velocity.

Table 11.4 Doppler indices

Indices	Formula for calculation
S/D ratio	Peak systolic velocity/peak diastolic velocity
PI	S – D/mean
RI	S – D/S

D, peak diastolic velocity; *PI*, pulsatility index; *RI*, resistance index; *S*, peak systolic velocity.

Umbilical artery Doppler

- In a normal fetus, the following are noted:
  - The placental resistance decreases with advancing gestation and UA diastolic flow increases.
  - UA shows a waveform with continuous flow during systole and diastole (Figure 11.4a).
  - Doppler shows a decrease in S/D ratio, RI, and PI (Figures 11.5 and 11.6).
- In FGR, the following are noted:
  - There is decrease in placental perfusion, increase in the resistance to flow, and decrease in the UA diastolic flow (Figure 11.4b).
  - Gradually the diastolic flow becomes absent [absent end-diastolic velocity (AEDV)] and then the flow reverses during diastole [reversed end-diastolic velocity (REDV; Figure 11.4c and d)].

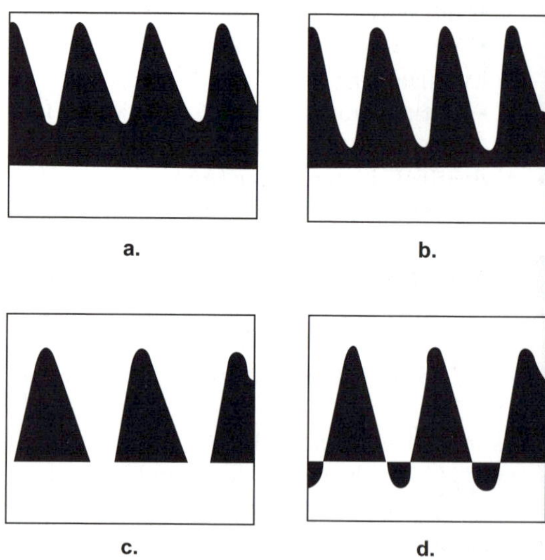

Figure 11.4 Umbilical artery Doppler waveforms. **a.** Normal. **b.** Reduced end diastolic flow. **c.** Absent end diastolic flow. **d.** Reversed end diastolic flow.

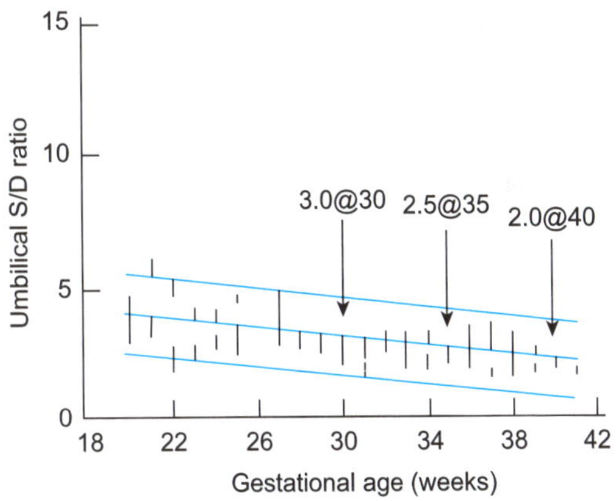

Figure 11.5 S/D ratio of umbilical artery Doppler.

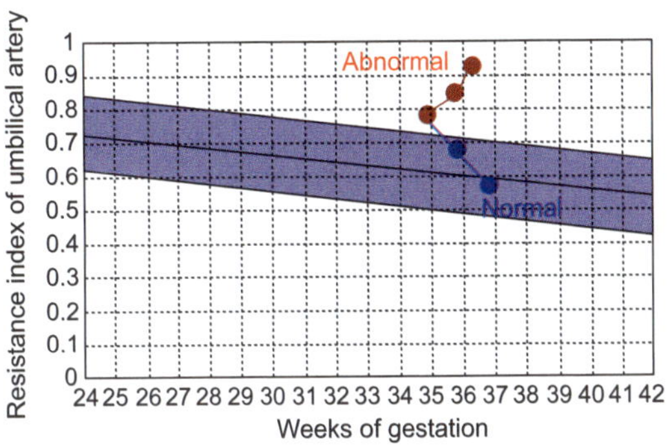

Figure 11.6 Resistance index of umbilical artery Doppler.

- Doppler shows an increase in S/D ratio, RI, and PI.
- With AEDV, the S/D ratio approaches infinity and the RI becomes 1.
- AEDV and REDV are associated with increased perinatal morbidity and mortality and require urgent intervention and delivery.

Extra edge

Interpretation of umbilical artery Doppler study values

- **S/D ratio of UA Doppler** is between 2 and 3 in the second and third trimesters. S/D ratio >3 indicates FGR.
- **PI of UA Doppler** is between 1.5 and 2 in the second trimester and between 1 and 1.5 in the third trimester.
- **RI of UA Doppler** decreases with advancing gestation and in late second and third trimesters it is around 0.5.

Middle cerebral artery Doppler

- In a normal fetus, at 28–32 weeks, middle cerebral artery (MCA) is characterized by high systolic velocity and minimal diastolic velocity resulting in a high PI value of >1.45.
- In a hypoxic fetus, the diastolic flow to MCA increases due to cerebral vasodilation that occurs as an adaptive mechanism, resulting in a decrease in PI value—MCA resistance decreases due to brain sparing effect.

Extra edge

Fetal decompensation cascade or Doppler sequence in FGR

- Increase in UA indices

↓

- Decrease in MCA resistance (brain-sparing effect)

↓

- Absent end-diastolic flow in UA

↓

- Reversed end-diastolic flow

↓

- Venous pulsations appear in IVC and ductus venosus

↓

- Umbilical vein pulsations

↓

- Constriction of cerebral circulation

↓

- Death of fetus

FGR → hypoxia → acidosis → death

Recent advance

Cerebroplacental ratio (CPR)

- The CPR is emerging as an important predictor of adverse pregnancy outcome and is used for assessment of fetal well-being in FGR.
- The CPR is calculated by dividing the Doppler indices of the MCA by the Doppler indices of the UA.
- Although the S/D ratio, RI, and PI have been used to calculate the CPR, PI is commonly used. CPR is calculated as the ratio of MCA PI and UA PI.
- MCA PI/UA PI ratio of <1.08 is a better predictor of fetal insufficiency than MCA PI or UA PI alone.

Venous Doppler changes These occur in late stages in fetuses with FGR, when there is fetal acidosis and compromised cardiac function. Increase in preload is manifested as follows:

- Pulsations in umbilical vein (UV)
- Reversed flow in the inferior vena cava (IVC) during atrial contraction
- Absence or reversal of flow in the ductus venosus (DV) during atrial contraction

Note *Venous Doppler changes are considered as preterminal changes that indicate urgent intervention and delivery. Doppler assessment of UV, IVC, and DV is used as a backup test in fetuses with AEDV and REDV in UA Doppler.*

Screening for FGR

- **Low-risk women (women without risk factors for FGR):** If FGR is suspected while performing clinical examination during routine antenatal visit, then serial USG is done to confirm the diagnosis.
- **High-risk women (women with risk factors for FGR):** Screening for FGR is done by clinical examination and by doing serial USG at regular intervals.

Classification of FGR

Clinical classification

See Table 11.5

Table 11.5 Clinical classification of FGR

Mild	Growth lag of <6 weeks
Severe	Growth lag of ≥6 weeks

Etiological classification

See Table 11.6

Table 11.6 Etiological classification of FGR

Etiology for FGR	Causes
Intrinsic causes	Due to fetal causes such as chromosomal abnormalities, congenital anomalies
Extrinsic causes	Due to maternal or placental causes such as uteroplacental insufficiency
Combined	Due to both intrinsic and extrinsic factors
Idiopathic	Cause not known

Classification based on symmetry of various anatomical structures

Causes and features of symmetric and asymmetric FGR are given in Table 11.7.

Table 11.7 Causes and features of symmetric and asymmetric FGR

	Symmetric FGR	Asymmetric FGR
Cause	Intrinsic: fetal causes—genetic, chromosomal, and congenital anomalies	Extrinsic: maternal causes, uteroplacental insufficiency
Fetal size	Uniformly small	Disproportionate—head is larger when compared to rest of the body
Onset	Starts early in pregnancy	Usually starts at >32 weeks
Cell number and size	Decreased cell number and size	Cell number normal, cell size decreased
Incidence	20%	80%
HC/AC	Normal	Increased
FL/AC	Normal	Increased
Ponderal index	Normal	Decreased
Postnatal prognosis	Poor prognosis	Good prognosis, if complications are managed

AC, abdominal circumference; *FL*, femur length; *HC*, head circumference.

Differences between small and healthy fetuses and FGR fetuses

See Table 11.8

Table 11.8 Features differentiating small and healthy fetuses and FGR fetuses

Feature	Small and healthy fetuses	FGR fetuses
Cause	Constitutionally small fetuses	Pathological restriction in growth
HC/AC	Normal	Increased
FL/AC	Normal	Increased
AC growth rate	Normal	Decreased
Ponderal index	Normal	Decreased
Liquor	Normal	Decreased
Subcutaneous fat	Normal	Reduced
Growth velocity	Normal	Reduced/flattened
Postnatal period	No complications	Complications anticipated

AC, abdominal circumference; *FL*, femur length; *HC*, head circumference.

Complications of FGR

Maternal complications

Maternal morbidity may be increased due to the following:

- The coexisting diseases that cause FGR such as preeclampsia
- Increased rate of CS in FGR

Fetal complications

The main problems are to the fetus.

Antepartum

- Oligohydramnios (reduced renal perfusion → decreased urine output → decreased liquor)
- Meconium aspiration
- Intrauterine death (uteroplacental insufficiency → chronic hypoxia → metabolic acidosis → intrauterine death)

Intrapartum

Uterine contraction during labor further compromises the uteroplacental circulation, leading to birth asphyxia.

Viva corner

Q1 Why is AC reduced in FGR?

- Depletion of liver glycogen and abdominal wall adipose tissue leading to decrease in AC
- Reduced oxygen transfer across placenta leading to fetal hypoxia → stimulation of chemoreceptors in carotid body → selective vasodilation and vasoconstriction in fetal circulation as described below

Vasodilation occurs in the blood supply to the following:

- Fetal brain (brain-sparing effect)
- Myocardium
- Adrenal glands—lead to increased corticosteroid and catecholamine synthesis (accelerated lung maturity in FGR)

Vasoconstriction occurs in blood supply to the following:

- Kidneys—lead to decreased urine production and oligohydramnios
- Splanchnic vessels
- Liver—reduced blood flow leads to reduction in liver mass and glycogen and reduced AC
- Peripheries

Q2 What is the importance of liquor assessment in FGR?

- Reduced liquor may indicate placental insufficiency or fetal anomalies such as renal agenesis and bilateral polycystic kidneys.
- Patients with FGR and reduced liquor should be followed up by more frequent surveillance.

(CONTD...)

(...CONTD)

Viva corner

- AFI ≤5 is associated with an increased rate of CS for fetal distress and low Apgar scores.

Q3 What are the gestational age–independent parameters in USG assessment of FGR?

- FL/AC ratio
- Fetal ponderal index
- Fetal transverse cerebellar diameter

Q4 What is the role of uterine artery Doppler in FGR?

- Defective placentation is associated with preeclampsia and FGR.
- Uterine artery Doppler has a role in prediction of preeclampsia and FGR. Persistent uterine artery diastolic notch in Doppler studies after 24 weeks of gestation indicates increased uterine vascular resistance and helps to identify women at risk for preeclampsia and FGR with 85% sensitivity (see figure below).

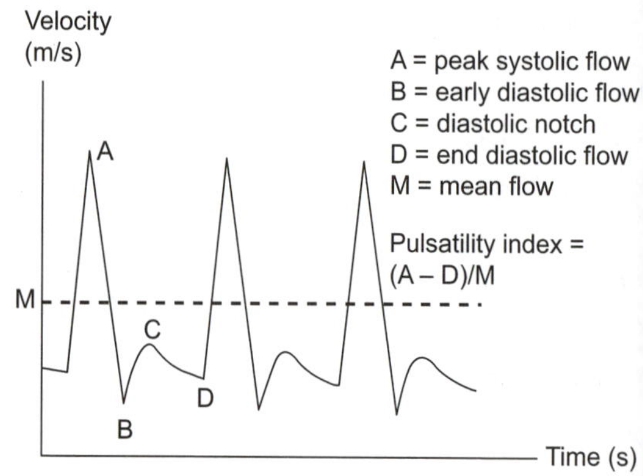

Figure Uterine artery Doppler showing persistent diastolic notch.

- Fetal distress (uteroplacental insufficiency → chronic hypoxia → metabolic acidosis → fetal distress → increased CS rate)
- Meconium aspiration
- Low Apgar
- Increased perinatal mortality

Postnatal

- Meconium aspiration syndrome (MAS)
- Hypoxic ischemic encephalopathy (due to birth asphyxia)
- Metabolic abnormalities
  - Hypothermia—due to reduced subcutaneous fat and energy stores
  - Hypoglycemia—due to reduced glycogen stores in liver
  - Hypocalcemia—perinatal hypoxia and acidosis → relative hypoparathyroidism → hypocalcemia
  - Hyperbilirubinemia—due to RBC destruction
  - Hyperviscosity and polycythemia—chronic hypoxia → stimulates erythropoietin secretion → increased RBC synthesis (polycythemia can lead to thrombosis that can cause cerebrovascular accidents, pulmonary infarcts, and necrotizing enterocolitis)
  - Necrotizing enterocolitis—decreased splanchnic circulation → ischemia
  - Sudden infant death syndrome
- Persistent fetal circulation—perinatal hypoxia and acidosis → severe pulmonary vasoconstriction → persistent blood flow through ductus arteriosus
- Other complications—congenital anomalies and infections

Long-term sequelae in FGR babies

- Majority of FGR babies have catch-up growth after delivery.
- Asymmetric FGR babies grow faster and have better prognosis than symmetric FGR babies.
- FGR that develops in early gestation (decreased brain cell number) is associated with the following:
  - Increased chance of low IQ
  - Neurological problems
  - Learning and behavioral problems
- FGR babies are at an increased risk of developing hypertension, type 2 DM, obesity, and coronary artery disease later in life. (Barker's hypothesis: This hypothesis proposes that nutrition during fetal life, infancy, and early childhood changes the gene expression to future environment.)

Part 1

External appearance in FGR babies after birth (Figure 11.7)

- Wrinkled skin
- Reduced subcutaneous fat and muscle mass
- Old-man look
- Wide, open eyes
- Prominent ribs
- Scaphoid abdomen

Management of FGR

Major threat in continuing pregnancy in FGR is intrauterine hypoxia and death. At the same time, early delivery can lead to prematurity and its complications. Hence, the risk of prematurity has to be balanced against the risk of intrauterine death.

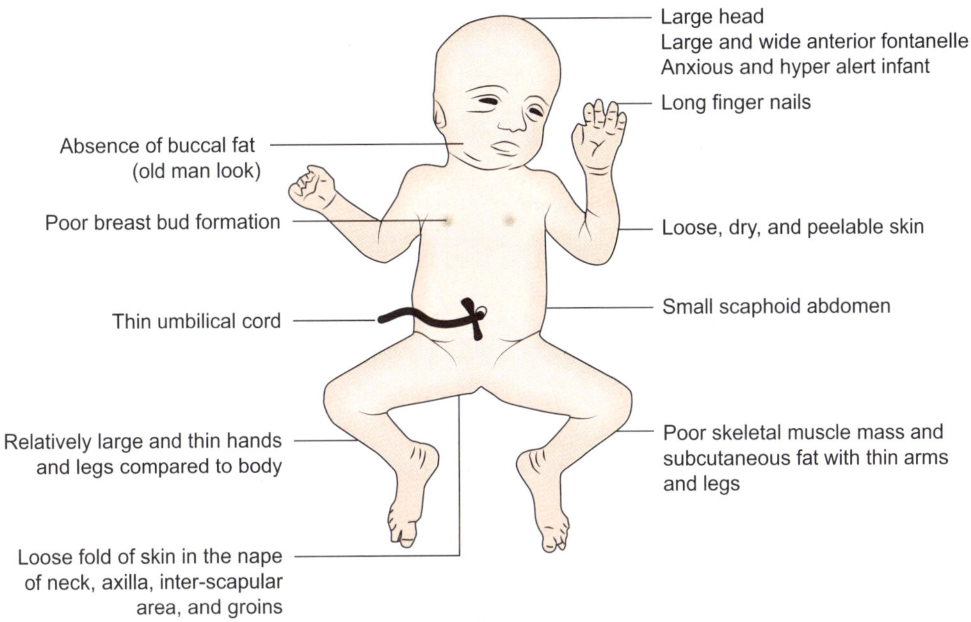

a.

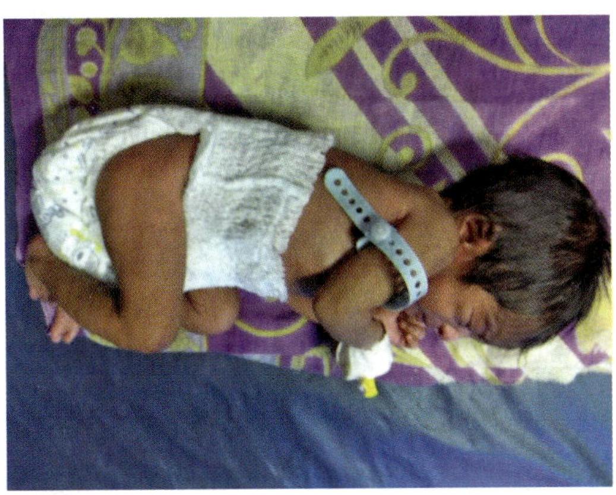

b.

Figure 11.7 Growth restricted baby at birth. **a.** Pictorial representation of features of FGR infant at birth. **b.** An FGR baby.

Extra edge

Royal College of Obstetricians and Gynaecologists (RCOG) (2002) recommendations on deciding the time of delivery in FGR fetuses

- The clinician needs to individualize each patient with FGR and decide the time for delivery, by weighing the risk of fetal demise due to delayed intervention against the risk of long-term disabilities resulting from preterm delivery due to early intervention.
- The two main parameters for deciding the optimal time of delivery include results on fetal surveillance tests and gestational age.
- Preterm delivery: It may be associated with future disabilities, intraventricular hemorrhage, sepsis, retinopathy of prematurity, etc.
- Delayed delivery: It may be associated with ischemic brain injury, periventricular leukomalacia, intraventricular hemorrhage, and IUD.

Management of pregnancy with FGR depends on the following:

- POG
- Fetal well-being
- Associated maternal and fetal complications

Investigations

- Routine antenatal investigations
- Investigations to identify the cause for FGR, if any
  - Complete blood count
  - Urine protein, sugar, and microscopy
  - Urine culture and sensitivity
  - Renal and liver function tests
  - VDRL and TORCH screening
  - USG—role of USG in FGR is
    - To diagnose FGR
    - To rule out anomalies
    - To assess fetal growth periodically
    - To assess AFI
    - To assess fetal well-being by doing Doppler studies and biophysical profile (BPP)

Antenatal management

- Most of the causes of FGR are not amenable to treatment and treatment may not improve fetal growth in FGR.
- Supportive care is given along with intensive antenatal surveillance and active intervention is done at optimal time.
- Antenatal surveillance is done by regular monitoring of fetal growth and fetal well-being by clinical and biophysical methods.

Monitoring of fetal growth

- Serial maternal weight gain
- Clinical examination—fundal height, SFH, and abdominal girth
- USG—serial USG every 2 weeks for assessment of fetal growth

Monitoring of fetal well-being

History

Daily fetal movement count (DFMC)

Clinical examination

- Fetal movements
- Amount of liquor
- FHR auscultation

Antenatal tests for assessment of fetal well-being

- Nonstress test (NST)—done weekly or twice weekly in severe FGR
- AFI—assessed weekly
- BPP—done weekly or twice weekly in severe FGR (Table 11.9). Modified BPP profile (NST and AFI) may be used to follow up FGR fetuses
- Doppler studies of fetal vessels
  - If Doppler studies are normal, it rules out fetal hypoxia and is repeated weekly.
  - Absent end-diastolic flow or reversal of flow in UA suggests imminent fetal death.

A detailed description of antepartum fetal surveillance is given in Part 3, Chapter 36, *Antepartum and Intrapartum Fetal Surveillance Tests.*

Table 11.9 Biophysical profile

Component	Normal	Score
Fetal body movement	3/30 min	2
Fetal breathing movement	1/30 min	2
Fetal tone	1/30 min	2
Amniotic fluid volume-Single deepest vertical pocket (SDP)	≥2 cm	2
Nonstress test	Reactive	2

Extra edge

Role of BPP in management of FGR fetuses

- Fetal hypoxemia is associated with progressive decline in liquor, fetal breathing, gross body movements, fetal tone, and NST.
- Fetal breathing is affected first followed by reduction in liquor and then FHR variability decreases. Loss of fetal movements and tone is a late event.
- Originally all parameters were given equal importance; however, it has been observed that oligohydramnios has an independent risk and its presence requires reassessment of management plan.
- Fetal death is rare in cases women with a normal BPP.
- BPP is usually done once a week and in severe cases it is done twice weekly or daily.

Biochemical tests that indicate fetal compromise

- Decrease in maternal estriol
- Decrease in human placental lactogen

Therapeutic measures in management of FGR

- Rest in left lateral position
  - Relieves IVC compression, thereby increases maternal cardiac output and uteroplacental perfusion
  - Decrease in physical activity diverts blood from peripheral to systemic circulation and thereby improves uterine blood flow
- Nutritious diet (advise on high-protein diet with iron, folic acid, and calcium supplementation)
- Correction of anemia
- Detection and management of associated medical conditions such as preeclampsia, gestational diabetes mellitus, and APLA
- Cessation of smoking, alcohol, and substance abuse

Management of FGR

Early onset FGR

If pre-viable (<500 g ± <24 weeks):

- Exclude congenital anomalies.
  - Offer genetic screening
  - Investigate for APLA
- Offer counseling by multidisciplinary health care team regarding fetal monitoring and obstetrical intervention until viability.
  - Obstetric intervention is done when the doppler abnormalities are severe enough indicating impending fetal death.
- Decision to deliver the fetus is individualized for the case, balancing the risk of intrauterine death with the risk of prematurity

If viable (>500 g and >24 weeks):

- Conduct initial ultrasound assessment: EFW, AFI, UA Doppler; in third trimester (~28 weeks) consider weekly BPP and growth every 2 weeks and manage as follows.

If growth continues along growth curve: conduct weekly BPP, UA Doppler and growth scan every 2 weeks → delivery at term (38 to 40 weeks), if no other issues.

If growth plateaus or stops <34 weeks:

- Administer corticosteroids; increase surveillance to 2–3 times per week; consider hospitalization
- If abnormal UA Doppler studies: add MCA and DV studies.
  - If abnormal UA, MCA, and DV Doppler studies and abnormal NST → deliver.
  - If abnormal Doppler studies and normal BPP and NST: continue intensive monitoring with BPP and Doppler studies 2–3 times per week

Extra edge

Role of drug therapy in FGR

- There are no significant benefits with drug therapy in FGR.
- There is no concrete evidence to evaluate benefits and risks of nutrient therapy, nitric oxide donors, antioxidants, plasma volume expanders, and oxygen therapy to the mother with FGR fetus.
- Combined aspirin and heparin therapy may benefit fetal outcome in women with APLA.

Role of low-dose aspirin in FGR

- Low-dose aspirin has been proved to be beneficial in women with previous H/o FGR and preeclampsia and in APLA syndrome, if started early in gestation.
- It acts by inhibiting thromboxane A2 synthesis and thereby prevents vasoconstriction and platelet aggregation in uteroplacental circulation.

Fetal therapy by injecting amino acids into amniotic fluid or umbilical cord is under research.

Predictors of FGR

- Reduced pregnancy associated plasma protein-A (PAPP-A) in first trimester screening.
- High resistance flow in uterine artery.

→ deliver if BPP or UA Doppler worsens or if MCA/DV doppler are abnormal

Late onset FGR

If >34 weeks and <37 weeks:

- Perform growth scan every 2 weeks
- Perform weekly surveillance of AFI, BPP, Doppler
- If normal AFI, BPP, and Doppler studies: conduct weekly surveillance → delivery or ongoing monitoring after 37 weeks.
- If AFI <5 cm, abnormal BPP, and/or Doppler studies: consider delivery.

If >37 weeks: Deliver

Note *Prior to delivery of fetus less than 32 weeks, magnesium sulphate is administered to the mother for fetal neuroprotection.*

Indications for immediate delivery in FGR

- UA Doppler showing REDF
- Doppler showing venous pulsations—pulsations in ductus venosus, IVC, and UV
- BPP score of <4
- Nonreassuring FHR

Mode of delivery

Mild FGR Cervical ripening and induction of labor can be done with intensive intrapartum monitoring. Intensive monitoring is required, as FGR fetuses are likely to develop fetal hypoxia during labor.

Severe FGR Cesarean section is commonly performed (though there is no current evidence supporting the use of routine cesarean section) for the following reasons:

- Severe fetal hypoxemia gets worsened during labor.
- Placental reserve is low and fetuses cannot withstand the stress of labor.
- Associated oligohydramnios can lead to cord compression and thick meconium stained liquor (MSL).

Intrapartum management

- Delivery should be conducted in a tertiary care hospital with facilities for the following:
  - Intensive intrapartum monitoring
  - Emergency CS
  - Intensive neonatal care

I stage

- The patient is put on labor room board
- Left lateral position
- Oxygen by mask
- Adequate labor analgesia
- Continuous electronic FHR monitoring preferred, otherwise intermittent auscultation of FHR every 15 minutes in the first stage and every 5 minutes in the second stage
- Oxytocin for augmentation of labor can be used

High-yield points

Role of artificial rupture of membranes (ARM)

As per WHO Labour Care Guideline 2020, the use of ARM alone for the prevention of delay in labor is not recommended.

- May help in augmentation of labor
- Early detection of meconium
- Scalp pH testing and scalp electrode insertion for better fetal monitoring is possible following ARM

Role of amnioinfusion

- Infusion of warm saline into uterine cavity is found to be beneficial in oligohydramnios with repeated variable deceleration.
  - Prevents cord compression
  - Dilutes the meconium (recent study reports mention that amnioinfusion does not prevent MAS in cases with MSL)

- Early decision for lower-segment cesarean section has to be taken, if there are signs of fetal compromise (FGR fetuses have poor capacity to tolerate labor)

II stage

- FHR monitoring should be done every 5 minutes in the second stage of labor.
- Delivery is usually not difficult as the baby is of small size. Delivery of the head should be gentle and slow to avoid rapid compression and decompression of the head.
- Routine forceps is not indicated. However, if there is a tendency of delay in the second stage, it is curtailed by low forceps to reduce the stress of labor on the fetus.

High-yield points

Comparison of FGR and preterm babies

	FGR	Preterm
Definition	BW <10th percentile with pathological restriction in growth	Delivery of the fetus before 37 completed weeks of gestation
Features		
Appearance	Wasted	Small but plump
Color	Pale pink	Red or very pink
Length	≥50 cm	<50 cm
Head circumference	≥35 cm	<35 cm
Skin	• Dry, loose, and thick • Dark, thick hair	• Shiny, transparent, thin, and edematous • Vernix ++, lanugo hair ++
Ears, breast, external genitalia	Mature	Premature
Tone	Good muscle tone	Floppy
Complications		
Risk of birth asphyxia	+	+
Hypothermia	+	+
Hypoglycemia	+	+
Hyperbilirubinemia	+	+
Meconium stained liquor	Common	Uncommon
Feeding problems	Uncommon	Common
Apneic spells	Uncommon	Common
Infections	Uncommon	Common
Intracranial hemorrhage	Uncommon	Common
Long-term sequelae	Uncommon, if complications are tackled	Common

Complications and long-term sequelae are more common in preterm babies than in term babies.

- Suctioning of oropharynx and nasopharynx is done as soon as the head is delivered to prevent meconium aspiration.
- Early cord clamping is done to avoid hypervolemia and hyperbilirubinemia.
- Neonatologist should be present at the time of delivery to resuscitate the newborn, as there is increased risk of birth asphyxia and meconium aspiration.

III stage

Active management of the third stage of labor to prevent postpartum hemorrhage (PPH; FGR is associated with preeclampsia where risk of PPH is high)

Following delivery

- NICU care may be required to prevent or treat complications.
- Early feeding is started to prevent hypoglycemia in the newborn.

Frequently asked viva questions

1. Summarize the case.
2. What is the diagnosis of the case?
3. How is FGR clinically diagnosed?
4. What is the role of USG in diagnosis and management of FGR?
5. What is the role of Doppler in FGR?

6. What treatment measures can you offer for FGR?
7. How will you manage the case during pregnancy? When will you terminate the pregnancy?
8. What is the mode of delivery in FGR cases? How will you manage the patient during labor?
9. Which is more difficult to manage, FGR or preterm babies?

12 Recurrent Pregnancy Loss

Introduction

Clinical discussion in a case of recurrent pregnancy loss (RPL) will mainly be focused on the details of previous pregnancies, etiological causes, investigations for evaluation of the cause, and the management of current pregnancy. RPL due to cervical incompetence and antiphospholipid antibody (APLA) syndrome are discussed in detail in this chapter.

Definition of RPL

Recurrent pregnancy loss (RPL) is defined as the loss of two or more pregnancies. It excludes ectopic pregnancy and molar pregnancy *(American Society of Reproductive Medicine (ASRM 2012); European Society of Human Reproduction and Embryology (ESHRE 2017))*.

Incidence of RPL

10–15% of the clinically recognizable pregnancies result in spontaneous miscarriages. Incidence of RPL is 1–2%.

Types of RPL

- **Primary RPL:** RPL without prior successful pregnancy
- **Secondary RPL:** RPL following a live birth
- **Recurrent "early" pregnancy loss:** When the RPL occurs prior to 10 weeks gestation, it is termed recurrent "early" pregnancy loss.
- **Recurrent "late" pregnancy loss:** When the RPL occurs after 10 weeks of gestation but before 20 weeks of gestation, it is termed recurrent "late" pregnancy loss.

Evaluation of RPL

Evaluation of RPL is usually started following two pregnancy losses in women without prior live births because the risk of further pregnancy loss after two or three pregnancy losses approaches similar values (30% and 33%, respectively).

Indications for starting the evaluation earlier

- Fetal cardiac activity documented prior to the pregnancy loss.
- Age of the female partner is >35 years.
- Patient with history of infertility.

Etiology of RPL

Factors implicated in the causation of RPL are mentioned in Table 12.1.

Genetic causes

- These account for 50% of sporadic abortions; however, they are not the most frequent cause of RPL.
- Abortion due to genetic causes usually occurs before 8 weeks of gestation.
- A blighted ovum (anembryonic pregnancy) is one of the leading causes for early pregnancy loss where only gestational sac is formed without any fetal pole—diagnosed by ultrasonography (USG) and absent fetal tissue on histopathology (Figure 12.1).
- Advanced maternal age is a predisposing factor for chromosomal abnormalities.
- Most frequent chromosomal abnormalities are autosomal trisomy, monosomy, and triploidy.

Table 12.1 Etiology of RPL

Etiology	Causes	Incidence (%)
Genetic	• Chromosomal abnormalities – Aneuploidy—trisomy, monosomy • Parental chromosomal rearrangements—balanced reciprocal or Robertsonian translocation	3–5
Anatomical	• Congenital causes: Mullerian anomalies (septate uterus, bicornuate uterus, cervical incompetence, etc.) • Acquired causes: Uterine synechiae, fibroid, cervical incompetence	10–15
Endocrine	• Corpus luteal insufficiency • Polycystic ovarian disease • Untreated hypothyroidism • Uncontrolled diabetes mellitus	15–20
Immunological	• Antiphospholipid antibody syndrome	20–30
Thrombotic factors	Inherited thrombophilias—factor V Leiden deficiency, protein C, and protein S deficiency	
Infections	*Chlamydia trachomatis*, *Ureaplasma urealyticum*, and *Mycoplasma hominis* have been associated with RPL	5
Miscellaneous	Smoking, alcohol, drugs, radiation, subchorionic hematoma	10
Unexplained	Cause not known	50

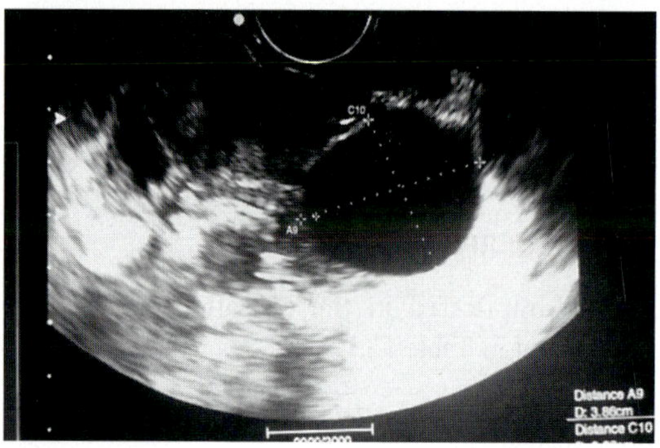

Figure 12.1 Anembryonic pregnancy. Mean gestational sac diameter of >25 mm without yolk sac or fetal pole.

Extra edge

Abortions with normal karyotyping are associated with a higher recurrence rate than abortions with abnormal karyotyping. Hence, in the presence of normal karyotyping of the abortus, the cause of pregnancy loss has to be evaluated.

Diagnosis of blighted ovum or anembryonic pregnancy

A pregnancy is said to be anembryonic if a transvaginal ultrasound reveals a gestational sac with a mean gestational sac diameter (MGD) >25 mm without yolk sac or fetal pole.

- The most common parental chromosomal abnormalities contributing to recurrent abortions are reciprocal or Robertsonian balanced translocations. The carriers of a balanced translocation are phenotypically normal, but are at an increased risk of miscarriages due to unbalanced chromosomal rearrangements.

Anatomical causes

Congenital causes

Failure of fusion of Mullerian ducts or incomplete reabsorption of septum results in uterine anomalies such as septate, bicornuate uterus, unicornuate uterus, uterus didelphys, and cervical incompetence. American Fertility Society classification of Mullerian anomalies is depicted in Figure 12.2.

- Anatomic abnormalities cause miscarriage by causing defective implantation and inadequate placentation.
- The septate uterus is the most common uterine abnormality associated with RPL.
- Renal anomalies are commonly associated with uterine anomalies.

Acquired causes

- **Asherman syndrome (uterine synechiae):** Abortion occurs due to reduced volume of

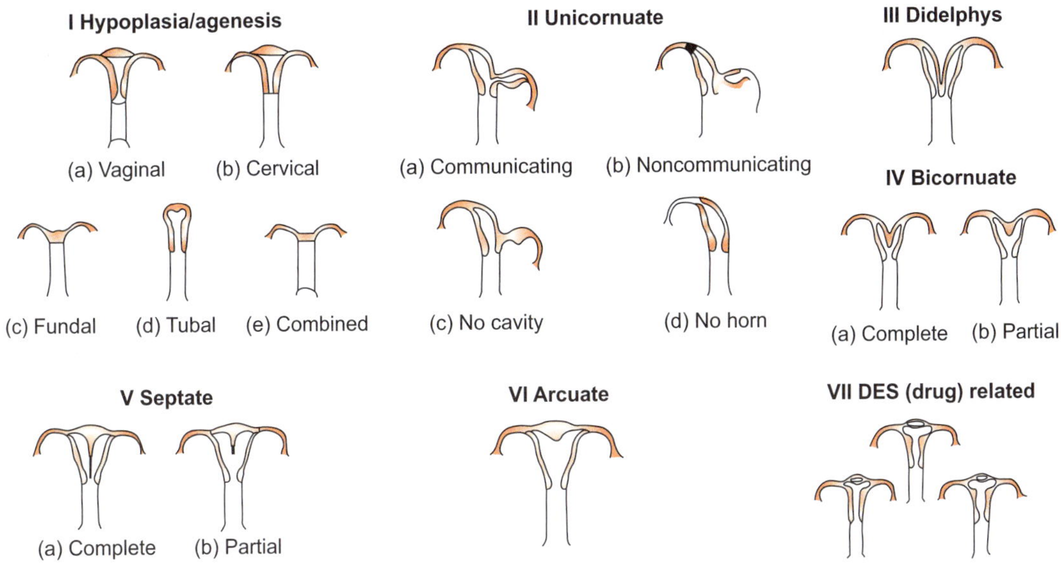

Figure 12.2 American Fertility Society classification of Mullerian anomalies. *DES*, diethylstilbestrol.

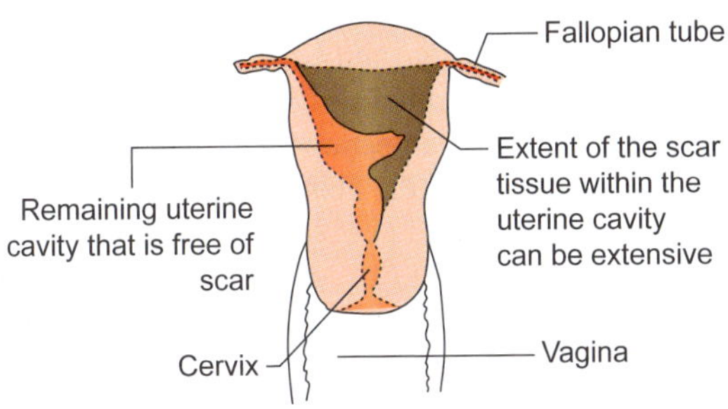

Figure 12.3 Pictorial representation of Asherman syndrome.

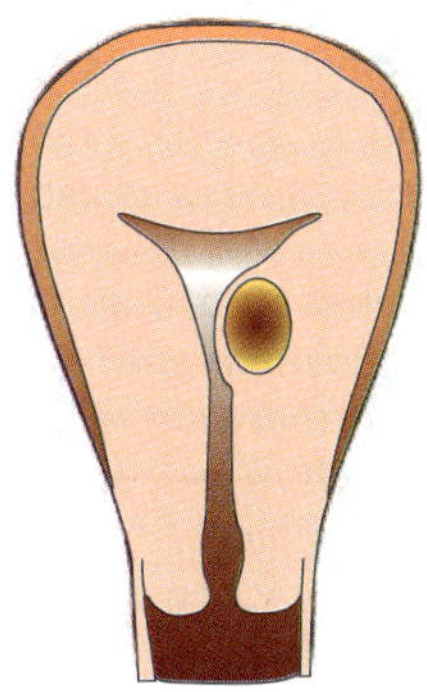

Figure 12.4 Submucous fibroid distorting the endometrial cavity.

uterine cavity or lack of sufficient endometrium (Figure 12.3).

- **Fibroid uterus**
  - *Submucous fibroid*: Distorts endometrial cavity affecting implantation (Figure 12.4)
  - *Large intramural fibroid*: Can cause uterine contractions leading to abortion
- **Cervical incompetence or insufficiency:** Cervical incompetence is the inability of the cervix to retain the pregnancy till term, in the absence of uterine contractions (Figure 12.5).
  - Cervical incompetence may be congenital or acquired following cervical amputation, conization, and laceration of cervix.
  - Cervical incompetence leads to midtrimester pregnancy losses/preterm births. It is not associated with early pregnancy loss.

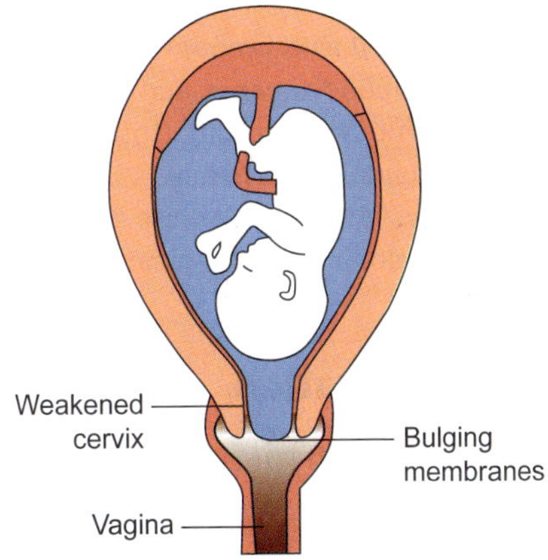

Figure 12.5 Cervical incompetence.

- Typical history is painless second-trimester abortion occurring within a short period of time.

Endocrine causes

- **Corpus luteal insufficiency [luteal phase defect (LPD)]:** Qualitative or quantitative corpus luteal dysfunction results in progesterone insufficiency, which is necessary for decidualization and implantation.
- **Polycystic ovarian disease (PCOD):** Raised levels of luteinizing hormone (LH) in follicular phase have an adverse effect on oocyte maturation and can cause abortion.
- **Uncontrolled diabetes mellitus (DM):** Women with diabetes who have elevated HbA1c levels in the first trimester are at a risk of abortion and fetal anomalies. However, the risk of abortion in well-controlled DM is similar to that in general population.
- **Abnormal thyroid profile:** It has not been conclusively demonstrated as a cause of RPL; however, in clinical practice, thyroid function test (TFT) is routinely done in all patients with RPL.

Note *The prevalence of DM and thyroid dysfunction in women with RPL is similar to that expected in the general population. Hence, routine screening for occult diabetes and thyroid disease in asymptomatic women with RPL is uninformative.*

Immunological causes

- **Autoimmune:** Antiphospholipid antibody (APLA) syndrome
  - It is associated with venous or arterial thrombosis, thrombocytopenia, and RPL.
  - RPL is due to placental thrombosis and uteroplacental insufficiency.
- **Alloimmune:** Immune response to antigens of individuals belonging to the same species
  - Fetus has half-paternal antigen that is foreign to the mother. Failure of development of immunotolerance by the mother results in rejection of the fetus

Thrombotic causes

Inherited thrombophilias

- It includes activated protein C resistance (commonly due to factor V Leiden mutation), protein C and protein S deficiency, hyperhomocysteinemia, and prothrombin gene mutation.
- Inherited thrombophilias are associated with venous thromboembolism and adverse pregnancy outcomes such as fetal loss, preeclampsia, intrauterine growth restriction (IUGR), and placental abruption.

Infections

- These are not proved to be a cause of RPL.
- Agents that are implicated in RPL but not proved are *Listeria monocytogenes*, *Mycoplasma hominis*, *Chlamydia*, and *Ureaplasma*.
- Toxoplasmosis, rubella, *Cytomegalovirus*, and herpes (TORCH) infections can cause abortions but do not cause RPL. Hence, routine screening for TORCH infections is not indicated as a part of investigation of RPL.

Miscellaneous

Other agents that can cause pregnancy losses include

- Environmental pollutants—heavy metal toxicity, benzene, and carbon tetrachloride
- Drugs such as methotrexate and inhalational anesthetic drugs
- Ionizing radiation
- Excess alcohol and smoking
- Chronic maternal illness—cardiac, renal, and hepatic disorders
- Subchorionic hematomas

Unexplained causes

These account for 50% of cases of RPL.

Case presentation

Salient points in history

Consider the following relevant points during history taking in cases of RPL.

Age of the patient

The risk of abortion is high in women >35 years of age. (women with advanced maternal age have increased

(CONTD...)

...CONTD)

rate of meiotic errors in oocyte development leading to increased aneuploidy and pregnancy losses).

H/o present pregnancy

The patient usually says that she has been admitted for evaluation of previous repeated pregnancy losses or has been admitted for safe confinement.

- H/o gestational diabetes mellitus (GDM), preeclampsia, and antepartum hemorrhage (APH)

Menstrual history

- H/o irregular cycles
- H/o PCOD has a higher rate of miscarriage

Marital history

- H/o consanguinity (genetic relationship between partners)
- Time since the couple has been attempting conception
- H/o infertility treatment

Past obstetric history

A detailed history of previous pregnancies has to be asked:

- Gestational age at which pregnancy was confirmed
- If H/o prior live pregnancy is present, ask the following:
  - Any history of GDM, preeclampsia, and APH
  - H/o preterm birth; if so, whether spontaneous or induced labor; if induced labor, reason for preterm induction of labor
  - If cesarean section indication and other details as mentioned in a case of previous cesarean pregnancy (refer to Part 1, Chapter 6, Postcesarean Pregnancy)
  - Any postpartum complication
- If H/o prior abortion is present, ask the following:
  - Whether spontaneous or induced abortion
  - Period of gestation (POG) at the time of abortion
  - Whether cardiac activity was confirmed by USG in that pregnancy
  - Pattern of pregnancy loss (typical H/o painless expulsion of products within a short time period in the second trimester is suggestive of cervical incompetence)
  - H/o dilatation and curettage
    - Forcible dilatation can cause cervical tear and weakness in future pregnancies.
    - Uterine synechiae can develop following vigorous curettage.
  - Whether products of conception were sent for histopathology; if so, content of the histopathology report
- If H/o intrauterine death (IUD)
  - Any antenatal complications such as preeclampsia, GDM, and APH
  - POG at which IUD occurred
  - Whether macerated or fresh stillbirth
  - Sex and weight of fetus, and H/o any congenital malformation in fetus
  - Whether autopsy was performed

Past history

- H/o chronic hypertension, DM, thyroid disorders, autoimmune disorders, and any other chronic illnesses
- H/o thrombosis
- H/o syphilis (ask for genital ulcer)
- H/o any surgical procedure on the cervix such as conization (can lead to midtrimester pregnancy losses)
- Previous diagnostic tests and treatment history

Personal history

- Any addiction such as smoking, alcohol, and drug abuse
- History of occupational and environmental exposures to organic solvents, medications, and ionizing radiation

Family history

H/o DM, hypertension congenital anomalies, and familial thrombotic history (indicates inherited thrombophilias).

Salient points in examination

Consider the following relevant points during examination in cases of RPL:

- General built and nutritional status
- Height, weight, and BMI
- Skin—hirsutism and acanthosis nigricans

(CONTD...)

(...CONTD)

- *Pallor and pedal edema*
- *BP*
- *Breast—galactorrhea*
- *Thyroid swelling*
- *P/A—obstetric examination as routine*
- *P/S—any abnormal discharge and cervix length*

Case summary

Some examples of writing summary and diagnosis in cases of RPL are given below.

Example 1 *Mrs. C, 28 years of age, G4P1L0A2, presents at 32 weeks for routine antenatal checkup. She has no specific complaints. She is perceiving normal fetal movements. There is no history suggestive of labor pains, leaking P/V, or bleeding P/V. She gives H/o cervical cerclage done at 14 weeks of gestation in present pregnancy. Her past obstetric history is suggestive of one preterm delivery at 30 weeks of gestation; the baby was alive but died on postnatal day 3 due to complications of prematurity. This was followed by two spontaneous pregnancy losses at about 20 weeks of gestation. In all the prior three pregnancies, she had H/o painless expulsion of abortus within a short time period. There is no significant medical or surgical history. On examination, there are no significant general examination findings. Her vitals are normal. Obstetric examination reveals a fundal height of 32 weeks with a singleton live fetus in cephalic presentation. Uterus is relaxed, liquor appears average, and FHR is 148 beats/min, regular.*

Example 2 *Mrs. T, 32 years of age, G4P0L0A3 at 28 weeks of gestation, presents for routine antenatal checkup. She has no specific complaints. She is perceiving normal fetal movements. There is no history suggestive of labor pains, leaking P/V, or bleeding P/V. She is on treatment with aspirin and heparin since early first trimester in present pregnancy. She gives H/o three consecutive spontaneous abortions at about 10 weeks of gestation over the past 3 years. The products of conception of her last abortion were sent for histopathology, but she does not know the details of the report. There is no significant medical or surgical history. On examination, there are no significant general examination findings. Her vitals are normal. Obstetric examination reveals a fundal height of 28 weeks with a singleton live fetus in cephalic presentation. Uterus is relaxed, liquor appears average, and FHR is 138 beats/min, regular.*

Case diagnosis

Example 1 *28 years of age, G4P1L0A2, at 32 weeks of gestation with recurrent midtrimester pregnancy losses probably due to cervical incompetence, with H/o cervical cerclage procedure done at 14 weeks of gestation, with a singleton live fetus in cephalic presentation, not in labor*

Example 2 *32 years of age, G4P0L0A3 at 28 weeks of gestation, probably a case of APLA syndrome on aspirin and heparin therapy with a singleton live fetus in cephalic presentation, not in labor*

Case discussion

Cervical incompetence and APLA syndrome are the two important causes of RPL that can be discussed in detail during clinical exams, and hence elaborated in the following sections.

CERVICAL INCOMPETENCE

Definition

Cervical incompetence refers to the inability of the cervix to retain the pregnancy till term in the absence of uterine contractions.

- It is characterized by painless cervical dilatation in the second trimester, with bulging of the membranes into vagina followed by rupture of membranes and expulsion of fetus.

Etiology

- **Congenital:** Associated with Mullerian anomalies and connective tissue disorders
- **Acquired**
  - Forcible dilation of cervix during medical termination of pregnancy (MTP)
  - Amputation of cervix
  - Conization of cervix

– Instrumental delivery in an incompletely dilated cervix
– Precipitate labor

Diagnosis of cervical incompetence

History suggestive of cervical incompetence

- H/o repeated midtrimester pregnancy loss
- Typical history of sudden rupture of membranes followed by painless expulsion of products of conception within a short time period
- H/o En masse expulsion of live fetus

Diagnosis during pregnancy

- **Speculum examination:** Dilatation of cervix with bulging of membranes can be seen.
- **USG criteria for diagnosis of cervical incompetence during pregnancy** (Figures 12.6 and 12.7):
  – Cervical length of <2.5 cm
  – Width of internal os >2 cm
  – Funneling of the internal os
  – Sacculation or bulging of membranes into the cervix either spontaneously or on applying fundal pressure

Note *Transvaginal ultrasonography (TVS) is better than transabdominal ultrasonography (TAS) in detecting cervical changes (full bladder required for TAS examination can compress the internal os, making it apparently appear closed).*

Diagnosis during nonpregnant state

- **No. 8 Hegar's dilator**: No. 8 Hegar's dilator can be passed easily through the internal os and there is absence of snapping closure while withdrawing the dilator from internal os
- **No. 14 Foley's catheter inflated with 2 mL saline inserted into uterus:** The catheter can be easily pulled out with traction force of less than 600 g
- **Hysterosalpingogram (HSG):** Premenstrual HSG shows funneling of the cervical canal
- **Hysteroscopy:** Cervical compliance index can be calculated based on the following parameters assessed in hysteroscopy (Table 12.2):
  – Canal/cannula ratio—upper cervical canal width compared with the hysteroscope width
  – Difficulty in passing No. 8 Hegar's through internal os
  – Traction required to pull out the No. 14 Foley's inflated with 2 mL saline from the uterus

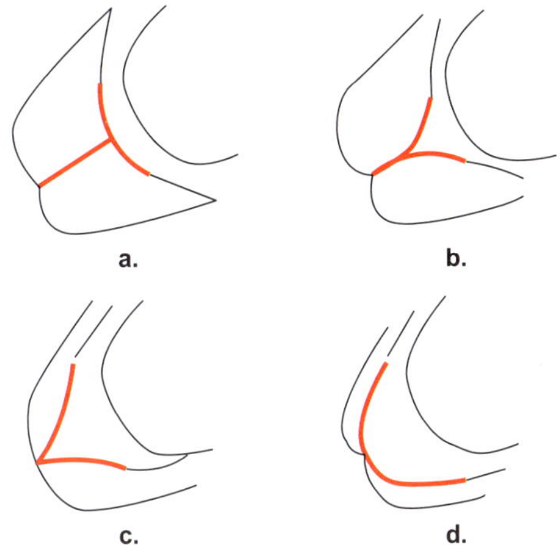

Figure 12.6 Pictorial representation of ultrasonography cervical findings in cervical incompetence. **a.** "T" sign. **b.** "Y" sign. **c.** "V" sign. **d.** "U" sign.

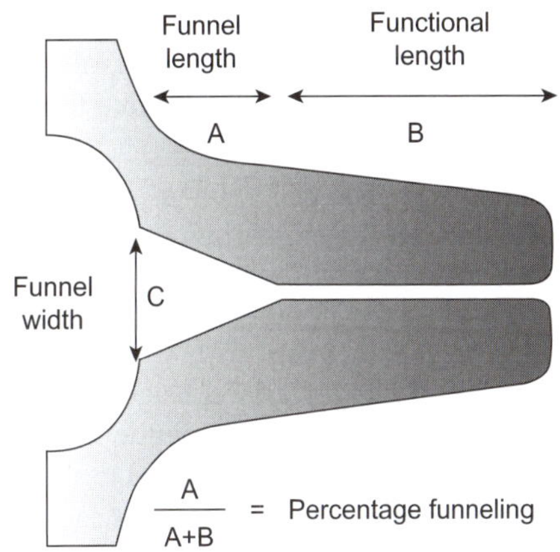

Figure 12.7 Pictorial representation of funneling of internal os in cervical incompetence.

Table 12.2 Cervical compliance index calculated based on the hysteroscopy findings

Finding	Score*		
	0	1	2
Canal/cannula ratio	<1.5	1.5–2	>2
No. 8 Hegar's	Will not pass	Passes with moderate force	Passes with little or no force
Catheter traction (g)	>600	<600	

*Score >2 is significant.

Part 1

Management of cervical incompetence

Cervical cerclage is the surgical procedure that is done for management of cervical incompetence.

Candidates for cervical cerclage

- Women with H/o at least three second-trimester pregnancy losses or three preterm births
- Women with H/o prior preterm delivery who have cervical length of <2.5 cm on ultrasound

Time period for doing a cerclage procedure

The cerclage procedure is performed at or after 14 weeks, usually around 14–16 weeks.

- **Prophylactic/elective cerclage/primary cerclage/ history-indicated cerclage:** Cerclage is placed in a pregnant woman who is at risk for cervical incompetence even before it has manifested, with the intention of carrying pregnancy till term (previous H/o of three or more spontaneous second-trimester pregnancy losses), that is, a prophylactic cerclage is applied before the cervix is dilated.
- **Therapeutic cerclage:** Cerclage is placed in a pregnant woman who is at risk for cervical incompetence with significant cervical changes (previous H/o one or more spontaneous midtrimester pregnancy losses with USG features of cervical shortening—cervical length of <2.5 cm at <24 weeks), that is, therapeutic cerclage is applied when the cervix has started to shorten.
- **Emergency/salvage cerclage:** Cerclage is placed in a pregnant woman who presents with advanced cervical dilatation. Success rate is less. The decision to place a rescue cerclage is made on individual basis considering the clinical circumstances, that is, emergency cerclage is applied when the cervix is short and dilated with bulging fetal membranes.

> **Viva corner**
>
> **Q1 Why is cerclage recommended at or after 14 weeks?**
>
> - By this time, chromosomally abnormal fetuses would have aborted spontaneously.
> - Major fetal anomalies can be detected or ruled out by USG at 14–16 weeks.
> - Cervical insufficiency does not manifest itself prior to mid-second trimester.
>
> **Note** *No literature indicates that early cerclage is advantageous over placement at 16 weeks.*

Methods of cervical cerclage

Cervical cerclage can be done through vaginal or abdominal route.

Cerclage methods done through vaginal route

McDonald's cerclage (Figure 12.8)

- Nonabsorbable suture (Prolene, or Mersilene tape) is placed like a purse string at junction of cervix and vagina and tied anteriorly.
- The 3 and 9 o'clock positions are avoided to prevent bleeding from descending cervical artery.
- Most commonly performed technique.
- Advantages and disadvantages of McDonald's cerclage are mentioned in Table 12.3.

Modified Shirodkar's cerclage (Figure 12.9)

- A small transverse incision is made at the cervicovaginal junction anteriorly and the bladder is pushed up.

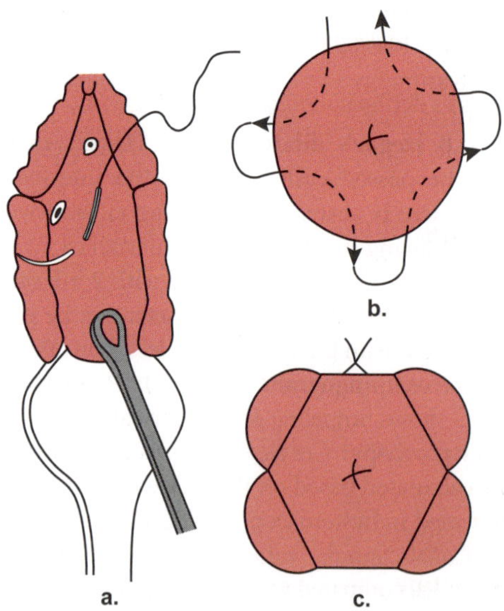

Figure 12.8 McDonald's cervical cerclage. **a-c.** A purse string suture using nonabsorbable synthetic suture material placed transvaginally high on the cervix.

Table 12.3 Advantages and disadvantages of McDonald's cerclage

Advantages	Disadvantages
• No incision is required • Easy to perform • Less bleeding • Suture removal is easy • Less cervical scarring and dystocia	• The cerclage is not placed at internal os where the actual defect is present and hence not anatomical • Exposed suture material can cause – Vaginal irritation and discharge – Bladder irritation

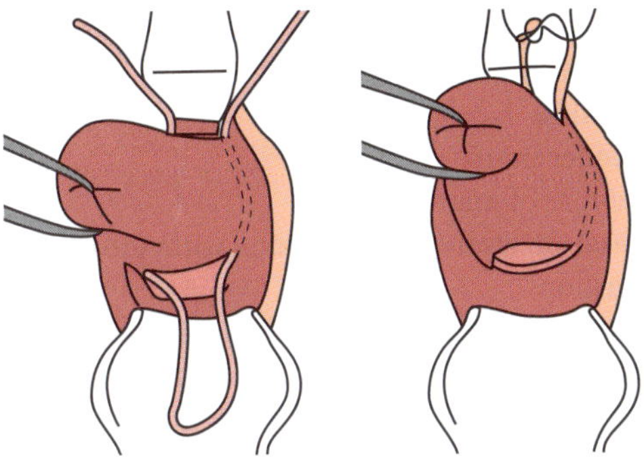

a. b.

Figure 12.9 Modified Shirodkar's cerclage. **a.** and **b.** The suture is placed at the level of the internal os after dissection of the vaginal mucosa and retraction of the bladder.

- Nonabsorbable suture is placed submucosally at the level of internal os and tied posteriorly (avoids bladder irritation).
- The anterior incision is then closed with absorbable suture material.
- Advantages and disadvantages of modified Shirodkar's procedure are mentioned in Table 12.4.

Note *In the original Shirodkar's procedure, the following were done:*
- *Fascia lata was used as suture material.*
- *Both anterior and posterior incisions were made.*
- *Aneurysmal needle was used.*
- *Knot was placed anteriorly.*

Table 12.4 Advantages and disadvantages of modified Shirodkar's cerclage

Advantage	Disadvantages
• More anatomical, as the suture is placed at the level of internal os	• Risk of bladder injury • May require anesthesia for removal of the suture

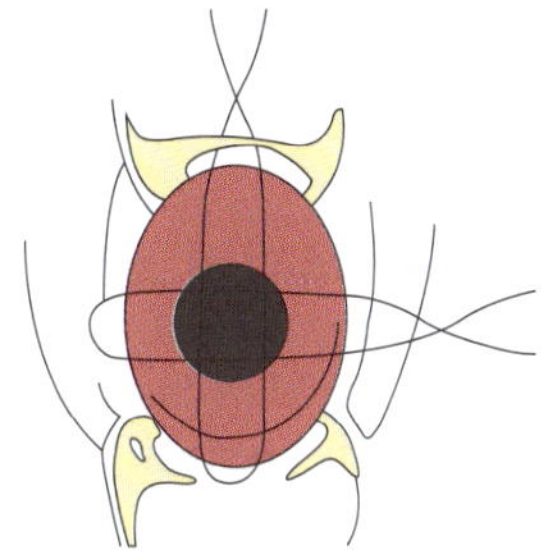

Figure 12.10 Wurm's cerclage. Two separate sutures are placed through the cervical tissue at right angles to each other and tied.

Wurm's procedure (Figure 12.10)

- Two separate sutures are placed through the cervical tissue at right angles to each other and tied.
- This cerclage is done especially when the cervix is dilated and membranes are bulging.

Extra edge

Techniques for reducing the bulging membranes during emergency cerclage

The main precaution is to avoid contact with the exposed membranes.

- Lithotomy with head-low position will help in reducing the bulging membranes.
- Intracervical Foley's catheter filled with 30 mL saline can be used to push the membranes into uterine cavity.
- Moistened swab held with sponge holding forceps can be used to push the membranes into uterine cavity.
- Transabdominal amniocentesis reduces the tension in the amniotic cavity and allows retraction of the membranes.
- Traction on cervical stay sutures can cause the membranes to fall back into the uterine cavity before placing the cerclage.
- Filling the bladder with 400 mL of normal saline may lead to retraction of the amniotic sac into the uterine cavity.

Part 1

Transabdominal methods of cervical cerclage

- To be done in preconception period and can be done via laparoscopy

Indications for abdominal cerclage

- Very short cervix
- Amputated cervix
- Deep cervical tears and traumatized cervix
- Previous failed vaginal method of cerclage

Benson and Durfee method of abdominal cerclage (Figure 12.11)

- A Pfannenstiel incision is given, uterovesical fold of peritoneum is incised, bladder is pushed down, and then a Mersilene tape is passed through the broad ligament at the level of isthmus and tied anteriorly.
- Advantages and disadvantages of abdominal cerclage are mentioned in Table 12.5.

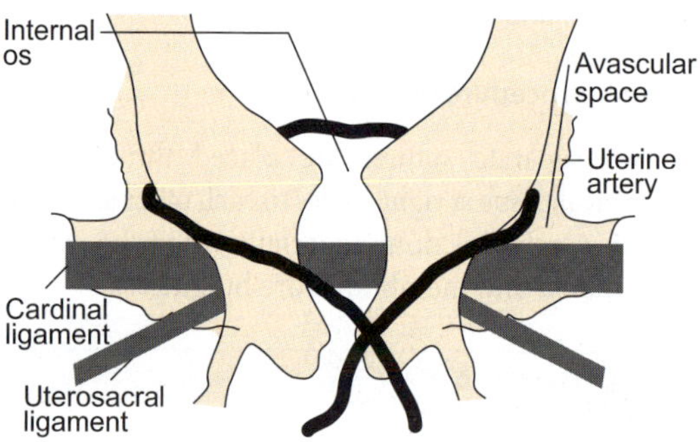

Figure 12.11 Abdominal cerclage. Mersilene tape is passed through the broad ligament at the level of isthmus and tied anteriorly.

Table 12.5 Advantages and disadvantages of abdominal cerclage

Advantages	Disadvantages
• Placement of cerclage is anatomical • It can be done in women where vaginal cervical cerclage is not possible—for example, very short cervix, amputated cervix, deep cervical tears, and previous failed cervical cerclage	• Laparotomy is required for placement of cerclage • Complications are more than in vaginal procedures—blood loss, risk of injury to ureter, uterine vessels, etc. • Removal of the suture is difficult in case of emergencies • Cesarean section is indicated following abdominal cerclage

Contraindications for cerclage

- Presence of uterine contractions
- Cervical dilatation of >4 cm
- Rupture of membranes
- Fetal anomalies/death
- Abruption/placenta previa (APH)
- Chorioamnionitis

Complications of cerclage

- Risk of anesthesia
- Bleeding
- Bladder injury
- Rupture of membranes
- Onset of uterine contractions with subsequent abortion
- Postoperative infections—chorioamnionitis
- Slippage/cut through/displacement of cervical sutures
- Fibrosis leading to cervical dystocia during labor
- Possibility of bucket-handle tear of cervix and rupture uterus, if stitch is not removed with onset of labor

Prerequisites before doing cerclage

- Perform USG to confirm a viable intrauterine pregnancy.
- Rule out lethal congenital anomalies.
- Perform vaginal swab culture sensitivity to rule out genital tract infections.
- Explain the potential complications of the procedure to the patient.
- Obtain informed written consent.
- Tocolytics can be started preoperatively.

Note *There is a paucity of published data on usage of perioperative tocolytics for cerclage. Tocolysis with indomethacin or beta-mimetics is used by some clinicians prior to and for a few days after cerclage procedure to minimize uterine irritability.*

Postoperative advice

- Bed rest is advised for at least 24 hours.
- Patient can be discharged on the second or third postoperative day.
- Tocolysis may be continued for a week to prevent uterine contractions due the procedure.
- Perioperative antibiotics are not routinely recommended. (Current evidence is insufficient

to recommend antibiotic prophylaxis for either prophylactic or emergency cerclage.)
- Supplemental progesterone is not routinely recommended.
- Abstinence from sexual intercourse is not routinely recommended.

Indications for removal of cerclage

- At 37 completed weeks
- At the onset of labor
- Rupture of membranes
- Clinical evidence of infection
- Abdominal cerclage removed during cesarean section, upon completion of family

ANTIPHOSPHOLIPID ANTIBODY SYNDROME

Definition

APLA syndrome is an autoimmune disorder characterized by the presence of antiphospholipid antibodies, recurrent vascular thrombosis, RPL, and thrombocytopenia.

Classification

- **Primary:** APLA in the absence of other autoimmune diseases
- **Secondary**: APLA associated with other autoimmune diseases such as SLE

Pathogenesis

- Autoantibodies are formed that are directed against phospholipids or plasma proteins bound to phospholipids. Many of these proteins are anticoagulants in clotting cascade and hence there is disruption of physiological anticoagulation.
- The basic pathological change is thrombotic microangiopathy involving multiple organ system.
- Placental damage resulting from thrombosis is thought to be the reason for pregnancy loss in patients with APLA syndrome.

Antibodies involved in APLA syndrome are the following:
- Anticardiolipin antibodies (ACA)
  - Detection is by direct method—by ELISA titers
- Lupus anticoagulant (LAC) antibody
  - Detection is by indirect method—by in vitro prolongation of coagulation studies
  - There is prolongation of the following:
    - Activated partial thromboplastin time (aPTT)
    - Prothrombin time (PT)
    - Russell viper venom test
    - Platelet neutralization procedure
    - Kaolin clotting time

Diagnostic criteria (Sapporo's criteria) for APLA syndrome

For diagnosis of APLA syndrome, one or more clinical and one or more laboratory criteria must be present.

Clinical criteria

- One or more episodes of venous or arterial thrombosis
- Presence of pregnancy complications
  - ≥3 consecutive spontaneous pregnancy losses at <10 weeks
  - ≥1 fetal death of morphologically normal fetus at >10 weeks
  - ≥1 preterm birth of morphologically normal fetus at <34 weeks, secondary to severe preeclampsia or placental insufficiency

Laboratory criteria

- Positive plasma levels of ACA on ≥2 occasions 6 weeks apart
- Detection of LAC on ≥2 occasions 6 weeks apart

Obstetric complications in APLA syndrome

- Recurrent first- or second-trimester pregnancy losses
- Early onset preeclampsia
- Uteroplacental insufficiency—IUGR
- Preterm labor
- Abruption
- IUD

Indications for testing for APLA syndrome

- Recurrent abortions
- Unexplained second- or third-trimester losses

Part 1

- Early onset severe preeclampsia
- Unexplained IUGR
- Venous or arterial thromboembolic events
- Autoimmune or connective tissue diseases
- False-positive serological test for syphilis
- Prolongation of coagulation studies

Treatment

Aim

- To improve maternal, fetal, and neonatal outcome
- To reduce the risk of thromboembolism

General measures

- Antenatal care in a tertiary care hospital
- Patient explained about complications, treatment options, and the need for regular antenatal care
- Advised on frequent antenatal visits once in 2 weeks
- Dating and anomalies scan done
- Serial obstetric scan done from 20 weeks
- Fetal surveillance from 28 weeks onwards with daily fetal movement count (DFMC), ultrasound with Doppler studies and nonstress test.

Specific treatment

Combined treatment with aspirin and heparin is recommended to reduce pregnancy loss and improve live birth rates in women with APLA.

Antepartum management

- Patients with APLA syndrome with H/o RPL, without prior history of thrombosis, should receive treatment with a combination of aspirin and heparin during pregnancy.
  - Low-dose aspirin should be started during attempted conception or with a positive pregnancy test. (Preconceptional aspirin has a possible beneficial effect on early stages of implantation.)
  - Prophylactic doses of unfractionated heparin (UFH) 5000–10,000 units administered subcutaneously every 12 hours or low-molecular-weight heparin (LMWH) such as enoxaparin 40 mg subcutaneously every 24 hours should be started when a viable intrauterine pregnancy is documented and continued until late third trimester.
  - In case the patient presents after conceiving, she should be immediately started on low-dose aspirin and heparin.
- Patients with APLA syndrome with a history of thrombosis should be fully anticoagulated with the following:
  - Adjust dose of UFH or LMWH administered subcutaneously every 12 hours for at least 6 months from the time of initial presentation with venous thromboembolism.
  - Consider reducing the dose of anticoagulation to prophylactic UFH or LMWH, if the patient reaches 6 months of anticoagulation during the pregnancy.
- Patients on LMWH changed to UFH (because of shorter half-life of UFH) at 36–37 weeks of gestation.

Intrapartum management

- Prophylactic heparin should be discontinued at least 12 hours prior to induction of labor or elective cesarean section.
- Adjusted-dose heparin should be discontinued 24 hours prior to induction of labor or elective cesarean section.

Postpartum management

Antithrombotic coverage during the postpartum period is recommended in all women with APLA, with or without previous H/o thrombosis to reduce the risk of postpartum deep vein thrombosis.

- Women with no H/o previous thrombosis—prophylactic dose heparin or LMWH therapy is recommended for 4–6 weeks after delivery.
- Women with H/o previous thrombosis—long-term anticoagulation is required, and it is preferred to change the treatment to warfarin, to reduce the risk of heparin-induced osteoporosis and bone fracture.

MANAGEMENT OF RPL

Evaluation of RPL

- Evaluation is individualized for each case.
- A planned and systematic approach should be adopted. Summary of evaluation and treatment of the causes of RPL is mentioned in Table 12.6.

Extra edge

Drugs used in APLA syndrome

Heparin prophylaxis

- It prevents thrombotic episodes and thrombosis in placental microcirculation.
- Heparin does not cross the placenta and is safe during pregnancy.
- Heparin therapy is monitored with aPTT and LMWH therapy is monitored with anti–factor Xa assay.

Complications of heparin therapy

- Bleeding
- Thrombocytopenia
- Osteoporosis and pathological fractures

Advantages of LMWH over UFH

- Less bleeding complications
- Decreased incidence of thrombocytopenia and osteoporosis
- Long half-life—less frequent dosing and monitoring
- Increased patient compliance

Low-dose aspirin

- Dose is 75–80 mg/day
- Decreases thromboxane A2
- No major side effects other than risk of small vessel bleeds during surgical procedures

Steroids

- Prednisolone
- Used only in secondary APLA syndrome

Immunoglobulins

Reserved for patients refractory to treatment with heparin and aspirin

Table 12.6 Summary of evaluation and treatment of the causes of RPL

Category	Evaluation	Treatment
Genetic causes	• Karyotyping of both parents • Ovarian reserve test	• Genetic counseling • Donor gametes • Preimplantation genetic diagnosis
Anatomic causes	• Ultrasound examination • Hysterosalpingogram • Hysterolaparoscopy • MRI	• No surgery possible in unicornuate, didelphys, arcuate uterus • Septate uterus—Jones and Tompkins' septoplasty, hysteroscopic resection of septum • Bicornuate uterus—Strassman's metroplasty • Cervical incompetence—cerclage • Fibroid—myomectomy/hysteroscopic resection of submucous fibroid
Endocrine causes	• Luteal phase defect—luteal phase endometrial biopsy • PCOD—LH, FSH levels, USG • DM—blood glucose, HbA1C • TSH, Sr. prolactin	• Progesterone supplementation • Metformin, clomiphene citrate • Insulin therapy • Thyroxine therapy, dopamine agonists (for prolactinomas)
Immunological and thrombotic causes	• APLA: LAC, ACA • Thrombophilias: Factor V Leiden, protein C, protein S, antithrombin III deficiency	• Heparin and aspirin
Infections	Endocervical culture: For *Chlamydia*, *Mycoplasma*, and *Ureaplasma*	Empirical antibiotics
Environmental causes	History	Behavioral modifications

ACA, anticardiolipin antibodies; *APLA*, antiphospholipid antibody syndrome; *DM*, diabetes mellitus; *FSH*, follicle-stimulating hormone; *LAC*, lupus anticoagulant; *LH*, luteinizing hormone; *PCOD*, polycystic ovarian disease; *TSH*, thyroid-stimulating hormone; *USG*, ultrasonography.

Evaluation during pregnancy in a woman with RPL

- Complete hemogram with platelet count
- Blood grouping and typing
- Urine analysis
- Glucose tolerance test (GTT)
- VDRL
- APLA titers—ACA and LAC
- Thyroid function test in case of clinical features suggestive of thyroid dysfunction (however, it is routinely done in clinical practice, although it is not indicated in the definitive tests for RPL)
- Cervical swab culture for *L. monocytogenes*, *M. hominis*, and *Ureaplasma urealyticum*
- USG—for cervical length, uterine malformations, and fibroid uterus
- Karyotyping of both the partners

Evaluation for RPL that can be done only in the interconceptional period

- **HSG:** Uses of HSG in RPL include the following:
  - To diagnose cervical incompetence
  - To study the endometrial cavity—endometrial polyps, submucous fibroid, and septate uterus
  - To diagnose uterine synechiae—Asherman syndrome
  - To check for tubal patency

However, HSG cannot differentiate a septate uterus from bicornuate uterus.

- **Hysterolaparoscopy:** Uses of hysterolaparoscopy in RPL include the following:
  - Detects uterine anomalies such as bicornuate/unicornuate/septate uterus
  - Differentiates a septate uterus (normal-looking uterine fundus) from bicornuate uterus (depression between the two horns)
  - Helps in identifying noncommunicating rudimentary horn of uterus
- **Luteal phase endometrial biopsy:** To identify LPD
- **Tests for diagnosis of cervical incompetence:** Passage of No. 8 Hegar's dilator without difficulty or HSG showing funnel-shaped cervical canal

Extra edge

Differentiating features between bicornuate uterus and septate uterus in USG

Bicornuate uterus	Septate uterus
Depressed fundus	Fundus appears normal
Uterine wall above the line joining the tips of tubal ostia is <5 mm	Uterine wall above the line joining the tips of tubal ostia is >5 mm
Angle between the two cavities is >90°	Angle between the two cavities is <90°

Ultrasound criteria to differentiate a bicornuate uterus from a septate uterus (see figure below)

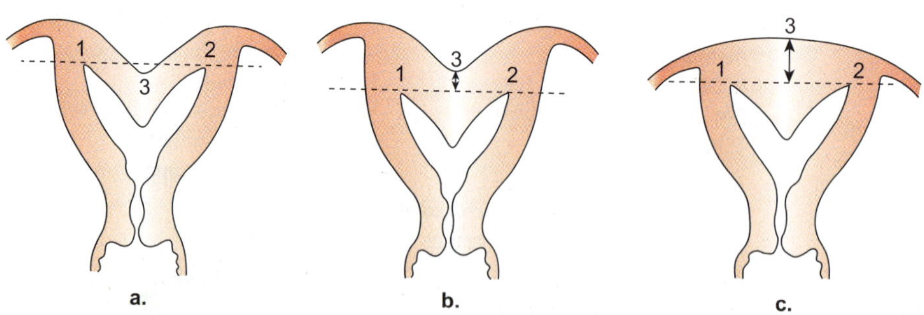

Figure Ultrasound criteria to differentiate a septate uterus from a bicornuate uterus. **a.** and **b.** When apex (3) of the fundus lies below a straight line joining the tubal ostia (1, 2) or <5 mm (arrow) above it, the uterus is bicornuate. **c.** When apex of the fundus is more than 5 mm (arrow) above the line, the uterus is septate.

Preconceptional management of a case with RPL

- Provide psychological support.
- Advise on lifestyle changes such as cessation of smoking and alcohol intake.
- Periconceptional folic acid is started.

Postconceptional management of a case with RPL

First trimester

- Management is individualized depending on the cause of RPL.
- Psychological support and reassurance is provided in the first trimester to alleviate anxiety.
- Confirm intrauterine viable pregnancy.
- Aspirin and heparin therapy are started in women with APLA.
- Continue folic acid prophylaxis.
- Progesterone therapy may be offered in women with diagnosed LPD and unexplained RPL. The doses of progesterone used in clinical practice are the following:
  - Dydrogesterone 10 mg BD oral till 20 weeks of pregnancy
  - Micronized progesterone—400 mg/day oral/vaginal till 20 weeks of pregnancy
- Oral glucose tolerance test (OGTT) is done.
- USG is done every 2 weeks up to the gestational age of previous abortion.
- In case of nonviable pregnancy, pregnancy is terminated and the abortus is sent for karyotyping.

Second trimester

- In suspected cases of cervical incompetence, transvaginal scan (TVS) is done to assess the cervical length and shape.
- Prophylactic cervical cerclage may be applied at 14–16 weeks in women with cervical incompetence, and those with previous ≥3 midtrimester abortion or spontaneous preterm delivery, after ruling out anomalies.
- A second trimester anomaly scan is done at 16–24 weeks of gestation.
- Repeat GTT at 24–28 weeks if previous test result was normal.
- Uterine artery Doppler at 22–24 weeks may be useful in predicting preeclampsia and IUGR in high-risk women.

Third trimester

- Serial growth scans and umbilical artery Doppler are indicated in patients with RPL, especially in women with APLA syndrome and thrombophilias due to the high risk for IUGR in these patients.

Part 1

Extra edge

Treatment modalities of doubtful or no value in RPL

- Bed rest
- Aspirin ± heparin in unexplained RPL and in thrombophilias
- Human chorionic gonadotropin (HCG) use
- Routine progesterone supplementation
- Immunotherapy

The role of progesterone supplementation in early pregnancy in women with RPL

- Progesterone induces secretary changes in the endometrium that is essential for endometrial maturation, endometrial stabilization, embryo implantation, and regulation of inflammatory mediators.
- Progesterone supplementation is recommended in pregnancy losses due to LPD.
- There is insufficient evidence to evaluate the effect of routine progesterone supplementation to prevent miscarriage in women with RPL.
- There might be some benefit with progesterone supplementation in women with unexplained losses.
- The argument for use of progesterone is that there is no evidence of harm and some evidence of benefit, although multicentric trial reports are still awaited. The decision should be based on clinician's discretion until strong evidence is available to recommend its routine use.
- There is no role of progesterone supplementation in normal healthy pregnant women for prevention of miscarriage.

- If patient is on aspirin, it should be stopped at about 32 weeks.
- If cervical cerclage has been done, then the stitch is removed at 37–38 weeks or earlier if the patient goes into labor.

Mode of delivery

- If there are no associated obstetric complications, there is no indication for intervention prior to 40 weeks. However, the pregnancy should not be allowed to go beyond expected date of delivery (EDD).
- RPL per se is not an indication for cesarean section (CS). CS is indicated only for any associated obstetric or medical complications.
- Mode of delivery has to be decided in consultation with the patient. Patients may request for elective cesarean section.
- Prophylactic heparin should be discontinued at least 12 hours prior to induction or elective CS. Adjusted-dose heparin should be discontinued 24 hours before induction or elective CS.

Puerperium

Postpartum thromboprophylaxis may be indicated in women with inherited thrombophilias and APLA syndrome.

Viva corner

Q1 How will you manage cases with RPL with karyotyping of the partners showing balanced translocation?

- Genetic counseling is offered regarding prognosis for future pregnancies and prenatal diagnosis.
- Various reproductive options include the following:
  - Proceeding to a natural pregnancy with or without prenatal diagnostic tests
  - Preimplantation genetic diagnosis in translocation carriers
  - Gamete donation

Q2 What is your further plan of management if a septum is found on hysterolaparoscopic evaluation of RPL?

- Hysteroscopic septal resection is done in the postmenstrual phase.
- The patient is started on OCPs postresection for 6 months that provide contraception and help in tissue healing.
- The patient can attempt conception after 6 months. Live birth success rate is 85%.
- There is no indication for routine cerclage as the causative factor has been addressed.
- TVS for cervical length is done at 14–16 weeks and if found to be <2.5 cm (associated factor), cerclage can be done.

Q3 How is LPD diagnosed and managed?

- Definition: LPD is defined as a lag of more than 2 days in the histological development of the endometrium when compared with the day of the cycle.
- Midluteal phase progesterone of <10 ng/mL or a sum of three random serum progesterone measurements <30 ng/mL measured during the luteal is suggestive of LPD.
- Progesterone supplementation is recommended in pregnancy losses due to LPD.

Q4 What is unexplained RPL and how is it managed?

Definition

- If no causative factor is identified in a woman with RPL, in spite of extensive investigations, then it is labeled as "unexplained" RPL.
- Unexplained causes account for nearly 50% of cases of RPL.

Management

- Patients are encouraged to continue attempts at pregnancy because studies have shown that these women have a high rate of live births with subsequent pregnancies.
- The most effective therapy for patients with unexplained RPL is antenatal counseling and psychological support.
- General advice is given on quitting smoking, avoiding excess alcohol and caffeine intake, and weight loss in obese women.

(CONTD...)

(...CONTD)

Viva corner

- Folic acid (400 μg/day) prior to attempting conception is indicated to prevent neural tube defects.
- There might be some benefit with progestogen supplementation in women with unexplained losses, although there is no strong evidence to support the use.

Prognosis for a successful pregnancy in cases of negative workup is 70% in women <35 years and 50% in women >35 years.

Causes of spontaneous abortions (may/may not cause RPL)

See Table 12.7

Table 12.7 Causes of spontaneous abortion

First-trimester abortion	Second-trimester abortion
• Chromosomal abnormalities of fetus (trisomy, monosomy) • Corpus luteal insufficiency (LPD) • Uterine anomalies and fibroid • Autoimmune diseases—APLA and thrombophilias • Endocrine disorders—thyroid dysfunction, PCOD • Maternal diseases—uncontrolled DM, renal hypertension, etc. • Infections • High-grade fever • Trauma • Radiation and drug intake	• Cervical incompetence • Uterine anomalies and fibroid • Intrauterine infections • Autoimmune diseases • Chronic maternal illness—renal diseases, etc. • Trauma

APLA, antiphospholipid antibody; *DM*, diabetes mellitus; *LPD*, luteal phase defect; *PCOD*, polycystic ovarian disease.

Frequently asked viva questions

1. Summary of the case.
2. What is the diagnosis of the case?
3. How will you evaluate the patient?
4. What is the plan of management for the patient?
5. What are the causes of RPL?
6. What are the points in history and examination which aids in diagnosis of cervical incompetence?
7. How will you manage a case of cervical incompetence?
8. What are the clinical features of APLA syndrome? How will you manage the patient?

Part 1

13 Preterm Labor

Introduction

Preterm labor is an important cause of perinatal morbidity and mortality. It may be spontaneous in onset or may be induced in view of medical conditions or pregnancy disorders in the mother or the fetus. Clinical discussion in a case of preterm labor will involve the following aspects:

- Risk factors
- Complications
- Management—role of antibiotics, steroids, and tocolysis

Definition of preterm labor

Onset of labor after the period of viability and before 37 completed weeks of gestation is termed preterm labor.

Note *The lower limit of this definition, that is, the period of viability, is not clearly defined. It is 22 weeks according to the WHO, 24 weeks in the United Kingdom, and 28 weeks in developing countries such as India.*

Classification of the time period of preterm labor based on the presumed lung maturity is

- **Early preterm delivery**—delivery between 28 and 34 weeks (lungs are not mature)
- **Late preterm delivery**—delivery after 34 weeks of gestation but before 37 completed weeks of gestation (lungs are presumed to be mature)

Incidence

It is 5–10% of all pregnancies. Preterm labor is a major cause of perinatal mortality and morbidity accounting for 50–70% of perinatal deaths.

RISK FACTORS FOR PRETERM LABOR

Demographic factors

- Maternal age <18 and >35 years
- Low socioeconomic status
- Low prepregnancy body weight

Behavioral factors

- Smoking, tobacco, and substance abuse—alcohol and cocaine
- Poor nutrition
- Stress
- Excessive physical activity

Obstetric factors

Maternal causes

- Grand multigravida
- Overdistended uterus—polyhydramnios and multiple pregnancy
- Uterine anomalies—septate uterus, bicornuate uterus, unicornuate uterus, and cervical incompetence
- Medical disorders—preeclampsia, anemia, cardiac disease, and hyperpyrexia
- Antepartum hemorrhage (APH)—placenta previa and abruption
- Preterm premature rupture of membranes (PPROM)—2/3rd cases of preterm labor are associated with PPROM
- Past history of preterm labor, second-trimester abortion, and recurrent abortions

Fetal causes

- Intrauterine death (IUD)
- Fetal anomalies

Miscellaneous

- Trauma
- Abdominal surgery during pregnancy

Infections

- Urinary tract infections
- Bacterial vaginosis
- Intrauterine infections

Iatrogenic

- Wrong estimation of gestational age (iatrogenic prematurity)
- Elective induction for fetal or maternal indication

Idiopathic

It occurs in 40–50% of cases (there is increasing evidence of subclinical infection in these cases).

DIAGNOSIS

Criteria for diagnosis of preterm labor

- Presence of preterm uterine contractions of at least four in 20 minutes, along with cervical changes showing the following:
  - Effacement of 80% or more
  - Dilatation of ≥1 cm

Preterm labor can be of two types:

- **Early preterm labor:** Cervical effacement is ≥80% and cervical dilatation is ≥1 cm, but <3 cm.
- **Advanced preterm labor:** Cervical dilatation is ≥3 cm.

Threatened preterm labor It refers to the presence of preterm uterine contractions but cervix is <80% effaced and <1 cm dilated and cervical length on ultrasound is <2.5 cm.

Note *Usually, the presence of uterine contractions in association with cervical changes is considered as preterm labor and the presence of uterine contractions without evidence of cervical changes is considered as threatened preterm labor.*

Part 1

Case presentation

Salient points in history

Consider the following relevant points during history taking in cases of preterm labor:

- *Age (common in <18 and >35 years)*
- *Socioeconomic status (SES)—common in low SES*
- *Occupation (long hours of standing and high-stress jobs are associated with preterm labor)*
- *Parity (common in grand multgravida)*
- *Last menstrual period (LMP), expected date of delivery (EDD), and period of gestation (POG)*

H/o present pregnancy

- *Lower abdominal pain, which increases in frequency, duration, and intensity as time progresses*
- *Associated low backache/pelvic pressure*
- *Whether perceiving normal fetal movements*
- *H/o leaking P/V or bleeding P/V*
- *H/o fever*
- *H/o urinary symptoms—suprapubic pain and burning micturition*
- *History suggestive of obstetric complications such as preeclampsia and anemia*
- *H/o trauma*

Menstrual history

Check for reliability of the patient's LMP—whether regular cycles, H/o OCP intake prior to conception, whether conceived following recent abortion or during lactation, etc.

Obstetric history

Elaborate on all previous pregnancies:

- *H/o preterm labor in past*

(CONTD...)

(...CONTD)

- *H/o second-trimester abortions*
- *H/o recurrent abortions*
- *Interpregnancy interval*

Past history

- *Any chronic medical illness*
- *Any surgery on cervix*

Personal history

H/o smoking, alcoholism, and drug abuse

Diet history

Calculate the protein and calorie intake (patient with poor nutritional status is more prone to preterm labor)

Salient points in examination

Consider the following relevant points during examination in cases of preterm labor.

General examination

- *Nutritional status (poor nutrition associated with preterm labor)*
- *Height, weight, and BMI (low BMI associated with preterm labor)*
- *Pallor and pedal edema*
- *Temperature, pulse, and BP*

Obstetric examination

- *Fundal height and symphysiofundal height*
- *Obstetric palpation—lie and presentation of fetus (malpresentations are more common)*
- *Uterus—relaxed or acting (if uterus is acting, watch for frequency, intensity, and duration of contraction)*
- *Feel of the uterus—whether uterus feels tense and tender (abruption)*
- *Auscultate fetal heart rate (FHR)*

Speculum examination

- *Look for any leaking P/V or bleeding P/V*
- *Check for cervical dilatation, length, and position*

Vaginal examination

- *Assess cervical position, consistency, dilatation, length or effacement, membrane status (±), station of presenting part (Bishop's score)*
- *Assess pelvis for vaginal delivery*

Note Speculum and vaginal examination are expected only from postgraduates.

Case summary

An example of writing summary in cases of preterm labor is given below.

Example *Mrs. O, 24 years of age, G2P1L1, at 32 weeks of gestation, presents with complaints of intermittent abdominal pain since morning. She says that the pain is progressively increasing in intensity and frequency since morning. There is no history of leaking or bleeding P/V. Her past obstetric history was uneventful. General examination findings are within normal limits: PR, 86/min; and BP, 120/70 mmHg. Obstetric examination reveals a single live fetus in cephalic presentation. Uterine contractions are present, two contractions in 20 minutes, each lasting for 15 seconds, and there is no uterine tenderness. FHR is 132 beats/min, regular heard in the left spinoumbilical line.*

Case diagnosis

An example of writing diagnosis in cases of preterm labor is given below.

Example *24 years of age, G2P1L1 at 32 weeks of gestation, with a singleton live fetus in cephalic presentation, with likely diagnosis of threatened preterm labor as suggested from history and clinical examination*

Case discussion

Complications of preterm labor

See Table 13.1

Table 13.1 Complications of preterm labor

Maternal	Fetal/neonatal
• Premature rupture of membranes • Chorioamnionitis • Placental abruption • Retained placenta • Postpartum hemorrhage • Endometritis	• Respiratory distress syndrome • Bronchopulmonary dysplasia • Intraventricular hemorrhage • Necrotizing enterocolitis • Jaundice • Sepsis • Hypothermia • Hypoglycemia • Hypocalcemia • Feeding difficulties • Retinopathy of prematurity • Patent ductus arteriosus • Long-term neurological problems

Management of preterm labor

- The patient should be admitted to labor ward.
- Speculum and vaginal examinations have to be done (if not performed earlier) to look for cervical changes to establish the diagnosis of preterm labor.
- Adequate rest is advised.
- Patient is counseled regarding risk of preterm delivery and the prognosis of preterm baby.
- Pulse and temperature charting should be maintained.
- Frequency and intensity of uterine contractions are monitored.
- Investigations that are done include
  - Hb, total and differential leucocyte count
  - Blood grouping and typing
  - Urine routine and microscopy, urine culture and sensitivity
  - High vaginal swab for culture sensitivity
  - C-reactive protein (CRP)—increased in the presence of infection
  - Ultrasonography (USG)—for fetal growth, estimated fetal weight, liquor, placental location, and fetal well-being
  - Cardiotocography (CTG) for FHR pattern
  - Other routine antenatal investigations done

Management depends mainly on the gestational age of fetus.

- **POG <34 weeks:** The patient should be managed conservatively up to 34 weeks of gestation or till fetal lung maturity, provided there are no indications for termination of pregnancy.
- **POG ≥34 weeks:** Labor should not be inhibited. Progression of labor and fetal well-being are monitored.

Contraindications for prolonging pregnancy in preterm labor

- POG >34 weeks
- Features of chorioamnionitis
- Nonreactive nonstress test (NST)
- Congenital anomalies
- Intrauterine death (IUD)
- Severe intrauterine growth restriction (IUGR)
- APH with hemodynamic instability
- Uncontrolled diabetes mellitus (DM)

Conservative management for preterm labor at POG <34 weeks includes the following therapy:

- Steroids for lung maturity
- Tocolysis to inhibit uterine contractions
- Antibiotics to treat infections

Antenatal corticosteroids (glucocorticoids)

- Steroid administration accelerates fetal lung maturity and reduces the incidence and severity of respiratory distress syndrome (RDS), thereby reducing neonatal morbidity and mortality.
- Dose: Inj. Betamethasone 12 mg IM two doses given 24 hours apart or dexamethasone 6 mg IM four doses given 12 hours apart are the standard regimen used.
- Optimal benefit begins 24 hours after therapy and lasts for 7 days.
- Benefit of repeated courses of glucocorticoids is doubtful and not currently recommended.
- Other advantages of steroids—it reduces the incidence of the following:
  - Necrotizing enterocolitis
  - Intraventricular hemorrhage (IVH)
  - Bronchopulmonary dysplasia
  - Patent ductus arteriosus

Mechanism of action

- Induces the enzyme system responsible for the synthesis of pulmonary surfactant
- Releases the surfactant stored in type II pneumocytes
- Increases lung compliance
- Potentiates the response to postnatal administration of surfactant

Steroids are used with caution in the following:
- Chorioamnionitis (may flare up infection)
- Uncontrolled diabetes (increases blood glucose levels)

Tocolysis

- Effectiveness of long-term tocolysis is not well established. However, short-term benefits of tocolysis have been proved.
- The primary purpose of tocolytic therapy is to delay delivery for at least 48 hours for the following reasons:
  - To allow maximum benefit of steroids to decrease the incidence of RDS
  - To delay the delivery for in utero transfer to a center with adequate neonatal facilities
  - To administer antibiotics to reduce neonatal infections, specifically Group B *Streptococcus* (GBS) infection
- Maintenance dose of tocolysis is not recommended in current practice.

Tocolytic agents

Various drugs used for the purpose are the following:
- Beta-mimetics (beta-adrenergic agonists)—isoxsuprine, ritodrine, and terbutaline
- Calcium channel blockers—nifedipine
- Magnesium sulfate
- PG synthetase inhibitors—indomethacin
- Nitric oxide donors—nitroglycerine
- Oxytocin receptor antagonists—atosiban

Contraindications to tocolytic therapy

- Advanced labor >4 cm dilatation
- Chorioamnionitis
- Severe preeclampsia
- Severe IUGR
- APH (abruption/placenta previa with hemodynamic instability)
- Fetal distress
- IUD
- Lethal fetal malformations
- Maternal cardiac disease
- Uncontrolled DM

Antibiotics

Prophylactic antibiotics are recommended in the management of preterm labor for the following:
- Treatment of subclinical intrauterine infections
- Prevention of Group B Streptococcal (GBS) infection in fetus
- Prophylaxis for genital tract infections, mainly bacterial vaginosis

Broad-spectrum antibiotics such as ampicillin + metronidazole or Inj. cefazolin IV are usually prescribed.

Note *It is suggested that in many cases of idiopathic preterm labor, subclinical infections may be responsible.*

Treatment of associated infections

Infections outside the uterus such as urinary tract infections, periodontal, and respiratory tract infections play an important role in causing preterm labor and should be treated with appropriate antibiotics.

Viva corner

Q1 What are the indications for tocolytic therapy?

- Preterm labor <34 weeks
- External cephalic version during labor
- Uterine hyperstimulation during labor

Intrapartum management

- Aim of intrapartum management is to prevent birth asphyxia and birth trauma.
- Delivery should be conducted in a tertiary care institute with adequate NICU facilities to minimize neonatal morbidity and mortality.

First stage

- Avoid ambulation to prevent preterm premature rupture of membranes (PPROM).
- Maintain adequate hydration.

- Administer adequate analgesia. Avoid strong sedatives.
- Provide antibiotic prophylaxis, especially in cases of group B streptococcal infection.
- Artificial rupture of membranes (ARM) is avoided as the bag of membranes acts as a protective factor preventing ascending infection
- FHR monitoring is done with CTG, if facilities are available. Otherwise intermittent auscultation should be performed every 15 minutes in the first stage.
- Repeated P/V examinations should be avoided to reduce the risk of infection.
- Speculum examination should be done following rupture of membranes, to rule out cord prolapse.

Second stage

- Delivery should be attended by an obstetrician and a trained neonatologist should be present at the time of delivery to resuscitate the preterm baby.
- Episiotomy is recommended to facilitate easy delivery by minimizing sudden compression and decompression of the head.
- Vacuum extraction is contraindicated—increases the risk of intracranial hemorrhage.
- Outlet forceps can be used if a delay in delivery is anticipated.
- Immediate cord clamping should be done to prevent hypervolemia in the baby.
- Inj. vitamin K is given to the baby, for the prevention of IVH.

Third stage

Active management of the third stage of labor is practiced. There is a risk of retained placenta in cases with preterm labor.

Role of cesarean section

- Cesarean section (CS) exclusively for preterm delivery is contraindicated.
- CS is indicated only for obstetric indications.
- If the lower segment is not well formed, a low vertical incision should be made (Kronig's incision).
- Vaginal delivery may be beneficial in preterm labor by expelling the lung fluid during delivery and thereby facilitating lung expansion.

Prediction of preterm labor (methods to identify women at risk for preterm labor)

Warning signs of preterm labor

- Abdominal cramps
- Dull low backache
- Feeling of pelvic pressure or heaviness
- Excessive vaginal discharge
- Leaking per vagina
- Frequent Braxton Hicks uterine contractions (contractions that occur in less than 10 minutes)
- Short cervix

Paperneik's risk scoring system for detection of women at risk for preterm labor

- This scoring system is based on socioeconomic factors, past medical history, daily habits, and certain aspects of current pregnancy.
- Score of 10 or more is considered as a high risk for preterm labor.
- The disadvantage is that the scoring system is not very useful as 50% of preterm deliveries occur in low-risk group.

Routine vaginal examination to assess the cervix at each antenatal visit

- **Disadvantages**
  - All patients may not prefer it.
  - It can by itself increase the risk of preterm labor.

Cervical length measurement by transvaginal scan

Transvaginal ultrasonography (TVS) for measurement of cervical length is done with an empty bladder during midtrimester (18—24 weeks). However, there is no evidence to support routine ultrasound cervical assessment for predicting preterm labor.

Indicators of high risk for preterm labor in transvaginal ultrasonography

- Cervical length <2.5 cm is taken as a cutoff value for short cervix predicting preterm labor. It has a high negative predictive value of 97%.
- Presence of funneling or widening of cervical canal.
- Bulging of membranes into the cervical canal.

Part 1

Home uterine activity monitoring (HUAM) by external tocodynamometer

- Uterine contractions are recorded by a tocodynamometer and transmitted by telemetry to the obstetrician on a daily basis.
- It is expensive.
- Role of HUAM is investigational at present.

Biochemical markers

- The presence of fetal fibronectin in cervicovaginal secretions after 24 weeks is a specific predictor of preterm delivery.
- Increased maternal salivary estriol can predict preterm labor.

Extra edge

Fetal fibronectin (fFN)

- fFN is a basement membrane protein secreted by chorionic tissue that acts as a glue between chorioamnion and decidua.
- It is present in cervicovaginal secretion up to 16–22 weeks, and then disappears and reappears after 37 weeks of gestation.
- Presence of fFN in cervical secretion after 24 weeks of gestation may indicate disruption between decidua and chorioamnion. Its presence between 24 and 37 weeks is an important marker of preterm labor.
- The test is performed by taking a high vaginal and cervical swab.
- A cutoff value of 50 ng/mL is considered positive.
- It has got a negative predictive value of 99.7%. Negative test excludes the risk of preterm delivery within the next 2–3 weeks.

Maternal salivary estriol levels

- Premature activation of fetal hypothalamic–pituitary–adrenal axis may result in an increase in the production of estriol from placenta and hence an increase in maternal serum and salivary estriol levels.
- This test has a poor sensitivity and specificity and a high false-positive rate.

Prevention of preterm labor

- Counseling high-risk patients regarding warning signs of preterm labor
- Identification and correction of possible risk factors
- Advise the following:
  - Adequate nutrition
  - Adequate rest
  - Avoid physical and mental stress
  - Avoid smoking and alcohol
- Cervical encerclage in proven cases of cervical incompetence (mentioned in detail in Part 1, Chapter 12, *Recurrent Pregnancy Loss*)
- Treatment of asymptomatic bacteriuria
- Treatment of bacterial vaginosis
- Accurate assessment of POG before induction of labor to avoid iatrogenic prematurity

Extra edge

Recent advances

Role of progesterones in prevention of preterm labor

- Progesterone decreases spontaneous activity of the myometrium.
- It decreases the number of oxytocin receptors and prevents formation of gap junctions.
- Progesterone therapy can be given in women with previous H/o >1 preterm delivery.

Progestogens (vaginal progesterone and intramuscular 17-hydroxyprogesterone acetate) are widely recommended for women at high-risk of preterm birth. Typical regimens include 17-hydroxyprogesterone caproate (250 mg intramuscularly weekly) or vaginal progesterone (200-mg micronized vaginal soft capsules) starting at 16–20 gestational weeks until 36 weeks for women with a singleton gestation and a history of spontaneous preterm birth, or for women with a short cervix (typically ≤25 mm).

Role of prophylactic cerclage

Women with previous history of recurrent midtrimester losses and a short cervix on ultrasound benefit with prophylactic cerclage.

Tests for assessing fetal lung maturity

- The tests are done on amniotic fluid collected by amniocentesis (Table 13.2).

Table 13.2 Tests for fetal lung maturity done in amniotic fluid

Parameter assessed	Value
Lecithin to sphingomyelin (L:S) ratio	A ratio of ≥2 is an indicator of fetal lung maturity
Phosphatidyl glycerol (PG)	Presence of PG in the amniotic fluid is a marker of fetal lung maturity
Dipalmitoylphosphatidylcholine (DPPC): It is the main component of pulmonary surfactant	DPPC >500 µg/dL is predictive of fetal lung maturity
Amniotic fluid optical density at 650 nm	Amniotic fluid optical density at 650 nm greater than 0.15 indicates lung maturity
Lamellar body count (it is the storage form of surfactant in amniotic fluid)	A lamellar body count >30,000/µL indicates pulmonary maturity
Orange-colored cells: Desquamated fetal cells obtained from the centrifuged amniotic fluid are stained with 0.1% Nile blue sulfate	Presence of orange-colored cells >50% suggests pulmonary maturity
Shake test or Foam test	It estimates the stability of bubbles that are formed after shaking a mixture of amniotic fluid and ethanol. It is a rapid bedside test to assess pulmonary maturity
Foam stability index (FSI): This test is a semiquantitative measurement of the surfactant in amniotic fluid. FSI is calculated by utilizing serial dilutions of amniotic fluid to quantitate the amount of surfactant present	FSI value of >48 assures fetal lung maturity

- Fetal lung maturity tests are indicated when maturity of the fetus is doubtful and termination of pregnancy is required.

PREMATURE OR PRELABOR RUPTURE OF MEMBRANES

PROM cases will not be usually kept for exams, but questions pertaining to this topic can be asked while discussing a case of preterm labor or during other case discussions.

Definition of PROM It is defined as spontaneous rupture of membranes, beyond 28 weeks of pregnancy, but before the onset of labor.

- **PPROM:** ROM occurring before 37 completed weeks of gestation
- **Term PROM:** ROM occurring beyond 37 weeks of gestation, but before the onset of labor
- **Prolonged ROM:** If the ROM is present for more than 24 hours before delivery

Clinical features

Symptoms

Escape of watery discharge per vaginum in the form of either a gush or a slow leak.

Signs

Speculum examination may show liquor leaking through the cervical os or collected in the posterior fornix.

Viva corner

Q1 What are the differential diagnosis for leaking P/V?

- Rupture of membranes
- Urine (stress incontinence and urge incontinence are common during pregnancy)
- Profuse vaginal discharge due to trichomonal infection or bacterial vaginosis
- Excessive cervical mucous secretion

Confirmation of diagnosis

The evaluation to confirm PROM is mentioned in Table 13.3.

Management of PROM

Management mainly depends on the gestational age (Table 13.4).

Expectant management may be considered at POG <34 weeks after ruling out contraindications for continuing pregnancy.

Contraindications for expectant management

- Acute chorioamnionitis
- Abruption
- POG >34 weeks
- POG <28 weeks (increased risk of fetal morbidity and mortality)
- Nonreassuring FHR
- Lethal congenital anomalies
- Women in advanced labor

Steps taken during expectant management

- The patient must be hospitalized.
- Strict bed rest is advised.
- Sterile vulval pad is given.
- Observe for signs and symptoms of chorioamnionitis (fever, tachycardia, uterine tenderness, foul-smelling vaginal discharge).
- Complete blood count and high vaginal swab should be done on a weekly basis.
- Antenatal corticosteroids are given to promote lung maturity.
- Prophylactic antibiotics are given to prevent infections.
- Short-term tocolysis is effective to gain time for steroids to act and in utero transfer of the patient to higher institute with better NICU facilities.

Table 13.3 Evaluation to confirm rupture of membranes

Procedure	Inference in premature rupture of membranes
Speculum examination	Liquor leaks through the cervical os
Vaginal pool fluid collected from the posterior fornix is examined for the following:	
• **Nitrazine test:** Detection of pH by litmus or nitrazine paper. Normal vaginal pH during pregnancy is 4.5–5.5 and that of liquor is 7–7.5	• Nitrazine paper turns from yellow to blue at pH >6
• **Fern test:** A slide smeared with the fluid is examined under microscope	• Characteristic ferning pattern due to amniotic fluid crystallization
• **Nile blue sulfate test:** Centrifuged cells stained with 0.1% Nile blue sulfate	• Orange blue coloration of the cells (exfoliated fat-containing cells from sebaceous glands of the fetus)
Ultrasound examination	May show decreased liquor

Table 13.4 Management of PROM depending on the POG

POG	Management
<28 weeks	• Prognosis is poor. Risk of pulmonary hypoplasia, deformities, and sepsis in the fetus • Termination of pregnancy by induction is done
28–34 weeks	Expectant management is given till fetal lung maturity is attained, after ruling out contraindications
34–37 weeks	Usually, lung maturity is achieved by 34 weeks. Hence, induction of labor is preferred. Antibiotics are administered. Steroids are given if there is a doubt regarding gestational age
>37 weeks	Term gestation and hence induction of labor is done. Spontaneous labor can be awaited for 6–12 hours after PROM if there is no indication for immediate delivery such as fetal distress or infection

POG, period of gestation; *PROM*, premature rupture of membranes.

- Frequent P/V examination should be avoided in patients with PROM to reduce the risk of infections.
- USG is done to assess the amount of liquor, to rule out anomalies, and to assess fetal well-being.
- Fetal surveillance with NST and biophysical profile (BPP) is done twice weekly.
- The patient should be delivered if:
  - Labor starts
  - Fetal distress occurs
  - Infection sets in
  - POG crosses 34 weeks
- CS is done only for obstetric indications.

Complications associated with PROM

Maternal complications

- Chorioamnionitis (increased risk of ascending infections if ROM is present for >24 hours)
- Preterm labor (in 80–90% of the cases, labor starts within 24 hours)
- Increased chances of cesarean section due to cord prolapse, abruption, oligohydramnios, and failed induction

Fetal/neonatal complications

- Nonreassuring FHR (the most common abnormality is variable decelerations due to umbilical cord compression as a result of oligohydramnios)
- RDS, bronchopulmonary dysplasia, and pulmonary hypoplasia
- IVH, cerebral palsy, neurodevelopmental delay, and hearing loss
- Hyperbilirubinemia and hypoglycemia
- Necrotizing enterocolitis
- Retinopathy of prematurity
- Patent ductus arteriosus (PDA) and pulmonary hypertension
- Water and electrolyte imbalance and acid–base disturbances

High-yield points

Chorioamnionitis

It is defined as inflammatory reaction of the fetal membranes, amnion, and chorion due to ascending vaginal infection.

Diagnosis of chorioamnionitis

- Temperature above 38.0°C (100.0°F) and presence of two out of the following five signs:
  - WBC count >15,000 cells/mm^3
  - Maternal tachycardia
  - Fetal tachycardia
  - Tender uterus
  - Foul-smelling vaginal discharge

PHYSICAL APPEARANCE OF A PRETERM BABY (FIGURE 13.1)

- Most preterm babies are of low birth weight (weight <2.5 kg).
- The preterm baby is usually deficient in subcutaneous fat—the baby's skin appears pink, thin, and transparent.
- There are abundant lanugo hair and vernix caseosa.
- Scalp hair is wooly and fuzzy.
- Elastic recoil of ears is absent.
- The nails are not grown up to the fingertips.
- Breast nodules are small.
- There is no flexion of extremities—weak muscle tone.
- The head circumference disproportionately exceeds that of the chest. (Normally, the head circumference is greater than the chest circumference at birth by about 1.5 cm.)
- Plantar deep creases are not visible before 34 weeks.
- The testicles may be undescended and scrotal rugosities are absent in male babies.
- The labia minora are exposed in female babies.

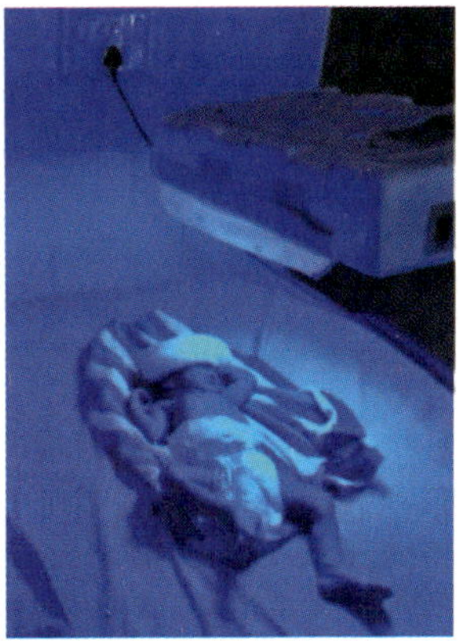

Figure 13.1 A preterm baby receiving phototherapy.

Part 1

High-yield points

Tocolytics

These are the drugs that inhibit uterine contractions.

Nifedipine

- It is a calcium channel blocker.
- It is a safe and effective tocolytic drug.
- Dose is 20–30 mg oral stat dose, followed by maintenance dose at 10–20 mg 6 hourly for 48–72 hours.
- Monitor pulse rate—dose is postponed if pulse rate is >100/min.
- Side effects include maternal hypotension, tachycardia, headache, dizziness, and facial flushing.
- Contraindications include maternal cardiac disease, maternal hypotension, and renal diseases.
- Concomitant use of nifedipine with magnesium sulfate is avoided.

Beta-agonists—terbutaline, isoxsuprine, and ritodrine

- **Terbutaline:** Administered subcutaneously as 0.25 mg every 3–4 hours
- **Isoxsuprine:** Four ampoules (40 mg) in 500 mL of 5% dextrose IV drip started at 0.2mg/min up to a maximum of 0.8 mg/min; continued for 24 hours, followed by maintenance dose of 10–20 mg oral or IM every 6–8 hours

Side effects of beta-agonists

- **Maternal:** Cardiac arrhythmias, pulmonary edema, hypotension, tachycardia, hyperglycemia, hypokalemia, tremors, nausea, and vomiting
- **Fetal:** Fetal tachycardia and fetal hypoglycemia

Recommended guidelines for monitoring IV beta-agonists

- Monitor pulse rate and the next dose is postponed if PR is >100/min.
- BP is checked every 15 minutes.
- Chest auscultation every 4 hours.
- Check maternal blood glucose every 4 hours.
- Maintain strict intake and output chart for fluid balance.

Magnesium sulfate

Magnesium sulphate is currently recommended for neuroprotection of preterm infants for women at risk of preterm birth at less than 32 weeks' gestation (ACOG recommendation).

Dose

4–6 g IV over 20 minutes followed by 2 g/h as continuous infusion for 24 hours. Monitor urine output, respiratory rate, and deep tendon reflexes.

Side effects

- **Maternal:** Flushing, headache, muscle weakness, respiratory depression, and pulmonary edema
- **Neonatal:** Lethargy and hypotonia

Nitroglycerine

- Dose is 100 μg IV bolus followed by IV infusion at 1 μg/kg/min. It can also be used as a transdermal patch.
- Side effects include headache and maternal and fetal hypotension.

Nonsteroidal anti-inflammatory drugs (NSAIDs)—indomethacin, ketorolac, and sulindac

Indomethacin

- Preferably used in preterm labor associated with polyhydramnios
- Dose—100 mg stat dose followed by 50 mg orally every 6–8 hours

Contraindications for NSAIDs

These include coagulation disorders, thrombocytopenia, and peptic ulcer disease.

Side effects of NSAIDs

- **Maternal:** Nausea, gastritis, and impairment of renal function
- **Fetal:** Premature closure of the ductus arteriosus, necrotizing enterocolitis, and risk of periventricular leukomalacia

Oxytocin antagonist

Atosiban is an oxytocin antagonist. The drug is currently not available in India.

Some of the frequently asked one liners on tocolytics during viva are as follows:

- **Tocolytic drug avoided in diabetics:** Beta-agonists as they cause hyperglycemia

(CONTD...)

...CONTD)

High-yield points

- **Tocolytic drug that is administered subcutaneously:** Terbutaline
- **Advantage of $MgSO_4$ for tocolysis in preterm labor:** It is neuroprotective
- **Absolute C/I for $MgSO_4$:** Myasthenia gravis
- **Main fetal complication of indomethacin:** Premature closure of ductus arteriosus

Frequently asked viva questions

1. Summarize the case.
2. What is the diagnosis of the case?
3. What is the plan of management for the case?
4. What investigations will you do for the patient with preterm labor?
5. What are the benefits of steroid therapy?
6. What are the drugs commonly used for tocolysis?
7. What precautions will you take during labor and delivery in a case of preterm labor?
8. What are the risk factors for preterm labor?

14 Liquor Abnormalities: Polyhydramnios and Oligohydramnios

Introduction

The fetus inside the amniotic cavity is surrounded by the amniotic fluid that is produced and reabsorbed continuously. Quantitative assessment of amniotic fluid by ultrasonography (USG) is an important test for fetal surveillance. Abnormalities of amniotic fluid may be markers for underlying fetal or maternal pathological conditions and are associated with increased perinatal morbidity and mortality.

Clinical cases such as gestational diabetes mellitus (GDM) and Rh incompatibility can be associated with polyhydramnios, whereas cases such as preeclampsia and intrauterine growth restriction (IUGR) can be associated with oligohydramnios. This chapter deals with case discussion on liquor abnormalities.

Source of amniotic fluid (secretion)

- **Early pregnancy:** Ultrafiltrate of maternal plasma across placenta
- **Second trimester:** Transudation across the fetal skin
- **From 20 weeks onward:** Fetal urine and fetal lungs are the main source of amniotic fluid
- **Amniotic fluid is kept in balance by the following mechanisms (absorption):**
  - Fetal swallowing, respiratory tract
  - exchange of fluids across chorionic plate, amnion, exchange between intervillous space and fetal capillaries
- Changes that affect fetal urine production, lung fluid secretion, fetal swallowing, and intramembranous flow can affect the amniotic fluid volume

Functions of amniotic fluid

- Acts as a shock absorber—protects the fetus
- Maintains an even temperature
- Allows movement and growth of fetus–prevents contractures
- Prevents cord compression
- Forms bag of membranes during labor that help in dilatation of cervix

Note *Amniotic fluid is not of much nutritive value.*

Assessment of amniotic fluid volume

The most practical method of assessment of amniotic fluid volume (AFV) is by USG. Two techniques are commonly used:
- Amniotic fluid index (AFI)
- Single deepest pocket (SDP)

Amniotic fluid index (Figure 14.1)

- Sum of the measurements of the deepest vertical pocket in all the four quadrants of the gravid uterus in centimeters
- Normal: 5–25 cm

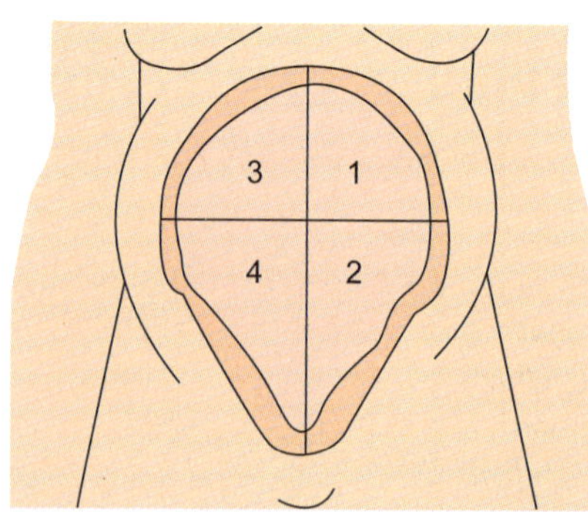

Figure 14.1 Amniotic fluid index. It is calculated as the sum of the measurements of the deepest vertical pocket in all the four quadrants of the gravid uterus in centimeters.

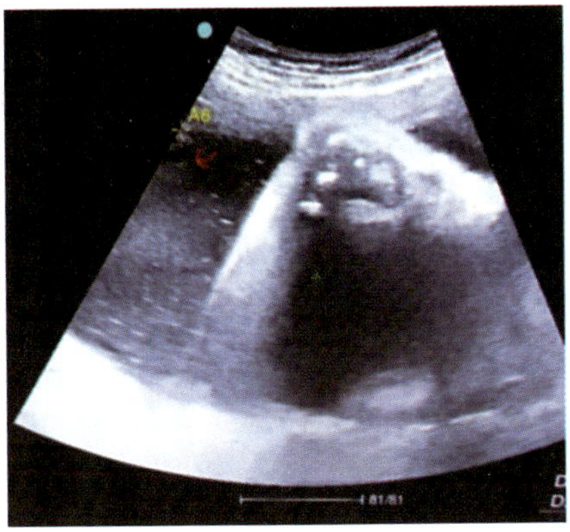

Figure 14.2 Ultrasound image showing liquor pocket.

Single deepest pocket (Figure 14.2)

- Measurement of the single largest cord-free vertical pocket in centimeter
- Normal: 2–8 cm

POLYHYDRAMNIOS

Definition

It refers to excessive volume of liquor of >2000 mL.

Ultrasonography definition

When the AFI is >25 cm or SDP is >8 cm, it is termed polyhydramnios.

Causes of polyhydramnios

See Table 14.1

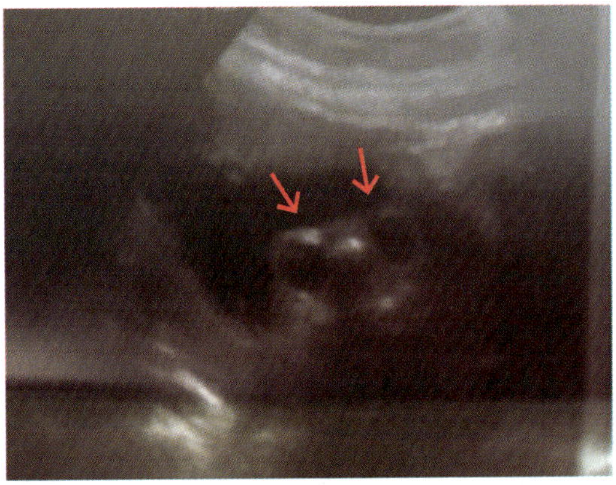

Figure 14.3 Ultrasound image of a fetus with anencephaly—absence of cranium and protruding eye balls (frog's eye sign).

Table 14.1 Causes of polyhydramnios

Maternal	Fetal	Placental	Idiopathic
• Maternal diabetes • Rh incompatibility	• Congenital malformations—anencephaly (Figure 14.3), spina bifida, esophageal, or duodenal atresia • Fetal hydrops • Fetal aneuploidy • Parvovirus B19 infection • Multiple pregnancy	Chorioangioma of circumvallate placenta	Accounts for 60% of cases (most common cause)

Case presentation

Salient points in history

Consider the following relevant points while taking history in cases of polyhydramnios:

- *Women with polyhydramnios may experience the following symptoms (due to uterine overdistension)*
  - *Difficulty in breathing*
  - *Pedal edema*
- *H/o present pregnancy*
  - *Blood group and Rh typing of the patient (to rule out Rh incompatibility)*
  - *Whether a diagnosed case of GDM (uncontrolled blood sugars associated with polyhydramnios)*
  - *Whether anomalies scan was done and told to be normal (to rule out fetal anomalies, multiple pregnancy)*

(CONTD...)

Part 1

(...CONTD)

Salient points in examination

Consider the following relevant points during examination of cases of polyhydramnios.

General physical examination

- *Patient may be uncomfortable at rest—may be dyspneic on lying down*
- *Weight (may have excessive weight gain)*
- *Pedal edema (preeclampsia is a complication of polyhydramnios; pedal edema may develop due to pressure effects in polyhydramnios)*
- *Varicosities in leg or vulva (due to pressure effects)*

Abdominal examination

Inspection

- *Abdomen appears overdistended*
- *The skin of the abdominal wall may be tense and shiny*

Palpation

- *Fundal height and symphysiofundal height (SFH) may be greater than the period of gestation (POG)*
- *Abdominal girth at the umbilicus is more than normal*
- *It may be difficult to palpate the uterus or the fetal parts (due to presence of excessive fluid)*
- *Fluid thrill may be present (in severe cases of polyhydramnios)*

Auscultation *Fetal heart rate (FHR) may appear muffled*

Vaginal examination

- *Cervix may be partially taken up and os may be slightly dilated*
- *Tense bulging membranes can be felt through the cervical os*

Case summary

An example of writing summary in cases of polyhydramnios is given below.

Example *Mrs. Y, 24 years of age, G2P1L1 at 30 weeks of gestation, presents with c/o breathlessness. Clinical examination reveals no pallor or pedal edema; PR, 90/min; BP, 120/70 mmHg; and CVS and RS examinations are within normal limits. Obstetric examination reveals overdistension of abdomen. Fundal height corresponds to 36 weeks of gestation; SFH measures 37 cm. There is difficulty in palpation of fetal parts. Fluid thrill is present. Clinically, liquor appears excess and uterus is relaxed. FHR is 132 beats/min, appears muffled.*

Case diagnosis

An example of writing diagnosis in cases of polyhydramnios is given below.

Example *24 years of age, G2P1L1 at 30 weeks of gestation and clinical examination reveals that abdomen is disproportionately enlarged in accordance with the POG calculated from last menstrual period (LMP), with a singleton live fetus, not in labor, probably a case of polyhydramnios*

Note *If diagnosis is doubtful, you can give a differential diagnosis of the causes of overdistended uterus and mention that exact diagnosis can be made after performing an ultrasound examination. Questions can be expected from all the causes of overdistended uterus.*

Case discussion

Differential diagnosis of fundal height >POG

The various differential diagnoses possible in these cases include:

- Wrong dates
- Full bladder
- Polyhydramnios
- Multiple pregnancy
- Macrosomia
- Pregnancy with pelvic mass (fibroid or ovarian)
- Concealed abruption
- Maternal ascites

Points in favor of polyhydramnios

- Overdistension of abdomen with tense and shiny skin
- Fundal height and SFH >POG
- Abdominal girth more than normal

- Difficulty in palpation of fetal parts
- Presence of fluid thrill
- Clinically excess liquor
- Fetal heart sounds appearing muffled
- Vaginal examination (cervix may be partially taken up and slightly dilated; tense bulging membranes can be felt through the cervical os)

Diagnosis

USG is required to confirm the diagnosis. AFI >25 cm confirms polyhydramnios.

Uses of ultrasonography in polyhydramnios

- Confirms diagnosis of polyhydramnios
- Diagnosis of fetal congenital malformations
- Excludes multiple pregnancy
- Confirms lie and presentation of fetus
- Placental localization

Specific investigations

- Blood grouping and Rh typing (to rule out Rh isoimmunization)
- Oral glucose tolerance test (OGTT)

Complications of polyhydramnios

Various complications (maternal and fetal) related to polyhydramnios are mentioned in Table 14.2.

Clinical types of polyhydramnios

Acute polyhydramnios

- Sudden onset, rapid accumulation of liquor
- Rare, usually occurs before 20 weeks of gestation
- Associated with twin-to-twin transfusion in multiple pregnancy and chorioangioma of placenta

Table 14.2 Complications of polyhydramnios

Maternal	Fetal
Antepartum • Respiratory compromise • Preeclampsia • Malpresentations • Premature rupture of membranes • Preterm labor • Placental abruption • Uterine dysfunction and inertia • Cord prolapse • Postpartum hemorrhage • Subinvolution	Increased perinatal morbidity and mortality due to • Congenital malformations • Prematurity

Chronic polyhydramnios

- Gradual onset, slow accumulation of liquor
- Most common type

Grades of polyhydramnios

Polyhydramnios can be graded as mild, moderate and severe based on ultrasound findings (Table 14.3).

Table 14.3 Grades of polyhydramnios

Grade	Amniotic fluid index	Single vertical pocket (cm)
Mild (most common)	25–30	8–11
Moderate	30–35	12–15
Severe	>35	>15

Extra edge

Reason for polyhydramnios in anencephaly and neural tube defects

- Transudation of fluid from exposed meninges
- Absent fetal swallowing reflex
- Suppression of fetal antidiuretic hormone (ADH) → excessive urination

Reason for polyhydramnios in esophageal and duodenal atresia

Absence of fetal swallowing results in polyhydramnios

Management

Antenatal management

Mild polyhydramnios usually resolves on its own without any treatment and no active intervention is required in patients with asymptomatic hydramnios.

In patients with severe polyhydramnios and in symptomatic cases, the objectives are to provide symptomatic relief, to find out the causative factor, and to avoid or manage complications.

- The patient is admitted.
- Investigations are done to look for any cause of polyhydramnios such as USG for fetal congenital

Part 1

malformations, OGTT for maternal diabetes, maternal blood grouping, and typing for rhesus incompatibility.
- If major fetal malformation is present, terminate the pregnancy after counseling the couple.
- If major fetal malformations are absent, pregnancy may be continued till term.
- Steroids are given for lung maturity in cases less than 34 weeks (as there is risk of preterm labor).
- Indomethacin therapy: 1.5–3 mg/kg/day can be given to reduce the amount of liquor (reduces fetal urine output); however, it should be stopped at 32 weeks (as it can cause premature closure of ductus arteriosus).
- If the patient is in respiratory distress or if the patient is not responding to medical therapy, decompression by serial amniocentesis at the rate of 500 mL/h; maximum up to 1–1.5 L/day under ultrasound guidance can be done, to relieve her symptoms [carries the risk of preterm labor, abruption, and premature rupture of membranes (PROM)].
- Manage other factors complicating pregnancy such as diabetes mellitus and Rh incompatibility.

Intrapartum management

- Delivery is planned after 37 completed weeks. Induction of labor is done based on the Bishop's score. If cervix is unfavorable, cervical ripening is done with Foley's catheter/PGE2. Stabilizing oxytocin is then started followed by controlled artificial rupture of membranes (ARM) to allow slow escape of liquor (controlled ARM is done to prevent cord prolapse).
- P/V should be done following rupture of membranes to rule out cord prolapse.
- Active management of third stage of labor (AMTSL) is practiced to prevent atonic postpartum hemorrhage.
- The newborn should be examined for any anomalies.

OLIGOHYDRAMNIOS

Definition

Liquor volume is deficient in amount (<200 mL at term).

Ultrasonography definition of oligohydramnios

- AFI <5
- Single deepest liquor pocket <2 cm

Causes of oligohydramnios

See Table 14.4

Table 14.4 Causes of oligohydramnios

Maternal	Fetal	Placental	Idiopathic
• Preeclampsia, chronic hypertension • Post-term pregnancy • Placental insufficiency (IUGR) • Premature rupture of membranes • Drugs: ACE inhibitors (**Hint:** *Remember four "P"*)	• Chromosomal anomalies • Congenital anomalies such as – Renal agenesis – Obstruction of urinary tract	• Amnion nodosum	• Most common cause of mild oligohydramnios

ACE, angiotensin-converting enzyme; *IUGR*, intrauterine growth restriction.

Case presentation

Salient points in History

Consider the following relevant points while taking history in cases of oligohydramnios.

Presenting complaints

- *The patient may give a history of perceiving reduced fetal movements*
- *H/S/o preeclampsia (preeclampsia is one of the causes for oligohydramnios)*
- *H/o leaking per vaginum (PROM is one of the causes for oligohydramnios)*
- *Whether anomalies scan was done and told to be normal (to rule out fetal anomalies as a cause of oligohydramnios)*

(CONTD...)

(...CONTD)

Salient points in examination

Consider the following relevant points during examination of cases of oligohydramnios.

General examination

- *Weight (reduced maternal weight gain)*
- *Pallor and pedal edema*
- *BP (preeclampsia is associated with oligohydramnios)*

Obstetric examination

- *Fundal height and SFH are less than POG*
- *Uterus appears full of fetus due to scanty liquor*
- *Evidence of IUGR may be present*

Case summary

An example of writing summary in cases of oligohydramnios is given below.

Example *Mrs. P, 25 years of age, primigravida at 32 weeks of gestation, came for routine antenatal checkup. Clinical examination reveals no pallor or pedal edema; PR, 80/min; BP, 120/80 mmHg; and CVS and RS examinations are within normal limits. Obstetric examination reveals fundal height corresponding to 28 weeks of gestation; SFH measures 29 cm. A single live fetus is present in cephalic presentation and clinically liquor appears reduced and uterus is relaxed. FHR is 132 beats/min.*

Case diagnosis

An example of writing diagnosis in cases of oligohydramnios is given below.

Example *25 years of age, primigravida at 32 weeks of gestation with clinical examination findings suggestive of reduced liquor, probably oligohydramnios with possible IUGR. USG is needed for confirmation of oligohydramnios and to rule out IUGR.*

Note *It may not be possible to differentiate cases of oligohydramnios and IUGR clinically as the two conditions may often coexist. Hence, it is always better to give a D/D of oligohydramnios and IUGR in cases with fundal height less than the POG.*

Case discussion

Differential diagnosis of fundal height <POG

- Wrong dates
- Oligohydramnios
- IUGR
- Intrauterine death
- Transverse lie

Points in favor of oligohydramnios in a case of fundal height <POG

- FH and SFH are <POG.
- Uterus feels "full of fetus."
- Clinically, liquor appears reduced.

Diagnosis

It is confirmed by USG. AFI <5 cm confirms oligohydramnios.

Uses of ultrasonography in oligohydramnios

- To confirm diagnosis
- To rule out anomalies
- To confirm lie and presentation
- Placental localization
- To assess serial fetal growth and fetal well-being by doing biophysical profile (BPP) and Doppler studies in cases of oligohydramnios associated with IUGR

Note *Due to lack of amniotic fluid and poor acoustic window, USG visualization of the fetal anatomy is often suboptimal in severe oligohydramnios. Transabdominal amnioinfusion may improve visualization.*

Complications

Complications related to oligohydramnios are given below.

Part 1

Maternal complications

- Increased operative interferences
- Complications due to associated medical conditions such as preeclampsia

Fetal complications

- Fetal deformities due to intra-amniotic adhesions (clubfoot, amputation of limb, skull deformity)
- Pulmonary hypoplasia
- IUGR
- Fetal distress
- Cord compression resulting in fetal hypoxia and asphyxia
- Meconium aspiration syndrome
- Increased perinatal mortality

Note

- *The severity of complications in oligohydramnios depend on the gestational age—the earlier the manifestation, the worse is the fetal prognosis.*
- *Oligohydramnios is a warning sign that placental reserve is low. Hence, there is a risk of fetal distress due to placental insufficiency or cord compression.*
- *Prognosis depends on the cause, POG, and severity of oligohydramnios.*

Management

Antepartum management

- If major fetal malformations are present: Terminate the pregnancy after counseling the couple.
- Isolated and late-onset oligohydramnios: Women with otherwise normal pregnancy who develop mild oligohydramnios near term probably require no treatment because in most of these cases, oligohydramnios will resolve by itself without any treatment. Conservative management is followed with antepartum fetal surveillance (APFS) up to term and delivered at 37 completed weeks.
- Hospitalization is required in severe cases of oligohydramnios for fetal surveillance.
- Reduced physical activity may improve liquor volume (no proven benefit).
- Maternal hydration may improve liquor volume.
- APFS: Fetal surveillance in the form of weekly ultrasound examination to measure AFI and tests for fetal well-being such as twice-weekly nonstress test and BPP, and fetal Doppler are done. If any of these tests shows abnormality, early delivery may be required.
- Management of other associated complications such as preeclampsia.
- The risk of preterm has to be balanced against the risk of intrauterine death in managing cases with severe oligohydramnios.

Mode of delivery

- Oligohydramnios at or near term—APFS is continued up to term and induction of labor is done at term.
- Elective cesarean section is usually preferred in severe oligohydramnios with IUGR.

Intrapartum management

- Careful monitoring of FHR is done with continuous electronic fetal monitoring, if facilities are available, or else by intermittent auscultation with stethoscope every 15 minutes in the first stage and every 5 minutes in the second stage.
- The chances of LSCS in labor are high because of fetal distress.
- Amnioinfusion during labor is found to be useful in cases with repeated variable decelerations by reducing cord compression.

Extra edge

Amnioinfusion

Amnioinfusion is infusion of normal saline through the cervix into the uterine cavity. It is found to be useful in cases of repeated variable decelerations during labor and reduces the need for cesarean section.

Benefits of amnioinfusion

Prophylactic or therapeutic amnioinfusion

- Prevents cord compression
- Dilutes or washes out the thick meconium
- Treatment of variable deceleration

Diagnostic amnioinfusion

USG-guided transabdominal amnioinfusion in the second trimester can be done in severe oligohydramnios, for better visualization of fetal parts.

Frequently asked viva questions

1. What are the causes of polyhydramnios?
2. What are the clinical features of polyhydramnios?
3. What are the complications of polyhydramnios?
4. How will you manage the patient with polyhydramnios?
5. What are the causes of oligohydramnios?
6. What are the clinical features of oligohydramnios?
7. What are the complications of oligohydramnios?
8. How will you manage the patient with oligohydramnios?

15 Antepartum Hemorrhage

Introduction

Hemorrhage during late pregnancy, also known as the antepartum hemorrhage (APH), is an obstetric emergency with potential risk to both the mother and the fetus. The condition needs to be managed with great care for optimal maternal and fetal outcome. Medical students need to be well versed with the causes and the management of APH. This chapter deals with the clinical case discussion on the two common causes of APH, namely placenta previa and abruption.

Definition of antepartum hemorrhage

It is defined as bleeding from or into the genital tract after the period of viability but before the delivery of fetus.

Causes of antepartum hemorrhage

- Placental causes (70%)—placenta previa and abruptio placentae
- Vasa previa
- Rupture uterus (in a case of previous cesarean pregnancy)
- Local lesions—cervical polyp, ectopy, erosion, cervical carcinoma, and local trauma
- Unexplained causes (25%)

The two main causes of APH are placenta previa (bleeding from abnormally located low-lying placenta) and abruptio placentae (bleeding due to separation of a normally located placenta).

PLACENTA PREVIA

Definition

When the placenta is implanted partially or completely over the lower uterine segment, it is termed placenta previa.

Types of placenta previa

Placenta previa is classified according to the proximity of placenta to the internal os as observed on transvaginal sonography (TVS) as follows (Figure 15.1):

- **Type I placenta previa (low-lying placenta):** The placenta is implanted in the lower uterine segment, but does not reach up to the cervix (**i.e., lower edge 0.5–2.0 cm from internal os**).
- **Type II placenta previa (marginal placenta previa):** The placenta reaches up to the edge of cervix but does not cover the internal os.
- **Type III placenta previa (partial placenta previa):** The placenta partly covers the internal os.
- **Type IV placenta previa (total or central placenta previa):** The placenta completely covers the internal os.

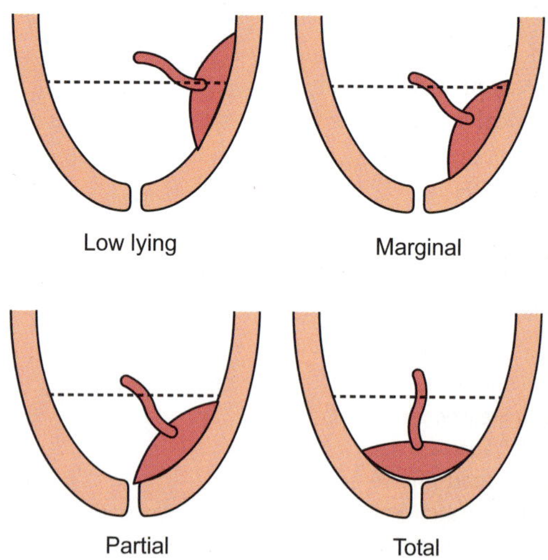

Figure 15.1 Types of placenta previa. Based on ultrasound findings, placenta previa is classified into four types: low lying, marginal, partial, and total.

Risk factors for placenta previa

- Multiparity
- Multiple pregnancy
- Previous cesarean section (CS)
- Previous H/o placenta previa

Clinical features of placenta previa

- H/o sudden-onset, painless, causeless, recurrent fresh vaginal bleeding is the hallmark of placenta previa.
- Pallor is proportional to the amount of visible blood loss.
- Signs of hemodynamic compromise (tachycardia, hypotension, features of shock) may be present in severe cases of placenta previa.
- Uterine size corresponds to the period of gestation (POG).
- Uterus is relaxed and nontender on palpation.
- The fetal presenting part is usually high up and cannot be pushed into the pelvic inlet due to the presence of placenta.
- Fetal malpresentations are common (e.g., breech, transverse lie).
- Fetal heart rate (FHR) is usually normal. Rarely, fetal distress or fetal death may occur as a result of maternal shock.

Vaginal examination

- Vaginal examination is contraindicated in APH with suspected diagnosis of placenta previa, as it may provoke further bleeding.
- Local inspection and per speculum examination can be performed to rule out local causes of APH.

Complications of placenta previa

Complications associated with placenta previa are mentioned in the Table 15.1.

Viva corner

Q1 What is "warning bleeding"?

It refers to small episodes of hemorrhage that occur prior to an episode of major hemorrhage in cases with placenta previa.

Q2 What is the cause of APH in placenta previa?

The inelastic placenta gets separated from the wall of the lower uterine segment (LUS) as the LUS progressively stretches in later months. This leads to opening up of the uteroplacental vessels and bleeding.

Q3 What is the cause for postpartum hemorrhage (PPH) in placenta previa?

- Failure of the lower segment to retract properly following delivery (lower segment does not have the same ability as the upper segment to retract following delivery).
- Risk of having a morbidly adherent placenta is more which can lead to PPH.

ABRUPTIO PLACENTAE (PLACENTAL ABRUPTION)

Definition of placental abruption

It refers to the premature separation of a normally implanted placenta before delivery of the baby.

Table 15.1 Complications of placenta previa

Maternal complications	Fetal complications
• Hemorrhage leading to shock • Preterm labor • Increased rate of cesarean section • Intrapartum hemorrhage • Postpartum hemorrhage • Increased risk of retained placenta due to morbidly adherent placenta → may require hysterectomy • Increased maternal mortality	• Prematurity • Low birth weight • Birth asphyxia • Intrauterine death • Risk of congenital malformations is more • Increased perinatal morbidity and mortality

Types of abruption (Figure 15.2a and b)

- **Revealed type**—when the bleeding comes out of the cervical canal and is visible externally (90%)
- **Concealed type**—when the hemorrhage is concealed (10%)
- **Mixed type**—includes both concealed and revealed abruption

Risk factors for abruptio placentae

- Hypertension in pregnancy
- Multiparity
- Increasing maternal age
- Thrombophilias
- Trauma
- Sudden decompression of uterus—premature rupture of membranes (PROM), polyhydramnios (following rupture of membranes) and following delivery of the first twin
- Smoking
- Short cord
- Folic acid deficiency
- Placental abnormalities (circumvallate placenta)

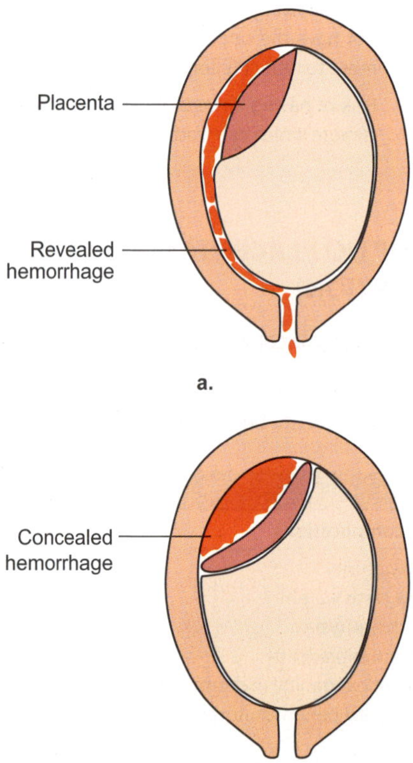

Figure 15.2 Placental abruption. **a.** Revealed hemorrhage. **b.** Concealed hemorrhage.

Clinical features

- H/o third-trimester bleeding associated with abdominal pain is present. History suggestive of preeclampsia may be present.
- Pallor may be out of proportion to the amount of blood loss in cases of concealed abruption.
- Signs of hemodynamic compromise such as tachycardia, hypotension, and shock may be present in severe abruption.
- There may be signs and symptoms suggestive of preeclampsia (increased BP, proteinuria, etc.).
- Fundal height may be more than the POG (in concealed hemorrhage).
- Uterus is tense and tender on palpation and it may feel woody hard due to persistent hypertonus.
- It may be difficult to feel the fetal parts due to uterine hypertonicity.
- Auscultation of FHR—severe grade of placental abruption may be associated with fetal bradycardia and absent FHR.

Vaginal examination

Although placental abruption is not a contraindication for vaginal examination, it is withheld in APH cases, until placenta previa is ruled out by ultrasonography (USG) examination.

Complications of abruptio placentae

Complications associated with abruption are mentioned in Table 15.2.

Table 15.2 Complications associated with abruption

Maternal complications	Fetal complications
• Hemorrhage leading to shock • Disseminated intravascular coagulation • Renal failure • Postpartum hemorrhage • Increased maternal mortality • Risk of abruption in future pregnancies (15%)	• Prematurity • Fetal hypoxia • Fetal death • Increased perinatal mortality

Extra edge

Cause for disseminated intravascular coagulation (DIC) in abruption

Placental abruption causes release of thromboplastin from the damaged tissue at placental site into maternal circulation resulting in large-scale consumption of clotting factors and DIC.

Note *DIC is a condition of inappropriate coagulation within the blood vessels, where there is large-scale consumption of clotting factors, resulting in the failure of the clotting mechanism at the site of bleeding. DIC triggers fibrinolysis and production of fibrin degradation products (FDPs) that reduce the efficiency of normal clotting.*

Causes for renal failure in placental abruption

- Massive hemorrhage results in impaired renal perfusion and acute tubular necrosis
- Coexistence of preeclampsia that is an important cause of renal vasospasm, increases the risk of renal failure

Causes of PPH in placental abruption

- **Atonic uterus:** Hemorrhage within the uterine musculature may prevent effective uterine contractions. Associated preeclampsia increases the risk.
- **Coagulation failure:** There may be failure of coagulation due to DIC (FDP prevents normal hemostasis at the placental site and inhibits myometrial contractions).

Case presentation

Salient points in history

Consider the following relevant points during history taking in cases of APH.

POG *Ascertain the accurate POG (management will depend on the diagnosis, clinical condition of the patient, and POG)*

Parity *Increased parity is a risk factor for both placenta previa and placental abruption*

Presenting complaints

Bleeding per vaginum

- *Amount of bleeding (soaked how many pads/cloth/garments, presence of clots, etc.)*
- *Whether painless bleeding or is associated with pain abdomen*
- *What initiated the bleeding—history of trauma, fall, sexual intercourse etc.*
- *Recurrent bleeding—whether the patient had similar episodes earlier in this pregnancy*
- *Color and character of the bleeding—whether it is bright red or dark altered blood*
- *Whether the bleeding has stopped or is still continuing*

Pain abdomen

Is bleeding associated with pain abdomen? If yes, determine the following:

- *Nature of pain—whether the pain is intermittent or continuous*
- *Intensity of pain*
  - *Intermittent colicky pain abdomen could be the onset of labor and the presence of blood mixed with mucous could be "show."*
  - *In concealed abruption, the pain is continuous and severe due to distension of the uterus by the retroplacental clot.*
  - *Severe pain that subsides dramatically with features of shock could be diagnostic of rupture uterus.*

Fetal movements

Is the patient perceiving fetal movements or any history of loss of fetal movements?

- *In concealed abruption and severe hemorrhage in abruption, the fetus may be dead.*
- *In placenta previa, the fetus is usually alive, except in cases with severe shock.*
- *In rupture uterus, the fetus may be dead or fetal distress may be present.*

(CONTD...)

(...CONTD)

Symptoms of preeclampsia

- *Any H/o high BP recordings in this pregnancy (one-third of women with abruption have symptoms of preeclampsia)*
- *H/o swelling of feet, sudden or excessive weight gain, and H/o imminent symptoms such as headache, blurring of vision, and epigastric pain*

Menstrual history

Whether her last menstrual period (LMP) is reliable to assess the POG.

Past obstetric history

- *H/o previous abortions—spontaneous or induced, whether D and E was done or not (surgical abortion methods increases the risk of placenta previa and morbidly adherent placenta)*
- *Mode of previous deliveries—vaginal or CS (the risk of placenta previa increases with the number of previous CS; risk of placenta accreta is greater in cases with placenta previa with previous CS than in cases with placenta previa with an unscarred uterus)*
- *H/o APH in prior pregnancies (there is risk of recurrence in cases of placenta previa and placental abruption)*

Personal history

H/o smoking and drug abuse (cocaine) (important etiological factors for both placenta previa and abruptio placentae)

Family history

H/o hypertension, diabetes mellitus, bleeding diathesis, and thrombophilias

Salient points in examination

Consider the following relevant points during examination in cases of APH

General physical examination

- *Whether patient is conscious and oriented or in shock*
- *Pallor and pedal edema are looked for*
- *Vitals—pulse, BP, respiratory rate, and temperature*
  - *Pallor, tachycardia, and hypotension are directly proportional to the blood loss in placenta previa.*
  - *Shock that is out of proportion to the visible blood loss is a feature of abruptio placentae, especially the concealed variety.*
  - *Edema and hypertension can also be associated with abruption, and hypertension can mask true hypovolemia.*
  - *Assess the vitals to determine the need for blood transfusion.*

Abdominal examination

- *Fundal height*
- *Uterine consistency, any tenderness (uterus will be "tense" and "tender" in abruption)*
- *Presentation of fetus*
- *Uterine contractions: The presence of uterine contractions indicates the onset of labor*
- *Auscultation of FHR: In placenta previa, FHR is usually present unless the patient is in shock. FHR may be absent in severe grades of abruption*

Examination of the vulva

It is done to ascertain whether bleeding is still continuing or has stopped, and to note the amount and color of bleeding.

Vaginal examination

***Vaginal examination is contraindicated** unless placenta previa is ruled out, as P/V examination can provoke torrential hemorrhage in placenta previa.*

Per speculum examination

- *A gentle speculum examination may be performed to rule out local causes of bleeding such as cervicitis, trauma, cervical polyp, and cervical malignancy. However, the presence of any of these does not rule out placenta previa.*

(CONTD...)

(...CONTD)

- *In severe bleeding, speculum examination need not be done as local findings may be obscured due to bleeding.*

Case summary 1

An example of writing summary in cases of APH due to placenta previa is given below.

Example *Mrs. M, 24 years of age, a primigravida, has been admitted at 34 weeks of gestation with H/o vaginal bleeding for the past 2 days. There is no H/o pain abdomen. There is a history of spotting P/V 2 weeks back. The patient's general physical examination reveals mild pallor; pulse, 92/min; and BP, 120/70 mmHg. Her CVS and RS examinations are normal. Obstetric examination reveals uterus corresponding to 32 weeks; uterus is relaxed with a single live fetus in cephalic presentation; FHR is 132 beats/min, regular. Vulval inspection reveals minimal fresh vaginal bleeding.*

Case diagnosis 1

An example of writing diagnosis in cases of APH due to placenta previa is given below.

Example *24 years of age, primigravida at 34 weeks of gestation with a singleton live fetus in cephalic presentation with APH. In this case, the history of painless, causeless, and recurrent bleeding favors the diagnosis of placenta previa. However, the diagnosis needs to be confirmed by ultrasound examination.*

Case summary 2

An example of writing summary in cases of APH due to abruptio placentae is given below.

Example *Mrs. Q, 30 years of age, G2 P1 L1 has been admitted at 34 weeks of gestation with H/o abdominal pain and vaginal bleeding for the past 4 hours. The patient's general physical examination reveals marked pallor and pedal edema is present; pulse, 106/min; BP, 140/90 mmHg. The patient's CVS and RS examination are normal. Obstetric examination reveals fundal height corresponding to 36 weeks; uterus is tense and tender on palpation. Symphysiofundal height (SFH) is 36 cm with single fetus in cephalic presentation; FHR is 100 beats/min. On vulval inspection, minimal dark-colored vaginal bleeding is present.*

Case diagnosis 2

An example of writing diagnosis in cases of APH due to abruptio placentae is given below.

Example *30 years of age, G2P1L1 at 34 weeks of gestation with a singleton live fetus in cephalic presentation with APH. The most likely diagnosis is abruption with fetal distress.*

Case discussion

All cases of APH need to be admitted. The first step in the management of APH is to stabilize the patient.

Clinical features of placenta previa and abruption, the two main differential diagnosis for APH are mentioned in Table 15.3.

- The clinical condition of the patient must be assessed.
- As the patient is likely to be hypovolemic, two wide bore IV cannula must be inserted and resuscitation with IV crystalloids are started.
- The patient's blood sample must be sent for complete hemogram, blood grouping and typing, and coagulation profile.
- Adequate blood need to be cross-matched and reserved, as urgent transfusion may be required at any time.
- Following stabilization of the maternal condition, the fetal condition must be assessed.
- Ultrasound is done to confirm placental localization, fetal presentation, and well-being.
- Placental localization helps in differentiating between the two most common causes of APH: placenta previa and abruptio placenta.
- Further management is decided based on the exact diagnosis.

PLACENTA PREVIA

If placenta previa is the diagnosis, then the management is as follows:

- The management is either active interference or expectant management depending on the maternal and fetal condition and the POG.

Table 15.3 Distinguishing features between placenta previa and abruptio placentae

Clinical features	Placenta previa	Abruptio placentae
Nature of bleeding	• Painless, causeless, and recurrent bleeding • Bleeding is always revealed	• Painful and is continuous; cause is often due to preeclampsia or trauma • Revealed, concealed, or mixed type of bleeding
Character of bleeding	Bright red	Dark colored
Pallor	Proportionate to visible blood loss	Out of proportion to the visible blood loss in concealed or mixed type
Features of preeclampsia	Not present	Present in one-third of cases
Abdominal examination		
Height of uterus	Proportionate to POG	May be greater than POG in concealed type
Feel of uterus	Soft and relaxed	May be tense, tender, and rigid
Malpresentations	The head is high floating and malpresentations are common	The head may be engaged
FHR	Usually present	Fetal distress may be present or absent FHR especially in concealed type
Ultrasonography	Placenta in lower segment	Placenta in upper segment

FHR, fetal heart rate; *POG*, period of gestation.

Indications for active interference in placenta previa

- Active vaginal bleeding continues.
- The patient is hemodynamically unstable.
- POG is ≥37 weeks.
- The patient is in labor.
- Fetus is dead.
- Fetus is congenitally malformed.

Expectant management in placenta previa

Aim

The aim is to delay delivery as much as possible to allow for fetal lung maturity and at the same time not to jeopardize the maternal condition. Only hemodynamically stable patients remote from term should be managed conservatively.

Objective

The objective is to reduce perinatal mortality and morbidity due to prematurity.

Prerequisites for expectant management—McAfee and Johnson's Regimen

- There is no active vaginal bleeding.
- The patient is hemodynamically stable.
- POG is <37 weeks.
- Fetal well-being is assured.

Steps taken during expectant management

- Admit the patient in labor room; sedation may be given.
- The patient is kept nil oral.
- Start an IV drip and send blood for investigations as mentioned earlier and adequate blood units are reserved.
- Monitor the patient's pulse and BP every 15 minutes initially and then hourly.
- Maintain an input/output chart.
- Assess the blood loss and transfuse if required (the aim is to maintain a hemoglobin level of 10 g/dL).
- Maintain an abdominal girth and fundal height chart to rule out abruption and concealed hemorrhage.
- Monitor FHR by auscultation or electronic fetal monitoring.
- Steroids are given for lung maturity—betamethasone 12 mg IM 24 hourly for two doses or Dexamethasone 6 mg IM 12th hourly for four doses.
- Women with Rh incompatibility require anti-D immunoglobulin prophylaxis.

The patient can be shifted to the ward if there is no bleeding for at least 24 hours.

- Advise on limitation of physical activity and adequate bed rest.

- Hematinics are prescribed to maintain hemoglobin within normal range.
- A speculum examination is done, after bleeding has stopped, to exclude any local pathology.

Follow-up Continued hospitalization is the best management option for patients with APH due to placenta previa who are managed conservatively. However, the patient can be managed on an outpatient basis if the following conditions are fulfilled:

- No bleeding for 72 hours during hospital stay
- Patient is hemodynamically stable
- Reactive nonstress test
- Patient is compliant with bed rest at home and regular follow-up
- Availability of transport and communication facilities between home and hospital

Patient is followed up every week till delivery or readmission.

Expectant management is abandoned in the following conditions:

- Pregnancy reaching 37 weeks
- Severe hemorrhage at any time endangering the life of the mother
- Fetus is dead or malformed
- Onset of labor or rupture of membranes

Mode of delivery

- CS is done in major degree placenta previa—types II (posterior), III, and IV.
- Vaginal delivery can be allowed in minor degree placenta previa—types I and II (anterior)
  - Induction may be done with oxytocin and/or artificial rupture of membranes (ARM) (in type I or type II anterior placenta previa)
  - All cases considered for vaginal delivery need close monitoring, as CS may be required any time, for obstetric indication or vaginal bleeding
- Steroid for lung maturity is given, if pregnancy is terminated at <37 weeks.

Precautions during cesarean section

- Prior arrangement for adequate blood reservation.
- It is better to plan an elective CS as there is increased perinatal morbidity and mortality following an emergency CS.
- CS should preferably be done by a senior obstetrician during working hours.
- A lower segment transverse incision on the uterus is given. The lower segment may be very vascular.
- In case of anterior placenta previa, placenta will be at the site of lower segment incision.

Part 1

Viva corner

Q1 What is double setup vaginal examination for placenta previa?

- It may be done when there are no facilities for ultrasound examination to confirm placenta previa. Double setup examination is rarely done nowadays due to the danger of provoking torrential hemorrhage.
- The double setup examination is done in operation theatre (OT) while all the preparations for an emergency CS are kept ready.

Double setup vaginal examination steps

- The patient is under general anesthesia or epidural anesthesia in lithotomy position.
- A per speculum examination is done to look for any local cause of bleeding.
- A careful digital examination is done. Two fingers are introduced gently into the vagina and the fornices are palpated for any bogginess felt through the vaginal fornix. There is a feeling of bogginess, if placenta is present.
- If there is no bogginess, the index finger is gently introduced into the cervical canal and a careful examination is done to feel for the placental edge.
  - If no placental edge is felt within 3 cm of the os, at term gestation, the membranes can be ruptured with the aim of conducting a vaginal delivery.
  - If the placental edge is felt at any point, the examination must be stopped and emergency CS needs to be performed.
  - If there is brisk vaginal bleeding during the procedure or there is excessive bleeding after membrane rupture, CS is performed.

Note *An organized blood clot can be mistaken for the placenta, but a blood clot is friable unlike the placenta that is firm and nonfriable.*

In such cases, the placenta may be cut through to deliver the baby, or separated up to its margin to rupture the membranes and deliver the baby.
- Anticipate morbidly adherent placenta.
- Anticipate postpartum hemorrhage (PPH) in all cases of APH.

Steps to control postpartum hemorrhage in cases with placenta previa

- Use of uterotonic agents such as oxytocin, methergin, PG F2 alpha, and misoprostol to reduce the blood loss
- Application of B-Lynch sutures or multiple CHO sutures (multiple square sutures involving the anterior and posterior walls of uterus) (refer to Part 1, Chapter 17(III), *Postpartum Hemorrhage)*
- Intrauterine compression packing
- Bilateral uterine artery ligation
- Internal iliac artery ligation
- Uterine artery embolization
- Cesarean hysterectomy is the final option to control bleeding, if all conservative measures fail and the patient continues to bleed

PLACENTAL ABRUPTION

Diagnosis

Abruption is mainly a clinical diagnosis. USG can neither confirm nor exclude the diagnosis of abruptio placentae. Retroplacental clot may be seen in USG in concealed hemorrhage. However, USG is done in all cases of APH to exclude placenta previa and to assess fetal well-being.

Clinical grading of abruption

Depending on the severity of clinical features, abruption is graded as follows:

Grade 0

- It is a retrospective diagnosis following the delivery of the baby.
- No obvious clinical features are present.

Grade 1 (mild)

- Slight external bleeding is present.
- Volume of retroplacental clot is <200 mL.
- Uterus may be irritable; uterine tenderness may or may not be present.
- Maternal shock is absent.
- FHR is good.

Grade 2 (moderate)

- The external bleeding is mild to moderate in amount.
- The volume of retroplacental clot may vary from 150 to 500 mL.
- The uterus is tender and abdominal pain is present.

Viva corner

Q1 What is Stallworthy's sign?

In cases of type II posterior placenta previa, when the head is pushed into the pelvis, there is slowing of FHR due to compression of the placenta, which is termed Stallworthy's sign.

Q2 What is dangerous placenta previa?

In type II posterior placenta previa, the placental thickness (about 2.5 cm) overlying the sacral promontory diminishes the AP diameter of the pelvic inlet, thereby preventing engagement of fetal presenting part. Hence, effective compression of the separated placenta cannot take place due to nonengagement of head and vaginal bleeding continues. Hence, type II posterior placenta previa is called dangerous placenta previa.

Q3 What are placenta accreta, increta, and percreta?

Abnormal trophoblastic invasion of placenta beyond the normal boundary established by the Nitabuch's fibrinoid layer results in morbidly adherent placenta or invasive placenta. The types of morbidly adherent placenta are as follows:

- **Accreta:** Placenta is attached to uterine myometrium, but does not invade it (*accreta* means "attaches").
- **Increta:** Placenta invades the myometrium (*increta* means "invades").
- **Percreta:** Placenta penetrates myometrium up to serosa (*percreta* means "penetrates").

- Maternal shock is absent; the patient may have tachycardia but no signs of hypovolemia.
- FHR is usually present; there may be signs of fetal distress.

Grade 3 (severe)

- Moderate to severe amount of revealed bleeding or concealed bleeding is present.
- More than half of the placenta separates and the volume of retroplacental clot is >500 mL.
- Tonic uterine contractions (tetany), abdominal pain, and marked uterine tenderness may be present.
- Features of maternal shock are present.
- Fetal death commonly occurs.
- Complications such as disseminated intravascular coagulation (DIC) and anuria may be present.

Management of abruption

- The initial step in the management is emergency resuscitation and stabilization of the patient as mentioned earlier.
- Once, placenta previa is ruled out and a clinical diagnosis of abruption is made, further management of the patient includes:
  - Blood sample is sent for complete hemogram, ABO blood grouping, typing and cross-matching, and coagulation profile [clotting time, fibrinogen levels, prothrombin time, activated partial thromboplastin time (aPTT), and platelet count]. Abnormal results of coagulation profile in cases of abruption with DIC complication are mentioned in Table 15.4.
  - Fresh frozen plasma (FFP) and whole blood for transfusion need to be urgently arranged and are usually required for effective resuscitation.
  - An indwelling urinary catheter is inserted to monitor urine output.
  - Delivery of the baby is the definitive treatment in abruption due to risk of complications.

Mode of delivery

- Delivery should be performed by the fastest possible route.
- If fetus is alive
  - Vaginal delivery can be allowed, if the patient is hemodynamically stable, if the Bishop's score of cervix is favorable and FHR is reassuring → ARM is done and oxytocin drip is started (ARM + oxytocin). CS is performed if Bishop's score of cervix is unfavorable or if fetal distress is present.
- If fetus is dead—allow for vaginal delivery.

Indications for emergency cesarean section

Indications for emergency CS in placental abruption are as follows:

- Appearance of fetal distress
- Bleeding continues to occur despite ARM and oxytocin infusion
- Nonprogress of labor
- Deterioration of maternal or fetal condition
- Fetal malpresentation
- Associated obstetric factors such as CPD
- Appearance of complication (DIC, oliguria, etc.)

Role of conservative management in placental abruption

- Conservative management is usually not practiced in abruption due to the associated complications.

Table 15.4 Abnormal results of coagulation profile in disseminated intravascular coagulation (DIC)

Test	Normal results	DIC
Fibrinogen	150–600 mg/dL	Reduced (<150 mg/dL)
Prothrombin time	11–16 seconds	Prolonged
Activated partial thromboplastin time	22–37 seconds	Prolonged
Thrombin time	15–25 seconds	Prolonged
Platelet count	1.2–1.5 lakh/mm^3	Reduced
D-dimer	<0.5 mg/L	Increased (>0.5 mg/L)
Fibrin degradation product	Less than10 µg	Increased (>10 µg/dL)

- The patient may be considered for expectant management with close monitoring until fetal maturity is achieved in the following situation:
  - Mild abruption at POG <34 weeks, if bleeding has stopped and fetal well-being is assured.

Viva corner

Q1 What is the role of ARM in abruption?

- Augments labor
- Decreases release of thromboplastin into circulation that is responsible for DIC

Q2 What is Couvelaire uterus?

It is a pathological condition of the uterus seen during CS following massive placental abruption. The uterus appears bluish in color due to widespread extravasation of blood into uterine musculature up to serosa.

Q3 Is Couvelaire uterus an indication of hysterectomy?

Couvelaire uterus may interfere with uterine myometrial contractions. However, Couvelaire uterus per se is not an indication of hysterectomy.

Q4 What are the causes of DIC in pregnancy?

- Intrauterine death with retained fetus
- Severe preeclampsia
- Abruption
- Amniotic fluid embolism
- Hemorrhagic shock
- Transfusion reaction

VASA PREVIA

Definition

Vasa previa is a rare condition in which the fetal blood vessels traverse the membranes overlying the internal os before getting attached to the placenta (Figure 15.3).

- Bleeding in vasa previa is mainly fetal in origin (unlike placenta previa where bleeding is mainly maternal) and is associated with a very high fetal mortality (75–100%).
- The fetal blood vessels are likely to get lacerated during membrane rupture leading to severe fetal bleeding.

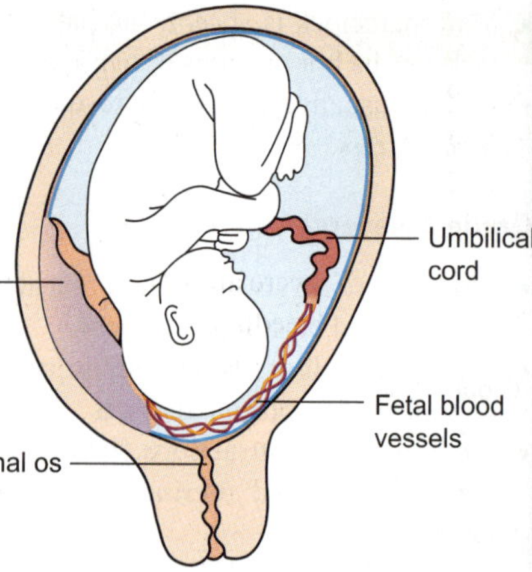

Figure 15.3 Vasa previa. Fetal blood vessels traverse the membranes overlying the internal os before getting attached to the placenta.

- During labor, the blood vessels may get compressed by the presenting part leading to fetal hypoxia.

Diagnosis of vasa previa

- Diagnosis of vasa previa is usually made when there is bleeding and fetal bradycardia following rupture of membranes.
- Apt test: It is a bedside test performed to find out whether the vaginal bleeding is of fetal or maternal origin by testing the ability of fetal hemoglobin to withstand alkali denaturation.

Management of vasa previa

Emergency CS must be done once diagnosis is made as the fetal mortality is very high.

ASSESSMENT OF SEVERITY OF BLOOD LOSS IN ANTEPARTUM HEMORRHAGE

See Table 15.5

Resuscitation of patients with severe bleeding

- Start a wide bore IV line, send blood for blood grouping and typing, cross-matching and reservation.

Table 15.5 Assessment of severity of blood loss in antepartum hemorrhage

Group	Amount of bleeding	Clinical features
Group I	Bleeding is mild, blood loss <750 mL (<15% of the intravascular volume is depleted)	No change in the vitals, urinary output, or central nervous system
Group II	Moderate bleeding, blood loss is between 750 and 1500 mL (15–30% of intravascular volume is depleted)	• Baseline tachycardia • Fall in BP of ≥10 mmHg DBP • Urine output is about 30 mL/h • Patient may be anxious and agitated
Groups III and IV	Severe bleeding, blood loss is 1500–2500 mL (30–40% of blood volume is depleted)	• Features of shock are present • Feeble pulse • Decreased or unrecordable BP • Oliguria or anuria • Patient is in confused state

- Crystalloids are given till blood is made available for transfusion. One liter of crystalloid solution expands the intravascular volume by approximately 250 mL.
- Packed red cells and specific blood components should be used for replacement of blood and clotting factors when required.
- Platelet transfusion should be given when counts are less than 50,000/mm^3. One unit of platelets will increase platelets by 10,000/mm^3.
- If there are alterations in prothrombin time (PT) or aPTT or DIC is suspected, then FFP should be given.
- For every 4 units of packed cells, 1 unit of FFP should be transfused.
- If patient is in a critical condition, it may not be possible to monitor the intravascular volume status with pulse and BP alone; central venous pressure (CVP) line may be required to monitor fluid replacement.
- Urine output measurement is an important aspect in the management of patients with severe bleeding and shock. A Foley's catheter is inserted to monitor urine output and the output should be maintained at 30 mL/h to prevent renal damage.
- The patients need to be managed in high dependency units or obstetric intensive care units.

Frequently asked viva questions

1. Summarize the case.
2. What is the provisional diagnosis of the case?
3. What are the initial steps in management of the case?
4. How will you confirm the diagnosis?
5. What are the clinical features differentiating placenta previa and abruption?
6. How will you manage a case of APH due to placenta previa?
7. What is the role of conservative management in placenta previa? What is the mode of delivery?
8. How will you manage a case of abruption? What is the mode of delivery?
9. What are the complications anticipated in abruption?

16 Primigravida with Mobile Head at Term

Introduction

Engagement of fetal head usually occurs during labor in a multigravida, while in a primigravida, it occurs before the onset of labor. Cephalopelvic disproportion (CPD) is an important cause of floating or mobile head at term, in a primigravida. Clinical discussion in a case of mobile head at term includes pelvic assessment, CPD, and trial of labor which are dealt in this chapter.

Causes of mobile head at term

These are mentioned in Table 16.1.

Table 16.1 Causes of mobile head at term

Maternal causes	Fetal causes
• Full bladder • Contracted pelvis • Cephalopelvic disproportion • Placenta previa • Polyhydramnios • Tumors in lower uterine segment—fibroid	• Deflexed head • Macrosomia • Prematurity • Multiple pregnancy • Short umbilical cord • Cord around neck • Congenital anomalies such as hydrocephalus

Terminologies

Cephalopelvic disproportion It means relative disparity between the maternal pelvis and the fetal head (it is a relative terminology).

CPD can be due to a normal-sized baby with a contracted pelvis or a large baby with a normal pelvis.

Contracted pelvis It means alteration in shape and size of pelvis to such a degree that it alters normal mechanism of labor even in an average-sized baby, resulting in difficulty in vaginal delivery (it is an absolute terminology).

- One or more diameters of the pelvis in one or more planes is shorter than normal. Contraction can be at the level of inlet, cavity, or outlet (absolute disproportion).

MOLDING

It is the alteration in the shape of the head of fetus to adapt itself to the resistant birth passage during the process of labor. During normal delivery, an alteration of 4 mm in skull diameter usually occurs due to molding (Figure 16.1). It occurs due to the following:

- Ununited sutures that help the bones to overlap during delivery
- Compressible nature of bones and fontanelles

Grades of molding

- **Grade 1:** The bones are touching each other, but not overlapping.
- **Grade 2:** The bones are overlapping, but can be easily separated.
- **Grade 3:** The bones are overlapping and cannot be separated (fixed overlapping).

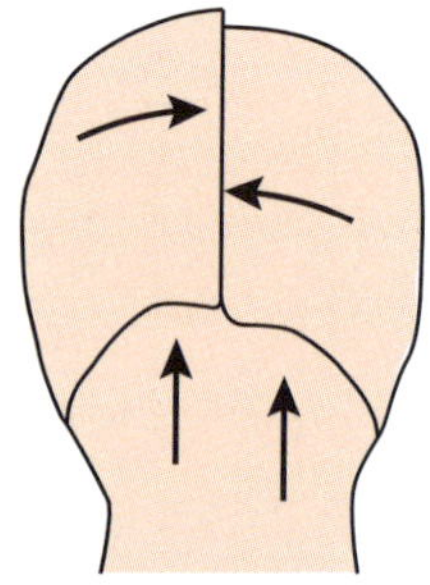

Figure 16.1 Molding of fetal head. Coming together or overlapping of skull bones, when resistance is encountered in the bony pelvis.

Clinical significance

- Slight molding is inevitable and beneficial as it enables the head to negotiate through the birth canal.
- Extreme molding is seen in disproportion and may produce severe intracranial hemorrhage due to tearing of tentorium cerebelli or subdural hemorrhage.
- Molding can provide information about the position of the head in the pelvis.

CAPUT SUCCEDANEUM

It is the formation of swelling due to stagnation of fluid in the layers of the scalp, beneath the girdle of contact of the head (Figure 16.2). As the head descends, it presses over the dilating cervix and the tissues in contact with the girdle of contact get compressed. This interferes with venous and lymphatic drainage leading to stagnation of fluid and appearance of swelling in the scalp.

- The swelling is diffuse and boggy, and is not limited by the suture line.
- It disappears spontaneously within 24 hours after birth.

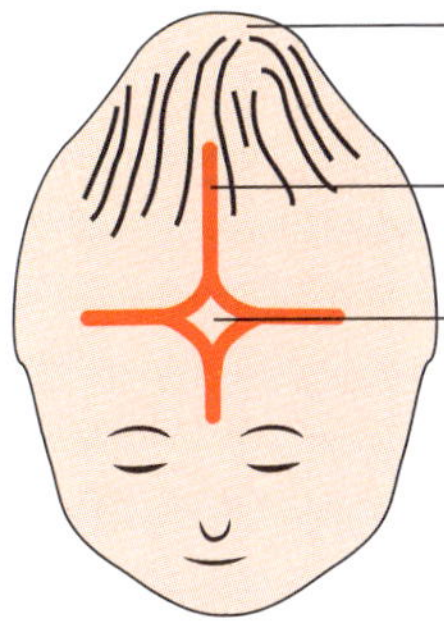

a.

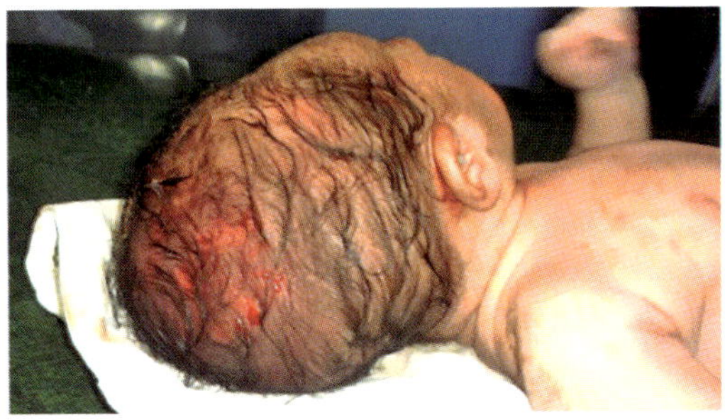
b.

Figure 16.2 Caput succedaneum. **a.** The area of the scalp that is pressed against the cervix becomes edematous. The fluid is superficial to the periosteum and crosses suture lines. **b.** Caput in a newborn.

Clinical significance

- It signifies static position of the head for a long period of time.
- Location of the caput gives an idea about the position of the head occupied in the pelvis and the degree of flexion achieved.

Case presentation

Salient points in history

Consider the following relevant points during history taking in cases of mobile head at term:

- *Age (teenage pregnancy—risk of contracted pelvis and CPD)*
- *Parity (primigravida—more risk for CPD)*
- *Period of gestation (POG)—confirm the dates (preterm head will be mobile)*

History of present pregnancy

- *Whether obstetric ultrasonography (USG) done and told to be normal (to rule out fetal anomalies, placenta previa, multiple pregnancy, polyhydramnios, and mass in lower uterine segment, etc.)*
- *H/o bleeding P/V in the third trimester (placenta previa is associated with mobile head)*
- *H/o gestational diabetes mellitus (GDM) (uncontrolled blood sugars may be associated with macrosomia)*

Past obstetric history

Note *In a multigravida, previous vaginal delivery of an average-sized baby excludes contracted pelvis but CPD can still be a possibility in certain situations.*

Ask for any history suggestive of CPD in previous delivery:

- *Duration of labor (H/o prolonged labor)*

(CONTD...)

(...CONTD)

- *Mode of delivery (any difficult instrumental delivery, cesarean section (CS) for II stage CPD)*
- *Apgar score (H/o severe birth asphyxia, stillbirth/early neonatal death)*
- *Weight of baby*
- *Any complications such as traumatic postpartum hemorrhage (PPH) and third-degree perineal tear*

Past history

- *H/o hypertension, DM, and tuberculosis*
- *H/o poliomyelitis, rickets, osteomalacia, and fractures involving pelvic joints (can lead to pelvic deformity)*

Salient points in examination

Consider the following relevant points during examination in cases of mobile head at term.

General examination

- *Height (height <145 cm is considered as short stature; short and stout women may have android pelvis, and tall women may have anthropoid pelvis)*
- *Weight*
- *BMI*
- *Gait*
- *Spine abnormalities (kyphosis, scoliosis)*
- *Any lower limb shortening/wasting/deformity*

Note *Obstetric examination should always be performed after the patient voids (distended bladder can be a cause for mobile head).*

Obstetric examination

- *Pendulous overhanging abdomen—may be suggestive of CPD*
- *Subumbilical flattening—suggestive of occipitoposterior position*
- *Fundal height and symphysiofundal height (SFH) may be >POG in big baby, multiple pregnancy, polyhydramnios*
- *Pelvic grips—head freely mobile with 5/5th of the head palpable*
- *Liquor—increased in polyhydramnios*
- *Estimated fetal weight—to assess whether it is a big size baby*

Case summary

An example of writing summary in cases of mobile head at term is given below.

Example *Mrs. L, 24 years of age, a primigravida has been admitted at 39+2 weeks of pregnancy for safe confinement. She is perceiving normal fetal movements. On general examination, her height is 148 cm, there is no pallor or pedal edema, pulse is 82/min and BP is 120/80 mmHg. Systemic examination revealed normal cardiovascular and respiratory systems. Spine examination is normal. Obstetric examination revealed a term size uterus with a singleton live fetus in cephalic presentation, 5/5th of the head is palpable per abdomen. Liquor volume is adequate and uterus is relaxed. On auscultation, fetal heart rate (FHR) is 146 beats/min and is regular.*

Case diagnosis

An example of writing diagnosis in cases of mobile head at term is given below.

Example *24 years of age, primigravida at 39+2 weeks of gestation with a singleton live fetus in cephalic presentation with mobile head at term, not in labor*

Case discussion

Differential diagnosis

Differential diagnosis includes all the causes of floating head at term as mentioned in Table 16.1.

MANAGEMENT APPROACH IN A PRIMIGRAVIDA WITH MOBILE HEAD AT TERM

- Evaluation should be done to rule out the possible causes of floating head.

- USG helps to rule out placenta previa, multiple pregnancy, polyhydramnios, uterine or fetal malformation, any space occupying lesion in LUS, and to assess the fetal weight.
- Pelvic assessment is done to rule out CPD, by performing a vaginal examination. A systematic assessment of pelvis is done—first the pelvic inlet is assessed, then the midpelvis, and then the pelvic outlet (Table 16.2).
- Evaluation of cervix (Bishop's score) and the presenting part is also done during the vaginal examination.
- Clinical methods to assess CPD are performed at or after 38 weeks or preferably at the onset of labor.

Note *CPD is best diagnosed in labor when there is slow progress of labor or failure to progress.*

Table 16.2 Parameters assessed in pelvic assessment

Inlet	Midcavity	Outlet
• Sacral promontory • Diagonal conjugate • Forepelvis	• Sacral curvature • Sidewalls • Sacrosciatic notch • Ischial spine • Interspinous distance	• Subpubic arch • Intertuberous diameter

Steps in pelvic assessment (Figure 16.3)

1. Start with the sacral promontory and then follow the curve of sacrum downwards along the midline (Figure 16.3a).
   a. In an adequate pelvis, the promontory cannot be easily palpated, the sacrum is well curved, and the coccyx cannot be felt.
   b. In an inadequate pelvis, the sacral promontory is easily palpated and prominent, the sacrum is straight, and the coccyx is prominent and/or fixed.
2. After assessing the sacrum, the fingers are then moved laterally, to feel the sacrospinous ligaments. If these ligaments are followed laterally, the ischial spines can be palpated. The interspinous distance is estimated by separating the index and middle fingers wide apart (Figure 16.3b, c).
   a. In an adequate pelvis, at least two fingers can be placed over the sacrospinous ligaments and the ischial spines are not prominent.
   b. In an inadequate pelvis, the sacrospinous ligaments usually allow less than two fingers and the ischial spines may be sharp and prominent.
3. Next, the retropubic area (forepelvis) is palpated by placing two fingers behind the symphysis pubis with the palm of the hand

Part 1

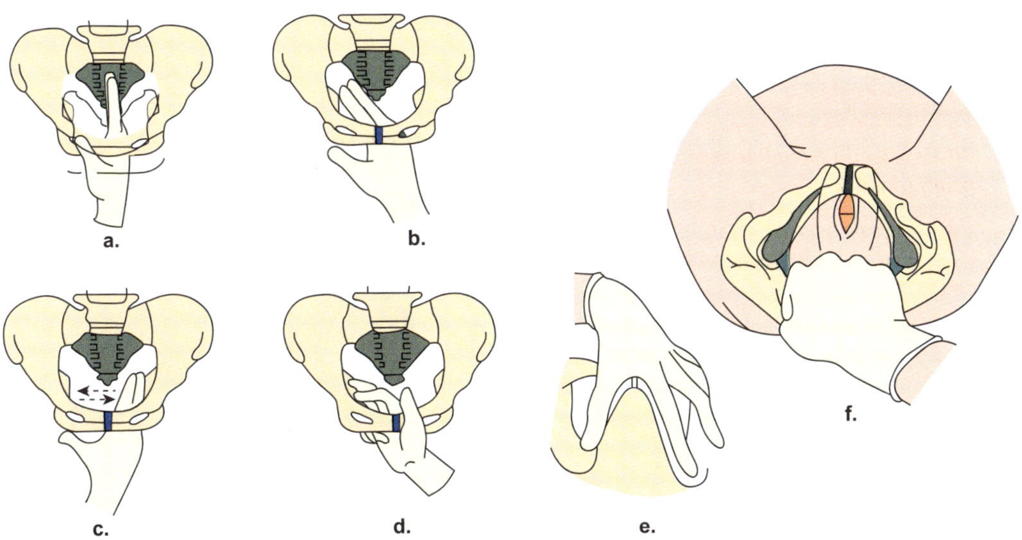

Figure 16.3 Steps in pelvic assessment. a. Assessing the sacrum. b. Assessing the sacrosciatic notch. c. Assessing the ischial spines and the interspinous distance. d. Assessing the forepelvis. e. Assessing the subpubic angle. f. Assessing the intertuberous diameter.

facing forwards. The fingers are then moved laterally to both sides (Figure 16.3d).

   a. In an adequate pelvis, the retropubic area is flat.
   b. In an inadequate pelvis, the retropubic area is angulated.

4. To measure the subpubic angle, the examining fingers are turned so that the palm of the hand faces upwards and the angle under the pubis is felt.
   a. In an adequate pelvis, three fingers can be placed under the pubis and the subpubic angle is about 90° (Figure 16.3e).
   b. In an inadequate pelvis, only two fingers can be placed under the pubis and the subpubic angle is about 60°.
5. The hand is then withdrawn from the vaginal introitus and the intertuberous diameter is assessed with the knuckles of the closed fist of the hand placed between the ischial tuberosities (Figure 16.3f).
   a. In an adequate pelvis, the intertuberous diameter allows four knuckles.
   b. In an inadequate pelvis, the intertuberous diameter allows less than four knuckles.

ASSESSMENT OF CEPHALOPELVIC DISPROPORTION

- Fetal head is the largest part of the fetus and it is the best pelvimeter in clinical practice.

> **Viva corner**
>
> **Q1 When will you do pelvic assessment in a primigravida?**
>
> The traditional teaching was to perform a vaginal examination at 38 weeks to assess the pelvis and to rule out CPD.
>
> In clinical practice, it is observed that engagement most often occurs at the onset of labor. Hence, in a low-risk primigravida, pelvic assessment can be postponed to 39–40 weeks or at the onset of labor.
>
> However, if a major degree of CPD is suspected like in case of short stature and pelvic deformity or if the pregnancy is associated with other medical or obstetric complications, pelvic assessment can be done at 38 weeks to decide on the mode of termination.

It is assessed whether the greatest diameter of the fetal head can pass through the different planes of the pelvis. Assessment of the relative size of the fetal head to the pelvis is more important than the absolute size of pelvis, that is, assessment of CPD is more important than assessment of the pelvis alone.

- Disproportion may be present in one or more planes. Assessment of the pelvis and assessment of the presence and degree of CPD are required while evaluating a case of mobile head at term.

Clinical methods for assessment of cephalopelvic disproportion

Prerequisites

- The bladder and bowel should be emptied.
- The patient should be in dorsal position with the legs flexed and slightly abducted.

Clinical methods for assessment of CPD are described below.

Abdominal method for assessment of cephalopelvic disproportion

Ian Donald method

Ian Donald method (abdominal method) (Figure 16.4)

Procedure

- Two fingers (index and middle) of the clinician's right hand are placed over symphysis pubis.
- Head is grasped by left hand and is pushed downwards and backwards into the pelvis.

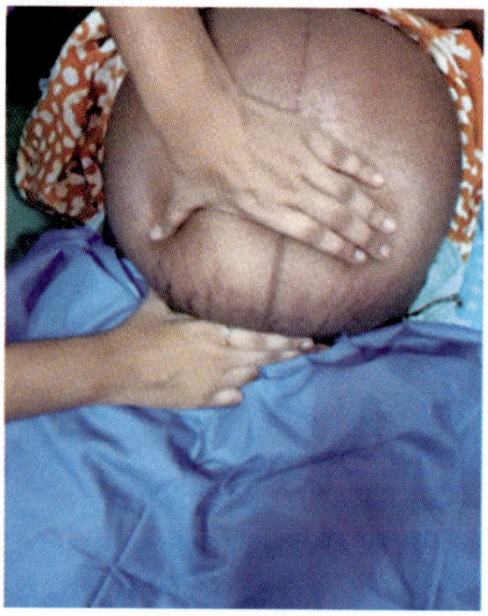

Figure 16.4 Ian Donald method for cephalopelvic disproportion assessment (abdominal method).

Inference

- If the head can be pushed down into pelvis without overlapping of the parietal bone on the symphysis pubis, it indicates no CPD.
- If the head can be pushed down a little but with slight overlapping of parietal bone on the pubic symphysis (evidenced by touch on the under-surface of the fingers of right hand), it indicates moderate CPD.
- If the head cannot be pushed down and the parietal bone overhangs the symphysis pubis displacing the fingers, it indicates severe CPD.
- The abdominal method for CPD assessment can be used as a screening procedure.

Abdomino-vaginal method for assessment of cephalopelvic disproportion

Munro Kerr–Muller method

Munro Kerr–Muller method (abdomino-pelvic method or bimanual method; Figure 16.5)

Bimanual method is superior to the abdominal method as pelvic assessment can be done simultaneously.

Procedure

- The fingers of the clinician's right hand are introduced into the vagina, with the fingertips placed at the level of ischial spines, to note the descent of the head and the thumb placed over the front of the pubic symphysis, to note the degree of overlapping.
- The fetal head is grasped by the left hand and is pushed downward and backward into the pelvis.

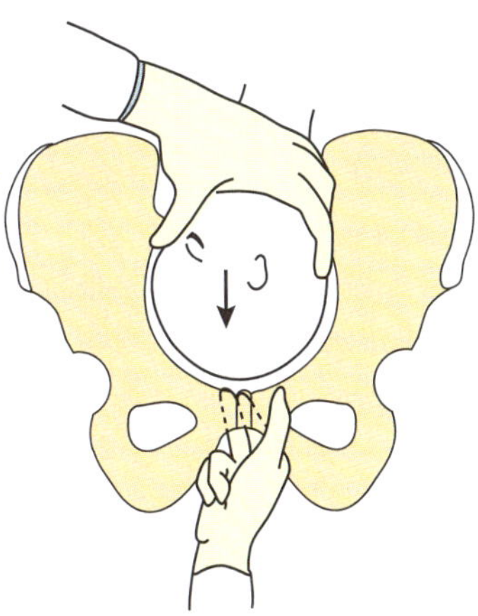

Figure 16.5 Munro Kerr–Muller method for cephalopelvic disproportion assessment.

Inference

- If the head can be pushed down, up to the level of ischial spines and there is no overlapping of the parietal bone over the symphysis pubis, it indicates no CPD.
- If the head can be pushed down but not up to the level of ischial spines and there is slight overlapping of the parietal bone, it indicates slight or moderate CPD. Vaginal delivery may or may not be achieved with molding.
- If the head cannot be pushed down and the parietal bone overhangs the symphysis pubis displacing the thumb, it indicates severe CPD. Vaginal delivery is not possible; needs cesarean delivery.

Limitations of cephalopelvic disproportion assessment methods

The clinical methods of CPD assessment during antenatal period are not used in modern obstetric practice for the following reasons:

- Practically, it is very difficult to push the head down into the pelvis in the presence of an unfavorable cervix, that is, when the patient is not in labor.

Extra edge

Role of USG in a patient with mobile head at term

- USG helps in excluding other causes of mobile head such as placenta previa, fetal anomalies, and pelvic tumors.
- Cephalometry: Accurate measurement of biparietal diameter (BPD) by USG or magnetic resonance imaging (MRI) will be useful to elicit its relation with the diameters of the pelvic planes through which it has to pass. The average BPD at term measures 9.4–9.8 cm and BPD more than this represents a big head.
- USG can be used to assess fetal weight by accepted formulas.

Role of MRI in assessing CPD

- MRI is useful to assess the pelvic capacity at different planes.
- It is useful to assess the fetal head size.
- It can assess the pelvic soft tissues that are also important for a successful vaginal delivery.
- However, MRI is very expensive and is rarely used for pelvic assessment.

- It may be difficult to elicit the tests in the presence of thick abdominal wall, irritable uterus, deflexed head, or high floating head.
- Only brim CPD can be detected by these methods. Disproportion at the level of midpelvis or outlet cannot be assessed by these methods.
- The CPD assessment methods does not take into consideration the main factors involved in successful trial of labor, such as the "give way" of pelvis, molding of the fetal head, and uterine contractions.
- As mentioned earlier, CPD is best diagnosed during labor.

CONTRACTED PELVIS

Maternal pelvis is described in detail in Part 3, Chapter 32, *Maternal Pelvis and Fetal Skull.*

Contracted pelvis It means that one or more diameters of the pelvis in one or more planes is shorter than normal. Contraction can be at the level of inlet, cavity, or outlet (absolute disproportion).

Contracted pelvic inlet

- Pelvic inlet is considered contracted when the obstetric conjugate (OC) is <10 cm or diagonal conjugate (DC) is <11.5 cm. Inlet contraction can be mild, moderate, or severe as described below.
  - *Mild*: OC 9.5–10 cm
  - *Moderate*: OC 7.6–9.4 cm
  - *Severe*: OC <7.5 cm

Contracted midpelvis

Midpelvis is considered contracted when the sum of the interspinous diameter (ISD) and posterior sagittal diameter of the midpelvis is <13 cm (normal: 10 + 5 = 15 cm).

- **ISD <10 cm:** Contracted midpelvis is suspected
- **ISD <8 cm:** Indicates contracted midpelvis

Note *There is no precise clinical method for midpelvic assessment.*

Suspect contracted midpelvis in case of the following:

- Ischial spines are prominent
- Side walls are converging
- ISD is less than average
- Sacrosciatic notch is narrow

Contracted outlet

Contracted outlet is suspected when intertuberous diameter (transverse diameter of outlet) is <8 cm.

Note *Isolated outlet contraction without midpelvic contraction is rare, that is, a contracted outlet is often associated with contracted midpelvis.*

Complications associated with cephalopelvic disproportion and contracted pelvis

During pregnancy

The general course of pregnancy is not much affected. However, the following may occur:

- Abdomen becomes pendulous and overhanging.
- Malpresentations and unstable lie are common.

During labor

Depending on the degree of CPD, the following may occur:

- Early rupture of the membranes
- Cord prolapse
- Late onset of labor, delayed cervical dilatation and descent
- Prolonged labor (due to incoordinate uterine action)
- In neglected cases, possibility of obstructed labor with features of exhaustion, dehydration, ketoacidosis, and sepsis
- Increased incidence of operative interference
- Increased incidence of PPH and sepsis
- Perineal injuries following delivery
- Fetal trauma and birth asphyxia leading to increased perinatal mortality and morbidity

Extra edge

Etiology of contracted pelvis

Deformities arising from faulty development

- Justo major pelvis
- Justo minor pelvis (generally contracted pelvis)
- Simple flat (nonrachitic)
- Naegele's pelvis (imperfect development of one sacral ala)
- Robert's pelvis (both sacral ala absent)
- Split pelvis (imperfect development of pubis)

(CONTD...)

(...CONTD)

Extra edge

Deformities arising from diseases of pelvic bones and joints

- Rickets
- Osteomalacia
- New bony growth
- Fractures
- Atrophy
- Diseases of sacroiliac/sacrococcygeal joints

Deformities arising from diseases of spinal column

- Kyphosis
- Scoliosis
- Spondylolisthesis

Deformities arising from diseases of lower extremities

- Coxitis
- Dislocation of one/both femurs
- Atrophy/loss of one limb

MANAGEMENT OF CPD

Management of brim CPD

- Minor degrees of brim CPD—do not give rise to any problem and the patients can be allowed for spontaneous vaginal delivery at term
- In case of moderate degree of brim CPD without any medical or obstetric complications—trial of labor can be given
- In case of moderate degree of brim CPD with medical or obstetric complications such as in an elderly gravida, conception after infertility treatment, preeclampsia, and previous cesarean pregnancy—CS is the preferred mode of delivery
- In cases with severe degree of brim CPD—elective CS is done
- In cases with malpresentations, significant midpelvis, and outlet contraction—CS is done

Trial of labor

Definition

It is the conduct of spontaneous labor in cases with moderate degree of brim CPD, in an institution under supervision with watchful expectancy, hoping for a vaginal delivery.

A trial of labor aims at avoiding an unnecessary CS.

Prerequisite

Arrangements should be made for emergency CS, if the need arises.

Contraindications for trial of labor

- Associated midpelvic and outlet contraction
- Presence of complicating factors such as elderly primigravida, malpresentation, postcesarean pregnancy, preeclampsia, and in medical disorders such as diabetes and heart diseases
- If facilities for performing emergency CS are not available

Advantages of trial of labor

- It eliminates unnecessary CS.
- A successful trial ensures a good future obstetric outcome (future vaginal deliveries) for the woman.

Disadvantages of trial of labor

- Test of disproportion remains unproved when CS is done for fetal distress or uterine dysfunction.
- There is increased perinatal morbidity and mortality due to birth asphyxia or intracranial hemorrhage when the trial ends in a traumatic vaginal delivery.
- There is increased maternal morbidity due to prolonged labor and/or operative delivery, and psychological morbidity when trial ends in a traumatic vaginal delivery or in CS.

Successful trial A trial is said to be successful if a healthy baby is born vaginally, either spontaneously or by forceps or ventouse, with the mother in a good condition.

Failure of trial Delivery by CS or delivery of a dead baby in a patient allowed for trial of labor is termed failure of trial.

Conduct of trial of labor (intrapartum management)

- Await spontaneous onset of labor. If the patient does not go into labor, induction of labor can be done.
- Avoid orals and maintain hydration with intravenous fluids (as there is increased chances of the patient being taken up for CS during labor).

Part 1

- Adequate analgesia is administered.
- The progress of labor is monitored with a partogram:
  - Progressive dilatation of the cervix
  - Progressive descent of the fetal head (station of the head)
  - Assessment of maternal and fetal condition
- FHR monitoring is done using continuous cardiotocography (CTG), if facilities are available or else by intermittent auscultation every 15 minutes in first stage and every 5 minutes in second stage of labor.
- Augmentation of labor may be done with oxytocin and/or artificial rupture of membranes (ARM) in case of inadequate uterine contractions. Controlled ARM should be done in case of free floating head.
- Pelvic examination should be done following rupture of membranes:
  - To exclude cord prolapse
  - To note the color of liquor
  - To note the dilatation and effacement of cervix and station of the fetal head
- To assess the pelvis during labor
- Watch out for unfavorable features such as th following:
  - Abnormal uterine contraction
  - Early rupture of the membranes
  - Cervix loosely applied to fetal head
  - Cervical dilatation <1 cm/h in the activ phase (protracted active phase)
  - Descent of fetal head <1 cm/h (pro tracted descent) in spite of regular uterin contraction
  - Arrest of cervical dilatation and nondescen of fetal head in spite of adequate uterin contractions
  - Formation of excessive caput or irreducibl (grade III) molding
  - Fetal distress
- Trial of labor may be continued as long as th progress is satisfactory (evidenced by descen of the fetal head and progressive cervical dilatation) and the maternal and fetal condition remain good. However, if any ominous features appear, trial of labor is terminated and th patient is taken up for CS.

Viva corner

Q1 What do you mean by generally contracted pelvis?

Shape of the pelvis remains unaltered (small gynecoid pelvis) but the diameters in different planes (inlet, outlet, cavity) are shortened.

Q2 Which type of CPD would be best suited for trial of labor?

Moderate degree of brim CPD with normal midpelvis and outlet is best suited for trial of labor. If the head negotiates through the brim by asynclitism, then vaginal delivery is possible.

Q3 Can trial of labor be allowed for outlet contraction?

No. In such cases, the true picture will be evident only in late labor. In addition, isolated outlet contraction is unlikely and is usually associated with contracted midpelvis.

Q4 Does a successful vaginal delivery in the past rule out the possibility of disproportion?

Previous successful vaginal delivery excludes contracted pelvis. However, disproportion can occur rarely because of the following:

- Increase in size of successive babies
- Spondylolisthesis and partial subluxation of sacral promontory that may reduce the pelvic capacity

In a multigravida:

- Prolonged labor due to inadequate uterine contraction is less likely. Other causes such as malpresentation and disproportion are to be ruled out.
- Oxytocin should be used judiciously.

Management of midpelvic and outlet disproportion

- CPD at the midpelvis is defined as one where the fetal head fails to pass through the interspinous diameter.
- Isolated outlet contraction without midpelvic contraction is rare.
- Clinical diagnosis of midpelvic and outlet disproportion can be made only after the head sufficiently comes down into the pelvis (unlike inlet disproportion).
- Elective CS is done if midpelvic and outlet contraction are suspected.

Frequently asked viva questions

1. Summarize the case.
2. What is the provisional diagnosis of the case?
3. List out the differential diagnosis for the case?
4. What are the clinical methods to assess CPD?
5. How will you manage a patient with brim CPD?
6. What is "trial of labor" and how will you conduct trial of labor?
7. List the possible causes of free floating fetal head at term.
8. How can you confirm the diagnosis for mobile head?
9. List the complications associated with free floating head.

17 Supplementary Topics

Section I: Elderly Gravida, Teenage Pregnancy, and Obesity in Pregnancy
Section II: Induction of Labor
Section III: Postpartum Hemorrhage
Section IV: Puerperium—Normal and Abnormal

There are four sections in this chapter and the information provided will be useful during clinical case discussion in obstetrics.

Section I: Elderly gravida, teenage pregnancy, and obesity in pregnancy

ELDERLY GRAVIDA

Definition

Women having pregnancy at >35 years are termed elderly gravida.

Complications in an elderly gravida

Maternal and fetal complications in an elderly gravida are mentioned in Table 17.1.

Incidence of Down syndrome according to maternal age

See Table 17.2

Table 17.2 Incidence of Down syndrome according to maternal age

Age (years)	Incidence of Down syndrome
<30	1:1000
30–35	1:250
40	1:70
45	1:20

Management

- Elderly gravida is a high-risk pregnanc requiring special antenatal care.
- Patient counseling and reassurance are require as these patients are very anxious.
- Prenatal diagnostic tests such as quadruple test noninvasive prenatal testing (NIPT), chorioni villi sampling, and amniocentesis should b offered to detect chromosomal anomalies.
- Regular ultrasonography (USG) and othe antenatal fetal surveillance tests are required.
- Vaginal delivery can be allowed with continuou intrapartum monitoring.

Table 17.1 Complications in an elderly gravida

Maternal complications			Fetal complications
During pregnancy	During labor	Postpartum	
• Abortions • Preeclampsia, chronic hypertension • Gestational diabetes mellitus, overt diabetes mellitus • Fibroid complicating pregnancy • Intrauterine growth restriction • Preterm labor	• Uterine inertia • Incoordinate uterine action • Operative interferences such as instrumental deliveries and cesarean section • Retained placenta due to uterine inertia and fibroid uterus	• Failed lactation	• Chromosomal abnormalities such as Down syndrome

- Operative delivery rates are higher. The need for postoperative care in high dependency units exists.

TEENAGE PREGNANCY

Definition

According to WHO, teenage pregnancy, also known as adolescent pregnancy, is pregnancy in a female under the age of 20 years.

Complications

Complications associated with teenage pregnancy are mentioned in Table 17.3.

Table 17.3 Complications of teenage pregnancy

Antenatal	Intrapartum	Postpartum
• Abortions • Anemia • Malnutrition • Preeclampsia • Intrauterine growth restriction • Preterm labor	• Contracted pelvis • Cephalopelvic disproportion • Increased rate of cesarean section • Perineal lacerations during delivery	• Failed lactation • Emotional unprepared (increased chance of postpartum blues and depression)

Table 17.4 Interpretation of BMI

BMI	Interpretation
19–25	Normal
<19	Undernourished
26–30	Overweight
>30	Obesity

Management

- Teenage pregnancy is a high-risk pregnancy requiring proper antenatal care.
- Psychological support and patient education are required.
- Contraception is advised following delivery for spacing of pregnancy.

OBESITY IN PREGNANCY

- Obesity in pregnancy—prepregnancy BMI >30
- BMI = weight (kg)/[height (m)]^2
- Interpretation of BMI is mentioned in Table 17.4
- Morbid obesity: Body weight >150% of ideal weight is termed morbid obesity.
- Calculation of BMI during pregnancy
  - Prepregnancy weight is used for calculation of BMI during pregnancy.
  - If prepregnancy weight is not available, initial weight during antenatal visit in the first trimester is used for calculation.
- Complications of obesity in pregnancy are mentioned in Table 17.5.

Management

- Regular antenatal care with stress on screening for gestational diabetes mellitus (GDM) and venous thromboembolism
- Calorie restriction and attempt to lose weight during pregnancy should be avoided.
- High-protein, low-fat, and low-carbohydrate diet is advised.

Table 17.5 Complications of obesity in pregnancy

Antenatal	Intrapartum	Postpartum

• Chronic hypertension and preeclampsia (15%)
• Overt diabetes and gestational diabetes mellitus
• Risk of cardiovascular disease, osteoarthritis, and venous thromboembolism
• Mechanical discomfort
• Difficulty in palpating fetal parts, fetal presentation, and fetal heart rate
• Prolonged pregnancy—due to sedentary lifestyle
• Macrosomia
	• Difficulty in getting veins for securing IV line
	• Incoordinate uterine action and uterine inertia
	• Difficulty in pelvic assessment and conducting delivery due to obesity, but bony pelvis is usually normal
	• More likely to have big baby → can lead to shoulder dystocia
	• Increased risk of operative interferences due to big baby and incoordinate uterine action
	• Postpartum hemorrhage
		• Failed lactation
		• Subinvolution
		• Deep vein thrombosis
		• Complications resulting from cesarean section
		  – Postoperative infection
		  – Wound gaping
		• May fail to lose the excess weight gained during pregnancy

Part 1

- Ultrasound may be frequently required to assess fetal presentation, fetal growth, and fetal well-being.
- Anticipate complications and problems due to obesity in pregnancy.

Section II: Induction of labor

INTRODUCTION

When the risk of continuation of the pregnancy either to the mother or the fetus is more, labor can be initiated aiming for a vaginal delivery and is termed induction of labor. Induction of labor may be required for pregnancy complications such as preeclampsia, gestational diabetes mellitus (GDM), Rh isoimmunization, intrauterine growth restriction (IUGR), post-term pregnancy etc., and questions related to this topic are invariably asked in most of the clinical case discussions.

Definitions

Induction of labor It refers to initiation of uterine contractions after the period of viability aiming for a vaginal delivery.

Augmentation of labor It refers to stimulation of uterine contractions that are already present but are ineffective.

Indications for induction of labor

Fetal indications

- **Post-term pregnancy:** Post-term pregnancy is associated with increased perinatal mortality. Induction is usually started at 41 completed weeks of gestation, aiming for delivery before 42 weeks.
- **GDM:** Induction is done at 38 completed weeks of gestation in women with GDM on insulin as there is an increased risk of sudden intrauterine death (IUD) in the last few weeks of pregnancy.
- **Rh isoimmunization**: Induction is done depending on the severity of affection in the fetus in isoimmunized cases. Rh-incompatible pregnancy should not be allowed to cross the expected date of delivery (EDD).
- **IUGR:** Induction is done depending on the severity of IUGR. The risk of preterm has to be weighed against the risk of IUD.
- **Major fetal malformations:** Induction is done in fetuses with major congenital malformations which are incompatible to survive after birth.

Combined (maternal and fetal) indications

- **Preeclampsia:** Induction is done at 37 completed weeks in mild preeclampsia and at 34 completed weeks in severe preeclampsia. Preeclampsia is a progressive disease that comes to a halt only with the delivery of the fetus. Hence, induction is planned once fetal maturity is achieved, as continuation of pregnancy increases the risk of maternal and perinatal morbidity.
- **Premature rupture of membranes (PROM)**: Majority of patients go into spontaneous labor within 24 hours of rupture of membranes without any intervention. However, induction of labor is done following PROM due to the risk of infectious morbidity in the mother and fetus.
- **Antepartum hemorrhage (APH)**
  - *Minor degree placenta previa*: Induction of labor can be done in cases of minor degree placenta previa (Type I and Type IIA).
  - *Abruption*: If the Bishops score is favorable and fetal well-being is assured, labor can be induced by artificial rupture of membranes (ARM) in cases with abruption.
- **Intrauterine death of fetus:** IUD is a definite indication for induction of labor.
  - There is risk of disseminated intravascular coagulation (DIC) in the mother due to thromboplastin released into maternal circulation from the dead fetus (likely to occur if the pregnancy continues beyond 3 weeks following the death of the fetus).
  - Continuation of pregnancy results in mental trauma to the patient.

> **Extra edge**
>
> **Advantages of ARM in abruption**
>
> - Helps in onset of labor
> - Decreases release of thromboplastin into maternal circulation, which is one of the causes for DIC in abruption
> - Further separation of placenta is reduced and bleeding gets controlled to some extent because of initiation of uterine contractions

Maternal indications

Progressively worsening maternal illnesses: These include maternal medical illnesses such as renal

Table 17.6 Bishop's score

Bishop Score = ... (total)			Date of Bishop Score: ..../..../....	
Score	0	1	2	3
Dilation	Closed	1–2	3–4	5
Length	>4	3–4	1–2	0
Consistency	Firm	Medium	Soft	—
Position	Posterior	Midline	Anterior	—
Head: station	−3	−2	−1, 0	+1, +2

diseases, liver diseases, and autoimmune diseases. Induction of labor is done if continuation of pregnancy carries a risk to the life of the mother.

Contraindications for induction

- Contracted pelvis/cephalopelvic disproportion
- Malpresentation
- Cord presentation
- Previous scars on the uterus
- Major degree placenta previa
- Pelvic tumors
- Active genital herpes
- Invasive carcinoma of cervix

Prerequisites for induction

- There should be a genuine indication for induction
- Contraindications should be ruled out
- Confirm dates/fetal maturity
- Assess fetal well-being
- Assess cervix (Bishop's score)
- Provide counseling and obtain informed consent of the patient

Success of induction depends on the degree of ripening of cervix.

- **Ripe cervix:** Indicates a *favorable cervix* for induction
- **Unripe cervix:** Indicates an *unfavorable cervix* for induction

Cervical ripening

It is a process by which cervix becomes soft and thin.

- Prior to onset of labor, the cervix becomes shortened, soft, and dilated, called a ripe cervix. A ripe cervix is likely to result in successful induction.
- Bishop's score is preinduction cervical assessment to assess the ripening of cervix (Table 17.6).
  - Bishop's score ≥6 indicates a favorable cervix
  - Bishop's score <6 indicates an unfavorable cervix

Modified Bishop's score In the original Bishop's scoring, cervical effacement was used in assessment of cervical ripening (Table 17.7). In modified Bishop's scoring, cervical length is used instead of cervical effacement (Table 17.6).

Methods of cervical ripening

Mechanical methods

- **Foley's catheter:** No. 22 F size Foley's catheter is inserted into the cervix and the balloon is inflated with 50 mL normal saline at the level of internal os (Figure 17.1).

Table 17.7 Scoring for cervical effacement in Bishop's score*

Factor	Score			
	0	1	2	3
Cervical effacement	0–30%	40–50%	60–70%	>80%

* All other scoring remains the same.

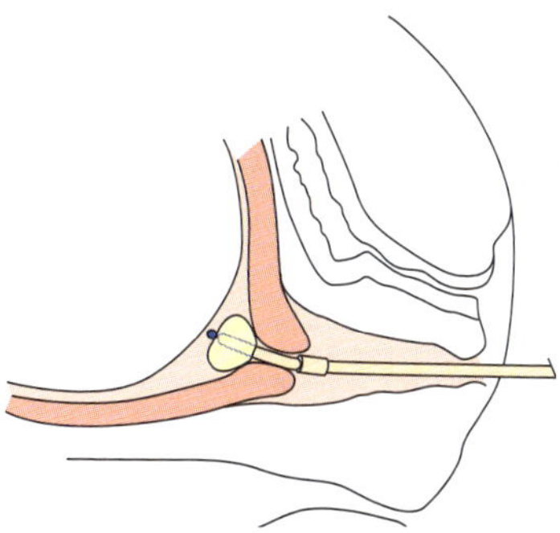

Figure 17.1 Foley's catheter for cervical ripening.

- Principle
  - Foley's catheter causes separation of membranes from the lower uterine segment and release of endogenous prostaglandins which help in dilatation of cervix and initiation of uterine contraction.
- Foley's catheter is removed after 24 hours, if not expelled.

- **Sweeping of membranes (stripping of membranes):** Membranes are stripped off from the lower uterine segment with the fingers introduced through the cervical canal (Figure 17.2).
  - *Principle*: Separation of membranes causes release of endogenous prostaglandins.

Medical methods

- **Dinoprostone gel:** PGE2 gel 0.5 g is given as intracervical application. Reassessment is done after 6 hours and not to exceed 3 doses in 24 hours.
- **Misoprostol tablet:** Misoprostol 25 μg placed vaginally in the posterior fornix or 50 μg is given orally. Dose can be repeated at 4- to 6-hour interval for up to four to six doses.

Methods of induction of labor

The agents used for cervical ripening can cause initiation of uterine contractions and thereby help in induction of labor.

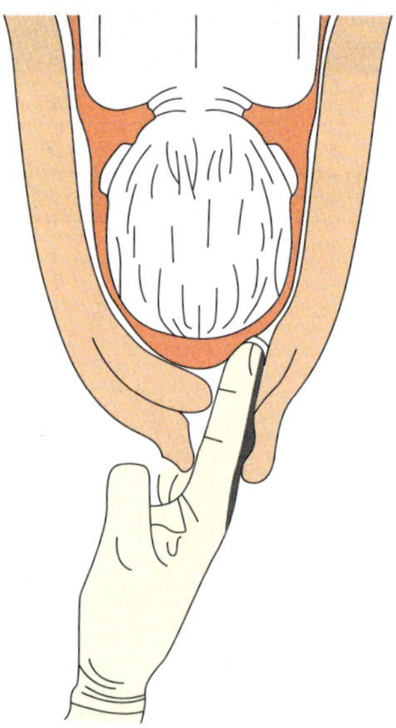

Figure 17.2 Sweeping of membranes.

Mechanical methods (discussed in the section *"methods for cervical ripening"*)

- Foley's catheter
- Sweeping of membranes

Surgical method

- **ARM:** It is the procedure by which the membranes are teased and ruptured with a Kocher's forceps to allow escape of liquor (Figure 17.3).

Advantages of ARM

- Color of the liquor can be made out.
- Intrauterine scalp pH monitoring can be done in case of fetal distress.
- Descent of fetal head can occur to some extent.

Disadvantages of ARM

- Once ARM is done, delivery is mandatory as the patient is committed to deliver
- Risk of cord prolapse

Viva corner

Q1 What are the things to be checked following ARM?

- Color of liquor
- Cord prolapse to be ruled out
- Vaginal bleeding (abruption can occur following sudden uterine decompression)
- Station of the presenting part
- Fetal heart rate (fetal distress can occur in cord compression and occult cord prolapse)

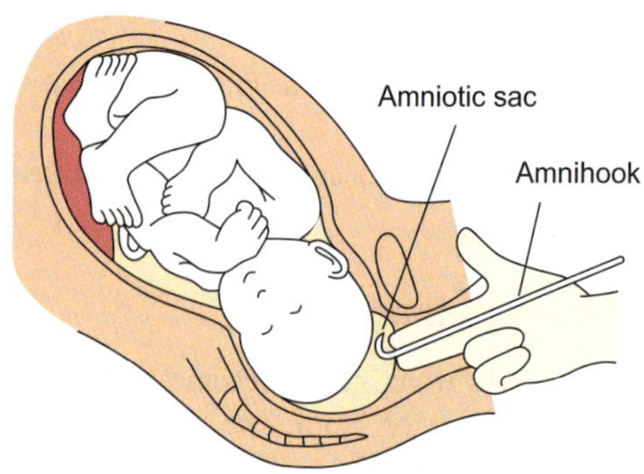

Figure 17.3 Procedure of artificial rupture of membranes.

- Risk of abruption
- Risk of infection

Contraindications of ARM

- IUD
- Cord presentation

Medical methods

- Prostaglandins
  - PGE2 and PGE1 (as discussed under *Medical Methods of Cervical Ripening*)
- Oxytocin
  - It is given as IV infusion.
  - Usually 2.5 units of oxytocin is mixed in 500 mL Ringer's lactate solution.
  - Oxytocin is started at 2.5 milliunits/min and titrated every 30 minutes till effective uterine contractions are established.
  - Infusion rate is calculated according to milliunits/min.

Complications of induction of labor

See Table 17.8

Table 17.8 Complications associated with induction of labor

Maternal risks	Fetal risks
• Failed induction • Increased incidence of cesarean section • Hyperstimulation • Antepartum hemorrhage (abruption)—especially following artificial rupture of membranes due to sudden decompression of uterus • Postpartum hemorrhage • Chorioamnionitis • Amniotic fluid embolism	• Iatrogenic prematurity • Birth asphyxia • Fetal infection • Cord prolapse

Failed induction

If the onset of labor does not start after attempting induction of labor, it is termed failed induction. According to ACOG, "*Failed induction is defined as failure to achieve regular uterine contractions (every 3 minutes) after attempting induction of labor by administrating oxytocin at least for 12 to 24 hours after rupture of membranes.*" Cesarean section (CS) is done in cases with failed induction of labor.

High-yield points

Condition in which ARM is the induction method of choice

Abruption

Viva corner

Q1 How will you calculate the dose of oxytocin when given in titrated dose?

- When 2.5 units of oxytocin is added to 500 mL Ringer lactate (RL) solution, it means that
  - 500 mL solution contains 2.5 units (2500 milliunits) of oxytocin.
  - 1 milliliter contains 5 milliunits of oxytocin (1 mL = 16 drops).
  - 16 drops contain 5 milliunits of oxytocin.
  - 8 drops contain 2.5 milliunits of oxytocin.
  - When the flow rate is started at 8 drops/min, it means that the dose of oxytocin is 2.5 milliunits/min. Oxytocin drip is titrated every 30 minutes by 8 drops/min (2.5 milliunits/min) till effective uterine contractions (see table below).

When effective uterine contractions are not achieved with 2.5 units oxytocin titrated up to 64 drops/min, then 5 units oxytocin in 500 mL RL drip is started at 32 drops/min and titrated.

- If RL solution 500 mL contains 5 units (5000 milliunits) of oxytocin
  - 1 milliliter (16 drops) contains 10 milliunits of oxytocin.
  - When drip is started at 32 drops/min, it is equivalent to 20 milliunits/min (equivalent to 2.5 units at 64 drops/min) and titrated till effective uterine contractions.

(CONTD...)

Part 1

(...CONTD)

Viva corner

Table **Titrated dose of oxytocin**

2.5 units oxytocin		5 units oxytocin	
Drops/min	Dose in milliunits/min	Drops/min	Dose in milliunits/min
8	2.5	32	20
16	5	40	25
24	7.5	48	30
32	10	56	35
40	12.5	64	40
48	15		
56	17.5		
64	20		

Section III: Postpartum hemorrhage

INTRODUCTION

Postpartum hemorrhage (PPH) is a major obstetric emergency commonly encountered in obstetric practice and is a leading cause of maternal morbidity and mortality. Questions from this topic are consistently asked in most of the clinical case discussions and has been discussed in detail in this section.

WHO definition of PPH

Amount of blood loss of 500 mL or more following vaginal delivery or blood loss of 1000 mL or more following CS is defined as PPH.

Clinical definition of PPH

Any amount of bleeding from or into the genital tract following delivery of the baby up to the end of puerperium that adversely affects the general condition of the mother is termed PPH.

Primary PPH Primary PPH is defined as abnormal bleeding from or into the genital tract that occurs within 24 hours of delivery of the baby.

Secondary PPH Secondary PPH is defined as abnormal bleeding from or into the genital tract that occurs 24 hours after delivery, up to 6 weeks postpartum.

Important causes of PPH

Acronym: Remember "four Ts"
- Tone (atonic uterus)—atonic PPH
- Trauma (genital tract injuries)—traumatic PPH
- Tissue (retained placental tissue)
- Thrombin (coagulopathy)

Atonic PPH

- Uterine atony is responsible for 90% cases of PPH.
- Uterine atony refers to the failure of the uterine muscles to contract normally following delivery of the baby and placenta.
- Separation of the placenta from the wall of the uterus results in shearing off, of the maternal blood vessels. Under normal circumstances, the contraction of uterine muscles causes compression of these blood vessels. However, if the uterine musculature does not effectively contract, the bleeding continues to occur resulting in atonic PPH.

Risk factors for atonic PPH

- Grand multiparity
- Overdistension of uterus—multiple pregnancy, hydramnios, and big baby
- Induction of labor
- Prolonged/precipitate labor
- Anesthesia (halogenated drugs like halothane)
- APH (placenta previa, abruption etc.)

Traumatic PPH

It occurs mainly due to injuries to the genital tract that occur during delivery.

Causes of traumatic PPH

- Episiotomy extension
- Tears and lacerations of perineum, vagina, or cervix
- Pelvic hematoma
- Rupture uterus
- More common following instrumental deliveries

Clinical features in PPH

- Patient bleeds profusely following delivery
- The general condition (pallor, pulse, BP) of the patient depends on the amount of blood loss
- Placing a hand on the uterus will reveal whether PPH is atonic or traumatic
  - *If the uterus is flabby:* It indicates atonic PPH
  - *If the uterus is well contracted:* It indicates traumatic PPH

Management of PPH

PPH can unexpectedly complicate even normal deliveries and hence all obstetricians should be prepared to prevent and treat this potential life-threatening emergency.

Preventive measures for PPH

Antenatal measures—preventive measures for PPH begin from the antenatal period

- Blood group and Rh typing is done for all antenatal women
- Correction of anemia
- Placental localization by ultrasound
- Women at risk for PPH should be identified

Intrapartum measures

- Blood should be cross matched and kept available.
- PPH should be anticipated in women at risk.
- Active management of third stage of labor (AMTSL) reduces postpartum blood loss. AMTSL as a prophylactic measure for PPH prevention has the following components (new WHO 2012 recommendations):
  - Uterotonic: Administration of uterotonics, preferably oxytocin (10 units IV/IM), immediately following the delivery of the baby
  - Delayed cord clamping: Delay clamping the cord for at least 1–3 minutes to reduce the risk of infant anemia
  - Delivery of the placenta by controlled cord traction (CCT)
  - Postpartum vigilance: Assessment of uterine tone to ensure a contracted uterus; continue to check every 15 minutes for 2 hours. If there is uterine atony, perform fundal massage and monitor more frequently.

Curative measures for PPH

Immediate steps Resuscitation of the patient and evaluation of cause and management of PPH should go hand in hand.

- Call for help.
- Check the vitals—pallor, pulse, and BP.
- Secure two wide-bore IV lines and start resuscitation with crystalloid solution infusion to restore the fluid volume until blood is available.
- Send blood for hemoglobin estimation, complete blood counts, blood grouping and typing, cross-matching and reservation, and transfuse blood if required.
- Whenever there is excessive bleeding after delivery, it is most often due to uterine atonicity. Therefore, it is prudent to administer oxytocics immediately.
- Empty the bladder by inserting an indwelling urinary catheter (distended bladder can interfere with uterine contractions).
- Palpate the uterus
  - *If uterus is relaxed*: Indicates atonic PPH
  - *If uterus is well contracted*: Indicates traumatic PPH (explore the genital tract)
- Further management depends on the cause for PPH.

Management of atonic PPH

- Administer oxytocic drugs (drugs which contract the uterus).
- Explore the uterine cavity for any retained placental bits or fragments (interferes with uterine contraction).
- Bimanual compression of the uterus—massage the uterus to aid in contraction of the uterine musculature (Figure 17.4).
- The vagina and cervix must be inspected for lacerations and tears (traumatic PPH may be coexisting with atonic PPH).

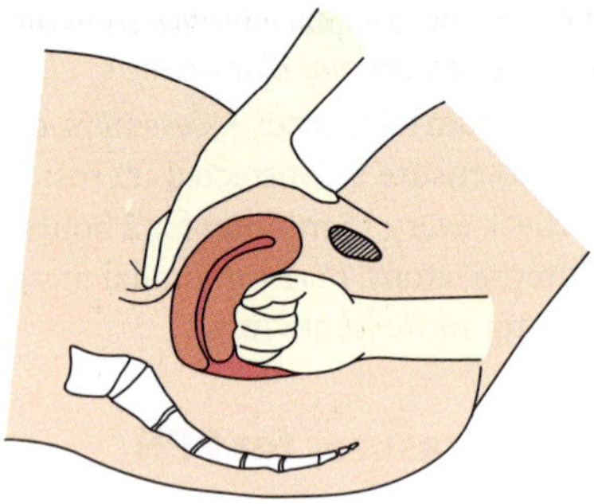

Figure 17.4 Bimanual uterine compression.

Oxytocics used in the medical management of PPH

- Start oxytocin IV infusion, 20 units in 500 mL normal saline at about 60 drops/min.
- Injection methergin 0.2 mg IV or IM can be repeated up to two doses.
- Injection carboprost (PGF2 alpha 250 µg IM) can be repeated at intervals of >15 minutes, up to a maximum of eight doses. Intramyometrial injection of carboprost 250 µg may be given.
- Misoprostol (PGE1) 800 µg can be given orally or placed per rectally *(WHO recommends PO 400/600 µg, GOI recommends 800 µg)*.

If all the conservative measures fail to control PPH, then surgical intervention must be considered for controlling PPH.

Surgical measures to control PPH

- Explore the uterus under general anesthesia.
- Repair any genital tract injuries in case of traumatic PPH.

Hemostatic compression sutures

B-Lynch compression sutures

- The B-Lynch suture is a uterine bracing suture that is secured vertically around the anterior and posterior uterine walls.
- It controls bleeding by compressing the anterior and posterior uterine walls together, thereby causing hemostatic compression of the uterine fundus and lower uterine segment.
- Prior to applying the B-Lynch suture, bimanual compression test must be performed—the uterus is bimanually compressed and if the bleeding is controlled temporarily, then B-Lynch sutures are likely to be effective.
- The sutures are first anchored in the anterio aspect of the lower uterine segment, passed ove the uterine fundus, anchored in the posterio aspect of the lower uterine segment, and then agai brought back anteriorly passing over the fundu of the uterus. These sutures are finally anchore near the entrance point on the anterior aspect o the lower uterine segment. Simultaneously, th uterus is massaged and manually compressed i order to reduce its size (Figure 17.5).
- Advantages: This technique is safe and effective and helps to retain future fertility.

Modified B-Lynch suture

It is a modification of the B-Lynch technique where separate sutures are placed compressin the anterior and posterior walls and sutures ar anchored over the uterine fundus to prevent fron slipping (Figure 17.6).

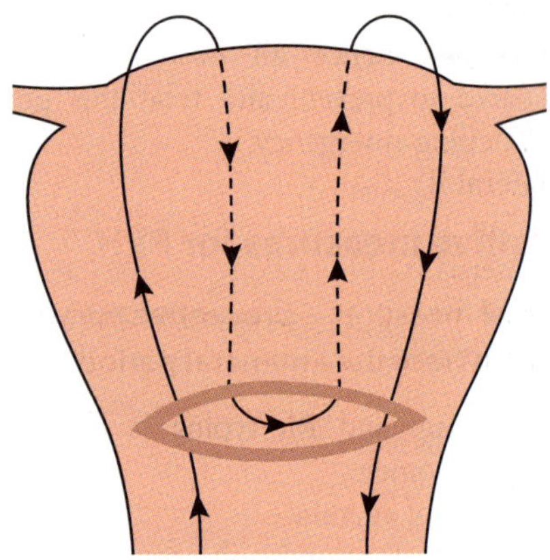

Figure 17.5 B-Lynch sutures.

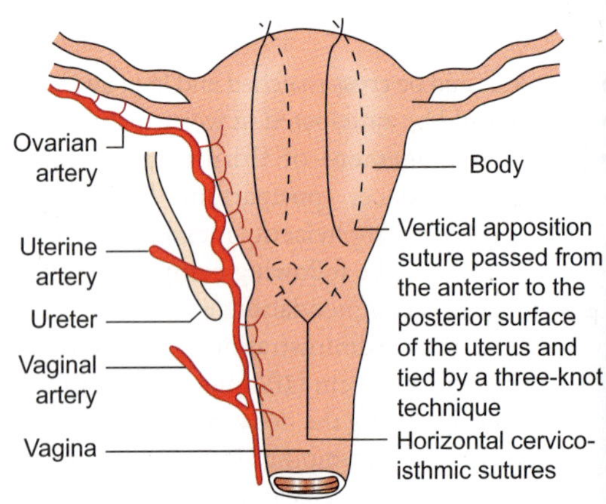

Figure 17.6 Modified B-Lynch sutures.

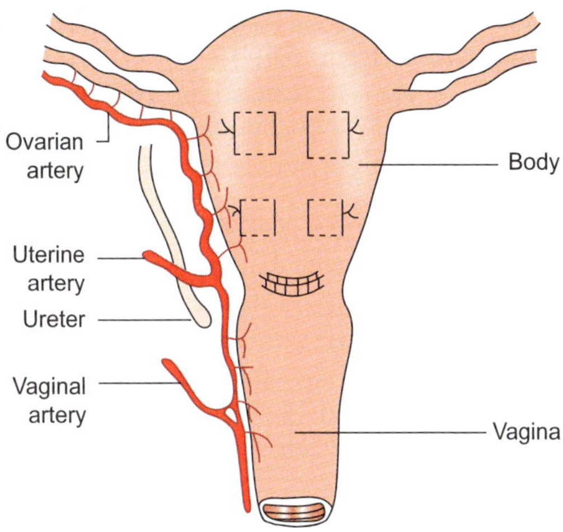

Figure 17.7 Cho sutures.

Multiple Cho sutures

This involves placement of multiple square sutures involving both the anterior and posterior walls of uterus (Figure 17.7).

Uterine devascularization procedures

- **Bilateral ligation of uterine vessels and utero-ovarian vessels:** 90% of the blood supply to the uterus is via the uterine artery. Ligation of uterine vessels at the level of uterine isthmus helps to control bleeding (Figure 17.8). If the bleeding still remains uncontrollable, ligation of utero-ovarian anastomosis just below the ovarian ligament is done.
- **Bilateral internal iliac artery ligation:** This method causes 85% reduction in pulse pressure in the arteries distal to the ligation and is highly effective in controlling PPH. Fertility is preserved.

(***Note:*** *Uterine artery is a branch from the anterior division of the internal iliac artery.*)

- **Uterine artery embolization:** In this procedure, angiographic embolization of bilateral uterine artery is done with small pellets of Polyvinyl alcohol (PVA) particles in Gelfoam, which acts as an occluding agent. An interventional radiologist is required to perform the procedure.
- **Uterine packing:** Packing of the uterine cavity can be considered in atonic PPH refractory to treatment. However, it is associated with complications such as concealed bleeding and infection.
- **Uterine tamponade:** Attempts have been made to control bleeding by uterine tamponade with hydrostatic balloon catheters (Ebb balloon tamponade system for uterine and vaginal tamponade, Sengstaken–Blakemore esophageal catheter, Bakri balloon and condom balloon tamponade can be used for uterine tamponade). The balloon is inflated inside the cavity with 200–500 mL saline and is kept for 12–24 hours to achieve hemostasis (Figure 17.9).
- **Hysterectomy:** Hysterectomy is the final step if the patient is not responding to the above-mentioned surgical methods.

Management of traumatic PPH

- Bleeding in spite of a contracted uterus points to traumatic PPH.
- Presence of tears and lacerations in the genital tract is an important cause for traumatic PPH.
- The genital tract is explored under illumination and anesthesia and hemostasis is achieved.

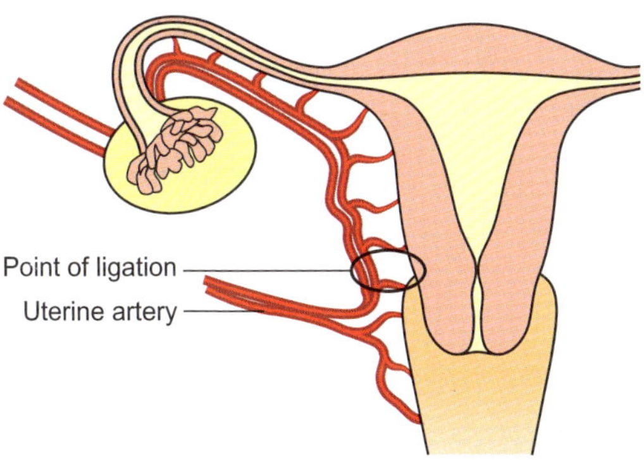

Figure 17.8 Uterine artery ligation.

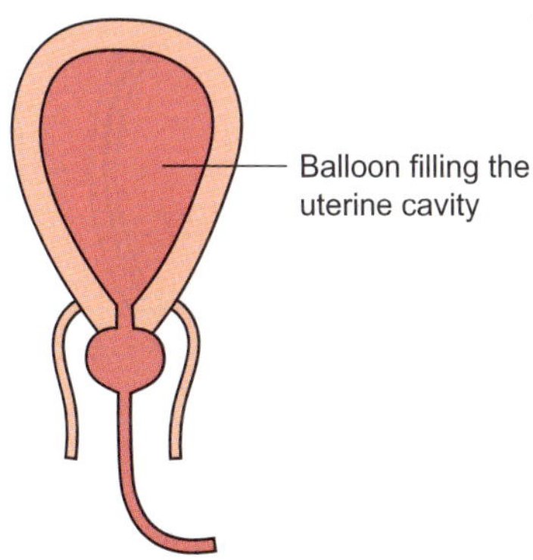

Figure 17.9 Ebb (uterine + vaginal) balloon tamponade.

Part 1

RETAINED PLACENTA

- The average time from delivery of the baby until placental expulsion is about 10 minutes.
- The placenta is said to be retained when it is not expelled even 30 minutes after the delivery of the baby (according to the WHO, 15 minutes).
- Longer intervals are associated with an increased risk of PPH.

Management of retained placenta

The following steps can be taken to facilitate the placental delivery:

- Uterine massage must be performed.
- Oxytocics can be repeated, e.g., oxytocin 10 IU given IV/IM.
- Bladder must be emptied.
- Controlled cord traction must be attempted to deliver the placenta.
- If the placenta appears to be trapped in the lower uterine segment, a vaginal examination may be performed to remove the placenta.
- If the placenta does not deliver even after 30 minutes of delivery of the baby, the patient is shifted to operation theatre for manual exploration of placenta under general anesthesia.
- Further management depends on whether a distinct cleavage plane between the placenta and the uterine wall can be located or not.
- If a distinct cleavage plane can be located, then manual removal of the placenta is done (described below).
- If a distinct cleavage plane cannot be located, diagnosis of morbidly adherent placenta should be considered. The various types of morbidly adherent placenta are placenta accreta, increta, and percreta (Figure 17.10).
- Steps of manual removal of placenta and management of morbidly adherent placenta are mentioned in the following subsections.

Steps of manual removal of placenta

- Under general anesthesia, the patient is placed in lithotomy position and bladder is catheterized.
- Uterus is stabilized with one hand placed over the abdomen and the other hand is introduced inside the vagina in a cone-shaped manner.
- The hand is passed into the uterine cavity along the umbilical cord.
- As the placental margin is reached, the ulnar border of the hand is used to gradually separate the placenta from the uterine wall.
- The placental tissue is gradually separated by using the sideways slicing movements of the fingers.
- Once the placenta has separated, it is grasped with the hand and gradually taken out.
  - The abdominal hand helps in stabilizing the fundus and in guiding the movements of the fingers within the uterine cavity, until the placenta has completely separated.

Management of morbidly adherent placenta

- In parous women, hysterectomy is indicated in case of morbidly adherent placenta.
- In patients desirous of fertility, conservative management includes clamping and cutting the umbilical cord as close as possible to its base, leaving the placenta behind, which gets autolyzed in due course of time.
- Appropriate antibiotics should be given.

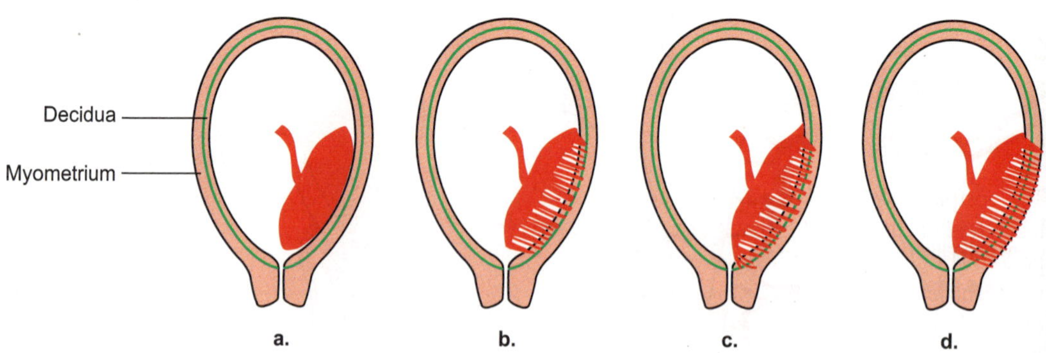

Figure 17.10 Adherent placenta. **a.** Normal placenta, the villi do not invade the myometrium. **b.** Placenta accreta, the villi attach to the myometrium. **c.** Placenta increta, the villi invade the myometrium. **d.** Placenta percreta, the villi invade the entire depth of the myometrium and extend to the serosa.

- Methotrexate therapy can be given in the postnatal period.
- Management of partial (focal) placenta accreta includes removal of the placental tissue as much as possible.

High-yield points

Causes of secondary PPH

- Retained bits of cotyledon or membranes (most common)
- Infection and separation of slough, thereby exposing bleeding vessels
- Endometritis and subinvolution of the placental site
- Secondary hemorrhage following CS usually occurs between 10th and 14th postoperative day (it is due to separation of slough exposing a bleeding vessel or bleeding from granulation tissue)

Complications due to PPH

Complications related to PPH include the following:
- Blood loss resulting in hypovolemic shock, DIC, septicemia, and death
- Acute renal failure
- Blood transfusion reaction
- Multiple organ failure associated with circulatory collapse and decreased organ perfusion
- Need for emergency surgical intervention including hysterectomy and loss of childbearing potential
- Puerperal sepsis
- Lactation failure
- Sheehan syndrome (Pan hypopituitarism)

Section IV: Puerperium—normal and abnormal

INTRODUCTION

The postpartum period in general tends to receive less attention than the antenatal and intrapartum period. The postpartum period is significant because the parturient and her newborn are vulnerable and can easily slip from "health" to "ill health." Hence, it is important to understand the changes that take place in normal puerperium, so that appropriate care can be instituted to the mother and baby in case of any deviation from normal.

Terminologies

Puerperium

Puerperium is the period following childbirth, extending up to 6 weeks postpartum. During this period the pelvic organs return to the prepregnant state. It is arbitrarily divided into
- Immediate—within 24 hours
- Early—within 7 days
- Remote—from 7 days to 6 weeks postpartum

Involution

Return of genital organs to the prepregnancy state following delivery is termed involution. Uterus is taken as a reference guide for involution because its size can be clinically measured (Figure 17.11).
- Immediately following delivery, uterine fundus is at the level of umbilicus.
- In the first 24 hours following delivery, there is no change in fundal height.
- From the second day onward, there is a steady decrease in fundal height by 1.25 cm (1/2 inch) per day.
- The uterus becomes a pelvic organ by 2 weeks postpartum. However, it takes about 6 weeks postpartum for all pelvic organs including the uterus to return to the normal prepregnant state.

Lochia

Lochia is the normal postpartum vaginal discharge with a characteristic fishy odor present for about 3–4 weeks following delivery. It contains shreds of decidua, RBCs, epithelial cells, leukocytes, and bacteria.

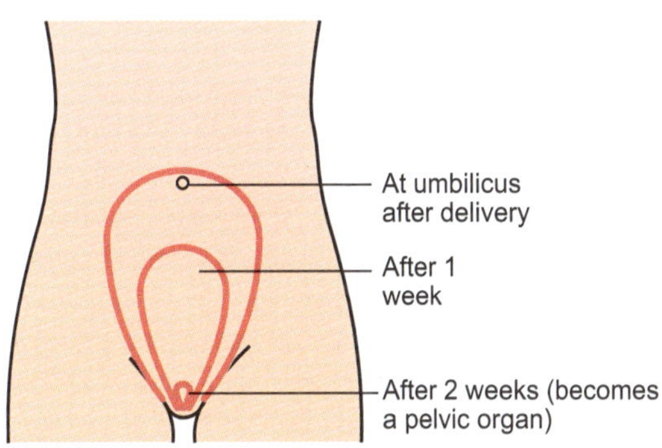

Figure 17.11 Involution of uterus.

Types of lochia

- **Lochia rubra:** Lochia in the first 3–4 days of puerperium is red in color. It consists of blood, shreds of fetal membranes and decidua, vernix caseosa, lanugo, and meconium.
- **Lochia serosa:** After 3–4 days, lochia becomes progressively pale and persists for about 1 week. It consists of less RBCs but more leukocytes, mucus, and bacteria.
- **Lochia alba:** Lochia is white in color and persists for 1–2 weeks. It contains plenty of leukocytes, mucus, epithelial cells, and bacteria.

Management of normal puerperium

The principles in management during puerperium are as follows:

- To restore the health of the mother
- To prevent infections
- To promote breastfeeding
- To motivate the couple for contraception

Postnatal care

It includes the following:

- **Monitoring vitals**
- **Early ambulation:** Early ambulation is encouraged as it reduces the risk of deep venous thrombosis.
- **Diet:** During lactation, calorie and protein requirements are more than those during the nonpregnant state (+550 kcal/day and +30 g/day proteins). Advise on adequate diet and plenty of fluid intake.
- **Bladder care:** The patient is encouraged to pass urine as early as possible following delivery. She may have acute retention of urine due to pain and spasm following bruising of the paraurethral and perineal region.
- **Care of the bowel:** Early ambulation, high-fiber diet, and fluids reduce constipation problems.
- **Episiotomy wound care:** The patient is advised to maintain personal cleanliness of vulval region. Analgesics are prescribed and sitz bath advised to relieve pain. In case of persistent perineal pain, a vaginal and rectal examination should be done to rule out vulval hematoma, wound gaping, and infection.
- **Care of the breasts:** Following normal delivery, breastfeeding should be started as early as possible. Initial frequency should be at 2–3 hours interval. The nipples should be cleaned and kept dry after each feed.
- **Breastfeeding:** Effective milk transfer from the breast into the mouth of the baby occurs when infant's mouth is wide open, chin touches the breast, and the nipple and areola are within the baby's mouth between the tongue and the palate. This is termed proper latching during breastfeeding (Figure 17.12).
- **Care of the neonate:** It includes keeping the baby warm and handling it with clean hands.
- **Postnatal exercises:** Exercises to improve tone of abdominal and pelvic muscles are advised.
- **Contraception advice:** Nonlactating women should be advised to start contraception after 3 weeks of delivery and the lactating women should start contraception after 3 months of delivery.
- **Drugs:** Analgesics for pain management during initial few days following delivery; hematinics should be continued for at least 3 months postpartum.
- **Discharge from the hospital:** Patient can be discharged after 24–48 hours following delivery.
- **Advice at discharge**
  - Advice on diet—increased calories and protein intake during lactation
  - Exclusive breastfeeding for 6 months
  - Iron and calcium supplementation for 3 months
  - Advise on contraception

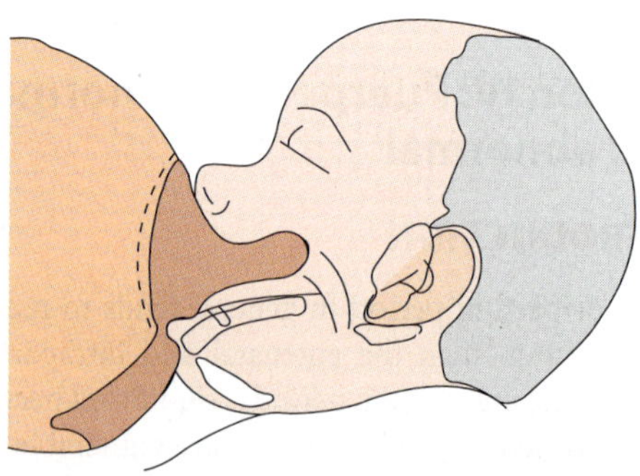

Figure 17.12 Proper latching during breastfeeding. The infant's mouth is wide open, chin touches the breast, and the nipple and areola are within the baby's mouth between the tongue and the palate.

– Postpartum exercises
– Immunization schedule for the baby
- **Postnatal checkup**: It is scheduled after 6 weeks or earlier in case of any complaints.

Choice of contraception during postpartum period

- Progesterone-only contraceptives: DMPA (injectable progestin) or progestin-only oral pill (minipill) can be advised at 6 weeks postpartum.
- Intrauterine contraceptive device (IUCD)
  – Postplacental IUCD insertion is safe and effective. However, expulsion rates are higher compared with interval insertion.
  – IUCD can be inserted at 6 weeks postpartum.
- OCPs interfere with milk secretion and hence are contraindicated in the initial 6 months in lactating women. They can be prescribed after 6 months following delivery.
- Barrier methods can be practiced but failure rate is high.
- Couples who have completed family should be encouraged to undergo sterilization procedure.

ABNORMAL PUERPERIUM

Complications during puerperium

- Postpartum hemorrhage and shock
- Puerperal sepsis
- Subinvolution
- Thromboembolism
- Breast complications—engorgement, mastitis, and abscess formation
- Urinary complications—infection, retention, and incontinence
- Postpartum blues, depression, and psychosis

Part 1

Viva corner

Q1 Why there is amenorrhea during puerperium?

Persistently elevated prolactin levels during lactation inhibit follicle-stimulating hormone (FSH) and luteinizing hormone (LH), thereby suppressing ovulation and causing amenorrhea.

- In a nonlactating woman, ovulation may return as early as 3 weeks postpartum.
- In a woman who is exclusively breastfeeding, the contraceptive protection due to anovulation remains up to 6 months postpartum in the majority of cases.

Q2 What are "after pains?"

It refers to spasmodic lower abdominal pain due to vigorous uterine contractions as a result of oxytocin release, commonly present during suckling.

Q3 What is "rooming-in?"

Rooming-in refers to keeping the baby with the mother after delivery.

Q4 What do you mean by exclusive breastfeeding (EBF)?

EBF means feeding the baby only with breast milk. Water or formula feeds are not allowed. EBF is recommended for the first 6 months following delivery.

Q5 What are the benefits of breastfeeding?

- Benefits to the baby
  – Contains all nutrients in appropriate and easily digestible form for the baby
  – Immunological protection—contains IgA that protects the baby from infections and diarrhea
  – Increases bonding between mother and baby
  – Less risk of allergies, DM, and cardiac diseases later in life
- Benefits to the mother
  – Helps in involution of uterus
  – Natural contraception
  – Helps in weight reduction
  – Protects against breast cancer

Q6 What is milk ejection or milk let-down reflex?

Suckling causes nipple and areola stimulation → ascending tactile impulse via thoracic sensory nerve (T4, 5, 6) to paraventricular and supraoptic nuclei of hypothalamus → release of oxytocin

(CONTD...)

(...CONTD)

Viva corner

from posterior pituitary → contraction of myoepithelial cells of the alveoli → milk let down and ejection occurs.

Q7 What are the conditions that require lactation suppression?

- Stillbirth
- Neonatal death
- Conditions where breastfeeding is contraindicated
  - Infant with galactosemia
  - Active, untreated tuberculosis
  - Maternal chemotherapy
- Drug for lactation suppression—cabergoline (bromocriptin analog)
  - *For lactation inhibition (lactation not yet established):* 0.5 mg two tablets stat
  - *For lactation suppression (established lactation):* 0.25 mg two tablets stat

Common complications encountered during the puerperium are discussed in the following subsections.

Puerperal pyrexia

Definition A rise in temperature of 100.4°F (38°C) or more on two separate occasions, 24 hours apart, within the first 10 days following delivery, excluding the first 24 hours following delivery is called puerperal pyrexia.

Common causes of puerperal pyrexia

- Puerperal sepsis
- Urinary tract infection
- Wound infection
- Breast engorgement and infection
- Pulmonary infection
- Thrombophlebitis

Puerperal sepsis

Definition Infection of the genital tract after delivery is termed puerperal sepsis. Primary sites of infection are perineum, cervix, vagina, and uterus.

Note *Puerperal pyrexia is considered to be due to puerperal sepsis, unless proved otherwise.*

Common predisposing factors for puerperal sepsis

- Anemia and malnutrition
- Premature rupture of membranes
- Prolonged rupture of membranes >18 hours
- Repeated vaginal examination
- Prolonged labor
- Traumatic instrumental delivery
- More common in cesarean than in vaginal delivery

Common organisms

- Aerobes—group A *Streptococcus* (GAS), *Staphylococcus*, *Enterococcus*, *Escherichia coli*, *Pseudomonas*, and *Klebsiella*
- Anerobes—*Peptococcus*, *Peptostreptococcus*, *Bacteroides*, and *Clostridium* species

Clinical features

Symptoms The patient may complain of the following:

- Fever
- Abdominal pain
- Foul smelling lochia
- Pain and discharge from wound sites
- Patient may have PPH (secondary PPH due to infection and nonepithelialization of placenta wound)

Clinical examination findings

- Rise in temperature
- Tachycardia
- Subinvoluted and tender uterus may be present on abdominal and bimanual examination if uterine infection has set in
- Lochia—may be unhealthy and foul smelling if there is uterine infection
- The episiotomy wound or abdominal wound in CS may appear red and indurated with purulent discharge, dehiscence may be present

Complications

Infection can spread outside the uterus leading to the following:

- Pelvic peritonitis
- Generalized peritonitis
- Thrombophlebitis
- Septicemia and shock
- Increased maternal morbidity and mortality

Management

Investigations

It depends on the clinical examination findings:

- Complete blood count
- Urine examination for pus cells, culture and sensitivity
- High vaginal swab for culture and sensitivity
- Pus from the wound for culture and sensitivity
- Blood culture and sensitivity, peripheral smear is checked for malarial and filarial parasites
- Coagulation profile if Gram-negative septicemia is suspected
- Pelvic ultrasound—to detect any retained bits inside the uterus, any foreign body inside the uterus and to rule out pelvic abscess
- Doppler USG study in suspected cases of deep venous thrombosis (DVT) to detect venous thrombosis

Treatment

- Monitor vitals.
- Maintain an intake and output chart.
- Maintain adequate fluid intake—oral fluids are encouraged. IV fluids may be required if patient is not tolerating orals or if dehydrated.
- Correct anemia—blood transfusion may be required if the patient is severely anemic.
- Antibiotics: Gentamicin (2 mg/kg IV loading dose followed by 1.5 mg/kg IV q 8H) and ampicillin (1 g IV q 6H) plus metronidazole (500 mg IV q 8H) should be started. Cefotaxime 1 g IV q 8H is an alternative to gentamicin plus ampicillin.
- Antibiotic regimen can be changed based on the culture and sensitivity report. The treatment is continued for at least 7–10 days.
- Symptomatic treatment with antipyretics and tepid sponging as required.

Other complications during puerperium are described below.

Subinvolution of uterus

It refers to arrest or delayed involution of uterus that normally occurs following delivery.

Causes for subinvolution of uterus

- Overdistension of the uterus (twins, polyhydramnios)
- Retained products of conception (placental bits)
- Puerperal sepsis
- Anemia and other maternal illness
- Fibroid uterus

Urinary problems in puerperium

- **Urinary tract infections:** These are common due to catheterization during labor or due to stasis of urine during puerperium.
- **Retention of urine:** It may be due to pain and spasm following bruising of paraurethral and perineal regions.
- **Incontinence of urine:** Stress incontinence is common. True incontinence can occur due to fistula formation in obstructed labor.
- **Vesicovaginal fistula (VVF):** VVF may occur as a complication of obstructed labor due to pressure necrosis of urinary bladder.

Breast problems during puerperium

Breast engorgement

Symptoms

Pain and feeling of tenseness or heaviness in both breasts, transient rise of temperature, and painful breastfeeding

Treatment

- Analgesics
- Breast support
- Putting the baby to breast regularly at frequent intervals
- Manual expression of any remaining milk after each feed

Cracked nipples

Nipples become painful during suckling. If infection sets in, it may spread to deeper tissue to cause mastitis.

Treatment

- Prevention is by local cleanliness during pregnancy and in puerperium to prevent crust formation over the nipples.
- Correct latching provides relief from pain and aids in rapid healing.
- Purified lanolin can be applied to hasten healing.
- In severe cases, breast pump or nipple shields can be used.

Retracted and flat nipples

- It is common in primigravida.
- **Treatment:** Most cases of retracted or flat nipple will not cause problem during breastfeeding. In severe cases, milk can be expressed out manually or by using a breast pump.

Acute mastitis

Clinical features

- Fever with chills, pain, and swelling in one quadrant of the breast (usually unilateral)
- On examination—swelling of the breast that is tense and tender, and the overlying skin becomes warm and flushed
- Common organisms—*Staphylococcus aureus*, *S. epidermidis*, and *Streptococcus viridians*
- If left untreated, it can lead to formation of breast abscess

Treatment

- Breast support
- Antibiotics
- Analgesics
- Breastfeeding can be continued

Breast abscess

- Clinical features are similar to mastitis but with marked tenderness and fluctuation.
- Treatment: Abscess should be drained under anesthesia. Breastfeeding is continued in the uninvolved side until infection resolves.

Deep vein thrombosis during puerperium

Risk factors

These include advanced age, obesity, anemia, operative delivery, immobility, smoking, and prior DVT.

Symptoms

These include rise in temperature, pain in the calf muscles, and edema of legs.

Examination findings

- Asymmetrical leg edema
- Positive Moses' sign—pain on squeezing the calf muscles
- Positive Homan's sign—pain in the calf on dorsiflexion of the foot

Investigations

- Doppler USG
- Magnetic resonance imaging (MRI)—most accurate in diagnosis

Treatment

This includes foot-end elevation, analgesics, antibiotics, and anticoagulant therapy with heparin.

Prophylaxis for venous thromboembolism (VTE)

- Prevention of trauma, sepsis, and anemia during pregnancy and labor
- Use of elastic compression stocking or pneumatic compression devices during surgery
- Leg exercises and early ambulation following operative delivery
- Low-molecular-weight heparin (LMWH) prophylaxis during pregnancy and 6 weeks postpartum in high-risk women with history of venous thromboembolism

Psychiatric illnesses during puerperium

Puerperal blues

- A transient state of mental illness, observed 4–5 days after delivery and lasting for few days
- Clinical features—depression, anxiety, insomnia, and negative feelings

Postpartum depression

- More gradual in onset over 4–6 months following delivery
- Clinical features—insomnia, social withdrawal, irritability, and suicidal tendency
- Recurrence is high in subsequent pregnancies

Viva corner

Q1 Can you list some puerperal emergencies?

- Postpartum hemorrhage
- Shock—hypovolemic or endotoxic shock
- Postpartum eclampsia
- Pulmonary embolism
- Acute inversion of uterus
- Postpartum cardiomyopathy

Postpartum psychosis (schizophrenia)

- Onset is relatively sudden, usually within 4 days of delivery. It is common in women with a past history of psychosis or with a positive family history.
- Clinical features: Fear, restlessness, confusion, hallucinations, delusions, suicidal, and infanticidal tendencies.
- Recurrence is high in subsequent pregnancies.

Psychiatric counseling and appropriate therapy should be instituted in patients with psychiatric illnesses during puerperium.

Frequently asked viva questions

1. What are the complications anticipated in an elderly gravida?
2. What difficulties will you encounter in managing an obese pregnant woman?
3. What are the various indications for induction of labor?
4. What are the various methods available for ripening of cervix?
5. What are the various methods available for induction of labor?
6. How will you start an oxytocin drip?
7. What are the various complications in an induced labor?
8. What are the risk factors for PPH?
9. What are the common causes of PPH?
10. What is active management of third stage of labor (AMTSL)?
11. What are the drugs available to control PPH?
12. How will you manage a patient who is bleeding profusely following delivery?
13. What are the various surgical interventions available in the management of PPH?
14. What advise will you give to a postnatal mother?
15. What are the common causes of puerperal fever?
16. What are the clinical features of puerperal sepsis and how will you manage the patient?

Part 2
Gynecology

18 History Taking and Examination

Introduction

Gynecology deals with the diseases of female genital organs. Gynecological problems commonly encountered in clinical practice include abnormal menstrual bleeding, pelvic pain, white discharge P/V, mass abdomen, mass descending P/V, infertility, and gynecological malignancies, etc. Taking a detailed history and performing a physical examination are of utmost importance for diagnosis of the gynecological problem and detection of underlying pathology. This chapter deals with history taking and examination in gynecology. It is important for the doctor to maintain good communication with the patient in order to elicit proper history because the gynecological history includes asking certain private and confidential questions to women, about which they may be reluctant while telling the history.

BASICS IN GYNECOLOGY

- **Menstrual cycle:** Menstruation is a cyclical physiological uterine bleeding due to shedding of the endometrium, as a result of interplay of hormones at hypothalamic–pituitary–ovarian axis.
  - It occurs from the time of menarche to menopause.
  - Menstrual cycles normally occur once in 28 days (range of 24–38 days) with blood loss of 5–80 mL and flow lasting 4–8 days.
  - The menstrual cycle has two phases:
    - Proliferative phase: Under influence of estrogen (first half of the cycle)
    - Secretory phase: Under influence of progesterone (second half of the cycle following ovulation, up to the start of the next menstrual cycle)
  - Variation in cycle length is due to variation in length of the proliferative phase, as the secretory phase (postovulatory phase) is fixed (14 days prior to the start of next menstruation).

Terminologies

- **Menarche:** It refers to the first menstrual period.
- **Perimenopause:** It refers to the years of transition before menopause, when the cycles become irregular. This period usually lasts for about 4 years before menopause occurs.
- **Menopause:** It refers to permanent cessation of menstruation at the end of reproductive life due to loss of ovarian follicular activity. It can be defined with certainty following stoppage of menstruation (amenorrhea) for 12 consecutive months without any other pathology.
- **Mittelschmerz:** It refers to the midcycle pain related to ovulation.
- **Abnormal uterine bleeding (AUB)**: It refers to the deviation in the normal frequency, duration, or amount of menstrual bleeding. Earlier, 28 days +/–7 days with duration of flow of 3–5 days was considered as normal menstrual cycle. International Federation of Gynecology and Obstetrics (FIGO) has slightly changed the nomenclature in 2018. The terminologies earlier used in AUB indicating abnormal bleeding patterns are represented in Table 18.1 and the FIGO 2018 nomenclature of symptoms of normal and abnormal bleeding is represented in Table 18.2.

Table 18.1 Terminologies earlier used in abnormal uterine bleeding

Menorrhagia	Excessive (>80 mL) or prolonged bleeding (>7 days) at regular intervals
Polymenorrhea	Bleeding at intervals of less than 21 days
Oligomenorrhea	Bleeding at intervals of 35 days or more
Hypomenorrhea	Scanty flow during periods at regular intervals
Metrorrhagia	Irregular acyclical bleeding
Menometrorrhagia	Prolonged and excessive bleeding at irregular intervals
Postmenopausal bleeding	Bleeding that occurs after the cessation of menses for a period of 12 months or more in a woman who is aged 40 years or above

Table 18.2 Normal and abnormal menstrual cycle (FIGO 2018)

Clinical parameter	Descriptive term	Normal limits (5th–95th percentiles)
Frequency of menses (days)	Normal Frequent Infrequent	24–38 <24 >38
Regularity of menses: Cycle-to-cycle variation in days over 12 months	Regular Irregular	Shortest to longest cycle variation ≤ 7–9 days Shortest to longest cycle variation ≥ 8–10 days
Duration of flow (days)	Normal Prolonged	Upto 8 days flow is considered normal >8 days
Volume of monthly blood loss (mL) *(Note: Amount of flow is more subjective depending on the impact on quality of life)*	Normal Heavy Light	5–80 80 <5
Intermenstrual bleeding (bleeding between regular menstrual cycles)	Absent Random Cyclical	– Unpredictable Predictable (early/mid/late cycle)
Heavy menstrual bleeding (HMB)	Excessive menstrual bleeding of volume which interferes with the woman's physical, social, emotional, and/or material quality of life (ACOG)	

Note *Irregular menstrual cycles are common in the first few years following menarche and in the perimenopausal period due to anovulation.*

- **Dysmenorrhea:** It refers to painful menstruation, usually lower abdominal cramps, referred to thighs and lower back.
- **Dyspareunia:** It refers to painful sexual intercourse.
  - *Superficial dyspareunia*: The pain can be on the external surface of the genitalia or vagina on penetration. It is most likely due to vaginal causes such as infections and episiotomy scar.
  - *Deep dyspareunia*: The pain is deeper in the pelvis on deep pressure against the cervix. The patient describes the pain as "deep inside" during intercourse. It is most likely due to pathology of the upper genital tract such as endometriosis.
- **Postcoital bleeding:** It refers to the bleeding following sexual intercourse.
- **Intermenstrual bleeding:** Spontaneous bleeding occurring between regular menstrual cycles (can be cyclical or random).
- **Postmenopausal bleeding (PMB):** Bleeding that occurs after the cessation of menses for a period of at least 12 months or more, in a woman who is aged 40 years or above.
- **Amenorrhea:** Absence of uterine bleeding for at least 6 months.
  - *Primary amenorrhea*: It refers to the failure to attain menarche. Evaluation should start by 15 years of age in the presence of secondary sexual characters and by 13 years in the absence of secondary sexual characters.

- *Secondary amenorrhea*: When there is no menstruation for at least 6 months in a woman who has established menstrual cycles, it is referred to as secondary amenorrhea.
- **Leucorrhea:** It refers to excess of normal vaginal discharge.
  - *Normal vaginal discharge*: Nonodorous, nonhomogenous with pH of 3.8–4.5
  - *During proliferative phase*: Vaginal discharge is thin, copious, and stretchable under estrogen influence
  - *During secretory phase*: Vaginal discharge is thick, viscid, and scanty under progesterone influence
- **Hirsutism:** It refers to excessive growth of hair in women, in the male distribution pattern. It is usually related to increased androgen production in the body.

COMMON GYNECOLOGICAL SYMPTOMS

- **Menstrual complaints:** Patient may complain of abnormal bleeding patterns such as menorrhagia, polymenorrhea, oligomenorrhea, hypomenorrhea, metrorrhagia, intermenstrual bleeding, postcoital bleeding, and PMB or may present with amenorrhea.
  - The various causes for menorrhagia/HMB are mentioned in Table 18.3.
  - The various causes for postcoital, intermenstrual, and PMB are mentioned in Table 18.4.
- **Dysmenorrhea**: Pain during menstruation is one of the common gynecological complaints. Dysmenorrhea may be classified as primary and secondary.
  - *Primary dysmenorrhea:* Dysmenorrhea in the absence of identifiable pelvic pathology
    - It is confined to ovulatory cycles.
    - It occurs in the adolescent age group.
    - The pain is related to prostaglandin-induced uterine contractions and uterine hypoxia.
  - *Secondary dysmenorrhea:* Dysmenorrhea in the presence of pelvic pathology
    - It occurs in 30–40 years age group.
    - The pain may be related to pelvic congestion or increased vascularity in the pelvic organs.
    - Common causes of secondary dysmenorrhea are as follows:
      - Fibroid uterus

Table 18.3 Causes of menorrhagia/heavy menstrual bleeding

Anatomical	Hormonal	Systemic	Drug-related
• Fibroid uterus • Adenomyosis • Endometriosis • Pelvic inflammatory disease • Tubercular endometritis (early stages) • Intrauterine contraceptive device • Functional ovarian tumors • Uterine A-V malformations	• Hypothyroidism • PCOS	• Thrombocytopenia • Leukemia	• Anticoagulants such as warfarin and heparin • Antiplatelet drugs such as aspirin

Table 18.4 Causes of postcoital, intermenstrual, and postmenopausal bleeding

Postcoital	Intermenstrual	Postmenopausal
Local lesions such as • Cervical carcinoma • Cervical erosion • Cervical polyp • Cervicitis	• Intrauterine contraceptive device usage • Breakthrough bleeding with oral contraceptive pill use • Decubitus ulcer in uterovaginal prolapse • Submucous fibroid polyp • Includes all causes mentioned under "postcoital bleeding"	• Cervical carcinoma • Endometrial carcinoma • Endometrial hyperplasia • Endometrial/cervical polyp • Atrophic endometritis • Atrophic vaginitis • Exogenous estrogen use • Hormone-secreting ovarian tumors such as granulosa cell tumor

Table 18.5 Types of dysmenorrhea

Spasmodic	Congestive
• Usually primary, i.e., in the absence of pelvic pathology	• Usually secondary dysmenorrhea, due to underlying pelvic pathology
• Pain starts with or just before menstruation and lasts for about 24–48 hours	• Pain starts a few days prior to the onset of bleeding and intensifies with menstruation. The onset and duration of pain depends on the underlying pathology
• Pain is spasmodic and confined to lower abdomen; may radiate to the medial aspect of thighs • May be associated with systemic discomfort like nausea, vomiting, diarrhea, and headache	• The pain is dull aching and may be present in the back and front

 - Adenomyosis
 - Endometriosis
 - Chronic pelvic infection
 - Pelvic congestion syndrome
 - Cervical stenosis
- Dysmenorrhea may be spasmodic or congestive in nature (Table 18.5)
- **Pelvic or lower abdominal pain:** Pain may or may not be related to the menstrual cycles. Pain may be acute or chronic in nature.
  - Chronic pelvic pain (CPP) is defined as noncyclic pain of at least 6-month duration, unrelated to menstruation, intercourse, or pregnancy.
  - Causes of acute and chronic pelvic pain are mentioned in Tables 18.6 and 18.7, respectively.
- **Mass abdomen:** Patient may present with slow or rapidly growing mass in the lower abdomen. The various causes of abdominopelvic mass in different age groups are mentioned in Table 18.8. The various causes of uterine enlargement are mentioned in Table 18.9.

Table 18.6 Causes of acute pelvic pain

Gynecological	Nongynecological
• Pregnancy-related causes—abortion, ectopic pregnancy • Adnexal pathology—acute pelvic inflammatory disease (PID), torsion or rupture of ovarian cyst • Uterine cause—red degeneration of fibroid	• Appendicitis • Cystitis • Renal calculi

- **Mass descending per vaginum:** Women may present with a sensation of something coming down through the vagina. The differential diagnosis for mass descending per vaginum includes the following:
  - Uterovaginal prolapse
  - Isolated cystocele
  - Isolated rectocele
  - Isolated enterocele
  - Congenital elongation of cervix
  - Fibroid polyp
  - Chronic inversion of uterus
  - Vaginal wall cysts such as Gartner's cyst

Table 18.7 Causes of chronic pelvic pain

Gynecological	Nongynecological
• Endometriosis • Adenomyosis • Pelvic inflammatory disease • Fibroid uterus • Ovarian tumor • Uterine displacement—retroverted fixed uterus, uterovaginal prolapse • Pelvic adhesions • Pelvic congestion syndrome • Intrauterine contraceptive device usage	• Gastrointestinal – Irritable bowel syndrome – Chronic constipation – Appendicitis – Diverticulitis • Urological – Cystitis – Calculi • Orthopedic – Diseases of the bones, ligaments, and muscles of the lumbosacral region • Neurological: Nerve entrapment or compression • Hernias: Inguinal, femoral, obturator hernia

Table 18.8 Common causes of abdominopelvic mass in various age groups

Premenarchal	Reproductive	Postmenopausal
Toddlers (up to 3 years of age) • Full bladder • Mucocolpos • Ovarian tumor **Prepubertal age group** • Full bladder • Hematocolpos • Ovarian tumor	• Full bladder • Pregnancy • Fibroid • Adenomyosis • Ovarian tumor • Chocolate cyst of ovary • Tubo-ovarian mass, ectopic pregnancy • Pelvic hematocele • Pelvic abscess • Encysted peritonitis	• Ovarian tumor • Pyometra • Sarcoma uterus

Table 18.9 Causes of uterine enlargement

Uniform uterine enlargement	Irregular uterine enlargement
• Pregnancy • Adenomyosis • Endometrial polyp • Pyometra, hematometra • Endometrial carcinoma	• Fibroid uterus

- **Vaginal discharge:** Vaginal discharge can be physiological or pathological. Pathological discharge may be associated with foul smell and pruritus. Common causes of vaginal discharge in different age groups are mentioned in Table 18.10.
- **Pruritus vulvae:** It refers to itching of the skin of the vulva. The common causes of pruritus vulva include the following:
  - Vulvovaginitis caused by candidiasis, trichomoniasis
  - Dermatitis
  - Pediculosis
  - Scabies
  - Psoriasis
  - Lichen planus, lichen simplex
  - Vulvar carcinoma
- **Urinary symptoms:** Women may present with the following symptoms:
  - *Symptoms of urinary tract infection*: These include dysuria, increased frequency and urgency of micturition.
  - *Stress incontinence*: The patient complains of leakage of a small amount of urine with increase in intra-abdominal pressure such as coughing, laughing, and sneezing.
  - *Urge incontinence*: The patient complains of a sudden sensation of urinary urgency and voids before she makes it to the toilet. Large volume of urine is passed.
  - *Voiding difficulties*: Patient with uterovaginal prolapse may have complaints such as, being able to pass urine only on reducing the mass, thin stream of urine and a sense of incomplete evacuation.
- **Bowel symptoms:** Women may present with the following symptoms:
  - Rectal tenesmus with increased frequency of bowel movement—may be present in pelvic abscess

Table 18.10 Common causes of abnormal vaginal discharge in various age groups

Premenarchal	Reproductive	Postmenopausal
• Foreign body in vagina • Sexual abuse • Poor perineal hygiene • Pinworm infestation • Skin lesions—eczema, psoriasis • Chemical irritants	• Bacterial vaginosis • Trichomonal vaginitis • Candidiasis • Chlamydial and gonorrheal infection • Cervicitis, cervical erosion • Chemical irritants	• Cervical carcinoma • Vulvar, vaginal, and endometrial carcinoma • Atrophic vaginitis • Forgotten pessary

- Constipation—may be due to rectocele or due to pressure symptoms in case of cervical or posterior wall fibroid
- Incontinence of feces and flatus—present in complete perineal tear (anal sphincter injury)

- **Infertility:** It is the inability to conceive after 1 year of unprotected regular sexual intercourse.
  - *Primary infertility*: The patient has never become pregnant.
  - *Secondary infertility*: The patient has previously been pregnant.
- **Sexual dysfunction:** Patient may present with dyspareunia, vaginismus, reduced libido, sexual arousal disorders, etc. The various causes for dyspareunia are mentioned in Table 18.11.
- **Premenstrual symptoms:** Women may experience a range of symptoms for few days prior to menstruation that get relieved with the onset of menstruation. Premenstrual symptoms include mood disturbances, breast tenderness, bloating, and headache, etc.
- **Postmenopausal symptoms:** Women may experience a range of symptoms following menopause termed postmenopausal symptoms. The symptoms include hot flushes, vaginal dryness, loss of libido, irritability, mood swings, insomnia, difficulty in concentration, and osteoporotic symptoms.

Table 18.11 Causes of dyspareunia

Superficial dyspareunia	Deep dyspareunia
• Vaginitis—*Candida, Trichomonas, Gonococcus* etc. • Prior scarred episiotomy • Vulvar skin lesions—lichen sclerosis, dermatitis etc. • Vulvodynia • Vestibulitis, Bartholin's cyst • Postmenopausal estrogen deficiency • Postradiation scarring • Psychogenic—sexual abuse, lack of sexual interest	• Endometriosis • Chronic pelvic inflammatory disease • Adnexal pathology • Ovaries prolapsed or adherent in the pouch of Douglas • Acutely retroverted uterus

Viva corner

Q1 How is it assessed whether the patient is having excessive menstrual bleeding?

Indicators of excessive menstrual bleeding are the following:

- Passage of big clots
- Use of double pad protection
- Flooding occurs during day and night
- Interference with work and social activity
- Symptoms of anemia (easy fatigability, tiredness, etc.)

Q2 What are the methods for assessment of menstrual blood loss?

Objective assessment:

- Based on specialized techniques that are time-consuming
- Not routinely done
- Methods are the following:
  - Alkali hematin method—highly precise method of measuring blood loss but it is cumbersome
  - Radioisotope Cr-51 labeling of human RBC

Subjective assessment:

- It includes simple nonlaboratory methods such as counting and weighing the number of stained tampons and sanitary pads.

Pictorial blood loss assessment (PBAC):

- A simple nonlaboratory scoring method for diagnosis of menorrhagia, based on the number of sanitary pads or tampons used each day and the degree of soiling (see figure below).
  - It is a simple method of assessment of the amount of blood loss with a scoring system
  - One standard tampon or sanitary pad that is soiled equals 5 mL of blood loss.
  - Pictorial score of ≥100 has a specificity and sensitivity of >80% for diagnosis of menorrhagia.

Other tests used to quantify menorrhagia: Estimation of hemoglobin, serum iron, and serum ferritin levels

(CONTD...)

Part 2

(...CONTD)

Viva corner

PBAC scoring system

Pads		
1 point	For each lightly stained pad	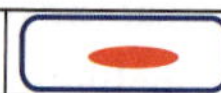
5 points	For each moderatelly stained pad	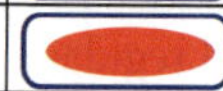
20 points	For each completely saturated pad	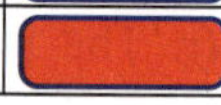
Tampons		
1 point	For each lightly stained tampon	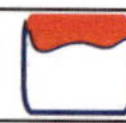
5 points	For each moderately stained tampon	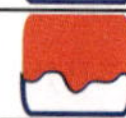
10 points	For each completely saturated tampon	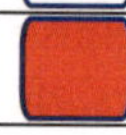
Clots/flooding		
1 point	For each small clot (Australian 5 cent coin)	
5 points	For each large clot (Australian 50 cent coin)	
5 points	For each episode of flooding	

Figure Pictorial blood loss assessment chart. It is used to assess the volume of menstrual blood loss. The chart has diagrams of pads and tampons. The number of pads/tampons used each day is marked and the total score calculated.

Q3 Why should menstrual blood loss be assessed?

Menorrhagia is defined as excessive or prolonged blood loss on a regular cyclical basis and objectively defined as menstrual blood loss of >80 mL.

- Some patients may exaggerate; some can tolerate heavy bleeding.
- Only 40% of women with a history of menorrhagia have >80 mL blood loss per cycle.
- Only 60% of women with blood loss of >80 mL consider their periods to be heavy.

Hence, blood loss has to be assessed to identify cases with excessive menstrual bleeding.

Q4 What is the significance of passage of clots during menstruation?

- It indicates that uterine bleeding is excessive and has exceeded the fibrinolytic activity of endometrium (Normally, menstrual blood is not clotted, as it undergoes fibrinolysis by the enzymes in the endometrium. However, when the bleeding is excessive, it exceeds the fibrinolytic activity and the blood gets passed out very quickly.)
- Passage of large clots is one of the parameters in PBAC and correlates with menorrhagia.

Proforma for history taking and examination in gynecological cases

The following is a detailed account of various elements that should be considered during history taking and clinical examination in gynecology. The case/disease-specific elements in history taking and clinical examination are discussed in respective chapters under the heading "Case Presentation."

The case presentation in subsequent chapters will include only the salient points pertaining to the specific case being discussed in order to avoid repetition of content.

A few examples of how to present a clinical case in gynecology during the viva voce examination

(CONTD...)

(...CONTD)

taken by undergraduate medical students are presented in Appendix.

History

Patent profile

She is Mrs. ______, W/o Mr. __________, at ____ years of age, residing at __________, educated up to ____, working as a _____, belonging to ______ socioeconomic class.

She is para ___ live ____, multiparous/ nulliparous woman (if multiparous, mention whether sterilized or not; if attained menopause, mention as "postmenopausal for __ years"), presenting with chief complaints of ____.

Presenting complaints

The presenting complaints should be recorded in chronological order. Common presenting complaints include the following:

- *Menstrual complaints*
- *Pain abdomen*
- *Mass abdomen*
- *Mass descending per vaginum*
- *Discharge per vaginum*
- *Urinary complaints*
- *Sexual dysfunction*
- *Any other*

History of presenting complaints

- *It includes details regarding onset, duration, and progression of the presenting illness up to the present state.*
- *Current treatment details should be mentioned, if the patient is under treatment or is an inpatient (treatment history).*

Menstrual complaints

- *Menstrual cycles—regularity, length of cycle, duration of flow, amount of bleeding, associated passage of clots, and number of sanitary pads used*
  - *An example of representing menstrual cycles— "4/30, moderate flow without clots" (indicates that the bleeding lasts for 4 days and occurs once in every 30 days and the flow is moderate in amount without any passage of clots)*
- *Any AUB such as menorrhagia, polymenorrhea, oligomenorrhea, hypomenorrhea, and metrorrhagia*
- *H/o preceding amenorrhea, in patients with prolonged and excessive bleeding*
- *H/o associated dysmenorrhea (±), whether spasmodic/congestive*
- *Last menstrual period (LMP) was on _____ (first day of LMP)*
- *H/o intermenstrual bleeding*
- *H/o postcoital bleeding*
- *H/o PMB in a postmenopausal woman should be asked for. If H/o PMB is present, it is mentioned as "She is postmenopausal for the past ___ years and presents with complaints of PMB"*

H/o pain abdomen

If the patient presents with pain in lower abdomen, the following details should be determined:

- *Duration of pain—acute/chronic*
- *Site of pain*
- *Whether continuous/intermittent*
- *Nature of pain (dull aching/pricking/colicky)*
- *Aggravating and relieving factors*
- *Relation of pain with other factors such as menstruation, sexual activity, micturition, and defecation*

H/o mass abdomen

- *Time period since when the mass is present or observed?*
- *Has the mass been increasing in size or has it remained static?*
- *H/o any associated pain*
- *H/o associated pressure symptoms such as increased urinary urgency, frequency, and constipation*

H/o vaginal discharge

Amount (scanty/profuse), color and consistency of discharge, whether associated with foul smell/ blood staining/ pruritus.

H/o mass descending per vaginum

History related to mass descending P/V is explained in detail in Part 2, Chapter 24, Pelvic Organ Prolapse.

(CONTD...)

H/o urinary complaints

H/o increased frequency, and urgency of micturition dysuria, hesitancy or difficulty in initiating micturition, and any stress/urge/true incontinence.

Menstrual history

- *Age at menarche*
- *H/o details of previous menstrual cycles—regularity, length of cycle, duration of flow, and amount of bleeding, and associated dysmenorrhea*
- *Any change in menstrual cycles from the past*
- *LMP*
- *If attained menopause, mention the age at menopause*

Marital and sexual history

- *Age at marriage*
- *The time since the patient has been married*
- *Consanguineous/nonconsanguineous marriage*
- *Whether she is sexually active. If yes, ask the following:*
  - *Number of sexual partners (present and past)*
  - *H/o recent change of partner in the past 3 months*
  - *H/o whether having protected or unprotected intercourse*
  - *H/o sexually transmitted diseases (STDs) in the past*
  - *Whether the patient is currently anxious to conceive*
  - *Whether the patient or her partner is experiencing any sexual dysfunction*
  - *H/o dyspareunia*
- *H/o any sexual abuse/intimate partner violence*

Note *Women are often hesitant to talk about sexual history and may complain of nonspecific symptoms till they are asked specifically about it.*

Obstetric history (Table 18.12)

Details of each pregnancy irrespective of the outcome should be recorded.

- *H/o details of previous live births, stillbirths, deaths, and miscarriages (both spontaneous and induced)*
- *Delivery details are recorded—mode of delivery (normal vaginal delivery or cesarean section (CS)) and H/o any obstetric complications such as postpartum hemorrhage and puerperal or postabortal sepsis*
- *Number of living children at present*
- *When was the last child birth?*

Contraception

- *Method of contraception in between pregnancies*
- *Whether sterilized or not (in multiparous woman)*
- *Whether the patient is currently using any method of contraception. If yes, type of contraceptive used and since how long it is being used?*

The obstetric history is summarized as follows: She is para___ live ___ abortion ___, sterilized/not sterilized and her last child birth was _____ years back.

In case of mass descending P/V, ask the following details with regard to the previous pregnancies (in addition to the above):

- *Place where the patient delivered*
- *The person who conducted the delivery (home deliveries may be conducted by untrained dais)*
- *Duration of labor pains*
- *H/o premature bearing down*

Table 18.12 Summary of obstetric history

S. No.	Year/place	Antenatal period	Period of gestation/mode of delivery	Live/ stillbirth	Weight/ sex	Puerperium	Breast-feeding	Present health

(CONTD...)

(...CONTD)

- H/o instrumentation prior to full dilatation of cervix
- H/o whether episiotomy was given or not/H/o perineal tears
- Whether episiotomy/perineal tears were repaired
- H/o any strenuous work during puerperium
- Whether the patient practiced postnatal exercises
- Spacing in between pregnancies

Past medical/surgical history

- H/o diabetes mellitus (DM)/hypertension (HT)
- H/o tuberculosis
- H/o jaundice
- Thyroid disorders
- H/o blood transfusion
- H/o previous surgeries such as CS, tubectomy, dilatation and curettage appendicectomy, ovarian cystectomy, and myomectomy are noted
- H/o sexually transmitted diseases
- H/o drug intake for any chronic medical illness

Personal history

- H/o alcohol intake, smoking/tobacco chewing, and drug addictions
- Sleep/appetite—whether normal or disturbed
- H/o any drug allergies

Family history

- H/o HT/DM
- H/o tuberculosis
- H/o genital malignancy

Examination of the patient

The examination of the patient includes the following:

- General and systemic examination
- Gynecological examination that includes:
  - Abdominal examination
  - Pelvic examination
    - Inspection of the external genitalia
    - Speculum examination
    - Bimanual examination
    - Rectal and rectovaginal examination

General and systemic examination

- Built—skeletal framework of the patient (tall/average built/short)
- Nourishment—well/average/poorly nourished
- Height
- Weight
- BMI
- Pallor
- Icterus
- Lymphadenopathy—especially the left supra-clavicular nodes, cervical nodes, axillary nodes, and inguinal nodes must be palpated for any enlarged lymph nodes
- Pedal edema
- Vitals—temperature, pulse, respiratory rate, and BP
- Any loose teeth (to be removed, if patient is planned for surgery)
- Features of hyperandrogenism such as hirsutism (presence of facial hair), acne, and deepening of voice may be present in chronic anovulatory state such as polycystic ovarian disease (PCOD) and in androgen-secreting ovarian tumors
- Secondary sexual characteristics—breast, axillary, and pubic hair development (especially in a case of primary amenorrhea)

Breast examination

Breast examination is an integral part of gynecological examination and should be performed in all women. Examination of both the breasts should be done in three positions:

- With the patient's hands on her hips
- With arms raised
- Supine position

Inspection

Check for symmetry of both the breasts, nipple retraction, and skin changes such as dimpling, retraction, or peau d'orange appearance.

Palpation

- Check for the presence of any mass or tenderness.

(CONTD...)

Part 2

(...CONTD)

- *Nipples are assessed for the presence of discharge, retraction.*
- *Axillary and supraclavicular regions are palpated for the presence of any lymphadenopathy.*

Thyroid examination

Check for any thyromegaly

Cardiovascular and respiratory system examination

Mention whether normal or any abnormality detected (any abnormality detected has to be evaluated before any surgical procedure)

Abdominal examination

Prerequisites

- *Bladder should be empty prior to abdominal and vaginal examination (the only exception to this rule is while checking for stress incontinence when the patient is asked to cough or strain with full bladder to look for escape of spurts of urine).*
- *Position of the patient: The patient should be in supine position with thighs flexed and slightly abducted (this position relaxes the abdominal muscles, making palpation easier).*
- *Ensure adequate lighting and privacy.*
- *Stand on the right side of the patient.*
- *A female attender should be present during examination by a male doctor.*

Inspection

- *Abdominal shape—symmetrical/asymmetrical*
- *Any visible mass or abdominal distension*
- *Umbilicus—position and whether it is inverted/flushed with skin surface/everted (umbilicus can become everted with increase in intra-abdominal pressure such as pregnancy, ascites, and intra-abdominal tumors)*
- *Any scars/sinuses (such as tubectomy and CS scar)*
- *Engorged veins, if any (may be due to inferior vena cava obstruction or portal hypertension)*
- *Any visible pulsations*
- *Hernial orifices (ask the patient to strain or cough and look for cough impulse; in case of previous abdominal surgeries, check for incisional hernia)*

Palpation

- *The clinician must warm his/her hands before palpation.*
- *Palpate with the flat of the hand gently and not with the tip of the fingers.*
- *Palpation is done from nontender to tender area.*
- *Palpate all the abdominal quadrants for the presence of organomegaly or palpable mass. Figure 18.1a shows the various quadrants of the abdomen.*
- *Check for tenderness and presence of any guarding, rigidity, or rebound tenderness.*

Note

- *Guarding is an attempt by the patient to prevent painful palpation.*
- *Rigidity means the abdominal muscles are firm and palpation is difficult.*
- *Rebound tenderness refers to pain on removal of the pressure (palpating fingers).All these may be indicative of underlying inflammation or peritonitis.*

- *If any mass is palpable, look for the following:*
  - *Site—in relation to the various abdominal quadrants*
  - *Size of the mass—abdominopelvic masses can be expressed in terms of the size of the gravid uterus in weeks. However, this is easier only for masses which arise centrally and from the pelvis. Hence, it is suggested that the size of the mass be measured by a measuring tape (Figure 18.1b)*
  - *Consistency—whether hard, firm, rubbery, soft, fluctuant, indentable, or pulsating (fibroid usually has a firm consistency benign ovarian mass usually has a cystic consistency; malignant ovarian tumor may have variegated consistency)*
  - *Surface—whether smooth/regular or nodular/irregular*
  - *Whether all borders are felt (lower border cannot be reached in a uterine mass (Figure 18.1c), but in an ovarian mass with a long pedicle, all borders may be felt; margins of a malignant tumor may be irregular and may not be well defined)*

(CONTD...)

..CONTD)

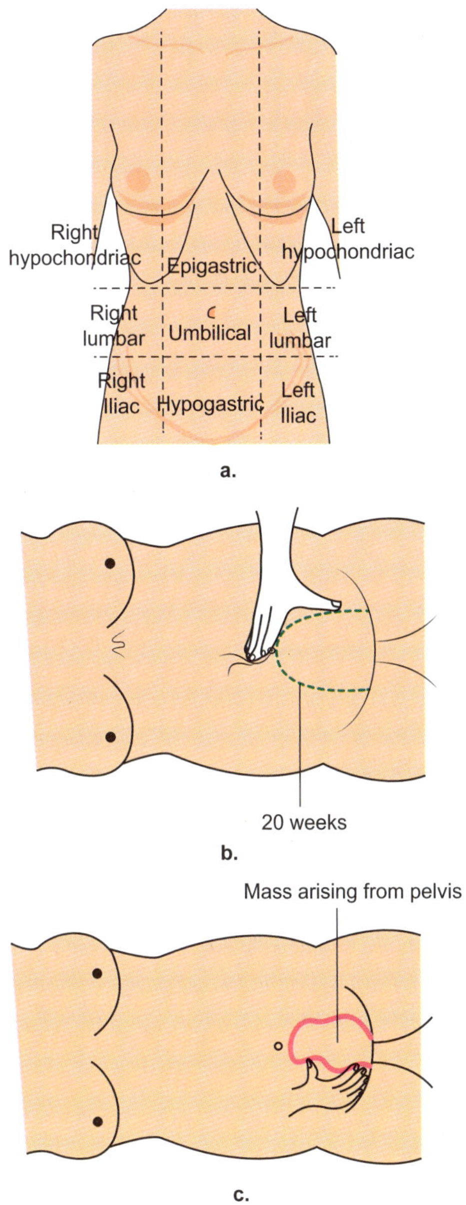

Figure 18.1 Abdominal examination. **a.** Quadrants of the abdomen. **b.** Mass in the lower abdomen corresponding to 20-week gravid uterus. **c.** Palpation of abdominopelvic mass. The lower border cannot be palpated in case of a mass arising from the pelvis.

- *Mobility—check for horizontal and vertical mobility (fibroid usually has only horizontal mobility; a benign ovarian tumor may be freely mobile; a malignant mass may be fixed or has restricted mobility)*
- *Tender/nontender (benign masses such as fibroids and benign ovarian cysts are usually nontender on palpation; tenderness may be associated with conditions such as pelvic inflammatory disease (PID), torsion of ovarian cyst, red degeneration of fibroid, and ectopic pregnancy; in acute peritonitis, guarding, rigidity, and rebound tenderness of the lower abdomen will be present). Abdominal tenderness is graded as mentioned in Table 18.13*
- *Fluid thrill—can be elicited in large-volume ascites and in an ovarian tumor that is huge and cystic*

Table 18.13 Grades of abdominal tenderness

Grade	Degree	Description
0	None	Palpation is not painful even when asked about it
1	Mild	Patient indicates that palpation is painful only when asked about it
2	Moderate	Patient indicates that palpation is painful by wincing during palpation
3	Severe	Patient withdraws her limbs at the time of examination or appears distressed during abdominal palpation

Demonstration of fluid thrill (Figure 18.2)

- *The patient is in supine position and the clinician places the palmar aspect of one hand on the flank on one side.*
- *An assistant or the patient herself is asked to place the ulnar aspect of her hand firmly in the midline of the abdomen.*
- *The clinician taps the opposite flank of the abdomen with his/her other hand.*
- *If gross ascites is present, the impulse generated by the tap will be transmitted to the clinician's other hand on the flank.*

(CONTD...)

(...CONTD)

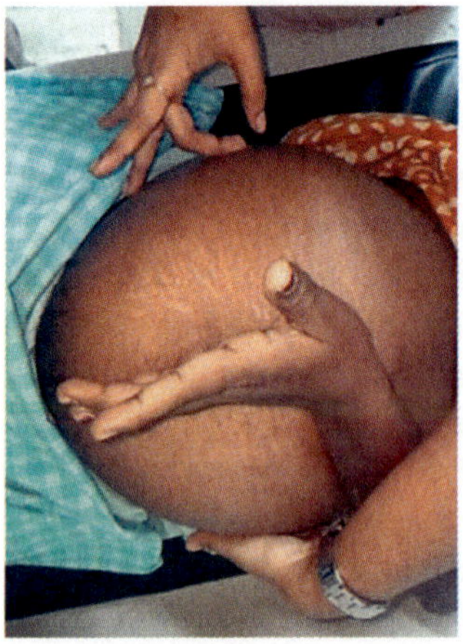

Figure 18.2 Demonstration of fluid thrill.

- *The hand on the abdomen helps in preventing the transmission of the impulse through the abdominal wall.*

Note *Normally abdomen is soft and nontender on palpation with no organomegaly or palpable masses.*

Percussion

Technique of percussion (Figure 18.3)

- *The fingers of the clinician's left hand are spread slightly and the palmar surface of the middle finger is placed flat over the area to be percussed.*
- *The distal two phalanges of the middle finger of the clinician's right hand are flexed and the tip of the finger is used to perpendicularly strike the middle finger of the left hand placed on the abdomen.*

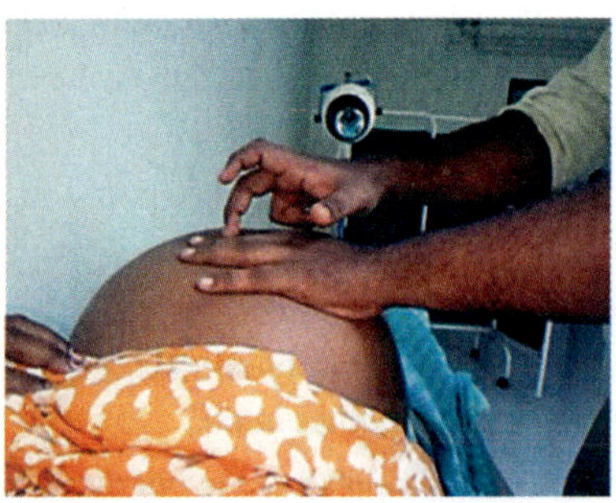

Figure 18.3 Demonstration of percussion of abdomen.

- *The stroke is delivered through flexion of the wrist and not through action of the elbow or shoulder.*
- *The striking finger must be withdrawn as soon as the stroke is delivered.*

Check for the following findings on percussion:

- *The percussion note is resonant over an area of air-filled bowel and is dull in the presence of fluid.*
  - *In case of ascites, resonance is present in the center with dullness in the flanks (Figure 18.4a and b).*
  - *In case of mass arising from pelvis, dullness is present in the center with resonance in the flanks (Figure 18.4c and d).*
- *Check for shifting dullness as described below.*

Demonstration of shifting dullness (Figure 18.5)

Presence of dullness in both flanks when the patient is supine, and dullness only in the dependent flank when the patient is on one/lateral side indicates the presence of ascites.

- *The patient is in supine position and the clinician starts percussing from the midline of the abdomen toward one of the flanks. The level at which the percussion note changes from resonance to dull is noted.*
- *The patient is then instructed to turn to the opposite side (the side away from the flank that is percussed).*
- *Allow time for the fluid to gravitate to the side of the dependent flank and perform the percussion again.*
- *The dependent flank where the fluid had gravitated will be dull to percussion, while the nondependent flank will be resonant.*
- *The steps are repeated on the other side.*

Note *Fluid thrill and shifting dullness are demonstrable only in the presence of a large volume ascites. Absence of shifting dullness or fluid thrill does not rule out the presence of a small volume of ascites.*

(CONTD...)

(...CONTD)

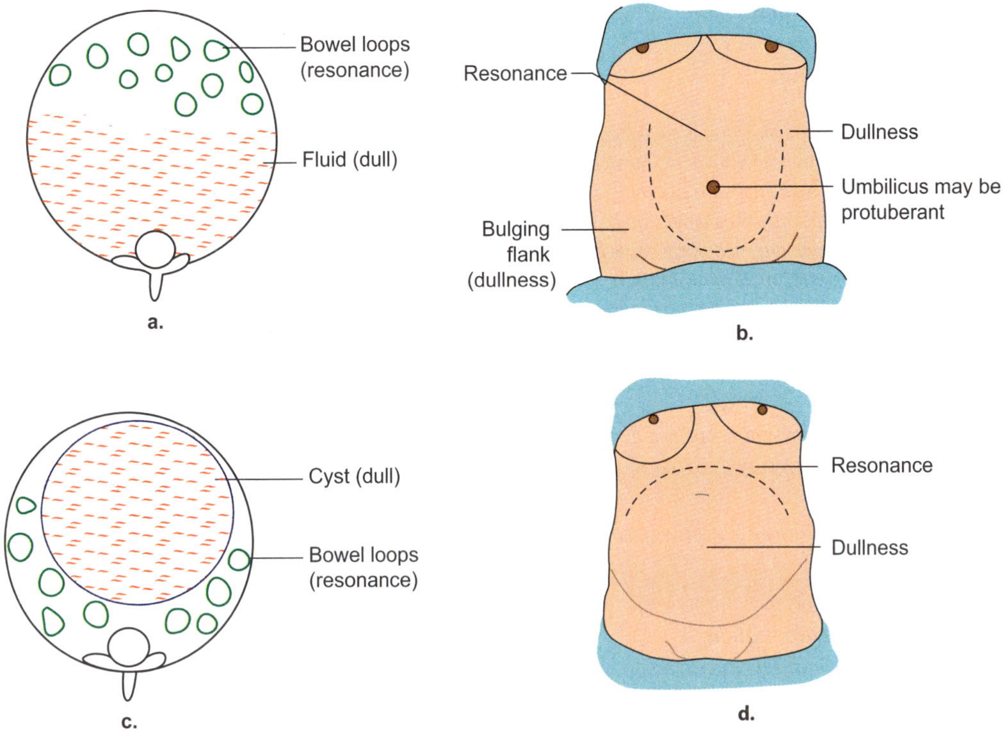

Figure 18.4 Difference between ascites and ovarian mass on percussion. **a** and **b.** Percussion in ascites. **c** and **d.** Percussion of ovarian mass.

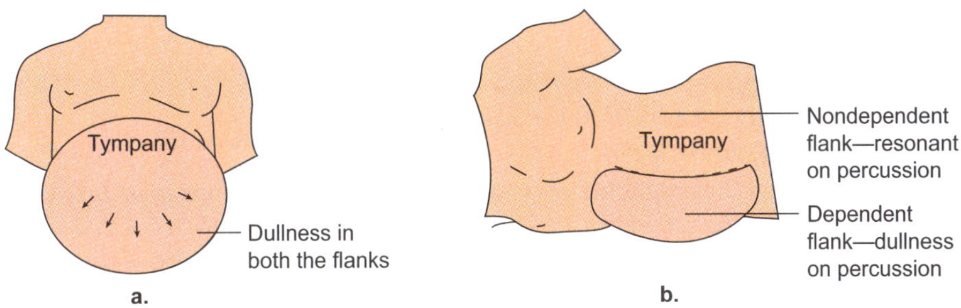

Figure 18.5 Demonstration of shifting dullness in a patient with ascites. **a.** Dullness elicited in both the flanks in supine position. **b.** Dullness in the dependent flank and resonance in the nondependent flank in lateral position.

Auscultation

Auscultate for bowel sounds produced by peristalsis and for any vascular sounds.

- *Bowel sounds*
  - *Paralytic ileus, peritonitis: Sluggish or absent bowel sounds*
  - *Intestinal obstruction: Hyperactive bowel sounds*
- *Bruit—may be heard in huge fibroids with increased vascularity and in uterine sarcomas*

Pelvic examination

It includes the following:

- *Inspection of the external genitalia*
- *Per speculum examination—inspection of the cervix and vagina*

(CONTD...)

Part 2

(...CONTD)

- *Bimanual pelvic examination*
- *Rectal examination*
- *Rectovaginal examination*

Note *Pelvic examination is expected to be performed only by postgraduates. Undergraduates are expected to perform only the inspection of external genitalia in gynecology cases and to perform clinical examination in a case of mass descending per vaginum.*

Prerequisites

- *Informed verbal consent is obtained (to examine a minor, consent from the parent or guardian is required).*
- *Bladder should be empty. Rectum should preferably be empty.*
- *A female attendant (chaperone) should be present during examination.*
- *A light source should be available.*
- *Ensure privacy of the patient.*
- *Stand on the right side of the patient.*
- *Sterile gloves, lubricant, speculum, sponge holding forceps, and swabs should be available.*

Position of the patient

- *Dorsal position (supine position with the thighs flexed and slightly abducted) is the usually preferred position (Figure 18.6a).*
- *Lithotomy position (supine position with legs on stirrups) is ideal for examination under anesthesia (Figure 18.6b).*
- *Left lateral position or Sims' position (patient in left lateral position with the left leg extended and right leg flexed at the hip and knee) is ideal for rectal examination (Figure 18.6c). This position is also useful for visualization of anterior vaginal wall and demonstration of enterocele, following insertion of Sims' speculum (the vagina gets distended with air when speculum is inserted into the introitus).*

Inspection of external genitalia

Inspect the following:

- *Distribution of pubic hairs*
- *Skin—any discoloration, lesions, ulcers, pigmentation, excoriation marks, etc.*
- *Clitoris, labia majora, and minora*
- *Labia minora separated to visualize the introitus, hymen, and urethral orifice*
- *Perineal body and anal orifice*

Note *The Bartholin's glands are normally not palpable. The openings of Bartholin's ducts are located on the inner aspect of labia minora at the junction of anterior two-third and posterior one-third. Swelling which is present at the junction of anterior two-third and posterior one-third of labia minora is most likely to be a Bartholin's cyst or abscess.*

Speculum examination

- *Speculum examination involves inspection of the vagina and cervix and should always be done prior to bimanual examination.*

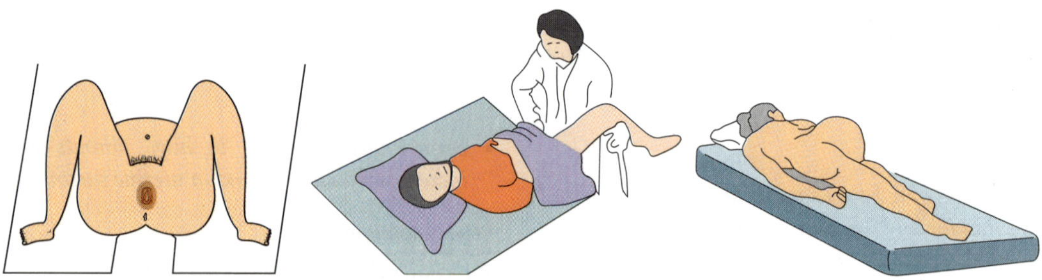

a. b. c.

Figure 18.6 Positioning the patient for pelvic examination. **a.** Dorsal position. **b.** Lithotomy position. **c.** Sims' position (patient in left lateral position; left leg is extended and right leg is flexed at the hip and knee).

(CONTD...)

(...CONTD)

- *Advantages of speculum examination prior to vaginal bimanual examination are as follows:*
  - *PAP smear can be taken*
  - *Vaginal discharge can be visualized and collected for examination before it gets contaminated with the lubricant used for vaginal examination*
  - *If cervical lesion is present, it may bleed during bimanual examination, making it difficult to visualize later*
- *Speculum examination is done using a Cusco's self-retaining vaginal wall speculum or a Sims' posterior vaginal wall speculum along with an anterior vaginal wall retractor (Figure 18.7). The patient should be brought to the edge of the couch to facilitate insertion of speculum.*
- *The vagina and cervix are examined for the following:*

Vagina
- *Color (normal vagina is pink, but can be erythematous in case of vaginitis)*
- *Vaginal rugosities*
- *Any lesion growth or ulcer*
- *Abnormal discharge*
- *Dryness (vagina is usually moist, but in postmenopausal women, vaginal dryness may be present due to estrogen deficiency)*
- *Check for the presence of cystocele (anterior vaginal wall prolapse), rectocele, and enterocele (posterior vaginal wall prolapse)*

Cervix
- *Color (cervix is normally dull pink in color)*
- *External os (external os is round in nulliparous women and is a transverse slit with anterior and posterior lips in multiparous women)*
- *Position and direction (cervix is normally located at the level of ischial spines; cervix points downwards in an anteverted uterus, and upwards in a retroverted uterus)*
- *Any cervical lesion—erosion, growth, ulcer, or polyp*
- *Any abnormal discharge*
- *Any bleeding through the os*
- *Pap smear, if indicated should be taken before withdrawing the speculum*

Bimanual pelvic examination

- *Lubricated index and middle fingers of the clinician's right hand are inserted into the vagina and the left hand is placed on the lower abdomen. Palpate the pelvic organs between the abdominal and vaginal hands—cervix, uterus, adnexa, pouch of Douglas (POD) (Figure 18.8)*

Palpation of the cervix *Note the following cervical findings:*
- *Cervical consistency (in nonpregnant state, cervix feels firm like that of "tip of the nose"; in pregnancy, it feels soft like that of "lips"); whether cervix is friable and bleeds on touch (features of malignancy)*
- *Cervical mobility*

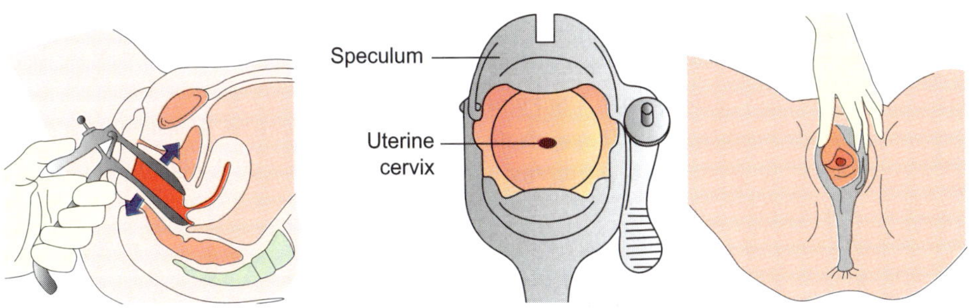

Figure 18.7 Speculum examination. **a.** Insertion of Cusco's speculum. **b.** Visualization of cervix after insertion of Cusco's speculum. **c.** Sims' posterior vaginal wall speculum used to retract the posterior vaginal wall.

(CONTD...)

Part 2

(...CONTD)

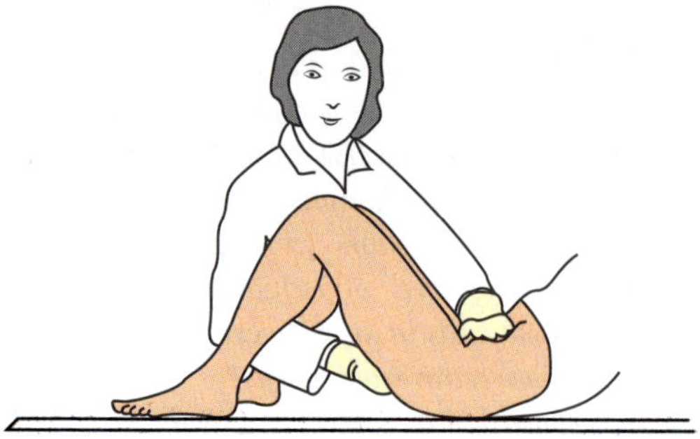

a.

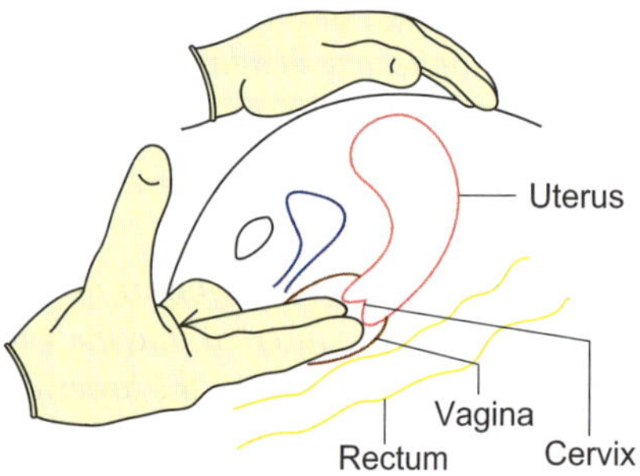

b.

Figure 18.8 Bimanual examination. **a.** Bimanual pelvic examination performed in a patient in dorsal position. **b.** The uterus and the adnexa are palpated between the abdominal and vaginal fingers.

- *Any cervical motion tenderness is noted (normally, the movement of cervix is not painful. Cervical motion tenderness may be present in PID and ectopic pregnancy)*

Palpation of uterus *The clinician's fingers in vagina are placed in the posterior fornix, the uterus is pushed toward the abdominal hand and the uterus is palpated between the two hands. Note the following findings on palpation of the uterus:*

- *Uterus size and shape*
- *Position—anteverted or retroverted (Figure 18.9)*
- *Mobility—mobile/restricted mobility/fixed (uterus is normally mobile; in endometriosis and malignancy, it may be fixed)*
- *Tenderness (uterine tenderness is present in infection, adenomyosis, endometriosis)*

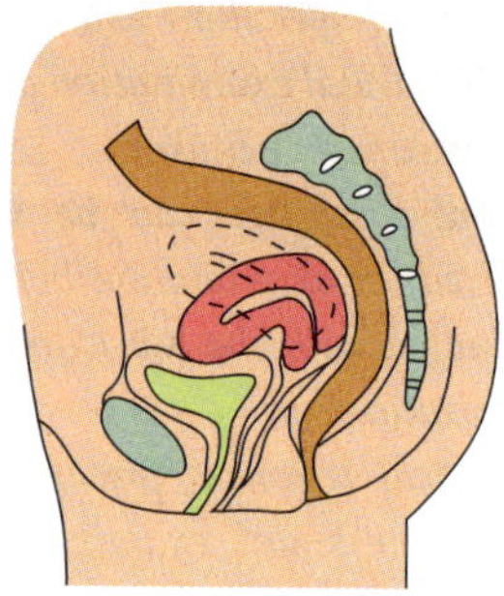

a.

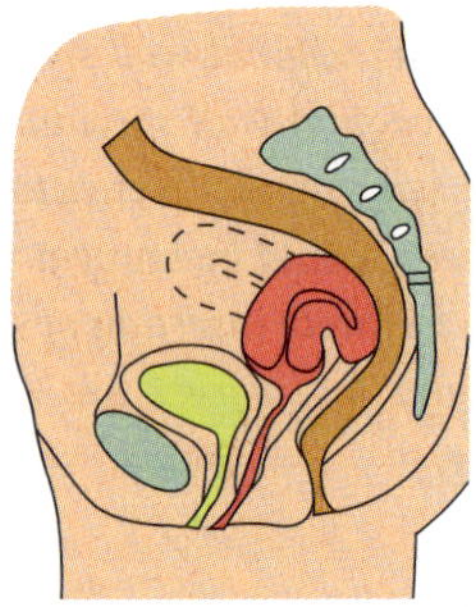

b.

Figure 18.9 Uterine palpation. **a.** Anteverted uterus. **b.** Retroverted uterus.

Note *Normally, the uterus is anteverted, midposition, pear shaped, firm in consistency, and mobile.*

Palpation of adnexa *The vaginal fingers are then moved to the lateral fornices and the adnexa are palpated between the two hands. Note the following adnexal findings:*

- *Any palpable adnexal mass*
- *Any adnexal tenderness*

Palpate for any mass *If any mass is palpable on bimanual examination, note the following:*

- *Site*
- *Size*
- *Shape*
- *Surface*
- *Consistency*
- *Mobility*
- *Tenderness*

(CONTD...)

...CONTD)

- Whether the mass is felt separate from the uterus (origin of the mass is most likely from the adnexa) or is felt continuous with the uterus (it probably arises from the uterus, like a fibroid)
- Whether movement of the mass is transmitted to the cervix (suggestive of uterine mass)

Palpation of POD through the posterior fornix

Note the following findings:

- *Any fullness or bogginess in POD (may indicate collection of fluid, pus or blood in the POD)*
- *Any nodules (nodules can be felt in POD in endometriosis and metastatic ovarian tumor)*
- *Any palpable mass (adherent ovary in POD, pelvic hematocele etc., can be felt)*

Assessment of the integrity of the perineal body

- *The perineal body is palpated between the vaginal fingers which are flexed posteriorly over the perineum and the thumb placed externally over the perineal body.*
- *Deficient perineum should be looked for (normally perineal length is 3–4 cm).*

Assessment of the integrity and tone of levator ani

The vaginal fingers are turned and placed laterally above the level of levator ani. The muscle is palpated between the vaginal fingers and the thumb placed externally, medial to the ischial tuberosity.

Rectovaginal examination

- *The procedure is done by inserting the clinician's index finger into the vagina and the middle finger into the rectum (Figure 18.10). The rectovaginal septum and parametrium can be palpated between the two fingers. Note the following:*
  - *Any tenderness, nodularity, or induration of rectovaginal septum and parametrium*

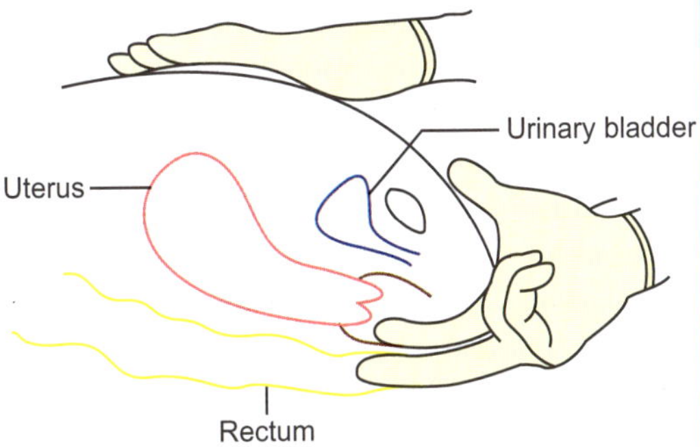

Figure 18.10 Rectovaginal examination.

Note *Some clinicians include rectovaginal examination as part of the routine pelvic examination, while others do this procedure only in specific cases (mainly done in carcinoma cervix, to assess involvement of parametrium and rectovaginal septum).*
While doing rectovaginal examination, the same finger should not be used to examine both the vagina and the rectum, to avoid transmission of human papillomavirus and fecal contamination.

Rectal examination

Lubricated index or middle finger is inserted into the rectum for rectal examination. Bowel should preferably be empty prior to examination (Figure 18.11). Note the following:

- *Any tenderness or nodularity of uterosacral ligament*
- *Any nodule or mass or bogginess in POD*
- *Any irregularity in the rectal mucosa*
- *The patient is asked to strain and the presence of rectocele should be noted*
- *Anal sphincter tone is assessed*

Case summary (summary of history and examination)

A summary is made at the end of history and examination which should include the patient's name, age, parity, whether adolescent/reproductive/

(CONTD...)

Part 2

(...CONTD)

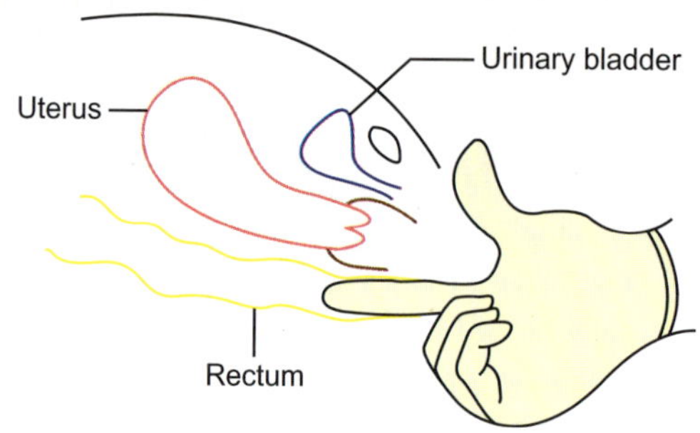

Figure 18.11 Rectal examination.

perimenopausal/postmenopausal, chief complaints, significant positive and negative history, any associated comorbidities, and salient points in general and gynecological examinations.

Provisional diagnosis/differential diagnosis

Based on the history and clinical examination, a provisional diagnosis or differential diagnosis is made.

- *Medical students should be prepared with the investigations required to confirm the diagnosis and an appropriate management plan for the case, depending on the suspected pathology (often the immediate questions following case presentation in clinical exams will be on these sections).*

SPECIFIC DISCUSSION POINTS IN HISTORY TAKING AND EXAMINATION IN GYNECOLOGY

Significance of age

Common gynecological problems in different age groups are mentioned in Table 18.14.

Significance of parity

- **Nulliparous:** Increased incidence of fibroid uterus, endometriosis, endometrial hyperplasia and carcinoma, and ovarian tumors
- **Multiparous:** Increased risk of cancer cervix, adenomyosis, and uterovaginal prolapse

Significance of menstrual history

- Early menarche and late menopause are risk factors for endometrial cancer
- To rule out pregnancy-related causes
- To identify abnormal bleeding patterns

Significance of marital and sexual history

- Evaluation of infertility may be required in women who have not conceived after 1 year of unprotected regular sexual intercourse
- Multiple sexual partners—risk of HIV, STDs, and carcinoma cervix
- To advise on safe sexual practices

Significance of obstetric and contraceptive history

- To know the parity status
- Recent delivery/abortion may be associated with sepsis, retained products of conception
- Pregnancy-related causes of bleeding should be ruled out in adolescent, reproductive, and perimenopausal age groups
- During lactation, women may experience amenorrhea or irregular menstrual cycles

Contraceptive history

- Intrauterine contraceptive device usage may be associated with AUB
- Use of oral contraceptive pills for >5 years protects against ovarian and endometrial cancer
- Use of injectable progesterones may be associated with amenorrhea or irregular cycles
- To provide contraceptive counseling

Significance of past medical history

Previous medical problems may have a bearing on the patient's presenting complaints.

- H/o DM could be responsible for vulvovaginal candidiasis and associated pruritus.

Table 18.14 Common gynecological problems in different age groups

Premenarchal age group	Adolescent and reproductive age groups	Perimenopausal age group	Postmenopausal age group
Newborn • White/blood-stained discharge (due to withdrawal of maternal estrogen) • Ambiguous genitalia • Ectopic anus **Infants** • Mucocolpos (imperforate hymen) **Toddlers** • Labial adhesions **5–11 years age group** • Pruritus vulvae—commonly due to pinworm infestation • Discharge per vaginum (can be physiological or due to worm infestation, vulvovaginitis, foreign body etc.) • Bleeding per vaginum (can be due to trauma, foreign body, sexual abuse, precocious puberty, hormone-secreting ovarian tumors)	• AUB • Vaginal discharge • Pregnancy-related conditions such as abortion, ectopic pregnancy • Infertility • Amenorrhea • STDs • Hirsuitism • Intersex problem	• AUB • Vaginal discharge • Pruritus vulva	• Vaginal discharge • Mass descending per vaginum • Postmenopausal bleeding • Postmenopausal symptoms • Pruritus vulva

AUB, abnormal uterine bleeding; *STDs*, sexually transmitted diseases.

Part 2

- Triad of DM, HT, and obesity is associated with an increased risk of endometrial carcinoma.
- Presence of thyroid dysfunction can cause menstrual irregularities.
- H/o severe anemia requires correction of anemia before undergoing surgery.
- H/o systemic illnesses such as heart disease, chronic obstructive pulmonary disease (COPD), or renal disease require evaluation and treatment prior to surgery and may require special anesthetic preparation.
- H/o STDs caused by chlamydia and gonorrhea may have an effect on future fertility.
- H/o PID or puerperal sepsis can cause gynecological problems such as menstrual disturbances, lower abdominal pain, and infertility.

Significance of past surgical history

- Previous abdominal surgeries may cause intra-abdominal adhesions that can cause difficulty during gynecological surgery.
- Previous pelvic surgeries may cause gynecological problems such as chronic pelvic pain, menstrual disturbances, and infertility.

Significance of family history

- Certain gynecological malignancies such as cancers of the ovary, uterus, and breast have familial predisposition. Ask for a positive family history of such cancers in the patient's first-degree relatives (especially mother and sister).
- Menstrual patterns such as age at menarche, frequency and regularity of cycles, and age of menopause may be similar among family members.
- Gynecological problems such as premature menopause may run in families.
- Thyroid dysfunction and coagulation disorders, which may produce gynecological problems, can be familial in nature.
- Family H/o DM, HT, and ischemic heart disease is important during evaluation of women of older age.

Significance of breast examination

- Staging of breast development is important in girls who have not attained sexual maturity. Tanner staging of breast and pubic hair development is used in clinical practice for documentation and follow-up of cases (Table 18.15; Figure 18.12).

- In women especially >30 years, breasts must be palpated for any mass. In India, breast carcinoma is the most common malignancy in women followed by carcinoma cervix.
- Galactorrhea may be due to hyperprolactinemia—important in infertility cases and in evaluation of oligomenorrhea and amenorrhea.
- Unilateral blood-stained nipple discharge may be associated with intraductal papilloma.

Significance of abdominal palpation

- To check for organomegaly
- To identify any abdominopelvic masses
- To check for tenderness, guarding, and rigidity

Significance of percussion

- Percussion helps to differentiate between a large ovarian cyst and ascites. In case of an ovarian cyst, the tumor is dull on percussion in the midline, whereas the flanks are resonant as occupied by the intestines. In ascites, the abdomen is resonant in the midline due to the presence of intestines, whereas the flanks are dull on percussion due to collection of ascitic fluid.
- Presence of ascites can be detected by eliciting fluid thrill and shifting dullness.
- Most intraperitoneal tumors arising from the pelvic organs are dull on percussion, whereas a retroperitoneal tumor usually has bowel loops in front of it, which may give a resonant note on percussion.
- Liver span can be assessed on percussion.

Table 18.15 Tanner staging of breast and pubic hair development

Stage	Breast development	Pubic hair development
Stage 1	Preadolescent; elevation of nipple only	No pubic hair
Stage 2	Breast bud stage; elevation of breast and nipple as a small mound; enlargement of areolar diameter	Sparse, long straight, only slightly curled hair along the labia
Stage 3	Further enlargement of the breast and areola with no separation of the contours	Dark, more coarse and curled hair extending sparsely spread over mons pubis
Stage 4	Further enlargement with projection of the areola and nipple to form a secondary mound above the level of the breast	Adult type abundant hair limited to the mons pubis
Stage 5	Normal mature breast	Adult type hair extending to the medial surface of the thighs

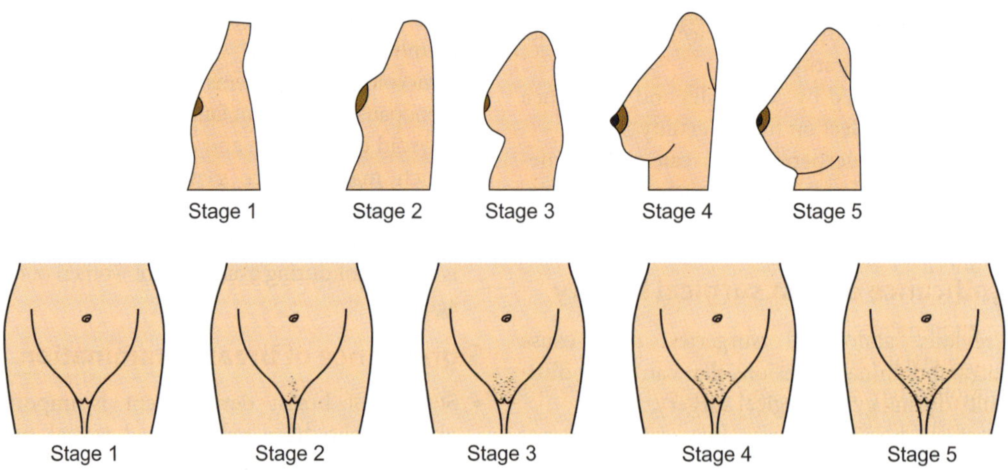

Figure 18.12 Tanner staging of breast and pubic hair development.

Extra edge

Signs of intraperitoneal and retroperitoneal hemorrhage on abdominal examination

- **Grey Turner's sign:** Discoloration (bruising) at the flanks (seen in cases with retroperitoneal hemorrhage)
- **Cullen's sign:** Periumbilical bruising (may be seen in ruptured ectopic pregnancy and in acute pancreatitis)

Differentiation between intra-abdominal mass and the mass arising from abdominal wall

Mass arising from the abdominal wall can be distinguished from intra-abdominal mass by asking the patient in supine position to tighten her abdominal wall muscles by lifting her head and looking at her toes. The following findings are noted:

- The mass arising from the abdominal wall will remain palpable, while the intra-abdominal mass will not be palpable (see figure below).

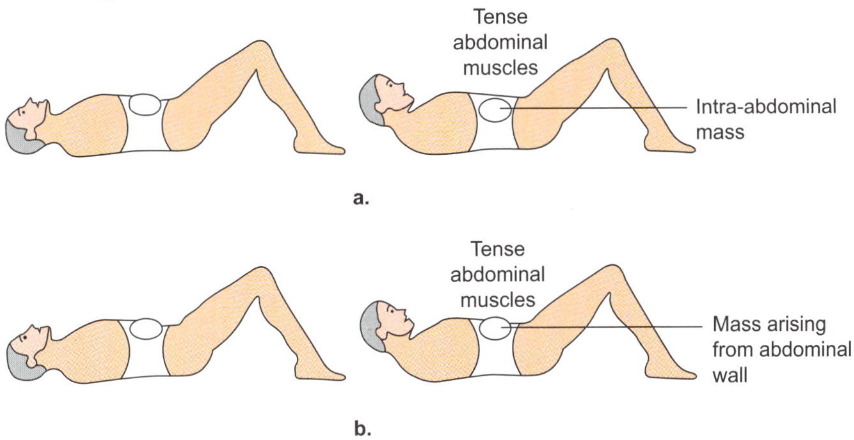

Figure Palpation of abdominal mass. **a.** Palpation of intra-abdominal mass. **b.** Palpation of mass arising from abdominal wall.

Significance of bimanual pelvic examination

- To ascertain uterine size, position, mobility, and presence of any adnexal mass and tenderness
- To differentiate a uterine mass from ovarian mass (discussed in Part 2, Chapter 20, *Fibroid Uterus*)

Significance of rectovaginal and rectal examination

- Tenderness or nodularity of uterosacral ligament and rectovaginal septum—may be present in endometriosis
- Parametrial and rectovaginal septum infiltration—may be present in carcinoma cervix (assessment is required for clinical staging of carcinoma cervix)
- Nodules in POD—may be due to endometriosis or secondary deposits in malignant ovarian tumor
- Bogginess in POD—present in case of collection of blood in ruptured ectopic pregnancy and collection of pus in pelvic abscess
- Retroverted uterus and ovary which is adherent in the POD can be felt as a mass in POD
- Rectal mucosal irregularity—may be present in case of lesion or growth in the rectum
- Rectocele can be diagnosed and differentiated from enterocele

Special indications for performing a rectal examination in gynecology

- In children and virgins, if indicated (vaginal examination is avoided)
- As an adjunct to vaginal examination

- If vaginal examination is painful
- Vaginal atresia
- Endometriosis—nodularity of uterosacrals and adherent ovaries can be appreciated
- Collection in POD—collection of pus in pelvic abscess and collection of blood in ruptured ectopic pregnancy are best made out in rectal examination
- Carcinoma cervix—parametrial, pelvic side wall, and rectal mucosal involvement can be made out
- Carcinoma ovary—secondary deposits in POD may be present
- In cases with rectocele and enterocele
- Patients having bleeding per rectum—to check for any intraluminal growth or lesion

PROCEDURES THAT CAN BE DONE DURING GYNECOLOGICAL EXAMINATION

- Pap smear—obtaining sample for cervical cytology
- Cervical biopsy can be taken in case of cervical lesion
- Collection of sample of vaginal discharge for microscopic examination
- Endometrial sampling in women with peri-menopausal or PMB can be taken on outpatient basis
- Culdocentesis—aspiration of collected pus or blood in POD

Gynecological diagnosis is made after careful analysis of the history, clinical examination, and results of various investigations. Management plans must be formulated and discussed with the patient. The various gynecological clinical exam cases are discussed in the successive chapters of this section.

Viva corner

Q1 What do you mean by anteverted and anteflexed uterus?

- The uterus makes an angle of 90° with that of vagina, termed anteversion. (**Hint:** *Remember as "v" for version—vagina*)
- The body of the uterus makes an angle of about 170° with that of the cervix, termed anteflexion (see figure below).

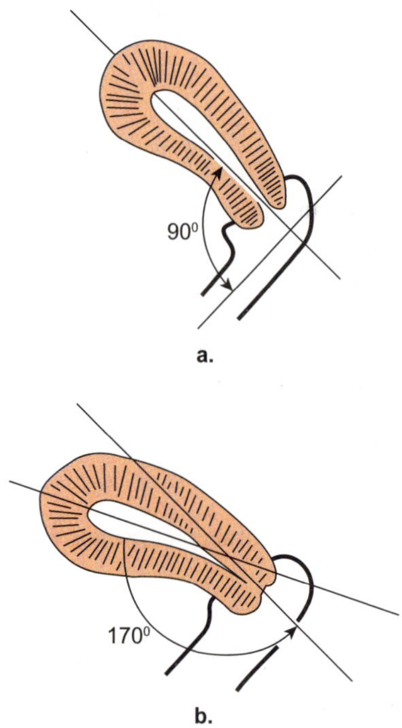

Figure Position of uterus. **a.** Anteversion—angle between uterus and vagina. **b.** Anteflexion—angle between the uterus and cervix.

Frequently asked viva questions

1. What is the importance of age in gynecology?
2. What is the importance of parity in gynecology?
3. What are the common causes of menorrhagia?
4. What are the common causes of PMB?
5. What are the common causes of postcoital bleeding?
6. What are the common causes of abdominopelvic mass?
7. What are the common causes of mass descending per vaginum?
8. What are the common causes of chronic pelvic pain?
9. What are the common causes of white discharge per vaginum?

19 Abnormal Uterine Bleeding

Introduction

Abnormal uterine bleeding (AUB) is a very common problem encountered in gynecology OPD. **AUB** can mean both heavy and irregular menstrual bleeding, and many patients experience a combination of both.

Gynecologists encounter several challenges when delivering medical care to these women due to multiple etiologies of AUB, as well as, numerous available medical and surgical treatment options for the condition. This chapter deals with history taking, clinical examination, evaluation, and management of a case of AUB.

AUB

- AUB is defined as any bleeding from the genital tract, which is a deviation from normal in frequency, cyclicity, quantity or duration of flow, and occurs in the absence of pregnancy.
- AUB includes organic and systemic causes.
- Dysfunctional uterine bleeding (DUB) is defined as AUB in the absence of pelvic pathology or systemic or endocrine causes. This terminology is no longer used (FIGO).

Normal and abnormal menstrual cycle

Earlier, 28 days ±7 days with duration of flow of 3–5 days was considered as normal menstrual cycle. International Federation of Gynecology and Obstetrics (FIGO) has slightly changed the nomenclature in 2018:

- **FIGO AUB system 1** is for nomenclature of symptoms of normal and abnormal bleeding (refer Table 18.2).
- **FIGO AUB system 2** is for classification of causes of AUB (PALM-COEIN). Once bleeding is defined as abnormal, the acronym PALM-COEIN is used for categorizing causes (Table 19.1):
  - *PALM:* Polyp, Adenomyosis, Leiomyoma, Malignancy (and hyperplasia)
  - *COEIN:* Coagulopathy, Ovulatory disorders, Endometrial, Iatrogenic, and Not otherwise classified

Table 19.1 PALM-COEIN classification system for causes of AUB in women of reproductive age group

PALM – structural causes	COEIN – nonstructural causes
• **P** - Polyp (AUB-P) (endometrial or cervical polyp) • **A** - Adenomyosis (AUB-A) • **L** - Leiomyoma (AUB-L) with subclassification system (refer Table 20.1) • **M** - Malignancy and hyperplasia (AUB-M)	• **C** - Coagulopathy (AUB-C): Inherited and acquired coagulopathy, von Willebrand disease, blood dyscrasias • **O** - Ovulatory dysfunction (AUB-O): Anovulatory causes, PCOS • **E** - Endometrial disorder (AUB-E): In women with regular ovulatory cycles with no structural uterine abnormalities, heavy bleeding can be due to a primary disorder at the endometrial level, endometritis • **I** - Iatrogenic (AUB-I): Iatrogenic causes, hormones, IUCD, hormonal contraceptives, anticoagulants • **N** - Not otherwise classified (AUB-N): Arteriovenous malformations (AVM), myohyperplasia, varicose veins of uterus, isthumocele

- The "PALM" components are assessed visually on imaging (structural)) and the "COEIN" are nonstructural components.

Refer Chapter 20, Table 20.1, for subclassification of AUB-L depending on the site of leiomyoma in relation to endometrium, myometrium, and serosa.

Terminologies earlier used in AUB

The terminologies earlier used in AUB indicating abnormal bleeding patterns are represented in Table 19.2 and Figure 19.1. However, these terms such as menorrhagia, metrorrhagia, oligomenorrhea, and DUB have been abandoned as per the FIGO 2018 guidelines. *(These terminologies are still being used by several gynecologists and may by asked in clinicals/viva voce!)*

Types of AUB

- **Chronic AUB:** Uterine bleeding that is abnormal in amount, regularity, and/or duration and has been present for majority of the cycles in the past 6 months
- **Acute AUB:** An episode of heavy bleeding that requires immediate intervention to reduce further blood loss

Agewise causes of AUB (differential diagnosis)

- **Prepubertal**
  - Trauma
  - Foreign body in vagina
  - Sexual abuse
  - Vulvovaginitis
  - Precocious puberty
  - Hormone-secreting ovarian tumors (granulosa cell tumor, germ cell tumor)
  - Exogenous hormones

Table 19.2 Terminologies earlier used in abnormal uterine bleeding *(still being used by several gynecologists)*

Menorrhagia	Excessive (>80 mL) or prolonged bleeding (>8 days) at regular intervals
Polymenorrhea	Bleeding at intervals of less than 24 days *(earlier defined as less than 21 days)*
Oligomenorrhea	Bleeding at intervals of 38 days or more *(earlier defined as 35 days or more)*
Hypomenorrhea	Scanty flow during periods at regular intervals
Metrorrhagia	Irregular acyclical bleeding
Menometrorrhagia	Prolonged and excessive bleeding at irregular intervals
Postmenopausal bleeding	Bleeding that occurs after the cessation of menses for a period of 12 months or more in a woman who is aged 40 years or above

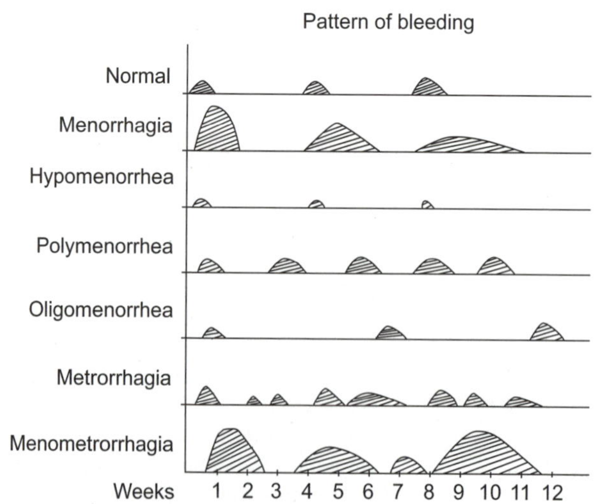

Figure 19.1 Pictorial representation of abnormal menstrual bleeding patterns.

- **Adolescent age group** (**Hint**: *Acronym—PACE^2 IN*)
  - Pregnancy-related causes
  - Anovulatory cycles (due to immature hypothalamo-pituitary ovarian axis)
  - Coagulation disorder—von Willebrand's disease (vWD) and idiopathic thrombocytopenic purpura (ITP)
  - Endocrinopathy—polycystic ovarian disease (PCOD) and thyroid dysfunction
  - Exogenous hormones
  - Infections—PID and genital tuberculosis
  - Neoplasms—hormone-secreting ovarian tumors
- **Reproductive age group**
  - Pregnancy and puerperium-related causes—abortions, ectopic pregnancy, secondary postpartum hemorrhage (PPH), etc.
  - Neoplasms—fibroid and adenomyosis
  - Anovulatory cycles
  - Endometrial causes (AUB-E)
  - Endocrinopathy—PCOD and thyroid dysfunction
  - Exogenous hormones and IUCD-related bleeding
  - Infections—PID and genital tuberculosis
- **Perimenopausal age group**
  - Anovulatory cycles (due to depletion of ovarian follicles)
  - Benign and malignant neoplasms—fibroid, adenomyosis, carcinoma cervix, endometrial hyperplasia and carcinoma
- **Postmenopausal age group**
  - Carcinoma cervix
  - Carcinoma endometrium
  - Endometrial hyperplasia
  - Atrophic endometritis
  - Atrophic vaginitis
  - Exogenous hormones

Ovulatory dysfunction (AUB-O)

- Formerly termed as "anovulatory DUB"
- Most common in adolescent girls and perimenopausal women, accounting for 80% of cases of AUB-O
- Ovulatory dysfunction results from abnormal functioning of HPO axis. In anovulatory cycles, there is no mid-cycle LH surge, resulting in anovulation and absence of progesterone production. Estrogen is the only hormone acting on the endometrium and may result in the following:

Viva corner

Q1 Why is anovulatory bleeding prolonged and excessive?

Pathophysiology of normal menstruation in ovulatory cycles versus anovulatory bleeding is mentioned in the table below that explains the reason for prolonged and excessive bleeding in anovulatory cycles.

Q2 Why is anovulatory bleeding painless?

In the absence of progesterone, there is a marked reduction in the ratio of PGF2-alpha and PGE2 (progesterone is responsible for the secretion of PGF2-alpha) and the lack of PGF2-alpha accounts for uncontrolled nature of bleeding and absence of uterine cramps.

Table Pathophysiology of normal menstruation versus anovulatory bleeding

Normal menstruation	Anovulatory bleeding
• Endometrium is structurally stable due to progesterone effect • Endometrial breakdown is a uniform event following the withdrawal of hormones • Self-limited bleeding due to estrogen-induced re-epithelization • Cessation of bleeding occurs by vasoconstriction, platelet plug formation, tissue collapse, and estrogen-induced tissue re-epithelization	• Endometrium is fragile without structural support due to lack of progesterone • Not a uniform breakdown—random breakdown of endometrium • Insufficient tissue loss to stimulate regeneration of endometrium. There is no healing effect of estrogen • No formation of thrombin plug, no orderly tissue collapse • Altered prostaglandin synthesis

- Threshold bleeding: Endometrium lacks stromal structural support without the growth-limiting effects of progesterone. The relatively low levels of estrogen cause focal areas of endometrial breakdown and shedding, resulting in frequent and prolonged bleeding
- Metropathia hemorrhagica: In some women with anovulation, estrogen production continues in the absence of ovulation → continuous, unopposed estrogen action on the endometrium leads to prolonged periods of amenorrhea of 2–3 months → when the endometrium outgrows its blood supply, bleeding occurs
    - It is also known as cystic glandular hyperplasia or Schroeder's disease.
    - It is common in the 40- to 45-year (perimenopausal) age group.
    - The most common clinical presentation is a bleeding pattern characterized by amenorrhea for 2–3 months followed by painless, profuse, and prolonged bleeding (**Hint:** *Remember "3Ps"*)
    - In some cases, the episode of heavy bleeding may be preceded by normal cycles or menorrhagic cycles.
    - Clinical examination may reveal mild uterine enlargement up to 8–10 weeks.
    - Histopathology of the endometrium shows cystic glandular hyperplasia with the glands showing cystic dilatation termed "Swiss cheese pattern" type of endometrium.

Viva corner

Q1 What is irregular ripening of corpus luteum and irregular shedding?

- **Irregular ripening:**
    - There is inadequate corpus luteal function leading to inadequate progesterone support to the endometrium. It presents as spotting before the start of menses.
    - Premenstrual endometrial sampling reveals incomplete secretory changes in the endometrium.
    - Treatment is to administer progesterone in the premenstrual phase.
- **Irregular shedding (Halban's disease):**
    - Persistent corpus luteum, persistence of progesterone secretion, irregular desquamation, and failed regeneration of endometrium.
    - The menstruation comes on time, bleeding is prolonged, but not heavy. Endometrial sampling on days 5–6 of menstruation reveals a mixed picture of proliferative and secretory endometrium.
    - Treatment is with nonsteroidal anti-inflammatory drugs (NSAIDs) and the condition is self-limiting.

Q2 What are the symptoms and signs of hypothyroidism?

- Fatigue, weakness
- Hair loss, coarse, dry hair
- Cold intolerance
- Muscle cramps
- Constipation
- Weight gain
- Memory loss
- Husky, low-pitched, and coarse voice
- Irregular menstrual cycles with increased menstrual flow
- Depression, irritability
- Pitting edema in the lower extremities

Q3 What are the symptoms and signs of hyperthyroidism?

- Palpitations
- Tachycardia
- Nervousness
- Heat intolerance
- Warm, moist skin
- Tremors in hands
- Insomnia
- Increased bowel movements
- Light or absent menstrual periods
- Weight loss
- Hair loss

Case presentation

Salient points in history

Consider the following relevant points during history taking in cases of AUB:

- *Age (cause for AUB may vary among different age groups)*
- *Socioeconomic status (SES; Ca. cervix is common in lower SES and Ca. endometrium in higher SES)*
- *Parity (fibroid and endometrial carcinoma are common in nulliparous women; adenomyosis and Ca. cervix are common in multiparous women)*

Presenting complaints *Examples of presenting complaints in AUB include:*

- *H/o excessive bleeding during periods (HMB)*
- *Irregular heavy bleeding*
- *Continuous bleeding for ___ days with preceding amenorrhea for ___ months*

Detailed history of the abnormal bleeding should be taken

- *Regularity of cycles, duration of flow, and amount of bleeding (excessive, average, scanty)*
- *Pattern of abnormal bleeding—menorrhagia, polymenorrhea, oligomenorrhea, hypomenorrhea, metrorrhagia, and menometrorrhagia*
- *Associated passage of clots*
- *Type of protection—sanitary pad/cloth*
- *How frequently pads are changed (number of pads changed may not correlate with the amount of blood loss)*
- *H/o preceding amenorrhea (may indicate anovulatory bleeding or pregnancy-related causes)*
- *Additional symptoms that may provide a clue to the underlying disease are the following:*
  - *H/o dysmenorrhea—fibroid, adenomyosis, endometriosis, and PID (anovulatory bleeding usually is not associated with pain)*
    - *Spasmodic dysmenorrhea—in ovulatory cycles*
    - *Congestive dysmenorrhea—in endometriosis and PID*
  - *H/o dyspareunia—endometriosis*
  - *H/o infertility—endometriosis, PID*
  - *H/o abdominal pain—PID*
  - *H/o vaginal discharge—PID*
  - *H/o postcoital bleeding (Ca. cervix, cervical polyp, cervical erosion, etc.)*
  - *H/o intermenstrual bleeding (submucous fibroid, Ca. cervix, cervical polyp, cervical erosion, endometrial polyp, etc.)*
  - *H/o combined oral contraceptive (COC) pill or IUCD usage*
  - *H/o use of any hormones and drugs (unless directly questioned, the patient may not reveal this history)*
  - *H/o easy bruising/prolonged bleeding from wounds, heavy bleeding after surgery or dental procedures (suggestive of bleeding disorder)*
  - *H/o fever/cough/night sweats (suggestive of tuberculosis)*
  - *H/o weight gain, lethargy, hair loss, hoarse voice, cold intolerance, and constipation (suggestive of hypothyroidism)*
  - *H/o weight gain/acne/hirsutism (suggestive of PCOD)*

Menstrual history

- *Age at menarche*
- *Previous cycles—regular/irregular*
- *Flow for ___ days*
- *Amount of bleeding—excessive, average, or scanty*
- *Associated dysmenorrhea and passage of clots*
- *Last menstrual period (LMP)*

Marital history

- *Married for _____ years*
- *H/o multiple sexual partners [risk of PID, sexually transmitted diseases (STDs), cervical carcinoma]*

Obstetric history

- *Parity*
- *H/o of infertility (may be due to anovulation, endometriosis, fibroid, etc., which are causes of AUB)*

(CONTD...)

(...CONTD)

- *Time of last childbirth*
- *Contraception used, if any (irregular intake of COC pills and IUCD usage may present with AUB)*

Past history

- *H/o diabetes mellitus (DM) and hypertension (to be controlled before surgery)*
- *H/o surgery*
- *H/o blood transfusion*
- *Thyroid disorder*
- *Tuberculosis*

Family history

- *Tuberculosis*
- *Any coagulation disorders*
- *Family H/o genital malignancy*

Salient points in examination

Consider the following relevant points during examination in cases of AUB.

General examination

- *Height, weight, and body mass index (obesity and weight loss are risk factors for ovulatory dysfunction)*
- *Hirsutism, acne, and acanthosis (features of PCOD) looked for*
- *Petechiae and ecchymosis (suggestive of coagulation disorder)*
- *Pallor—to know the severity of bleeding*
- *Lymphadenopathy (tuberculosis, leukemia, or lymphoma)*
- *Vitals—temperature, pulse, BP, respiratory rate*
- *Thyroid examination—any thyroid swelling*
- *Breast examination—galactorrhea (prolactinoma is associated with anovulation); any palpable mass (fibroadenoma is associated with hyperestrogenism)*

Abdominal examination

- *Palpate for organomegaly—splenomegaly in idiopathic thrombocytopenic purpura (ITP), hepatosplenomegaly in leukemia.*
- *Abdominopelvic mass may be palpable in structural causes of AUB such as fibroid and adenomyosis.*

Pelvic examination

Inspection of external genitalia

Whether healthy or presence of any lesion/ulcers to be noted

Per speculum examination

Any cervical and vaginal pathology (cervical growth, cervical polyp, cervicitis, any abnormal discharge, etc.) (Per speculum and bimanual examination are expected in case presentation by postgraduate students only. Per speculum and bimanual pelvic examination should not be done in adolescent girls who are not sexually active.)

Bimanual pelvic examination

- *Uterus size (enlarged in pregnancy, fibroid, adenomyosis, etc.)*
- *Uterine tenderness (present in PID, adenomyosis, etc.), cervical motion tenderness in PID*
- *Adnexal mass (ovarian cyst, ovarian tumor, tubo-ovarian mass, ectopic pregnancy, etc.)*
- *Adnexal tenderness (PID, endometriosis, ectopic pregnancy)*

Per rectal examination

Nodularity can be felt in POD and along the uterosacral ligament in endometriosis.

Case summary 1

An example of writing summary in cases of AUB in adolescent age group is given below.

Example *Ms. O, 15 years of age, presents with H/o heavy menstrual bleeding for the past 5 days. She gives H/o irregular cycles with heavy menstrual bleeding since menarche. On examination, pallor is present, vitals are stable, and abdomen is soft on palpation, and on local examination, bleeding per vaginum is present; per speculum and vaginal examination not done.*

(CONTD...)

(...CONTD)

Case diagnosis 1

An example of writing diagnosis in cases of AUB in adolescent age group is given below.

Example *15 years of age, adolescent girl with AUB, most probably puberty menorrhagia due to anovulatory* AUB (AUB-O)

The possible differential diagnoses are as follows:

- *Coagulation disorders*
- *Genital tuberculosis*

Case summary 2

An example of writing summary in cases of AUB in reproductive age group is given below.

Example *Mrs. Q, 34 years of age, multiparous, sterilized woman, presents with complaints of irregular cycles with heavy menstrual bleeding for the past 1 year. Her previous cycles were regular 3/30 days. On examination, pallor is present, vitals are stable, and abdomen is soft on palpation. Speculum examination reveals healthy cervix and vagina. Bimanual examination reveals that the uterus is bulky, mobile, and nontender. There is no adnexal mass or tenderness.*

Case diagnosis 2

An example of writing diagnosis in cases of AUB in reproductive age group is given below.

Example *34 years of age, multiparous and sterilized woman with AUB for further evaluation.*

The possible differential diagnoses include the following:

- *AUB-O*
- *AUB-P, AUB-A, AUB-L (structural causes)*

Case summary 3

An example of writing summary in case of AUB in perimenopausal age group is given below.

Example *Mrs. M, 45 years of age, multiparous and sterilized woman, presents with complaints of irregular cycles with heavy menstrual bleeding for the past 10 months. Her previous cycles were regular 5/30 days. On examination, mild pallor is present and vitals are stable. Speculum examination reveals a healthy cervix and vagina. Bimanual examination reveals uterus uniformly enlarged up to 8 weeks size, mobile, and nontender, and no adnexal mass is palpable.*

Case diagnosis 3

An example of writing diagnosis in cases of AUB in perimenopausal age group is given below.

Example *45 years of age, multiparous and sterilized, perimenopausal woman with AUB for further evaluation.*

The possible differential diagnoses include the following:

- *Perimenopausal anovulatory AUB (AUB-O)*
- *AUB-P, AUB-A, AUB-L, AUB-M (structural causes)*

Note

- *If no structural pathology can be identified on clinical examination, present the case as "AUB for further evaluation," as further evaluation is required to identify or rule out structural causes of AUB.*

Part 2

Case discussion

Investigations in a case of AUB

Appropriate investigations are done based on the case scenario. In majority of cases, history and physical examination will limit the differential diagnosis and lead to logical selection of investigations and diagnostic procedures to identify the cause of AUB.

- Hemoglobin (to determine the severity of bleeding)
- Complete blood count (CBC)—total count (TC), differential count (DC), platelets (to look for any hematological cause for bleeding)
- Blood grouping and typing (patients with severe anemia may require blood transfusion)

- Coagulation profile—bleeding time, clotting time, prothrombin time (PT), and activated partial thromboplastin time (aPTT; indicated in adolescent AUB to rule out coagulation disorders)
- Urine pregnancy test (to rule out pregnancy-related causes)
- Thyroid function test (indicated in adolescent AUB and women with history suggestive of thyroid dysfunction)
- Manteaux test, erythrocyte sedimentation rate (ESR), and chest X-ray in suspected tuberculosis
- Liver and renal function tests (to rule out systemic causes of bleeding)
- Serum FSH, LH, prolactin, testosterone, fasting insulin, and fasting lipid profile (in PCOS cases)
- Pelvic ultrasound [transabdominal sonography (TAS)/transvaginal sonography (TVS)]—to look for endometrial thickness (ET), uterine and adnexal pathology
- Pap smear to be done (carcinoma cervix is one of the causes of AUB; cervical cancer screening with PAP or LBC to be performed once bleeding stops to rule out preinvasive lesions of cervix)
- Fractional curettage or endometrial sampling—especially indicated in perimenopausal women with AUB to rule out endometrial hyperplasia and endometrial carcinoma

MANAGEMENT OF AUB

Treatment is individualized based on the following factors:

- Age of the patient (<40 years, treatment is usually conservative)
- Severity of bleeding
- Etiology or cause
- Desire for fertility and preservation of uterus
- Need for contraception
- Previous treatment details
- Medical comorbidities

General measures

- **Correction of anemia:** Oral iron therapy is sufficient for most women with mild and moderate anemia. Patients with profuse bleeding and severe anemia require packed cell transfusion.
- **Lifestyle modification:** Obese women are advised on weight reduction by regular exercise and intake of healthy diet.

Definitive treatment in AUB

It consists of medical or surgical management and is initiated after identifying the etiology or cause of AUB such as the following:

- **AUB-P:** Polypectomy, hysteroscopic resection
- **AUB-L:** Medical management/myomectomy/hysterectomy
- **AUB-A:** May require hysterectomy
- **AUB-M:** Endometrial hyperplasia without atypia—medical management; atypical endometrial hyperplasia and endometrial carcinoma—hysterectomy indicated; type of hysterectomy for endometrial or cervical carcinoma depend on the staging
- **AUB-C:** Usually responds to medical management with nonhormonal and hormonal therapy
- **AUB-O:** Usually responds to medical management with nonhormonal and hormonal therapy. Levothyroxine in hypothyroidism and Cabergolin in hyperprolactenemia
- **AUB-E:** Usually responds to medical management with nonhormonal therapy. Specific therapies await further delineation of underlying mechanisms for AUB-E; antibiotics prescribed for endometritis
- **AUB-I:** The specific iatrogenic cause of AUB needs to be addressed
- **AUB-N:** Embolization for AV malformation

Thus, the cause for AUB has to be identified and treated accordingly. Medical therapy is the first line of management for women with AUB and surgery is indicated when medical treatment fails.

Management of three different case scenarios, namely, AUB in adolescent age group, reproductive age group, and perimenopausal age group, are discussed in the subsequent sections.

AUB IN ADOLESCENT AGE GROUP

Investigations

- CBC (Hb, TC, DC, platelets) with peripheral smear
- Urine pregnancy test
- Coagulation profile—bleeding time, clotting time, PT, and aPTT
- Thyroid function test
- Renal and liver function tests (to R/o systemic causes of bleeding)

- Mantoux test, ESR, and chest X-ray in suspected case of tuberculosis
- Ultrasonography (USG) pelvis (look for ET, uterine and adnexal pathology)

Special investigations

- Menstrual blood is investigated for tuberculosis polymerase chain reaction (TB PCR) test, if there is a strong suspicion of tuberculosis.
- Special hematological investigations in indicated cases are the following: vWD antigen assay, vWD ristocetin cofactor activity, factor VIII and IX assay, platelet function tests, and bone marrow assay.
- Endometrial aspiration may be considered only in obese girls with persistent anovulatory cycles for 2–3 years despite treatment, to rule out endometrial hyperplasia and carcinoma.

Treatment

Anovulatory AUB is the most common cause for adolescent AUB. The following treatment is initiated, if all other causes are ruled out.

Patients can be divided into three categories on the basis of severity of anemia and treated accordingly.

Mild anemia (Hb 10–11 g)

- The patient is reassured.
- Hematinics are prescribed.
- NSAIDs can be prescribed during menstruation to reduce pain and bleeding.
- The patient is advised to maintain a menstrual calendar.
- The patient is kept under observation with regular follow-up. Usually, regular cycles will ensue in most cases.
- If symptoms persist, cyclical COC pills can be prescribed for 3–6 months.

Moderate anemia (Hb 7–10 g)

- Hematinics are prescribed.
- Nonhormonal therapy is usually prescribed that includes the following:
  - NSAIDs such as mefenamic acid 500 mg BD or TDS during menstruation
  - Tranexamic acid 500 mg TDS during menstruation
- Hormonal therapy is advised if the patient is not responding to nonhormonal therapy.
  - Cyclical progesterone treatment [medroxyprogesterone acetate (MPA) 10 mg/day from day 5 to 25 or day 15 to 25]
  - Cyclical COC pills for 3–6 months

Severe anemia (Hb <7 g)

- The patient should be admitted.
- If the patient is in hypovolemic shock, resuscitate with IV fluids and blood transfusion.
- Hormonal therapy is given to stop an acute episode of bleeding. The following drugs can be used:
  - IV conjugated equine estrogen (25 mg q 4 hours) till bleeding stops, followed by cyclical oral progesterone or COC pills
  - Oral progesterones—norethisterone or medroxy progesterone acetate (MPA) (10 mg q 8 hours—till bleeding stops and then the dose tapered gradually over 3–4 weeks
  - COC pills q 6–8 hours till bleeding stops and then the dose tapered gradually over 3–4 weeks
    - Following treatment of an acute episode of bleeding, hormonal therapy is continued with cyclic progesterones or COC pills for 3–4 cycles
- Hematinics are prescribed to correct anemia.
- Menstrual calendar should be maintained.
- Weight reduction is advised for obese girls.
- The patient should be followed up regularly to check for compliance and improvement of the condition.
- Treatment can be stopped after 3–6 months to ascertain whether cycles have regularized with normal flow or else treatment can be continued.
- Genital tuberculosis should be excluded if the patient is not responding to medical therapy.

AUB IN REPRODUCTIVE AGE GROUP

Investigations

- Complete hemogram—to assess the severity of bleeding.
- Urine pregnancy test (if the woman is not sterilized).
- Ultrasound (TVS is better than TAS) is done to assess the ET and for any pelvic pathology such as fibroid, adenomyosis, endometrial polyp, tubo-ovarian masses, and endometrioma.
- The detection of focal pathology within the uterine cavity such as polyp and submucous fibroid

can be enhanced by performing saline infusion sonography (SIS).
- Pap smear should be done.

Treatment

Treatment depends on the cause of AUB.

Treatment of AUB-E: Ovulatory bleeding

Ovulatory disorder usually responds to nonhormonal therapy. Therapy includes the following:
- NSAIDs—mefenamic acid, ibuprofen, naproxen
- Antifibrinolytics—tranexamic acid
- Ethamsylate
- COC pills and progesterones are also effective in stopping bleeding
- Follow-up to see the response to therapy

Treatment of AUB-O: anovulatory bleeding

- **If the patient requires additional contraceptive benefit:**
  - COC pills are prescribed.
  - If COC pills are not tolerated or contraindicated, cyclical progesterones (MPA or norethisterone 10 mg OD) can be prescribed from day 5 to 25. Alternatively, MPA 150 mg q 3 monthly depot IM injection can be given.
- **If the patient does not require contraception (has undergone sterilization):**
  - Cyclical progesterones can be given as brief course from day 15 to 25 or 21 to 25.
- **If fertility is desired:**
  - Ovulation induction can be done with drugs such as clomiphene citrate or gonadotropins.

Treatment of structural causes

- **AUB-P:** Polypectomy
- **AUB A:** Hysterectomy may be needed
- **AUB-L:** Hysterectomy/myomectomy may be needed

AUB IN PERIMENOPAUSAL AGE GROUP

Investigations

- Complete hemogram—to assess severity of bleeding
- USG—to assess ET and to rule out pelvic pathology
- Diagnostic endometrial sampling—is mandatory in perimenopausal women with AUB to rule out endometrial hyperplasia and carcinoma
- Should perform Pap smear

Treatment

Treatment depends on the cause for AUB.
- **AUB-P:** Polypectomy
- **AUB A:** Hysterectomy may be needed
- **AUB-L:** Hysterectomy/myomectomy may be needed
- **AUB-M:** Type of hysterectomy depends on stage of malignancy (described in Part 2, Chapter 23, *Carcinoma Endometrium;* Chapter 22, *Carcinoma Cervix*).
- **AUB-O:** Progesterones [cyclical MPA or norethisterone/depot MPA injections/LNG-IUD] are the first choice of therapy for AUB-O in perimenopausal age group, provided endometrial malignancy has been excluded.
- In case of failure of medical therapy, endometrial ablation or hysterectomy is done.

ROLE OF USG IN EVALUATION OF AUB

USG provides information on the following:
- ET
- Uterine pathology such as fibroid and adenomyosis
- Endometrial polyp and submucous fibroid [intracavitary lesions are best appreciated in SIS]
- Associated ovarian pathology such as tumor, cyst, and PCOS
- Documentation of ovulation—evidenced by collapse of the dominant follicle with minimal fluid collection in POD

ROLE OF ENDOMETRIAL SAMPLING IN EVALUATION OF AUB

- It provides histopathology of the endometrium for individualization of treatment.
- Endometrial hyperplasia and carcinoma can be detected/ruled out.
- It helps to look for any evidence of endometritis and tuberculosis.
- Ovulation can be confirmed by premenstrual secretory endometrium.

Viva corner

Q1 What is progesterone withdrawal bleeding?

- It refers to bleeding that follows withdrawal of progesterones.
- Progesterone withdrawal bleeding occurs only in an estrogen-primed endometrium.
- Amount of bleeding depends on the previous estrogen-stimulated endometrial proliferation.
  - *Low estrogen levels*: Bleeding light and scanty
  - *Sustained high estrogen levels*: Heavy and prolonged bleeding, but self-limiting
- Examples include bleeding in normal menstruation and in women receiving cyclical progesterone therapy.

Q2 What is progesterone breakthrough bleeding?

- It refers to intermittent bleeding that can occur during continuous treatment with exogenous progesterones.
- Bleeding is of variable duration and is usually light.
- Examples include bleeding that occurs with minipill usage, OCP usage, and progestin IUDs and implants.

Q3 What is estrogen withdrawal bleeding?

- It refers to bleeding that follows sudden withdrawal of estrogen.
- Examples:
  - *Bleeding following B/L oophorectomy during follicular phase*
  - *Midcycle bleed coinciding with abrupt fall in estrogen levels just prior to ovulation*

Q4 What is estrogen breakthrough bleeding?

- It refers to bleeding that follows continuous estrogen exposure as in a case of anovulation.
- Amount and duration of bleeding depends on the duration of unopposed estrogen stimulation.

- Dating of endometrium can be done by premenstrual endometrial sampling (to identify luteal phase defect).
- Pregnancy-related complications can be identified.
- It stops an acute episode of bleeding temporarily (therapeutic curettage).

Indications for endometrial sampling in AUB

- Women with AUB at >40 years (perimenopausal AUB)—to exclude endometrial hyperplasia and carcinoma
- Women of reproductive age with persistent anovulatory AUB (>6 months), associated with risk factors such as obesity, PCOD, or tamoxifen therapy
- Ultrasound showing increased ET (>12 mm) in perimenopausal women
- Postmenopausal bleeding
- Women not responding to medical therapy

Methods for endometrial sampling

- **Fractional curettage (dilatation and curettage):** Requires anesthesia, cervical dilatation and is a blind procedure
- **Endometrial aspiration biopsy:** Anesthesia and cervical dilatation are not required and is a blind procedure
- **Hysteroscopy-directed endometrial biopsy:** Gold standard method for evaluation of endometrial pathology as it allows direct visualization of the endometrium and targeted biopsies

The endometrial histopathology in AUB can be of the following types

- Normal endometrium 50% (proliferative or secretory—most common histology)
- Endometrial hyperplasia 30%
- Irregular shedding 5–10%
- Irregular ripening <5%
- Atrophic endometrium <5%
- Chronic endometritis 1–2%

Types of endometrial hyperplasia (WHO 2014 classification)

- Endometrial hyperplasia without atypia
- Endometrial hyperplasia with atypia

Endometrial hyperplasia has been elaborated in Part 2, Chapter 23, *Carcinoma Endometrium*.

ROLE OF HYSTEROSCOPY IN EVALUATION OF AUB

- It provides direct visualization of endometrium—identifies endometrial polyp and submucous fibroid.
- Endometrial polyp and submucous fibroid can be treated in the same sitting by hysteroscopic resection.
- Hysteroscopy-directed endometrial biopsy can be done in the same sitting and has a better diagnostic yield than a blind biopsy.

Viva corner

Q1 Why is premenstrual endometrial sampling preferred over proliferative phase sampling for dating of endometrium?

Proliferative phase endometrial sampling is not done for dating of endometrium due to the following reasons:

- Proliferative phase is highly variable.
- Proliferative phase changes are not as discrete as changes seen in secretory phase.

Q2 How is luteal phase defect diagnosed?

If the endometrium lags behind by more than 2 days than the expected endometrial picture for that particular day in a premenstrual endometrial biopsy, it is suggestive of luteal phase defect.

Q3 What are the causes of undatable endometrium?

It may not be possible to accurately date the endometrium in the following conditions:

- **If endometrium is under the influence of hormones:** Exogenous hormones, anovulation, and pregnancy
- **If endometrium is affected by organic causes:** Chronic inflammation, hyperplasia, carcinoma, and polyps
- **Sampling errors:** Inadequate tissue obtained (lack of surface epithelium)

ROLE OF SALINE INFUSION SONOGRAPHY IN EVALUATION OF AUB

Procedure

Ultrasound (TVS) is performed after introducing saline into the uterine cavity. It is helpful in the diagnosis of intracavitary lesions.

Indications

- In cases with focal endometrial abnormality in USG
- Cystic or heterogeneous endometrium in ultrasound
- To differentiate submucous fibroid from endometrial polyp

Advantages

- Done as an outpatient procedure
- Cost-effective and avoids unnecessary hysteroscopy
- Tubal patency can be made out by looking for appearance of fluid in POD (but the tube from where spillage occurred cannot be made out)

Disadvantages

- The patient may experience pain during the procedure.
- Risk of infection is present.
- Malignancy cannot be ruled out.

MEDICAL AND SURGICAL TREATMENT OPTIONS FOR MANAGEMENT OF AUB

The treatment options for AUB are listed in Table 19.3. Treatment options depend on the cause for AUB, age, parity, desire for fertility, and associated factors.

Drugs available for medical management of AUB

Nonhormonal

- **NSAIDs** (mefenamic acid 500 mg TDS for 3–5 days during menstruation reduces bleeding by 20–40%)

Extra edge

Features differentiating an endometrial polyp from submucous fibroid are mentioned in the table below.

Table Features differentiating endometrial polyp from submucous fibroid

	Endometrial polyps	Submucous fibroid
Ultrasonography appearance	Echogenic	Hypoechoic
	Lesion projects into endometrial cavity	Lesion distends endometrial cavity
Saline infusion sonography	Pedicle can be identified	Broad base
	Polyp appears more echogenic relative to hypoechoic myometrium	Submucous fibroid can be delineated against the echogenic endometrium
Doppler	Pedicle may be vascular	Peripheral vessels may be seen around the fibroid

Table 19.3 Available medical and surgical treatment for AUB

Medical	Surgical
• Nonhormonal – NSAIDs—mefenamic acid, ibuprofen – Antifibrinolytics—tranexamic acid – Capillary fragility inhibitor—ethamsylate • Hormonal – Progesterones – COC pills (estrogen + progesterone therapy) – Estrogen-only therapy in acute bleeding – Androgenic steroids—danazol and gestrinone – GnRH analogues – LNG IUD – Ormeloxifene—selective estrogen receptor modulator	• Therapeutic curettage • Minimal invasive surgery (endometrial ablation) • Hysterectomy

AUB, abnormal uterine bleeding; *COC*, combined oral contraceptive; *LNG IUD*, Levonorgestrel Intrauterine device; *NSAID*, nonsteroidal anti-inflammatory drug.

- *MOA*: Inhibits cyclooxygenase and thus reduces prostaglandin synthesis
- *Other NSAIDs*: Ibuprofen and ketorolac

- **Antifibrinolytics** (tranexamic acid 500 mg TDS reduces bleeding by 50%)
  - *MOA:* Tranexamic acid inhibits tissue plasminogen activator. In anovulatory bleeding, tissue plasminogen activator, which is a fibrinolytic enzyme, is increased, causing menorrhagia.
- **Ethamsylate** 500 mg TDS
  - *MOA:* It reduces capillary fragility, and thereby prevents capillary breakdown and decreases bleeding.

Hormonal

- **Progesterones:** These are used to arrest bleeding and regulate menstrual cycles.
- Norethisterone and MPA are commonly used.
  - *MOA:*
    - Antimitotic and antigrowth effect on the endometrium
    - Inhibits expression of growth oncogenes and estrogen receptors
  - *To arrest bleeding:* MPA or norethisterone 10 mg TDS is prescribed till bleeding stops and then tapered over 3–4 weeks.
  - *To regularize cycles:* Cyclical MPA or norethisterone 10 mg OD can be given from day 5 to 25 or day 15 to 25 or day 21 to 25 of a menstrual cycle for three to six cycles.
- Injectable progesterones such as depot MPA 150 mg IM injection every 3 months can be used.

However, injectable progesterone is not a popular treatment because bleeding can be irregular and unpredictable, and some women experience amenorrhea.

- **COC pills**
  - *MOA*: COC pills limit endometrial growth and cause orderly regression of endometrium.

- *To arrest bleeding*: High-dose COC pill is prescribed TDS till bleeding stops, and then the dose is tapered gradually over 3–4 weeks.
- *To regularize cycles*—cyclical COC pills for three to six cycles. They reduce blood loss by 50%.
- Seasonale (extended-use COC pills)
  - Prescribed continuously for 84 days followed by a gap of 6 days during which menstruation occurs
  - Improvement in hemoglobin because of prolonged period of amenorrhea
  - Used in severe anemia cases and in chronic systemic illness such as renal causes of AUB to stop bleeding for few months

- **Estrogen-only therapy:** High-dose estrogen therapy can be used to control acute bleeding episodes.
  - *MOA*: It acts by promoting rapid endometrial growth to cover the denuded endometrial surface.
  - It is a very effective method, usually given if other hormonal therapy fails to control acute heavy bleeding.
  - *Intravenous estrogen*: 25 mg conjugated equine estrogen (Premarin) q 4 hours for 24 hours or until bleeding reduces significantly is the usual regimen.
  - *Oral estrogen*: High doses of oral estrogen (2.5 mg conjugated estrogen or 2 mg micronized estradiol q 4–6 hours for 24 hours) usually control bleeding, and then the dose is tapered.
  - Estrogen therapy should be followed by cyclical progesterone therapy or COC pills to stabilize the estrogen-stimulated endometrial growth.
- **Danazol:** Dose is 200–400 mg OD taken oral.
  - *MOA*: It has antiestrogen and antiprogesterone effects—inhibits endometrial growth and blood loss.
  - Danazol has androgenic side effects and hence is not usually recommended. It is used for short-term therapy before surgery.
- **Gestrinone:** Dose is 2.5 mg twice weekly.
  - It inhibits endometrial growth and reduces blood loss.
  - Side effects are similar to but less than those of danazol.
- **GnRH analogues:** Leuprolide 3.75 mg monthly IM depot injection is given.
  - *MOA*: It causes amenorrhea by inhibiting pituitary production of gonadotropins.
  - It is a very effective drug.
  - Main indications
    - While waiting for surgery to buy time to improve hemoglobin preoperatively
    - Prior to endometrial ablative procedures to reduce ET
    - In patients with renal failure and blood dyscrasias for short-term relief from bleeding problem
  - Disadvantages
    - Expensive
    - Causes menopausal symptoms such as hot flushes
    - Causes irreversible osteoporosis if used for more than 6 months
- **LNG IUD:** Levonorgestrel impregnated IUD contains 52 mg levonorgestrel and releases 20 μg/day.
  - *MOA*: Antagonizes the proliferative effects of estrogen and suppresses endometrium, thereby reduces blood loss and dysmenorrhea
  - Provides effective contraception
  - Effective for 5 years following insertion
  - Disadvantages
    - Insertion may be difficult.
    - It takes 3 months to show decrease in bleeding. Hence, it cannot be used to control an acute bleeding episode.
    - Amenorrhea may occur in 25% of cases, hence not advised in young girls.
- **Ormeloxifene:** Newer drug that is a selective estrogen receptor modulator
  - *MOA*: It inhibits estrogen action on uterus and breast and prevents uterine and breast cancers.
  - A substantial reduction in bleeding has been observed when used as 60 mg twice weekly for 12 weeks and then once weekly for 12 weeks.

Adverse effects of the commonly used drugs in the treatment of AUB

See Table 19.4

Table 19.4 **Adverse effects of the commonly used drugs in the treatment of AUB**

Drug	Adverse effects
NSAIDs	Gastritis, autoimmune hemolytic anemia, thrombocytopenia, diarrhea
Tranexamic acid	Nausea, vomiting, diarrhea, thrombosis, abdominal pain
Ethamsylate	Nausea, abdominal pain, headache, rash
COC pills	Nausea, headache, hypertension, hyperglycemia, thrombosis, liver and gallbladder disease, hepatoma, breast cancer
Progesterones	Weight gain, depression, headache, abnormal lipid profile, acne
Danazol and gestrinone	Acne, hirsutism, fluid retention, weight gain, mood changes, breast atrophy
GnRH analogues	Menopausal symptoms, osteoporosis, loss of libido, irritability

AUB, abnormal uterine bleeding; *COC*, combined oral contraceptive; *NSAID*, nonsteroidal anti-inflammatory drug.

Viva corner

Q1 How will you manage a case of acute profuse uncontrollable bleeding?

- History taking and clinical examination are done to assess the blood loss and to exclude structural abnormalities and coagulopathies.
- A wide-bore IV line is secured.
- Blood investigations are done—hemoglobin, blood grouping, typing, and coagulation studies.
- Blood transfusion is indicated in severe anemia (hemoglobin <7 g/dL).
- Urine pregnancy test is done to rule out pregnancy-related causes.

Majority of the cases are anovulatory AUB and hormonal therapy controls bleeding in 24 hours.

Drugs to control an acute bleeding episode in AUB

Progesterone therapy

It is commonly used to arrest bleeding as majority of the cases are due to anovulatory causes and hence respond to progesterone therapy.

- **Dose:** MPA or norethisterone 10 mg TDS till bleeding stops, followed by BD for 7 days, followed by OD for 7 days

Progesterone therapy may not be effective in the following situations :

- Endometrium completely exhausted from prolonged sloughing (thin endometrium in USG)
- Presence of organic cause for bleeding
- Preexisting secretory endometrium

High-dose COC pills

Alternatively, high-dose COC pills can be given to arrest bleeding.

- **Dose:** COC pill TDS till bleeding stops, followed by BD for 7 days, followed by OD for 7 days or till rest of the pill pack gets over.

High-dose estrogen therapy

Alternatively, high-dose estrogen therapy can be prescribed.

- **Dose:** It includes one of the following:
  - Conjugated estrogen (Premarin) 2.5 mg oral dose q 4–6 hours
  - Estradiol 2 mg oral dose q 4 hours
  - Conjugated estrogen (Premarin) 25 mg IV q 4 hours
  - Continued for 24 hours or till bleeding stops followed by OD dose for 7–10 days

Most importantly, arrest of an acute bleeding episode should always be followed by cyclical COC pills or cyclical progesterones for three to four cycles.

Therapeutic curettage

Perimenopausal women with heavy bleeding and women who do not respond to medical management may benefit from therapeutic curettage. It helps in the following ways:

- Controls bleeding temporarily
- Provides tissue for histopathology

Surgical options for management of AUB

Dilatation and curettage

- It serves both therapeutic and diagnostic purposes.
- **Therapeutic purpose:** It reduces bleeding temporarily by removing the structurally fragile, bleeding endometrium. This allows restoration of normal hemostatic events and regeneration of the endometrium.
- **Diagnostic purpose:** The endometrial sample is sent for histopathology to identify endometrial pathology such as endometrial hyperplasia, carcinoma, and tuberculosis.

Endometrial ablation (minimal invasive surgery)

- Endometrial ablation involves destruction of the endometrium by resection or thermal energy.
- Endometrial ablation is a safe and effective minimally invasive surgical procedure that has become a well-established alternative to medical treatment or hysterectomy to treat abnormal uterine bleeding in select cases.

Indications

- Failed medical therapy in AUB
- Poor surgical candidates for hysterectomy
- Patients who do not want surgery
- Women with a desire to preserve the uterus

Endometrial ablation is especially beneficial in perimenopausal age group women who are not desirous of fertility or menstrual function.

Contraindications

- Premalignant or malignant lesion of the cervix and endometrium
- Acute pelvic infection
- Previous upper segment uterine scar (chance of perforation)
- Uterine size >12 weeks
- Uterine malformations
- Desire for future fertility

Advantages

- Less morbid procedure
- Short recovery time

Preoperative preparation

Prior therapy with GnRH analogues or danazol or MPA for 4–6 weeks reduces endometrial thickness that facilitates the procedure (it is easier to resect a thin endometrium).

Various techniques

- **First-generation techniques:** Resectoscopic endometrial ablation
  - Transcervical resection of endometrium (TCRE)
  - Rollerball endometrial ablation (REA)
  - Laser endometrial ablation (LEA)—Nd:YAG laser commonly used
- **Second-generation endometrial ablation:** Nonresectoscopic endometrial ablation
  - Thermal balloon ablation
  - Hydrothermal ablation
  - Microwave endometrial ablation
  - Radio-frequency–induced endometrial ablation
  - Cryotherapy
  - Photodynamic therapy

Outcome

- Improvement in symptoms occurs (reduced rate of dysmenorrhea, blood loss) in 90% of cases.
- Amenorrhea following the procedure occurs in 40–50% of cases.
- Success is not absolute and symptoms may recur or persist—20% of cases may require surgery later.

Viva corner

Q1 Why is pregnancy contraindicated following endometrial ablation?

Endometrium has tremendous regenerative capacity. Although extensive destruction of endometrium is done during endometrial ablation, there is still a chance of persistence or regeneration of endometrium. Complications of pregnancy are more in cases of pregnancy following the procedure.

High-yield points

Advantages of resectoscopic endometrial ablation methods

- Requirement of endometrial preparation is less as it is visually resected.
- Endometrial tissue is obtained for histopathology.
- Other uterine pathology such as polyps and submucous fibroid can be resected in the same sitting.

Disadvantages of resectoscopic endometrial ablation methods

- Require skilled personnel
- Need general anesthesia
- Distension media used, which has its own disadvantages (fluid overload)
- Complications such as uterine perforation, hemorrhage, and thermal injuries to adjacent structures
- Expensive

Advantages of nonresectoscopic endometrial ablation methods

- Can be done in OPD under local anesthesia
- No distension media used (complications due to their usage are avoided)
- No bleeding during surgery
- Duration of the procedure less compared with that in hysteroscopic methods

Disadvantages of nonresectoscopic endometrial ablation methods

Endometrial tissue is not obtained for histopathology.

Complications of endometrial ablation

- Uterine perforation
- Hemorrhage
- Fluid overload (specific to resectoscopic endometrial ablation)
- Intrauterine scarring
- Pelvic infection
- Increased risk of complications if pregnancy occurs following the procedure

Uterine artery embolization (UAE)

- Can be performed in cases of severe uncontrolled bleeding wherein conventional treatment has failed
- Advantage: 90% decrease in bleeding

(Details of the UAE procedure are mentioned in Part 2, Chapter 20, *Fibroid Uterus.*)

Hysterectomy

Indications

- Chronic AUB not responding to medical treatment
- Premalignant conditions such as atypical endometrial hyperplasia
- Associated pelvic pathology that needs concomitant surgery
- Failed endometrial ablation

Routes of surgery

- Abdominal hysterectomy
- Vaginal hysterectomy (VH)
- Laparoscopic-assisted VH (LAVH)
- Laparoscopic hysterectomy (hysterectomy procedure is described in Part 3, Chapter 38, *Common Gynecological Surgical Procedures*)

Advantage

Most effective treatment for control of bleeding

Disadvantages

- Perioperative complications may be present.
- Duration of hospital stay, complications, and recovery period are more compared with those in other treatment modalities.
- We end up removing a normal uterus in one-third of cases.

Frequently asked viva questions

1. Summarize the case.
2. What are the differential diagnoses for the given case?
3. Define AUB. What is PALM- COEIN classification?

4. What are the causes of AUB in different age groups?
5. What investigations do you want to do for the given case?
6. What are the drugs used for medical management of AUB?
7. How will you control acute profuse bleeding in AUB?
8. How will you manage AUB in the perimenopausal age group?
9. What is the role of endometrial ablation in AUB?
10. When is hysterectomy indicated in AUB?

20 Fibroid Uterus

Introduction

Fibroids or leiomyomas are estrogen-dependent benign neoplasms of the uterus that arise from the smooth muscles of the myometrium. Fibroids are one of the important causes of menorrhagia in women belonging to the reproductive age group.

Risk factors

- Age—more common in the third and fourth decades
- Nulliparity (chronic estrogen exposure)
- Obesity (increased conversion of androgens to estrogens)
- Early menarche (prolonged years of estrogen exposure)
- Diabetes and hypertension (HT)
- Strong family history

Protective factors

- Multiparity
- Progesterone-only pills

Anatomical types of fibroid (Figure 20.1)

- **Intramural (70%):** Most common type of fibroids with growth of the fibroid centered within the uterine myometrium
- **Submucous (15%):** Fibroids with growth directed into the endometrial cavity
- **Subserous (15%):** Fibroids with growth directed outwards into serosal layer of uterus

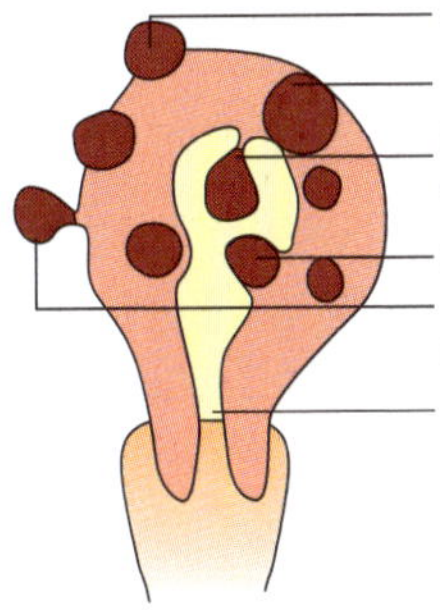

Figure 20.1 Anatomical types of fibroid.

Note

- *All fibroids originate initially as intramural fibroids.*
- *When the fibroid becomes pedunculated with a small stalk attaching the fibroid to the uterus, it is termed as a pedunculated fibroid.*

Other sites of fibroid

- Cervical fibroid [ultrasonography (USG) finding: "lantern on the dome of St. Paul's cathedral" appearance] (Figure 20.2)
- Broad ligament fibroid

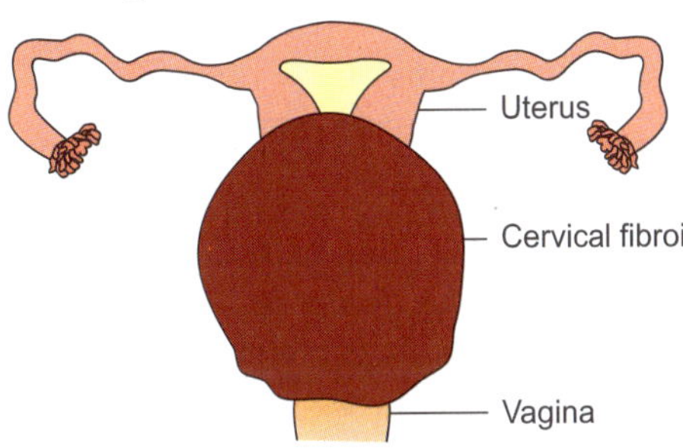

Figure 20.2 Cervical fibroid.

Table 20.1 Subclassification of leiomyoma (FIGO 2018)

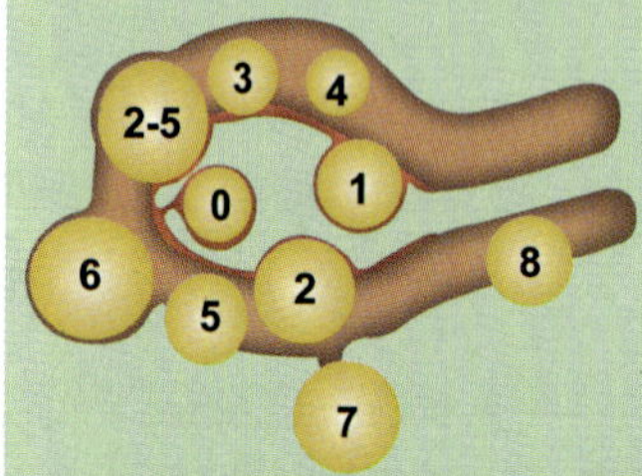	**SM: Submucosal**	0	Pedunculated intracavitary
		1	<50% intramural
		2	≥50% intramural
		3	Contacts endometrium; 100% intramural
	O: Other	4	Intramural
		5	Subserosal ≥50% intramural
		6	Subserosal <50% intramural
		7	Subserosal pedunculated
		8	Other (specify, e.g. cervical, parasitic)
	Hybrid leiomyomas (impact both endometrium and serosa)	Two numbers are listed separated by a hyphen—the first refers to the relationship with the endometrium while the second refers to the relationship to the serosa. *Example:*	
		2–5	Submucosal and subserosal, each with less than half the diameter in the endometrial and peritoneal cavities, respectively.

FIGO 2018 subclassification of leiomyoma depending on the site of fibroid in relation to endometrium, myometrium, and serosa is given in Table 20.1.

Clinical features

- More than 50% of fibroids are asymptomatic
- The patient may present with the following symptoms:
  - Symptoms of anemia—tiredness, easy fatigability, palpitation, etc.
  - Menstrual symptoms
  - Dysmenorrhea
  - Pain abdomen
  - Pressure symptoms
  - Mass abdomen
  - Infertility/subfertility

Menstrual symptoms

Menorrhagia

Causes are as follows:
- Increased surface area of endometrium from where the bleeding occurs
- Increased vascularity of uterus
- Venous congestion—due to compression of veins by the fibroid
- Associated endometrial hyperplasia (both fibroid and endometrial hyperplasia are due to hyperestrogenism)
- Interference with uterine contractility
- Altered prostaglandin metabolism

Polymenorrhea

Causes are as follows:
- Ovarian hyperemia (uterine hyperemia → ovarian hyperemia → early maturation of oocytes)
- Associated pelvic inflammatory disease (PID) (10–15%)
- Associated endometriosis (30%)

Metrorrhagia

Causes are as follows:
- Infection/ulceration of pedunculated submucous fibroid, which may cause acyclical bleeding
- A coincidental presence of endometrial hyperplasia/endometrial carcinoma/endometrial polyp (related to hyperestrogenism)
- Fibroid undergoing sarcomatous change

Note *Irregular bleeding is not a characteristic symptom of fibroid. Hence, in case of irregular or continuous bleeding, endometrial pathology has to be ruled out by doing an endometrial sampling.*

Dysmenorrhea

Spasmodic dysmenorrhea

- Associated with pedunculated submucous fibroid —attempt to expel the fibroid with uterine contractions
- Fibroid at uterotubal junction

Congestive dysmenorrhea

Due to increased vascularity and pelvic congestion

Pain abdomen

- Dull aching pain or heaviness of lower abdomen is the usual complaint.
- Fibroids may give rise to pain in the following conditions:
  - Degeneration and infection of fibroid
  - Torsion of pedunculated subserous fibroid
  - Expulsion of pedunculated submucous fibroid
  - Fibroid outgrowing its blood supply—causing necrosis
  - Fibroid causing pressure on sacral plexus and obturator nerve—backache
  - Fibroid undergoing sarcomatous change
  - Associated endometriosis and PID

High-yield points

Causes for acute pain abdomen in fibroid

- Torsion
- Hemorrhage
- Red degeneration
- Sarcomatous change (rare)
- Infection
- Capsular rupture

Pressure symptoms

These are due to pressure on the surrounding structures such as the following:

- **Bladder**
  - Increased diurnal frequency due to bladder irritability, and urgency
  - Urinary retention—caused by cervical fibroid and fibroid impacted in POD
- **Bowel:** Rectal tenesmus and constipation
- **Ureter:** Possibility of hydroureter and hydronephrosis because of compression by broad ligament or cervical fibroid
- **Spinal nerves:** Backache due to pressure on sacral plexus and obturator nerve (pain radiating to thigh)
- **Veins and lymphatics:** Edema and varicosities of lower limbs

Extra edge

Urological problems in fibroid

- Fibroid may pull up the urethrovesical angle and cause stress urinary incontinence.
- Retention of urine may be present in cervical fibroid and fibroid impacted in POD.
- Hydroureteronephrosis: Broad ligament fibroid and big fibroid may compress the ureter leading to hydronephrosis.

Mass abdomen

Fibroid may present as a slow-growing mass in the abdomen.

Infertility

- Fibroid is the sole cause of infertility only in 3–5% of patients. Also, fibroids more commonly occur in nulliparous women (nulliparous women → uninterrupted estrogen stimulation → fibroid). Hence, fibroids can be the cause or the effect of infertility.
- Extent to which a fibroid can influence fertility depends on the position, number, and size of fibroid.

Note *Mere presence of fibroid in patients with infertility is not considered as the cause of infertility unless all other causes have been ruled out (rule out other causes such as male factor, tubal and ovarian causes).*

Causes of infertility in fibroid

- Fibroids are estrogen dependent and are associated with anovulation and infertility.
- Distortion of endometrial cavity interferes with normal implantation. Submucous > intramural > subserosal fibroid in distorting the endometrial cavity.
- Abnormal uterine contractions due to the presence of fibroid interfere with the following:
  - Sperm ascent
  - Ovum transport
  - Implantation
- Cervical fibroid causes displacement of cervix → prevents sperm ascent.
- Fibroids at intramural portion of fallopian tube interfere with ovum and sperm transport.
- Inflammatory mediators due to the presence of fibroid cause defective implantation and infertility.
- Associated endometriosis may be present.

Part 2

Case presentation

Salient points in history

Consider the following relevant points during history taking in cases of fibroid uterus:
- *Age (more common in reproductive and peri-menopausal age groups)*
- *Parity (more common in nulliparous/infertile women)*

Presenting complaints

Menstrual complaints

Menstrual history has to be taken in detail:
- *Duration of bleeding*
- *Pattern of bleeding (regular/irregular)*
- *Amount of flow*
- *No. of pads changed per day*
- *Associated passage of clots*
- *Associated dysmenorrhea*
- *Last menstrual period (LMP; to rule out pregnancy related causes for bleeding)*
- *H/o intermenstrual bleeding/postcoital bleeding*

Mass abdomen

- *Site*
- *Onset—sudden or gradual increase in size*
- *H/o associated pain*

Pain

- *Site*
- *Duration*
- *Nature/type of pain*
- *Relation of pain to menstrual cycle*
- *Radiation of pain*
- *Aggravating factors/relieving factors*

H/o urinary complaints

- *H/o increased frequency of micturition*
- *H/o acute retention of urine*
- *H/o stress incontinence*
- *H/o symptoms of urinary tract infection (UTI) (dysuria, increased frequency and urgency)*

H/o any vaginal discharge

- *Onset and duration*
- *Quantity, consistency, and color*
- *H/o associated foul smell/itching/blood staining*

H/o infertility

- Since how long is she married?
- Has she been evaluated for infertility earlier? If so, the details of evaluation, if available.

If menorrhagia is one of the chief complaints, ask for important histories such as the following:

- *H/o symptoms of anemia*
- *History suggestive of coagulation disorder*
- *H/o thyroid dysfunction*
- *H/o intake of medications—hormones, anticoagulants, etc.*

If mass abdomen is one of the chief complaints, ask for important negative histories such as the following:

- *Symptoms suggestive of ovarian tumor such as H/o dyspepsia, loss of weight, loss of appetite, hematemesis, and melena*
- *H/o tuberculosis and pelvic inflammatory diseases (patient may have a tubo-ovarian mass)*
- *Family H/o tuberculosis/genital tract malignancy*

Menstrual history

- *Age at menarche*
- *Characteristics of previous menstrual cycles*
  - *Previous cycles—regularity/duration/quantity*
  - *H/o menstrual disturbances in the past*
  - *LMP*

Obstetric history

- *Parity (fibroid common in nulliparous women)*
- *Time since last childbirth*
- *H/o infertility*
- *H/o contraceptive usage*
- *Future plan for fertility and contraception—to plan management*

Past history

- *Diabetes and HT*
- *Tuberculosis*

(CONTD...)

(...CONTD)

- *Surgery (ask for any surgery for similar complaints—myomectomy)*
- *Blood transfusion*

Salient points in examination

Consider the following relevant points during examination in cases of fibroid uterus:

- **Weight:** *Fibroid is more common in obese individuals.*
- **General examination:** *Pallor may be present due to prolonged and heavy bleeding.*
- **Breast examination:** *Fibroadenoma occurs due to increased estrogen and may coexist with fibroids.*

Abdominal examination

Inspection

- *Any distension or visible mass*
- *Umbilicus position*
- *Any scars/sinuses/engorged veins*
- *Cough impulse checked for at hernial orifices*

Palpation

- *Mass is palpable per abdomen if uterine size is more than 12 weeks.*
- *Description of the mass*
  - *Site of the mass (gynecological masses are usually described as "mass arising from pelvis")*
  - *Size (size corresponding to weeks of a gravid uterus)*
  - *Condition of overlying skin (any tenderness, warmth, fixity to mass)*
  - *Borders (inability to reach the lower limit of the mass)*
  - *Consistency (firm/soft)*
  - *Mobility (check for sideways and vertical mobility)*
  - *Margins of the mass (whether well-defined/ill-defined margins)*
  - *Surface of the mass (smooth/bosselated/irregular)*
  - *Any tenderness on palpation*
- *Example: "Mass arising from pelvis up to 16 weeks in size, firm in consistency, with irregular surface; margins well defined; upper and lateral borders clearly made out but lower border is not felt, with side-to-side mobility, and is nontender on palpation."*

Note
- *A degenerated fibroid may be soft and cystic on palpation.*
- *It may be difficult to differentiate a subserous fibroid from an ovarian mass.*

Percussion

- *Fibroid has a dull note on percussion.*
- *Check for the presence of free fluid—may be present in malignant ovarian tumor (which is a differential diagnosis for mass abdomen)*

Auscultation

Abnormal sounds (bruits)—heard in sarcoma uterus (due to increased vascularity)

Genital examination

External genitalia Inspect whether external genitalia is healthy or any lesion is present

Per speculum examination
- *Vaginal mucosa—whether healthy or any discharge/inflammation/lesion present*
- *Cervix—position and whether healthy or presence of any lesion*

Note *Cervix may be pulled high up and hitched behind pubic symphysis in large cervical and posterior wall fibroids.*

Bimanual examination (expected only in postgraduate case presentation)
- *Described as a mass arising from pelvis up to __ weeks in size*
- *In case of uterine mass, the following findings may be present:*
  - *Movement of the mass is transmitted to the cervix (ovarian mass—movement of the mass is not transmitted to cervix).*
  - *Mass is felt in continuity with uterus, that is, no groove is felt between the mass and the*

(CONTD...)

Part 2

(...CONTD)

uterus (ovarian mass—uterus separately felt, groove felt between uterus and mass).

Case summary

An example of writing summary in cases of fibroid uterus is given below.

Example *Mrs. J, 41 years of age, P2L2, sterilized, presents with chief complaints of menorrhagia and dysmenorrhea for the past 8 months. On examination, pallor is present and vitals are stable. Cardiovascular and respiratory systems are within normal limits. Abdominal examination reveals that there is a mass arising from pelvis, enlarged up to 16 weeks size. On speculum and bimanual examination, cervix and vagina are healthy. There is an irregularly enlarged mass up to 16 weeks in size, firm in consistency, side-to-side mobility present, and nontender on palpation. Uterus is not felt separately and movement of the mass is transmitted to the cervix.*

Case diagnosis

An example of writing diagnosis in cases of fibroid uterus is given below.

Example *41 years of age, multiparous and sterilized woman with history and clinical features suggestive of fibroid uterus (AUB-L).*

Case discussion

Differential diagnosis for abdominopelvic mass

The various differential diagnoses for abdominopelvic mass in gynecology are mentioned in Table 20.2.

Note

- *Mention the differential diagnosis specific to a case, taking history and examination findings into consideration.*

Table 20.2 Differential diagnosis for mass abdomen

Differential diagnosis	Explanation
Uterine fibroid	History and clinical examination findings in the example given in the section *"case presentation"* are suggestive of fibroid uterus
Pregnancy	Pregnancy to be ruled out in patients with history of preceding amenorrhea before evaluating for other gynecological causes of mass abdomen
Full bladder	Always examine the patient after she voids to rule out full bladder as a cause of mass abdomen
Adenomyosis	• Patients are usually multiparous with history of menorrhagia and dysmenorrhea • On examination, uterus does not exceed 14 weeks in size, is uniformly enlarged, and on P/V, the uterus is tender on palpation (hence ruled out as D/D in the given case where the uterus is enlarged up to 16 weeks size)
Ovarian tumor	History and clinical examination will help to differentiate an ovarian tumor from a fibroid uterus
Pyometra, hematometra	History and examination will be suggestive of cervical cancer, cervical amputation, tubercular endometritis, etc., that can result in cervical stenosis, leading to pyometra and hematometra
Endometrial carcinoma	Endometrial carcinoma usually presents in early stages with AUB and such marked enlargement of the uterus as in the given case is not seen (hence ruled out as D/D in the given case example)
Tubo-ovarian mass	History suggestive of pelvic inflammatory disease, genital tuberculosis may be present. Tender adnexal mass may be present on examination

AUB, abnormal uterine bleeding; *LMP*, last menstrual period.

Features differentiating a fibroid from adenomyosis are mentioned in Table 20.3.

Table 20.3 Features differentiating a fibroid from adenomyosis

Features	Fibroid	Adenomyosis
Age	Reproductive age group	Perimenopausal age group
Parity	Common in nulliparous women	Usually occurs in multiparous women
Symptoms	Menorrhagia mainly, along with dysmenorrhea	Dysmenorrhea along with menorrhagia is the common symptom
Examination of uterus	Variable enlargement of uterus	Uterus not enlarged more than 14 weeks
	Nontender on palpation	Uterus tender on palpation
	May be irregularly enlarged	Uniformly enlarged
Ultrasonography	Well-circumscribed lesion within the myometrium	Not a well-circumscribed lesion, heterogeneous or coarse myometrium
MRI	Well-circumscribed lesion	Presence of myometrial cysts, asymmetrical thickening of uterine walls, loss of clear endomyometrial border
Surgical option	Myomectomy possible	Difficult to remove adenomyotic lesion as it is not well circumscribed; hysterectomy is the treatment of choice; segmental resection may be possible in isolated lesion in nulliparous women

Clinical features differentiating a fibroid from an ovarian mass are mentioned in Table 20.4.

Table 20.4 Clinical features differentiating a fibroid from an ovarian mass (Figure 20.3)

Feature	Fibroid	Ovarian mass
Age group	Reproductive and perimenopausal	Any age
History	Predominantly menstrual symptoms	Menstrual symptoms usually absent
Examination	Midline mass, arising from pelvis	May be midline or on either side
Mobility	Horizontal mobility only	Both vertical and horizontal mobility may be present
Consistency	Firm	Variable
Ascites	"No ascites"	May have associated ascites/free fluid in malignant ovarian tumor
Bimanual examination	Movement of the mass is transmitted to the cervix	Movement of the mass is not transmitted to the cervix
	Uterus not felt separately from the mass	Uterus felt separately from the mass
	No groove felt between uterus and mass	Groove felt between uterus and mass
		Mass may be tipped through the fornix

Investigations

Most of the cases of fibroid uterus can be readily diagnosed from the patient's symptoms and clinical examination findings. Ultrasound is required to confirm the diagnosis and to exclude ovarian mass and adenomyosis.

- **Transabdominal sonography (TAS)** is preferred when uterus is enlarged and distorted.
- **Transvaginal sonography (TVS)** is preferred when uterus is not palpable. It helps in detection of small fibroids.
- Fibroid appears as a well-defined hypoechoic lesion within the myometrium distorting the uterine contour. It can be intramural or protrude into the endometrial cavity (submucous fibroid) or protrude outwards as a subserous fibroid. It has a

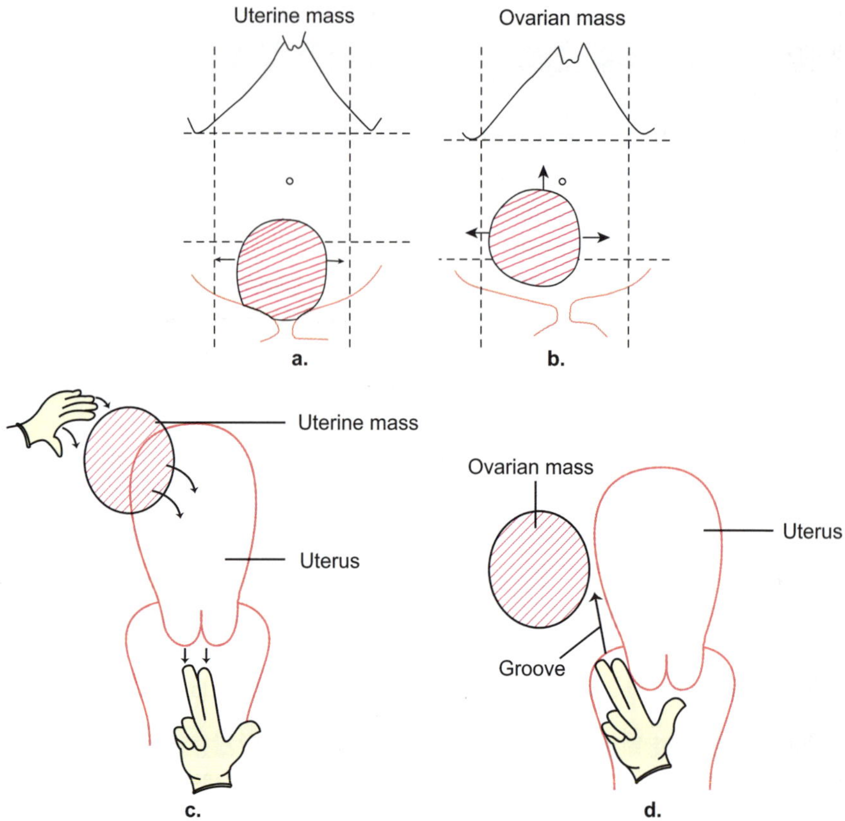

Figure 20.3 Differentiating uterine mass from ovarian mass. **a.** Uterine mass is usually in midline and has only horizontal mobility. **b.** Ovarian mass may be in one of the sides and may have both horizontal and vertical mobility. **c.** Movement of the mass is transmitted to the cervix in case of uterine mass. **d.** A groove is felt between the uterus and the mass in case of ovarian mass.

Viva corner

Q1 How is a true broad ligament fibroid differentiated from a pseudo broad ligament fibroid?

See table below

Table Features differentiating a pseudo and a true broad ligament fibroid

Pseudo broad ligament fibroid	True broad ligament fibroid
Arises from lateral wall of uterus and bulges between the layers of broad ligament	Arises from broad ligament (muscle fibers in parametrium)
Uterine vessels are displaced lateral to the fibroid	Uterine vessels lie medial to the fibroid (see figure below)
Ureter is displaced lateral to the fibroid	Course of ureter is variable in relation to the fibroid. May lie medial or lateral to fibroid

Significance during surgery

Dissection should be limited to within the capsule in case of broad ligament fibroid and the course of ureter has to be delineated before clamping uterine vessels in order to avoid ureteric injury.

(CONTD...)

(...CONTD)

Viva corner

Q2 What are other gynecological conditions that can be associated with fibroid uterus?

Fibroids may be associated with other estrogen-dependent conditions such as the following:

- Anovulation and follicular ovarian cysts
- Endometrial hyperplasia
- Endometrial carcinoma
- Endometriosis
- Adenomyosis

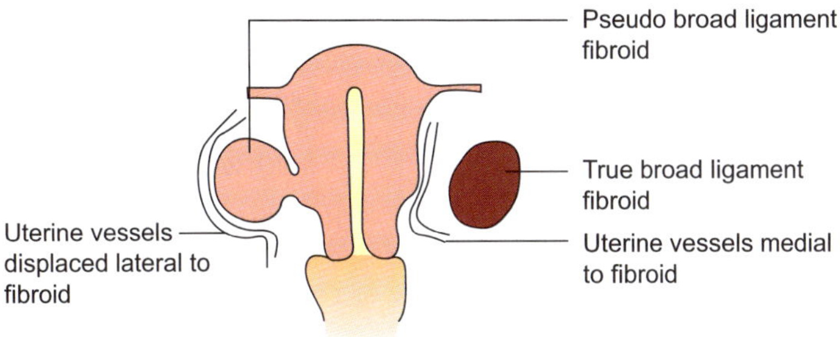

Figure Broad ligament fibroid. True broad ligament fibroid displaces the uterine vessels medially, but the pseudo broad ligament fibroid displaces the uterine vessels laterally.

pseudocapsule formed by the surrounding compressed myometrium that merges with the normal myometrium.

- Degenerative changes in fibroid may produce different echogenic patterns:
  - Irregular central anechoic areas are seen in cystic degeneration.
  - Hyperechogenicity with posterior shadowing is seen in calcified fibroids.
- On Doppler, a fibroid shows a characteristic circumferential flow pattern (vascular ring—vascularity in the periphery and a relatively avascular center).

Uses of USG in fibroid uterus

- To assess uterine size and contour
- To assess number, size, and location of fibroids
- To assess endometrial thickness
- To look for adnexal pathology
- To look for pressure changes such as hydroureter and hydronephrosis in large fibroids
- A preoperative USG guides the surgeon during surgery, laparoscopy, or hysteroscopy for treatment of fibroid
- To differentiate from adenomyosis—which appears as a diffuse lesion with coarse myometrium, more prominently visualized during or just after menstruation
- Saline infusion sonography (SIS) useful in delineating submucous fibroid

Other investigations

- Hemoglobin—to assess the severity of bleeding, and as a part of preoperative workup
- Blood grouping and typing
- Bleeding time and clotting time
- Should perform Pap smear in all cases
- Fractional curettage [endocervical curettage (ECC) and endometrial curettage (EMC)]—indicated in patients with irregular bleeding in perimenopausal age group to rule out associated endometrial pathology
- Intravenous pyelography (IVP) is recommended in cases of large fibroids, cervical , and broad ligament fibroids to look for displacement of the ureter and for any signs of compression such as hydroureter and hydronephrosis
- If surgery is planned, other preoperative investigations required are the following:
  - Urine—albumin, sugar, and microscopy
  - Blood sugar
  - Blood urea and serum creatinine
  - HIV and HBsAg
  - ECG and chest X-ray (if >35 years)

High-yield points

Special investigations other than USG used in the evaluation of fibroid:

MR imaging

- It is currently considered as the most accurate imaging technique for the detection and localization of leiomyomas. Superior to USG in diagnosis of fibroid, but very expensive
- An MRI pelvis may be required for accurate mapping of fibroids, especially in cases planned for myomectomy
  - Can detect small fibroid (<5 mm)
  - Can detect fibroid in unusual locations
  - Differentiates fibroid from adenomyosis
  - Differentiates subserous fibroid from adnexal pathology
  - Definitive diagnosis of adenomyosis and leiomyosarcoma

Role of MR imaging in treatment of fibroids:

- Helps in surgical planning prior to myomectomy
- To monitor the response to medical therapy
- To predict and assess the response to uterine artery embolization
- **Hysteroscopy**
  - Can visualize and remove submucous fibroid and endometrial polyps (diagnostic and therapeutic)
  - To differentiate submucous fibroid and endometrial polyps (which is difficult in USG)
- **Saline infusion sonography (SIS):** Evaluation of endometrial cavity is enhanced by infusion of saline into endometrial cavity.
  - Differentiates submucous fibroid from endometrial polyps
  - Diagnosis of uterine synechiae
  - Can assess tubal patency as evidence of spillage of saline into peritoneal cavity (free fluid in POD which was not visualized prior to saline infusion)
- **Hysterosalpingography (HSG):** In cases of infertility:
  - Filling defects and distortion of endometrial cavity—noted in submucous fibroid and endometrial polyps
  - To check for tubal patency
- **Laparoscopy**
  - Subserous fibroids can be resected.
  - Tubal patency can be checked in infertility cases.
  - PID and endometriosis can be diagnosed.
- **X-ray:** Calcified fibroids can be seen as "egg shell calcification" in pelvic X-rays taken for another purpose such as HSG or IVP.

Complications of fibroid

- Torsion (common in subserosal pedunculated fibroid)
- Hemorrhage into fibroid
- Infection (submucous fibroids are prone to infection and ulceration)
- Degeneration
- Uterine inversion—can rarely occur in a submucous fibroid
- Malignant change (very rare)

Secondary changes in fibroid

- Atrophy—occurs during menopause
- Degeneration
  - Hyaline degeneration (most common)
  - Fatty degeneration
  - Cystic degeneration
  - Calcareous degeneration—seen in old patients with long-standing fibroid (phosphates and carbonates are deposited along the course of the vessels and visualized in X-ray)
  - Red degeneration (common during pregnancy)
- Sarcomatous change
  - 0.2% incidence
  - Presents as sudden increase in size of fibroid, postmenopausal bleeding, and tenderness on palpation
  - Absence of capsule and increased vascularity in USG

Viva corner

Q1 What is a wandering fibroid?

A subserous fibroid can undergo torsion and may detach completely from the uterus and receive blood supply from an adjacent structure; such a fibroid is termed a parasite or wandering fibroid.

Treatment

Treatment for fibroid is based on the following:
- Patient's age
- Severity of symptoms
- Desire for future fertility
- Patient's preference

Treatment options include the following:
- **Conservative or expectant management:** Asymptomatic fibroids may be treated conservatively
- **Medical management:** Not curative, only a temporary therapy
- Commonly used drugs
  - Nonsteroidal anti-inflammatory drugs (mefenamic acid)
  - Hemostatic agents (tranexamic acid, ethamsylate)
  - Combined hormonal contraceptives and progestins appear to have limited efficacy in the treatment of uterine leiomyomas
  - Antiprogestogens (mifepristone)
  - GnRH agonists (leuprolide, naferelin, goserelin)
  - GnRH antagonists (cetrorelix, ganirelix)
  - Androgenic steroids (danazol, gestrinone)
- Newer drugs
  - Selective estrogen receptor modulators (raloxifene, ormeloxifene)
  - Selective progesterone receptor modulators (ulipristal acetate, asoprisnil)
  - Aromatase inhibitors (anastrozole)
- **Surgical management:** Definitive treatment
  - *Hysterectomy*: Abdominal, vaginal, laparoscopic-assisted vaginal hysterectomy (LAVH), and laparoscopic hysterectomy
  - *Myomectomy*: Abdominal, vaginal, hysteroscopic, and laparoscopic myomectomy
- **Minimally invasive techniques:** Destruction of fibroid by various methods such as the following:
  - Myolysis
  - Uterine artery embolization (UAE)
- **Noninvasive procedure:** Magnetic resonance-guided focused ultrasound (MRFUS)

The various treatment options are described next.

Expectant management

Indications

- Asymptomatic fibroids
- Fibroids detected in postmenopausal age group

Prerequisites

- Diagnosis is certain and other causes of pelvic mass excluded.
- The patient is willing to come for regular follow-up.

Follow-up during expectant management

- Initial assessment of size, number, and location of fibroids by ultrasound is done.
- The patient is advised to maintain a menstrual calendar.
- The patient is followed up every 6 months to 1 year.
  - Any fresh symptoms are noted.
  - Bimanual examination and USG are done to determine the growth of fibroid.
  - Interfere or treat when required.

Medical management

Medical management can alleviate symptoms and reduce the size of fibroid. However, medical therapy can be used only for short duration due to side effects of drugs. Hence, medical therapy is not curative, and is only a temporary substitute for definitive surgical therapy.

Indications for medical therapy

- Symptomatic fibroids (menorrhagia, dysmenorrhea)
- Emergency control of heavy bleeding
- Correction of anemia before surgery
- Temporary postponement of surgery
- Women unwilling for surgery
- In patients who are medically unfit for surgery [e.g., uncontrolled diabetes mellitus (DM), HT]
- To minimize the size and vascularity of fibroid prior to surgery
  - Before myomectomy
  - Converts the route of surgery [abdominal to vaginal hysterectomy (VH)]
- Women nearing menopause (perimenopausal women as fibroids reduce in size following menopause)

Table 20.5 Nonhormonal medical therapy for fibroid uterus

Prostaglandin synthetase inhibitor—Mefenamic acid	
Mechanism of action	Inhibits PG synthetase
Dose	500 mg TDS
Advantages	Decreases dysmenorrhea and blood loss (20%)
Disadvantage	No decrease in the size of fibroid
Side effects	Nausea, vomiting, gastric discomfort, diarrhea
Hemostatic agents	
Tranexamic acid	
Mechanism of action	Inhibits tissue plasminogen activator, an antifibrinolytic enzyme
Dose	500 mg TDS (PO) or 10–15 mg/kg body weight IV q8 hourly
Advantage	Reduces blood loss by 50%
Disadvantage	No decrease in the size of fibroid
Side effects	Nausea, dizziness, abdominal pain, and diarrhea
Ethamsylate	
Mechanism of action	Reduces capillary fragility → prevents breakdown of capillaries
Dose	500 mg TDS
Advantage	Reduces blood loss
Disadvantage	No decrease in the size of fibroid
Side effects	Nausea, headache, and abdominal pain

Drugs used for medical management of fibroid

Iron therapy

Correction of anemia with oral iron therapy

Nonhormonal therapy

The drugs used for nonhormonal therapy are mentioned in Table 20.5.

Hormonal therapy

Low-dose COC pills

Low-dose COC pills may be useful in some women with heavy menstrual bleeding (HMB), but they do not appear to be effective in decreasing bulk symptoms.

- **Mechanism of action (MOA):** Causes endometrial atrophy and decreases prostaglandin production
- **Advantage:** Reduces HMB

Progestins

Progestin therapy for medical management of fibroids has shown mixed results and further studies are necessary to evaluate the current and long-term effects of these therapies.

- Progestins cause endometrial atrophy and thus provide relief of menstrual bleeding-related symptoms. Hence, may be considered for treatment of mild symptoms.
- *LNG-IUD* is one of the options as a local treatment for menorrhagia and symptomatic myoma.
- The effectiveness of progestin implants, injections, and pills for treatment of fibroids is still controversial.
- **Levonorgestrel IUD**
  - *MOA:* Levonorgestrel that is released causes thinning of endometrium → decreases blood loss.
  - *Advantages*
    - Reduces blood loss
    - Reduces uterine volume
    - Provides additional contraceptive benefit
  - *Disadvantages*
    - Expensive
    - Cannot be used in fibroids that distort endometrial cavity and when uterine size is >12 weeks
    - Side effects—breakthrough bleeding and amenorrhea

GnRH agonists These include leuprolide, nafarelin, goserelin, and buserelin (Table 20.6).

GnRH antagonists These include cetrorelix and ganirelix (Table 20.7).

Androgenic steroids These include danazol and gestrinone (Table 20.8).

Antiprogesterone This includes RU 486 (mifepristone) (Table 20.9).

Table 20.6 GnRH agonists in medical management of fibroid

Mechanism of action	Continuous GnRH exposure → initial flare reaction followed by downregulation of pituitary gonadotropin receptors → decrease in GnRH release → suppression of estrogen and progesterone synthesis (hypogonadism or pseudo or medical menopause state)
Dose	• Leuprolide 3.75 mg IM q monthly for 3–6 months • Goserelin 3.6 mg SC q monthly for 3–6 months • Nafarelin 200 mg nasal spray daily
Advantages	• Reduce fibroid size (50%) • Reduce menorrhagia, causes amenorrhea, and restores hemoglobin level • Reduce the vascularity—decreases blood loss during surgery → decreased need for transfusion • The fibroid reduces in size so that the route of hysterectomy can be changed (the need for abdominal hysterectomy can be changed to VH or LAVH. The need for vertical skin incision can be changed to transverse skin incision)
Disadvantages	• Expensive • Hypoestrogenic side effects • Can cause thinning of fibroid capsule and enucleation becomes difficult during myomectomy (loss of surgical planes during surgery) • Possibility of small seedling fibroids going unnoticed during surgery and recurring later • Increase in size of fibroid after stopping the drug
Side effects	• GnRH analogues not to be used for more than 6 months • Prolonged use leads to hypoestrogenic side effects—menopausal symptoms such as hot flushes, weight gain, mood swings, depression, vaginal dryness, and osteoporosis – All the menopausal symptoms are reversible on stopping the drug except bone demineralization (osteoporosis) that is irreversible – Add-back therapy is used to decrease the risk of osteoporosis – Drugs used for add-back therapy include combined estrogen + progestins, tamoxifen, raloxifene, tibolone, and bisphosphonates (alendronate)

LAVH, laparoscopic-assisted vaginal hysterectomy; *VH*, vaginal hysterectomy.

Table 20.7 GnRH antagonists in medical management of fibroid

Mechanism of action	Rapid decrease in gonadotropins → hypoestrogenic state → decrease in fibroid size
Dose	Cetrorelix 60 mg IM dose, repeated after 3–4 weeks
Advantages	• No initial flare effect

Note: These drugs require further evaluation. GnRH antagonists appear to be less reliable than GnRH agonists in studies.

Table 20.8 Androgenic steroids in medical management of fibroids

Mechanism of action	Androgenic steroids such as danazol and gestrinone have antigonadotropin activity → decrease in LH and FSH → decrease in estrogen → decrease in fibroid size
Dose	• Danazol: 400–800 mg/day for 6 months • Gestrinone: 2.5 mg twice per week for 6 months

(CONTD...)

Table 20.8 *(CONTD...)*	
Advantages	• Reduce the size of fibroid and improves menorrhagia • Halt rapid regrowth of fibroid following discontinuation of therapy (unlike GnRH analogues)
Side effects	Androgenic and hypoestrogenic side effects (side effects are more with danazol than with gestrinone): Acne, hirsutism, weight gain, edema, hair loss, deepening of voice, flushing, sweating, and vaginal dryness

FSH, follicle-stimulating hormone; *LH*, luteinizing hormone.

Table 20.9 Mifepristone in the medical management of fibroid	
Mechanism of action	Acts by blocking progesterone receptors in fibroid
Dose	10–25 mg/day for 3 months
Advantages	• Causes amenorrhea and decrease in size of fibroid by 50% • No decrease in bone density and no menopausal symptoms (unlike GnRH) • Growth rate of fibroid after stopping the drug is less compared with that of GnRH analogues
Disadvantages	• Causes endometrial hyperplasia, which is a major concern • Expensive

Newer drugs

- **Selective progesterone receptor modulators:** Asoprisnil and ulipristal acetate
  - *MOA*: They demonstrate progesterone specific agonist or antagonist activity which is dependent on target tissue
  - *Dose*: Ulipristal acetate 5–10 mg or Asoprisnil 5–10 mg PO daily for 12 weeks causes amenorrhea and reduces menstrual blood loss and fibroid volume
  - *Advantage*: No endometrial hyperplasia (unlike progesterone receptor antagonist mifepristone)
- **Selective estrogen receptor modulators:** Raloxifene, ormeloxifene
  - *MOA*: They are nonsteroidal agents that bind to estrogen receptor and modulate its effects. They exhibit either agonist or antagonist effects depending on the target tissue.
  - *Dose*: Raloxifene 60 mg/day for 12 months has been shown to cause a significant decrease in uterine size and myoma size.
- **Aromatase inhibitors:** Fadrozole and anastrozole→ reduce fibroid size and bleeding.
  - *MOA*: Inhibit aromatase enzyme that converts estrogen to active estradiol, which plays a role in fibroid growth (aromatase enzyme is highly expressed in fibroid when compared with normal myometrium). Further research is needed into the use of this class of drugs in women of reproductive age.

Main disadvantage of medical therapy

All medical therapies are only temporary. Symptoms recur and the size of fibroid may increase after stopping medical treatment.

Surgical management

Surgery is the definitive treatment for fibroid.

Indications for surgical management of fibroid

- Symptomatic fibroids—menorrhagia, pain, pressure symptoms, and anemia due to blood loss
- Asymptomatic fibroid causing pressure on ureters and hydroureteronephrosis, such as broad ligament fibroid
- Failure to respond to medical management
- Infertility, if other causes have been ruled out
- Habitual abortion caused by submucous fibroid
- Pedunculated subserous fibroids because they can undergo torsion
- Growth of fibroid after menopause
- When nature of the mass cannot be ascertained or rapidly growing fibroids (defined as a gain of 6 weeks or more in uterine size within a year or less—high suspicion of malignancy)

Extra edge

Earlier it was believed that surgical intervention was required for fibroids >12 weeks size for the following reasons:

- Potential compression of adjacent structures with further increase in size
- Greater surgical risk if fibroid becomes larger in size
- Inability to accurately assess ovaries if fibroid is more than 12 weeks in size
- Possible malignancy of the pelvic mass

Current recommendation: Expectant management can be offered to asymptomatic fibroids of any size with radiological monitoring and patient counseling.

Intervention on the basis of size of fibroid alone is not advised for the following reasons:

- Surgery for larger fibroids is not associated with increased morbidity.
- Fibroids may continue to remain without producing any symptoms.
- Risk of malignant change is extremely low.

Hence, there is no definite size above which surgery is recommended, and each case has to be judged individually.

Hysterectomy (Figure 20.4)

Indications

- Age >40 years
- Multiparous women who have completed family
- Other treatment options for fibroid being contraindicated or having failed
- Uncontrolled bleeding during myomectomy

Routes of surgery

- Abdominal hysterectomy
- VH
- Total laparoscopic hysterectomy (TLH)
- LAVH

Factors to be considered before deciding the route of surgery

- Uterine size
- Presence of other associated gynecological conditions or diseases
- Location, number, and size of fibroids
- H/o previous abdominal surgeries
- Mobility and descent of uterus

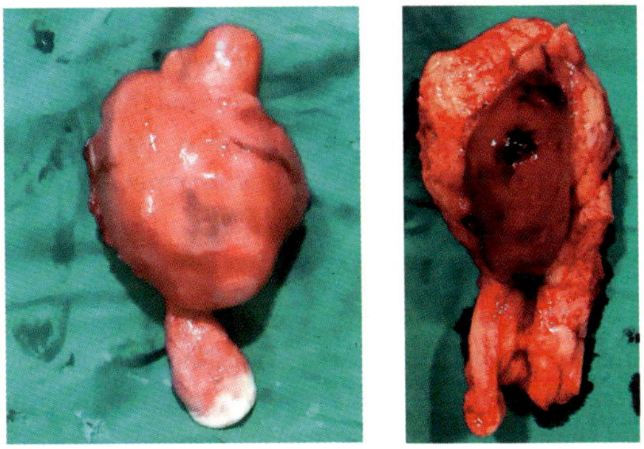

a. b.

Figure 20.4 Hysterectomy specimens. **a.** Hysterectomy specimen showing multiple fibroid uterus. **b.** Hyterectomy specimen cut open to show submucous fibroid.

Prerequisites for vaginal hysterectomy

- Uterine size of 12–14 weeks
- No previous surgeries
- No adnexal pathology
- No other pelvic pathology such as endometriosis
- No suspicion of malignancy
- Mobile uterus
- Laxity of vagina, descent of cervix, and wide subpubic angle—serve as helpful factors during surgery

Advantages of VH

- Faster postoperative recovery
- Shorter hospital stay

Surgical procedure of abdominal and vaginal hysterectomy is discussed in Part 3, Chapter 38, *Common Gynecological Surgical Procedures.*

Procedures to remove big fibroids during VH

- Myomectomy with a myoma screw
- Morcellation (to remove in piecemeal)
- Bisection/bivalving (dividing into two halves)
- Coring

All these procedures are tried after opening UV fold and POD and only after clamping of uterine vessels.

Total laparoscopic hysterectomy

TLH includes laparoscopically detaching the uterine body and cervix from the surrounding supporting structures and suturing the vaginal cuff. It includes bivalving, coring, or morcellating the excised tissues, as required. The uterus is then removed through the vagina or abdomen (uterine vessels are clamped abdominally through the laparoscopic port).

Laparoscopy-assisted vaginal hysterectomy

LAVH includes laparoscopically detaching the uterine body from the surrounding upper supporting structures. The vaginal portion of the procedure is then performed, uterine vessels are clamped, and the cervix and uterus are detached from the remaining supporting structures. The uterus is then removed through the vagina (uterine vessels are clamped through vaginal route).

Contraindications for TLH or LAVH

- Broad ligament fibroid and cervical fibroid
- Associated endometriosis and pelvic adhesions

Complications of hysterectomy

- Anesthetic complications
- Intraoperative
  - Hemorrhage
  - Injury to bladder, ureter, bowel, etc.
- Immediate postoperative
  - Hemorrhage
  - Sepsis
  - Paralytic ileus and intestinal obstruction
  - Thrombosis, pulmonary embolism, and chest infection
  - Burst abdomen
- Late postoperative
  - Dyspareunia—due to adhesions and short vagina
  - Chronic pelvic pain
  - Incisional hernia
  - Residual ovarian syndrome
  - Vault granuloma
  - Vault prolapse
  - Early onset menopause due to atrophy of ovaries following decreased vascularity

Myomectomy

It is a term used for removal of the fibroid alone while preserving the uterus.

Viva corner

Q1 What is the role of prophylactic oophorectomy during hysterectomy?

Prophylactic oophorectomy is the removal of healthy ovaries in high-risk women to reduce future risk of ovarian and/or breast carcinoma. The procedure has fallen into controversy as it is frequently being performed in women with average/low risk, along with hysterectomy for benign causes.

Pros:

- Reduces future risk of ovarian and/or breast carcinoma
- Eliminates the potential for further surgery for benign disease

Cons:

- The removal of healthy ovaries deprives the benefits of endogenous estrogens in premenopausal women and benefits of endogenous androgens in postmenopausal women thereby increasing the mortality from cardiovascular diseases.
- It may also result in problems such as osteoporosis, cognitive impairment, sexual dysfunction, and parkinsonism.
- The risks, costs, and benefits of prophylactic oophorectomy in the absence of genetic markers and at the time of hysterectomy for benign lesions have not been fully evaluated.
- The number needed to treat for prophylactic bilateral oophorectomy in women at low risk for developing ovarian cancer is 300.

Interpretation:

Prophylactic oophorectomy is associated with a decreased risk of breast and ovarian cancer but an increased risk of mortality due to cardiovascular diseases.

Current recommendation:

- Women with a strong family history of ovarian and/or breast cancer and those who carry germline mutations (BRCA-1 and BRCA-2) have a significantly increased lifetime risk for developing

(CONTD...)

(...CONTD)

Viva corner

ovarian cancer. Hence, prophylactic oophorectomy is recommended in these women.

- It has been suggested that for women at low risk of ovarian cancer, ovarian conservation until at least till age 65 years seems to benefit long-term survival. Hence, the current opinion is for a thoughtful scrutiny of the practice of prophylactic oophorectomy for women at all ages, who are not known to be at increased risk for ovarian cancer.

Indications

- Younger age group
- Women with symptomatic fibroid desiring fertility
- Patient who wishes to retain her uterus
- Submucous, subserous, and pedunculated fibroids
- When in vitro fertilization (IVF) is indicated (if fibroid distorts uterine cavity)

Extra edge

ACOG criteria for myomectomy in patients with infertility

Indications for myomectomy in patients with infertility or recurrent pregnancy loss:

- Presence of fibroid of sufficient size or specific location as a probable factor for infertility
- No other likely explanation existing for failure to conceive or recurrent pregnancy loss other than the fibroid
- Steps prior to the procedure
  - Evaluate other causes of male and female infertility or recurrent pregnancy loss.
  - Evaluate the endometrial cavity and fallopian tubes (by doing a hysterosalpingogram).
  - Counsel regarding complications and that the myomectomy procedure may end up in hysterectomy to control heavy bleeding during the surgery.

Routes of myomectomy

- Abdominal myomectomy
- Laparoscopic myomectomy
  - *Indications*: Can remove fibroids <10 cm in diameter and <5 in number by laparoscopy
  - *Advantages*: Less postoperative pain, faster recovery, short hospital stay, and cosmetically better
  - *Disadvantages*
    - Prolonged operative time
    - Requires expertise
    - May need to be converted to laparotomy in case of complications and hemorrhage
    - Increased postoperative adhesions
    - Risk of uterine rupture in subsequent pregnancy, as approximation is not perfect as in abdominal myomectomy
    - High recurrence (a small fibroid not recognized at laparoscopy can regrow later)
- Hysteroscopic myomectomy
  - *Indications*: Submucous fibroid with less than 50% extension into myometrium, and submucous fibroid polyp
  - *Complications*
    - Uterine perforation
    - Hemorrhage
    - Fluid overload due to distension media used for hysteroscopy

Preoperative preparation for myomectomy

- Correction of anemia and adequate arrangement of crossmatched blood prior to surgery
- USG to note number, site, and size of fibroids
- Preoperative GnRH/danazol/mifepristone to decrease size and vascularity of fibroid
- In cases of infertility and recurrent pregnancy loss —rule out other causes
- Surgery planned in the postmenstrual phase to reduce blood loss
- The patient counseled regarding the following aspects:
  - The patient may require hysterectomy in case of excessive hemorrhage—consent for hysterectomy to control hemorrhage during the procedure is taken.
  - There is 40–60% chance of pregnancy after myomectomy.
  - There is 30–50% chance of recurrence/persistence of fibroid after myomectomy.
  - There is 1–5% chance of persistence of menorrhagia after myomectomy.
  - There is 20–25% risk of relaparotomy after myomectomy.

Part 2

Principles of myomectomy

- Anesthesia: Controlled hypotensive anesthesia (less popular) may be used. Sodium nitroprusside or nitroglycerine is used to maintain mean BP of 60 mmHg.
- Trendelenburg position facilitates venous drainage and decreases BP at the operative site.
- After the abdomen is entered, uterine anatomy is identified by noting position of the round ligaments. The adnexa and ureters are identified.
- Steps taken for prevention of intraoperative hemorrhage
  - Local injection of vasoconstrictive agents such as vasopressin (20 units of vasopressin diluted in 200 mL of NS) or adrenaline infiltration over operating planes
  - Occlusion of uterine vessels (at the level of uterine isthmus) and ovarian vessels (around the infundibulopelvic ligament) by using either a tourniquet or Bonney's myomectomy clamp (Figure 20.5)

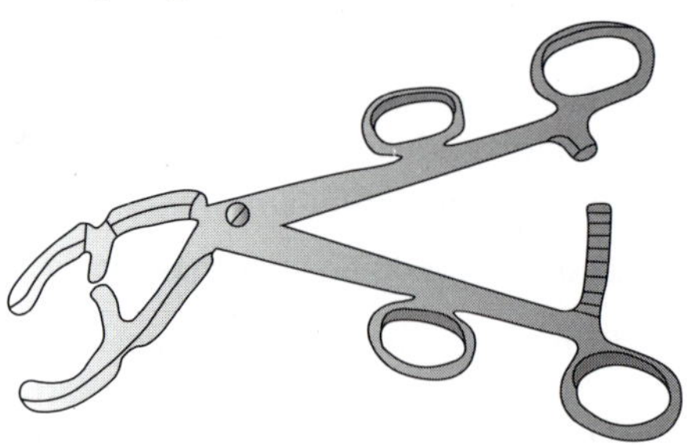

Figure 20.5 Bonney's myomectomy clamp.

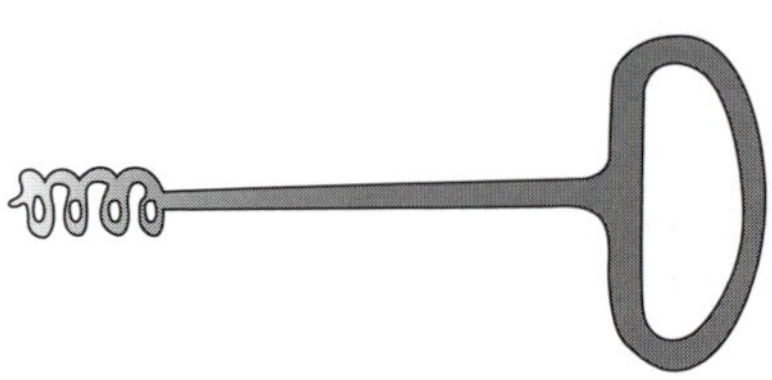

Figure 20.6 Myoma screw.

- A longitudinal incision is given on the anterior wall of uterus over the most prominent part of the fibroid and deepened till the plane between the capsule and the fibroid is reached and tunneling incision is proceeded with to reach other fibroids. The fibroid is separated from the capsule by sharp and blunt dissection and is removed with a myoma screw (Figure 20.6).
- All fibroids should be attempted to be removed through a single incision or fewer incisions as far as possible. Posterior wall fibroids are removed through an anterior incision by transcavity approach.
- Posterior incision is avoided (increases adhesions which may impede future fertility).
- Avoid injury to tubes, uterine vessels, and endocervical canal.
- Myometrial dead space is obliterated in layers with meticulous hemostasis.
- Bonney's hood is used for posterior wall fibroid near fundus (Figure 20.7).
- Ensure patency of the endometrial cavity if the cavity has been opened—this can be done by either inserting a dilator through the cervix or staining the endometrium using methylene blue prior to surgery.
- Microsurgical techniques used to minimize postoperative adhesions
  - Use of suction, irrigation, and floatation techniques
  - Use of fine instruments and sutures
  - Use of adhesive barriers

Complications of myomectomy

- Hemorrhage
- Trauma to bladder, ureter, and bowel
- Infection
- Adhesions and intestinal obstruction
- Recurrence of fibroids and persistence of symptoms

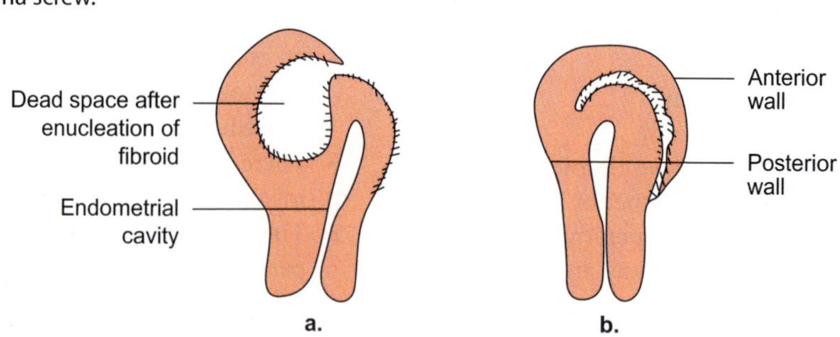

Figure 20.7 Bonney's hood. **a.** A posterior fundal incision made to enucleate the fibroid. **b.** After closing dead space, the excess serosa is drawn across the fundus and fixed to anterior surface of uterus.

Postoperative advice after myomectomy

- Patients should wait for 4–6 months after myomectomy to allow the uterus to heal before pregnancy. Fibroids can grow back, and hence it is better to try conception as early as possible, after a period of 4–6 months following myomectomy.
- The discharge slip should contain details of the procedure including whether endometrial cavity has been entered or not. Elective cesarean section is indicated in the subsequent pregnancy at 37 completed weeks of pregnancy, if cavity has been entered.

Extra edge

Bonney's myomectomy clamp

- It is used for clamping the uterine vessels at the level of isthmus to decrease vascularity at the site of fibroid during myomectomy (see figure below).
- The blades are covered with rubber to prevent damage to the blood vessels that are clamped.

Bonney's clamp

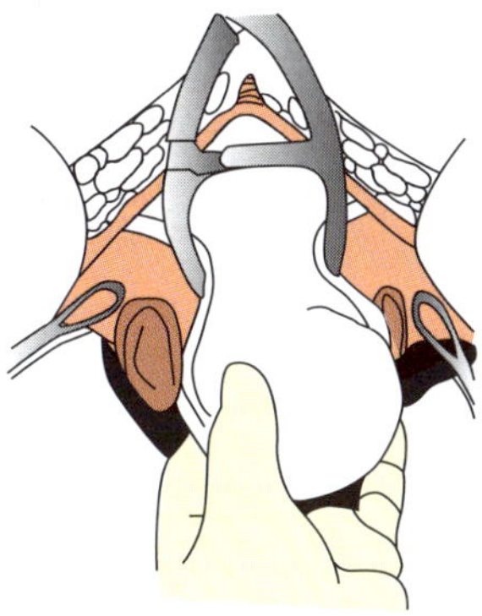

Figure Application of myomectomy clamp.

- Round ligaments are clamped along with uterine vessels at isthmus to prevent blades from slipping down into cervix and thereby losing compression effect on uterine vessels.
- Clamps are released every 15 minutes to prevent hypoxic injury leading to release of tissue degradation products such as histamine that can lead to anaphylactic shock.

Bonney's hood

- It is used to remove a posterior wall fibroid near fundus. This procedure allows a posterior approach but avoids a posterior defect.
- A transverse posterior fundal incision is made and the posterior wall fibroid is enucleated.
- The flap raised is sutured over the uterine wall anteriorly, such that the final scar is on the anterior uterine wall. This prevents a posterior wall scar and the related adhesions to rectum, bowel, and omentum.

Bonney's test

It is used for the diagnosis of stress urinary incontinence. Absence of leakage of urine following bladder neck elevation is indicative of beneficial outcome following surgical repair.

Viva corner

Q1 What can be used if Bonney's clamp is not available to decrease blood loss?

- Rubber tourniquet or suction catheter passed through holes in broad ligament on either sides of isthmus and tied anteriorly
- Local injection of vasopressin (acts as a medical tourniquet)

Q2 What are the various techniques to prevent adhesion formation?

- Vertical anterior incision
- Minimal number of incisions
- Avoiding posterior incision (maximum chance of adhesions)
- Bonney's hood technique for posterior wall fibroids
- Meticulous hemostasis
- Microsurgical techniques
- Round ligament plication
- Use of adhesive barriers—interceed, Gore-Tex, etc.

RECENT ADVANCES IN MANAGEMENT OF FIBROID

Laparoscopic myolysis

It is a laparoscopic procedure that destroys the fibroid using laser, cryotherapy, or electrosurgical energy.

- Nd:YAG laser or long bipolar needle electrodes are passed under laparoscopic guidance into the fibroid and multiple holes are drilled into the substance of the fibroid. The fibroid is destroyed by decrease in vascularity and tissue necrosis and is later absorbed.
- It is not recommended for women desiring future fertility because of the following:
  - There is increased scar tissue formation leading to uterine wall weakness and rupture in future pregnancy.
  - Fertility and pregnancy rates following this procedure are not well known.
- Indications
  - Perimenopausal symptomatic fibroid
  - Less than four fibroids, and fibroid size between 4 and 10 cm

Cryomyolysis

Liquid nitrogen cryoprobe is used to bring about freezing of selective tissue, leading to cell death.

Magnetic resonance–guided focused ultrasound

It is a noninvasive outpatient procedure that uses magnetic resonance–guided, high-intensity focused ultrasound waves to ablate the fibroid tissue. Tissue destruction is caused by thermal ablation.

Indications

- Woman who has completed her family but wants to preserve menstrual function
- Perimenopausal age group
- Fibroids between 4 and 10 cm in size

Procedure

- An interventional radiologist uses MRI to provide a three-dimensional view of the targeted tissue, which allows precise focusing and delivery of the ultrasound energy.
- Ultrasound energy is focused at a specific point, leading to marked heating and destruction of tissue by denaturation of proteins.
- Symptoms reduce within 3 months of the procedure.

Advantages

- Rapid recovery
- Reduction in symptoms seen in 70% of patients within 6 months

Disadvantage

Chance of skin burns in 5% of patients

Uterine artery embolization

It is a minimally invasive procedure used as an alternative to a major surgical procedure.

Principle

Minimally invasive angiographic interventional procedure that delivers polyvinyl alcohol (PVA) particles into both uterine arteries → decreases myometrial blood flow and results in ischemia and necrosis of fibroid. Normal myometrium is revascularized by the development of collateral circulation.

Indications

It is mostly suited for multiparous women:

- Who are unfit for surgery
- Who want to retain their uterus and are not willing for a major surgery

Contraindications

- Pregnancy
- Acute pelvic infections
- Undiagnosed pelvic mass
- Pedunculated subserous fibroids (fibroids disintegrate and may become free in peritoneal cavity after UAE, causing peritoneal irritation and infection, thereby leading to peritonitis and bowel adhesions)
- Patients desirous of future fertility (fertility rate decreases after the procedure)
- Adenomyosis—poor response to UAE
- Arteriovenous malformations
- Malignancy

Procedure (Figure 20.8)

- It is performed by an interventional radiologist under fluoroscopic control.
- It is done under deep sedation or local anesthesia.
- Percutaneous catheter is passed into right femoral artery → negotiated into external iliac

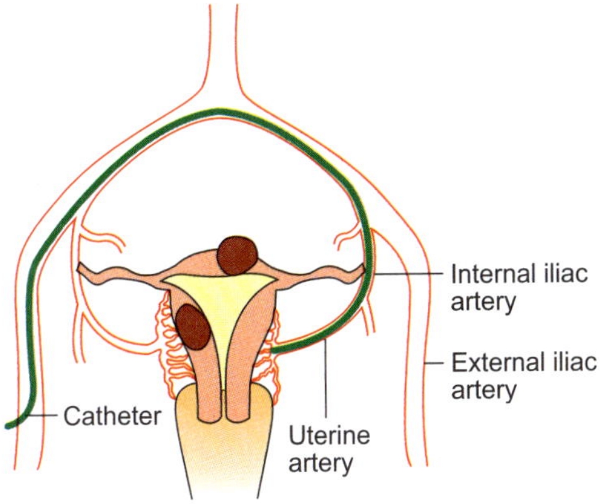

Figure 20.8 Diagrammatic representation of uterine artery embolization procedure.

vessels → common iliac artery → opposite-side common iliac artery → internal iliac artery → opposite-side uterine artery → embolized with PVA pellets. This is followed by catheterization and embolization of the same-side uterine artery.

- IV antibiotics are given after the procedure.

Success rate

- There is 70–100% improvement in symptoms.
- There is 50% decrease in uterine size.
- Benefits are seen in 3–6 months.

Complications

- Allergy to contrast medium
- Puncture site bleeding, hematoma, and infection
- Postembolization syndrome
- Persistent vaginal discharge
- Radiation exposure to ovary
- Infection (especially in submucous fibroid)
- Risk of occurrence of premature ovarian failure and amenorrhea because of nontarget embolization of ovarian arterial circulation
- Increased risk of complications, if pregnancy occurs following the procedure—spontaneous abortions, placental insufficiency, preterm delivery, postpartum hemorrhage (PPH), and uterine rupture

Advantages

- It is a minimal invasive procedure that avoids surgery.
- It involves shorter hospital stay and recovery.
- Major complications are less.

Viva corner

Q1 Why is UAE not suitable for women desirous of future fertility?

UAE is not suitable for women desirous of future fertility for the following reasons:

- It can lead to amenorrhea and ovarian failure.
- Data on future reproductive potential are limited.
- There is risk of complications such as spontaneous abortions, placental insufficiency, preterm delivery, PPH, and uterine rupture during future pregnancy.

Q2 What is postembolization syndrome?

- **C/F:** Pain, low-grade fever, nausea, and vomiting seen 1–3 weeks following UAE procedure in 40% of cases
- **Cause:** Due to release of inflammatory mediators from fibroid
- **Hemogram:** Shows leukocytosis
- **Management:** Hydration, analgesics, and antibiotics

Postembolization syndrome has to be differentiated from infection where fever and pain last for a longer duration and there is leukocytosis with left shift.

Disadvantages

- It is not suitable for women desirous of preserving their fertility, as data are still lacking.
- An interventional radiologist is required to do the procedure.

FIBROID DURING PREGNANCY

Effect of fibroid on pregnancy

See Table 20.10

Effect of pregnancy on fibroid

- Size and consistency of fibroid—may increase in size or remain the same size in early pregnancy; tends to decrease in size in the third trimester; fibroid may be softer in consistency during pregnancy
- Red degeneration
- Torsion of subserous fibroid
- Infection

(**Hint**: *Remember as "RTI"*)

Part 2

Table 20.10 Effect of fibroid on pregnancy

Pregnancy	Labor	Puerperium
• Infertility	• Nonengagement of head (if fibroid is in LUS)	• Subinvolution
• Abortion	• Uterine inertia	• Sepsis
• Malpresentation	• Increased rate of LSCS	• Secondary PPH
• Preterm labor	• PPH— due to adherent placenta, imperfect retraction	
• IUGR • Abruption		

IUGR, intrauterine growth restriction; *LSCS*, lower-segment cesarean section; *LUS*, lower uterine segment; *PPH*, postpartum hemorrhage.

Viva corner

Q1 What is the role of myomectomy during pregnancy?

- It is avoided during pregnancy except in cases of torsion of fibroid with intractable pain.
- Myomectomy during lower-segment cesarean section (LSCS) is contraindicated due to increased morbidity from excessive hemorrhage (there is increased vascularity of fibroid during pregnancy).

Q2 How will you manage patients with red degeneration of fibroid during pregnancy?

- Red degeneration of fibroid is common in midpregnancy.
- Cause: It occurs due to rapid growth of the fibroid leading to ischemic necrosis and release of inflammatory mediators.
- Clinical features: Patients present with fever, nausea, vomiting, and acute abdominal pain. Examination reveals localized tenderness over the fibroid. The condition has to be differentiated from other causes of pain abdomen during pregnancy such as abruption.
- Management is conservative and consists of bed rest and analgesics. There is no role for surgery.

Q3 What will you do if fibroids are encountered during cesarean section?

- Fibroids encountered during cesarean section should not be removed due to risk of excessive bleeding. Surgery, if indicated, can be done 3 months after delivery.

Q4 What are the factors that reduces the size of fibroid?

- Postmenopausal regression in size of fibroid.
- Treatment with drugs such as GnRH agonists and antagonists, danazol, gestrinone, mifepristone, selective estrogen receptor modulators (SERM) such as raloxifene and ormiloxefene, selective progesterone receptor modulators (SPRM) such as asoprisnil and ulipristal, and aromatase inhibitors such as fadrozole.

Frequently asked viva questions

1. Summarize the case.
2. What is the differential diagnosis for the case?
3. How will you differentiate a fibroid from adenomyosis?
4. How will you confirm the diagnosis?
5. What investigations do you want to do for your case?
6. How will you manage the case?
7. What are the available treatment options?
8. What are the drugs used for the medical management of a fibroid?
9. What are the indications for hysterectomy?
10. What are the indications for myomectomy?
11. What steps will you take to reduce bleeding during myomectomy?
12. What are the recent advances in the management of a fibroid?
13. What are the complications of fibroid uterus?

21 Ovarian Mass

Introduction

There can be various causes for presence of an abdominopelvic mass in a patient presenting to the gynecological OPD. Ovarian mass is one of the differential diagnoses for an abdominopelvic mass and has been primarily discussed in this chapter.

- Ovarian cysts are the most common ovarian masses encountered among women belonging to the reproductive age group.
- Ovarian cysts can be either non-neoplastic or neoplastic in nature.
- Non-neoplastic cysts, also known as functional cysts of ovary, are very common and can occur at any age (early reproductive age until perimenopause).
- Ovarian neoplasms (tumors) can be benign or malignant in nature.
  - Most ovarian tumors (80%) are benign and occur in women between 20 and 45 years of age.
  - Malignant ovarian tumors are common in the postmenopausal age group.
- Symptoms of ovarian malignancy are nonspecific and nongynecological and hence ovarian malignancies are usually detected in advanced stages.

Non-neoplastic cysts of ovary (functional cysts or cystic ovaries)

Non-neoplastic cysts of ovary are very common and can occur from adolescence to perimenopausal age. The term includes the following: follicular cysts, corpus luteal cysts, and theca lutein cysts.

Features of the functional cysts

- Related to temporary hormonal disturbances
- Usually not more than 5–8 cm in diameter
- Unilocular
- Contain clear fluid except when hemorrhage occurs
- Usually asymptomatic
- Usually regress spontaneously

A brief description of the functional cysts of the ovary is given next.

Follicular cysts

- Most common functional cysts
- Usually <5 cm size
- Can be single or multiple cysts
- Usually asymptomatic; can undergo torsion, hemorrhage, and rupture, and can present with symptoms of acute abdomen
- Disappear spontaneously within few weeks to few months

Theca lutein cysts

- Usually bilateral
- Associated with excessive human chorionic gonadotropin (hCG) secretion such as in gestational trophobastic tumors and with hCG and clomiphene therapy for infertility
- Usually regresses spontaneously following the treatment of gestational trophoblastic tumors
- May present with local pain and tenderness

Corpus luteal cysts

- Usually occur due to overactivity of corpus luteum leading to hemorrhage inside the corpus luteum
- May present with amenorrhea or delayed periods
- May present similar to threatened abortion or the cyst may rupture leading to intraperitoneal hemorrhage, simulating a ruptured ectopic pregnancy
- May be associated with pregnancy and can persist for about 12 weeks
- Spontaneous regression usually occurs, unless complicated

Ovarian neoplasms/tumors

- Benign tumors—80% of all ovarian tumors
- Malignant tumors—20% of all ovarian tumors, of which 80% are primary ovarian tumors and 20% are secondaries from other sites such as gastrointestinal tract (GIT)
  - Ninety percent of primary ovarian tumors—epithelial ovarian tumors
  - Ten percent of primary ovarian tumors—nonepithelial ovarian tumors

Note
- *Ovarian tumors in adolescent and postmenopausal age group are mostly malignant.*
- *Ovarian malignancy accounts for 5% of all gynecological cancers in India.*

WHO CLASSIFICATION OF OVARIAN TUMORS (NINE MAJOR GROUPS)

- Epithelial tumors (may be benign, borderline malignant, or malignant)
  - Serous tumors
  - Mucinous tumors
  - Brenner tumor
  - Clear cell tumor
  - Endometrioid tumors
  - Mixed epithelial tumor
  - Undifferentiated carcinoma
  - Unclassified
- Sex cord stromal tumors
  - Granulosa cell tumors and theca cell tumors
  - Androblastomas
  - Gynandroblastomas
  - Unclassified
- Germ cell tumors
  - Dysgerminoma
  - Endodermal sinus tumor
  - Embryonal cell carcinoma
  - Polyembryoma
  - Choriocarcinoma
  - Teratoma
  - Mixed forms
- Gonadoblastoma—pure/mixed with germ cell
- Lipid cell tumors
- Soft-tissue tumors
- Secondary (metastatic) tumors
- Unclassified
- Tumor-like conditions

COMMON BENIGN OVARIAN TUMORS

- Serous cyst adenoma
- Mucinous cyst adenoma
- Dermoid cyst

RISK FACTORS FOR EPITHELIAL OVARIAN CANCER

- Age group 50–70 years (uncommon below 45 years)
- Obesity
- Nulliparity (Continuous ovulation associated with nulliparity increases the risk of epithelial ovarian malignancy. Ovulation is a process of hormone-induced injury on the surface of ovary, involving trauma and repair, with possibilities for DNA damage. Protective factors include conditions that suspend ovulation, such as pregnancy, lactation, and oral contraceptive use.)
- Early menarche
- Late menopause
- Family history of ovarian malignancy (hereditary ovarian cancers occur a decade earlier than sporadic cases)

PROTECTIVE FACTORS FOR OVARIAN CANCER

- Multiparity
- Breast feeding
- Oral contraceptive pills (OCP use for 5 years—50% risk reduction)
- Salpingectomy

High-yield points

Significance of age in ovarian tumor

- More than 80% of epithelial ovarian cancers occur in postmenopausal women, usually between 50 and 70 years of age.
- Thirty percent of ovarian tumors in postmenopausal age group are malignant, whereas only 7% in premenopausal age group are malignant.
- Seventy percent of ovarian tumors that occur in women <20 years of age are germ cell tumors.

(CONTD...)

(...CONTD)

High-yield points

- Hereditary ovarian cancers occur one decade earlier than sporadic cases. If a malignant ovarian tumor occurs in the premenopausal age group, detailed family history and screening of other family members are to be done.

Familial ovarian cancer syndromes

- **Lynch syndrome:** Hereditary nonpolyposis colorectal cancer (HNPCC) or Lynch syndrome is an autosomal dominant genetic condition that has a high risk of colon cancer as well as other cancers including endometrial (second most common), ovarian, stomach, small intestine, and hepatobiliary tract cancers. Average age at diagnosis is 40 years.
- **Breast and ovarian cancer syndrome:** A diagnosis of hereditary breast and ovarian cancer syndrome (HBOC) is considered when there are multiple cases of breast cancer and/or ovarian cancer on the same side of the family. It usually occurs in association with BRCA1 or BRCA2 mutation. Average age at diagnosis is 50 years.

Part 2

Case presentation

Salient points in history

Consider the following relevant points during history taking in cases of ovarian mass:

- **Age:** *Ovarian cancer is more common in women belonging to the age group between 50 and 70 years (postmenopausal age group).*
- **Parity:** *Women with a history of nullparity or low parity are at an increased risk of ovarian cancer.*

Note *Symptoms of ovarian cancers are usually nonspecific and nongynecological. Early stage ovarian malignancy can be asymptomatic and hence ovarian malignancies are usually detected in advanced stages (a silent killer).*

Presenting complaints

- *H/o mass abdomen—onset, duration, and whether gradual or sudden increase in size (malignant tumor has a rapid progression)*
- *H/o vague nonspecific symptoms such as pain abdomen, abdominal discomfort, bloating sensation, early satiety, dyspepsia, and indigestion—can be present in mass of any origin but are frequently present in ovarian malignancy*
- *H/o loss of weight and appetite—may indicate malignancy*
- *H/o urinary retention, constipation, and pedal edema—pressure symptoms due to large abdominal mass*
- *H/o breathlessness—may be due to abdominal distension with tumor or ascites or due to pleural effusion*
- *H/o hirsutism, change in voice, irregular bleeding, postmenopausal bleeding, etc.—may be present in hormone-secreting ovarian tumors*
- *H/o acute pain abdomen—may be due to rupture or torsion of ovarian tumor*

Menstrual history

- *Age at menarche [patients with H/o early menarche (<12 years) and late menopause (>52 years) are associated with an increased risk for ovarian cancer].*
- *Menstrual cycles—duration, regularity, and amount of flow (most ovarian tumors do not affect the menstrual cycles; the tumors that can cause menorrhagia are granulosa cell tumors and theca cell tumors)*
- *Age at menopause*
- *H/o postmenopausal bleeding—may be present in hormone-secreting ovarian tumors such as granulosa cell tumor and in benign Brenner tumors*

Marital and obstetric history

- *Married at __ years*
- *Parity*
- *H/o infertility and treatment for infertility with ovulation induction drugs*

(CONTD...)

(...CONTD)

- *Last childbirth*
- *H/o breastfeeding (reduces risk)*
- *History regarding contraception (H/o using OCPs or tubal ligation acts as a protective factor)*

Past history

- *H/o diabetes and hypertension*
- *H/o surgery*
- *H/o blood transfusion*
- *H/o tuberculosis*
- *H/o breast malignancy (increases risk for ovarian cancer)*

Family history

- *H/o ovarian cancer in the family (women who have a mother, daughter, or sister with ovarian cancer are at an increased risk of developing ovarian tumor)*
- *H/o genital tract malignancy, breast or GIT malignancy (may be present in familial cancer syndromes)*

Salient points in examination

Consider the following relevant points during examination in cases of ovarian mass.

General examination

- *Built*
- *Nourishment*
- *Height, weight, and BMI (obese women may have an increased risk of developing ovarian cancer)*
- *Pallor*
- *Icterus*
- *Pedal edema*
- *Lymphadenopathy (especially left supraclavicular nodes)*
- *Vitals (temperature, pulse, BP, and respiratory rate are checked)*
- *Breast and thyroid examinations done*

Note *Findings on general physical examination such as unexplained weight loss, pallor, pedal edema, and lymphadenopathy, are suggestive of malignant disease.*

CVS and RS examinations

CVS and RS examinations are done to exclude any coexisting medical disorders (to be treated prior to surgery). Breath sounds are absent or reduced in case of associated pleural effusion in malignant tumors.

Abdominal examination

Inspection

Look for the following findings:
- *Abdominal distension*
- *Umbilicus—normal/flushed with skin/everted*
- *Stretched and shiny skin*
- *Dilated veins*
- *Scars/sinuses*
- *Cough impulse at hernial orifices (present/absent)*

Palpation

Palpate all the quadrants of the abdomen.
- *If there is a palpable mass, note the following:*
  - *Mass—arising from pelvis "up to _ weeks size" or "occupying the _ quadrants of the abdomen"*
  - *Size—approximate size of the mass*
  - *Surface—smooth or irregular*
  - *Consistency—soft/firm/cystic/hard (in ovarian malignancy, consistency may be hard or variable*
  - *Borders—whether all borders are felt (the lower border is usually not palpable in mass arising from pelvis, except in case of an ovarian cyst with a long pedicle)*
  - *Mobility in vertical and horizontal directions (benign cysts can be moved from side to side; cyst with a long pedicle may be mobile in both horizontal and vertical directions; malignant tumors usually have restricted mobility or they are fixed)*
  - *Any tenderness on palpation*
- *Any organomegaly (palpable liver/spleen)*
- *Fluid thrill is checked for (present in tense or large-volume ascites)*

Percussion

- *On percussion, there is usually dullness over the mass and resonance in flanks (bowels are displaced to sides).*

(CONTD...)

(...CONTD)

- *Shifting dullness is demonstrable if associated ascites is present.*

Auscultation

- *Any bruit (may be heard in highly vascular tumors)*
- *Bowel sounds*

Pelvic examination

Inspection of external genitalia

Whether external genitalia are healthy or any lesion present is determined (inspect for any growth/ulcer/abnormal pigmentation)

Speculum examination

Cervix and vagina are inspected for any abnormal discharge or lesions.

Bimanual pelvic examination

- *Uterine size, position (anteverted/retroverted), and mobility are determined.*
- *Any palpable adnexal mass—whether any mass is felt through the fornices is determined.*
- *Any nodules in POD (may be present in malignant ovarian tumor)*
- *In case of ovarian mass, the following findings are noted:*
  - *Ovarian mass is felt separately from the uterus.*
  - *Movement of the mass via abdomen is not transmitted to the cervix.*
  - *A groove may be felt between the mass and the uterus.*

Rectal and rectovaginal examination

- *Check for the following:*
  - *Any nodules or deposits in POD*
  - *Whether rectal mucosa is free or involved*

Case summary

An example of writing summary in cases of ovarian mass is given below.

Example *Mrs. N, 63 years of age, para 1 live 1, sterilized, postmenopausal woman, presents with complaints of progressively increasing abdominal distension for the past 2 months associated with loss of appetite and loss of weight. There is no history of postmenopausal bleeding. On examination, the patient is obese with a BMI of 30, mild pallor is present, there are no other significant general examination findings, the patient's vitals are stable, and CVS and RS examinations are normal. Abdominal examination reveals a mass arising from pelvis up to 20 weeks in size, which is ill-defined and nontender with variegated consistency. Surface of the mass is irregular and mobility is restricted. On per vaginal examination, cervix and vagina are healthy and the mass is tipped through the right lateral fornix. The mass is felt separately from the uterus and the movement of the mass is not transmitted to the cervix. Rectal and rectovaginal examinations are normal.*

Case diagnosis

An example of writing diagnosis in cases of ovarian mass is given below.

Example *63 years of age, para 1 live 1, postmenopausal woman with abdominopelvic mass. Considering her history and examination findings, it is most likely to be a case of malignant ovarian tumor.*

Case discussion

Differential diagnosis of abdominopelvic mass

Gynecological causes of abdominopelvic mass

- Ovarian tumor—benign or malignant
- Tubo-ovarian mass
- Paraovarian cyst
- Fibroid uterus
- Adenomyosis (uterus not enlarged >14 weeks)
- Pyometra, hematometra
- Pelvic hematocele

Nongynecological causes of abdominopelvic mass

- Pregnancy
- Full bladder

- Encysted ascites
- Diverticulitis
- Appendicular abscess
- Mesenteric cyst
- Retroperitoneal tumors
- Cecum and sigmoid colon tumor
- Secondary tumors from breast, GIT

Differentiating clinical features

- Clinical features differentiating abdominal distension due to ascites from that due to ovarian mass are given in Table 21.1.
- Clinical features differentiating fibroid and ovarian mass—refer to Part 2, Chapter 20, *Fibroid Uterus,* Table 20.3.
- Clinical features differentiating a benign ovarian mass from a malignant ovarian mass are mentioned in Table 21.2.

Investigations

Investigations done to evaluate the nature of the mass

- **Ultrasound of the abdomen and pelvis:** This is the first step in the evaluation. Transabdominal and transvaginal ultrasonography (TAS and TVS) should be performed.

- **Uses of USG in evaluation of ovarian mass**
  - Origin of the mass can be confirmed.
  - A benign ovarian mass can be differentiated from a malignant ovarian mass (Table 21.3).
  - Morphology of other pelvic organs can be assessed.
  - Enlarged pelvic and para-aortic nodes, ascites and metastasis to other intra-abdominal organs and omental caking, if any, can be assessed.

Table 21.1 Clinical features differentiating ascites from ovarian mass (refer to Part 2, Chapter 18, *History Taking and Examination,* Figure 18.3)

Ascites	Ovarian mass
Abdomen is transversely distended	Abdomen is longitudinally distended
Percussion findings—dullness in flanks (fluid) and resonance in center (bowel)	Percussion findings—dullness in center (mass) and resonance in flanks (bowel displaced to sides)
Shifting dullness and fluid thrill may be demonstrable in large-volume ascites	Shifting dullness and fluid thrill are not demonstrable
No definite mass is palpable	Definite mass is palpable

Table 21.2 Clinical features differentiating a benign from a malignant ovarian mass

Feature	Benign ovarian mass	Malignant ovarian mass
Age	Younger age group	Extremes of age (<20 and >50 years)
Duration of progression of illness	Slow	Rapid progression within a short period of few months
Cachectic symptoms (loss of weight and appetite)	Absent	Present
Palpation	Smooth surface, borders well defined, cystic consistency, mobile mass	Irregular surface, borders may be ill defined, variable consistency (due to presence of solid areas), restricted mobility or fixed mass
Site	Unilateral (80%)	Bilateral (70%)
Ascites	Absent	Present
POD deposits	Absent	May be present

Table 21.3 Ultrasound features differentiating a benign ovarian tumor from a malignant ovarian tumor

Benign ovarian tumor	Malignant ovarian tumor
Usually unilateral	Usually bilateral
Unilocular	Multilocular
Thin cyst wall	Thick cyst wall
Thin septations	Thick septae
Anechoic	Mixed echogenicity due to solid areas (Figure 21.1), papillary projections from inner wall of cyst may be present
No ascites, no lymphadenopathy	• Presence of ascites and pelvic and para-aortic lymphadenopathy suggest malignancy • Hepatosplenomegaly and omental thickening or caking may be present in advanced tumors
High-resistance flow pattern in Doppler	Doppler shows low-resistance flow pattern (increased vascularity)

In a suspected malignant ovarian mass, further investigations that are done include:

- **Doppler flow studies:** Increased vascularity with low resistance index indicates malignancy.
- **Tumor marker**: Carcinoma antigen (CA) 125-CA 125 levels are elevated in nonmucinous epithelial ovarian tumors.
  - Levels are useful in differentiating benign from malignant lesions.
  - Sensitivity is high in postmenopausal women.
  - CA 125 is also useful to check response to therapy and for early diagnosis of recurrence.
  - CEA and CA 19-9 are the common tumor markers elevated in patients with gastrointestinal or colon cancers.
- **CT and MRI**: These are done if ultrasonography (USG) is not conclusive in detecting the origin of tumor, to identify spread of tumor, and to identify enlarged pelvic or para-aortic nodes.
- **Ascitic fluid for malignant cytology:** If ascites is present, ascitic fluid can be collected for malignant cytology by abdominal paracentesis or culdocentesis.
- **Chest X-ray**: It is done to exclude pleural effusion and lung metastasis.
- **Stool occult blood, upper GI endoscopy, and colonoscopy**: These are done to rule out primary GIT malignancy.
- **Pap smear** is done.
- **Intravenous pyelogram**: It is done to detect any ureteric obstruction and deviation in course of ureters in large tumors where normal anatomy may be distorted.

If history, clinical examination, and evaluation are suggestive of ovarian malignancy, the next step is to proceed with exploratory laparotomy.

Note *History, clinical examination, imaging studies, and CA 125 levels can be suggestive of malignancy, but the confirmation of diagnosis of malignancy can be established only by exploratory laparotomy and surgical staging (staging laparotomy).*

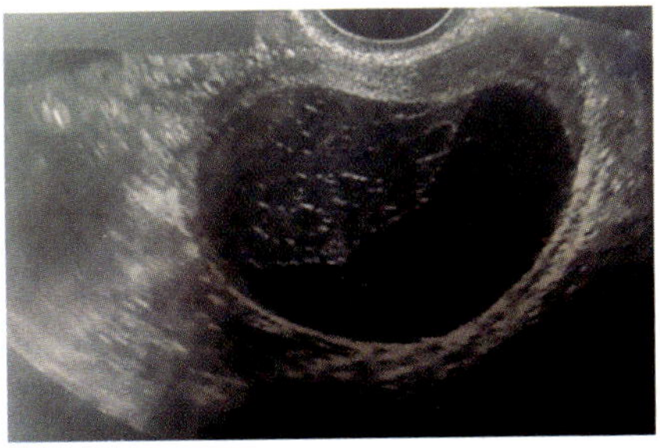

Figure 21.1 Ultrasound image showing solid component within an ovarian mass.

Preoperative investigations

In addition to the evaluation mentioned above, other preoperative investigations that are required include the following:

- Hemoglobin
- Complete blood count
- Blood grouping and typing
- Urine routine and microscopy
- Blood sugars
- Renal function tests
- Liver function tests
- HIV and HBsAg (in high-risk cases)
- ECG
- Chest X-ray

MANAGEMENT OF MALIGNANT OVARIAN TUMORS

Surgery is the mainstay of treatment. Most of the patients require a staging laparotomy followed by chemotherapy.

Principal steps of staging laparotomy

- **Incision:** Vertical midline skin incision is made (it minimizes chances of tumor rupture and facilitates better exploration of peritoneal cavity).
- **Aspiration cytology:** Aspiration of ascitic fluid or peritoneal washing for cytology is done (peritoneal washing is taken from paracolic gutters, pouch of Douglas, and undersurface of diaphragm by instilling 10–20 mL of normal saline or distilled water).
- **Pelvic exploration:** It is done to note the gross physical characteristics of the tumor and condition of the contralateral ovary, uterus, and tubes.
- **Systematic palpation of entire peritoneal structures:** It is done starting from cecum, ascending colon, hepatic flexure, undersurface of diaphragm, transverse colon, splenic flexure, descending colon, sigmoid colon, omentum, liver, spleen, pelvic lymph nodes, and para-aortic lymph nodes. This is done for staging and assessment of operability of the tumor.
- **Procedure done:** Total abdominal hysterectomy (TAH) with bilateral salpingo-ovariectomy (BSO) and infracolic omentectomy is performed.
- **Peritoneal biopsies:** Multiple biopsies are taken from suspicious areas in peritoneal cavity (cul-de-sac, pelvic walls, paracolic gutters, mesentery, etc.), and scrapings are taken from the undersurface of the diaphragm.

Viva corner

Q1 Which ovarian tumor can present with menstrual irregularities and postmenopausal bleeding?

- Granulosa cell tumor
- Theca cell tumor
- Brenner tumor (benign tumor)

Q2 Which ovarian tumors can present with precocious puberty?

- Granulosa cell tumor
- Immature teratoma
- Embryonal cell carcinoma
- Polyembryoma
- Choriocarcinoma

Q3 What are the causes of nodules in POD in P/R examination?

- Malignant ovarian tumor
- Endometriosis

Q4 What is the pattern of spread of epithelial ovarian tumors?

- **Transcoelomic spread:** Through exfoliation of the cancer cells that get implanted on the peritoneal cavity and follow the circulatory path of peritoneal fluid (metastases are seen on the posterior cul-de-sac, paracolic gutters, right hemidiaphragm, liver capsule, and peritoneal surfaces of the intestine, mesentery, and omentum)
- **Direct spread:** To adjacent organs such as uterus and fallopian tubes
- **Lymphatic spread:** Through involvement of pelvic and para-aortic group of lymph nodes (lymphatic spread above the diaphragm results in involvement of supraclavicular lymph nodes)
- **Hematogenous spread:** Less common mode of spread, can occur to organs such as lungs

Q5 What is risk malignancy index (RMI)?

- RMI is used to differentiate between malignant and benign ovarian tumors.
- It is calculated using the product of ultrasound score, menopausal status, and serum CA 125 level (units/mL).

$RMI = U \times M \times CA\ 125$

where U is the ultrasound score (1 point each for multilocular cyst, solid areas, metastasis, ascites, and bilateral lesion); $M = 1$ if premenopausal, and 3 if postmenopausal; and CA 125 level is noted in units per milliliter.

- The risk of cancer is 75% when the RMI value is >250.

FIGO staging of ovarian cancer (revised surgical staging, 2014)

Table

FIGO	Surgical-pathologic findings
I	Tumor confined to ovaries
IA	Tumor limited to 1 ovary (capsule intact); no tumor on ovarian surface; no malignant cells in the ascites or peritoneal washings
IB	Tumor limited to both ovaries (capsules intact); no tumor on ovarian surface; no malignant cells in the ascites or peritoneal washings
IC	Tumor limited to 1 or both ovaries, with any of the following
IC1	Surgical spill
IC2	Capsule ruptured before surgery or tumor on ovarian surface
IC3	Malignant cells in the ascites or peritoneal washings
II	Tumor involves 1 or both ovaries with pelvic extension (below pelvic brim) or primary peritoneal cancer
IIA	Extension and/or implants on uterus and/or fallopian tubes
IIB	Extension to other pelvic intraperitoneal tissues
III	Tumor involves 1 or both ovaries, with cytologically or histologically confirmed spread to the peritoneum outside the pelvis and/or metastasis to the retroperitoneal lymph nodes
IIIA1	Positive retroperitoneal lymph nodes only (cytologically or histologically proven)
IIIA1(i)	Metastasis up to 10 mm in greatest dimension
IIIA1(ii)	Metastasis more than 10 mm in greatest dimension
IIIA2	Microscopic extrapelvic (above the pelvic brim) peritoneal involvement with or without positive retroperitoneal lymph nodes
IIIB	Macroscopic peritoneal metastasis beyond the pelvis up to 2 cm in greatest dimension, with or without metastasis to the retroperitoneal lymph nodes
IIIC	Macroscopic peritoneal metastasis beyond the pelvis more than 2 cm in greatest dimension, with or without metastasis to the retroperitoneal lymph nodes (includes extension of tumor to capsule of liver and spleen without parenchymal involvement of either organ)
IV	Distant metastasis excluding peritoneal metastases
IVA	Pleural effusion with positive cytology
IVB	Parenchymal metastases and metastases to extra-abdominal organs (including inguinal lymph nodes and lymph nodes outside of the abdominal cavity)

FIGO, International Federation of Gynecology and Obstetrics

- **Lymph node sampling:** Pelvic and para-aortic lymph node sampling is done in all cases.
- Appendicectomy is performed in case of mucinous tumors.

Treatment of malignant epithelial ovarian tumor

Stage IA (Grade 1)—low grade, low risk

- Primary treatment for stage I epithelial ovarian cancer is surgical staging and doing a TAH with BSO with infracolic omentectomy (Figure 21.2).

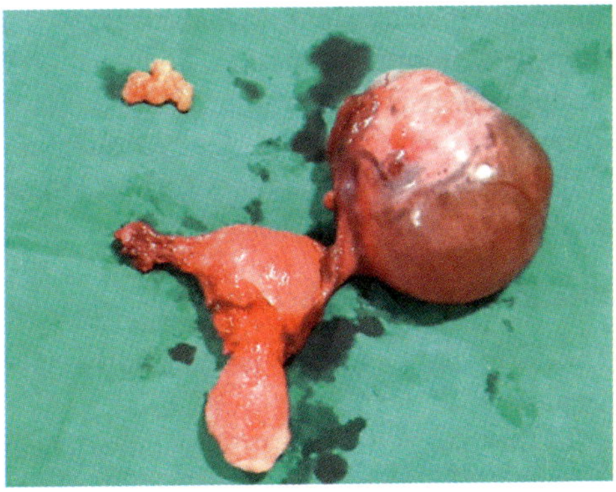

Figure 21.2 Specimen of uterus with ovarian tumor.

- In women who desire to preserve their fertility, the uterus and contralateral ovary can be preserved in stage IA, Grade 1. The patient must be periodically monitored with routine pelvic examination, USG, and determination of serum CA 125 levels.

Stages IA (Grades 2 and 3), IB, and IC: high grade, high risk

Staging laparotomy is performed (TAH + BSO + infracolic omentectomy) followed by adjuvant chemotherapy.

Stages II, III, and IV

- Primary debulking surgery or cytoreductive surgery is performed which includes staging laparotomy with the removal of as much disease as possible (TAH + BSO + total omentectomy + resection of all macroscopic disease in abdomen) followed by postoperative chemotherapy/radiotherapy.
- When tumor masses <1 cm diameter are left behind, it is known as optimal debulking.
- When large tumor masses of >1 cm in diameter are left behind, it is known as suboptimal debulking.

Benefits of cytoreduction in women with epithelial ovarian cancer

- **Improves general condition:** Removal of the tumor bulk helps to rapidly improve the disease-related symptoms such as abdominal pain, abdominal distension, dyspnea, and early satiety, and improves the quality of life.
- **Increases chemosensitivity:** Removal of the tumor bulk reduces the tumor burden, thereby maximizing the effect of chemotherapeutic agents (the residual lesions become well perfused and therefore mitotically active).
- **Improves immune function:** Removal of the tumor bulk may help to improve host immune competence by reducing the production of immunosuppressive cytokines such as interleukin-10 by the tumor tissue.

Indications for chemotherapy

- In stage IA, Grade 1, no chemotherapy is required.
- All other stages require postoperative chemotherapy. After surgery, women with ovarian cancer are offered chemotherapy to destroy the remaining cancer cells, which couldn't be completely removed by surgery.

Adjuvant chemotherapy Chemotherapy given after surgery.

- Platinum and taxane-based combination therapy is recommended as the first-line treatment for epithelial ovarian tumors. Chemotherapy agents usually administered are either cisplatin or carboplatin in combination with either paclitaxel or cyclophosphamide for three to four cycles.

Note *The renal and gastrointestinal toxicities of carboplatin are modest when compared with those with cisplatin. Hence, patients treated with carboplatin do not require prehydration as required by those treated with cisplatin.*

Neoadjuvant chemotherapy (NACT) It refers to chemotherapy given before surgery (chemotherapy for three cycles followed by interval cytoreductive surgery).

Indications for neoadjuvant chemotherapy

- Very poor general condition of the patient
- Stage III ovarian tumor with the following:
  - Irresectable pelvic mass
  - Extensive peritoneal disease
  - Perisplenic involvement
  - Nodes at porta hepatis
  - Involvement of diaphragm

Advantages of NACT

- Rapid subjective improvement of symptoms
- Subsequent surgery becomes easier
- Less postoperative complications

Palliative chemotherapy It refers to chemotherapy given to patients with stage IV cancer with distant metastasis.

Assessment of response to treatment

Regular follow-up is essential for all patients with ovarian cancer after treatment. Recurrence usually develops within the first 2 years after treatment. Assessment during follow-up visits includes:

- **Clinical assessment**: History and examination are done.

High-yield points

Significance of tumor marker CA 125

- Carcinoma antigen (CA) 125 is a surface glycoprotein used for screening and diagnosis of nonmucinous epithelial ovarian tumors.
- It is also used for monitoring response of patients to chemotherapy and follow-up for detecting recurrence after treatment.
- CA 125 levels may be raised in other malignancies such as carcinoma breast, lung, colon, and endometrium and also in some benign conditions such as endometriosis, pelvic inflammatory disease, tuberculosis, and peritonitis and in 1% of normal women.
- Estimation of CA 125 levels has low specificity and hence CA 125 test should not be used as a stand-alone test to diagnose ovarian cancer.
- Values of CA 125 >35 IU/mL are present in majority of cases with nonmucinous epithelial ovarian tumors.

Tumor markers in ovarian tumors

Ovarian tumor	Tumor marker
Dysgerminoma	Placental alkaline phosphatase, LDH
Yolk sac tumor (endodermal sinus tumor)	AFP and alpha-1 antitrypsin
Embryonal cell carcinoma	hCG and AFP
Polyembryoma	hCG and AFP
Choriocarcinoma	hCG
Teratoma	hCG negative and AFP negative
Nonmucinous malignant epithelial tumors	CA 125
Mucinous ovarian tumors	Carcinoembryonic antigen (CEA), CA 19-9

AFP, alpha-fetoprotein; *hCG*, human chorionic gonadotropin; *LDH*, lactic acid dehydrogenase.

- **Radiological assessment**: USG, CT, and MRI are done.
- **Tumor marker CA 125 levels**: Levels usually become undetectable following initial surgery and one or two cycles of chemotherapy. Often the CA 125 levels will rise before any symptoms suggestive of cancer recurrence develop. On follow-up with CA 125 levels, if levels:
  - *Decrease*: Indicates good response
  - *Persists*: Indicates presence of resistant clones
  - *Increase*: Indicates treatment failure

Follow-up

- Patients should be examined every 3 months for the first 2 years, and thereafter, every 4–6 months.
- During each visit, serum CA 125 level should be checked. If CA 125 level increases, further evaluation such as CT scan and MRI may be performed.

Second-look laparotomy/laparoscopy

Definition

Second-look laparotomy is performed in a patient who has no clinical evidence of disease (on physical examination, CA 125, CT scan) after a prescribed course of treatment, to determine the response to therapy.

Procedure

- Second-look laparotomy is similar to surgical staging.
- Multiple biopsies are taken.
- Pelvic and para-aortic nodes are dissected, if not done previously
- Second-look laparoscopy is less invasive, but false-negative rates are high due to adhesions.

Role of second-look laparotomy/laparoscopy

- Not shown to influence patient survival
- To be performed only in research settings

Secondary debulking or cytoreduction

Definition

Cytoreductive surgery that is done in patients with a persistent or recurrent tumor after primary therapy is termed secondary debulking.

Goal

The goal is to remove all residual tumor burden to <1 cm.

Persistence/recurrence of disease

- **Progressive/persistent disease:** Disease-free interval of less than 6 months following primary therapy
- **Recurrence of disease:** Disease-free interval of more than 6 months following primary therapy

Second-line chemotherapy agents These are used in ovarian tumors resistant to platinum-based therapy. The agents used are doxorubicin, topotecan, etoposide, gemcitabine, docetaxel, vinorelbine, ifosfamide, and 5-fluorouracil.

> **Extra edge**
>
> **Treatment modalities for ovarian tumors other than staging laparotomy with adjuvant chemotherapy**
>
> - **Intraperitoneal chemotherapy:** As the spread of disease is mainly transperitoneal, intraperitoneal chemotherapy provides high concentration of the drug at the site of tumor. Intraperitoneal chemotherapy is administered through a specially designed port. However, this method is not useful in large-volume residual disease. Toxicity is higher. It is, therefore, useful in women with stage III disease who have optimal cytoreduction.
> - **Immunotherapy:** Use of interferons and monoclonal antibodies (Herceptin) is under trial.
> - **Hormonal therapy:** Progesterones can be used in recurrent, well-differentiated endometrioid carcinoma.
> - **Radiotherapy (salvage therapy):** Radiotherapy can be used for palliation in advanced metastatic ovarian carcinoma—pulmonary, bone metastasis, etc.

SALIENT POINTS OF SPECIFIC OVARIAN TUMORS

Borderline ovarian tumors/tumors of low malignant potential

Definition

Epithelial ovarian tumors having characteristics in between those of benign and malignant tumors are termed borderline ovarian tumors (BOTs).

Features

- BOTs present one decade earlier than malignant ovarian tumors.
- These tumors do not have good response t chemotherapy or radiotherapy.
- Recurrence is common after 15–20 years.

BOTs are differentiated from benign tumor by the following features (at least two of thes should be present to term as BOTs):

- Nuclear atypia
- Cellular pleomorphism
- Increased mitotic activity
- Microscopic papillary projections

Note *BOTs do not have stromal invasion.*

Management

- Staging laparotomy is done.
- The resected ovarian tumor is sent for froze section; if BOT is identified, further management includes:
  - TAH + BSO is done, if the patient has com pleted family.
  - If the patient is desirous of fertility, U/L ovariotomy is performed and completion of surgery (removal of other ovary and uterus) is done after completion of family.
- Lymph node sampling is not required.

Surface epithelial tumors

Serous cystadenoma

- It arises from the totipotent surface epithelium of the ovary.
- It accounts for 40% of ovarian tumors (most common ovarian tumors).
- It is bilateral in 40% of cases.
- Risk of malignancy is 40% (serous cystadenocarcinoma).
- The cysts are not very large unlike mucinous cystadenoma.
- The wall is smooth, shiny, and grayish white.
- It may be unilocular or multiloculated.
- The content fluid is clear and rich in serum proteins.

Mucinous cystadenoma

- It arises from the totipotent surface epithelium of the ovary.
- It accounts for 20–25% of all ovarian tumors.

- It is bilateral in 10% of cases.
- Risk of malignancy is 10% (mucinous cystadenocarcinoma).
- It may enlarge to a huge size and is the largest benign ovarian tumor.
- The wall is lobulated with whitish or bluish white hue.
- The cyst is multiloculated and cut section shows honeycomb pattern.
- The contents are thick, viscid, and mucinous.
- Rupture of the cyst can result in pseudomyxoma peritonei.

Endometrioid tumor

- Mostly malignant
- Associated with endometrial cancer in 20% of cases

Clear cell carcinoma

- Also called mesonephroid tumor
- Highly malignant

Brenner tumor

- Uncommon tumor
- Resembles fibroma of ovary
- Generally seen in postmenopausal women and presents with postmenopausal bleeding
- Occasionally associated with pseudo-Meigs syndrome—Brenner tumor in association with ascites and pleural effusion

Germ cell tumors

Germ cell tumors are the most common ovarian tumors in young girls.

Dysgerminoma

- Corresponds to seminoma of testis
- Seen in young girls/children
- Bilateral in 20% of cases
- Malignant in 30–50% of cases
- Most common malignant germ cell tumor
- Most common malignant ovarian tumor associated with pregnancy
- Common in women with abnormal gonads
- Highly chemosensitive and radiosensitive
- Has a peculiar elastic rubbery consistency with a smooth capsule
- Secretes placental alkaline phosphatase and lactate dehydrogenase
- Chemotherapy regimens—bleomycin, etoposide, and cisplatin (BEP regimen) or vinblastine, bleomycin, and cisplatin (VBP regimen)

Teratoma

It is of the following types:
- Mature teratoma (benign—dermoid cyst)
- Immature teratoma (malignant—solid)
- Monodermal or highly specialized teratomas—for example, struma ovarii and carcinoid tumors

Dermoid cyst

- Dermoid cyst arises from the germ cells of ovary.
- It constitutes 95% of teratomas (most common teratoma).
- It accounts for 30–40% of ovarian tumors.
- It is bilateral in 15–20% of cases.
- Risk of malignancy is 1–2%. Squamous cell carcinoma is the most common malignancy.
- It is the most common ovarian tumor associated with pregnancy.
- Torsion is the most common complication.
- The cyst is of moderate size and the capsule is smooth.

Viva corner

Q1 What are the differentiating features between germ cell tumor and epithelial ovarian tumors?

See table below

Feature	Germ cell tumor	Epithelial ovarian tumor
Age of presentation	Young age group	Mostly postmenopausal
Stage at presentation	Mostly stage I	Usually in advanced stages
Treatment	Both chemosensitive and radiosensitive	Staging laparotomy followed by chemotherapy
Prognosis	Good	Poor

- It contains structures from all three germ layers. The content is predominantly sebaceous material and may contain hair, teeth, and bones.

Yolk sac tumor

- Seen in young women
- Secretes alpha-fetoprotein and alpha-1-antitrypsin
- Has rapid growth and poor prognosis

Nongestational choriocarcinoma

- Seen in prepubertal girls
- Secretes hCG
- High metastatic potential to bone, lung, liver, and brain

Embryonal cell carcinoma

- Presents with precocious puberty and menstrual irregularities
- Secretes both hCG and alpha-fetoprotein
- Highly malignant

> **High-yield points**
>
> **Indications for chemotherapy in germ cell tumors**
>
> All cases need postoperative chemotherapy except the following:
>
> - Stage IA dysgerminoma
> - Stage IA, Grade 1 immature teratoma
>
> **Role of conservative surgery in the management of ovarian cancers**
>
> In women who want to preserve fertility, U/L salpingo-oophorectomy can be done in the following cases:
>
> - Stage I epithelial ovarian cancers (Grade 1)
> - Stage I germ cell tumors
> - Sex cord stromal tumors that are unilateral

Sex cord stromal tumors

Feminizing tumors

Granulosa cell tumor

- It secretes estrogen.
- Clinical presentation
  - *Prepubertal age group*: Precocious puberty
  - *Adults:* Amenorrhea followed by prolonge
    bleeding
  - *Postmenopausal:* Postmenopausal bleeding
- May be associated with carcinoma endometriun

Theca cell tumor

- Usually develops in postmenopausal women
- Presents with postmenopausal bleeding
- May be associated with endometrial carcinoma

Virilizing tumors

Sertoli–Leydig cell tumor

- It secretes androgen.
- Women present with complaints of altered body contour, flattening of breasts, irregular menstruation and amenorrhea, hirsutism, enlargemen of clitoris, and change in voice.
- All of the above changes are reversible after removal of the tumor except change in voice.

Tumors of connective tissue

Ovarian fibroma

- Solid benign ovarian tumor
- Meigs syndrome—association of ovarian fibroma with ascites and pleural effusion

> **Note** ***Pseudo-Meigs syndrome:*** *When ascites and pleural effusion are seen in conditions other than ovarian fibroma such as Brenner tumor and granulosa cell tumor, it is termed pseudo-Meigs syndrome.*

Metastatic carcinoma

Secondaries in ovary

- Mostly from GIT
- Solid tumor with irregular surface and is bilateral
- Ascites present
- Spreads by surface implantation or retrograde lymphatics

Krukenberg tumor

It is a metastatic tumor of ovary with special features:
- Bilateral
- Smooth surface
- Solid, waxy consistency
- Structure of the ovary maintained
- Freely mobile in pelvis
- Mostly from primary site in GIT and breast
- Characteristic signet ring cells in histology

> **Extra edge**
>
> **Specific histopathology cell types in ovarian tumor**
> - **Papillary cystadenoma:** Psammoma bodies
> - **Brenner tumor:** Walthard's inclusion bodies
> - **Clear cell tumor:** Hobnail cells
> - **Granulosa cell tumor:** Call–Exner bodies and coffee bean nuclei
> - **Leydig cell tumor:** Reinke crystal
> - **Yolk sac tumor:** Schiller–Duval bodies
> - **Krukenberg tumor**: Signet ring cells

SCREENING FOR OVARIAN CANCER

- Research is being done to assess whether ovarian cancers can be detected at an early stage, so that effective treatment can be provided.
- Some of the tests in various research trials include estimation of CA 125 levels and performing a transvaginal sonography (TVS).
- Currently, there exists no screening program for ovarian cancer, as it is not known whether these screening tests could help in early detection of ovarian cancers.

Management of high-risk women with familial ovarian cancers

- Genetic counseling is given.
- BRCA1 and 2 genetic mapping is done.
- If the woman is desirous of fertility, TVS and CA 125 levels are done at regular intervals combined oral contraceptive (COC) pills can be prescribed.
- On completion of family, prophylactic salpingo-oophorectomy is performed.
- Annual mammography can be done in women older than 30 years.

Prevention of ovarian cancers

- OCP intake for ≥5 years decreases risk by 50%.
- Having two children + OCPs for ≥5 years decreases risk by 70%.
- Prophylactic salpingo-oophorectomy on completion of family is recommended in high-risk patients such as those with familial ovarian cancers.

MANAGEMENT OF ADNEXAL CYSTS

Symptomatic ovarian cysts

Symptomatic cysts often need surgical intervention as the symptoms are usually due to complications or large size of the cyst.

Asymptomatic ovarian cysts

Management of asymptomatic ovarian cysts depends on the following:
- Age of the patient
- Menopausal status
- Size of the cyst
- Ultrasonography features
- Tumor marker levels

Management of asymptomatic ovarian cysts is outlined in Flowchart 21.1.

Surgical treatment

Ovarian cystectomy/ovariotomy

- It is done in young women.
- Cystectomy involves enucleation of cyst leaving behind normal ovarian tissue.
- If cystectomy is not possible, ovariotomy is done by clamping, cutting, and ligating the infundibulopelvic ligament.

Laparoscopic ovarian cystectomy/ovariotomy

Laparoscopic cystectomy is performed by aspiration of fluid from the cyst followed by dissection of the cyst.

Part 2

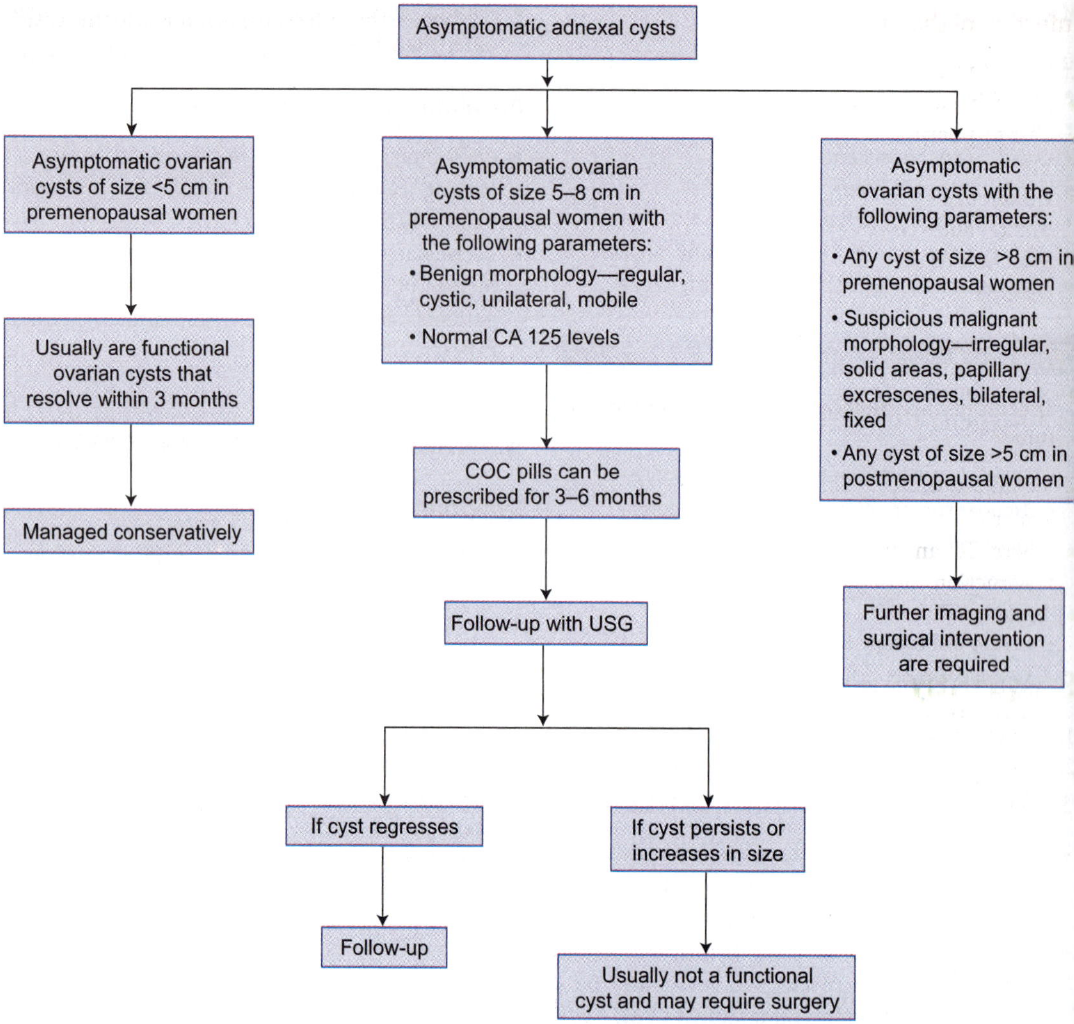

Flowchart 21.1 Management of asymptomatic adnexal cysts. *COC,* combined oral contraceptive pills; *USG,* ultrasonography.

COMPLICATIONS OF OVARIAN TUMORS

Torsion

- It is the most common complication of ovarian cysts or tumors.
- Torsion occurs commonly in dermoid cysts (as they are filled with fat and are heavy) and mucinous cystadenomas.
- Patient usually presents with severe abdominal pain.

Hemorrhage into the cyst/tumor

- This occurs most commonly into a corpus luteal cyst, and less often in a follicular cyst. Bleeding into corpus luteum results in the formation of a hemorrhagic cyst of the ovary.
- Patient usually presents with pain abdomen.

Rupture

It can occur in the following instances:
- Following trauma and bimanual examination
- Can occur spontaneously in case of mucinous cystadenomas

nfection of the tumor

t can occur in the following instances:

- Following acute salpingitis
- During puerperium—due to ascending infection
- Adherence to adjacent intestines following torsion and subsequent infection
- Infection of dermoid cyst containing sebaceous material

Pseudomyxoma peritonei

- It develops following rupture of mucinous cystadenocarcinoma of ovary or carcinoma of appendix/large intestine.
- Peritoneal cavity becomes filled with mucinous material.
- There is an increased chance of intestinal obstruction.
- Prognosis is poor.

Frequently asked viva questions

1. Summarize the case.
2. What is the diagnosis/differential diagnosis of the case?
3. What are the differential diagnoses for the case?
4. How will you differentiate a fibroid from an ovarian mass?
5. How will you differentiate an ovarian mass from ascites?
6. How will you differentiate a malignant ovarian mass from a benign ovarian mass?
7. Classify ovarian tumors.
8. What are the risk factors for epithelial ovarian tumors?
9. What are the complications of ovarian tumors?
10. What are the steps of staging laparotomy?
11. What is the role of CA 125 in management of ovarian tumors?
12. What do you mean by second-look laparotomy and secondary debulking surgery?
13. What are the chemotherapy agents used in the management of ovarian tumors?

22 Carcinoma Cervix

Introduction

Carcinoma cervix is the most common genital malignancy in developing countries such as India and often presents with abnormal uterine bleeding (AUB) or postmenopausal bleeding (PMB). Cervical intraepithelial neoplasia (CIN) is the preinvasive stage of the disease and there is a long latent period between CIN and invasive carcinoma of cervix that can be detected by screening. With the availability of HPV vaccination, effective screening tests and treatment modalities to diagnose and treat preinvasive lesions, cancer cervix is now considered as a preventable disease. This chapter deals with carcinoma cervix and its preinvasive lesions. Carcinoma cervix can be discussed during case presentation of AUB or PMB in clinical exams.

Causes of postmenopausal bleeding

- Carcinoma cervix
- Carcinoma endometrium
- Endometrial hyperplasia
- Benign lesions of cervix—polyp, cervicitis, tuberculosis of the cervix, and decubitus ulcer
- Benign conditions of endometrium—senile endometritis and atrophic endometritis
- Vaginal causes—senile vaginitis, atrophic vaginitis, forgotten pessary and rarely carcinoma vagina
- Hormone-secreting ovarian tumors—Brenner tumor, granulosa cell tumor, and theca cell tumor
- Hormone replacement therapy

Risk factors for cancer cervix [Hint: acronym (CM PIS)[2]]

- Coitus at an early age (<16 years)
- Childbirth at early age (<20 years)
- Multiparity
- Multiple sexual partners

Extra edge

Human papillomavirus (HPV)

- It is the major etiological agent in preinvasive lesions of cervix and carcinoma cervix.
- HPV infection is detected in 99% of preinvasive and invasive carcinoma cervix.
- HPV belongs to the Papovaviridae family of DNA viruses.
- More than 100 types of HPV are identified, of which about 40 types cause infection of the genital tract.
- Depending on the risk for causing cervical cancer, HPV are grouped as mentioned in the table below.
- E6 and E7 oncoproteins in the high-risk group play an important role in the molecular pathogenesis of cervical cancer.

Table Grouping of HPV types as per the risk of causing cervical cancer

Risk category	HPV types	Lesions caused
Low-risk group	HPV 6, 11	Causes low-grade squamous intraepithelial lesion (LGSIL) and genital warts
High-risk group	HPV 16, 18, 31, 33, 45, 52, 58	Causes high-grade squamous intraepithelial lesion (HGSIL) and cervical cancer. HPV 16 and 18 cause about 70% of cervical cancers and preinvasive cervical lesions

- Pills—combined oral contraceptive (COC) pills (COC pill usage for >5 years increases the risk of endocervical carcinoma); exposure to diethyl stilbesterol during fetal life
- Human papillomavirus (HPV 16, 18)—major etiological agent in cervical cancer
- Infections
  - HIV and sexually transmitted diseases (STDs) (Ca. cervix is an AIDS-defining cancer)
  - HSV-2 and *Chlamydia trachomatis*—act as cofactors
- Immunosuppression
- Socioeconomic group—low socioeconomic status (SES), poor local hygiene
- Smoking cigarettes (smoking for 20 years doubles the risk for Ca. cervix)
- Smegma from uncircumscribed partners (increased incidence of Ca. cervix is seen among African Americans and decreased incidence is seen among Jews and Muslims who undergo circumcision)

Symptoms of cancer cervix

- Carcinoma cervix usually occurs in multiparous women between the age group of 35 and 65 years.
- It may be asymptomatic in early stages.
- AUB is the most common presentation, which can manifest in various forms as below:
  - PMB
  - Metrorrhagia/heavy menstrual bleeding (HMB)
  - Postcoital bleeding
  - Intermenstrual bleeding

  (uncontrolled bleeding may occur when the growth erodes a vessel)
- Vaginal discharge
  - Blood-stained discharge
  - Foul-smelling purulent discharge (due to infection of necrotic tissue in the growth)
- Back pain: It is a late symptom due to infiltration of sacral nerves.
- Cachexia and weight loss may be present in advanced stages.
- Invasion of surrounding structures can present with signs/symptoms such as the following:
  - *Hematuria*: Bladder involvement
  - *Tenesmus and bleeding per rectum*: Rectal involvement
  - *Renal failure and uremia*: Compression of ureters (uremia is the most common cause of death in carcinoma cervix)
  - *Pain radiating to legs*: Sciatic nerve involvement
  - *Edema of lower limbs*: Lymphatic and venous compression

Signs

- Cancer cervix will have the following features on speculum examination:
  - The cervical lesion may be exophytic (cauliflower like proliferative growth), endophytic (hard, barrel-shaped cervix), or ulcerative.
  - The lesion will have the following characteristic features—friability, bleeding on touch, induration, and fixity (Figure 22.1).
- Rectal and rectovaginal examinations should be done in all cases of suspected carcinoma cervix, to check for parametrial involvement, involvement of pelvic side walls, and rectal mucosal and rectovaginal septum involvement

Note *Preinvasive and microinvasive lesions of cervix cannot be diagnosed by naked eye examination. They can be diagnosed only on histopathology examination.*

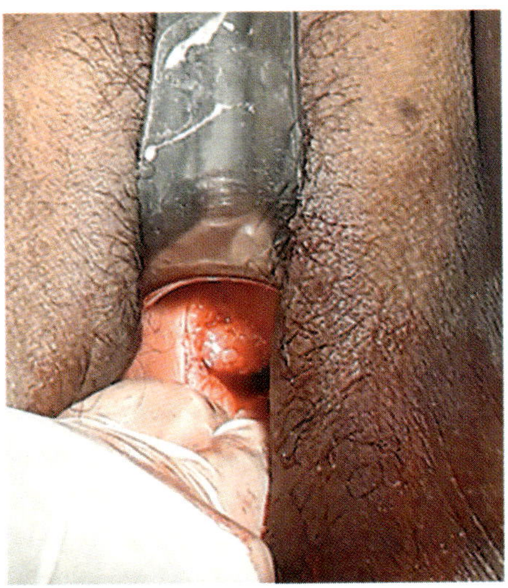

Figure 22.1 Suspicious cervix for evaluation.

Part 2

Case presentation

Salient points in history

Consider the following relevant points during history taking in cases of carcinoma cervix:

- *Age (most common in the age group between 35 and 65 years)*
- *SES (more common in low socioeconomic group)*
- *Parity (more common with increased parity)*

Presenting complaints

- *Menstrual abnormalities—PMB, HMB, irregular bleeding, intermenstrual bleeding, and postcoital bleeding*
- *Discharge P/V—whether blood stained/foul smelling*
- *H/o hematuria, tenesmus, and bleeding per rectum (involvement of bladder and rectum)*
- *H/o cachectic features such as loss of weight and loss of appetite*

Menstrual history

- *Age at menarche*
- *Previous menstrual cycles—pattern, amount, and duration of bleeding*
- *Age at menopause (if postmenopausal)*

Marital history

- *Married at the age of ___ years; married for the past ___ years*
- *H/o prolonged usage of COC pills*
- *H/o multiple sexual partners*

Obstetric history

Parity (increased parity associated with Ca. cervix)

Past history

- *H/o PID and STDs*
- *Whether Pap smear has been done earlier?*
- *H/o circumcision in the male partner*

Family history

Family H/o of genital malignancy

Personal history

Addictions such as smoking and alcohol

Salient points in examination

Consider the following relevant points during examination in cases of carcinoma cervix.

General examination

- *Built and nourishment*
- *Pallor*
- *Pedal edema*
- *Icterus (may be present in case of secondaries in liver)*
- *Lymphadenopathy—palpate for left supraclavicular nodes (metastasis) and inguinal nodes*
- *Breast and thyroid examination*
- *Systemic examination (pulmonary metastasis may be present in advanced stages)*

CVS and RS examinations

- *CVS and RS examinations are done to identify any coexisting medical disorders that need to be evaluated and treated prior to therapy.*
- *Breath sounds may be reduced or absent in pleural effusion.*

Abdominal examination

Inspection

Any distension or visible mass

Palpation

- *Check for hepatomegaly (may be present in case of advanced disease with metastasis).*
- *Check for uterine enlargement and tenderness (may be present in associated pyometra).*

Pelvic examination

Per speculum examination

- *If an obvious lesion is present (ulcerative/proliferative/endophytic lesion), describe the lesion, for example, "Cervix is replaced by an ulceroproliferative growth "or" a growth measuring ___ × ___ cm is present in the anterior or posterior lip of cervix."*

(CONTD...)

...CONTD)

- *Check whether the lesion is:*
  - *Friable*
  - *Bleeds on touch*
  - *Indurated*
  - *Fixed*
- *Check whether vaginal walls are involved.*
  - *If involved, extent of involvement—upper two-third only or involves the lower one-third as well*

Bimanual pelvic examination

- *Whether uterus is normal sized or enlarged (in pyometra)*
- *Whether uterus is mobile/fixed/has restricted mobility (sometimes all the pelvic structures are matted together and fixed with the uterus, which is termed "frozen pelvis")*

Per rectal and rectovaginal examination

- *Whether parametrium is involved or not [if parametrium is involved, check if it is involved up to pelvic side walls (parametrial induration will be nodular in carcinoma cervix and smooth in case of inflammation)]*
- *Rectal mucosa—whether free or involved*
- *Rectovaginal septum—whether free or involved*

Case summary

An example of writing summary in cases of carcinoma cervix is given below.

Example *Mrs. R, 52 years of age, P5L5, comes to the OPD with a history of PMB and foul-smelling discharge P/V for the past 1 month. On examination, her general examination findings and vitals are normal. Abdomen is soft and on per speculum examination, the cervix is replaced by an ulceroproliferative growth, which is friable, indurated, and bleeds on touch, with involvement of the upper one-third of the anterior vaginal wall. On rectal and rectovaginal examinations, bilateral parametrium involved up to pelvic side walls.*

Case diagnosis

An example of writing diagnosis in cases of carcinoma cervix is given below.

Example *52 years of age, multiparous, postmenopausal woman presents with PMB. History and clinical examination findings are suggestive of carcinoma cervix. Provisional diagnosis is carcinoma of the cervix, stage IIIB. Diagnosis has to be confirmed by histopathological examination of cervical biopsy.*

Note

- *Undergraduate medical students are usually not expected to do speculum and bimanual examination. Hence, the differential diagnosis will include all the causes of postmenopausal bleeding. Either endometrial carcinoma or carcinoma cervix can be discussed.*
- *If questioned about the next step in evaluation, it should be mentioned that a speculum examination is required to look for any lesion in cervix and vagina, followed by bimanual, rectal, and rectovaginal examinations.*

Case discussion

Differential diagnosis of cervical lesion

- Carcinoma of cervix
- Cervical polyp
- Cervical fibroid
- Cervical papilloma or warts
- Tubercular ulcer of cervix
- Syphilitic ulcer
- Retained products of conception in the cervical canal

Confirmation of diagnosis

Cervical biopsy is the first step in evaluation of a cervical lesion. Cervical punch biopsy should be taken from the edge of the lesion, using a cervical punch biopsy forceps and sent for histopathology.

Note

- *Cervical cancer is a clinical diagnosis confirmed by biopsy.*
- *Biopsy should not be taken from the center of ulcer or growth because it would contain only necrotic tissue due to reduced blood supply.*
- *When an obvious growth is visible, cervical biopsy is taken directly, and Pap smear is not necessary.*

Macroscopic or naked eye appearance of cervical cancer

It is of three types:

1. **Exophytic:** A proliferative, cauliflower-like growth arises from the cervix with rough, granular, bleeding surface (Figure 22.1).
2. **Infiltrative or endophytic:**
   - Lesion infiltrates the cervical stroma without any obvious growth.
   - It arises mostly from endocervical canal.
   - Cervix is barrel shaped on bimanual examination
3. **Ulcerative:** Lesion excavates the cervix like an irregular crater.

Histopathological types of cervical cancer

- **Squamous cell carcinoma:** It arises from the squamous epithelium of cervix (squamocolumnar junction) and is the most common type (80–90%).
  It is of three types:
  - *Large cell keratinizing:* Shows foci of keratinization with keratin pearls
  - *Large cell nonkeratinizing:* No keratin pearls
  - *Small cell carcinoma:* Poorly differentiated carcinoma
- **Adenocarcinoma:** It arises from columnar cells lining the endocervical canal.
  - It occurs in 10–20% of cases.
  - Prognosis is poor when compared with that of squamous cell carcinoma.

Staging of carcinoma cervix [International Federation of Obstetrics and Gynecology (FIGO) staging, 2018]

Until 2018, the FIGO staging was based on clinical examination with the addition of certain procedures that were allowed by FIGO to change the staging.

In 2018, this has been revised by the FIGO Gynecologic Oncology Committee to allow imaging and pathological findings, where available, to assign the stage.

Table Staging of Carcinoma of the Cervix (FIGO, 2018)[a]

Stage I	**The carcinoma is strictly confined to the cervix uteri (extension to the corpus should be disregarded)**
IA	Invasive carcinoma that can be diagnosed only by microscopy, with maximum depth of invasion <5 mm[b]
IA1	Measured stromal invasion <3 mm in depth
IA2	Measured stromal invasion ≥3 mm and <5 mm in depth
IB	Invasive carcinoma with measured deepest invasion ≥5 mm (greater than stage IA), lesion limited to the cervix uteri[c]
IB1	Invasive carcinoma ≥5 mm depth of stromal invasion and <2 cm in greatest dimension
IB2	Invasive carcinoma ≥2 cm and <4 cm in greatest dimension
IB3	Invasive carcinoma ≥4 cm in greatest dimension
Stage II	**The carcinoma invades beyond the uterus, but has not extended onto the lower third of the vagina or to the pelvic wall**
IIA	Involvement limited to the upper two-third of the vagina without parametrial involvement
IIA1	Invasive carcinoma <4 cm in greatest dimension

(CONTD...)

(...CONTD)

Table *(CONTD...)*	
IIA2	Invasive carcinoma ≥4 cm in greatest dimension
IIB	With parametrial involvement but not up to the pelvic wall
Stage III	**The carcinoma involves the lower third of the vagina and/or extends to the pelvic wall and/or causes hydronephrosis or non-functioning kidney and/or involves pelvic and/or paraaortic lymph nodes[d]**
IIIA	Carcinoma involves the lower third of the vagina, with no extension to the pelvic wall
IIIB	Extension to the pelvic wall and/or hydronephrosis or non-functioning kidney (unless known to be due to another cause)
IIIC	Involvement of pelvic and/or paraaortic lymph nodes, irrespective of tumor size and extent (with r and p notations)[d]
IIIC1	Pelvic lymph node metastasis only
IIIC2	Paraaortic lymph node metastasis
Stage IV	**The carcinoma has extended beyond the true pelvis or has involved (biopsy proven) the mucosa of the bladder or rectum. A bullous edema, as such, does not permit a case to be allotted to stage IV**
IVA	Spread of the growth to adjacent organs
IVB	Spread to distant organs

[a] *Int J Gynecol Obstet.* 2018;143:43–991.

[b] Imaging and pathology can be used, when available, to supplement clinical findings with respect to tumor size and extent, in all stages.

[c] The involvement of vascular/lymphatic spaces does not change the staging. The lateral extent of the lesion is no longer considered.

[d] Adding notation of r (imaging) and p (pathology) to indicate the findings that are used to allocate the case to stage IIIC. For example, if imaging indicates pelvic lymph node metastasis, the stage allocation would be stage IIIC1r and, if confirmed by pathological findings, it would be Stage IIIC1p.The type of imaging modality or pathology technique used should always be documented. When in doubt, the lower staging should be assigned.

The following amendments to the staging classification of carcinoma of the cervix were made by the FIGO Committee for Gynecologic Oncology in 2018:

1. *Allowing the use of any imaging modality and/or pathological findings for allocating the stage*
2. *In stage I, amendments to microscopic pathological findings and to size designation, allowing the use of imaging and/or pathological assessment of the size of the cervical tumor*
3. *In stage II, allowing the use of imaging and/or pathological assessment of size and extent of the cervical tumor*
4. *In stages I through III, allowing assessment of retroperitoneal lymph nodes by imaging and/or pathological findings and, if deemed metastatic, the case is designated as stage IIIC (with notation of method used for stage allocation)*
5. *No recommendations for routine investigations, which are to be decided on the basis of clinical findings and standard of care*

General recommendations:

1. *The revised staging system does not mandate the use of a specific imaging technique, lymph node biopsy, or surgical assessment of the extent of tumor. In low-resourced conditions, clinicians can continue to assess the patient clinically as done earlier.*
   a. *The size of the primary tumor can be assessed by clinical evaluation, (pre- or intra-operative) imaging, and/or pathological measurement.*
   b. *Identification of lymph node metastasis to be accomplished using imaging*

(CONTD...)

(...CONTD)

technique(s) and/or pathological assessment methods available to the provider, and the choice of technique depends on its availability.

2. *It is recommended that the method used for imaging (e.g., ultrasound, computed tomography (CT), magnetic resonance imaging (MRI), position emission tomography [PET], PET-CT. MRI-PET, etc.) and/or the pathological technique used (e.g., evaluation of the operative specimen, lymph node biopsy, or fine needle aspiration cytology), and the results thereof, should be recorded, so that subsequent data analysis can be performed. The imaging method can be used for the following:*
   a. *For measurement of the primary tumor size*
   b. *For assessment of extension into the surrounding tissues and adjacent organs*
   c. *For assessment of location and characteristics of the retroperitoneal lymph nodes.*
3. *It is recognized that there will be limitations for imaging findings in low-and lower-middle-income countries as a result of paucity, non-availability, or inadequate access to extensive imaging services.*
4. *As in the previous staging, when in doubt, the lower staging should be assigned.*

Staging of Carcinoma Cervix (FIGO, 2009), which was in clinical practice for several years, is given below to appreciate the changes made in the new FIGO 2018 staging:

- *Stage I: Cancer is confined to cervix.*
  - *IA: Microinvasive cancer (diagnosed only on microscopy)*
  - *1B: Clinically visible lesion*
  - *IA1: Depth of stromal invasion ≤3 mm and horizontal extension of ≤7 mm*
  - *IA2: Depth of stromal invasion >3 mm and ≤5 mm, horizontal extension of ≤7 mm*
  - *IB1: Clinically visible lesion of ≤4 cm*
  - *IB2: Clinically visible lesion of >4 cm*
- *Stage II: Cancer spreads beyond cervix, but not to pelvic side walls or lower one-third of vagina.*
  - *IIA: Involves upper two-third of vagina without parametrial involvement*
  - *IIB: Parametrium involved but not up to pelvic side walls*
- *Stage III: Cancer extends to pelvic side walls and/or involves lower one-third of vagina and/or causes hydronephrosis or nonfunctioning kidney.*
  - *IIIA: Involves lower one-third of vagina but not the pelvic side walls*
  - *IIIB: Extends to pelvic side walls and/or hydronephrosis or nonfunctioning kidney*
- *Stage IV: Cancer extends beyond true pelvis or involves mucosa of bladder or rectum.*
  - *IVA: Involves mucosa of adjacent organs—bladder and rectum*
  - *IVB: Distant metastasis*

The standard staging procedures which were earlier accepted by FIGO 2009 for cancer cervix staging include the following:

- *Per speculum examination, bimanual pelvic examination, and rectal examination to assess tumor size, vaginal extension, and parametrial invasion*
- *Colposcopy, cervical biopsy, endocervical curettage, or conization*
- *Cystoscopy and proctoscopy to look for bladder and rectal involvement*
- *Hysteroscopy in endocervical lesions and to detect extension to uterus*
- *Intravenous pyelography (IVP) to detect hydroureteronephrosis*
- *Chest X-ray to detect lung metastasis*

Note ***Cervical cancer was clinically staged earlier because*** *cervix can be completely visualized and palpated and carcinoma cervix is predominantly a disease of low-resource settings where imaging and surgical staging may not be feasible or cost-effective. However, accurate assessment of parametrial infiltration, lymph node metastasis, tumor volume, and distant metastasis is not possible only by clinical staging. Hence, the need for incorporation of imaging modalities in the new FIGO 2018 CA cervix staging*

Uses of investigation modalities for staging

- **Ultrasonography:** To assess tumor volume, hydroureteronephrosis, liver metastasis, and associated gynecological pathology
- **CT scan:** To assess lymph nodes, hepatic and distant metastasis
- **MRI:** To assess parametrial infiltration, lymph nodes, tumor volume, hydroureteronephrosis, and vaginal extension (MRI is the best investigation for assessment of local invasion and parametrial involvement)
- **Positron emission tomography (PET) scan:** To assess lymph nodes and distant metastasis
- **Sigmoidoscopy:** To assess large bowel involvement
- **Sentinel node biopsy:** To assess lymph node involvement

Note

- *In cases of suspected pelvic inflammation, a course of antibiotic should be given prior to clinical staging.*
- *If any doubt exists as to which stage to be assigned, the lower stage should be chosen.*
- *Once assigned, the stage remains the same. Staging cannot be changed once therapy has begun.*

Viva corner

Q1 What information is obtained on doing a rectal examination in a case of suspected carcinoma cervix?

- Parametrial involvement
- Involvement of pelvic side walls
- Infiltration of rectovaginal septum/rectal mucosa
- Can help in diagnosis of endophytic growth with barrel-shaped cervix

Q2 What are the causes of nodularity of uterosacral ligament?

- Endometriosis
- Carcinoma cervix infiltrating the parametrium

Q3 What are the causes of POD deposits?

- Endometriosis
- Secondary deposits from ovarian tumor

Q4 How will you take a cervical biopsy?

- If the lesion is small, excision biopsy of the entire lesion is taken, which should also include a portion of the healthy tissue.
- If the lesion is big, cervical biopsy is taken with a punch biopsy forceps from the edge of the lesion.
- In early stages where there is no visible lesion, colposcopy-directed biopsy or cone biopsy is taken or large loop excision of transformation zone is done (LLETZ).

Q5 How is bleeding managed after taking biopsy in carcinoma cervix?

There may be brisk hemorrhage after biopsy, which is usually self-limiting or can be effectively controlled by giving compression. If bleeding continues, the following measures can be done:

- Tight packing of the vagina
- Application of Monsel's paste (ferric subsulfate solution)
- Hemostatic radiotherapy

Q6 What is the lymphatic drainage of cervix?

- Lymphatics from parametrial and paracervical nodes → obturator nodes → external iliac nodes → common iliac and internal iliac nodes → para-aortic nodes
- Lymphatics from posterior cervix → uterosacral and rectal lymph nodes

Q7 What is the risk percentage of ovarian metastasis in carcinoma cervix?

- Squamous cell carcinoma of the cervix—0.5%
- Adenocarcinoma of cervix—1.7%

Mode of spread of carcinoma cervix

- Contiguous spread to uterus, vagina, bladder, rectum, and parametrium
- Lymphatic spread to parametrial, obturator, external iliac, common iliac, internal iliac, and para-aortic lymph nodes
- Hematogenous spread to distant organs

Complications of carcinoma cervix

- Hemorrhage (uncontrolled bleeding can occur if the lesion infiltrates a blood vessel)
- Pyometra—especially with endocervical cancer
- Hydronephrosis and pyelonephritis
- Vesicovaginal fistula (VVF)
- Rectovaginal fistula (RVF) (RVF is comparatively rare because of the interposition of the POD; the rectum is involved either through the uterosacral ligament or through the rectovaginal septum)

Causes of death in cancer cervix

- **Uremia:** This occurs due to ureteric obstruction following parametrial involvement, leading to hydroureteronephrosis. Infection sets in, thereby compromising renal function. Uremia is the most common cause of death in carcinoma cervix.

Viva corner

Q1 What is a microinvasive lesion?

- Stage IA1 cervical cancer where the depth of extension into stroma is ≤3 mm is called microinvasive lesion.
- Lymphatic and vascular involvement is not seen at this depth of invasion and hence termed microinvasive lesion.
  - *Depth of invasion ≤3 mm*: Lymph node metastasis rare
  - *Depth of invasion >3 to ≤5 mm*: 5% involvement of lymph nodes

Q2 What do the terms early stage and locally advanced disease mean?

- The term "early-stage disease" is used for stages IA, IB, and IIA.
- The term "locally advanced disease" is used for stages IIB–IVA.
- Carcinoma in situ is not included in FIGO staging.

Extra edge

Disadvantages of clinical staging

- It is difficult to assess the lymph node involvement on clinical examination, which is a main factor determining prognosis.
- There is difficulty in differentiating inflammatory and malignant induration of the parametrium. In cases of suspected pelvic inflammation, a course of antibiotic should be given prior to clinical staging.
- In inflammation, the induration is smooth.
- In malignancy, the induration is nodular.

Recent advancement in investigation of cervical cancer

Fluoro-2-deoxy-glucose (FDG) PET scan: This test is based on the fact that malignant cells exhibit glycolysis more than normal cells and FDG accumulates in malignant cells. FDG PET scan is a gold standard investigation for carcinoma cervix but very expensive.

Tumor marker

Squamous cell carcinoma (SCC) antigen is a serum marker for carcinoma cervix. Although the antigen is not specific, it has been found to be useful to monitor treatment response and to predict tumor recurrence.

Sentinel lymph node sampling

- Sentinel lymph node (SLN) is the first node that drains a primary tumor. This node can be detected by intraoperative lymphatic mapping. This is done by injecting methylene blue dye into the tumor or by lymphoscintigraphy using technetium-99.
- It is studied in Ca. breast, Ca. vulva, and Ca. cervix, Ca. penis.

- **Hemorrhage:** The bleeding from the growth may be brisk or continuous, leading to severe anemia.
- **Sepsis:** Pelvic or generalized peritonitis may occur as a consequence of pyometra.
- **Cancer cachexia:** Depressant action of cancerous tissues on the general metabolism leads to cachexia.
- **Metastases to the distant organs:** Metastases to the distant organs such as liver, lung, lymph nodes, and bones occur in advanced stages.

Pretreatment evaluation

Investigations

- Complete hemogram—to detect and correct anemia before surgery or chemoradiation
- Blood grouping and typing
- Urine albumin, sugar, and microscopy examination (to detect RBCs)
- Renal function test (to detect renal failure, to obtain a baseline value prior to starting therapy)
- Liver function test (to obtain a baseline value prior to starting therapy; may be abnormal in advanced malignancy with metastasis)
- Tests for HIV and HBsAg

TREATMENT OF CANCER CERVIX

The two main modalities of treatment are surgery and radiotherapy (RT). Treatment depends on the following:

- Stage of the cancer
- Age of the patient
- Associated comorbidities
- Associated gynecological problems (fibroid, ovarian tumor)
- Facilities and expertise available
- Patient's choice

Treatment options include the following:

- **Surgery:** Surgery is reserved only till stage IIA.
- **RT:** Stages IIB to IVB, primary chemoradiation is the treatment of choice. However, RT can be given in all stages

Treatment options for various stages of carcinoma cervix are mentioned in Table 22.1.

Pretreatment preparation

General health of the patient must be improved prior to therapy by correcting anemia and malnutrition for the following reasons:

- To make the patient sufficiently fit to withstand surgery

Table 22.1 Treatment of cancer cervix

Stage	Options	Procedure
IA1 without LVSI	Surgery/RT	• If fertility is desired, therapeutic conization can be done. Further management is based on histopathology: – If margins are negative: Follow-up – If margins are positive: Radical trachelectomy • If patient has completed her family, type I hysterectomy is done
IA1 with LVSI	Surgery/RT	• If fertility is desired, radical trachelectomy with PLND is done • If patient has completed family, type II hysterectomy with PLND is done
IA2	Surgery/RT	• If fertility is desired, radical trachelectomy with PLND is done • If patient has completed family, type II hysterectomy with PLND is done • Patients may require postoperative chemoradiation
IB1	Surgery/RT	• Type III hysterectomy with PLND with postoperative adjuvant chemoradiation • If fertility is desired, radical trachelectomy with PLND can be considered in highly selected cases
IB2 and IIA	Surgery/RT	• Type III hysterectomy with PLND and para-aortic LND with postoperative adjuvant chemoradiation (or) • Primary chemoradiation

(CONTD...)

Table 22.1 (CONTD...)

Stage	Options	Procedure
IB3 and IIA	Surgery/RT	• Type III hysterectomy with PLND and para-aortic LND with postoperative adjuvant chemoradiation (or) • Primary chemoradiation is a better option in these cases
IIB, IIIA, IIIB	RT	• Chemoradiation is the treatment of choice
IVA	RT	• Chemoradiation is the treatment of choice • Pelvic exenteration surgery is rarely done
IVB	Palliative chemotherapy/RT	• Symptomatic treatment with least morbidity is the main concern in these patients

LVSI, lymphovascular space involvement; *PLND*, pelvic lymph node dissection; *RT*, radiotherapy.

Viva corner

Q1 What are the factors based on which decision for postoperative chemotherapy/radiotherapy is decided upon?

Patients with high- and intermediate-risk factors are associated with an increased risk of recurrence and hence require adjuvant chemotherapy/radiotherapy.

High-risk factors—40% recurrence within 3 years:

- Positive lymph nodes
- Positive margins
- Microscopic parametrial involvement

(**Hint:** *Remember as "LMP"*)

Intermediate-risk factors—30% recurrence within 3 years:

- Large tumor size
- Lymphovascular space involvement (LVSI)
- Cervical stromal invasion

The most important variable associated with survival is the status of lymph node involvement.

- To improve tissue oxygenation for effective ionizing effect of RT

Role of surgery in cancer cervix

Indications

Surgery is limited to stage I up to stage IIA lesions.

Surgical options for Ca. cervix

These include the following:

- Cone biopsy
- Radical trachelectomy
- Extrafascial or type I hysterectomy
- Radical hysterectomy—modified radical hysterectomy (MRH), radical hysterectomy (RH) and extended RH with bilateral pelvic lymphadenectomy
- Recent advances—nerve-sparing surgery and laparoscopic radical hysterectomy

Advantages of surgery

- Ovaries may be preserved.
- A more pliable vagina is retained for sexual intercourse.
- Bladder and bowel complications associated with RT are avoided.
- Pelvic lymph nodes can be removed.
- There is the psychological benefit of the disease being removed.
- Quality of life and patient satisfaction are better with surgery.
- Specimen is obtained for histopathological examination.

Disadvantages of surgery

- Not applicable to all stages
- Anesthetic complications
- Complications due to surgery (Table 22.2)

Table 22.2 Complications associated with surgical management of carcinoma cervix	
Intraoperative complications	**Postoperative complications**
• Hemorrhage • Injury to surrounding structures such as bowel, bladder, and ureter	• Immediate/acute complications: Hemorrhage, intestinal obstruction, sepsis, febrile morbidity, pulmonary embolism, vesicovaginal fistula • Late/chronic complications: Bladder atony/hypotony, lymphocyst formation

Role of radiotherapy in cancer cervix

Indications

- It is a primary treatment modality that can be used for all stages.
- Postoperative RT indicated in high- and intermediate-risk cases as follows:
  - Positive margins
  - Positive lymph nodes
  - Microscopic parametrial involvement
  - Large tumor size
  - Lymphovascular space involvement (LVSI)
  - Cervical stromal invasion

Viva corner

Q1 What are the conditions where surgery is preferred over RT for treating carcinoma cervix?

- Associated PID
- Associated fibroid, ovarian tumor, prolapse uterus, and endocervical carcinoma
- Stump carcinoma
- Adenocarcinoma of cervix (radioresistant)
- Young patients
- Recurrence after radiation therapy

Q2 What is radical trachelectomy?

- It is a conservative treatment option for carcinoma cervix in women who desire preservation of uterus for fertility.
- It involves the removal of cervix almost up to the internal os along with the paracervical tissue (see figure below)
- It can be done in the following stages:
  - Stage IA1
  - Stages IA2 and IB1
- It can be done via abdominal/vaginal route.
- PLND and cervical encerclage are done along with the procedure.
- Long-term outcome is uncertain, as experience with this procedure is limited.
- There are limited data on pregnancy outcome—increased risk of abortions, preterm labor, and premature rupture of membranes.
- If recurrence occurs, definitive treatment with surgery/RT is necessary.

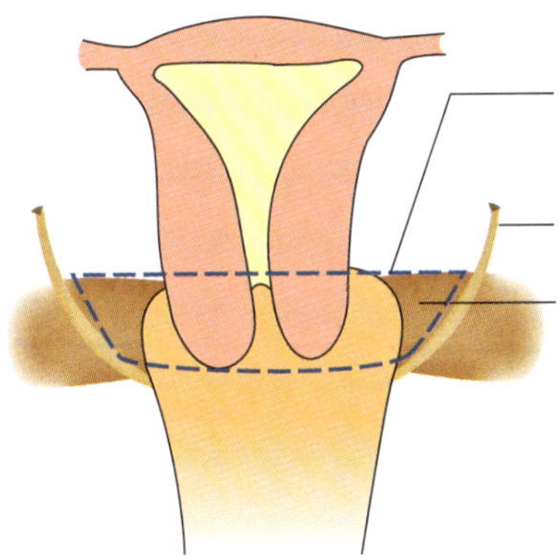

Figure Diagrammatic representation of radical trachelectomy. Ectocervix and parametrium medial to ureter are removed.

Q3 What are the types of hysterectomy?

Piver classification (see figure below):

- **Type I:** Simple or extrafascial hysterectomy
- **Type II:** Modified radical hysterectomy or Wertheim hysterectomy
  - Uterine artery is ligated at the level of ureter, preserving the ureteric branch to ureter.
  - Ureter is not dissected from vesicouterine ligament.

(CONTD...)

(...CONTD)

Viva corner

- Parametrium: The medial half of parametrium is removed.
- Vagina: A small margin of vagina is removed.

- **Type III:** Radical hysterectomy or Meigs hysterectomy
  - Uterine artery is ligated at its origin.
  - Ureter is dissected from vesicouterine ligament.
  - Parametrium: The entire parametrium is removed.
  - Vagina: The upper one-third of vagina is removed.
- **Type IV:** Extended radical hysterectomy; structures removed in addition to type III hysterectomy are as follows:
  - Periureteric tissue
  - Superior vesical artery
  - Vagina—three-fourth of vagina removed
- **Type V:** Pelvic exenteration surgery
  - Distal ureter and segment of bladder and rectum are removed.

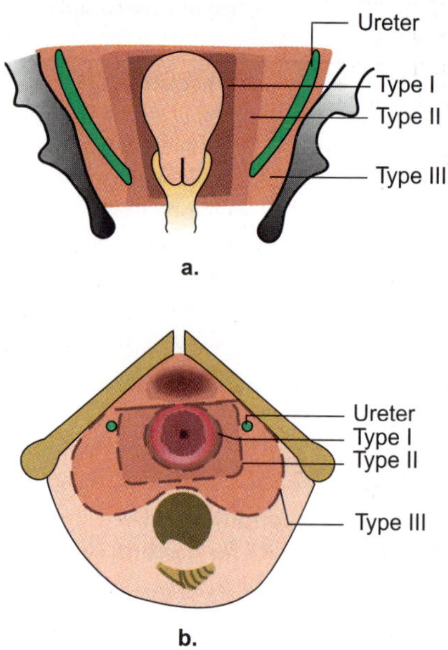

Figure Diagrammatic representation of the types of hysterectomy. **a.** Frontal view. **b.** Cross-sectional view. The innermost line indicates type I hysterectomy, the middle line type II hysterectomy, and the outer line type III hysterectomy.

- In case of recurrence following surgery, RT can be given.
- Hemostatic RT can be given to control brisk hemorrhage.

Advantages

- It can be given in all stages of cancer cervix.
- It can be given as an OPD procedure.
- Patients with comorbid conditions who are unfit for surgery can be treated by RT.
- Complications due to surgery are avoided.
- Survival rates are similar to those for surgery.

Disadvantages

- Urinary fistulas and strictures can develop following RT.
- Radiation fibrosis of bowel and bladder can occur.
- RT causes stricture and shortening of vagina, leading to dyspareunia.
- It leads to ovarian destruction.
- It can lead to avascular necrosis of femur head.
- There is a possibility of secondary sarcomas because of destruction of the surrounding normal structures.
- Patient satisfaction is less (tumor lesion is not removed).
- Quality of life is poor with RT.

Methods of administration

Technique of RT

- Radiation dose is expressed in rad (radiation absorbed dose) or Gray.
- 1 Gray = 100 rad; hence, 1 rad = 1 cGy (centigray).
- Radiation obeys the "inverse square law," that is, the dose of radiation at a given point is inversely proportional to the square of distance of that point from the radiation source.
- RT is of the following types:
  - External beam RT (EBRT; teletherapy)
  - Intracavitary RT (brachytherapy)

In early stages: Brachytherapy is given first followed by EBRT.

In advanced stages: EBRT is given first to shrink the primary tumor and make the insertion of intracavitary source feasible, followed by brachytherapy.

Teletherapy

- Radiation is given from a distance targeting the lesion and the draining nodes.
- The aim is to deliver the maximum tolerated dose to the tumor, while avoiding damage to the surrounding normal tissues.
- EBRT is given by a linear accelerator, which can deliver a high dose of radiation to deep tissues with relative sparing of superficial structures such as skin.

Brachytherapy

- The tumor and surrounding areas are treated by direct contact with high-energy sources placed in the vagina or cervix.
- Radioactive sources commonly used are cesium-137 and iridium-192.
- Intracavitary radiation is delivered by using a tandem inserted into the uterus and vaginal ovoids inserted into the vagina (Figure 22.2).
- Procedure: After cervical dilatation, a hollow tube (tandem) is inserted into the cervical canal. Two ovoids (hollow, round applicators) are put, one in each lateral fornix. Roller gauze is packed between them and both vaginal walls. Cesium or iridium is then transferred to the applicators by "Afterloading" remote technique. "Afterloading technique" is used to avoid radiation hazard to hospital staff.

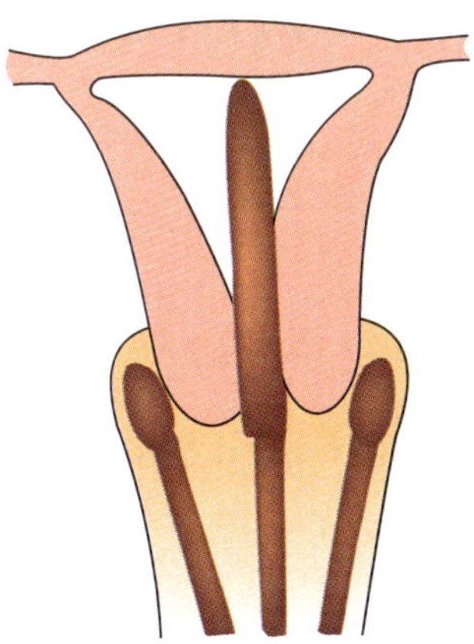

Figure 22.2 Uterine tandems and ovoids in position for brachytherapy—uterine tandem inserted into the uterine cavity and vaginal ovoids used for intracavitary radiation.

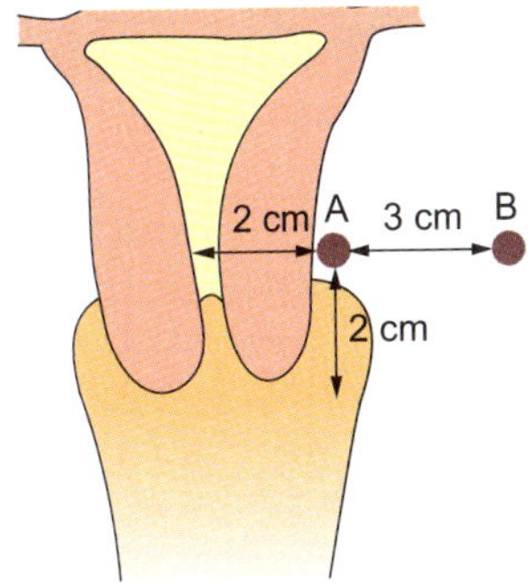

Figure 22.3 Points A and B used in radiotherapy. Point A is 2 cm above and lateral to the external os. Point B is 3 cm lateral to point A.

Calculation of radiation dose

The radiation dose is calculated according to the amount of radiation received at two arbitrary points (Figure 22.3):

- **Point A:** It is 2 cm above and lateral to external os—corresponds to the point of crossing of uterine artery with ureter in the parametrial tissue.
- **Point B:** It is 3 cm lateral to point A—corresponds to obturator nodes on lateral pelvic wall.
- The total dose of RT is 80–85 Gy at point A and 50–65 Gy at point B. This dosage to points A and B limits the bladder and rectal dose to less than 60 Gy.
- EBRT and brachytherapy administered for treatment of carcinoma cervix are mentioned in Table 22.3.

Complications of RT

Complications associated with RT are given in Table 22.4.

Note *Late toxicity following RT is due to gradually increasing ischemia and fibrosis, owing to progressive obliterative endarteritis caused by chronic effects of radiation on tissues.*

Part 2

Part 2

Table 22.3 Radiotherapy in cancer cervix

External beam radiotherapy	Intracavitary RT
Delivers uniform dose of radiation to the tumor and entire pelvis	Delivers maximum dose to the tumor, parametrium, and paravaginal tissue, and the radiation diminishes toward the lateral pelvic wall
It is administered using linear accelerator	Uterine tandems and vaginal ovoids are used as applicators
It is administered in fractions, 5 days/week for 5 weeks (25 fractions)	The dose is delivered as follows: • Low-dose rates over 36–48 hours using cesium-137 (or) • High-dose rates—once a week for 2–3 weeks using iridium-192

Table 22.4 Complications associated with radiotherapy

Early complications	Late complications
• Uterine perforation at the time of insertion of applicators in brachytherapy • In teletherapy, nausea, vomiting, diarrhea, and abdominal cramps • Skin rashes and bone marrow depression	• Vaginal stenosis • Vesicovaginal fistula and rectovaginal fistula • Cystitis • Proctitis leading to diarrhea, tenesmus, and rectal bleeding • Small bowel obstruction and strictures • Premature menopause due to ovarian failure

Chemotherapy

- It is used for adjuvant therapy and palliative therapy.
- Drugs used include cisplatin, bleomycin, 5-flurouracil (5-FU), vincristine, mitomycin, and adriamycin.
- Neoadjuvant chemotherapy: Chemotherapy prior to radical surgery or RT improves treatment outcome.
- Chemoradiation: It is the concomitant administration of chemotherapy along with RT. Chemotherapy acts as a radiosensitizer and the synergistic action of the two therapies gives better results.
- The drug used is cisplatin 40 mg/m^2, administered weekly for 6 weeks in combination with RT.
- Chemoradiation is the treatment of choice for cervical cancer stages IIB to IVA.

Extra edge

Radiosensitivity

It is the response of tumor cells to radiation.

Factors affecting radiosensitivity

- **Oxygenation:** Tissue hypoxia reduces radiosensitivity.
- **Tumor histology:** Squamous cell carcinomas and dysgerminomas are highly radiosensitive unlike adenocarcinomas.
- **Tumor volume:** Smaller tumor volume requires lesser radiation dose.
- **Cell cycle:** Mitotic cells and cells in G2 phase are radiosensitive.
- **Radiosensitizers:** These are agents that increase radiosensitivity.

  Radiosensitizers include the following:
- Chemotherapeutic agents such as cisplatin, bleomycin, and 5-FU
- Oxygen
- Tumor necrosis factor (TNF)
- Interferons

Prognostic factors in cancer cervix

- Stage of the disease
- Lymph node metastasis
- Parametrial involvement
- Tumor volume
- Histological type
- Tumor differentiation (grade)

Follow-up of treated cases

- The patient is followed up every 3 months for the first 2 years and then annually for the rest of the life.
- During follow-up visits, H/o symptoms such as bleeding P/V, discharge P/V, and pelvic pain are noted.

Examination includes the following:
- Speculum examination of the vaginal vault
- Bimanual and rectal examination to palpate for any recurrence of disease

Investigations
- Pap smear of the vault during every visit; chest X-ray is done every year.
- Other investigations are done depending on the clinical findings and resources available.

Disease persistence Persistent cervical cancer refers to the cancer lesion that has not completely regressed after 3 months of RT.

Disease recurrence Disease recurrence refers to a new lesion that develops 6 months after completion of primary therapy.

PREVENTION OF CANCER CERVIX

Primary prevention

- Prophylactic HPV vaccine is recommended for women in the age group 9–26 years.
- Use of condom to prevent STDs, increasing the age at marriage and of first childbirth, limitation of family size, maintenance of local

High-yield points

Management of cancer cervix in a pregnant woman

- Cervical cancer is the most common gynecological malignancy in pregnancy.
- Vaginal bleeding is the usual presenting symptom.
- The safety and complications of procedures used for diagnosis and treatment of cancer cervix in pregnant women are listed in Table A below.
- Management of carcinoma cervix in pregnancy depends on the stage of the disease and is mentioned in Table B below.
- Cesarean section is preferred over vaginal delivery. Vaginal delivery is associated with an increased risk of spread of the tumor.

Table A Safety and complications of procedures in cervical cancer in pregnancy

	Procedure	Safety/complications
Diagnostic procedures	Colposcopy	Safe
	Cervical biopsy	Bleeding tends to be more
	Endocervical curettage	Rupture of membranes
	Conization	Increased risk of abortion, preterm labor
Imaging modalities	Ultrasonography, MRI	Safe
	CT scan	Fetal radiation
Treatment modalities	Surgery	Bleeding tends to be more
	Chemotherapy	Abortion, congenital malformation, fetal death
	Radiotherapy	Abortion, fetal death

Table B Management of cervical cancer during pregnancy

Stage	Management during pregnancy
Stage IA1	Pregnancy can be followed till term and vaginal delivery can be allowed. Hysterectomy can be done, 6 weeks later
Stage IA2	Continue pregnancy till fetal maturity. Do cesarean section and modified radical hysterectomy with PLND
Stage IB1	Do not delay treatment for more than 4 weeks to attain fetal maturity. Do classical cesarean section and radical hysterectomy with PLND
Stages II–IV	If the fetus is viable, deliver by classical cesarean section followed by chemoradiation

PLND, pelvic lymph node dissection.

hygiene, and treatment of STDs are other steps in prevention.

- Removal of cervix during hysterectomy for benign conditions helps in prevention of stump carcinoma (Incidence is 1%).

Secondary prevention

Secondary prevention is the prevention of progression of CIN to invasive cancer. This consists of screening, and appropriate management of preinvasive cervical lesions, and follow-up.

PREMALIGNANT LESIONS OF CERVIX OR CERVICAL INTRAEPITHELIAL NEOPLASIA

Definition

- CIN is a premalignant condition involving the cervix, where the cellular abnormalities are limited to the surface epithelium and do not extend beyond the basement membrane.
- Dysplasia refers to the abnormal maturation of the cells of stratified squamous epithelium of cervix. Dysplasia is described as mild, moderate, and severe dysplasia and carcinoma in situ based on the involvement of basal, intermediate, and superficial cells or the full thickness of the epithelium. As dysplasias of all grades can progress to invasive cancer, this terminology has been replaced by the term CIN in histological grade.
- CIN has the potential to develop invasive carcinoma over time. However, there is a long latent period between CIN and invasive carcinoma which can be detected by screening.
- CIN is classified into three histological grades as mentioned in Table 22.5.
- Bethesda system is a cytological grading that includes the following terminologies: low-grade squamous intraepithelial lesion (LSIL) for CIN 1 and high-grade squamous intraepithelial lesion (HSIL) for CIN 2 and 3.

Screening methods for diagnosis of preinvasive lesions of the cervix

- Screening is done to identify individuals with a high probability of having or developing a disease

Extra edge

Q1 Describe the HPV vaccine for prevention of cervical cancer.

Cervical cancer accounts for >90% of all HPV-related cancers. HPV vaccines are used to prevent HPV infection and therefore cervical cancer. They also prevent other HPV-related cancers that include anal, vaginal, vulval, and oropharyngeal cancers.

- **The vaccines are available as bivalent, quadrivalent, and nanovalent vaccines.**
  - Bivalent vaccine offers protection against HPV 16, 18 (Cervarix).
  - Quadrivalent vaccine offers protection against HPV 6, 11, 16, 18 (Gardasil).
  - Nanovalent vaccine offers protection against HPV 6, 11, 16, 18, 31, 33, 45, 52, 58.
- **Age of administration** (girls and boys) is 9–14 years. Catch-up vaccination is recommended at 15–26 years. There is no recommendation regarding the use of vaccine after 26 years of age.
- **Dosage:** Two doses at 0, 6–12 months in 9–14 years age group. Three doses at 0, 1–2, and 6 months in 15–26 years age group are administered.
- The vaccines are prophylactic, not therapeutic. If infection by HPV is acquired before administration of vaccine, it cannot be cured by the vaccine.
- The vaccine is most effective if it is given before the start of sexual activity. However, HPV vaccine can be given in women who had sexual activity, when the vaccine will prevent acquisition of new infections, although it cannot act against infections that are already established.
- Vaccination of men prevents genital warts and penile cancers and transmission of the virus to the sexual partner.
- **Screening with cytology (Pap smear) must continue:** The vaccine covers only some high-risk HPV types. Hence, screening is recommended to detect other HPV infection-related cytological abnormalities.

Table 22.5 Grades of CIN

CIN classification				Bethesda system
Histological grade	**Corresponding dysplasia**	**Description**	**Cause and progression**	**Corresponding terminology**
CIN 1	Mild dysplasia	Atypical changes are limited to lower one-third of epithelium	• CIN 1 represents low-grade lesion • CIN 1 lesions are caused by HPV during the infectious phase • Most CIN 1 lesions regress spontaneously • Progression to invasive cancer occurs infrequently (1%)	Low-grade squamous intraepithelial lesion (LSIL) for CIN 1
CIN 2	Moderate dysplasia	Atypical changes extend to middle one-third of epithelium	• CIN 2 and 3 lesions represent high-grade lesions • They are caused by persistent HPV infection • They are not necessarily preceded by CIN 1 • Progression to invasive cancer occurs more often (5% and 12% respectively in CIN 2 and CIN 3 lesions)	High-grade squamous intraepithelial lesion (HSIL) for CIN 2 and 3
CIN 3	Severe dysplasia and carcinoma in situ	Atypical changes are severe and extend through the entire thickness of epithelium. Basement membrane is intact		

CIN, cervical intraepithelial neoplasia.

It is a public health intervention based on the population at risk or target population.

- Screening for cervical cancer has reduced its incidence. Screening for cervical cancer is easy to perform because of the following reasons:
  - The cervix can be easily visualized and tests can be performed.
  - Cervical cancer goes through premalignant changes and there is a long latent period of 10–20 years before the disease progresses from a premalignant lesion to a malignant lesion.
- Several screening modalities are available, but Pap smear (exfoliative cytology) is a time-tested

High-yield points

Pathogenesis of CIN

- The ectocervix and the vagina are lined by squamous epithelium and the endocervix by columnar epithelium. The junction between the two is known as the squamocolumnar junction (SCJ).
- SCJ of cervix is a dynamic point that keeps moving up and down in relation to different phases of life (see figure below).
- At birth, SCJ is located on the ectocervix and is called the original SCJ (Figure a).
- Under the influence of estrogen at puberty and pregnancy, the endocervix everts to expose the columnar epithelium (Figure b). Under the influence of estrogen, the columnar epithelium becomes filled with glycogen and lactobacilli colonize the epithelium. *Lactobacillus* acts on the glycogen to produce lactic acid, thereby reducing the vaginal pH.
- Reduced vaginal pH stimulates the columnar epithelium to undergo metaplasia and converts it into immature squamous and later mature squamous epithelium.
- Metaplasia advances cephalad from original SCJ toward external os. This process establishes an area called transformation zone (TZ), which extends from the original SCJ to the new SCJ (new SCJ is the junction between the metaplastic squamous epithelium and the columnar epithelium) (see Figure c).
- The entire TZ with early metaplastic cells is susceptible to oncogenic effects leading to CIN. Most cervical malignancies occur in the region of TZ.
- Metaplasia is more likely to begin following menarche or pregnancy when metaplasia is most active.
- In postmenopausal women, the new SCJ moves further cephalad and lies within the endocervical canal (Figure d).

(CONTD...)

(...CONTD)

High-yield points

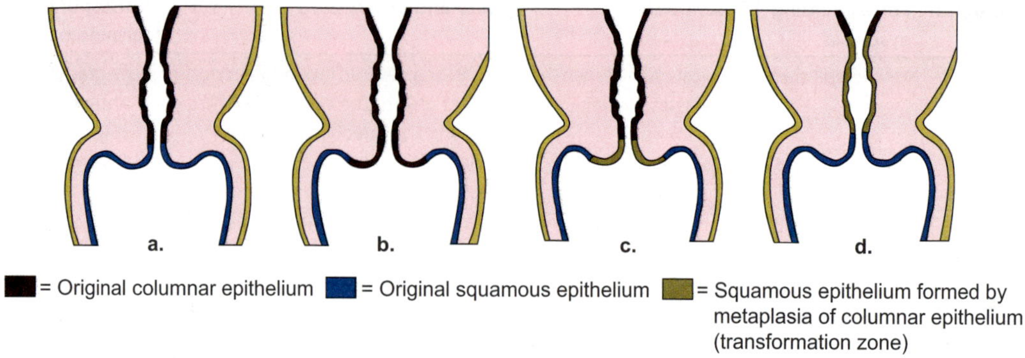

Figure Dynamic squamocolumnar junction of the cervix. **a.** Before puberty, the ectocervix is covered with squamous epithelium. **b.** Increased estrogenic activity during puberty exposes the columnar epithelium onto the ectocervix. **c.** Replacement of columnar epithelium by squamous epithelium to form the transformation zone (TZ). New squamocolumnar junction is situated at or slightly outside the external os during reproductive period. **d.** Indrawing of the squamocolumnar junction and the TZ into the cervical canal following menopause.

method of screening for cervical cancer and is most widely used.
- **Screening methods include the following:**
  - Pap smear
  - ThinPrep—liquid-based cytology (LBC)
  - HPV DNA testing
  - Visual inspection after acetic acid (VIA)
  - Visual inspection after Lugol's iodine (VILI)

Screening guidelines

The American Cancer Society (ACS) has updated its cervical cancer screening guidelines in 2020 with some distinct changes in comparison with previous and other guidelines (Table 22.6). The American Cancer Society (ACS) 2020 recommendations are as follows:
- Cervical cancer screening starting at age 25 years with primary human papillomavirus (HPV) testing every 5 years through age 65 years (preferred)
- If primary HPV testing is not available, then screened with cotesting (HPV testing in combination with cytology) every 5 years or cytology alone every 3 years (acceptable)
- The ACS recommends that individuals aged >65 years with no history of cervical intraepithelial neoplasia grade 2 (CIN 2) or more severe disease within the past 25 years, and who have documented negative screening in the prior 10 years, discontinue all cervical cancer screening
- New guideline retains the recommendation to continue screening of women who have received the HPV vaccine
- Follow-up for individuals who screen positive for HPV and/or cytology should be in accordance with the 2019 American Society for Colposcopy and Cervical Pathology (ASCCP) risk-based management consensus guidelines for abnormal cervical cancer screening tests and cancer precursors.

Changes made in the ACS 2020 cervical cancer screening recommendations: The new screening recommendations differ in important aspects in comparison with previous and other guidelines as follows:
- The preferred screening strategy is primary HPV testing every 5 years, with cotesting or cytology acceptable only where access to primary HPV testing is not yet available.
- The recommended age to start screening is 25 years rather than 21 years.
- Primary HPV testing is recommended starting at age 25 years rather than age 30 years.

Table 22.6 Summary of cervical cancer screening recommendations

Age	ACS (2020)	ACOG (2016, 2018)	USPSTF & AAFP (2018)
<21 years	Not recommended	Not recommended	Not recommended
21–29	***Start at 25 years*** Primary HPV testing alone every 5 years (preferred) **OR** Co-testing every 5 years **OR** Cytology alone every 3 years	***Start at 21 years*** Cytology alone every 3 years	***Start at 21 years*** Cytology alone every 3 years
30-65	Primary HPV testing alone every 5 years (preferred) **OR** Co-testing every 5 years **OR** Cytology alone every 3 years	Cytology alone every 3 years **OR** Primary HPV testing alone every 5 years **OR** Co-testing every 5 years (preferred)	Cytology alone every 3 years **OR** Primary HPV testing alone every 5 years **OR** Co-testing every 5 years
>65	Not recommended[a]	Not recommended[b]	Not recommended[b]
Hysterectomy (with no history of cervical cancer or high-grade precancerous lesion)	Not recommended	Not recommended	Not recommended

AAFP, American Academy of Family Physicians; *ACOG*, American College of Obstetrics and Gynecology; *ACS*, American Cancer Society; *USPSTF*, U.S. preventive services task force.

[a] No CIN 2 or greater within 25 years and documented negative screening in prior 10 years.

[b] History of adequate screening: 3 consecutive negative cytology results or 2 consecutive negative co-testing results within 10 years with the most recent test within 5 years

- The guideline is transitional, i.e., options for screening with cotesting or cytology should be phased out once full access to primary HPV testing for cervical cancer screening is available.
- No changes have been made in recommendations for screening intervals, age or criteria for screening cessation, screening based on vaccination status, or screening after hysterectomy.

Concerns on the new recommendations:

- There is limited availability of FDA-approved primary HPV testing tests.
- Significant laboratory infrastructure changes are required to switch to this screening method.
- Limited access to primary HPV testing in rural and under-resourced countries which have disproportionately high rates of cervical cancer incidence, morbidity, and mortality.
- Hence, until primary HPV testing is widely available and accessible, cytology-based screening methods should remain as options in cervical cancer screening guidelines.

Note *Cervical cancer screening guidelines are difficult to implement in developing countries and hence the WHO has recommended a minimum requirement of one adequate Pap smear per lifetime in women older than 35 years of age in low-resource settings. If multiple smears can be performed, screening intervals can be increased to 10 years. The incidence of cervical cancer can be reduced remarkably even with such infrequent testing.*

Screening procedures

Pap smear

- **Principle:** It is a conventional cytological technique based on exfoliative cytology. The abnormal cells of the cervix exfoliate that can be collected, smeared, and stained.

Extra edge

What is primary HPV testing?

- A primary HPV test is an HPV test that is done by itself for screening without cytology. The US Food and Drug Administration (FDA) has approved certain tests to be primary HPV tests.
- Other HPV tests are approved only as part of a cotest, when HPV test and Pap test are done together.
- As primary HPV testing is not easily available, a cotest every 5 years or a Pap test every 3 years are still good options for cervical cancer screening.

Why does the new ACS 2020 guidelines recommend a primary HPV test over a Pap test or HPV/Pap cotest?

Primary HPV testing has proven to be highly sensitive in detecting cervical precancer and cancer. Hence, ACS new guidelines advocates primary HPV testing as the preferred mechanism of testing.

Why does the new ACS 2020 guidelines recommend screening starting at age 25 instead of age 21?

ACS in 2020 noted that the benefits of cervical cancer screening do not outweigh the harms for women aged 21 to 24 years of age, based on emerging evidences as follows:

- HPV vaccine administration has led to a drop in HPV infections and cervical precancer in this age group.
- In young women, HPV infections are mostly self-limiting and go away without any treatment. Screening people in this age group often leads to unnecessary treatment.

Why do the guidelines for cervical cancer screening keep changing?

HPV vaccination, newer technologies like HPV testing, and emerging new evidences from large studies have resulted in more accurate predictions of developing cervical precancer and cancer, which has led to continual changes in the guidelines for cervical screening.

Viva corner

Q1 How is a Pap smear taken?

Prerequisites for taking a Pap smear: 48 hours prior to taking a Pap smear, the woman:

- Should not use vaginal cream
- Should not do vaginal douching
- Should not have sexual intercourse

Procedure:

- The cervix is visualized by placing a Sims' or Cusco's speculum.
- Sample is taken prior to use of lubricants and bimanual examination to prevent dislodgement of exfoliative cells.
- The ectocervix is scraped using an Ayre spatula by rotating the spatula 360° at external os (see figure below) and endocervix scraped with a Cytobrush.
- The cells are smeared on a glass slide and fixed with liquid fixative or fixative spray. Fixation is done immediately to avoid air drying that can lead to artifacts.
- The slides are stained using Papanicolaou stain and examined.
- Fixatives used are the following:
  - Ethyl alcohol 95% (1:1 mixture of 95% ethanol and ether)
  - Isopropyl alcohol 85%
  - Methanol
  - Surgical spirit

Q2 What are the uses of Ayre spatula?

Ayre spatula can be used for the following:

- To take a Pap smear
- To take surface cytology in carcinoma cervix
- To take smear for hormonal cytology—smear taken from lateral vaginal wall
- To take a vault smear—follow-up of cases for recurrence following treatment with surgery/RT
- To take a buccal smear

(CONTD...)

..CONTD)

Viva corner

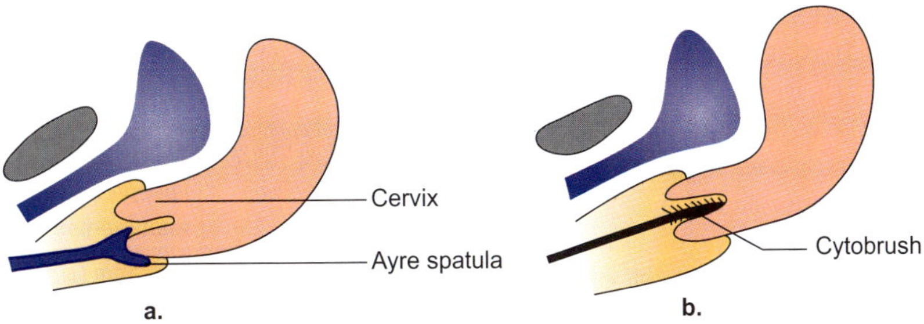

Figure Technique of taking Pap smear. **a.** Ayre spatula. **b.** Endocervical cytobrush.

Ayre's wooden spatula and Cytobrush are used for the procedure.

- **Efficacy of Pap smear:** Pap smear has a high specificity (98%) but low sensitivity (60%) and high false-negative rate (50%).
- **False-negative values occur due to the following:**
  - Sampling error
  - Fixation error
  - Interpretation error
- **Advantages of Pap smear as a screening test are as follows:**
  - Easy to perform on an OPD basis
  - Reasonable sensitivity and specificity
  - Not very expensive

ThinPrep—liquid-based cytology

- **Principle:** Monolayer preparation of cells using a liquid-based medium to collect the sample
- **Procedure**
  - Sample from cervix is collected in the usual way using a spatula and endocervical brush or by using a special broom sampling device.
  - Sample is rinsed in a vial containing liquid-based medium—80–90% cells are transferred to the liquid medium and transported to the laboratory.
  - Cells are separated by passing the liquid through a filter that traps large epithelial cells.
  - Thin monolayer of cells is prepared, fixed, and is interpreted by a cytologist.
- **Advantages**
  - Decreases sampling and preparation errors
  - Eliminates artifacts due to air drying
  - Removes blood and other cells that interfere with interpretation
  - Low false-negative rates
  - High specificity
  - Fewer unsatisfactory smears
  - Can use the residual sample for HPV testing
- **Disadvantages**
  - It is expensive.
  - Laboratory staff need special training to do the procedure.

HPV testing

- Tests for detection of high-risk HPV DNA are commonly used.
- In women <30 years, prevalence of HPV infection is high and transient. Hence, the test has poor sensitivity in this age group.
- In women >30 years, HPV testing may be done along with cytology. The screening interval can be increased to 5 years, if HPV co-testing is negative.

Visual inspection after acetic acid (VIA)

- When acetic acid 5% is applied to the cervix, abnormal areas turn acetowhite. Biopsy can be taken from abnormal areas.
- **Principle:** Abnormal cells have increased chromatin density and are rich in protein that get coagulated with acetic acid and hence turn white, while normal cells containing glycogen remain normal. Areas of CIN, neoplasia, and HPV-related changes turn acetowhite with acetic acid application.

- **Advantages**
  - Health workers can be trained to identify abnormal areas after application of acetic acid on cervix. If VIA is positive, the patient has to be referred to a higher institution for colposcopic evaluation.
  - This method has been extensively studied in developing countries including India and is currently recommended as the primary screening test for cancer cervix in developing countries.
- **Disadvantages**
  - Specificity of the test is less (80%) and the false-positive rate is high, resulting in large number of referrals for further evaluation.

Visual inspection after Lugol's iodine

When Lugol's iodine or Schiller's iodine is applied on the cervix, normal cervical epithelium, which is rich in glycogen, stains mahogany brown (Schiller test). The abnormal areas rich in protein do not take up the iodine and appear mustard yellow. Advantages and disadvantages are similar to those of VIA.

Lugol's iodine It consists of 10% potassium iodide with 5% iodine.

Reporting of cervical cytology

The Bethesda system of reporting the cytology smear classifies the epithelial cell abnormalities as given in Table 22.7.

Table 22.7 Bethesda system of classification of epithelial cell abnormalities

Squamous cell abnormalities	Glandular cell abnormalities
• Atypical squamous cells of undetermined significance (ASCUS) • Atypical squamous cells high grade (ASC-HG) • Low-grade squamous intraepithelial lesion (LSIL) • High-grade squamous intraepithelial lesion (HSIL) • Squamous cell carcinoma	• Atypical endocervical cells • Atypical endometrial cells • Atypical glandular cells (AGC) • Endocervical adenocarcinoma in situ • Adenocarcinoma

CIN, cervical intraepithelial neoplasia.

Evaluation and management following cytology report

The Bethesda system assures uniformity of reporting and provides clear guidelines for further evaluation and management (Table 22.8).

Table 22.8 Evaluation following cytology report

Cervical cytology	Further evaluation/ management
Normal	Continue screening as usual
Atypical squamous cells of undetermined significance	HPV testing (or) repeat cytology after 6 months to 1 year
Atypical squamous cells—high grade	Colposcopy
LSIL	Colposcopy
HSIL	Colposcopy
AGC	Colposcopy, ECC
Adenocarcinoma in situ	Colposcopy, ECC, and endometrial sampling, if >35 years

AGC, atypical glandular cells; *HSIL*, high-grade squamous intraepithelial lesion; *LSIL*, low-grade squamous intraepithelial lesion; *ECC*, endocervical curettage.

Colposcopy

- Colposcopy is visualization of the cervix, vagina, and vulva under a low-magnification microscope to detect premalignant and malignant lesions. It helps in localization of abnormal areas and taking biopsy. Acetic acid 5% and Lugol's iodine can be applied and biopsies are taken from acetowhite areas/areas without Iodine uptake. Colposcope also uses a green filter to appreciate the vascular changes and color tone because the unfiltered white/yellow light may reduce the contrast between the terminal vessels and the surrounding tissue (Figure 22.4).
- Satisfactory colposcopy is indicated by visualization of the squamocolumnar junction (SCJ), transformation zone, and the columnar epithelium.
- It is complementary and not a substitute for cytology (Table 22.9).

Indications

- Abnormal Pap smear.

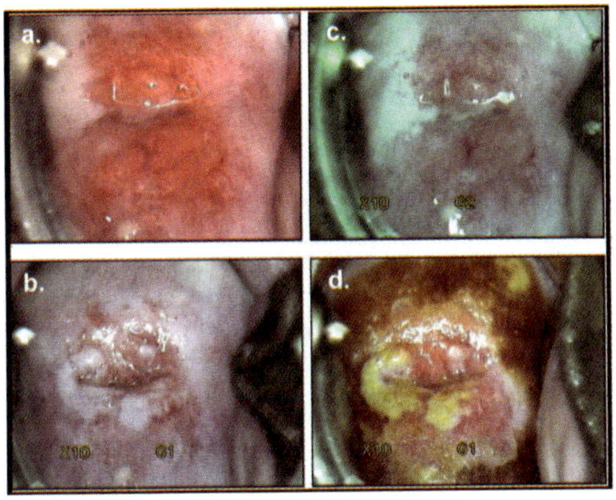

Figure 22.4 Colposcopy images of cervix. **a.** Magnified view. **b.** Acetowhite areas after 5% acetic acid application. **c.** Examination under green filter. **d.** Examination after application of Lugol's iodine.

Table 22.9 Comparison of cytology and colposcopy for cancer cervix screening

Cytology	Colposcopy
Laboratory method of detection	Clinical method of detection
Cytology evaluates the morphological changes of the exfoliated cells	Colposcopy evaluates the changes in the terminal vascular network of the cervix that reflect the biochemical and metabolic changes in the tissue
Cytology identifies cases that require further evaluation by colposcopy	Colposcopy identifies the sites from where biopsies are to be taken

- Cervix looks suspicious but Pap smear is normal.
- Lesion is not clinically detected—to locate abnormal areas and to study the extent of lesion.
- It is done to plan conservative surgery under colposcopic guidance.
- It is done for follow-up of patients who are conservatively managed.

Abnormal colposcopic findings

- Mosaic pattern
- Acetowhite areas
- Abnormal vessels
- Punctate lesions

(**Hint:** *Remember as M A^2 P*)

- **Reid's colposcopic index (RCI):** It is a systematic, objective method of colposcopically grading the severity of premalignant cervical lesions. The index consists of four colposcopic variables each with scores (0–2): lesion margin, color of acetowhitening, blood vessels, and iodine staining. Maximum score is 8.
- **Swede's colposcopic index (SCI):** This includes lesion size as a variable to be scored in addition to the 4 variables found in the Reid colposcopic index, along with few modifications to definitions of the scores for the other variables. Maximum score is 10.

Management of preinvasive lesions of cervix

- Colposcopy is performed in indicated cases following screening with cytology. The lesion has to be confirmed by histopathological examination of the cervical biopsy specimen prior to definitive treatment.
- Preinvasive lesions are classified as low-grade squamous intraepithelial lesion (LSIL) or high-grade squamous intraepithelial lesion (HSIL) according to the recent terminology (Bethesda system) and as CIN 1, 2, and 3 according to CIN terminology.

Treatment modalities for CIN lesions

Currently available treatment modalities are ablative and excision procedures that are mentioned in Table 22.10.

Management of CIN 1

- Most cases of CIN 1 regress spontaneously over time. Risk of progression to invasive cancer is <1%.
- **In women <25 years of age**—repeat cytology at 12 and 24 months. If cytology shows persistent LGSIL, then colposcopy and biopsy are indicated.
- **In women >25 years of age**—management options include the following:
  - Follow-up with cytology/HPV cotesting at 12 and 24 months. If cytology is positive or HPV testing is positive, colposcopy and biopsy are indicated

Part 2

Table 22.10 Treatment modalities available for cervical intraepithelial neoplasia lesions

	Ablative procedures	Excision procedures
Procedures	• Cauterization (thermoablation) • Cryotherapy (Figure 22.5) • Laser ablation	• Cold knife conization (Figure 22.6) • Laser conization with CO_2 laser • Large loop excision of transformation zone (LLETZ) • Loop electrosurgical excision procedure (LEEP)
Advantages	• Easy to perform • No risk of excessive bleeding • Useful in low-resource settings	• Specimen obtained for histopathological examination • Can identify occult microinvasive lesion or adenocarcinoma of endocervix (tissue biopsy obtained)
Disadvantages	• These procedures cause local destruction of tissue and hence no tissue is obtained for histopathology • Cryotherapy can cause profuse watery discharge for 2–4 weeks	• Cold knife conization can be associated with immediate complications such as hemorrhage and infection and late complications such as cervical stenosis, cervical incompetence, recurrent pregnancy loss, and preterm labor • Laser conization equipment is expensive and expertise is required for performing the procedure

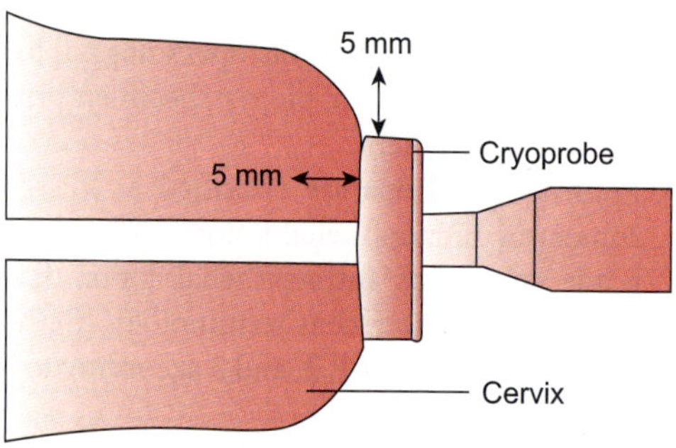

Figure 22.5 Cryotherapy.

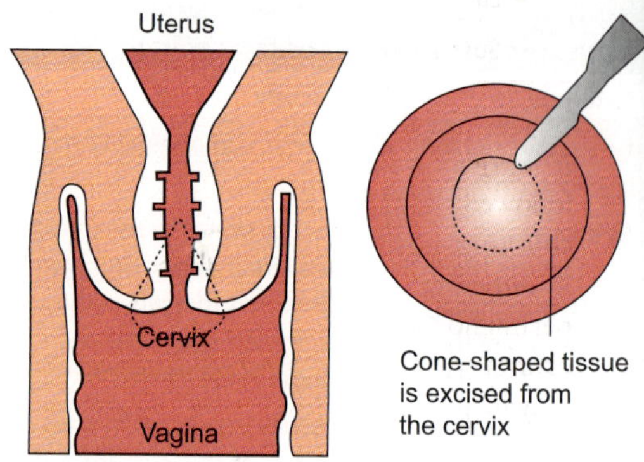

Figure 22.6 Cold knife conization.

- Treat with excision/ablative procedure, if patient cannot be followed up

Management of CIN 2 and 3 (histology)

- Risk of progression of CIN 2 to invasive cancer is 5% and of CIN 3 to invasive cancer is 12%. Therefore, colposcopy and prompt treatment is mandatory.
- **In women who have completed family, manage as follows:**
  - If colposcopy is satisfactory, excision or ablation procedure is recommended; excision preferred.
  - If colposcopy is unsatisfactory, excision procedure is recommended.
- **In young women desirous of future reproductive function, mange as follows:**
  - If colposcopy is satisfactory, options are as follows:
    - Follow up with cytology and colposcopy every 6 months and HPV cotesting after 1 year. If HSIL persists, repeat biopsy.
    - Treat with excision procedure.
  - If colposcopy is unsatisfactory, excision procedure is recommended.

Management following treatment of CIN 2 and 3 lesions

- Excisional procedures such as conization serve as both diagnostic and therapeutic procedures. Subsequent management depends on histological examination of the margins of excised specimen.

Viva corner

Q1 When do you prefer excisional procedure over ablative procedure for CIN lesions?

- Efficacy is similar for both excisional and ablation procedures.
- Choice of the procedure depends on the need for tissue specimen, availability, cost, and desire for future childbearing.
- Excision procedure is preferred in the following situations:
  - High-grade lesions and endocervical lesions, since it provides tissue for histological confirmation and for evaluation of the margins
  - Unsatisfactory colposcopy
  - Lesion extending into endocervical canal
  - Large lesions
  - Suspected microinvasive cancer

Q2 What is conization procedure and what are its indications?

- It refers to excision of a cone-shaped tissue from the cervix, with the base of the cone at the ectocervix and apex in the endocervical canal close to the internal os.
- The procedure is done under anesthesia.

Indications for diagnostic conization

- Unsatisfactory colposcopy—entire limits of the lesion or the transformation zone not visible in colposcopy
- Lesion extending into the endocervical canal
- Large lesions
- Suspected microinvasive cancer
- Cytology—histology discordance (cytology shows more severe grade lesion)
- Histological diagnosis of adenocarcinoma in situ

- *If margins are negative*: The patient can be followed up with cytology and HPV cotesting.
- *If margin is positive for CIN 3*: In women in perimenopausal age group and women who cannot come for follow-up, hysterectomy may be performed.

Viva corner

Q1 What are the indications for hysterectomy in CIN lesions?

Hysterectomy is not a primary procedure for management of CIN. Indications for hysterectomy in CIN are as follows:

- CIN 3 with cone margins involved
- Recurrent high-grade lesion
- Adenocarcinoma in situ

DOWNSTAGING FOR CERVICAL CANCER (WHO)

- It is defined as "detection of the disease at an earlier stage when it is still curable. Detection is done by nurses and other paramedical health workers using a simple speculum for visual inspection of the cervix."
- The "downstaging screening" is an alternative to regular cytological screening in the developing countries, where effective mass screening cannot be extended and majority of carcinoma cervix cases are diagnosed at an advanced stage.
- This method is suboptimal when compared with cytological screening. However, in places where prevalence of cancer is high and cytological screening is not available, "downstaging screening" is useful.
- This strategy can minimize the cancer death through early detection.

Downstaging procedure

- A female primary healthcare worker is trained for 2–3 weeks to perform speculum examination and to distinguish a normal cervix from an abnormal cervix.
  - *Characteristics of a normal cervix*: Pink in color, smooth surface, and does not bleed on touch
  - *Characteristics of an abnormal cervix*: Reddish, patchy red or white areas, presence of growth or ulcer on the surface, bleeding on touch, and friable lesion

Extra edge

Lymph node involvement and 5-year survival rate in carcinoma cervix

See table below

Table Lymph node involvement and 5-year survival rate in carcinoma cervix

Stage	Pelvic lymph nodes (%)	Para-aortic lymph nodes (%)	5-year survival (%)
IA1	0.5–1	0	95–100
IA2	5	<1	
IB	15	8	80–90
IIA	25	10	65–70
IIB	35	20	40–45
III	45	30	20–40
IV	55	40	15–20

- Once any abnormality is suspected, the case i referred to a center where diagnosis and treatment of premalignant and malignant lesions ar done.

Frequently asked viva questions

1. Summarize the case.
2. What is the diagnosis of the case?
3. What are the causes of postmenopausal bleeding?
4. What are the risk factors for carcinoma cervix?
5. How will you evaluate the case?
6. How will you manage the patient?
7. What are the advantages of surgical treatment?
8. What are the indications for radiotherapy?
9. How will you screen for cancer cervix?
10. What are the methods available for screening?
11. How will you treat preinvasive lesions of cervix?

23 Carcinoma Endometrium

Introduction

Endometrial carcinoma and cervical carcinoma account for one-third of the cases of postmenopausal bleeding. Abnormal perimenopausal or postmenopausal bleeding should always be taken seriously and be properly evaluated. Carcinoma endometrium is the most common genital malignancy in Western countries, while in developing countries such as India, it ranks third among genital malignancies next to carcinoma cervix and ovary. A case of abnormal uterine bleeding (AUB) in perimenopausal age group or a case of postmenopausal bleeding (PMB) can be discussed along the lines of endometrial carcinoma and has been discussed in this chapter.

Uterine causes of postmenopausal bleeding

The various causes of PMB have been mentioned under the heading "*introduction*" in Part 2, Chapter 22, *Carcinoma Cervix*. The uterine causes of PMB are mentioned in Table 23.1.

Endometrial hyperplasia

- It is a premalignant disease of the endometrium characterized by abnormal proliferation of the endometrial glands.

Table 23.1 Uterine causes of postmenopausal bleeding

Cause of bleeding	Percentage
Endometrial atrophy (most common)	60–80
Estrogen replacement therapy	15–25
Endometrial polyps	2–12
Endometrial hyperplasia	5–10
Endometrial carcinoma	10

- It occurs commonly in 40- to 55-year (perimenopausal) age group.
- It occurs as a result of unopposed estrogen action on the endometrium.
- Risk factors for endometrial hyperplasia are similar to those for endometrial carcinoma (mentioned in the subsequent text).
- Clinical presentation: Perimenopausal women present with AUB; older women present with PMB.

Risk factors for endometrial carcinoma

- Early age at menarche
- Late age at menopause (>52 years—2.5-fold increased risk)
- Age group: 55–70 years (majority of endometrial carcinoma occur in this age group)
- Diabetes mellitus (DM) and hypertension (HT)
- Obesity
- Nulliparity
- Chronic anovulation like in polycystic ovarian disease (PCOD)
- Endometrial hyperplasia
- Long-term unopposed estrogen exposure such as estrogen hormone replacement therapy (HRT)
- Tamoxifen therapy
- Family history of endometrial, ovarian, and colon cancer
- Hereditary nonpolyposis colorectal cancer (HNPCC) (women with HNPCC have a 40–60% lifetime risk of endometrial carcinoma)
- Women with germline mutations (*PTEN*, *p53*, and *BRCA* genes)

Factors that reduce the risk for endometrial carcinoma

- Early age at menopause

- Multiparity
- Oral contraceptive pill (OCP) usage
- Consumption of a high-fiber diet
- Physical activity

Clinical features of endometrial carcinoma

Symptoms

- PMB
- AUB in perimenopausal age group such as
  - Periods of amenorrhea followed by prolonged and heavy bleeding
  - Intermenstrual bleeding
- Abnormal vaginal discharge
- Pelvic pain

Signs

- Enlarged uterus
- Pyometra

Viva corner

Q1 What is corpus cancer syndrome?

It is the combination of DM, obesity, and hypertension with carcinoma of endometrium.

Q2 What is Simpson's pain?

- It refers to the unique nature of pain seen in patients with Ca. endometrium that is mild, appears at the same time every day lasting for 1–2 hours, in hypogastric region and bilateral iliac fossa.
- This pain is seen in 15% of cases and is attributed to expulsive nature of uterine contraction.

Q3 What are type I and type II endometrial cancer?

Endometrial cancers are of two types, type I and type II. The pathogenesis and clinical behavior are different in the two types of cancers (see table below).

Table Differentiating features of type I and type II endometrial cancer

Type I endometrial cancer	Type II endometrial cancer
• Endometrial cancers that are typically low grade	• Endometrial cancers that are typically high grade
• Associated with exposure to unopposed estrogens	• Estrogen independent and often are papillary serous or clear cell type
• These are diagnosed at an early stage and have an excellent prognosis. They account for 90% of endometrial cancers	• They tend to be diagnosed at a later stage and have a poor prognosis

Case presentation

Salient points in history

Consider the following relevant points during history taking in cases of carcinoma endometrium.

Patient profile

- *Age (as the age advances, risk of endometrial cancer increases)*
- *Socioeconomic status (SES) (Ca. endometrium is common in higher SES; Ca. cervix is common in lower SES)*
- *Parity (Ca. endometrium is common in nulliparous women; Ca. cervix is common in multiparous women)*

Presenting complaints

- *H/o continuous bleeding or irregular heavy bleeding in a perimenopausal woman*
- *H/o postmenopausal bleeding in a postmenopausal woman*
- *The following noted—onset of bleeding, duration, amount of bleeding*

(CONTD...)

(...CONTD)

- *H/o intermenstrual bleeding*
- *H/o postcoital bleeding*
- *H/o discharge P/V*
  - *Onset*
  - *Duration*
  - *Amount—profuse or scanty*
  - *Whether blood stained/foul smelling*
  - *Associated symptoms such as pain and fever (may be present in associated pyometra)*
- *H/o HRT (estrogen use without progestins in postmenopausal women increases the risk of endometrial cancer)*
- *H/o tamoxifen therapy (used for the treatment of hormone receptor–positive breast cancer)*
- *H/o change in bowel and bladder habits (ask H/o hematuria, bleeding per rectum, and painful defecation to find out whether bleeding is due to nongynecological causes)*
- *H/o whether the patient is on regular Pap smear screening (carcinoma cervix is another important cause of postmenopausal bleeding)*

Menstrual history

- *Age at menarche*
- *Previous menstrual cycles—pattern, amount, and duration of bleeding (ask for any treatment for PCOD, irregular cycles and any H/o prolonged estrogen use, as endometrial cancer is more common in women with prolonged unopposed estrogen exposure*
- *If attained menopause, mention as "attained menopause at ___ years and is postmenopausal for the past ___ years" (in women with late menopause, the risk of endometrial carcinoma is increased)*

Marital history

- *Married at the age of ___ years; married since ___ years*
- *H/o prolonged usage of combined oral contraceptive (COC) pills (increased risk of adenocarcinoma of cervix)*
- *H/o multiple sexual partners (increased risk of carcinoma cervix)*

Obstetric history

Parity (nulliparous—risk of endometrial and breast carcinoma; multiparous—risk of cervical carcinoma)

Past history

- *H/o DM and HT (associated with corpus cancer syndrome)*
- *H/o any drug intake for chronic illness and use of HRT*
- *H/o surgery*
- *H/o blood transfusion*
- *H/o tuberculosis*
- *H/o treatment received for any other carcinoma such as breast cancer*

Family history

Family H/o genital/breast/colon malignancy (to identify cases of familial cancer syndromes)

Personal history

- *H/o addictions—smoking and alcohol*
- *Sleep and appetite (decreased appetite and early satiety occur in malignancy)*

Salient points in examination

Consider the following relevant points during examination in cases of carcinoma endometrium.

General examination

- *BMI (obesity increases risk of endometrial cancer because androstenedione produced from adrenals and ovaries is converted into estrone in peripheral fat)*
- *Pallor*
- *Pedal edema*
- *Icterus (secondaries in liver)*
- *Lymphadenopathy (especially check for left supraclavicular node and inguinal nodes)*
- *Blood pressure (HT is a risk factor for endometrial carcinoma)*
- *Breast examination—any palpable mass*
- *Thyroid examination*

(CONTD...)

(...CONTD)

CVS and RS examination

CVS and RS examinations are done to exclude coexisting medical disorders (coexisting medical disorders should be evaluated and treated prior to surgery).

Abdominal examination

Inspection

- *Any distension/engorged veins*
- *Any visible mass*
- *Scars or sinuses*

Palpation

- *Organomegaly*
- *Any mass/ascites (uterus may be enlarged in pyometra)*
- *Any tenderness on palpation*

Pelvic examination (expected only in postgraduate case presentation)

Inspection of the external genitalia

Any growth or ulcer should be noted.

Per speculum and rectovaginal examinations

- *Cervix and vagina inspected (look for any abnormal discharge, ulcer, growth)*
- *Any bleeding through cervical os*

Bimanual examination

- *Uterine size, mobility, tenderness*
- *Any adnexal mass*

Per rectal and rectovaginal examinations

Check for parametrial infiltration, rectal mucosal, rectovaginal septal involvement (in carcinoma cervix), and any nodularity in POD.

Case summary

An example of writing summary in cases of carcinoma endometrium is given below.

Example *Mrs. Y, 62 years of age, nulliparous, postmenopausal woman, presents with complaints of bleeding per vaginum, on and off for the past 15 days. She attained menopause at 52 years and she is a known hypertensive. On examination, the patient is obese, BMI is 32, mild pallor is present, and BP is 140/90 mmHg. Abdomen is soft and speculum examination reveals that cervix is healthy, and bleeding through os is present. On bimanual examination, uterus is anteverted, normal size, mobile, and fornices are free. On rectal and rectovaginal examinations, parametrium and POD are free.*

Case diagnosis

An example of writing diagnosis in cases of carcinoma endometrium is given below.

Example *62 years of age, nulliparous, postmenopausal woman with postmenopausal bleeding for evaluation. Endometrial carcinoma would be the first probable differential diagnosis in this case as the patient is nulliparous, obese, and hypertensive (risk factors for carcinoma endometrium).*

Note *Endometrial cancer presents early with abnormal bleeding; therefore, most cases are stage I or II at diagnosis (early diagnosis in the initial stages is possible unlike ovarian malignancies that are in advanced stages at the time of diagnosis).*

Case discussion

Differential diagnosis for postmenopausal bleeding

- Endometrial carcinoma
- Endometrial hyperplasia
- Cervical carcinoma
- Atrophic endometrium
- Atrophic vaginitis
- Endometrial polyp
- Estrogen-producing ovarian tumors

Diagnosis

Histopathological examination of endometrial biopsy specimen is the gold standard for diagnosis of endometrial cancer.

Note *Undergraduates are not expected to do speculum and bimanual examination. Hence, the differential diagnosis will include all the causes of postmenopausal bleeding such as carcinoma cervix, carcinoma endometrium, endometrial hyperplasia, atrophic endometritis, and endometrial polyp. Either endometrial carcinoma or carcinoma cervix can be discussed. If questioned about the next step in evaluation, it should be mentioned that a speculum examination is required to look for any lesion in cervix and vagina followed by bimanual, rectal, and rectovaginal examinations.*

Investigations

- **Transvaginal ultrasound (TVS):** The initial evaluation of postmenopausal bleeding is to do a TVS to look for endometrial thickness (ET). TVS can also identify endometrial polyps, pyometra, and any other pelvic pathology.
  - Postmenopausal ET ≥5 mm is taken as cutoff for endometrial sampling.
- **Endometrial sampling:** It is usually performed as an outpatient procedure using Vabra aspirator/Pipelle/Novak curette. This procedure requires no cervical dilatation or anesthesia and has a high sensitivity and specificity of 98%.
- **Dilatation and curettage (D&C) or fractional curettage:** In women with a high index of suspicion of endometrial carcinoma, if the result of endometrial sampling is negative or inconclusive, or if tissue is inadequate, then fractional curettage is done. Endocervical curettage (ECC) should be done first, followed by dilatation and endometrial curettage (EMC), and the samples should be sent for histological examination separately. ECC is done to rule out endocervical extension of endometrial cancer or a primary endocervical cancer.
- **Pap smear:** It is sensitive only in 50% of cases of endometrial carcinoma (Pap smear is done in all cases presenting with perimenopausal or postmenopausal bleeding, to rule out carcinoma cervix—if cervix has an obvious growth, take cervical biopsy and workup for Ca. cervix as mentioned in Part 2, Chapter 22, *Carcinoma Cervix*).
- **Hysteroscopy-directed biopsy:** It is considered as the gold standard for evaluation of endometrial pathology. It is indicated when ultrasonography (USG) shows focal endometrial abnormality.
- **Saline infusion sonography (SIS):** It is helpful in women with suspected endometrial polyps on USG but is not used as a routine in the evaluation of endometrial carcinoma.

INDICATIONS FOR ENDOMETRIAL SAMPLING

- Women with postmenopausal bleeding
- Postmenopausal women on estrogen therapy
- Women with HNPCC syndrome
- Premenopausal women with AUB with risk factors such as chronic anovulation, polycystic ovarian disease (PCOD) obesity, and metabolic syndrome

Part 2

INDICATIONS FOR FRACTIONAL CURETTAGE OR DILATATION AND CURETTAGE

- Recurrent bleeding with negative endometrial sampling
- Recurrent bleeding with ET <5 mm
- Complex atypical hyperplasia in endometrial sampling

Viva corner

Q1 What are the USG characteristics suspicious of endometrial carcinoma?

- Endometrial thickness ≥5 mm in a postmenopausal woman (TVS has a sensitivity of 100% and specificity of 96% for identifying endometrial abnormalities)
- Nonhomogenous echo texture of endometrium
- Irregular and poorly defined margins
- Polypoidal endometrial growth
- Fluid collection within the endometrium (pyometra)

Q2 Why is 5 mm taken as cutoff for endometrial thickness in postmenopausal women?

- Incidence of endometrial cancer is <0.5% in postmenopausal women with ET <5 mm.

(CONTD...)

(...CONTD)

Viva corner

- At 5 mm thickness, sensitivity of TVS for endometrial pathology is almost 95%.

Q3 What is the ET guideline for premenopausal women?

ET guidelines have not been established for premenopausal women. However, a persistent finding of ET >12 mm, irrespective of the day of menstrual cycle, requires further evaluation.

Q4 What is the role of hysteroscopy in suspected endometrial carcinoma?

- Fluid distension media used in hysteroscopy can cause dissemination of cancer cells into peritoneal cavity. Hence, it is not recommended in suspected endometrial carcinoma.
- Hysteroscopy-directed biopsy can be taken if USG shows focal endometrial abnormalities.

MANAGEMENT

If histopathology of endometrial biopsy is reported as endometrial hyperplasia or endometrial carcinoma, it is managed accordingly, as mentioned in the following subsections.

Management of endometrial hyperplasia

The WHO (1994) has classified endometrial hyperplasia based on the cytological and architectural features in histopathology as given in Table 23.2.

- According to the WHO latest classification in 2014, endometrial hyperplasia is classified into two categories:
  - Hyperplasia without atypia
  - Atypical hyperplasia/endometrioid intraepithelial neoplasia (EIN)
- Management of endometrial hyperplasia depends on the type of hyperplasia and the age of the patient.
- High-dose progesterone therapy is effective in reversing hyperplastic changes with or without atypia.

Table 23.2 Types of endometrial hyperplasia—based on architecture and cellular atypia (WHO 1994)

Type of hyperplasia	Risk of progression to endometrial carcinoma (%)
Simple hyperplasia without atypia	1
Complex hyperplasia without atypia	3
Simple hyperplasia with atypia	8
Complex hyperplasia with atypia	29

Management of endometrial hyperplasia without atypia [Royal College of Obstetricians and Gynaecologists (RCOG) 2016 guidelines]

Hyperplasia without atypia at all ages can be treated with progesterone therapy—both continuous oral progesterones [medroxyprogesterone acetate (MPA) or norethisterone] and local levonorgestrel-releasing intrauterine device (LNG-IUD)-Mirena are effective.

Premenopausal women

LNG-IUD or continuous progesterones (MPA or norethisterone 10–20 mg/day) are prescribed for 6 months.

Postmenopausal women

Progesterone therapy can be given as in premenopausal women.

Response to medical therapy

- Endometrial sampling is repeated after 6 months to assess response to therapy.
- Repeat sampling will show histological regression of endometrial pathology in majority of cases.
- Cases with persistence of hyperplasia are treated with high-dose progesterones—MPA 200 mg/day or megestrol acetate 160 mg/day.
- In case of refractoriness to therapy, hysterectomy is done.

Indications for hysterectomy in endometrial hyperplasia without atypia

- Progression to atypical hyperplasia during follow-up
- No histological regression of hyperplasia despite 12 months of therapy
- Relapse of endometrial hyperplasia after completing progesterone treatment

- Persistence of bleeding symptoms
- Refusal by the woman to undergo endometrial surveillance or comply with medical treatment

Management of endometrial hyperplasia with atypia

Hyperplasia with atypia is usually a complex hyperplasia.

In women who have completed family

- Hysterectomy is the treatment of choice for the following reasons:
  - Associated endometrial carcinoma may be present in 40% of women.
  - There is increased risk of progression to endometrial carcinoma.

In younger women desirous of future childbearing

- LNG-IUD or high-dose continuous progesterone therapy may be prescribed for 9 months after counseling about the risks of underlying malignancy and subsequent progression to endometrial cancer.
- Endometrial sampling every 3 months is mandatory to assess response to therapy.
  - If there is regression of endometrial pathology, the patient is kept under surveillance with periodic endometrial sampling. Hysterectomy is performed on completion of family.
  - If there is no regression, hysterectomy is done.

Extra edge

RCOG 2016 recommendations on management of endometrial hyperplasia

Endometrial hyperplasia without atypia

- LNG-IUD should be the first-line therapy because it has a higher disease regression rate, more favorable bleeding profile, and fewer adverse effects when compared with oral progesterones.
- Cyclical progesterones should not be used because they are less effective in inducing regression of endometrial hyperplasia without atypia.
- Treatment with oral progesterones or the LNG-IUD should be for a minimum of 6 months in order to induce histological regression of endometrial hyperplasia without atypia.
- Endometrial ablation is not recommended for the treatment of endometrial hyperplasia because complete and persistent endometrial destruction cannot be ensured, and intrauterine adhesion formation may preclude future endometrial histological surveillance.
- Hysterectomy should not be considered as a first-line treatment for hyperplasia without atypia because progesterone therapy induces histological and symptomatic remission in the majority of women, and avoids the morbidity associated with major surgery.

Women with atypical endometrial hyperplasia

- Women with atypical hyperplasia should undergo a total hysterectomy because of the risk of underlying malignancy or progression to cancer.
- Women desirous of further childbearing, who are treated conservatively and having evidence of histological regression of the disease, should be followed up with endometrial biopsy every 6–12 months, until hysterectomy is performed.

Management of endometrial carcinoma

Histological types of endometrial hyperplasia

- Endometrioid: >75% (most common histological type)
- Serous: 5–10%
- Clear cell: 5%
- Mucinous: 1–2%
- Undifferentiated: 1–2%
- Squamous

Pretreatment evaluation

Once endometrial carcinoma is diagnosed by histopathology, investigations are required to assess the extent of lesion, fitness for surgery, and other comorbid conditions.

Investigations to assess the extent of disease

- Renal and liver function tests
- Chest X-ray—to look for pulmonary metastasis and evaluate the cardiorespiratory status
- Ultrasound abdomen and pelvis—to look for ascites, liver metastasis, pelvic and para-aortic

Part 2

lymphadenopathy, myometrial invasion, extension to cervix, and ovarian metastasis (it is not as sensitive as CT/MRI)

- MRI—to assess myometrial invasion, parametrial extension, and lymph node metastasis
- CA 125 is elevated in advanced stages and in papillary serous endometrial carcinoma
- Barium enema, colonoscopy, and proctosigmoidoscopy—done in cases with suspected HNPCC

Other routine preoperative investigations

- Hemoglobin
- Complete blood count
- Blood grouping and typing
- Blood sugar
- Urine analysis
- Lipid profile
- ECG, chest X-ray
- HIV, HBsAg (in high-risk cases)
- Pap smear

Staging of Ca. endometrium (FIGO, 2009)

Endometrial carcinoma is surgically staged. Clinical staging significantly understages the disease and is done only in women who are not fit for surgery.

Stage I

It is confined to corpus uteri.

- **1A:** No or less than half of myometrium involved
- **1B:** Invasion of more than or equal to half of myometrium

Stage II

It involves cervical stroma but does not extend beyond uterus.

Stage III

There is local and/or regional spread of tumor.

- **IIIA:** Involves serosa/adnexa
- **IIIB:** Vaginal/parametrial involvement
- **IIIC:** Metastasis to pelvic and para-aortic nodes

Stage IV

It involves bladder/bowel mucosa/distant metastasis.

- **IVA:** Involves bladder or bowel mucosa
- **IVB:** Distant metastasis including intra-abdominal metastasis/inguinal nodes

Histological grading

- **Grade 1:** <5% nonsquamous or nonmorular growth pattern (G1)
- **Grade 2:** 6–50% nonsquamous or nonmorular growth pattern (G2)
- **Grade 3:** >50% nonsquamous or nonmorular growth pattern (G3)

Note

- *Endocervical glandular involvement: Stage I*
- *Endocervical stromal involvement: Stage II*
- *Positive peritoneal cytology reported separately, and is not included in staging*

Steps of surgical staging

- Midline vertical incision is given.
- Ascitic fluid is collected for cytology. If there is no ascites, peritoneal wash with 50–100 mL of normal saline is done and the peritoneal washings are collected for cytology.
- Systematic exploration of the abdomen and pelvis is done.
  - Paracolic gutters, ascending colon, hepatic flexure, liver, hemidiaphragm, transverse colon, splenic flexure and spleen, descending colon, omentum, and kidneys should be inspected and palpated.
  - Any suspicious lesion should be biopsied.
- Extrafascial hysterectomy and bilateral salpingo-oophorectomy (BSO) is performed (Figure 23.1).
- The uterus specimen should be cut opened to assess tumor size, depth of myometrial invasion, and cervical extension.

(CONTD...)

(...CONTD)

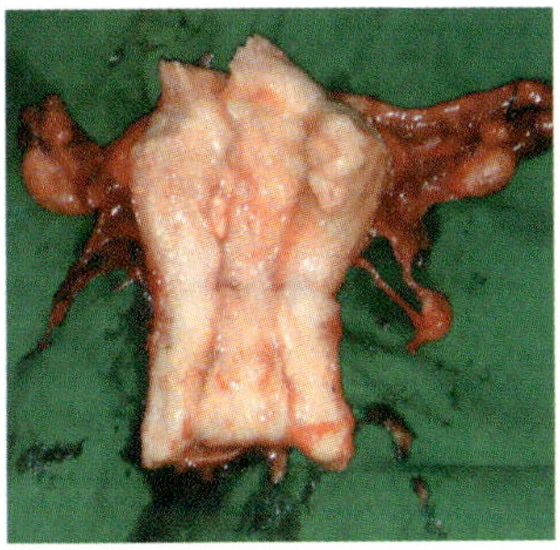

Figure 23.1 Carcinoma endometrium—extrafascial hysterectomy specimen.

- Pelvic and para-aortic lymphadenectomy is recommended in all women except those with preoperative diagnosis of grade 1 endometrioid tumors, with tumor size <2 cm, and myometrial invasion <50%.
- Infracolic omentectomy, peritoneal biopsies, and diaphragmatic scrapings should be done in addition, in cases with papillary serous, clear cell, and mixed Mullerian tumors (due to high risk of intra-abdominal spread and upper abdominal recurrence).

High-yield points

Indications for pelvic and para-aortic lymph node sampling

- Clear cell, serous, and squamous tumors
- G2 and G3 endometrioid tumors
- Tumor size >2 cm
- Myometrial invasion >50%
- Cervical involvement
- Extrauterine spread (adnexal or pelvic extension of disease)

In other words, pelvic and para-aortic lymphadenectomy is indicated in all cases, except in stage I endometrial carcinoma with the following characteristics:

- G1 endometrioid tumors
- Myometrial involvement <50%
- Tumor size <2 cm

Management of stage I endometrial carcinoma

Stage I endometrial carcinoma is managed by extrafascial hysterectomy + bilateral salpingo-oophorectomy BSO + pelvic and para-aortic lymph node sampling followed by postoperative radiotherapy (RT).

Management of stage II endometrial carcinoma

Two approaches may be used for management in stage II:

1. **Initial surgical staging followed by RT (the best approach)**
   - A surgical staging is done and modified radical hysterectomy with bilateral salpingo-oophorectomy, and pelvic and para-aortic lymphadenectomy is performed. Some prefer to do only extrafascial hysterectomy, as postoperative RT is required.
   - Surgical staging is followed by postoperative pelvic or extended field radiation.
2. **Initial RT followed by surgery**
   - Indications: It is done in patients who are unsuitable for extensive surgery (obese, elderly, those with medical problems).
   - The preferred approach is initial RT followed within 6 weeks by less extensive surgery [total abdominal hysterectomy (TAH) with BSO].

Management of stage III endometrial carcinoma

- Surgery is performed to determine the extent of the disease and to remove the tumor bulk, if possible.
- Preferred treatment is extrafascial hysterectomy with BSO, peritoneal biopsy from suspicious areas, pelvic and para-aortic lymphadenectomy, and partial omentectomy.
- Postoperative RT is given.
- Treatment outcomes are better in patients treated with both surgery and RT than in those treated with RT alone.

Management of stage IV endometrial carcinoma

- The primary aim is to provide palliative relief of symptoms.

- It usually involves a combination of surgery, RT, and systemic hormonal or chemotherapy.

Postsurgical treatment of endometrial cancer based on surgical–pathological staging (Table 23.3)

Postoperative RT is required in all stages except stage IA, grades 1 and 2. The various RT modalities used in treatment of endometrial carcinoma are the following:

- **Vault radiation**: Reduces vault recurrence from 15% to 1–2% (vaginal vault is a common site of recurrence)
- **External pelvic radiation**: Reduces pelvic lymph node recurrences in women who are at high risk, such as those with cervical extension, adnexal involvement, grade 3 tumors, and deep myometrial invasion
- **Extended-field radiation**: Indicated in women with histologically positive para-aortic nodes. It includes irradiation of pelvic, common iliac, and para-aortic nodes.
- **Whole abdominal radiation**: Indicated in women with stage III and IV disease. The entire abdomen is irradiated shielding the kidneys.

Table 23.3 Postsurgical treatment based on surgical–pathological staging

Surgical–pathological staging	Postoperative treatment
Stage IA, G1, 2	None
• Stage IA, G3 • Stage IB, G1, 2	Vaginal cuff radiation
• Stage IB, G3 • Isthmus, cervical, and pelvic extension (stage II)	Pelvic irradiation + vaginal cuff boost
Positive para-aortic/common iliac lymph nodes	Pelvic irradiation + vaginal cuff boost + extended field radiation
Adnexal/parametrial involvement	Whole abdominal radiation or chemotherapy
Positive peritoneal cytology	Progestins
Stage IV	Palliative RT

G1, grade 1; *G2*, grade 2; *G3*, grade 3 ; *RT*, radiotherapy.

High-yield points

Simplified version of treatment of endometrial carcinoma

- **Stage I:** Extrafascial hysterectomy + B/L salpingo-oophorectomy + pelvic and para-aortic lymph node sampling followed by postoperative RT
- **Stage II:** Radical hysterectomy + B/L salpingo-oophorectomy + pelvic and para-aortic lymphadenectomy followed by postoperative RT or else RT followed by TAH + BSO
- **Stage III:** Debulking of the tumor (TAH with BSO + selective lymphadenectomy + biopsy of suspicious areas + omental biopsy) followed by RT
- **Stage IV:** Palliative chemotherapy, RT, and progesterones

Role of fertility-sparing therapy in endometrial carcinoma

- It can be offered only in stage IA, grade 1 with no myometrial invasion, in young nulliparous women who wish to retain their reproductive potential, after adequate counseling about the risks associated with conservative management.
- Megestrol acetate 160 mg or MPA 200 mg OD is given for 3 months and endometrial biopsy is repeated. Nonresponse or progression of the disease requires surgical management.
- If there is response, endometrial biopsy is repeated every 3 months till two consecutive biopsies are negative. The patient may then be allowed to conceive. TAH + BSO is done on completion of family.

Role of hormonal therapy in endometrial carcinoma

Surgery is the treatment of choice; hormonal therapy is used where surgery cannot be done due to poor general condition of the patient or as an adjuvant to surgery.

Indications

- Advanced endometrial carcinoma
- Metastasis
- Recurrence—progesterones are currently recommended as initial treatment for all patients with hormone receptor–positive recurrent endometrial tumors

Agents used

- Oral MPA 200 mg/day
- Megestrol acetate 160 mg/day

Role of chemotherapy in endometrial carcinoma

Indications

- Mainly for palliation in advanced or metastatic disease
- Agents used: Paclitaxel, cisplatin/carboplatin, doxorubicin, and cyclophosphamide
- Response better with combination chemotherapy

Follow-up of patients treated for endometrial carcinoma

- The American College of Obstetricians and Gynecologists (ACOG) recommends follow-up of patients every 3–4 months for 2–3 years, and then every 6 months. After 5 years, patients can have annual follow-up. Patients with recurrence often present with symptoms.

Routine post-treatment surveillance is as follows:

- Patient education is given regarding symptoms of recurrence such as vaginal bleeding and pelvic pain.
- During each visit, history for any fresh complaints is taken, and clinical examination including a pelvic examination should be done.
- USG, CT scan, MRI, and intravenous pyelogram (IVP) are done only if they are clinically indicated.
- CA 125: Elevated levels are seen in advanced and recurrent disease. CA 125 is helpful in follow-up of patients with uterine papillary serous carcinoma and those with previously elevated levels.

Extra edge

Role of vaginal hysterectomy and laparoscopy in endometrial carcinoma

- Vaginal and laparoscopic surgeries are associated with less postoperative morbidity, early ambulation, and better wound healing.
- May be performed in women with stage IA, grade 1 endometrial carcinoma who are obese.
- Peritoneal washings are taken while the pouch of Douglas is opened.

Disadvantages

- Complete staging is not possible.
- Approach to upper abdomen and para-aortic lymph nodes is compromised.
- Laparoscopy can lead to port site metastasis.

Role of hormone replacement therapy after surgery for endometrial carcinoma

- Estrogens are withheld for initial few years (1–3 years) following surgery, which is the most common time period for recurrence.
- Alternatively, topical estrogens can be used to treat vaginal symptoms such as dryness.
- Symptomatic relief of hot flushes can be achieved by giving nonhormonal agents such as clonidine.
- Selective estrogen receptor modulators (SERMS) such as raloxifene and weight-bearing exercises can help to reduce bone loss.

Extra edge

Q1 What is the incidence of synchronous endometrial and ovarian cancer?

The incidence of synchronous endometrial and ovarian cancer is 1.5–3.5%. In most of the cases, both endometrial and ovarian cancers are well-differentiated adenocarcinoma with excellent prognosis.

Q2 Why do ovaries have to be removed during surgical staging of carcinoma endometrium?

- Chance of micrometastasis to the ovaries
- Risk of ovarian carcinoma developing later

Q3 What is the role of tumor markers in carcinoma endometrium?

- Various tumor markers include CA 125, CA 19-9, and CA 15-3.
- Tumor markers have no role in screening—not cost-effective.
- CA 125 is useful in predicting myometrial invasion and extrauterine spread, and in follow-up of patients with advanced and recurrent cancer.

Factors affecting survival in endometrial carcinoma

- Poor histological grade
- Clear cell and squamous type

Part 2

- Advanced stage at presentation
- Large tumor size
- Myometrial invasion
- Cervical extension
- Lymphovascular space involvement
- Positive peritoneal cytology
- DNA aneuploidy (worse prognosis)
- Estrogen and progesterone receptor status—positive receptor status has good prognosis

Five-year survival rate in endometrial carcinoma

- **Stage I:** 80–90%
- **Stage II:** 60–80%
- **Stage III:** 50%
- **Stage IV:** 20%

RECURRENCE OF ENDOMETRIAL CARCINOMA

- Recurrence occurs in about 25% of the patients treated for endometrial carcinoma.
- Majority of recurrence occurs within 3 years of initial treatment.
- In patients treated with surgery alone, most recurrences tend to be vaginal or pelvic.
- Patients treated with combined surgery and RT tend to have distant metastasis involving lung, liver, brain, and bone.
- Vaginal bleeding is the most common symptom associated with local recurrence and pelvic pain is often present with pelvic recurrence.

Management

- Pelvic or vaginal recurrence in patients who have not received prior pelvic irradiation is best treated with external irradiation followed by brachytherapy vaginal boost.
- Role of surgery in recurrent endometrial carcinoma
  - Surgical resection of a metastatic vaginal nodule >2 cm prior to radiation may improve local control.
  - In patients with isolated pelvic recurrence after irradiation, exploratory laparotomy and pelvic exenteration may be done.
  - Patients with intraperitoneal recurrence may need surgery to relieve intestinal obstruction.
- Lung metastasis: It is managed by long-term progesterone therapy.

ROLE OF SCREENING FOR ENDOMETRIAL CARCINOMA

- Routine screening for endometrial cancer is not cost-effective and is not recommended.
- There is lack of an appropriate, cost-effective and acceptable screening test for endometrial carcinoma.
- Screening for endometrial carcinoma is not warranted, as >95% of patients are symptomatic and present with vaginal bleeding at an early stage.
- Only 50% of endometrial cancers have malignant cells in Pap smear. Therefore, this cannot be used as a screening test.
- Screening by TVS and endometrial sampling is expensive and is recommended only for high-risk women, such as those with a family history of Lynch syndrome II (HNPCC).

Frequently asked viva questions

1. Summarize the case.
2. What is the diagnosis of the case?
3. How do you want to evaluate the case?
4. What are the causes of postmenopausal bleeding?
5. What are the various histological types of endometrial hyperplasia?
6. How will you manage a case of endometrial hyperplasia?
7. What are the risk factors for endometrial carcinoma?
8. How will you manage a case of endometrial carcinoma diagnosed by endometrial biopsy?
9. What is the role of screening in endometrial carcinoma?

24 Pelvic Organ Prolapse

ntroduction

'elvic organ prolapse, commonly termed as terovaginal prolapse, is a common clinical problem n gynecological practice, especially seen among arous women. It is a form of hernia that includes the escent of the vaginal wall and/or the uterus. This is ne of the common cases kept for clinical examination nd has been discussed in detail in this chapter.

)efinition of pelvic organ prolapse

'elvic organ prolapse refers to protrusion of pelvic rgans into or out of the vagina, which occurs due o failure of the anatomical supports.

The pathophysiology of prolapse can be better nderstood if the surgical anatomy is known.

;upports of uterus

t includes the muscular and fibromuscular upports of uterus.

Auscular supports

- Pelvic diaphragm (levator ani)
- Urogenital diaphragm
- Perineal body

Fibromuscular supports

- Pubocervical ligament
- Transverse cervical ligament (otherwise termed Mackenrodt's ligament or cardinal ligament)
- Uterosacral ligament

The muscular and fibromuscular supports are described in the next subsections.

Muscular supports

Pelvic diaphragm (levator ani muscle; Figure 24.1)

It has three divisions:

- Pubococcygeus
- Iliococcygeus
- Ischiococcygeus

Medial fibers of pubococcygeus form a sling around rectum called puborectalis that provides sling support to the rectum.

Urogenital diaphragm (Figure 24.2)

It contains the following muscles:

- Sphincter urethrae
- Deep transverse perineal muscles

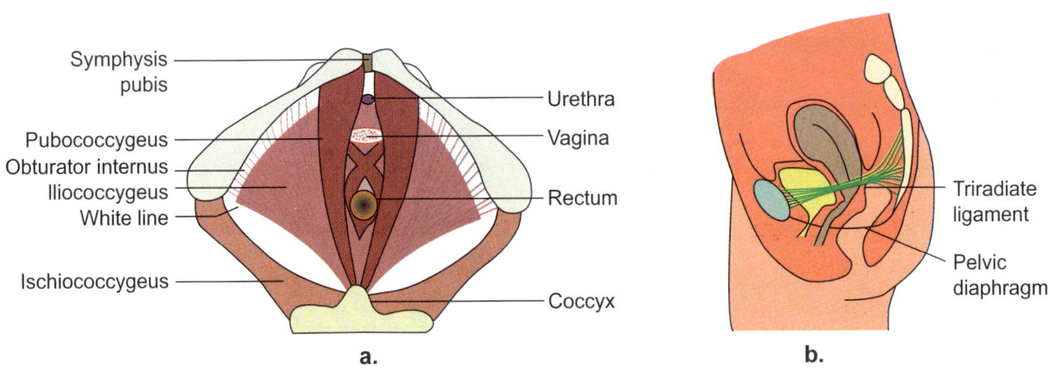

Figure 24.1 Levator ani or the pelvic diaphragm. **a.** Diagram of levator ani or the pelvic diaphragm. **b.** The muscle orms the pelvic floor and supports the lower part of the vagina.

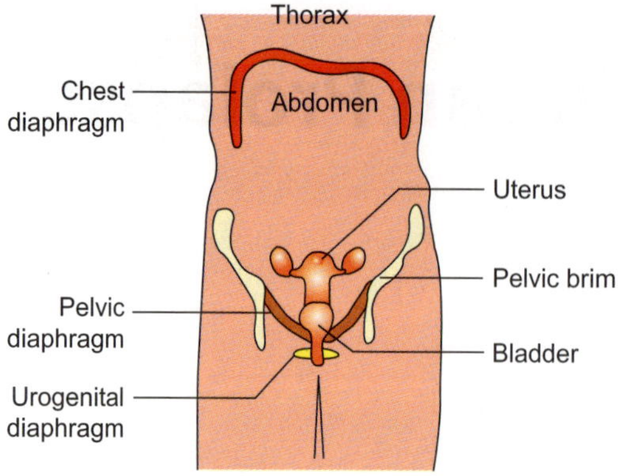

Figure 24.2 Relationship of pelvic diaphragm and urogenital diaphragm.

Perineal body

It consists of a confluence of the following nine muscles between the introitus and the anus and measures about 4 × 4 × 4 cm:

- Levator ani (paired)
- Superficial transverse perineal muscles (paired)
- Deep transverse perineal muscles (paired)
- Fibers of external anal sphincter
- Longitudinal muscle coat of rectum
- Bulbospongiosus

Fibromuscular supports of uterus (Figure 24.3)

Pericervical ring

It consists of triradiate condensation of three ligaments at the pericervical region forming suspension support to the cervix:

- **Anterior:** Pubocervical ligament or bladder pillar (not well developed)

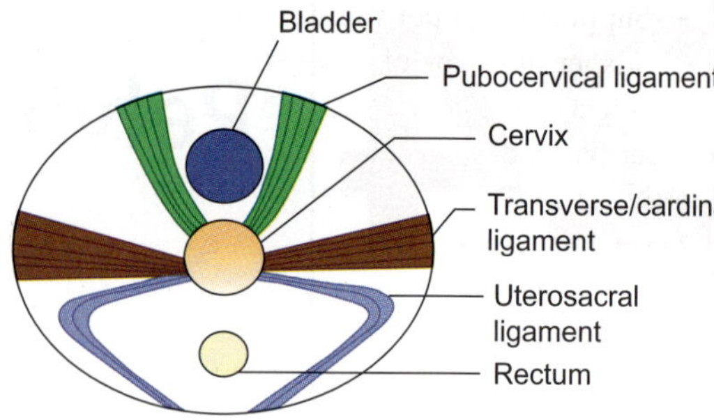

Figure 24.3 Triradiate ligament.

- **Posterior:** Uterosacral ligament or rectal pillar.
- **Lateral:** Mackenrodt's ligament or cardinal ligament or transverse cervical ligament

The triradiate ligament forms a fibroelastic collar around the supravaginal cervix, stabilizing the cervix at the level of ischial spines.

- Ligaments are formed as a condensation of endopelvic fascia.
- Endopelvic fascia is the pelvic connective tissue that forms the loose areolar tissue, nerve sheath, septa, and ligaments. It forms a covering or sheath for the pelvic organs.

Supports of vagina—De Lancey's concepts

Vaginal supports are important in holding the vagina, bladder, urethra, and rectum in their position. Vaginal supports are divided into three levels (Figure 24.4):

- **Level 1**
  - Mackenrodt's and uterosacral ligaments

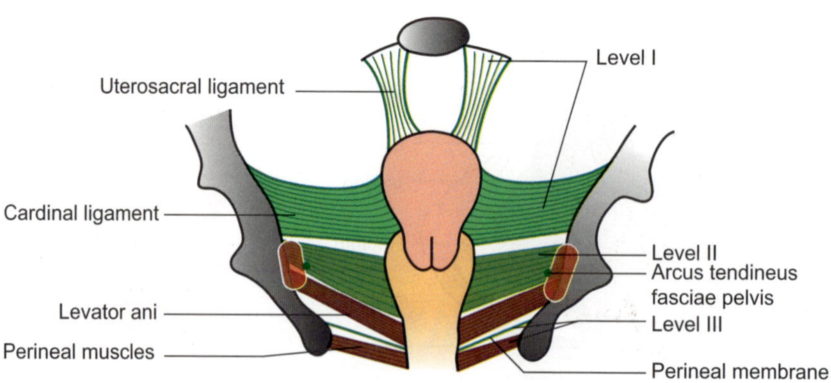

Figure 24.4 Supports of the vagina described as level I, II, and III supports.

- Support for upper vagina
- Suspension type of support

Defect in level 1 vaginal supports lead to uterovaginal prolapse, vault prolapse, and enterocele.

- **Level 2**
  - Rectovaginal and pubocervical fascia
  - Support for midvagina
  - Lateral support

Defect in level 2 vaginal supports lead to paravaginal and pararectal defects.

- **Level 3**
  - Perineal body and urogenital diaphragm
  - Support for distal vagina
  - Fusion support

Defect in level 3 vaginal supports lead to urinary incontinence, gaping introitus, and deficient perineum.

BIOMECHANICS PREVENTING PROLAPSE (BONNEY'S ANALOGY OF VAGINAL PROLAPSE)

The vagina is in the same relationship to the abdominal cavity as the in-turned finger of a surgical glove is to the rest of the glove (Figure 24.5a). An increase in abdominal pressure forces the vagina to prolapse, similar to the way in which an increase in pressure in the glove forces the finger to protrude downwards (Figure 24.5b). Biomechanics including a combination of constriction, suspension, and flap valve effect prevents vaginal prolapse with increase in intra-abdominal pressure.

- **Constriction:** It occurs by levator ani. With an increase in intra-abdominal pressure, the lower end of the vagina is held closed by the constriction of pelvic floor muscles, that is, the levator ani, thereby preventing prolapse (Figure 24.5c).
- **Suspension:** Suspension of the vagina to the pelvic walls is by the uterosacral and Mackenrodt's ligaments (Figure 24.5d).
- **Flap valve effect:** The uterosacral ligament maintains the uterus in anteverted position against the levator plate. With increase in the intra-abdominal pressure, the uterus flexes further over the levator plate, thereby pinning it in place (Figure 24.5e).

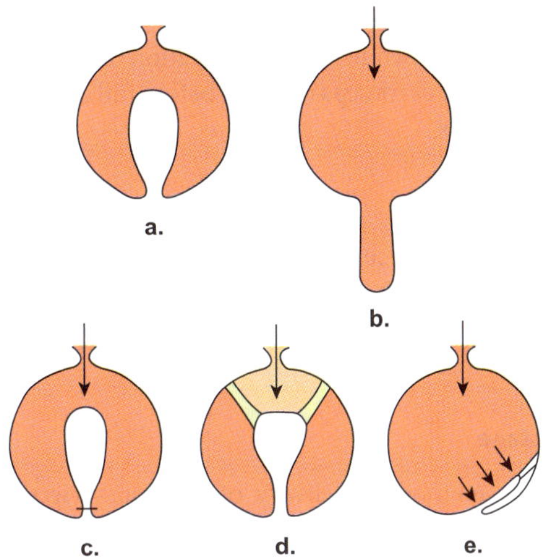

Figure 24.5 Biomechanics of pelvic support. **a.** Relationship of vagina to abdominal cavity. **b.** Vagina may prolapse with increase in intra-abdominal pressure, if it is not supported. **c.** Constriction support by levator ani. **d.** Suspension support by uterosacrals and Mackenrodt's ligament. **e.** Flap-valve effect due to the anteverted position of uterus maintained by uterosacrals.

Etiology/risk factors for prolapse

Primary or predisposing factors

- Trauma due to vaginal delivery, leading to weakness of pelvic organ supports
- Postmenopausal estrogen deficiency, leading to asthenia and atrophy of pelvic floor supports
- Congenital or inherent weakness of pelvic floor supports

Secondary factors

This includes the factors that lead to increase in intra-abdominal pressure.

The primary and secondary risk factors for prolapse are described below.

Primary or predisposing risk factors

Obstetric factors (trauma due to childbirth)

- Home delivery by untrained dais
- Increased number of pregnancies (increased parity)
- Rapid succession of pregnancies (decreased interpregnancy interval)

I stage

- Big baby

- Prolonged labor
- Bearing down before full dilatation of cervix
- Vacuum or forceps delivery before full dilatation of cervix

II stage

- Prolonged second stage
- Precipitate labor
- No timely episiotomy
- Inadequate repair of perineal injuries

III stage

Crede method of delivery of placenta—vigorous push on uterus to expel placenta

Puerperium

- Early return to strenuous work
- Postnatal pelvic floor exercises not practiced

Postmenopausal estrogen deficiency

- Estrogen deficiency
  - Leads to asthenia and atrophy of pelvic floor muscles
  - Leads to reduction in collagen synthesis
- Postmenopausal estrogen deficiency leads to aggravation of injuries to pelvic fascia that occurred during childbirth and manifestation of prolapse.

Congenital or inherent weakness of pelvic floor muscles

- Congenital or inherent weakness of pelvic floor muscles may be present in the following conditions:
  - Spina bifida and split pelvis
  - Muscular dystrophies
  - Connective tissue disorders—Marfan syndrome and Ehlers–Danlos syndrome
- Prolapse occurs at a young age (nulliparous prolapse) in such cases.
- Trauma following childbirth may act as a precipitating factor.

Secondary risk factors

Long-standing cases of increase in intra-abdominal pressure can lead to prolapse in the presence of other factors such as weakness of pelvic floor support.

- Smoking
- Chronic cough
- Chronic constipation
- Obesity
- Large intra-abdominal tumors and ascitis
- Lifting heavy weights—laborers

SYMPTOMS OF PROLAPSE

Postural symptoms

- Mass descending per vaginum
- Feeling of something coming out
- Pelvic pressure and heaviness
- Dragging sensation in lower abdomen

Urinary symptoms

- Stress urinary incontinence (SUI): It refers to involuntary passage of a small amount of urine with increase in intra-abdominal pressure, such as coughing, sneezing, and laughing (SUI may be present if prolapse is associated with descent of urethrovesical junction).
- Difficulty in initiating micturition: The patient finds it difficult to empty the bladder and the difficulty increases with straining, as bladder base and trigone descend below the level of urethra with straining. The patient can empty the bladder only after reducing the mass digitally (takes the bladder base up).
- Sense of incomplete evacuation of bladder: There is a strong desire to pass urine after micturition (because of inadequate empting of bladder in associated cystocele).
- Rarely, retention of urine can occur.
- Increased frequency and urgency of micturition, and dysuria are symptoms suggestive of cystitis that may be present in prolapse (incomplete emptying of bladder and urinary stasis lead to increased risk of cystitis).

Rectal symptoms

Incomplete evacuation of feces (more the patient strains, more prominent the bulge becomes and more is the difficulty in defecation; the patient learns to avoid this by passing two fingers into the vagina and support the posterior vaginal wall for evacuation of feces, termed digital splinting)

Vaginal discharge

- Excessive white discharge (leukorrhea)—may be present due to congestion, leading to an increased activity of cervical glands
- Whether blood-stained discharge—blood-stained discharge may be present due to:
  - Decubitus ulcer
  - Carcinoma cervix rarely (carcinoma cervix is rarely associated with prolapse)
- Whether foul-smelling discharge (decubitus ulcer with secondary infection may produce foul-smelling vaginal discharge)
- Whether discharge is associated with pruritus and irritation (may be present in associated infections such as candidiasis and trichomoniasis)

Backache

Backache is present in standing position (while ambulating) and reduces on lying down. Pain is due to stretching of nerve fibers in uterosacral ligaments (uterosacral strain).

Subfertility

It may be present in young women with prolapse due to the following reasons:

- H/o difficulty in coitus: Huge prolapse may interfere with coitus.
- Seminal pool is deposited away from external os.
- Vaginal and cervical infections can be hostile to sperms.

Part 2

Case presentation

Salient points in history

Consider the following relevant points during history taking in cases of uterovaginal prolapse:

- ***Age***: *More common in postmenopausal women*
- ***Occupation***: *Lifting heavy weights (e.g., construction worker)—risk factor for prolapse*
- ***Parity***: *More common in multiparous women*

Presenting complaints

- *Mass descending per vaginum*
- *Urinary symptoms*
- *Defecation problems*
- *Vaginal discharge*
- *Backache*
- *Difficulty in walking*
- *Coital difficulties*

History of presenting complaints

Mass descending per vaginum

- *Onset*
- *Duration*
- *Progression*
- *Mass reducible or irreducible (irreducibility of prolapse indicates long-standing nature of the problem and is due to congestion, edema, and hypertrophy of the prolapsed uterus)*
- *Aggravating factors—increase in size with coughing, sneezing, and straining*
- *Relieving factors—decrease in size on lying down*
- *Inconvenience during walking/carrying out regular activities—mechanical difficulty*

Urinary complaints

- *Stress incontinence*
- *Difficulty in initiation of micturition*
- *Manual reduction of prolapse to empty the bladder*
- *Weak stream of urine*
- *Sense of incomplete emptying of bladder*
- *Increased frequency and urgency of micturition and dysuria*

Defecation problems

- *Digital splinting to evacuate stools*
- *Incomplete emptying*
- *Digital evacuation of stools*

Vaginal discharge

- *Profuse/scanty*
- *Associated foul smell/blood staining/pruritis*

Low backache

Worsens as day progresses and improves on lying down

(CONTD...)

(...CONTD)

H/o infertility (in young patients)

H/o other precipitating factors

- *H/o strenuous work*
- *H/o chronic cough (chronic bronchitis, asthma)*
- *Mass abdomen and ascites*
- *H/o chronic constipation*

(These precipitating factors need to be taken care of before surgical treatment, so as to reduce the risk of recurrence following surgery.)

Menstrual history

- *Menstrual cycles: Menorrhagia may be present (because of pelvic congestion in prolapse).*
- *H/o postcoital bleeding/intermenstrual bleeding /postmenopausal bleeding may be present (if decubitus ulcer is present).*
- *Find out the age at menopause in a postmenopausal woman and any H/o postmenopausal bleeding (deficiency of estrogen following menopause can result in weakening of connective tissue and aggravation of prolapse).*

Obstetric history

- *Parity and desire to preserve fertility in young women should be noted as it will affect the choice of treatment option.*
- *Details of previous pregnancies*
  - *Antenatal period—H/o anemia and poor nutrition*
  - *H/o home deliveries conducted by untrained dais*
  - *Duration of labor—prolonged labor/difficult labor*
  - *H/o premature bearing down*
  - *H/o instrumentation before full dilatation of cervix*
  - *Weight of the baby*
  - *Episiotomy given or not/any perineal tears*
  - *H/o unrepaired episiotomy/perineal tears*
  - *Postnatal—strenuous work during puerperium*
  - *H/o postnatal exercises to strengthen pelvic floor practiced or not*
  - *Interpregnancy interval (pelvic floor weakened, no time for involution in case of frequent pregnancies)*
  - *Contraception details*

Past history

- *H/o diabetes and hypertension (HT)—to be controlled before surgery*
- *Chronic obstructive pulmonary disease (COPD) (chronic cough—precipitating factor and may lead to vault prolapse after surgery)*

Family history

Inherent weakness of fibromuscular tissues can have familial inheritance.

- *Family H/o prolapse*
- *Family H/o muscular dystrophies and connective tissue disorders such as Marfan syndrome and Ehlers–Danlos syndrome*

Personal history

Smoking (aggravating factor)

Salient points in examination

Consider the following relevant points during examination in cases of uterovaginal prolapse.

General examination

- *Built and nourishment (the patient may be obese; postmenopausal women may be asthenic)*
- *Pallor*
- *Respiratory system (crepts/rhonchi)*

P/A

- *Check for divarication of rectus abdominis.*
- *Palpate for mass abdomen and free fluid.*
- *Check inguinal orifices for cough impulse.*

Spine examination

Check for any spine deformity—to rule out spina bifida (results in defect in nerve supply to pelvic floor muscles).

Pelvic examination

Inspection of the external genitalia

- *Inspect whether the external genitalia are healthy or whether there are any signs of estrogen deficiency in postmenopausal women*

(CONTD...)

(...CONTD)

such as vulvar atrophy/dryness, decreased labial pad of fat, and sparse pubic hair.

- *Look for gaping introitus (introitus is measured from the midpoint of urethral meatus to the midpoint of posterior fourchette).*
- *Inspect the perineum for any evidence of old healed perineal tears and measure the length of perineal body—from posterior fourchette to midpoint of anus. Normal length of perineal body is 3–4 cm.*
- *Stress urinary incontinence: If the patient complains of SUI, it has to be checked in full bladder at the beginning of examination, by asking the patient to cough and looking for escape of urine from urethra. If SUI is present, then Bonney test is performed by elevating bladder neck with index and middle fingers on either side, which should stop leakage of urine on stress (indicates good surgical outcome). Rest of the examination is done after the patient voids.*

The patient is asked to strain or cough and the following are noted (if there is no prolapse on lying down position, ask the patient to stand or squat):

- *Degree of prolapse: The degree of prolapse should be assessed after maximum straining. Mention as "cervix is seen __ cm outside the introitus/at the level of introitus" (cervix is identified by identifying external os with anterior and posterior cervical lips).*
- *Look for cervical and vaginal wall changes such as the following:*
  - *Cervix—hypertrophy/congestion/edema/erosion*
  - *Loss of vaginal rugosities/dry vaginal mucosa (in postmenopausal women)*
  - *Keratinization of vaginal wall*
  - *Decubitus ulcer: If present, describe the ulcer—number, size, site, base, and edges [e.g., decubitus ulcer of size 2 × 2 cm is seen in the anterior vaginal wall with healthy granulation tissue/slough (greenish yellow in color) at the base of the ulcer, with healing edges]*
  - *Any discharge*
- *Visible bulge in the anterior vaginal wall with impulse on coughing—indicates the presence of cystocele.*

Palpation

- *Determine if it is possible to get above the fundus of uterus—able to approximate fingers above the fundus indicates procidentia.*
- *Determine whether mass is reducible or not.*
- *After reducing the mass, posterior vaginal wall examination is done.*
  - *Position of the patient: In dorsal position with thighs flexed and abducted or in Sims' position (left lateral position with left leg extended, right leg and thigh flexed).*
- *Retract the posterior vaginal wall with Sims' speculum.*
- *Cervix is held away from the field by an anterior vaginal wall retractor or vulsellum.*
- *Ask the patient to strain and slowly withdraw the speculum from the posterior vaginal wall.*
  - *The bulge that appears in the upper one-third of the posterior vaginal wall is enterocele.*
  - *The bulge that appears in the lower two-third of the posterior vaginal wall is rectocele.*

(For example, "the mass is reducible and on examination of the posterior vaginal wall, enterocele and rectocele are present.")

Bimanual examination

- *Uterine size—normal/atrophied (in postmenopausal women, uterus is usually atrophic)*
- *Uterine position—anteverted/retroverted (usually uterus becomes retroverted in prolapse due to weakening of uterosacral ligaments)*
- *Mobility of uterus*
- *Fornices—free or any tenderness/mass felt on palpation*

Examination of perineum

Levator ani *Feel for the bulk and tone of levator muscle*

Assessment of levator bulk and tone

- *A finger is placed 2–3 cm inside the vagina at 4 or 8 o'clock position and thumb outside on the skin over the perineum.*

(CONTD...)

Part 2

(...CONTD)

- *Ask the patient to contract her perineal muscles as though she is trying to stop urine flow or flatus and feel for the levator tone. Tone is graded from 0 to 5. It is usually mentioned as "levator tone is good/average/poor."*

Case summary

An example of writing summary in cases of uterovaginal prolapse is given below.

Example *Mrs. G, 64 years of age, para 4 live 4, presents to gynecology OPD with the complaints of mass descending per vaginum for 2 years associated with difficulty in walking and difficulty in micturition. On examination, general examination findings are normal and vitals are stable; on local examination, cervix is seen 4 cm outside the introitus, vaginal mucosa is atrophic, cystocele is present, and the mass is reducible; and on examination of the posterior vaginal wall, enterocele and rectocele are present. Introitus is gaping and levator tone is poor.*

Case diagnosis

An example of writing diagnosis in cases of uterovaginal prolapse is given below.

Example *64 years of age, multiparous, postmenopausal woman with third-degree uterovaginal prolapse with cystocele, rectocele, and enterocele*

Case discussion

Classification of prolapse

Shaw's classification

This is the simplest and most widely used classification. It classifies prolapse into four stages and uses ischial spine as the reference point.

- Grading of uterine descent (Figure 24.6)
  - *First degree*: Descent of cervix below ischial spines, but not up to introitus
  - *Second degree*: Descent of cervix up to introitus
  - *Third degree*: Descent of cervix outside introitus
  - *Fourth degree or procidentia*: Entire uterus present outside introitus
- Anterior vaginal wall
  - *Upper two-third descent*: Cystocele
  - *Lower one-third descent*: Urethrocele
- Posterior vaginal wall
  - *Upper one-third descent*: Enterocele
  - *Lower two-third descent*: Rectocele

The other classification systems for prolapse are explained below.

Jeffcoat's classification

- **First degree:** Descent of cervix up to introitus (Shaw's first and second degrees)
- **Second degree:** Descent of cervix below the level of introitus
- **Third degree:** Procidentia

Pelvic organ prolapse quantification system classification

- It is approved by the International Continence Society and is now widely recommended.
- This classification objectively quantifies the prolapse.
- It allows an accurate quantification of pelvic supports for scientific comparisons and is reproducible.
- In this system, positions of nine sites are measured in centimeter in relation to hymen (negative number for proximal and positive number for distal sites) and recorded in grid form (Figure 24.7a).

The nine sites in the grid are mentioned in Table 24.1 and example of pelvic organ prolapse quantification (POPQ) grid is given in Figure 24.7b.

Pelvic organ prolapse quantification system staging of prolapse

Based on measurements at the nine sites mentioned in Table 24.1, prolapse is staged from I to IV according to the most distal position of prolapse (Table 24.2; Figure 24.8).

Baden–Walker halfway system classification

- Descent of six anatomic sites in relation to hymen during maximal straining is described (Figure 24.9).

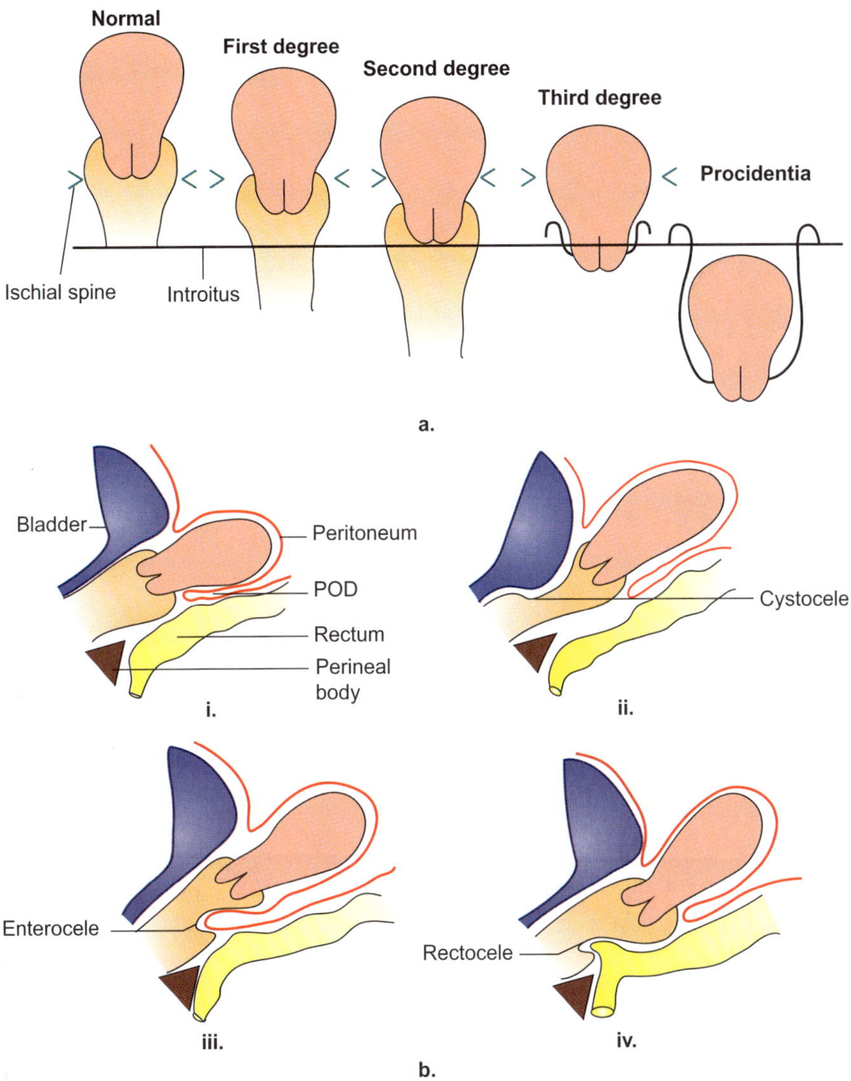

Figure 24.6 Shaw's classification for prolapse. **a.** Descent of uterus. **b.** Anterior and posterior vaginal wall prolapse. **(i).** Normal anatomy. **(ii).** Prolapse of the upper two-third of the anterior vaginal wall with the bladder (cystocele). **(iii).** Prolapse of the upper one-third of the posterior vaginal wall, drawing the pouch of Douglas (POD) with it (enterocele). **(iv).** Prolapse of the lower two-third of the posterior vaginal wall with the rectum (rectocele).

- Six anatomic sites: Urethral, vesical, uterine, cul-de-sac, rectal, and perineal body
  - *First degree*: Descent halfway up to hymen
  - *Second degree*: Descent up to hymen
  - *Third degree*: Descent halfway through the hymen
  - *Fourth degree*: Maximum progression through the hymen

Malpas classification

It is an etiological classification of prolapse and is classified as follows:

- Anterior vaginal wall prolapse
- Posterior vaginal wall prolapse
- Uterovaginal prolapse
- General prolapse
- Nulliparous prolapse
- Posthysterectomy vault prolapse

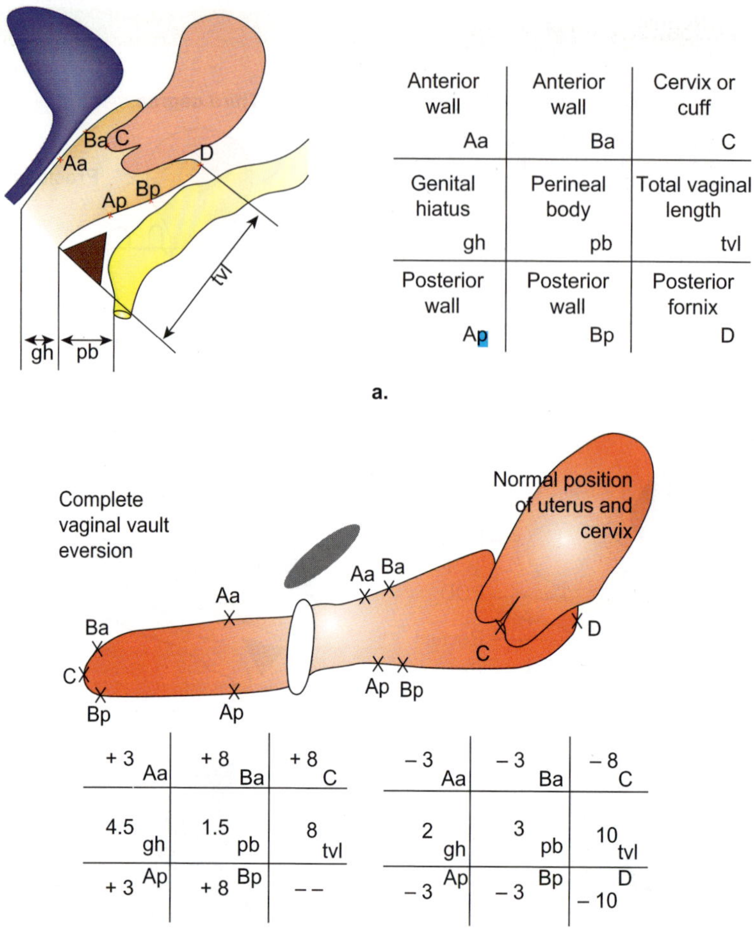

Figure 24.7 Pelvic organ prolapse quantification system. **a.** Classification. **b.** Example of grid for prolapse.

Table 24.1 POPQ system grid variables	
Aa	Point 3 cm proximal to urethral meatus on anterior vaginal wall
Ba	Most dependent portion of anterior vaginal wall
C	Cervix or vaginal cuff
D	Posterior vaginal fornix
Ap	Point 3 cm proximal to hymen on posterior vaginal wall
Bp	Most dependent position on posterior vaginal wall
gh	The diameter of genital hiatus (measured from middle of external urinary meatus to posterior midline of hymen)
pb	Width of perineal body (measured from posterior midline of hymen to the midanal opening)
tvl	Total vaginal length (greatest depth of vagina in centimeter after reducing the prolapse)

POPQ, pelvic organ prolapse quantification.

Table 24.2 POPQ system staging of prolapse	
Stage 0	No prolapse is demonstrated
Stage I	The criteria for stage 0 are not met, but the prolapse is >1 cm above the hymen (quantification value is < −1 cm)
Stage II	Within 1 cm of hymen (quantification value is > −1 but < +1)
Stage III	More than stage II, but 2 cm less than total vaginal length [quantification value > +1 but < +(tvl − 2)]
Stage IV	Complete eversion of genital tract [quantification value > +(tvl − 2)]

POPQ, pelvic organ prolapse quantification.

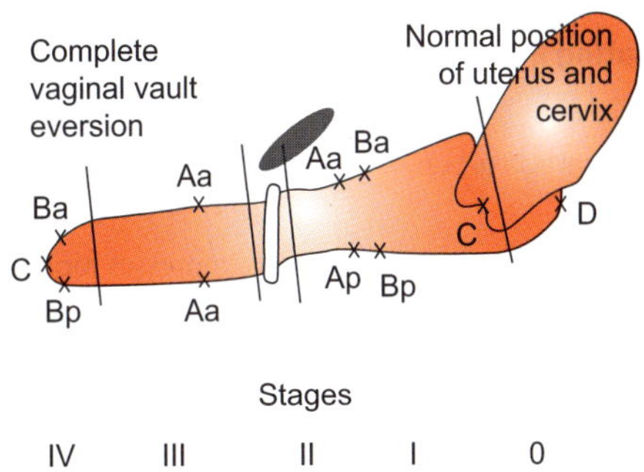

Figure 24.8 Pelvic organ prolapse quantification staging.

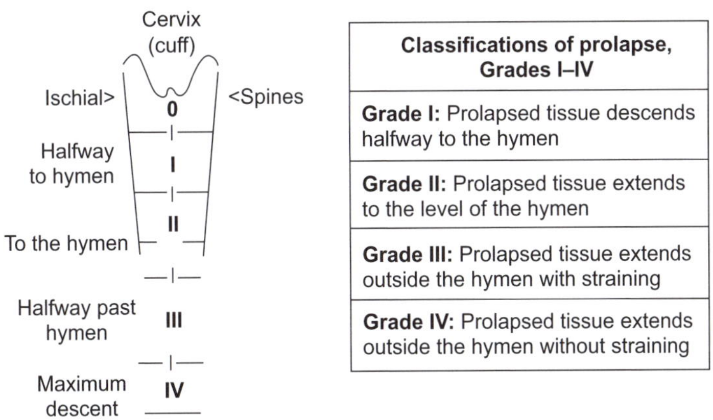

Figure 24.9 Baden–Walker halfway system.

Viva corner

Q1 How will you perform POPQ staging in a patient with prolapse?

- The patient is placed in lithotomy position.
- Ayre spatula is used for measurement.
- A grid with three columns and three rows is drawn and labeled with the patient's name.
- Measurement of genital hiatus and perineal body is done first and entered in the grid.
- Speculum is then inserted and tvl is measured with spatula.
- Points C and D are next measured during maximal Valsalva maneuver.
- Finally, points Aa, Ba, Ap, and Bp are measured.
- Record whether the measurements were taken in lithotomy or standing position, and whether on straining or applying traction.

Viva corner

Q1 What is dominant prolapse?

The dominant prolapse is the first part to descend on straining or the most dependent part of prolapse and provides clue about the site where the most significant fascial damage is located.

Q2 How is uterovaginal prolapse differentiated from general prolapse?

See table below

Table Features differentiating a uterovaginal prolapse from general prolapse

Uterovaginal prolapse	General prolapse
• Seen in young/perimenopausal age group	• Seen in postmenopausal women due to asthenia and atrophy of pelvis support
• Slow progress	• Progresses rapidly
• Cervix is the leading part followed by eversion of vagina	• Vagina is the leading part followed by the cervix
• Supravaginal elongation of cervix is present	• Supravaginal elongation of cervix is not present usually
• May/may not be associated with cystocele/rectocele/enterocele	• Always associated with other components such as cystocele/rectocele/enterocele
• Normal-sized uterus on palpation	• Atrophic uterus on palpation
• Descent is usually first or second degree	• Procidentia is more common

Q3 Prolapse is uncommon in a woman with old complete perineal tear (CPT). Why?

A patient with CPT continuously contracts the puborectalis part of levator ani to maintain continence, that is, to prevent defecation—this leads to strengthening of pelvic floor muscles that prevents prolapse.

Differential diagnosis for uterovaginal prolapse

- Isolated cystocele
- Isolated rectocele
- Isolated enterocele
- Congenital elongation of cervix
- Fibroid polyp
- Chronic uterine inversion
- D/D for cystocele, which includes Gartner cyst and urethral diverticulum

Clinical features

Clinical features differentiating congenital elongation of cervix from uterovaginal prolapse are mentioned in Table 24.3 (Figure 24.10).

Table 24.3 Clinical features differentiating congenital elongation of cervix from uterovaginal prolapse

Congenital elongation of cervix	Uterovaginal prolapse
• Seen in young women	• Seen in older women
• Not associated with urinary or rectal symptoms as there is no descent of vaginal wall	• Usually associated with urinary or rectal symptoms due to associated vaginal wall descent
• Vaginal part of cervix is elongated	• Supravaginal elongation of cervix may be present (as the cervix descends, the Mackenrodt's ligament attached to the supravaginal part of the cervix pulls it upwards, causing supravaginal elongation)
• Fornices are deep and narrow	• Fornices are shallow (as vaginal walls prolapse with descent of cervix)
• Not associated with cystocele/rectocele/enterocele	• Usually associated with cystocele/rectocele/enterocele

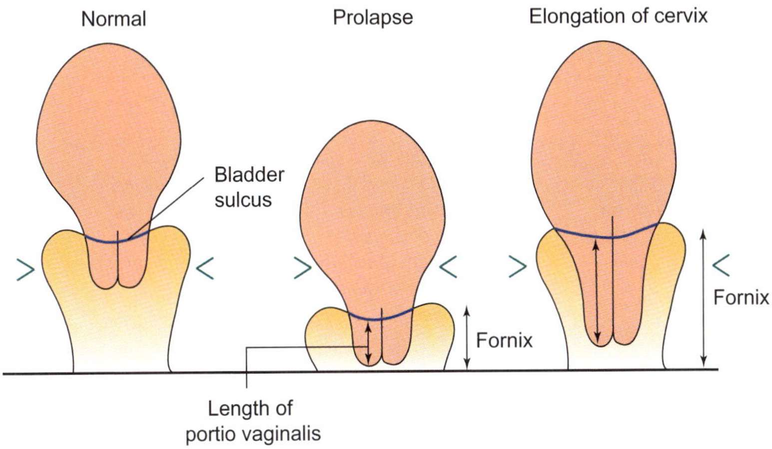

Figure 24.10 Differences between prolapse and elongation of cervix; normal state is also shown.

Clinical features differentiating an enterocele from a rectocele are mentioned in Table 24.4.

Clinical features differentiating a chronic uterine inversion from uterovaginal prolapse are mentioned in Table 24.5.

Clinical features differentiating fibroid polyp from chronic inversion are mentioned in Table 24.6.

Clinical features differentiating a cystocele from an anterior vaginal wall cyst are mentioned in Table 24.7.

Table 24.4 Clinical features differentiating an enterocele from a rectocele

Examination performed	Enterocele	Rectocele
Posterior vaginal wall examination	• Bulge is seen in the upper one-third of posterior vaginal wall • Gurgling sensation and visible peristalsis may be present	Bulge is seen in the lower two-third of posterior vaginal wall
Per rectal examination: A lubricated finger is inserted into rectum and the patient is asked to cough	Enterocele bulge will hit the tip of the finger	• Rectocele bulge will move away from the finger • In case of rectocele, it is possible to hook the finger into the vagina through the rectocele bulge

Table 24.5 Clinical features differentiating a chronic inversion from uterovaginal prolapse

Chronic inversion	Uterovaginal prolapse
• Cervix is not the leading point (no opening is seen in the leading part; see Figure 24.11) • The leading point is broad and shaggy (fundus of uterus) • Cervical rim may be palpable all around the mass	• Cervix is the leading point in prolapse—identified by visualization of external os with anterior and posterior lips of cervix
• Fundus of uterus may not be palpable on bimanual examination	• Fundus of uterus is palpable
• Uterine sound cannot be inserted into uterine cavity	• Uterine sound can be inserted

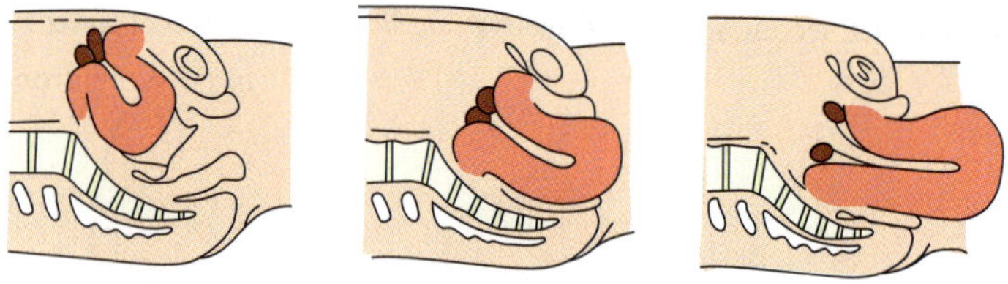

First degree
Inverted fundus up to cervix

Second degree
Body of uterus protrudes through cervix into vagina

Third degree
Prolapse of inverted uterus outside vulva

Figure 24.11 Degrees of chronic inversion of uterus.

Table 24.6 Clinical features differentiating fibroid polyp from chronic inversion

Fibroid polyp	Chronic inversion
• Leading part is broad and no opening is seen in the leading part	• Leading point is broad and shaggy
• Cervical rim is palpable above the polyp; peduncle can be seen coming through the cervical os	
• Fundus of uterus is palpable in normal position in bimanual examination	• Fundus of uterus may not be palpable on examination
• Uterine sound can be inserted into the uterine cavity	• Uterine sound cannot be inserted into uterine cavity

Table 24.7 Clinical features differentiating a cystocele from an anterior vaginal wall cyst (Gartner cyst)

Cystocele	Gartner cyst
• It is seen as a bulge in midline in the upper two-third of the anterior vaginal wall	• It is seen as a visible bulge in anterolateral vaginal wall
• It is not well defined	• It is well defined
• Cough impulse is present	• No cough impulse is present
• Female metal catheter inserted into urethra can be felt through the cystocele	• Female metal catheter inserted into urethra does not enter the cyst
• Cystocele is reducible	• Cyst is not reducible

Viva corner

Q1 How is third-degree prolapse differentiated from procidentia?

To differentiate third-degree prolapse from procidentia, try to get above the level of the swelling.

- It is not possible to approximate the fingers above the swelling in third-degree prolapse.
- It is possible to approximate the fingers above the swelling in procidentia.

Decubitus ulcer

It usually appears in the dependent part of the cervix.

Causes of decubitus ulcer

- Venous congestion leading to circulatory changes such as anoxia, ischemia, and edema
- Disturbances in blood supply (kinking of the uterine vessels leads to decrease in blood flow)
- Due to friction

Symptoms

- Excessive white discharge
- Blood-stained vaginal discharge

- Foul-smelling discharge (if secondary infection is present)

Management

- The prolapse is reduced (restores blood flow and prevents congestion).
- Vaginal tampon soaked in acriflavine and glycerine is inserted (glycerine has a hygroscopic action → reduces edema; acriflavine has an antiseptic effect).
- Tampon has to be changed daily.
- Nonirritant pessary can also be used to reduce the prolapse.
- Estrogen cream can be applied twice daily if vaginal walls are dry and atrophic, as in postmenopausal women.
- Anemia is corrected.
- The decubitus ulcer is expected to heal in a week, with these measures.
- If the ulcer is not showing signs of healing with the above-mentioned measures, a biopsy from the ulcer margin is taken, to rule out causes of nonhealing ulcer such as the following:
  - Cervical carcinoma
  - Syphilitic ulcer
  - Tubercular ulcer
- Diabetes has to be ruled out in patients with nonhealing decubitus ulcers.

Irreducible prolapse

When the prolapsed cervix and vagina become so congested and edematous that the prolapse becomes irreducible, it is termed irreducible prolapse.

Causes

- Long standing prolapse
- Carcinoma cervix—infiltration of parametria prevents reduction
- Associated fibroid
- Large pelvic mass/ascites

Clinical features

- Difficulty in urination or retention of urine
- Prolapse becoming irreducible
- Congested and edematous cervix

Complications

- Kinking of ureters → hydronephrosis
- Decubitus ulcer

Management of decubitus ulcer in an irreducible prolapse

- Elevate the foot end of the patient.
- Catheterize the bladder.
- Apply ice pack to the prolapse.
- Cover the prolapse with a gauze pad soaked in acriflavine and glycerine.
- The edema and congestion significantly decreases, and the mass becomes reducible in about a week with these measures.

MANAGEMENT OF PROLAPSE

Treatment options

- Expectant management
- Nonsurgical management—pessary
- Surgical management

Expectant management

- Kegel's exercise is advised.
  - This exercise is to strengthen pelvic floor muscles.
- The patient is taught to voluntarily contract her pelvic floor muscles lasting for at least 15-second duration, about 15 contractions and relaxations per cycle, for at least 6 cycles per day.
- Indications are as follows:
  - Minor degrees of uterovaginal prolapse (UVP)
  - During 6 months following delivery

Nonsurgical—pessary treatment

A pessary is a device placed inside the vagina to support the prolapsed vaginal walls. It can be used to relieve symptoms of prolapse and urinary stress incontinence. However, pessary provides temporary treatment only—supports the vagina but does not prevent progression of prolapse.

Indications for pessary

- During pregnancy
- Lactation
- Poor surgical candidates—uncontrolled HT, diabetes mellitus (DM), etc.

- Patient refusing surgery
- For healing of decubitus ulcer

Insertion of pessary

Types of pessary These are ring pessary, dough-nut pessary, gel horn pessary, and Hodge pessary.

Ring Pessary It is commonly used (Figure 24.12).

- Initial fitting: The distance between the lower border of pubic symphysis and the top of posterior fornix is measured by doing P/V examination. Long diameter of the pessary should be 1.5 cm less than the measured distance.
- Ring pessary is available in small, medium, and large sizes.
- The pessary is folded and the leading edge is lubricated.
- It is inserted by directing it toward the sacrum, and it is unfolded above the pelvic floor with the anterior edge just beneath the pubic symphysis.
- A fingerbreadth distance should be present between the pessary edge and the pubic symphysis anteriorly, and between the sides of the pessary and the vaginal walls.

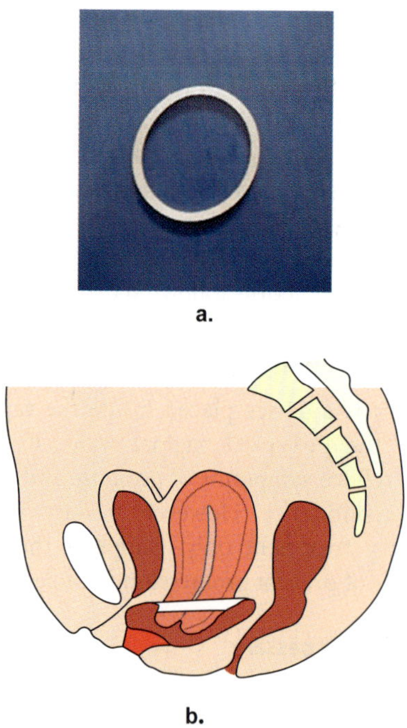

Figure 24.12 Ring pessary. **a.** Image of a ring pessary. **b.** Ring pessary in position.

- Once the pessary is inserted, the patient should ambulate in the clinic and perform activities such as squatting and Valsalva maneuver to ensure that it does not fall out.
- Ensure that the patient voids before leaving the clinic.

> **Extra edge**
>
> **Criteria for well-fitting pessary**
>
> - The patient should feel comfortable after insertion.
> - The pessary should be retained despite ambulation and straining.
> - The patient should be able to void freely.
> - Digital palpation around the pessary should ensure that a finger can be easily inserted in between the pessary and the vagina.

Follow-up after pessary insertion

- Follow up the patients at 3-month interval.
- Ask H/o vaginal bleeding, foul-smelling discharge, discomfort, and urinary tract infection (UTI) symptoms.
- Examination: Pessary is palpated to verify proper positioning.
- Pessary is removed and vaginal walls are inspected for any erosions and abrasions. If these are absent, the pessary is reinserted after cleaning it with soap and water.

Advantages of pessary

- Minimally invasive
- Provides immediate relief of symptoms

Disadvantages

- It is only a temporary treatment of symptoms due to prolapse.
- Pessary needs to be removed, inspected, and reinserted at least every 3 months.
- It can dislodge, if vagina orifice is patulous.
- It can cause dyspareunia.
- It can lead to complications such as the following:
  - Mucosal erosion and ulceration
  - Vaginitis
  - Chances of fistula formation and vaginal carcinoma because of prolonged uninterrupted pessary use

Viva corner

Q1 What is a pessary test?

Pessary test is used to differentiate backache due to prolapse from backache due to orthopedic origin. Following insertion of pessary, backache due to prolapse gets relieved, while backache of orthopedic origin will persist.

Surgical treatment for prolapse

Principles of surgery in treatment of prolapse

- To relieve symptoms
- To repair all defects
- To restore normal anatomy
  - To maintain normal length of vagina
  - Suspension of vault in normal posterior direction toward hollow of sacrum
  - To restore coital functions

Factors that determine the choice of surgical treatment

- Age of the patient
- Parity
- Desire to retain childbearing function
- Desire to retain menstrual function
- Degree and components of prolapse
- Presence of uterine or adnexal pathology such as fibroid and ovarian tumors

Preoperative evaluation

Investigations are done to assess surgical and anesthetic fitness:

- Blood—hemoglobin, grouping, and typing
- Urine—albumin, sugar, and deposits
- Blood sugar
- Blood urea and serum creatinine
- Chest X-ray
- ECG
- HIV, HBsAg (in high-risk cases)

To rule out related pathology, the following investigations are done:

- Pap smear (should be done in all cases)
- Pelvis ultrasonography (USG; especially if the patient has menstrual complaints)
- USG kidneys to look for changes such as hydroureteronephrosis in long-standing cases of prolapse

Ward Mayo surgery

Vaginal hysterectomy (VH) with pelvic floor repair. Pelvic floor repair includes anterior colporrhaphy and posterior colpoperineorrhaphy

Indications

- It is suitable for women aged more than 40 years who have completed family.
- Age limit can be relaxed to 35 years if there are associated problems such as fibroid or adenomyosis.

Note *Details of the Ward Mayo surgery procedure are mentioned in Part 3, Chapter 38, Common Gynecological Surgical Procedures.*

Manchester operation

Indications

- Suitable for women younger than 40 years of age, who have completed their family with the intention of preserving menstrual function
- Second or third-degree uterine prolapse with cystocele/rectocele, with or without supravaginal elongation of cervix

Principal steps

- Preliminary dilatation and curettage
- Amputation of cervix
- Shortening of Mackenrodt's and anchoring it in front of cervix
- Neocervix creation by taking Sturmdoff suture
- Anterior colporrhaphy
- Posterior colpoperineorrhaphy

Disadvantages

- Cervical incompetence leading to the following:
  - Habitual abortions
  - Preterm deliveries
- Cervical stenosis leading to the following:
  - Dystocia during labor
  - Hematometra
- Can lead to infertility as the cervical epithelium is replaced by vaginal epithelium (acidic vaginal secretion inhibits sperm migration)

Disadvantages are mainly due to cervical amputation. Hence, Manchester operation is usually preferred in women who have completed family.

Advantages

It preserves the following:
- Menstrual function
- Childbearing function (although the procedure preserves childbearing function, it is associated with many disadvantages)

Note *Details of the Manchester procedure are mentioned in Part 3, Chapter 38, Common Gynecological Surgical Procedures.*

Shirodkar's modification of Manchester procedure

- It is done to overcome the disadvantages of cervical amputation done in Manchester repair.
- Cervix is not amputated.
- Uterosacral and Mackenrodt's ligaments are dissected, crossed in the front of cervix, and sutured to the opposite side.

Indications

Women younger than 40 years with prolapse, those who want to conceive, where sling surgery is not possible, or as an alternative to sling surgery

Abdominal sling operations

Objective

To strengthen the supporting ligaments using substitutes such as rectus sheath or Mersilene tape

Indications

- Nulliparous prolapse
- If a woman desires childbearing function
- Specially designed for young women with second- or third-degree prolapse, with no or minimal cystocele/rectocele and no supravaginal elongation of cervix

The various sling surgeries are described below.

Shirodkar's sling operation (Figure 24.13)

- Mersilene tape (originally fascia lata was used) is fixed to the posterior aspect of the isthmus and to the anterior longitudinal ligament of the sacral promontory.
- Sling is taken through a psoas loop on the left side due to the presence of sigmoid colon on the left.

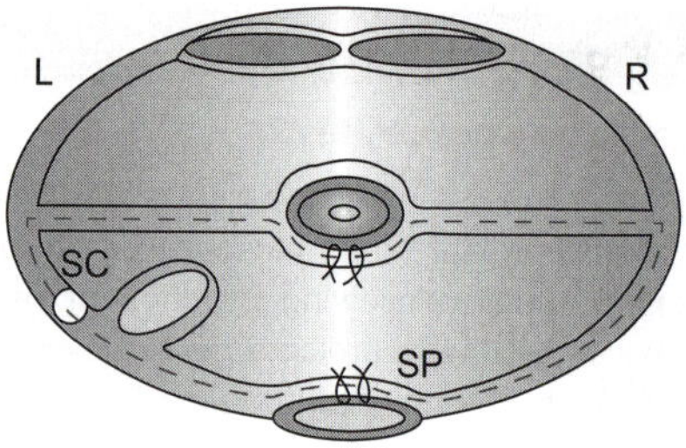

Figure 24.13 Shirodkar's sling operation. *SC*, sigmoid colon; *SP*, sacral promontory.

Purandare's sling

- Mersilene tape is fixed anteriorly to the isthmus of cervix and brought between leaves of broad ligament to emerge at the lateral border of rectus abdominis on either side and fixed to the rectus sheath on either side.
- Plication of round ligament is done.

Khanna's sling operation

Mersilene tape fixed to the isthmus of cervix posteriorly and fixed to the anterior superior iliac spine on either sides

Extra edge

Shirodkar's stitch and Shirodkar's needle: Used in cervical incompetence

Le Fort's operation (partial colpocleisis)

Indication

Very elderly women with prolapse who are unfit for surgery

Principal steps

- Perform Pap smear and pelvic scan to R/o any pelvic pathology prior to the procedure.
- Le Fort's operation can be performed under local anesthesia.
- Rectangular flaps of anterior and posterior vaginal walls are excised and raw areas are opposed with catgut sutures with a small tunnel on either side to permit drainage.

Limitations

- Limits sexual function
- Inability to evaluate any bleeding from genital tract
- Enterocele formation

High-yield points

Surgical procedures done for cystocele and enterocele repair

Route of surgery	Cystocele repair	Enterocele repair
Vaginal route	Anterior colporrhaphy	McCall culdoplasty • Uterosacral ligaments are approximated in midline, taking bites through posterior peritoneum . Enterocele sac is dissected free, excised at the neck, and the sac is obliterated
Abdominal route	• Macleod's method: V-shaped anterior vaginal flap is excised after pushing the bladder down and then the vault is closed • Martin's method: The vault is plicated with paravesical fascia at the level of trigone	• Halban's method: Anterior to posterior closure of enterocele sac incorporating the uterosacral ligaments • Moscowitz's method: Concentric purse string sutures to obliterate the sac incorporating the uterosacral ligament

Kelly's stitch This procedure is done for correction of stress urinary incontinence. Plication of paraurethral tissues over proximal urethra is done to elevate the urethrovesical angle.

Contraindications

- Menstruating women
- Diseased cervix or uterus

Prophylactic measures for prevention of prolapse during vaginal delivery

- Prevention of anemia
- Institutional delivery
- Prevention of premature bearing down
- Instrumental delivery by trained personnel
- Timely episiotomy and proper repair of episiotomy and perineal tears
- Prevention of early return to strenuous work during puerperium
- Postnatal exercises
- Spacing of pregnancy

Viva corner

Q1 Is hysterectomy always necessary for the treatment of prolapse?

Removal of uterus alone, without repair of other defects, will not correct the prolapse. However, hysterectomy facilitates repair of other defects.

VAULT PROLAPSE

Definition

Vault prolapse refers to descent of vaginal cuff following abdominal hysterectomy or VH (Figure 24.14).

Causes

- Wrong choice of surgery
- Poor surgical technique
- Uncorrected defects
- Uncorrected enterocele

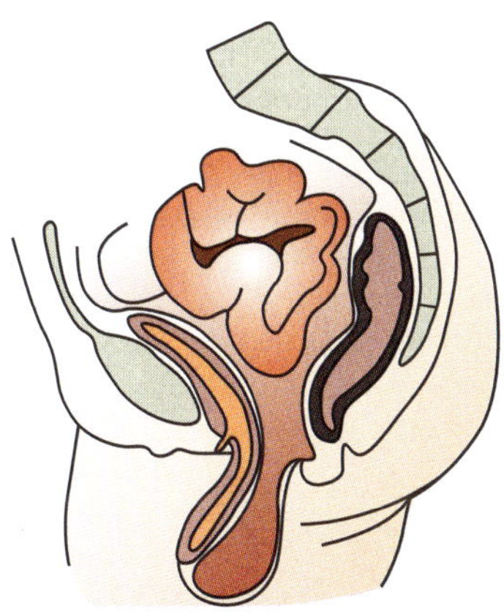

Figure 24.14 Vault prolapse.

- Failure to suspend vault to Mackenrodt's ligament
- Failure to suspend vault above the levator plate directed toward hollow of sacrum
- Conditions that increase intra-abdominal procedure
- Inherent weakness of support

Treatment for vault prolapse

Vaginal route

- Sacrospinous ligament fixation
- Uterosacral ligament suspension

Abdominal route

Sacral colpopexy

Mesh repair

- Transabdominal sacral colpopexy (Figure 24.15)
- Transvaginal tape (TVT)

Steps to prevent vault prolapse during surgery

- Repair of all defects
- Repair of enterocele
- Suspension of vault in normal direction, toward the hollow of sacrum
- Anchoring vault to the Mackenrodt's ligament

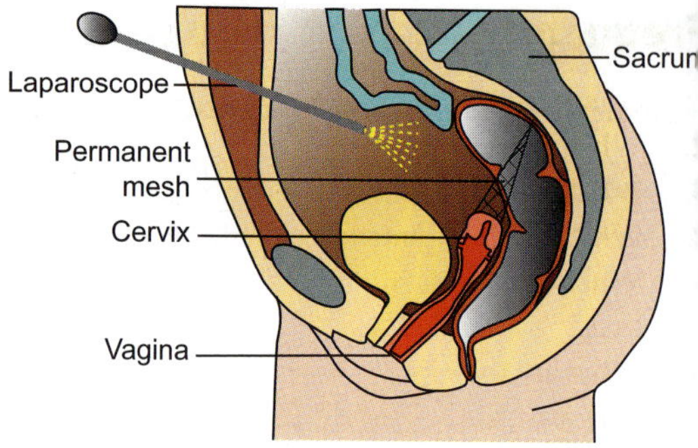

Figure 24.15 Transabdominal sacral colpopexy using surgical mesh.

Pregnancy with prolapse

- Surgery is avoided during pregnancy.
- Prolapse is reduced and maintained in position with pessary in the first trimester.
- Uterus enlarges and becomes an abdominal organ with advancing pregnancy when the prolapse will be taken up, which then reappears following delivery.
- During labor, there may be delay in dilatation of cervix.
- It is advisable to do cesarean section for pregnancies following repair of defects and sling surgery.

Extra edge

Clinical examination for divarication or diastasis of rectus abdominis

- Ask the patient to lie in dorsal position with knees flexed. Place your fingers in midline just above umbilicus.
- Ask the patient to lift her head and neck slightly off the floor and press down with your fingertips. If you feel a gap between the recti, it indicates divarication of rectus abdominis.

Grading of the tone of pelvic floor muscles

See table below

Table Grading used for assessment of the tone of pelvic floor muscles

International Continence Society grading	Modified Oxford scale grading
• 0: Absent contraction • 1: Weak contraction • 2: Moderate contraction • 3: Strong contraction	• 0/5: No pelvic floor muscle contraction • 1/5: A flicker or pulsation under the examination finger (weak contraction) • 2/5: An increase in muscle tension without any lift/squeeze of examination fingers (weak contraction) • 3/5: Some degree of lifting of posterior vaginal wall, squeezing of fingers, and indrawing of perineum (moderate contraction) • 4/5: Elevation of posterior vaginal wall against resistance and indrawing of perineum (good contraction) • 5/5: Elevation of posterior vaginal wall against strong resistance (strong contraction) • Grade of ≥3/5 can be seen on visual inspection of perineum

Frequently asked viva questions

1. Summarize the case.
2. What is the diagnosis?
3. What is the differential diagnosis for the case?
4. What are the supports of uterus?
5. What is the plan of management for the case?
6. What are the causes of uterovaginal prolapse?
7. How will you treat decubitus ulcer?
8. What are the indications for pessary?
9. What is Ward Mayo procedure?
10. Who are the candidates for Manchester procedure?
11. What are the various sling procedures?
12. What are the causes for vault procedure?
13. What are the steps to prevent vault prolapse following hysterectomy?
14. What are the common complications during prolapse surgery?

25 Infertility

Introduction

Infertility usually results from diseases of the reproductive system, in either the male or the female, which inhibits the ability to conceive. Evaluation of infertility includes a detailed history taking and examination of both the partners and specific diagnostic tests. Treatment must be aimed at correcting the underlying etiology. This chapter deals with the case discussion on infertility.

Definition

Infertility is defined as the failure of the couple to conceive within 1 year of regular unprotected sexual intercourse.

- Prevalence of infertility is about 10–15% in couples of reproductive age group.
- About 80% of women conceive within 1 year of marriage and 90% within 2 years.

Terminologies

The various terminologies used in infertility are mentioned in Table 25.1.

Initiation of evaluation for infertility

Couples who are not able to conceive after 1 year c regular unprotected sexual intercourse should b evaluated.

However, evaluation may be started earlier i the following instances:

- Age of the woman >35 years
- Women with irregular menstrual cycles
- H/o oligomenorrhea or amenorrhea
- Known or suspected uterine/tubal diseas endometriosis, or diminished ovarian reserve
- Male partner with known poor semen quality c suspected infertility

Causes of infertility

Infertility can be due to problems in the male, femal or both the partners. In some couples, etiology i unknown, referred to as unexplained infertility. Th various causative factors are mentioned in Table 25.2

Female factors for infertility

The female factors for infertility may be due t problems in the ovaries, fallopian tubes, uterus cervix, or peritoneum (Table 25.3).

Table 25.1 Terminologies used in infertility

Terminology	Description
Cycle fecundability	It is the probability that a single cycle will result in pregnancy (20–25% in normal couples)
Cycle fecundity	It is the probability that a single cycle will lead to live birth
Infertility versus sterility	Infertility implies apparent failure of the couple to conceive. Sterility implies absolute failure of the couple to conceive
Primary infertility	Inability to conceive in a couple with no prior pregnancies
Secondary infertility	Inability to conceive in a couple with at least one prior conception, irrespective of pregnancy outcome (pregnancy may have resulted in a live birth, stillbirth, abortion, or ectopic pregnancy)

Table 25.2 Causes of infertility

Cause for infertility	Percentage
Male factor	25–40
Female factor	40–55
Both	10
Unexplained	10

Table 25.3 Causes of female infertility

Causative factor	Percentage	Problems that lead to infertility
Ovarian causes	30–40	• Ovulatory dysfunction such as anovulation and decreased ovarian reserve • Luteinized unruptured follicle (LUF) syndrome
Tubal causes	30–40	• Salpingitis— due to tuberculosis, gonorrhea, chlamydia, puerperal sepsis • Endometriosis leading to peritubal adhesions • Previous tubal surgeries • Cornual fibroid
Uterine causes	10	• Uterine anomalies such as bicornuate uterus and septate uterus • Submucous fibroid • Endometrial polyps • Intrauterine adhesions (Asherman syndrome) • TB endometritis
Cervical causes	5	• Congenital cervical stenosis • Postsurgical cervical stenosis following procedures such as conization, amputation, cryotherapy • Infections • Immunological causes such as antisperm antibodies
Peritoneal causes	5	Peritoneal adhesions caused by pelvic inflammatory disease and pelvic endometriosis
General causes		• Diabetes • Hypothyroidism • Tuberculosis • Smoking

Extra edge

Causes of infertility in endometriosis

- Distortion of tubo-ovarian relationship due to peritubal and periovarian adhesions
- Elevated levels of cytokines, macrophages, prostaglandins, and TNF-alpha—affect fertilization, embryo development, and implantation

Infertility in women with fibroid uterus

- Fibroids can be a cause or an effect of infertility.
  - Uterine fibroid as a sole cause for infertility occurs only in 3–5% of patients.
  - Fibroids are more common in nulliparous women (postponement of pregnancy → uninterrupted estrogen stimulation → fibroid).
- Rule out other causes such as male factor, tubal, and ovarian causes before attributing fibroid as the cause for infertility.
- The extent to which a fibroid can influence fertility depends on the position, number, and size of the fibroids.
- Pregnancy rate following myomectomy is 40–60%.

(CONTD...)

(...CONTD)

Extra edge

Causes of infertility in fibroid

- Fibroids are estrogen dependent—associated with anovulation and infertility.
- Fibroids can cause distortion of endometrial cavity—interfere with normal implantation (more common with submucous fibroid).
- Abnormal uterine contractions due to the presence of a fibroid interfere with sperm ascent, ovum transport, and nidation.
- Cervical fibroid prevents sperm deposition at the os.
- Fibroids at the intramural portion of fallopian tube interfere with ovum transport.
- Associated endometriosis may be present.
- Inflammatory mediators due to the presence of fibroid can lead to infertility.

Male factors for infertility

- For fertilization to occur, the following male factors are required:
  - Structurally and functionally normal sperms should be produced.
  - Sperms should be produced in sufficient numbers.
  - Sperms should be deposited in the vagina during the time of ovulation.
- Any defect in the sperm production, maturation, and/or transport can lead to infertility.
- Male factors for infertility are classified into pretesticular, testicular, or post-testicular causes (Table 25.4).

Unexplained infertility

- Unexplained infertility accounts for 10% of cases of infertility.
- Unexplained infertility is the term used when a couple has failed to establish a pregnancy despite no abnormality detected on completion of the basic workup for infertility that includes the following:
  - History and examination of both partners
  - Semen analysis
  - Assessment of ovulation
  - Hysterosalpingogram (HSG) or laparoscopy for assessment of tubes

Table 25.4 Causes of male infertility

Cause for infertility	Underlying problem	Examples
Pretesticular causes (hypogonadotropic hypogonadism)	Disorders at the level of hypothalamus/pituitary or other peripheral organs	• Hypothalamic disorders—tumors, infiltrative diseases such as tuberculosis and sarcoidosis • Pituitary disorders—tumors, radiation
Testicular causes (hypergonadotropic hypogonadism)	• Testicular spermatogenesis or testosterone production is affected • Most men with these disorders have oligospermia or azoospermia	• Chromosomal abnormalities—Klinefelter syndrome, Y chromosome microdeletion, mixed gonadal dysgenesis • Local conditions—varicocele, cryptorchidism, trauma, mumps orchitis, radiation, tight underclothing • Substance abuse—alcohol, smoking, caffeine • Occupational exposure to heat and toxins
Post-testicular causes	• The problem may be in sperm motility, transport, or ejaculation • Spermatogenesis is normal	• Abnormalities of epididymis • Congenital bilateral absence of vas deferens • Acquired blocks in the ejaculatory ducts due to infection and trauma • Antisperm antibodies • Erectile and ejaculatory dysfunction

Viva corner

Q1 What is the importance of age in fertility?

Females

- Fertility decreases gradually after 30 years of age because the number of oocytes decreases with age.
- There is an increased risk of chromosomal abnormalities with advanced maternal age.

Males

- Testosterone level tends to decrease after 50 years.

Q2 What is the effect of smoking in fertility?

Females

- Chemicals in smoke are toxic to germ cells in ovaries.
- Smoking increases risk of abortion (due to vasoconstriction and uteroplacental insufficiency caused by the chemicals in smoke).
- It stimulates hepatic metabolism and reduces the blood level of sex steroids.

Males

- Reduces sperm count and motility

Case presentation

Both male and female partners should be evaluated.

Salient points in history from the female partner

Consider the following relevant points during history taking from the female partner in cases of infertility:

- *Age (fertility decreases with advancing maternal age)*
- *Occupation (to identify occupational hazards that may affect conception)*

Presenting complaints

The patient may say that she is married for the past __ years, is not able to conceive since then, and is anxious to conceive.

Menstrual history

- *Age at menarche*
- *Regularity of menstrual cycle—regular/irregular*
- *Amount and duration of flow—profuse/moderate/scanty, flow for __ days*
- *Any recent change in menstrual pattern/flow*
- *Associated dysmenorrhea (anovulatory cycles are usually painless; congestive dysmenorrhea is present in fibroid and endometriosis)*
- *Associated midcycle pain (Mittelschmerz) and premenstrual symptoms such as mastalgia and bloating sensation (indicates ovulation)*
- *Last menstrual period*

Marital history

- *Age of the male partner*
- *Number of years married*
- *Consanguineous or nonconsanguineous marriage*
- *Whether cohabiting with husband*
- *Contraception used, if any*

Sexual history

- *Age of the male partner*
- *Frequency of coitus per week*
- *H/o coital difficulties such as the following:*
  - *H/o dyspareunia*
  - *H/o retrograde ejaculation/premature ejaculation in the male partner*
- *Whether aware of ovulation and fertile period of a menstrual cycle*
- *Whether having protected/unprotected sexual intercourse*

Obstetric history

- *Details of previous pregnancies, if any (indicates secondary infertility)*
- *H/o complications such as severe postpartum hemorrhage (PPH) and postabortal/puerperal sepsis (severe PPH can lead to Sheehan syndrome—postpartum pituitary necrosis)*
- *H/o any curettage done*

(CONTD...)

(...CONTD)

Part 2

Past history

- *H/o any evaluation for infertility done earlier such as semen analysis, HSG, laparoscopy, and the results of evaluation*
- *H/o any treatment such as ovulation induction, intrauterine insemination (IUI), and in vitro fertilization (IVF)*
- *H/o any surgery*
- *H/o tubal and ovarian surgeries (ovarian drilling)*
- *H/o thyroid disorders*
- *Any other chronic medical illnesses such as diabetes and hypertension*
- *H/o sexually transmitted diseases (STDs)*
- *H/o pelvic inflammatory disease (PID) (ask H/o fever, vaginal discharge, and pain abdomen)*
- *H/o of tuberculosis or contact with tuberculosis*
- *Whether a known case of polycystic ovarian disease (PCOD), fibroid, or endometriosis*

Personal history

- *H/o alcohol, smoking, and drug addiction*
- *H/o intimate partner violence*

Family history

- *Family H/o infertility in siblings (suggestive of chromosomal anomalies)*
- *Family H/o congenital anomalies, and early menopause*

Salient points in examination of the female partner and distribution

Consider the following relevant points during examination of the female partner in cases of infertility.

General examination

- *Built and nourishment*
- *Height, weight, and BMI (extremely low or high BMI may be associated with infertility)*
- *Any stigmata of Turner syndrome (short stature, low-set ears and hairline, webbed neck, etc.)*
- *Signs of androgen excess—hirsutism, acne, acanthosis nigricans*
- *Pallor, lymphadenopathy (tuberculosis)*
- *Temperature, pulse, BP (fever and tachycardia may be present in acute PID)*
- *Thyroid swelling, if any*
- *Breast—any evidence of galactorrhea*
- *Secondary sexual characteristics—axillary and pubic hairs (suspect hypopituitarism in case of loss of axillary and pubic hairs)*

Abdomen

- *Any scars (previous surgical scars, subumbilical laparoscopy scar)*
- *Any palpable mass and tenderness*

Pelvic examination (expected only from postgraduates)

Inspection of the external genitalia

Whether normal or presence of any lesion/ulcer

Per speculum and vaginal examination

Look for the following:

- *Vaginismus (vaginal spasm) while attempting P/V examination*
- *Vagina—any abnormal vaginal discharge, vaginal septum*
- *Cervix—erosion, discharge, stenosis, scarring*

Bimanual examination

- *Uterine size, position, and tenderness*
- *Any adnexal mass (ovarian cyst, tubo-ovarian mass)*
- *POD—any nodules in POD (endometriosis)*

Rectal examination

Nodularity of uterosacral ligament (may be present in endometriosis)

Salient points in history from the male partner

Consider the following relevant points during history taking from the male partner in cases of infertility:

- *Age*
- *Occupation (radiation exposure and hot environment can impair sperm production)*

(CONTD...)

..CONTD)

Sexual history

- *H/o any coital difficulties such as the following:*
  - *H/o erectile dysfunction*
  - *H/o premature ejaculation*
  - *H/o retrograde ejaculation (may be present in diabetic neuropathy)*

Medical history

- *H/o mumps in childhood (can cause mumps orchitis)*
- *H/o STDs*
- *H/o tuberculosis/contact with tuberculosis*
- *H/o trauma to genital parts*
- *H/o chemotherapy/radiotherapy in the past*
- *H/o surgeries for varicocele, inguinal hernia, hydrocele, and undescended testis, if any*
- *H/o chronic medical illness such as renal disease, hypertension, diabetes, and thyroid disorders*
- *H/o drug intake for any chronic illness*

Personal history

H/o smoking, alcohol, and drug addiction (marijuana use is associated with reduced testosterone levels and sperm count)

Salient points in examination of the male partner

Consider the following relevant points during examination of the male partner in cases of infertility.

General physical examination

- *Height, weight, and BMI*
- *Body habitus*
- *Secondary sexual characteristics—hair growth and distribution*
- *Temperature, pulse, BP*
- *Check for gynecomastia*

Genital examination

- *Any inguinal hernia (check for cough impulse at hernial orifices)*
- *Any congenital anomalies—cryptorchidism and hypospadias or epispadias*
- *Penis—length of shaft*
- *Urethral meatus—any stenosis or diverticulum*
- *Testis—location, size/volume, and consistency*
- *Epididymis—volume and consistency (check for fullness/tenderness/thickening)*
- *Vas deferens (check for the presence and consistency of vas deferens)*
- *Any varicocele (long-standing varicocele leads to testicular atrophy)*
- *Any other lesion or mass*

Note The male partner should be evaluated along with the female partner. However, during gynecology clinical exams, only the female partner will be present. Hence, it should be mentioned that the history taking and examination of the male partner is pending or yet to be done.

Case summary

An example of writing summary in cases of infertility is given below.

Example *Mrs. V, 27 years of age, W/o Mr. G, 32 years of age, presents with complaints of not being able to conceive for the past 3 years since marriage. Her menstrual cycles are regular 4/30-day cycle with no dysmenorrhea. She is cohabiting with her husband and there are no coital difficulties. Her husband is a social drinker and smokes occasionally. On examination, her vitals are stable, breast and thyroid examination are normal, and abdomen is soft. External genitalia appear healthy; on speculum examination, cervix and vagina are healthy; and on bimanual examination, uterus is anteverted and normal sized with no forniceal tenderness. History taking and examination of the male partner has to be done.*

Case diagnosis

An example of writing diagnosis in cases of infertility is given below.

Example *A couple—female partner at 27 years of age, nulligravida, and male partner at 32 years of age—with diagnosis of primary infertility for evaluation*

Case discussion

INVESTIGATIONS

Investigations in workup of infertility

- A detailed history and examination from both the partners is the first step in evaluation.
- The cause for infertility can be multifactorial. Hence, a systematic approach is followed and includes evaluation of both the partners.
- Evaluation should start from simple tests (e.g., semen analysis, pelvic ultrasound) and proceed to more complex and invasive tests (e.g., laparoscopy) (refer to Table 25.8 for summary of investigations).

Investigations of the female partner

- Tests for ovulation
- Tests for tubal patency
- Tests for uterine pathology
- Tests for cervical factors
- Tests for peritoneal factors

Tests for ovulation

Whether a menstrual cycle is ovulatory or anovulatory can be assessed by the methods of evaluation given in the next subsections.

Menstrual history

Regular cycles, midcycle pain (Mittelschmerz), and primary dysmenorrhea during menstruation confirm ovulation. Five days before and the day of ovulation is termed "fertile window" of 6 days. However, women with irregular cycles require tests to assess whether ovulating and to ascertain the cause of anovulation.

Basal body temperature

- Ovulatory cycles produce a characteristic biphasic pattern of basal body temperature (BBT) due to thermogenic effect of progesterone.
- Following ovulation, BBT increases by 0.5°F over the preovulatory temperature (Figure 25.1).
- The patient records her oral temperature each morning before rising from bed, prior to eating or drinking anything. There is an increase of 0.5°F over the baseline temperature following ovulation.

Cervical mucus study

Ovulatory cervical mucus is thin and profuse, and withstands stretching up to 10 cm (spinnbarkeit test). This phenomenon can be assessed by the patient herself, in which case it is called Billings test.

Fern test

- Sodium chloride levels in the cervical mucus, secreted under the influence of estrogen, are high during ovulation. Sodium chloride undergoes crystallization when the mucus is dried upon a glass slide producing a typical ferning pattern (Figure 25.2).
- Disappearance of the fern pattern and elasticity that were present in the midcycle is suggestive of ovulation.
- Insler scoring: It is a scoring method for assessing favorability of ovulation that is determined

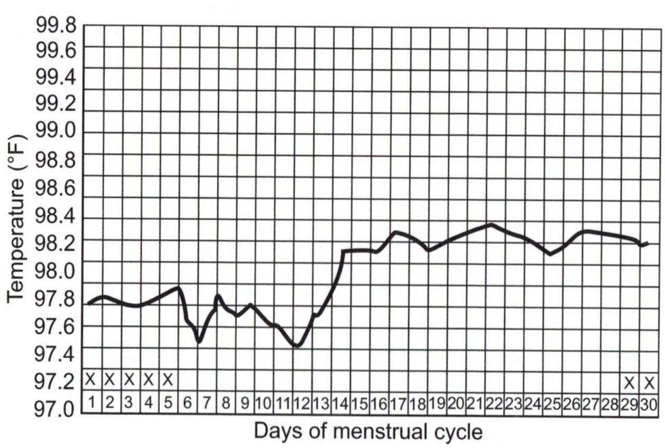

Figure 25.1 Basal body temperature chart. The ovulatory pattern is biphasic with a rise of temperature of about 0.5°F after ovulation.

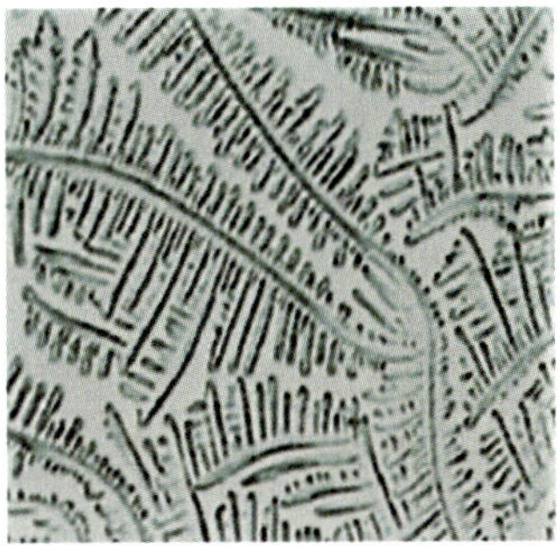

Figure 25.2 Ferning pattern of cervical mucus under estrogen influence.

based on ferning, spinnbarkeit, amount, viscosity, and cellularity of cervical mucus.

Urinary LH excretion

- Luteinizing hormone (LH) surge occurs prior to ovulation. Ovulation occurs 34–36 hours after onset of LH surge and 10–12 hours after the LH peak.
- The first voided urine in the morning is checked for LH using LH detection kit.
- LH level of >40 mIU/mL indicates a surge.

Serum progesterone concentration

Serum progesterone level of >3 ng/mL on days 21–23 of a 28-day cycle confirms ovulation.

Transvaginal sonography

- Serial sonographic examination of the ovaries is done to visualize the development of the dominant follicle and its subsequent collapse after ovulation.
- Transvaginal sonography (TVS) is performed from day 10 and the follicular growth is monitored (follicular monitoring).
- Ovulation occurs when the follicle enlarges to 18–20 mm. Collapse of the dominant follicle and appearance of fluid in POD imply ovulation.
- Measurement of endometrial thickness (ET) is done to assess the endometrial preparation for implantation. ET of >8 mm is considered favorable.
- This test is expensive and is mainly used to monitor follicular growth during ovulation induction.

Endometrial biopsy

- Progesterone secretion following ovulation causes secretory changes in the endometrium.
- Endometrial biopsy is done on days 21–23 of the menstrual cycle.
- Secretory endometrium is diagnostic of ovulation.
- Histological dating is done to identify luteal phase defect (LPD).
- Endometrial sample should also be subjected to acid-fast bacilli (AFB) staining and culture to rule out TB endometritis.

Note *Urinary LH detection kits and day 21 progesterone measurement and follicular monitoring with TVS are the tests commonly used for assessing ovulation.*

Tests for tubal patency

- Tests for tubal pathology are done in preovulatory phase because postovulatory phase insufflation may result in the following:
  - Disturbance of fertilized ovum
  - Pelvic endometriosis

Hysterosalpingogram

HSG is used as the primary test for tubal evaluation, unless there is a history of prior pelvic surgery, PID, or endometriosis.

Procedure

- HSG is done during the follicular phase (between days 4 and 11), after menstrual bleeding stops (postovulatory phase HSG is not done in order to avoid exposure to radiation and disruption of pregnancy, in case the woman has conceived during that cycle).
- It is performed by injecting a radio-opaque water or oil-soluble dye through the cervix and taking X-ray films under fluoroscopy. As the dye is injected, it flows through the uterus and tubes and spills into the peritoneal cavity. Tubal patency is indicated by spillage of the dye into the peritoneal cavity (Figure 25.3).
- An antispasmodic administered before the procedure reduces pain and relieves tubal spasm.
- HSG can diagnose uterine anomalies, endometrial polyps, tubal patency, site of tubal block, tubal rigidity and beading, and hydrosalpinx.

Advantages

- There is no need of anesthesia.
- HSG can identify intrauterine pathology such as submucous fibroid, endometrial polyps, and intrauterine adhesions.

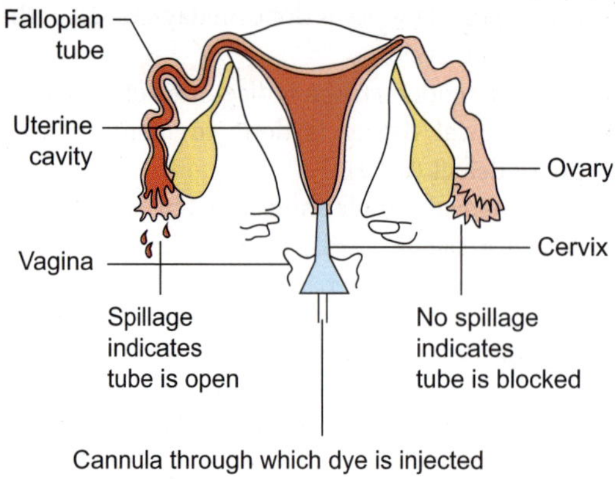

Figure 25.3 Pictorial representation of HSG depicting tubal spillage on one side and cornual block on the other side.

- It can detect uterine anomalies (unicornuate, septate, bicornuate, and didelphys uterus).
- It is 85–100% sensitive in detecting tubal block.
- The site of tubal block can be made out.
- HSG also has a therapeutic effect since it flushes the tubes, and may dislodge mucus and cellular debris blocking the tubes, thereby relieving tubal block.
- It provides a permanent record for tubal testing.

Disadvantages

- It is not reliable for detection of peritubal adhesions or tubal function.
- Tubal spasm due to pain may show a false block
- Radiation exposure

Contraindications

- Uterine bleeding
- Pregnancy
- Active pelvic infection, hydrosalpinx
- Suspected genital tuberculosis
- Allergy to contrast media

Complications

- During the procedure:
  - Vasovagal attack
  - Anaphylaxis to contrast media
  - Uterine cramps
  - Uterine perforation
  - Bleeding
  - Radiation exposure
  - Possibility of occurrence of venous intravasation of the dye if performed during menstruation
- Following the procedure:
  - Women may experience mild to moderate pain following the procedure.
  - There can be flare-up of genital infections (women found to have dilated tubes should be given doxycycline 100 mg BD orally for 5 days after the procedure).
  - False-positive cornual block can be reported due to cornual spasm.

Laparoscopic chromopertubation

Procedure Methylene blue dye is injected through the cervix with a Leech Wilkinson cannula and spillage of dye into peritoneal cavity is visualized under laparoscopic guidance (Figure 25.4).

Extra edge

Oil-based media and water-soluble media in HSG

See table below.

Table Difference between oil-based media and water-soluble media used in hysterosalpingogram

Characteristics	Oil-soluble dye	Water-soluble dye
Example	Lipiodol	Meglumine diatrizoate
Pain during and following the procedure	Minimal	More pain
Anaphylaxis	May occur	Very rare
Uterine contour	Well defined	Less well defined
Absorption of the dye	Delayed	Within hours
Granuloma formation	May occur rarely	Usually does not occur

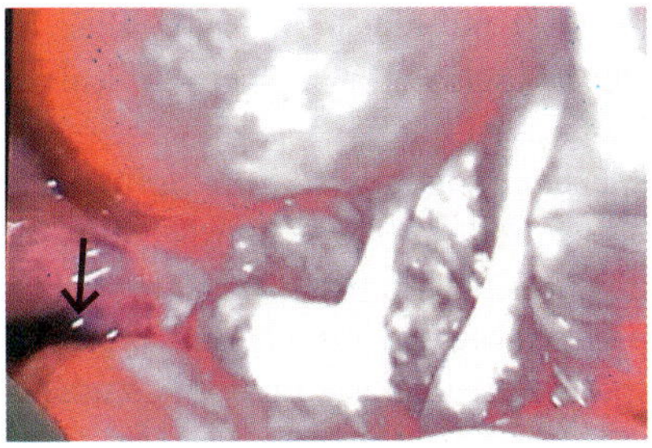

Figure 25.4 Laparoscopic chromopertubation—methylene blue dye in pouch of Douglas visualized through a laparoscope (arrow).

Note *It is not included as a part of initial evaluation because the procedure needs anesthesia and hospitalization and is more invasive and expensive than HSG.*

Indications

- Women with a history suggestive of PID, endometriosis, and prior pelvic surgery
- Women who fail to conceive after initial therapy
- Women with unexplained infertility

Advantages

- Pelvis and peritoneal cavity can be directly visualized.
- Peritubal, ovarian, and peritoneal factors can be evaluated. Laparoscopy helps in identifying peritubal adhesions, endometriosis, and tubo-ovarian mass (not possible in HSG).
- Therapeutic procedures such as adhesiolysis, excision, or ablation of endometriosis and ovarian drilling can be done in the same sitting.

Disadvantages

- Requires general anesthesia
- Invasive
- Cannot determine site of tubal block, abnormalities in tubal lumen, and uterine cavity (possible in HSG)
- Complications due to the procedure such as injury to bowel and hemorrhage

Sonohysterosalpingography or saline infusion sonography

Infusion of saline through the cervix into the uterine cavity and visualization by TVS is known as saline infusion sonography (SIS) or sonohysterosalpingography.

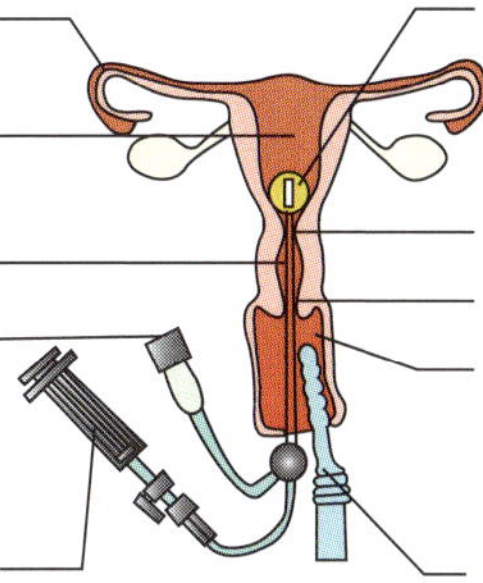

Figure 25.5 Saline infusion sonography.

Procedure

- Normal saline is instilled into cervix via No. 8 Foley's catheter and TVS is done simultaneously (Figure 25.5).
- Tubal patency is indicated by observation of the saline flow as a shower through the fimbrial end and appearance of free fluid in POD.

Advantages

- It is easy to perform.
- Checking for tubal patency can be combined with ultrasound evaluation of ovaries and uterus.
- It can identify endometrial polyp and submucous fibroid.

Viva corner

Q1 What are the uses of laparoscopy in infertility?

- Visualization of pelvis, uterine surface, fallopian tubes, ovaries, and POD
- Diagnosis and treatment of endometriosis and adhesions
- Diagnosis and treatment of ovarian cysts, and ovarian drilling for PCOD
- Chromopertubation for detection of tubal patency

Q2 What are the common causes of tubal blockage?

- Infections—PID and tuberculosis
- Endometriosis
- Tubal surgeries
- Postpartum and postabortal sepsis

Falloposcopy and salpingoscopy

These are the latest techniques to visualize the interior of fallopian tube. These are not done as a routine.

Tests for uterine factors

Various tests to diagnose uterine abnormalities include the following:

- **TVS:** Can detect uterine abnormalities such as endometrial polyp, synechiae, uterine anomalies, fibroid, and adenomyosis
- **HSG:** Can detect abnormalities in endometrium such as submucosal fibroid, endometrial polyp, synechiae, and uterine anomalies
- **SIS:** Provides enhanced visualization of the endometrium and detects intrauterine pathology such as submucous fibroid and endometrial polyp better than TVS and HSG
- **Hysteroscopy:** Best test for visualizing the uterine cavity; is recommended when ultrasound and HSG suggest intrauterine pathology and following IVF failure; can also perform resection of septum and polypectomy in the same sitting
- **Laparoscopy:** Can detect uterine anomalies and fibroid uterus
- **Endometrial biopsy:** Premenstrual sampling helps in detection of the following:
  - Ovulation—secretory phase endometrium
  - Luteal phase defect
  - Genital tuberculosis
  - Chronic endometritis

Tests for cervical factors

Postcoital test (Sims-Huhner test)

- This test is done to look for antisperm antibodies and to assess the quality of cervical mucus.
- The couple is advised to have sexual intercourse 1–2 days prior to the predicted time of ovulation.
- Cervical mucus is aspirated within few hours (2–12 hours) and studied for the following:
  - Quantity and quality of cervical mucus (ferning and spinnbarkeit indicate preovulatory estrogen effect)
  - Number of motile sperms per high-power field (HPF)
    - Normal sperm–mucus interaction indicated by presence of >5 motile sperms/HPF
  - Presence of antisperm antibodies checked for by performing sperm-cervical mucous contact test
  - Sperm penetration can be detected by performing Miller-Kurzrok test—cervical mucus is placed on a glass slide alongside the partner's semen sample and penetration of sperms through the mucus is studied under the microscope
- This test lacks reproducibility and sensitivity

Note *An abnormal postcoital test does not alter the management of unexplained infertility and is currently not used in the evaluation of infertility.*

Tests for peritoneal factors

Laparoscopy helps in identifying peritoneal factors for infertility such as peritubal adhesions, endometriosis, and tubo-ovarian mass.

Other investigations in female partner

Additional tests may be required in some women that include the following:

- Women with anovulation—serum follicle-stimulating hormone (FSH) and LH
- Women with signs of hyperandrogenism—testosterone, dehydroepiandrosterone (DHEA), 17(OH) progesterone
- Women with clinical features of hypothyroidism—thyroid function tests
- Women with galactorrhea—prolactin, thyroid-stimulating hormone (TSH)
- Women with obesity, PCOD—blood sugar, lipid profile
- History and examination suggestive of infection—cervical swab for *Chlamydia trachomatis*
- In women >35 years of age—assessment of ovarian reserve
- Mantoux test, chest X-ray, and endometrial sampling for AFB staining and culture in suspected genital TB
- Karyotyping in case of premature ovarian failure

Investigations of the male partner

Male partner should be thoroughly evaluated by a reproductive medicine specialist, or a clinical andrologist.

Extra edge

WHO classification of disorders of ovulation

See table below

Table WHO classification of disorders of ovulation

Type	Description	FSH and LH	Serum estradiol
Type I: hypogonadotropic hypogonadism	Hypothalamopituitary failure (5–10% of cases)	Low	Low
Type II: normogonadotropic hypogonadism	Hypothalamopituitary dysfunction (70–85% of cases)—polycystic ovarian disease	Normal	Normal
Type III: hypergonadotropic hypogonadism	Ovarian failure (10–30% of cases)	High	Low

FSH, follicle-stimulating hormone; *LH*, luteinizing hormone; *WHO*, World Health Organization.

Common causes for anovulation Advanced age, obesity, very low BMI, PCOD, hypothyroidism, galactorrhea, premature ovarian failure, radiotherapy or chemotherapy, pituitary/hypothalamic causes

Ovarian reserve

"Ovarian reserve" means the number of eggs the ovary has in reserve. Fertility decreases with decreasing ovarian reserve. The main reasons for reduced ovarian reserve are advancing maternal age, primary ovarian insufficiency (POI), and resistant ovary.

The tests for assessment of ovarian reserve are mentioned in the table below.

Table Tests to determine ovarian reserve

Parameter	Indicator of reduced ovarian reserve
Serum FSH on day 3	>15 mIU/mL
Estradiol on day 3	<80 pg/mL
Serum inhibin produced by developing antral follicles	<400 pg/mL
Serum anti-Mullerian hormone (normal value >1 ng/mL)	• <1 ng/mL • Levels >3 ng/mL seen in polycystic ovarian disease
Antral follicle count by transvaginal ultrasound	<10 follicles of 2–10 mm diameter
Clomiphene citrate challenge test—clomiphene 100 mg from day 5 to 9; FSH measured on days 3 and 10	Day 3 and Day 10 FSH >15 mIU/mL

FSH, follicle-stimulating hormone.

Semen analysis

- Semen analysis is a simple noninvasive test in males and is the single most important test in the evaluation of male fertility.
- History, physical examination, and semen analysis can identify majority of the conditions causing male infertility.

Procedure

- Semen sample is collected through masturbation, after a period of abstinence of 2–5 days. Avoid use of lubricants or condoms.
- Semen is collected in a container that is nontoxic to sperms.
- Ideally, the specimen must be collected at the same andrology laboratory where analysis is to be done.
- If the sample is collected at home, it should be transported to the laboratory at room temperature within 30 minutes to ensure accuracy of results.
- Normal semen parameters according to the World Health Organization (WHO, 2010) are listed in Table 25.5.
- The semen analysis must be repeated after 3 months if any of the parameters are abnormal or as soon as possible in case of gross deficiencies.

Table 25.5 Semen analysis parameters—lower reference limits (95% CI) in fertile men (WHO, 2010)

Parameter	Normal range
Volume	1.5 mL (1.4–1.7 mL)
Sperm concentration	15 (12–16) million/mL or greater
Total sperm count	• 39 (33–46) million sperms per ejaculate or more
Motility	• 40% total motility (progressive + nonprogressive motility) • 32% forward progression
Morphology	>4% of normal sperms
Vitality	58% (55–63%) or more alive

CI, confidence interval; *WHO*, World Health Organization.

Commonly used terminologies in semen analysis

See Table 25.6

Table 25.6 Terminologies used in semen analysis

Terminology	Description
Oligospermia	Reduced sperm count
Asthenospermia	Reduced sperm motility
Teratospermia	Increase in abnormal forms of sperms
Oligoasthenoteratospermia	All sperm variables subnormal
Azoospermia	No sperms in semen
Necrospermia	All sperms nonviable or nonmotile
Leukocytospermia	Increase in WBCs in semen (>1 million WBCs/mL)

WBC, white blood cell.

Other investigations in the male partner

Additional tests that may be required for the male partner include the following:

- Endocrine profile
  - Serum FSH level (low FSH level indicates hypothalamo pituitary failure)
  - Serum testosterone
  - Serum prolactin
- Ultrasound of scrotum
  - To look for testicular size and volume
  - Color flow Doppler and scrotal thermography for varicocele
- Transrectal ultrasound
  - To look for ejaculatory duct obstruction
- Vasography
  - To assess patency of vas deferens
- Postejaculatory urine examination: Retrograde ejaculation indicated by the presence of sperms in urine
- Sperm pelleting: Centrifuged sperm pellet examined for sperms prior to confirming azoospermia
- Karyotyping if azoospermia is present
- Genetic testing for cystic fibrosis and Y chromosome microdeletion
- Enzyme-linked immunosorbent assay (ELISA) and radioimmune assay tests to determine antisperm antibodies
- Sperm function tests
- Testicular biopsy: Indicated in cases with azoospermia and for diagnosis of genital tuberculosis [the tissue can be cryopreserved and the spermatozoa can be used for intracytoplasmic sperm injection (ICSI) in IVF procedures)
- Evaluation of patients with azoospermia given in Table 25.7

Table 25.7 Evaluation of patients with azoospermia

Cause for azoospermia	FSH and LH	Testosterone	Further evaluation
Pretesticular—hypogonadotropic hypogonadism	Decreased	Decreased	• Serum prolactin levels • CT/MRI of pituitary fossa
Testicular—hypergonadotropic hypogonadism	Increased	Decreased	• Karyotyping • Testicular biopsy
Post-testicular	Normal	Normal	• Perform vasography that detects obstruction or absence of vas deferens • Assess seminal fructose and pH—low values indicate absence/obstruction of vas deferens

FSH, follicle-stimulating hormone; *LH*, luteinizing hormone.

Viva corner

Q1 What are the causes of retrograde ejaculation?

- Diabetes
- Spinal cord diseases
- Transurethral surgeries causing damage to bladder neck
- Drugs—alpha-adrenergic blockers and reserpine

Baseline investigations indicated in both partners

- Hemoglobin
- Blood grouping and typing
- Urine—routine and microscopy
- Blood sugar values
- Serology—VDRL, HBsAg, and HIV

Summary of the investigations for evaluation of infertility in both the partners is given in Table 25.8.

Table 25.8 Summary of the investigations for evaluation of infertility in both the partners

Investigation of the female partner					
Tests for ovulation	**Tests for tubal patency**	**Tests for uterine factors**	**Test for cervical factor**	**Tests for peritoneal factor**	**Additional evaluation**
• Menstrual history • Basal body temperature • Urinary LH secretion • Day 21 serum progesterone • Cervical mucus study • Fern test • TVS for follicular monitoring • Premenstrual endometrial biopsy	• HSG • Laparoscopic chromopertubation • Saline infusion sonography • Falloposcopy and salpingoscopy	• TVS • HSG • Saline infusion sonography • Laparoscopy • Hysteroscopy • Endometrial biopsy	Postcoital test	Laparoscopy	• Serum FSH and LH • Serum testosterone, DHEA, 17(OH) progesterone • Thyroid function tests • Serum prolactin • Blood sugar, lipid profile • Cervical swab for *C. trachomatis* • Assessment of ovarian reserve • Mantoux test, chest X-ray, and endometrial sampling for acid-fast bacilli staining and culture in suspected genital tuberculosis • Karyotyping in cases with premature ovarian failure

Investigations of the male partner	
Initial evaluation	**Additional evaluation**
Semen analysis	• Endocrine profile—serum FSH, LH, testosterone, prolactin • Ultrasound of scrotum for testicular size and volume and for varicocele • Transrectal ultrasound for ejaculatory duct obstruction • Vasography—to assess patency of vas deferens • Postejaculatory urine examination for sperms in cases with retrograde ejaculation • Karyotyping in azoospermia cases • Genetic testing for cystic fibrosis and Y chromosome microdeletion • Enzyme-linked immunosorbent assay and radioimmune assay tests to determine antisperm antibodies • Sperm function tests • Testicular biopsy in cases with azoospermia and for diagnosis of genital tuberculosis

DHEA, dehydroepiandrosterone; *FSH*, follicle-stimulating hormone; *HSG*, hysterosalpingogram; *LH*, luteinizing hormone; *TVS*, transvaginal sonography.

MANAGEMENT OF INFERTILE COUPLE

Management decisions are based on the following factors:

- Age of both the partners
- Duration of infertility
- Cause of infertility
- Prior treatment failure

Couples should be advised on the following:

- To reduce weight to maintain optimum body weight (weight reduction of 5–10% of body weight can restore ovulation and result in pregnancy in obese women)
- To stop smoking and alcohol
- To avoid stress
- Counsel regarding the fertile period [advise young couples with infertility on timing of intercourse during the fertile period. The fertile period extends from 5 days prior to ovulation to the day of ovulation (6 days). Urinary LH kits can be used to determine the timing of ovulation].

Treatment of female factors for infertility

Treatment of ovarian factor for infertility

- In women with ovulatory dysfunction, the most appropriate treatment is to begin with ovulation induction.
- The treatment can be started even before other potential causes of female infertility have been investigated.

Drugs used for ovulation induction

- Clomiphene citrate (CC)
- Gonadotropins
  - Human menopausal gonadotropin (hMG) contains FSH and LH.
  - Human chorionic gonadotropin (hCG) has only LH activity.
  - Recombinant FSH has specific FSH activity.
- Aromatase inhibitors—letrozole [not yet approved by the Food and Drug Administration (FDA)]
- Drugs used to facilitate ovulation (adjuvant therapy)
  - Insulin sensitizers such as metformin
  - Bromocriptine
  - Glucocorticoids—dexamethasone

Clomiphene citrate

Mechanism of action It has both estrogenic and antiestrogenic effects. It binds with estrogen receptors in hypothalamus and competitively inhibits the negative feedback of estrogen on the hypothalamus, thus increasing GnRH production. This stimulates pituitary gonadotropin secretion and ovulation.

Indications for ovulation induction with CC

- Oligo-ovulation or anovulation due to HPO axis dysfunction [WHO Type II ovulatory disorder–polycystic ovarian disease (PCOD)]
- Cannot be used in hypothalamopituitary failure (WHO Type I ovulatory disorder) and primary ovarian failure (WHO Type III ovulatory disorder)

Ovulation induction with CC

- Baseline TVS is done on days 1–3 to rule out any ovarian cysts.
- CC is started at a dose of 50 mg/day. It can be started from days 2 to 5 of menstrual cycle and given for 5 days.
- Follicular monitoring is done with TVS from Day 10.
- Dominant follicular size of 18–20 mm on days 13–14 indicates good ovarian response. Ovulation is detected by ultrasonography (USG) changes such as collapse of the dominant follicle and appearance of fluid in POD.
- If there is no increase in size of follicle during follicular monitoring, dose can be increased to 100 and 150 mg in subsequent cycles.
- CC dose of >150 mg and >6 cycles are not recommended.
- CC failure: There is anovulation with maximum dose or failure to conceive despite ovulation

Disadvantage

- Ovulation occurs in 80% of cases but pregnancy rate is only 40%. Pregnancy rates are lower with clomiphene due to antiestrogenic action on the endometrium and cervical mucus.
- CC can lead to complications such as multiple pregnancy and ovarian hyperstimulation syndrome (OHSS).

Gonadotropins

Indications

- Hypogonadotropic hypogonadism (first-line drugs for WHO Type I ovulation dysfunction)
- CC failure
- Unexplained infertility
- Assisted reproductive technology (ART)—to achieve superovulation
- Success rate: Ovulation occurs in 90% cases

Disadvantages

- Gonadotropins are expensive.
- They can lead to complications such as multiple pregnancy and OHSS.

Drugs used to facilitate ovulation induction

Metformin

- It is a biguanide that reduces insulin resistance and helps in weight reduction in women with PCOD.
- It is used along with CC to improve pregnancy rates.
- The dose is 500–850 mg TDS.

Note *Insulin resistance plays a major role in the pathophysiology of PCOD, which is the most common cause of anovulatory infertility. Insulin sensitizers such as metformin may restore normal ovarian function in these women.*

Viva corner

Q1 What is the difference between ovulation induction (OI) and superovulation (SO)?

Ovulation induction

- Stimulation of growth of a single follicle
- Done in anovulatory cycles to stimulate ovulation

Superovulation

- Stimulation of growth of multiple follicles
- Done in IVF cycles so that multiple oocytes are available for retrieval

Q2 What is the risk of multiple gestation with CC and gonadotropins?

- **CC:** 5–8%
- **Gonadotropins:** 15%

Glucocorticoids Dexamethasone can be used along with CC in women with PCOD.

Dopamine agonists Bromocriptine or cabergoline is used for ovulation induction in women with anovulatory infertility associated with hyperprolactinemia.

Polycystic ovarian disease

PCOD is the most common cause of chronic anovulation.

Definition

It is a syndrome characterized by the following:

- Oligo-ovulation or anovulation
- Features of androgen excess
- USG appearance of multiple cysts in the ovaries

Rotterdam's criteria for diagnosis of PCOD Two of the following must be present to diagnose PCOD:

- Oligo-ovulation or anovulation
- Clinical (acne, hirsutism, androgenic alopecia) or biochemical (increased testosterone, androstenedione, DHEAS) features of hyperandrogenism
- Polycystic ovaries—12 or more peripherally arranged follicles measuring 2–9 mm in size or increase in ovarian volume of >10 cm^3 (Figure 25.6)

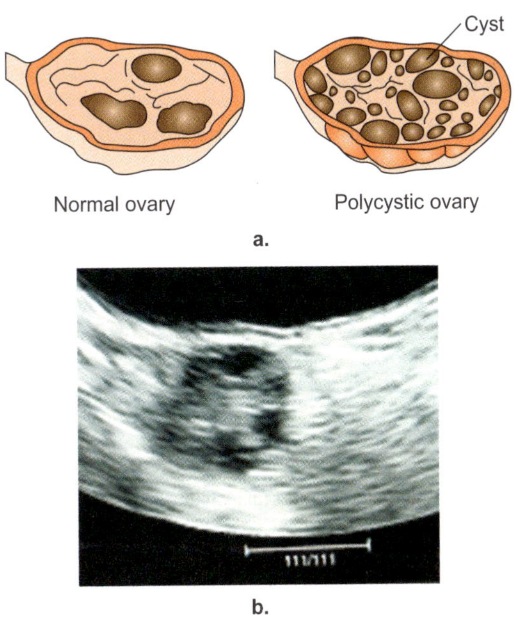

Figure 25.6 Polycystic ovaries. **a.** Pictorial representation of normal and polycystic ovaries. **b.** Ultrasound image of polycystic ovary.

Biochemical abnormalities in PCOD

- Hyperinsulinemia
- Hyperlipidemia
- Hyperprolactinemia
- Hyperandrogenism
- Hyperestrogenism
- Increased LH and low FSH (LH:FSH ratio >3)
- Low progesterone

High-yield points

Complications of PCOD

- Anovulatory infertility
- Diabetes mellitus (DM) due to insulin resistance
- If the patient conceives, increased risk of abortion and gestational diabetes mellitus (GDM)
- Endometrial hyperplasia and carcinoma due to unopposed estrogen
- Cardiovascular abnormalities

Treatment of PCOD

Aim of treatment

- To facilitate fertility
- To control hirsutism
- To prevent endometrial hyperplasia
- To prevent the long-term consequences of insulin resistance

Treatment options

- Weight reduction through diet and exercise
- Ovulation-inducing drugs such as CC and insulin-sensitizing agents (metformin) in women who are anxious to conceive
- Surgery—ovarian drilling in women who do not respond to CC
- Combined oral contraceptive (COC) pills or cyclic progesterone therapy can reduce the risk of endometrial hyperplasia and carcinoma

Note *The treatment must be individualized according to the need of the patient.*

Treatment of tubal factor for infertility

- Tubal factors may be in the form of adhesions or tubal block. Tubal occlusion can be a proximal occlusion or distal occlusion (fimbrial end).
- The success is low and the risk of ectopic pregnancy is high in the treatment of women with severe tubal disease. IVF is recommended in women with severe tubal disease.
- Procedures to treat tubal occlusion are the following:
  - Proximal tubal occlusion
    - Tubal microsurgery such as resection anastomosis and tubocornual anastomosis

Viva corner

Q1 How does weight loss help in PCOD?

- Lowers androgen levels
- Regularizes menstrual cycles
- Resumes ovulation
- Reduces insulin resistance

Q2 How does ovarian drilling help in PCOD?

Reduces the androgen levels by releasing the androgen-rich follicular fluid during drilling

Q3 How does metformin help in PCOD?

- Increases peripheral insulin sensitivity
- Reduces hepatic glucose production
- Reduces intestinal absorption of glucose

Q4 What is ovarian hyperstimulation syndrome (OHSS)?

- OHSS is an iatrogenic complication of controlled ovarian hyperstimulation.
- It is directly related to the number of stimulated follicles and is hCG dependent.
- **Pathogenesis:** Vasoactive mediators such as prostaglandins, cytokines, renin, angiotensin, and endothelins are released from ovaries, which cause endothelial injury and vasodilatation leading to third-space fluid collection and circulatory dysfunction.
- **Clinical features:** These include variable degree of ovarian enlargement, ascites, pleural effusion, oliguria, hemoconcentration, thromboembolism, and electrolyte disturbances that may be life-threatening.
- **Management:** OHSS is managed conservatively with fluid replacement.

Viva corner

Q1 What is the effect of hydrosalpinx on infertility?

Hydrosalpinx decreases pregnancy rate and increases abortion rate due to the following reasons:

- Hydrosalpinx fluid contains microorganisms, endotoxins, and cytokines that are embryotoxic.
- Oocyte or sperms can be phagocytosed by the macrophages in the hydrosalpinx fluid.
- The endometrial receptivity is reduced due to disturbances in the cytokine cascade.

Hence, removal of the diseased tube or occlusion of cornual end has to be done in hydrosalpinx in order to increase fertility outcome.

    - Hysteroscopic tubal cannulation
    - ART
  - Distal tubal occlusion—fimbrioplasty or ART
  - Hydrosalpinx—ART (if hydrosalpinx is >3 cm, resection of the hydrosalpinx followed by IVF is recommended)
  - Peritubal adhesions—laparoscopic adhesiolysis
  - Sterilized women wanting reversal of procedure—tubal recannulation
  - IVF done if tubal surgeries fail to achieve pregnancy

Treatment of uterine factors for infertility

- **Fibroids:** May require treatment if other causes of infertility have been ruled out
- **Endometrial polyps**: Removed by hysteroscopic polypectomy
- **Uterine synechiae:** Hysteroscopic adhesiolysis
- **Uterine anomalies:** Surgical correction
  - *Septate uterus*: Septoplasty or hysteroscopic lysis of septum
  - *Bicornuate uterus*: Metroplasty
  - *Unicornuate, didelphys, and arcuate uterus*: These are irreparable uterine defects
- **LPD:** Treated with luteal phase progesterone supportive therapy

Treatment of cervical factor for infertility

- Chronic cervicitis is treated with antibiotics.
- The most successful treatment option for cervical cause for infertility is intrauterine insemination (IUI).
- If IUI is unsuccessful, IVF is the next option.

Treatment of peritoneal factors for infertility

Adhesions caused by PID or endometriosis can be released by laparoscopic adhesiolysis, but IVF is the best option in many of these women.

Treatment of male factors for infertility

The patient is advised on the following.

- To stop smoking and to abstain from alcohol
- To avoid excessive heat exposure to scrotum
- To avoid tight underclothing
- Control of blood sugars in DM

Treatment of the factors causing male infertility includes the following:

- **Retrograde ejaculation:** Occurs in neuropathic disorders [may respond to α-sympathomimetic drugs (phenylpropanolamine, imipramine).; sperms can be collected from the urine, washed, and used for IUI or IVF]
- **Varicocele:** Surgical ligation of internal spermatic vein
- **Erectile dysfunction:** Phosphodiesterase type 5 inhibitor (sildenafil)
- **Mild/moderate oligospermia:** IUI or IVF
- **Azoospermia:** Treatment is based on the cause for azoospermia, whether it is pretesticular, testicular, or post-testicular cause (Table 25.9)

Table 25.9 Treatment of various causes of azoospermia

Pretesticular causes	Testicular causes	Post-testicular causes
• Hypothalamic cause—GnRH analogues • Pituitary cause—gonadotropins	Surgical retrieval of sperms for IVF, or assisted reproductive technology with donor sperms	• Obstructive azoospermia: Surgical anastomosis depending on the site of obstruction or surgical retrieval of sperms for IVF can be done

IVF, in vitro fertilization.

Note *Treatment has poor results in azoospermia and in conditions such as Klinefelter syndrome and other chromosomal abnormalities.*

Treatment of unexplained infertility

- Chances of spontaneous pregnancy are high in unexplained infertility. The couple is explained about the fertility period and a wait and watch policy is adopted for at least 6 months.
- If conception does not occur, further treatment is required. IUI with superovulation increases the available number and proximity of healthy gametes.
- IUI with superovulation using CC for three cycles, followed by IUI with controlled ovarian hyperstimulation (COH) using gonadotropins for another three cycles, is tried.
- If these approaches fail to achieve pregnancy, then IVF is the next option.

ARTIFICIAL INSEMINATION

Definition Artificial insemination refers to the procedure by which the sperm suspension is injected into the uterine cavity or cervical canal, to increase the chances of fertilization (Figure 25.7).

- The procedure may be performed with partner's semen or donor semen.
- The procedure may be performed as intracervical insemination (ICI) or intrauterine insemination (IUI)—IUI has a better success rate and is more widely used.
- The procedure may be performed during a natural cycle (unstimulated IUI) or following ovulation induction (stimulated IUI).

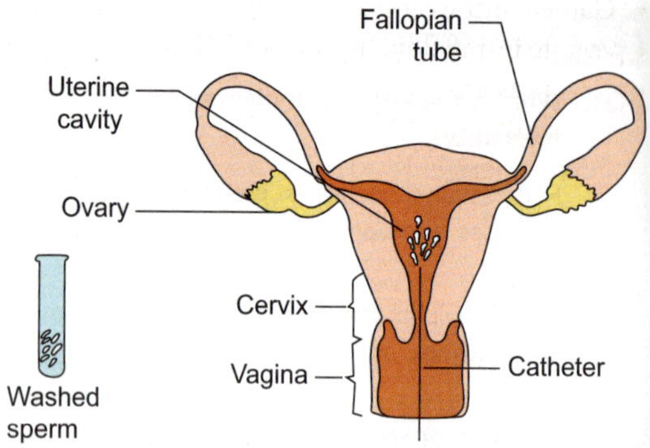

Figure 25.7 Pictorial representation of intrauterine insemination procedure.

Indications for IUI

- Unexplained infertility
- Male factor infertility such as oligospermia, asthenospermia, ejaculatory failure, and retrograde ejaculation
- Mild to moderate endometriosis
- Cervical factor for infertility such as cervical stenosis, and antisperm antibodies
- Failure to conceive with ovulation induction

ASSISTED REPRODUCTIVE TECHNOLOGY

Definition

ART refers to the procedures that handle gametes and embryos in vitro for the purpose of assisting in conception of couples.

The various ART procedures include the following:

- IVF
- Assisted fertilization techniques such as ICSI and assisted hatching (AH)

Viva corner

Q1 How does IUI increase the chance of conception?

The chance of conception increases following IUI for the following reasons:

- The semen is processed prior to IUI to remove semen proteins and concentrate the sperms.
  - Sperm washing helps to eliminate toxins and induces acrosomal reaction.
  - Sperm migration or density gradient techniques are used to select motile sperms.
- The procedure overcomes cervical mucus hostility.
- The procedure increases the number of sperms deposited into uterine cavity.

Q2 What are the indications for donor insemination?

- Azoospermia and severe oligospermia in male partner
- Failed intracytoplasmic sperm injection (ICSI)
- Risk of genetic transmission from male partner

- Gamete intrafallopian transfer (GIFT)
- Zygote intrafallopian transfer (ZIFT)
- Cryopreservation of sperms, oocytes, and embryos
- Donor sperms, oocytes, and embryo
- Gestational surrogacy

Complications of ART

- Multiple gestation
- OHSS
- Ectopic pregnancy
- Increased risk of prematurity, low birth weight (LBW), and possible neurodevelopmental delay in the offsprings

IVF

Indications for IVF

- Tubal factors for infertility
- Endometriosis—if pregnancy is not achieved with IUI + COH
- Unexplained infertility
- Severe male factor infertility
- Cervical or immunological factor for infertility
- Failure to conceive with IUI (three cycles)
- Failure of ovulation
- Cryopreservation of embryos for future use

IVF procedure

IVF procedure includes:

- Retrieving preovulatory oocytes from the ovary
- IVF of sperm and ovum
- Subsequent embryo transfer into the endometrial cavity

All patients should be assessed for ovarian reserve before enrolling for assisted reproductive techniques.

Steps of IVF procedure

Ovarian stimulation Ovarian stimulation protocols are used to increase the number of recruited ovarian follicles that get transformed into dominant follicles. COH is by downregulation with GnRH analogues and ovulation induction with gonadotropins. GnRH antagonists are also being used for downregulation.

Follicular aspiration The oocytes are aspirated from the ovary under ultrasound guidance on the day when the follicles are 17–18 mm in size.

Oocyte classification Following aspiration, the oocytes are graded according to the appearance of the corona–cumulus complex.

Semen preparation and oocyte insemination Semen preparation involves the following:

- Removal of certain components of the ejaculate (i.e., seminal fluid, excess cellular debris, leukocytes, morphologically abnormal sperms, etc.)
- Retention of the motile fraction of sperms
- Motile sperms in media added to the oocytes (oocyte insemination)

Embryo culture

- The inseminated oocytes are incubated for fertilization to occur.
- Criteria to ascertain fertilization include the presence of two pronuclei and extrusion of second polar body (occur approximately 18 hours following insemination).
- The fertilized embryos are transferred into growth media and incubated.
- A four-to eight-cell-stage, embryo is observed approximately 36–48 hours following insemination.

Embryo transfer

- Embryo transfer into endometrial cavity is done within 72 hours after oocyte insemination, when the embryo is approximately 8–16 cells in size.
- The transfer is usually performed transcervically under transabdominal ultrasound guidance.
- Luteal phase support is provided with vaginal progesterone.

Embryo cryopreservation Several eggs can be retrieved in a single cycle and fertilized, but only two or three embryos are transferred to the uterus. The remaining embryos can be cryopreserved and used in subsequent cycles.

Part 2

Viva corner

Q1 What are the indications for intracytoplasmic sperm injection?

ICSI is an assisted reproductive technology involving the direct injection of a single live sperm into an oocyte.

Indications for ICSI are as follows:

- Severe defects in semen quality (severe oligospermia/asthenospermia/teratospermia)
- Obstructive and nonobstructive azoospermia
- Failure of previous IVF cycles
- Ejaculatory failure
- Surgically retrieved/cryopreserved sperms
- Immotile cilia syndrome

Q2 What are the indications for oocyte donation?

- Ovarian failure
- Reduced ovarian reserve
- Gonadal dysgenesis
- Patient who underwent oophorectomy
- Previous failed IVF
- Women with genetically transmitted diseases

Q3 What are the indications for gestational surrogacy?

- Absent uterus
- Uterine pathology that is not able to support pregnancy
- Medical conditions where pregnancy is unsafe

Frequently asked viva questions

1. Summarize the case.
2. What is the provisional diagnosis?
3. How do you want to evaluate the case?
4. What are the normal semen analysis parameters?
5. How will you test for tubal patency?
6. How will you confirm ovulation?
7. What are the advantages and disadvantages of laparoscopy and HSG in workup for infertility?
8. How will you manage anovulation?
9. How will you manage tubal factors for infertility?
10. What is unexplained infertility?
11. How will you manage the case?
12. What are the indications for IUI?
13. What are the indications for IVF?

26 Amenorrhea

Introduction

Basic factors involved in the onset and continuation of normal menstruation are the following:

- Normal female chromosomal pattern (46, XX)
- Coordinated hypothalamopituitary–ovarian (HPO) axis
- Responsive endometrium
- Anatomical presence and patency of the outflow tract
- Active support of thyroid and adrenal glands.

Amenorrhea can develop as a result of problems in any of the factors mentioned above. Evaluation of a case of amenorrhea is briefed in this chapter.

Definition

Amenorrhea refers to the absence of menstruation or abnormal cessation of menstruation.

Classification of amenorrhea

Amenorrhea can be due to physiological or pathological causes as mentioned in Table 26.1.

Table 26.1 Classification of amenorrhea

Physiological amenorrhea	Pathological amenorrhea

• Prepubertal age group
• During pregnancy, lactation, and after menopause
	• Cryptomenorrhea
	• True amenorrhea
	  – Primary amenorrhea
	  – Secondary amenorrhea

- **Cryptomenorrhea:** Periodic shedding of the endometrium occurs, but the menstrual blood does not come out of the genital tract due to outflow tract obstruction. It usually presents as primary amenorrhea
- **Primary amenorrhea**: It refers to nonattainment/absence of menarche by 13 years of age in the absence of development of secondary sexual characteristics, or nonattainment/absence of menarche by 15 years of age with normal development of secondary sexual characteristics.
- **Secondary amenorrhea:** It refers to the absence of menstruation for at least 6 months, or for a period three times the length of previous menstrual cycles in a woman who was previously menstruating, in the absence of pregnancy.

Viva corner

Q1 What are the causes of cryptomenorrhea and how will you treat?

Causes of cryptomenorrhea are as follows:

- Congenital causes
  - Imperforate hymen
  - Transverse vaginal septum
  - Atresia of vagina and cervix
- Acquired causes
  - Stenosis of the cervix following amputation, cauterization, and conization

Treatment

- Imperforate hymen a cruciate incision is given under aseptic precautions to let out the retained blood collection
- Transverse vaginal septum—excision of the vaginal septum
- Cervical stenosis— dilatation of the cervix
- Vaginal atresia—vaginal reconstructive surgery to maintain the patency of outflow tract

PRIMARY AMENORRHEA

Causes of primary amenorrhea

Primary amenorrhea is usually the result of genetic or anatomic abnormality. However, all causes of secondary amenorrhea can present as primary amenorrhea. Causes of primary amenorrhea include those given in the next subsections.

Hypogonadotropic hypogonadism

- **Constitutional delay:** Delayed puberty due to delayed gonadotropin-releasing hormone (GnRH) pulse activation
- **Hypothalamo pituitary dysfunction:** Due to stress, weight loss, anorexia nervosa, chronic illness, and Kallmann syndrome (deficiency of GnRH)
- **Hypothalamopituitary lesion/pathology:** Pituitary adenoma, prolactinoma, and following radiotherapy

Hypergonadotropic hypogonadism

Premature ovarian failure or primary ovarian insufficiency: It may be due to Turner syndrome leading to gonadal dysgenesis, autoimmune diseases, or idiopathic causes.

Abnormal chromosomal pattern

- Turner syndrome (45, XO)
- Pure gonadal dysgenesis (46, XX or 46, YY)
- Androgen insensitivity syndrome (AIS), otherwise termed testicular feminization syndrome (TFS) (46, XY)

Developmental defect

Absence of uterus—Mullerian agenesis [Mayer-Rokitansky-Kuster-Hauser syndrome (MRKHS)]

Case presentation

Salient points in history

Consider the following relevant points during history taking in cases of primary amenorrhea:

- *Age*
- *Childhood growth and development (growth charts, if available)*
- *Age at menarche of the patient's mother and siblings*
- *H/o cyclical abdominal pain or H/o difficulty in emptying the bladder or acute retention of urine—features of Mullerian tract obstruction*
- *H/o vigorous exercise and dieting*
- *H/o recent weight gain or weight loss*
- *H/o headache and visual changes (pituitary adenoma*
- *H/o galactorrhea (prolactinoma)*
- *H/o thyroid symptoms*
- *H/o anosmia (Kallmann syndrome)*
- *H/o any chronic illness, tuberculosis*
- *H/o previous surgeries*
- *H/o radiotherapy, chemotherapy, and any other medications*

Salient points in examination

Consider the following relevant points during examination in cases of primary amenorrhea:

General examination

- *Height (short stature is a feature of Turner syndrome; tall stature may be seen in AIS)*
- *Weight*
- *Body mass index (BMI)—underweight or obese*
- *Hirsutism*
- *BP*
- *Stigmata of Turner syndrome—short stature, webbed neck, low hairline, low-set ears, broad chest ("shield" chest) with widely spaced nipples, undeveloped breasts, epicanthal folds, micrognathia, and an increase in carrying angle of the elbows*
- *Anorexia nervosa—cachexia, bradycardia, hypotension, hypothermia, and BMI <18 present*
- *Breast—[assess Tanner staging; check for galactorrhea (delayed puberty is associated with underdeveloped breasts; Mullerian agenesis and*

(CONTD...)

(...CONTD)

AIS are associated with well-developed breasts; hyperprolactinemia may present with galactorrhea)]

- *Axillary and pubic hairs—[assess Tanner staging (delayed puberty is associated with sparse pubic hair; Mullerian agenesis and Mullerian tract obstruction—normal axillary and pubic hair; AIS—absent or sparse axillary and pubic hair)]*
- *Field of vision and sense of smell checked for (field of vision may be affected in pituitary adenoma; anosmia is associated with Kallmann syndrome)*

CVS and RS examinations

Cardiac murmur may be present in Turner syndrome.

Abdominal examination

- *Palpate for any abdominal mass.*
  - *Palpate inguinal region: Testes may be palpable as inguinal swelling.*
  - *Imperforate hymen with hematometra: Uterus may be enlarged.*

Pelvic examination

Check for patency of vagina and cervix; presence of uterus by rectal examination

- *Pelvic examination (helps in detection of imperforate hymen, vaginal septum, congenital absence of the vagina/uterus).*
  - *Imperforate hymen: Bluish bulging membrane is seen at introitus.*
  - *Mullerian agenesis: The vagina is absent or short, with a rudimentary uterus or absent uterus.*
  - *AIS: The vagina is short and uterus is absent; testes may be palpable in the inguinal region.*
  - *Uterine enlargement: Hematometra due to imperforate hymen can present with uterine enlargement and primary amenorrhea. Pregnancy must be excluded.*

Case summary

An example of writing summary in cases of primary amenorrhea is given below.

Example *Ms. T, 15 years of age, was brought by her mother with a history of not having attained menarche. On examination, her height is 135 cm, breast development is absent, and webbing of neck is present. Abdominal examination is normal and hymen is patent.*

Case diagnosis

An example of writing diagnosis in cases of primary amenorrhea is given below.

Example *15 years of age, with primary amenorrhea for evaluation. Considering her clinical features, it could probably be a case of Turner syndrome.*

Case discussion

Evaluation of primary amenorrhea (Flowchart 26.1)

Rule out cryptomenorrhea due to imperforate hymen or transverse vaginal septum.

Check for the presence/absence of breast development (by clinical examination) and for the presence/absence of uterus (by ultrasonography)

If breasts are well developed, but uterus is absent Only two conditions are possible—AIS or MRKHS (Mullerian agenesis). Do karyotyping.

- AIS: Karyotyping is 46, XY.
- MRKHS: Karyotyping is 46, XX.

If breast development is present and uterus is present It implies that the patient has been exposed to estrogen in the past. Workup is similar to a case of secondary amenorrhea as mentioned in Flowchart 26.2.

If breast development is absent and uterus is present It implies that the patient has never been exposed to estrogen. It could be due to primary ovarian failure or failure of pituitary gonadotropin secretion. Workup is as follows:

- An endocrine evaluation is done. Serum follicle-stimulating hormone (FSH), luteinizing hormone (LH), thyroid-stimulating hormone (TSH), and prolactin are checked.
- Elevated FSH and LH levels (hypergonadotropic hypogonadism) imply gonadal dysgenesis or premature ovarian failure (POF).

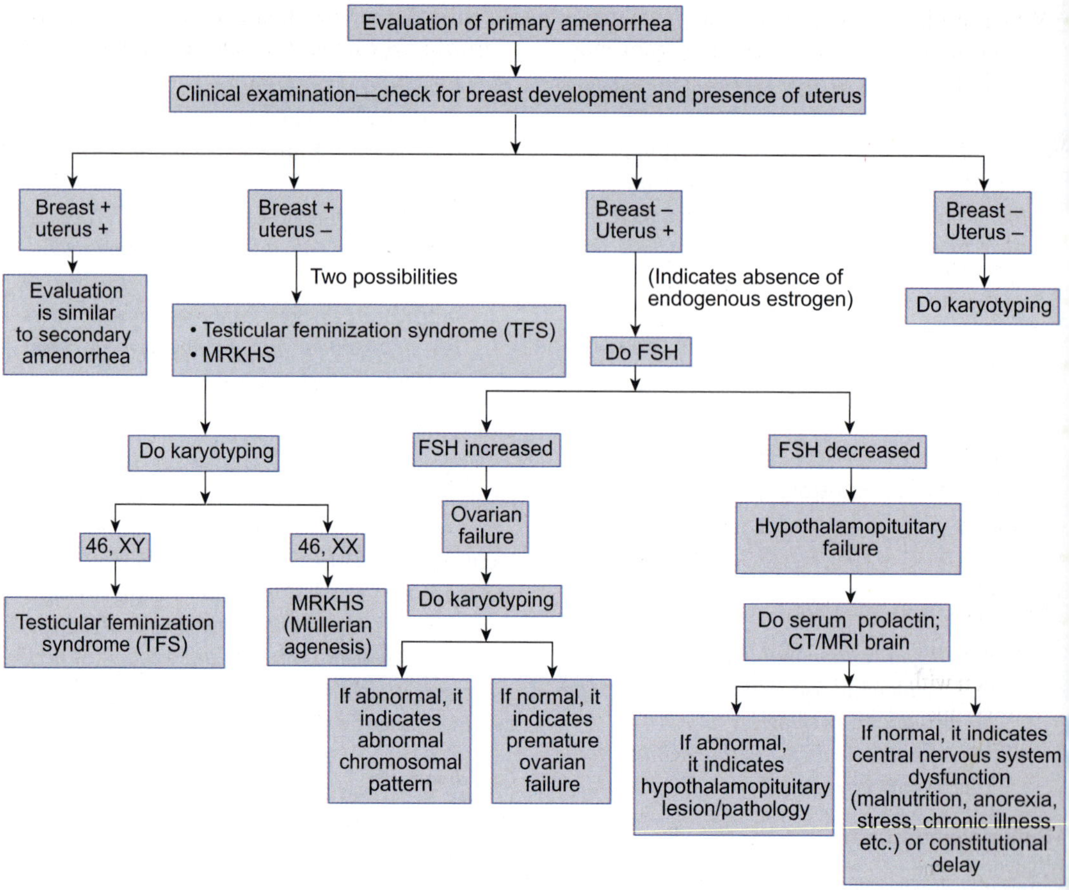

Flowchart 26.1 Evaluation of primary amenorrhea. *FSH,* follicle-stimulating hormone; *MRKHS,* Mayer-Rokitansky-Kuster-Hauser syndrome.

Turner syndrome (45, XO karyotype) is the most common cause of gonadal dysgenesis.

- Low FSH and LH levels imply constitutional delay of puberty or hypothalamic or pituitary failure (hypogonadotropic hypogonadism).
  - *Do MRI brain*: Detects central nervous system (CNS) tumors or empty sella syndrome where pituitary is affected causing decreased gonadotropin secretion.
  - *Do bone age radiograph*: Helps to distinguish a case of constitutional delay from hypogonadotropic hypogonadism.
- If signs or symptoms of hyperandrogenism are present, check serum testosterone, dehydroepiandrosterone sulfate (DHEAS), and 17-hydroxyprogesterone—to assess for congenital adrenal hyperplasia (CAH) or any androgen-secreting tumor of the ovary.

Management of primary amenorrhea

It depends on the cause of primary amenorrhea. Management of some of the specific causes of primary amenorrhea is described below.

Management of primary amenorrhea due to hypogonadotropic hypogonadism

- Constitutional delay, anorexia, and hypothyroidism are reversible causes—will respond to intervention.
- Any organic lesion—surgical removal is done.
- Cases with absent sexual development—treated by pubertal induction with low incremental doses of estrogen, followed by cyclical estrogen–progesterone therapy to correct hypoestrogenism and to provide regular withdrawal bleed.

- When fertility is required, ovulation induction can be done by administration of exogenous gonadotropins or pulsatile GnRH therapy.

Management of primary amenorrhea due to premature ovarian failure (hypergonadotropic hypogonadism)

- POF may present with primary or secondary amenorrhea.
- It is diagnosed on the basis of amenorrhea and elevated serum FSH levels (>40 IU/L).
- Karyotyping is done to identify Turner syndrome (45,XO).
- Most of the cases are idiopathic. Autoimmune disorders may coexist with POF, especially thyroid disorders that need evaluation and management.
- POF is managed with hormone replacement therapy.
- Estrogen plus progesterone replacement is required until the age of normal menopause (women with POF are at increased risk of osteoporosis due to low estradiol levels).
- Infertility can be treated with oocyte donation or else adoption can be done.

Management of Turner syndrome

- Turner syndrome (45,XO) is associated with ovarian dysgenesis and premature ovarian failure.
- Health issues in Turner syndrome include growth failure, cardiovascular disease, gonadal failure, and learning disabilities.
- Hormonal replacement therapy should be given to facilitate pubertal induction and continued until 50 years of age.
- Estrogen therapy should be coordinated with growth hormone therapy to optimize both growth and pubertal development.
- These patients have an increased risk of cardiovascular and renal problems. Echocardiography should be done every 5–10 years and hypertension should be treated.
- Infertility can be treated with oocyte donation.

Extra edge

Indications for surgical intervention in patients with primary amenorrhea

- Surgery is required in patients with congenital anatomic lesions (Mullerian agenesis) and those with Y chromosome (AIS).
  - Absence of vagina—reconstruction of an artificial vagina. The most common technique used is McIndoe vaginoplasty.
  - AIS (46,XY)—gonadectomy is performed to prevent gonadal malignancy (usually gonadoblastoma). Gonadectomy is delayed until puberty to ensure proper breast development, which occurs due to peripheral aromatization of testosterone (secreted by the testis) to estrogen.
- Androgen-secreting tumor of ovary or adrenal gland—surgical removal is done.

Part 2

SECONDARY AMENORRHEA

Causes of secondary amenorrhea

Various causes of secondary amenorrhea are mentioned in Table 26.2. Pregnancy should be excluded in all cases with secondary amenorrhea.

Table 26.2 Causes of secondary amenorrhea

Hypothalamic causes	Pituitary causes	Ovarian causes	Uterine causes	Other causes
• Stress • Weight loss or weight gain • Athletes (physical overactivity) • Granulomas due to tuberculosis and sarcoidosis • Tumors • Trauma • Chronic illness	• Pituitary necrosis (Sheehan syndrome) • Tuberculosis • Pituitary adenomas • Prolactinoma	• Polycystic ovarian disease • Primary ovarian insufficiency	• Intrauterine adhesions • Tuberculosis • Cervical stenosis	• Hypothyroidism • Cushing disease • Congenital adrenal hyperplasia

Case presentation

Salient points in history

Consider the following relevant points during history taking in cases of secondary amenorrhea:

- *Age*
- *Parity*
- *Duration of amenorrhea*
- *H/o previous menstrual cycles—regularity, duration, and amount of flow; dysmenorrhea*
- *Symptoms suggestive of hyperandrogenism—acne, hirsutism, and deepening of voice*
- *H/o vigorous exercise, weight loss or gain, vigorous dieting and H/o recent stress or illness*
- *H/o galactorrhea, headache, and visual field defects (may indicate CNS lesion)*
- *History suggestive of thyroid dysfunction*
- *History suggestive of tuberculosis*
- *Symptoms of menopause—hot flushes, vaginal dryness, sleep disturbances, mood changes, and decreased libido*
- *Obstetric history—H/o severe postpartum hemorrhage (PPH) with lactation failure (which indicates Sheehan syndrome)*
- *H/o endometrial curettage (curettage may cause endometritis and scarring of the endometrial lining and possible Asherman syndrome)*
- *Contraceptive history—H/o COC pill intake or depot medroxyprogesterone acetate (MPA) injections (may cause amenorrhea)*
- *Past history—surgery, tuberculosis, chronic diseases, radiotherapy, and chemotherapy*
- *Drug history (drugs such as danazol, metoclopramide, and antipsychotics such as phenothiazine can cause menstrual irregularities or amenorrhea)*
- *Family history—H/o autoimmune diseases, diabetes mellitus*

Salient points in examination

Consider the following relevant points during examination in cases of secondary amenorrhea:

General examination

- *Height, weight, and BMI [BMI >30 kg/m² is seen in 50% of women with polycystic ovarian disease (PCOD); patients with BMI <18.5 kg/m² may have hypothalamic dysfunction]*
- *BP*
- *Examination for signs of hyperandrogenism—hirsutism, acne*
- *Checking for signs of insulin resistance—acanthosis nigricans*
- *Examination for stigmata of Cushing disease—striae and easy bruising*
- *Neurological examination for visual field defects*
- *Breast—checking for galactorrhea, atrophy*
- *Thyroid examination—any thyroid swelling*

Abdominal examination

Palpate for any mass and tenderness

Pelvic examination

Check the following: loss of pubic hair, vulvar and vaginal atrophy (indicate hypoestrogenism); cervical stenosis; uterine size.

Case summary

An example of writing summary in cases of secondary amenorrhea is given below.

Example *Ms. R, 20 years of age, unmarried, presents with amenorrhea of 7 months' duration. She attained menarche at the age of 13 years and has irregular cycles since menarche. On examination, her height is 160 cm, weight is 78 kg, hirsutism is present, vitals are stable, breast and thyroid examinations are normal, and systemic and abdominal examinations are normal. External genitalia are healthy.*

Case diagnosis

An example of writing diagnosis in cases of secondary amenorrhea is given below.

Example *20 years of age, unmarried girl with secondary amenorrhea. Her history and clinical examination findings are suggestive of anovulatory dysfunction, probably due to PCOD.*

Case discussion

Evaluation of secondary amenorrhea (Flowchart 26.2)

- Secondary amenorrhea can occur as a result of problem in the hypothalamus, pituitary, ovary, uterus, or endocrine systems such as the thyroid.
- Rule out pregnancy by doing a urine pregnancy test.
- Once pregnancy is ruled out, TSH and prolactin levels are checked.
- After thyroid disease and hyperprolactinemia are eliminated, the remaining causes of secondary amenorrhea are classified as hypogonadotropic hypogonadism, hypergonadotropic hypogonadism, and normogonadotropic amenorrhea, each associated with specific etiologies.
- **The patient is then evaluated as follows:**
  - *The next step is to do a progestogen challenge test*—it helps to evaluate for a functioning endometrium and to detect endogenous estrogen that acts on the endometrium. MPA 10 mg is given for 5 days and withdrawal bleeding is awaited. If the patient has withdrawal bleeding, it indicates presence of endogenous estrogen and a functioning endometrium. Anovulation as in PCOD is the most common cause of amenorrhea in such cases. A negative progestogen challenge test indicates either an endometrial pathology or inadequate endogenous estrogen.
  - *The next step is to do an estrogen plus progestogen challenge test*— it can differentiate secondary amenorrhea due to endometrial pathology from that due to inadequate endogenous estrogen. The test involves administration of estrogen and progesterone in a sequential manner—conjugated equine estrogen 0.625 mg/day for 21 days and MPA 10 mg in the last 10 days.
  - A negative estrogen plus progestogen challenge test indicates a nonfunctioning endometrium such as in Asherman syndrome. Proceed with hysteroscopy or HSG in such cases. A positive test indicates absence of endogenous estrogen as in disorders of the hypothalamic–pituitary axis or the ovaries.
- The source of abnormality (whether hypothalamic–pituitary axis or the ovaries) for the absence of endogenous estrogen can be determined by estimation of gonadotropin levels. Normal or low FSH or LH levels suggest a pituitary or hypothalamic abnormality (hypogonadotropic hypogonadism). Elevated FSH and LH levels suggest an ovarian abnormality (hypergonadotropic hypogonadism).
- In case of hypogonadotropic hypogonadism, MRI brain is done to rule out pituitary tumor or an empty sella syndrome. Normal MRI indicates a hypothalamic dysfunction as the cause of amenorrhea such as stress, eating disorders, and vigorous exercises.
- Patients <40 years of age with secondary amenorrhea and elevated FSH levels (>40 IU/L) are considered to have POF.
- Patients with POF should undergo investigation of the other endocrine organs (particularly thyroid) as they can have other associated endocrinopathies.
- Karyotyping should be considered in women with secondary amenorrhea at age ≤30 years to rule out chromosomal abnormalities. Turner mosaics can have normal appearance and childbearing, but subsequently develop ovarian failure and secondary amenorrhea. These women are at risk for cardiac problems and should be investigated for CVS anomalies.

Management of secondary amenorrhea

It depends on the underlying cause such as the following:

- Treatment of hypothyroidism
- Treatment of hyperprolactinemia
- Weight loss and treatment for anovulation associated with PCOD
- Cyclical estrogen and progesterone therapy should be given in women with estrogen deficiency due to hypothalamopituitary or ovarian failure, till the normal age of menopause

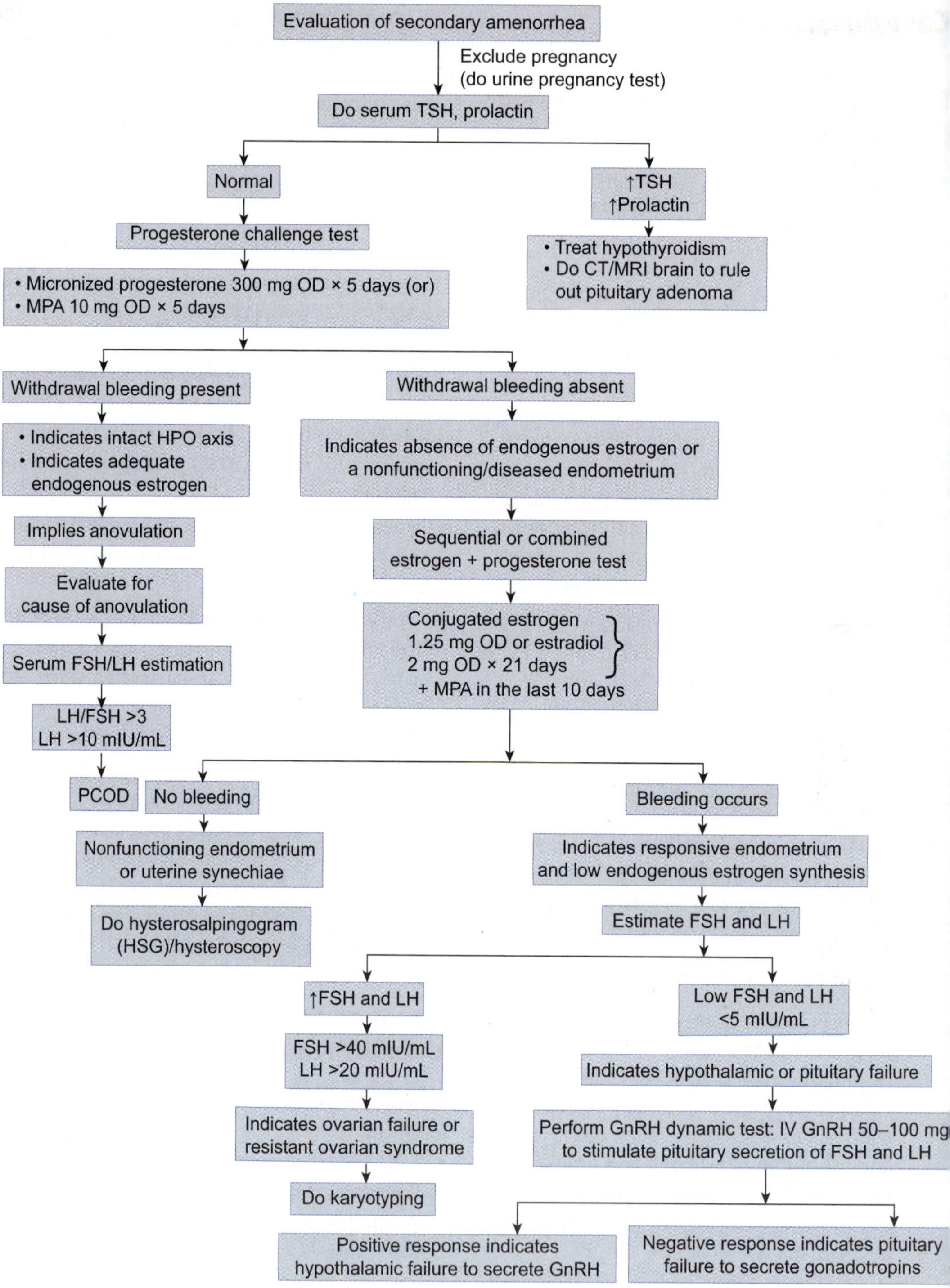

Flowchart 26.2 Evaluation of secondary amenorrhea. *FSH*, follicle-stimulating hormone; *GnRH*, gonadotropin-releasing hormone; *LH*, luteinizing hormone; *MPA*, medroxyprogesterone acetate; *PCOD*, polycystic ovarian disease; *TSH*, thyroid-stimulating hormone.

Extra edge

Management of hyperprolactinemia

- Rule out use of medications that may cause hyperprolactinemia (e.g., antipsychotics, antidepressants, antihypertensives, opiates). Medications raise prolactin levels, but to less than 100 ng/mL.
- A prolactin level >100 ng/mL suggests a prolactinoma and MRI should be performed.
  - Microadenomas (smaller than 10 mm) are slow growing and rarely malignant. Treatment of microadenomas should focus on management of infertility and galactorrhea. Dopamine agonists such as bromocriptine and cabergoline help to relieve symptoms and to restore fertility.
  - Macroadenomas are treated with dopamine agonists or removed by transsphenoidal resection, if necessary.
- Bromocriptine: Start with 2.5 mg at bedtime to minimize side effects (orthostatic hypotension, nausea, headache, fainting), and then slowly increase the dose to 7.5–10 mg/day as required.
- Cabergoline: Start with 0.25 mg once a week and then increase up to 3 mg weekly, as required.

Management of some of the specific causes of secondary amenorrhea is described below.

Management of secondary amenorrhea due to hypothalamopituitary causes (hypogonadotropic hypogonadism)

Hypothalamic amenorrhea

It is associated with abnormalities in GnRH secretion. Excessive weight loss, exercise, and stress are the most common causes.

Treatment of hypothalamic amenorrhea depends on the etiology.

- Women with excessive weight loss should be screened for eating disorders such as anorexia nervosa or bulimia nervosa. Menstruation usually resumes when a healthy body weight is achieved.
- Young athletes may develop a triad that includes eating disorder, amenorrhea, and osteoporosis. Menstruation usually resumes after a modest increase in caloric intake or a decrease in athletic training.
- In patients with amenorrhea caused by eating disorders or vigorous exercise, COC pills may decrease bone turnover and reverse bone loss.

Sheehan syndrome (pituitary amenorrhea)

Secondary amenorrhea can occur as a result of postpartum pituitary necrosis (Sheehan syndrome), following massive PPH.

Diagnosis

- Patients present with characteristic H/o massive PPH, failed lactation, and loss of pubic and axillary hair.
- Levels of estradiol, FSH, and LH are decreased.
- Serum levels of other anterior pituitary hormones should also be checked.

Treatment

- Hormone replacement with estrogen and progesterone restores menstrual function.
- Other anterior pituitary hormones [particularly TSH and adrenocorticotropic hormone (ACTH)] may be deficient and require replacement with thyroid hormone and corticosteroid.
- Pregnancy can be achieved by ovulation induction with exogenous gonadotropins.

Management of secondary amenorrhea due to premature ovarian failure (hypergonadotropic hypogonadism)

- POF is characterized by amenorrhea, hypoestrogenism, and increased gonadotropin levels (FSH >40 IU/L) occurring at less than 40 years of age.
- Karyotyping is done in women with secondary amenorrhea at less than 30 years to rule out complete or partial deletion of the X chromosome.
- Women with POF are at an increased risk of osteoporosis due to hypoestrogenism. Hence, estrogen–progesterone replacement is required to correct hypoestrogenism and to restore menstrual function. The treatment should be continued till the normal age of menopause.
- POF can be associated with autoimmune endocrine disorders such as hypothyroidism, Addison disease, and diabetes mellitus, and hence periodic screening is required.
- Fertility is possible through oocyte donation and in vitro fertilization (IVF).

Management of secondary amenorrhea due to polycystic ovarian disease and Asherman syndrome (normogonadotropic secondary amenorrhea)

Polycystic ovarian disease

It is the most common cause of chronic anovulation. Insulin resistance is thought to be the fundamental etiology in PCOD.

Diagnosis

- To diagnose PCOD, any two of the following three criteria should be present:
  - Oligomenorrhea/amenorrhea
  - Signs of androgen excess
  - Presence of polycystic ovaries on ultrasound (≥12 follicles of 2–9 mm in size, with increased ovarian volume ≥10 mL)
- In cases with hyperandrogenic symptoms, serum testosterone and other androgens should be ascertained.
- Screening for Cushing syndrome is done by doing a dexamethasone suppression test in women with characteristic features such as striae, buffalo hump, central obesity, easy bruising, hypertension, and proximal muscle weakness.

Treatment of polycystic ovarian disease

Treatment depends on the presenting complaints.

- Cyclical progesterones or COC pills are given to cause cyclical endometrial shedding to protect against endometrial hyperplasia.
- Weight loss through diet and exercise: Modest weight loss can lower androgen levels, improve hirsutism, normalize menstruation, and decrease insulin resistance.
- Insulin-sensitizing agents such as metformin (500–850 mg BD) can reduce insulin resistance and improve ovulatory function.
- Patients with hirsutism require management with antiandrogens such as spironolactone and cyproterone acetate.
- Infertility due to PCOD is managed with ovulation induction with clomiphene or gonadotropins. In resistant cases, laparoscopic ovarian drilling may be done.
- There is increased risk of diabetes mellitus due to insulin resistance—glucose tolerance test should be performed.

Asherman syndrome

Asherman syndrome refers to intrauterine adhesions.

Causes

- Following dilatation and curettage procedure (especially during postpartum period when the endometrium is highly susceptible to adhesions)
- Following endometrial ablation
- Uterine infections—genital tuberculosis

Diagnosis

- There is absence of normal endometrial strip on pelvic ultrasound.
- Hysteroscopy, HSG, or saline infusion sonography (SIS), can confirm the diagnosis.

Treatment

- Hysteroscopic lysis of intrauterine adhesions may be helpful.
- Long-term treatment with estrogen and progestogen may stimulate regrowth of the endometrium.

Women who become pregnant after treatment of Asherman syndrome are at a high risk of obstetric complications such as abortion, preterm labor, spontaneous uterine rupture, placenta accreta, intrauterine growth restriction (IUGR), and PPH.

Frequently asked viva questions

1. What are the common causes of primary amenorrhea?
2. How will you evaluate a patient with primary amenorrhea?
3. What are the common causes of secondary amenorrhea?
4. How will you evaluate a case of secondary amenorrhea?

27 Abnormal Vaginal Discharge

Introduction

Discharge per vaginum (P/V) is one of the common gynecological complaints that can be discussed during clinical case presentation in gynecology and has been briefed in this chapter.

Leukorrhea refers to excess of normal vaginal discharge. Normal vaginal secretion is nonodorous and nonhomogenous, with pH of 3.8–4.5, and varies with the menstrual cycle.

- **Proliferative phase:** Thin, copious, stretchable discharge under estrogen influence
- **Secretory phase:** Viscid, scanty discharge under progesterone influence

Causes of leukorrhea

- **Physiological causes:** Increased vaginal secretions occur during puberty, pregnancy, ovulation, and premenstrual phase.
- **Cervical causes:** These include cervical ectopy, ectropion, and cervical mucus polyp.
- **Vaginal causes:** Increased transudation of fluid from the vaginal epithelium occurs when there is pelvic congestion such as in uterovaginal prolapse, retroverted fixed uterus, and combined oral contraceptive (COC) pill usage.
- **Ill health:** Any chronic illness can cause excessive exfoliation of superficial cells → excess vaginal discharge.

ABNORMAL VAGINAL DISCHARGE

Abnormal vaginal discharge is characterized by a change of color, consistency, volume, or odor and may be associated with symptoms such as itch, soreness, dysuria, pelvic pain, or intermenstrual and postcoital bleeding.

Common causes of abnormal vaginal discharge

See Table 27.1

Causes of abnormal vaginal discharge in various age groups

See Table 27.2

Table 27.1 Common causes of abnormal vaginal discharge

	Cause	Nature of discharge
Infective	• Trichomonal vaginitis • Candidal vaginitis • Bacterial vaginosis • Cervicitis caused by chlamydia and gonorrhea	• Greenish yellow discharge with pruritis • Curdy white flakes with pruritis • Frothy white discharge • Mucopurulent discharge
Atrophic	Postmenopausal atrophic vaginitis	Irritation is more than the discharge
Foreign body	Forgotten pessary, tampons	Offensive, purulent, blood-stained discharge
Chemicals	Douches, latex condoms, deodorants	Irritation is more than the discharge
Neoplasms	Infected fibroid polyp, carcinoma cervix	Serosanguinous, often offensive discharge
Contamination	Fecal and urine contamination	Offensive discharge with pruritis

Table 27.2 Causes of abnormal vaginal discharge in various age groups

Premenarchal	Adolescent and reproductive age groups	Postmenopausal age group
• Foreign body in vagina • Sexual abuse • Poor perineal hygiene • Chemical irritants—lotions, bubble baths • Pinworm infection • Skin lesions—eczema, psoriasis	• Chlamydial and gonorrheal infections • Bacterial vaginosis • Trichomonal vaginitis • Candidiasis • Chemical irritants	• Atrophic vaginitis • Cervicitis • Cervical carcinoma • Vulvar, vaginal, or endometrial carcinoma

Case presentation

Salient points in history

Consider the following relevant points during history taking in cases of discharge P/V.

Age of the patient

- ***Newborn:*** *Withdrawal of maternal estrogen causes mucoid or blood-stained discharge.*
- ***Premenarchal:*** *Worm infestation is common; foreign body should be ruled out in case of blood-stained, foul-smelling discharge.*
- ***Adolescent and reproductive age groups:*** *Infective causes are common.*
- ***Postmenopausal:*** *Carcinoma cervix and pyometra have to be ruled out.*

Presenting complaints

Discharge per vaginum

Duration *The presentation is acute in case of infective vaginal discharge.*

Amount of discharge *The discharge is scanty in candidiasis.*

Color of discharge

- *Trichomoniasis—profuse, thin, and creamy or greenish yellow discharge*
- *Candidiasis—thick curdy white discharge*
- *Bacterial vaginosis—frothy white homogenous discharge*
- *Blood stained in cervical erosion and malignancy*

Odor

- *Foul smell is present in pathological discharge.*
- *Fishy odor is present in bacterial vaginosis.*

Associated pruritis

- *Trichomoniasis—moderate itching with profuse discharge*
- *Candidiasis—intense itching with scanty discharge*
- *H/o pruritus and discomfort especially at night is typically suggestive of pinworm infection*

Associated symptoms

- *Discharge in relation to menstrual cycles (physiological discharge varies during the menstrual cycle; if postmenopausal, atrophic vaginitis is a common cause of vaginal irritation and discharge)*
- *H/o dysuria, increased frequency and urgency of micturition (urinary symptoms may be frequently associated with vaginitis)*
- *H/o superficial dyspareunia—may be present in vaginitis*
- *H/o fever and lower abdominal pain—may be suggestive of pelvic inflammatory disease (PID)*
- *H/o postmenopausal or postcoital bleeding—suggestive of malignancy*
- *H/o intrauterine contraceptive device (IUCD) usage*
- *H/o COC pill usage—may cause leukorrhea*
- *H/o similar episodes in the past (may be suggestive of infection)*
- *H/o intake of antibiotics in recent past—may predispose to vulvovaginal candidiasis*
- *H/o diabetes—prone to develop vulvovaginal candidiasis*
- *H/o HIV infection—prone to develop vulvovaginal candidiasis*

(CONTD...)

...CONTD)

Hygiene practices

- *Frequent vaginal douching increases the risk of bacterial vaginosis.*
- *Regular use of chemical irritants such as soaps, spermicides, perfumes, and creams can cause vulvovaginitis.*
- *Tight-fitting, synthetic, and nylon undergarments can retain the moisture and predispose to infection.*
- *Wiping the anus from posterior to anterior while using toilet paper increases the risk of vaginitis.*

Sexual history

- *H/o multiple sexual partners*
- *H/o recent change of partner in the past 3 months*
- *H/o similar symptoms in the partner (e.g., dysuria, urethral discharge, ulcers)*
- *H/o whether having protected or unprotected intercourse*
- *H/o sexually transmitted diseases (STDs) in the past*

Past Medical History

- *Any history of experiencing similar symptoms in the past*
- *Use of any antibiotics in recent past (act as a predisposing factor for development of candidal vulvovaginitis)*
- *History of a systemic disease that could affect the vulvovaginal area (e.g., HSV and Behçet's disease can cause vulvovaginal ulcers; women with diabetes or HIV infections are prone to develop VVC*

Salient points in examination

Consider the following relevant points during examination in cases of discharge P/V.

General examination

- *Nutritional status*
- *Pallor*
- *Temperature, pulse (fever, tachycardia may be present in acute PID)*

Abdominal examination

Check for any lower abdominal tenderness (may be present in PID and cystitis).

Pelvic examination

External genitalia

Inspect for the following:

- *Scratch marks/excoriations*
- *Vulvar erythema and edema (indicate vulvitis)*
- *Any ulcer/growth*

Speculum examination

Look for the color, odor, and amount of discharge.

Vagina

Look for the following:

- *Signs of vaginal mucosal inflammation such as erythema and punctate hemorrhages—may be due to candidiasis or trichomoniasis*
- *Thin vaginal mucosa with loss of mucosal rugosities—seen in atrophic vaginitis in postmenopausal women*
- *Strawberry spots in vagina—seen in trichomoniasis*
- *Curdy white patches that may bleed on peeling—seen in candidiasis*

Cervix

Look for the following:

- *Cervicitis, cervical erosion, polyp, and any growth*
- *Mucopurulent discharge through cervix—in acute PID*

Bimanual pelvic examination

Palpate for the following:

- *Uterus size and position*
- *Uterine, forniceal, or cervical tenderness—may be suggestive of PID*
- *Any palpable adnexal mass*
- *Any forniceal tenderness (PID)*

Case summary

An example of writing summary in cases of discharge P/V is given below.

(CONTD...)

(...CONTD)

Example *Mrs. R, 28 years of age, multiparous, sterilized woman, presents with complaints of discharge per vaginum for the past 2 weeks. The discharge is profuse, foul smelling, and associated with pruritis. There is no history of pain abdomen, and fever. Her menstrual cycles are regular 4/30, with moderate flow, and her last menstrual period (LMP) was 10 days back. On examination, general examination is normal and vitals are stable. Abdomen is soft, external genitalia is healthy, and per speculum examination reveals profuse greenish yellow discharge. Cervix is normal and bimanual examination reveals a normal-sized, anteverted uterus and fornices are free.*

Case diagnosis

An example of writing diagnosis in cases of discharge P/V is given below.

Example *28 years of age, multiparous, sterilized woman with history and clinical examination suggestive of abnormal vaginal discharge due to trichomonal vaginitis.*

Case discussion

Vaginal infections

The common causes of vaginal discharge are bacterial vaginosis, trichomonal vaginitis, and candidal vaginitis which are described below.

Bacterial vaginosis

Causative agent

- Bacterial vaginosis is caused due to the alteration of normal vaginal flora, resulting in a decrease in lactobacilli and proliferation of organisms that are normally not present in vaginal flora. It is a polymicrobial infection with organisms such as *Haemophilus*, *Gardnerella*, *Mycoplasma*, *Prevotella*, and *Mobiluncus*.
- It is not sexually transmitted; about 50% of the patients are asymptomatic carriers.

Clinical features

The patient presents with vaginal discharge without associated pruritis.

On examination

Thin, grayish homogeneous discharge with an unpleasant "fishy" odor

Diagnosis

- pH >4.5.
- Microscopy—presence of "clue cells" (vaginal epithelial cells appear fuzzy as they are coated with coccobacilli); very few lactobacilli are seen (Figure 27.1).
- Amine test or whiff test is positive (fishy odor emanates when 10% KOH is added to the discharge).

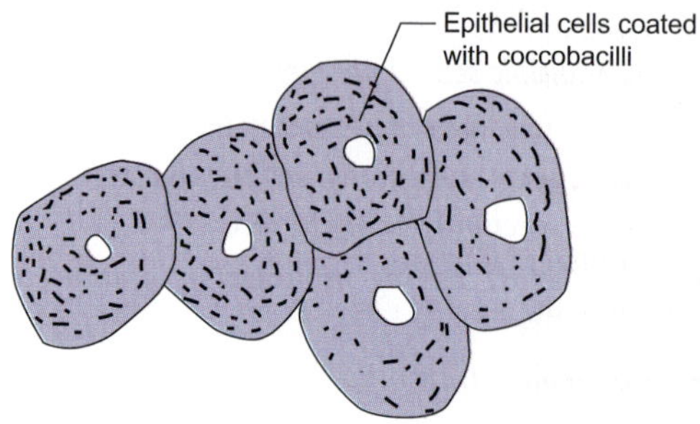

Figure 27.1 Clue cells in bacterial vaginosis.

- Amsel's diagnostic criteria for bacterial vaginosis: Three of the following four criteria must be met to establish the accurate diagnosis of bacterial vaginosis:
  - Thin, homogeneous discharge
  - Positive "whiff test"
  - Presence of "clue cells" > 20% on microscopic examination (highly significant criterion)
  - Vaginal pH >4.5

Treatment

It includes one of the following:

- Metronidazole 400 mg orally BD for 7 days
- Metronidazole gel 0.75% (5 g) once-daily vaginal application for 5 days
- Tinidazole 2 g orally for 2 days
- Tinidazole 1 g orally for 5 days
- Clindamycin 300 mg oral dose BD for 7 days
- Clindamycin 2% vaginal cream once-daily application for 7 days
- Clindamycin 100 mg vaginal suppository for 3 days

Extra edge

Nugent scoring system for bacterial vaginosis combines bacterial morphotypes with Gram staining properties to reflect the overall character of the vaginal microbiota.

Nugent scoring is given on a scale of 0 to 10 and has three components:

- A score of 0–4 reflecting the presence of rod-shaped Gram-positive lactobacilli where 0 indicates highest numbers.
- A score of 0–4 reflecting the numbers of Gram-negative and Gram-variable bacteria where 4 indicates highest numbers (Gardnerella/ bacteroides).
- A score of 0–2 reflecting the presence of curved rods (*Mobiluncus*).

Trichomonal vaginitis

Trichomonal vaginitis is the most common cause of vaginitis in the reproductive age group.

Causative agent

- *Trichomonas vaginalis*, a pear-shaped flagellated protozoa
- Transmitted through sexual contact

Clinical features

- There is profuse and offensive yellow-green-colored vaginal discharge.
- It may be associated with itching, vaginal irritation, dyspareunia, and urinary symptoms such as dysuria.

On examination

- Thin, greenish yellow, and frothy offensive discharge
- Vulvar and vaginal erythema
- Red and inflamed vaginal walls with multiple punctate hemorrhagic spots giving the appearance of "strawberry vagina"

Diagnosis

- pH >4.5
- Identification of motile, flagellated trichomonads (Figure 27.2) by wet mount preparation

Treatment

It includes one of the following:

- Metronidazole 400 mg BD orally for 1 week

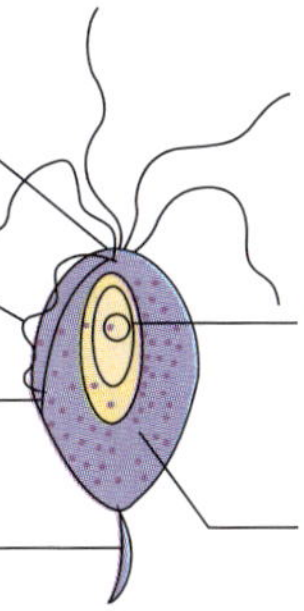

Figure 27.2 Motile, flagellated trichomonad seen under microscopy.

- Metronidazole 2 g oral single dose
- Tinidazole 2 g oral single dose
- Secnidazole 2 g oral single dose
- Refractory cases—Tinidazole 2 g orally OD for 14 days
- Should treat the partner simultaneously

Candidal vaginitis (moniliasis)

Causative agent

Candida albicans, a Gram-positive, yeast-like fungus

Predisposing factors for candidal vaginitis

- Diabetes
- Pregnancy
- Broad-spectrum antibiotics
- COC pill usage
- Immunosuppression—HIV and drugs such as steroid intake
- Obesity

Clinical features

Thick, curdy white discharge with intense vulvovaginal pruritus

On examination

- Thick, curdy white discharge (cottage cheese type) is present, often adherent to the vaginal walls.
- Vulvar and vaginal erythema may be present.
- Vaginal examination may be painful and removal of curdy white flakes reveals multiple oozing spots.

Diagnosis

- pH <4.5

Part 2

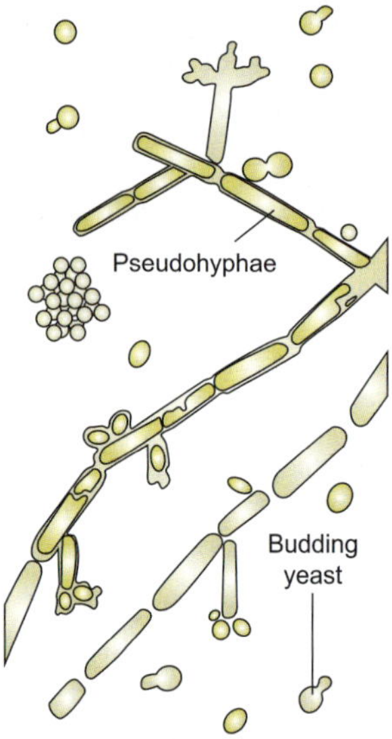

Figure 27.3 Pseudohyphae seen in candidiasis.

- Wet smear preparation with 10% potassium hydroxide (KOH) [pseudohyphae can be seen under the microscope (Figure 27.3)]
- Culture in Sabouraud media

Treatment

- Fluconazole 150 mg single oral dose
- Local application—miconazole, clotrimazole, and butoconazole intravaginal application for 7–10 days

Antifungal intravaginal cream preparations

See Table 27.3

Antifungal intravaginal suppository

See Table 27.4

Recurrent vulvovaginal candidiasis (VVC) If four or more episodes of symptomatic VVC occur annually, it is termed recurrent VVC.

Treatment of recurrent VVC It consists of oral Fluconazole 150 mg every 3 days for 9 days, followed by weekly for 6 months.

Cervicitis

Neisseria gonorrhoeae and *Chlamydia trachomatis* are the common causes of cervicitis leading to mucopurulent discharge from endocervical canal and referred to as "mucopus."

Table 27.3 Antifungal intravaginal cream preparations

Drug	Dosage application
Clotrimazole 1%	5 g/day intravaginally for 7–14 days
Miconazole 2%	5 g/day intravaginally for 7 days
Butoconazole 2%	5 g/day intravaginally for 3 days
Tioconazole 5%	5 g intravaginally single application
Terconazole	
0.4%	5 g/day intravaginally for 7 days
0.8%	5 g/day intravaginally for 3 days

Table 27.4 Antifungal intravaginal suppository

Drug	Dosage application
Clotrimazole	
100-mg vaginal tablet	1 tablet/day intravaginally for 6 days
200-mg vaginal tablet	1 tablet/day intravaginally for 3 days
500-mg vaginal tablet	1 tablet single-dose intravaginal application
Miconazole	
200-mg vaginal suppository	1 tablet/day intravaginally for 3 days
100-mg vaginal suppository	1 tablet/day intravaginally for 6 days
Nystatin 100,000-unit vaginal tablet	1 tablet/day intravaginally for 14 days
Terconazole 80 mg vaginal suppository	1 suppository per day for 3 days

Gonorrhea

Causative agent

- The causative agent is *N. gonorrhoeae*, a Gram-negative diplococcus.
- The incubation period is 3–7 days.
- The organism affects the columnar and transitional epithelium of the genitourinary tract.
- The organism may be localized to the lower genital tract to produce urethritis, bartholinitis, or cervicitis, or may ascend up along the spermatozoa in piggyback fashion to produce endometritis and salpingitis. Rarely, it may produce perihepatitis and septicemia.

Note
- *Squamous epithelium is resistant to gonococcal invasion; hence, it does not cause vaginitis.*
- *Infection with N. gonorrhoeae is often present along with other STDs.*

Clinical features

- Gonorrhea is nonspecific and asymptomatic in most cases.
- The patient may present with dysuria, mucopurulent vaginal discharge, and dyspareunia.
- Gonococcal septicemia is characterized by low-grade fever, polyarthralgia, tenosynovitis, septic arthritis, meningitis, endocarditis, and skin rash.

Diagnosis

Secretions are collected from urethra, Bartholin gland, and endocervix.

- Nucleic acid amplification testing (NAAT) of urine or endocervical discharge—highly sensitive and specific
- Gram stain—Gram-negative intracellular diplococci
- Diagnosis confirmed by culture in Thayer-Martin medium

Complications

PID, infertility, ectopic pregnancy, chronic pelvic pain, tubo-ovarian mass, and Bartholin abscess

Treatment [Centers for Disease Control and Prevention (CDC) 2010 treatment guidelines]

Recommended regimen

- Ceftriaxone 250 mg IM in a single dose PLUS
- Azithromycin 1g orally in a single dose OR
- Doxycycline 100 mg oral twice daily for 7 days

Alternative regimens

- Ceftizoxime 500 mg IM OR
- Cefoxitin 2 g IM with probenecid 1 g orally OR
- Cefotaxime 500 mg IM OR
- Cefixime 400 mg orally in a single dose PLUS
- Azithromycin 1 g orally in a single dose
- Simultaneous treatment of male sexual partner

Note *Gonococcal and chlamydial infections often coexist and it is difficult to rule out chlamydial infections. Hence, azithromycin 1 g single dose or doxycycline 100 mg twice daily for 7 days should be added to any of the treatment regimens for gonorrhea.*

Chlamydial infection

Causative agent

- The causative agent is *C. trachomatis*, an obligatory intracellular Gram-negative bacterium.
- Incubation period is 6–14 days (longer than that of gonorrhea).
- The organisms affect the columnar and transitional epithelium of the genitourinary tract.
- The infection is mostly localized to the urethra, Bartholin gland, and cervix. The infection can spread upwards to cause endometritis and salpingitis.

Note *Chlamydia does not cause deeper penetration and hence the symptoms may not be apparent.*

Clinical features

- Nonspecific and asymptomatic in most cases
- May present with dysuria, dyspareunia, and mucopurulent discharge P/V

Diagnosis

Samples are collected from the urethra and endocervix.

- Chlamydial NAAT and detection by polymerase chain reaction (PCR) is a highly sensitive and specific test.
- Chlamydia lipopolysaccharide antigen can be detected by enzyme-linked immunosorbent assay (ELISA) test.
- Tissue culture is 100% specific but is expensive and technically difficult, and it takes 3–7 days to obtain results.

Complications

- It causes tubal scarring resulting in infertility and ectopic pregnancy.

Part 2

- It is a more common cause of perihepatitis (Fitz-Hugh–Curtis syndrome) than gonorrhea.

Treatment (CDC, 2010 treatment guidelines)

Recommended regimens
- Azithromycin 1 g orally in a single dose OR
- Doxycycline 100 mg orally twice a day for 7 days

Alternative regimens
- Erythromycin base 500 mg orally four times a day for 7 days OR
- Erythromycin ethylsuccinate 800 mg orally four times a day for 7 days OR
- Levofloxacin 500 mg orally once daily for 7 days OR
- Ofloxacin 300 mg orally twice a day for 7 days

Investigations in a case of abnormal vaginal discharge

Microscopic examination

If history and/or physical examination are suggestive of vaginitis, a sample of the vaginal discharge may be obtained for microscopic examination.

Normal vaginal discharge It shows squamous epithelial cells, polymorphonuclear leukocytes, and *Lactobacillus* species.

Pathological vaginal discharge
- Presence of candidal buds or hyphae in candidal infection
- Presence of motile trichomonads in trichomonal vaginitis
- Presence of clue cells in bacterial vaginosis
- Presence of a large number of polymorphonuclear cells without any evidence of candidal species, trichomonads, or clue cells is suggestive of cervicitis

KOH preparation

This test is particularly useful in the diagnosis of candidal vaginitis.
- A drop of vaginal secretion is placed on a slide with a drop of 10–20% KOH.
- A coverslip is placed on the slide and air dried prior to examination under the microscope.
- KOH dissolves the nonfungal elements for detection of candidal hyphae and spores.

Whiff test

A positive whiff test/amine test is suggestive of bacterial vaginosis.
- Smell (whiff) the slide immediately after applying KOH. Fishy (amine) odor is useful for the detection of bacterial vaginosis.

Nitrazine pH paper

It helps to evaluate the vaginal pH.
- Normal vaginal pH ranges between 3.8 and 4.2.
- pH >4.5 is present in bacterial vaginosis and frequently in patients with trichomoniasis.
- pH <4.5 is present in candidiasis.

Cervical culture

In case of mucopurulent discharge, culture of cervical secretions is important to establish the diagnosis of cervicitis due to *N. gonorrhoeae* or *C. trachomatis*.

Viva corner

Q1 What is the cause of fishy odor in the whiff test?

Fishy odor in the whiff test for bacterial vaginosis is due to liberation of amines and organic acids produced from the alkalization of anaerobic bacteria.

Treatment of vaginal discharge

- Normal physiological vaginal discharge usually requires no treatment.
- Discharge associated with infections requires specific treatment (described earlier).
- If infections such as gonorrhea, chlamydia, or trichomoniasis are suspected, the woman's sexual partner must also be tested and treated.

General measures

- Advise to wear loose-fitting cotton undergarments.
- The patient must be advised to wipe her genital parts from anterior to posterior while using toilet paper.
- Vaginal irritants such as bubble baths and creams should be avoided.

- Advice on safe sex; use of condoms (barrier contraceptive) protects against HIV and sexually transmitted diseases.

SYNDROMIC APPROACH FOR TREATMENT OF STDs

Definition

A syndrome is a set of symptoms and signs that characterize a clinical condition. Syndromic management implies an approach in which clinical algorithms are used in case management of commonly presenting signs and symptoms.

In syndromic management, diagnosis and treatment are not based on specific testing for diseases, but are based on syndromes, that is, a group of clinical findings.

The symptoms selected for the syndrome are reasonably consistent and easy to recognize.

Components of syndromic management of STDs

- Client selection
- Chemical treatment
- Compliance of treatment
- Counseling
- Condom promotion
- Contact tracing and management
- Coming back for review

Examples of STDs treated by syndromic approach are mentioned in Table 27.5.

Table 27.5 STDs treated by syndromic approach

Syndrome	Common causes
Vaginal discharge	• Vaginitis (trichomoniasis, candidiasis, bacterial vaginosis) • Cervicitis (gonorrhea, chlamydia)
Urethral discharge	Gonorrhea, chlamydia
Genital ulcer	Syphilis, chancroid, herpes
Lower abdominal pain	Gonorrhea, chlamydia, mixed anaerobes
Scrotal swelling	Gonorrhea
Inguinal bubo	Lymphogranuloma venereum, chancroid
Neonatal conjunctivitis	Gonorrhea, chlamydia

Syndromic diagnosis and treatment

- Health workers and accredited social health activists (ASHA) identify the symptoms in patients and refer them to primary health centers (PHCs) and community health centers (CHCs) or to specialists at designated STI/RTI clinics in district hospitals and medical colleges.
- Seven kits that are color coded specifically for each syndromic diagnosis are supplied free to the PHCs, CHCs, and district hospitals by NACO (National AIDS control organization).
- Once syndromic diagnosis is made, the kits are used for treatment (Figure 27.4).

Frequently asked viva questions

1. What are the common causes of vaginal discharge?
2. How will you differentiate vaginal discharge due to candidiasis, trichomoniasis, and bacterial vaginosis?
3. What is syndromic approach in the management of vaginal discharge?

Part 2

Clinical condition	Kit to be prescribed	Drugs included	Color code
Urethral or anorectal or cervical discharge	KIT 1: Gray	• Tab azithromycin 1 g (1 tab) • Tab cefixime 400 mg (1 tab)	
Vaginal discharge (vaginitis)	KIT 2: Green	• Tab secnidazole 2 g (1 tab) • Tab fluconazole 150 mg (1 tab)	
Genital ulcer disease (nonherpitic)	KIT 3: White	Inj. benzathine penicillin 2.4 mu (1 vial) + tab azithromycin 1 g (kit also contains 10 mL disposable syringe + 21 gauge needle + 1 vial of 10 mL sterile water)	
Genital ulcer disease (nonherpitic) in patient allergic to penicillin	KIT 4: Blue	• Tab doxycycline 100 mg (1 tab BD for 14 days) • Tab azithromycin 1 g × 7 days	
Genital ulcer disease (herpetic)	KIT 5: Red	Tab acyclovir 400 mg × 1 tab TDS × 7 days	
Lower abdominal pain (pelvic inflammatory disease)	KIT 6: Yellow	• Tab cefixime 400 mg × 1 tab • Tab metronidazole 400 mg × (1 BD 14 days) tab doxycycline 1 g (1 BD 14 days)	
Inguinal bubo	KIT 6: Black	• Tab doxycycline 100 mg (1 BD × 21 days) • Tab azithromycin 1 g × 1 tab	

Figure 27.4 Drugs and kits used in syndromic treatment of STDs.

Part 3

Practical Viva Voce Topics

28 Instruments

Introduction

Each specialty has its own set of specific instruments with specific uses, and this section deals with the instruments used in obstetrics and gynecology. A medical student is expected to know the following features of each instrument:

- Identification of the instrument
- Parts of the instrument
- Indications for use
- Technique of use
- Advantages and disadvantages

In practical exam, once the candidate identifies the given instrument, he/she will usually be questioned regarding the indications for usage, theoretical aspect of the disease/condition, and the surgical management.

RED RUBBER CATHETER (FIGURE 28.1)

Description

- It is a non–self-retaining urinary catheter made of rubber, available in different sizes.

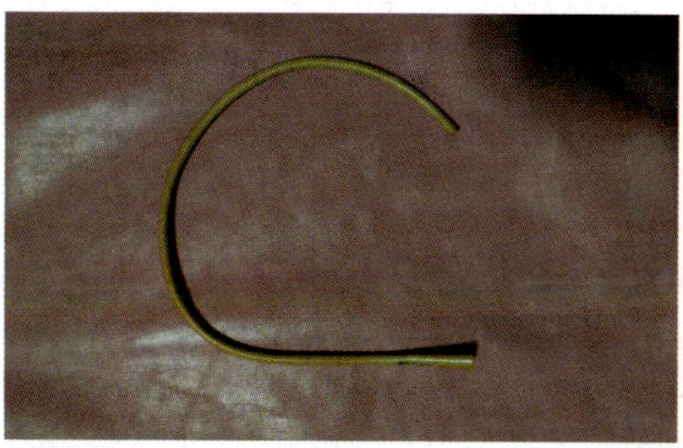

Figure 28.1 Red rubber catheter.

- One end is blunt and rounded with subtermin opening for drainage of urine and the other er is open and slightly expanded.
- It can be reused following sterilization by boiling
- It is used for intermittent urethral catheterizatio

Uses in obstetrics and gynecology

Red rubber catheter is used for draining urine the following situations:

- Acute retention of urine during pregnancy
- During labor (full bladder prevents uterir contraction and descent of fetal head)
- Before operative interventions such as force and vacuum delivery
- Management of postpartum hemorrhage (fu bladder prevents uterine retraction)

Viva corner

Q1 What are the other uses of red rubber catheter?

- As a tourniquet to collect blood samples
- As a tourniquet during myomectomy operation to reduce vascularity at operative site
- To administer O_2 when nasal catheter is not available
- As a mucus sucker—when attached to a mechanical or electric suction apparatus

FOLEY'S SELF-RETAINING CATHETER (FIGURE 28.2)

Description

- It is a self-retaining urinary catheter made c silicon rubber.
- It is available in a sterile package and should b disposed after single use.

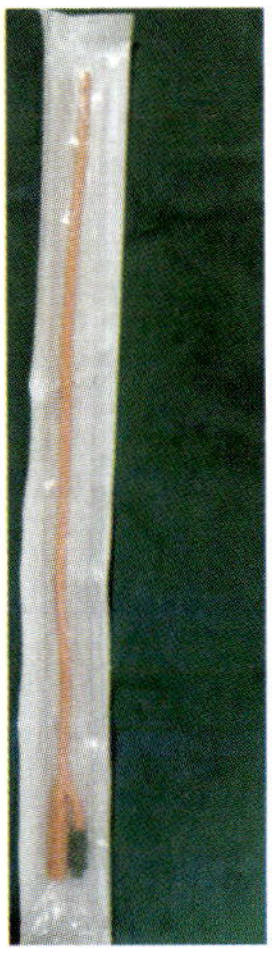

gure 28.2 Foley's self-retaining catheter.

The tip of the catheter has a subterminal opening for drainage of urine. Below this is a balloon that can be inflated, which makes the catheter self-retaining.

There are two channels within the catheter: the main channel is for drainage of urine and the other channel is for inflation of the balloon. The balloon is usually inflated with saline or distilled water and the volume of fluid recommended to inflate the balloon is marked on the catheter.

The catheter is available in different sizes [mentioned in "French (F)," e.g., 14Fr, 16Fr].

It is used for continuous drainage of urinary bladder.

ses in obstetrics and gynecology

is used for continuous bladder drainage in the llowing situations:

Acute/chronic retention of urine

Major obstetric and gynecologic surgeries—cesarean section, cesarean hysterectomy, hysterectomy, and laparotomy

Patients with severe preeclampsia and eclampsia to monitor urine output

Obstructed labor (prolonged catheterization may be required following cesarean section)

Following repair of bladder injury

During labor to empty the bladder

Before ventouse/forceps application

Incontinence of urine

Unconscious patients

Neurogenic bladder

Viva corner

Q1 What are the other uses of Foley's catheter?

- For Foley's cervical ripening prior to induction of labor
- For extra-amniotic instillation of ethacridine lactate in second-trimester medical termination of pregnancy (MTP)
- As a condom catheter for tamponade in cases of atonic PPH
- To perform saline infusion sonography
- Hysterosalpingography as an alternative to Leech-Wilkinson cannula (to instill the dye into uterine cavity)

Q2 What are the indications for prolonged catheterization?

- Following cesarean section for obstructed labor
- Following bladder injury repair
- Following repair of huge cystocele
- Following radical hysterectomy (which leads to bladder hypotonia)

FEMALE METAL CATHETER (FIGURE 28.3)

Description

It is a metal catheter; one end is curved with a blunt tip and there is a subterminal opening near the tip for urinary drainage.

Uses

- A female metal catheter is used for intermittent bladder catheterization when red rubber catheter is not available.
- It is also used to empty bladder before operative procedures such as vaginal hysterectomy and cystocele repair.

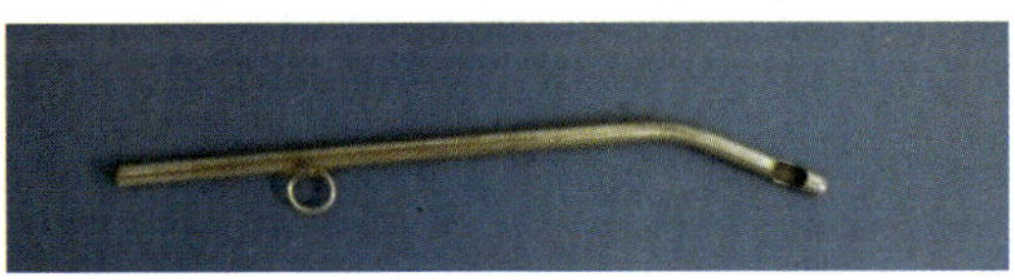

Figure 28.3 Female metal catheter.

SIMS' DOUBLE-BLADED POSTERIOR VAGINAL WALL SPECULUM (FIGURE 28.4)

Description

- It was designed by Marion Sims.
- It is a non–self-retaining vaginal speculum.
- It is available in different sizes.
- The ends of the blades are rounded to avoid trauma. The blades at both ends are of unequal sizes (one smaller than the other) to facilitate introduction into the vagina depending on the space available.
- The speculum has a concave groove in the center for the purpose of drainage and collection of blood, secretions, etc.
- It is used for retraction of posterior vaginal wall.

Uses

It is mainly used for inspection of the cervix and vagina in the situations given in the next subsections.

Obstetric uses

- To inspect cervix and vagina for discharge, leaking, bleeding, etc.
- To inspect cervix and vagina for any injuries following delivery
- Repair of cervical tear
- During dilatation and evacuation (D&E)
- During cervical cerclage

Gynecology uses

- To perform routine gynecological examination to inspect for the following:

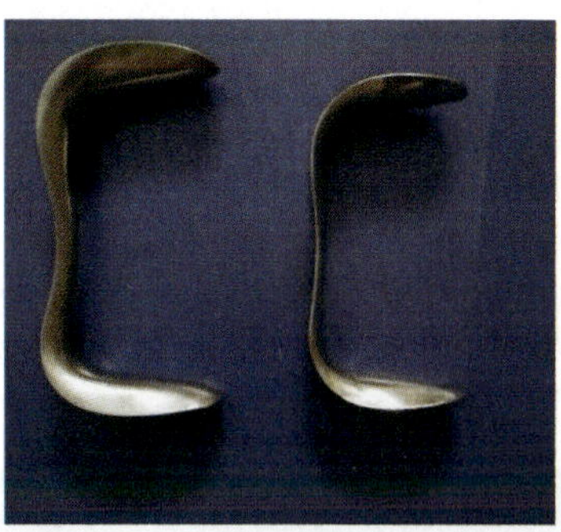

Figure 28.4 Sims' double-bladed posterior vaginal wall speculum.

  - Inspection of cervix for abnormalities such any growth, erosion, and discharge
  - Inspection of vagina for abnormalities su as vaginitis, cystocele, rectocele, enteroce and vesicovaginal fistula (VVF)
- To perform cervical procedures such as t following:
  - Cervical biopsy and conization of cervix
  - Polypectomy
  - Dilatation of cervix
- To perform uterine procedures such as t following:
  - Dilatation and curettage (D&C)
  - Endometrial biopsy (EB)
  - Intrauterine contraceptive device (IUC insertion
  - Hysteroscopy
  - Hysterosalpingography
- During major gynecological procedures such the following:
  - Vaginal hysterectomy
  - Anterior colporrhaphy and posterior colp perineorrhaphy
  - Manchester repair
  - VVF repair

Technique of insertion of speculum

- The patient should be lying with the buttoc at the edge of the table in dorsal position wi thighs flexed or in lithotomy position.
- Lubricate the blades of the speculum.
- Separate the labia and insert the transverse ax of blade along the long axis of introitus.
- Once inside the vagina, rotate the blade by 90° retract the posterior vaginal wall.
- The cervix and vaginal walls are examined.
- The posterior vaginal wall that is cover by the speculum is examined as the blade withdrawn.

Disadvantages

- The patient needs to be at the edge of the tab for insertion of the speculum.
- As it is not a self-retaining speculum, assistant is required to hold the speculu while doing procedures such as Pap smear ar cervical biopsy.

Extra edge

Sims' position

Sims' position, also called the lateral recumbent position, is the position in which the patient is asked to lie on his or her left side, with left leg straight and the right hip and right knee bent. It is used for performing rectal examination, posterior vaginal wall examination for rectocele and enterocele, and for giving enema.

Sims' sigmoid catheter

Sims' retention catheter was designed for use in women when continuous drainage by means of an indwelling catheter was required.

Sims' postcoital test

It is a test in the evaluation of infertility. The test examines interaction between sperm and mucus of the cervix.

CUSCO'S BIVALVED, METALLIC, SELF-RETAINING, VAGINAL SPECULUM (FIGURE 28.5)

Description

- It has two blades joined by screws that allow the blades to open and close. The handle has a rod and screw system designed to open and close the blades and to adjust the space between the blades.
- The speculum is self-retaining and hence does not need any assistant to hold it in position.
- It is used for retraction of vaginal walls.

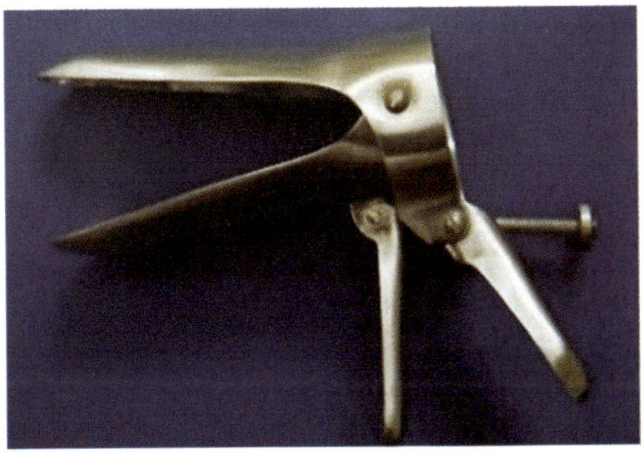

Figure 28.5 Cusco's bivalved, metallic, self-retaining, vaginal speculum.

Uses

Cusco's bivalved, metallic, self-retaining, vaginal speculum is used for retraction of cervix and vagina in those described in the next subsections.

Obstetrics

To inspect the cervix and vagina for any bleeding P/V, discharge P/V, and leaking P/V

Gynecology

- Routine speculum examination in gynecology
- Colposcopy
- Cervical procedures—Pap smear, biopsy, etc.
- Uterine procedures such as endometrial sampling
- IUCD insertion and removal
- During intrauterine insemination (IUI) procedure

Technique of insertion of speculum

- The blades of the speculum are lubricated.
- The labia are gently separated and the speculum is inserted with closed blades into the vagina, along the long axis of introitus.
- Following insertion, the speculum is rotated by 90°; the blades are then opened to retract the anterior and posterior vaginal walls and depending on the amount of exposure needed, fixation screw is tightened.
- While removing the speculum, the fixation screw is unscrewed; the blades are closed and then removed.

Disadvantages

- Anterior and posterior vaginal walls are covered by speculum and cannot be visualized.
- The speculum is space occupying and hence provides limited view of vagina and less maneuverability.

SIMS' ANTERIOR VAGINAL WALL RETRACTOR (FIGURE 28.6)

Description

- It is a long instrument having a shaft and oval fenestrated ends on both sides with transverse serrations.

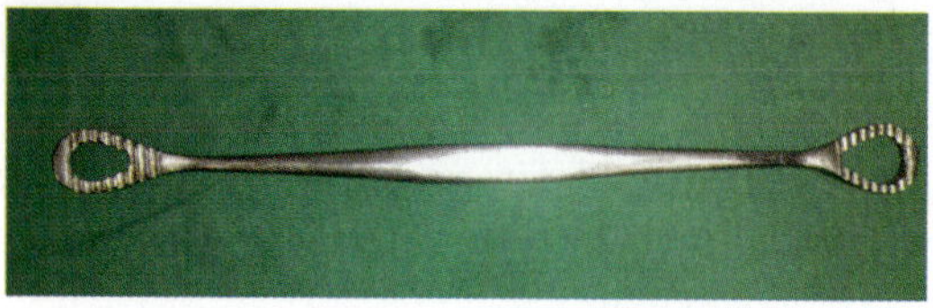

Figure 28.6 Sims' anterior vaginal wall retractor.

- The ends are at an angle of 15° to the shaft.
- It is used for retraction of the anterior vaginal wall.

Uses

- It is used to retract the anterior vaginal wall in conjunction with Sims' speculum, to visualize the cervix and vagina.
- Indications are similar to those for Sims' speculum.

Extra edge

Other uses of anterior vaginal wall retractor

It may be used as a blunt curette following delivery, to remove placental bits and membranes.

RAMPLEY'S SPONGE HOLDING FORCEPS (FIGURE 28.7)

Description

- It is a long metallic instrument with fenestrated rings having transverse serrations on the inner side, and a handle with ratchet and catch.
- The sponge holding forceps is used for holding gauze pieces during surgical procedures.

Uses

General indications

- To clean and prepare skin before start of surgery
- To swab cavities such as vagina and pelvic cavity

Obstetrics

- To hold pregnant cervix (as it is less traumatic when compared with a vulsellum or tenaculum) during procedures such as D&E and cervical encerclage
- To identify and repair cervical tears
- Can be used to remove products of conception from uterine cavity in abortion, when ovum forceps is not available

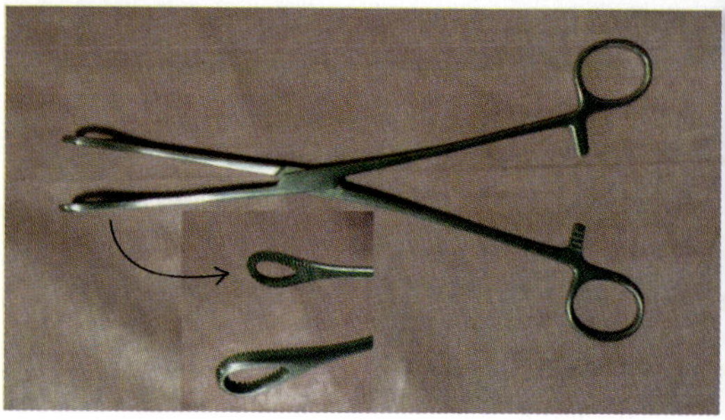

Figure 28.7 Sponge holding forceps.

Gynecology

- To check for hemostasis
- To apply pressure over bleeding points during surgery
- To keep omentum and bowel away from the operative field
- To perform polypectomy

ALLIS TISSUE HOLDING FORCEPS (FIGURE 28.8)

Description

- It is an instrument with sharp, serrated, multiple teeth at one end and a handle at the other end with the provision of a ratchet and catch.
- It is used for grasping or retracting tough tissues such as fascia.

Uses

Obstetrics

- To hold the rectus sheath while incising and closing the rectus sheath

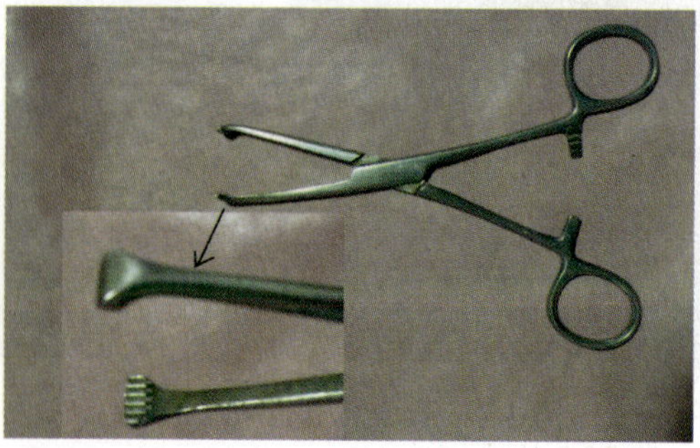

Figure 28.8 Allis tissue holding forceps.

- To hold the angles of uterine incision in cesarean section, as an alternative to Green-Armytage hemostatic clamp
- To hold the vaginal apex during episiotomy repair

Gynecology

- To hold the vaginal flaps
  - In vaginal hysterectomy
  - During closure of vault in abdominal
  - hysterectomy
  - In anterior colporrhaphy and colpoperineorrhaphy
  - During repair of VVF/rectovaginal fistula

Extra edge

Q1 What are the other uses of Allis forceps?

- To hold the anterior lip of cervix during procedures such as fractional curettage, as an alternative to vulsellum
- Can be used along with a sponge to clean the surgical site, as an alternative to sponge holding forceps

KOCHER'S FORCEPS (FIGURE 28.9)

Description

- It is a long metallic instrument with a tooth at the tip of one blade and a corresponding groove on the other blade. The handle has a ratchet and catch.
- It is of two types: straight and curved Kocher's forceps.
- The instrument holds tissues firmly when locked and slippage is less.

Uses

Obstetrics

- To do artificial low rupture of membranes
- Clamping the umbilical cord following delivery

Gynecology

- To hold the uterus near cornual end during abdominal hysterectomy
- To clamp pedicles
- To remove pedunculated fibroid polyps (polypectomy)

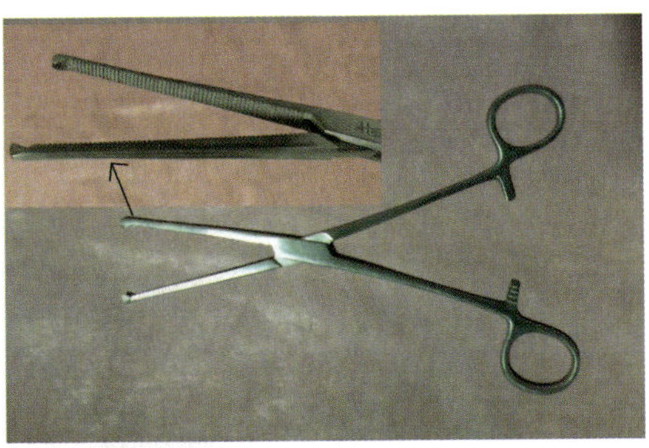

Figure 28.9 Kocher's forceps.

NEEDLE HOLDER (FIGURE 28.10)

Description

- It is an instrument used to grasp the needle while suturing during surgeries.
- The inner surface of the tip has serrations and a small groove for proper grasp of the curved needle.
- To maintain a firm grip on the needle, the jaws are textured and short, compared to the shank (increasing the applied force following the principle of a lever).

Use

To hold the needle during surgical suturing—pronation supination action is needed to pass the needle in its curve.

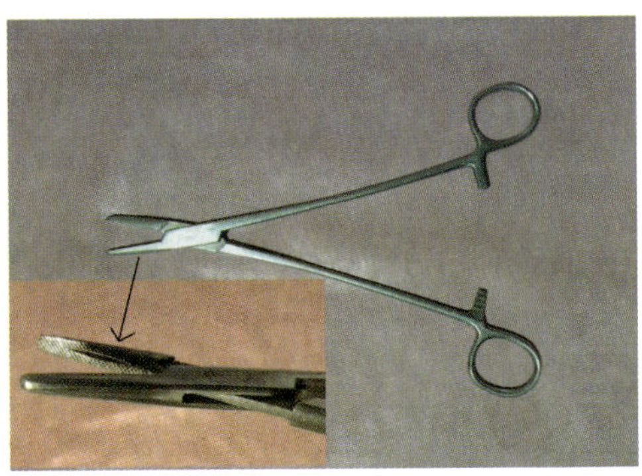

Figure 28.10 Needle holder.

Part 3

CURVED ARTERY AND STRAIGHT ARTERY HEMOSTATIC FORCEPS (FIGURE 28.11)

Description

- The instrument has blades with transverse serrations on the inner surface and a handle with a ratchet and catch.

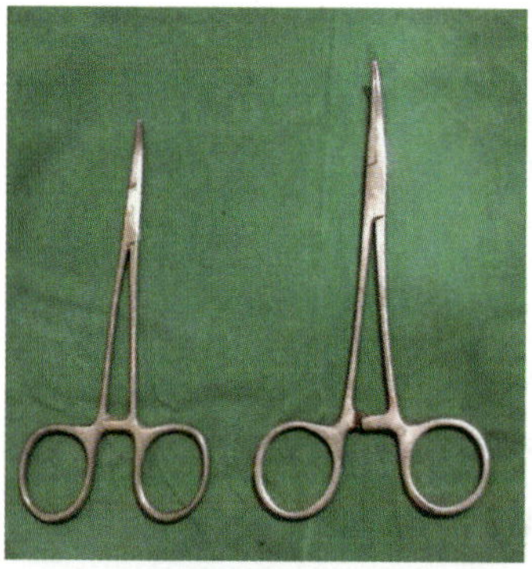

a.

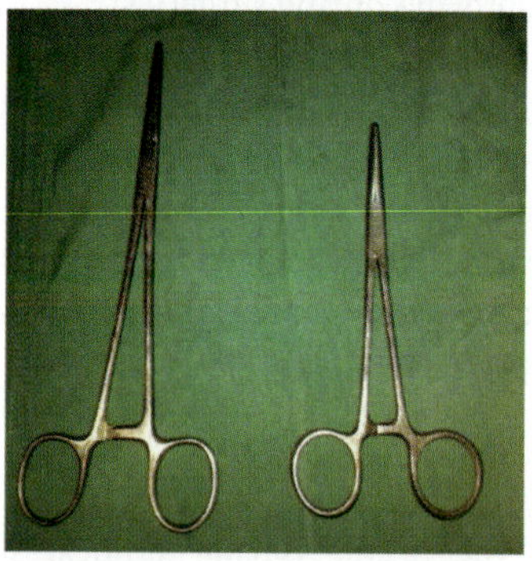

b.

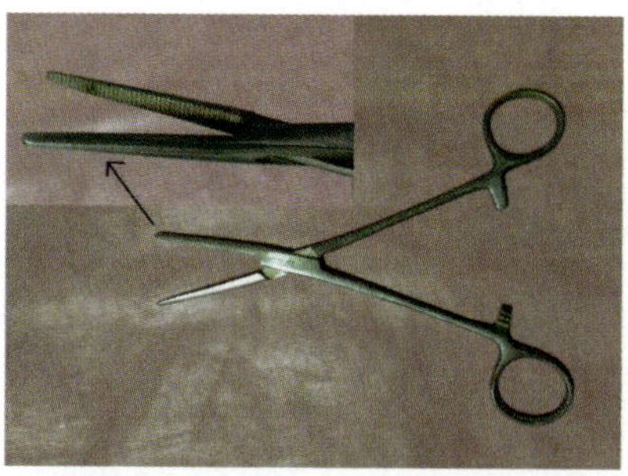

c.

Figure 28.11 Curved and straight artery hemostatic forceps. **a.** Small curved and long curved artery forceps. **b.** Long straight and small straight artery forceps. **c.** Transverse serrations on the inner aspect of artery forceps.

- It is of two types: curved and straight artery forceps.
- Both straight and curved artery forceps are available in two sizes: small and long
- The small curved forceps is used as a hemostat and the small straight forceps is commonly used for holding stay sutures.
- The long curved and long straight artery forceps are used as hemostatic clamps.

Uses in obstetrics and gynecology

- To secure hemostasis
- To clamp the pedicles before cutting and ligation
- To hold and ligate sutures
- To hold the stay sutures
- To hold structures such as peritoneum and rectus sheath during operative procedures
- To clamp the umbilical cord following delivery of baby

SHARP CURVED MOSQUITO HEMOSTAT (FIGURE 28.12)

Description

This is a small variety of artery forceps.

Uses

- To secure hemostasis
- To hold stay sutures in abdominal and vaginal surgeries
- To open cavity of abscesses

BABCOCK FORCEPS (FIGURE 28.13)

Description

- The instrument has triangular curved blades and when locked has a space in between the two blades to contain tissue.

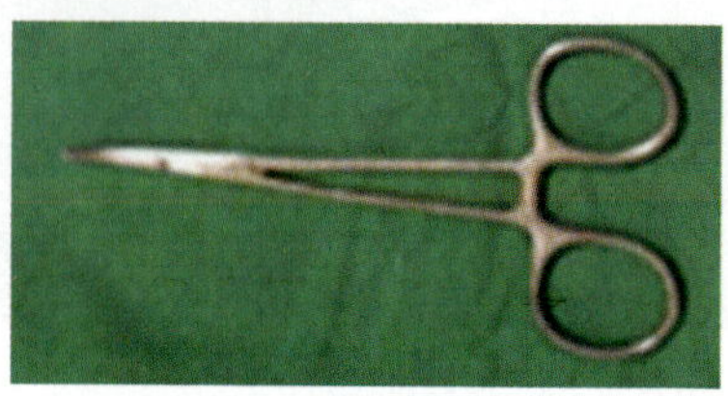

Figure 28.12 Sharp curved mosquito hemostat.

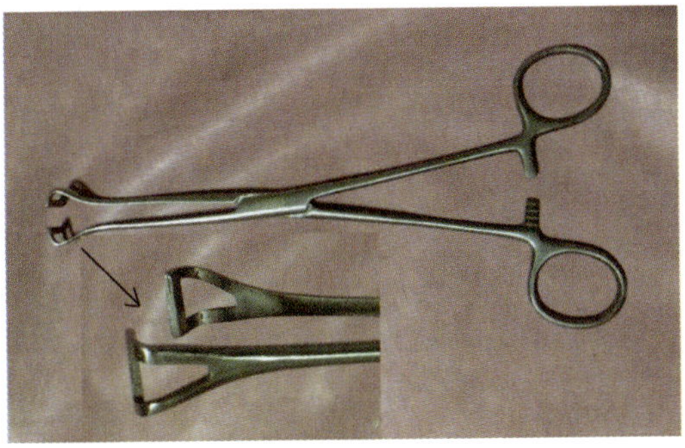

Figure 28.13 Babcock forceps.

- It is atraumatic and is used for holding tubular structures such as fallopian tube, appendix, intestine, and ureter without compressing them.

Uses

- To hold fallopian tubes during tubal sterilization and tubal ectopic pregnancy
- To hold vas deferens in vasectomy
- To hold appendix during appendicectomy
- To hold round ligament during hysterectomy
- To hold ureter during Wertheim's hysterectomy

GREEN-ARMYTAGE FORCEPS (FIGURE 28.14)

Description

- The instrument has triangular-shaped wide edges that help in compression of a wide area of tissues held.
- It is used to secure hemostasis.

Uses

- To hold the angles of uterine incision in cesarean section
- To clamp the bleeding uterine vessels in case of angle extension in lower-segment cesarean section (LSCS)

DEBAKEY ATRAUMATIC TISSUE FORCEPS (FIGURE 28.15)

Description

Forceps are instruments used for grasping and holding tissues during surgical procedures.

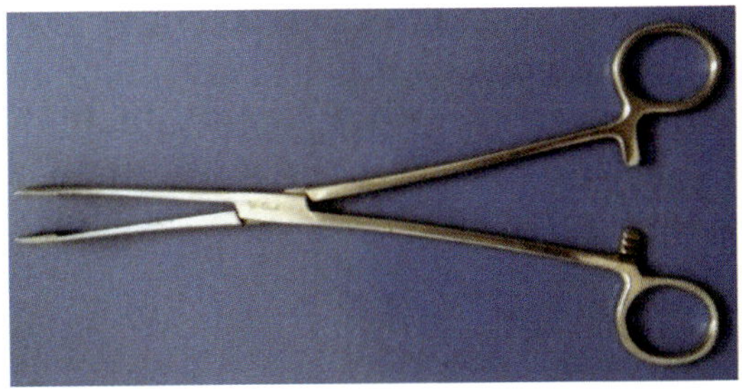

a.

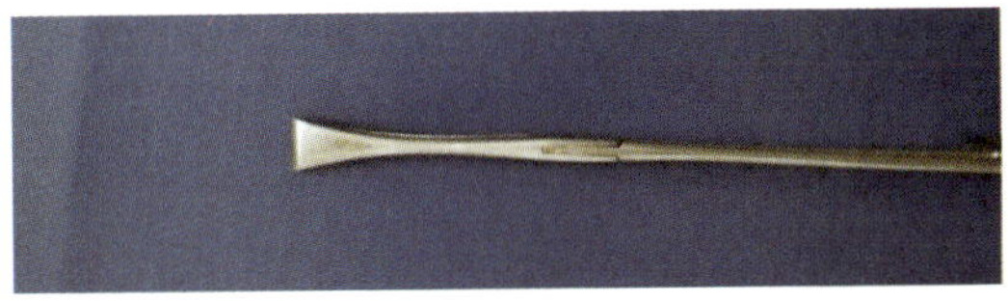

b.

Figure 28.14 Green-Armytage forceps. a. Full view. b. Close-up view.

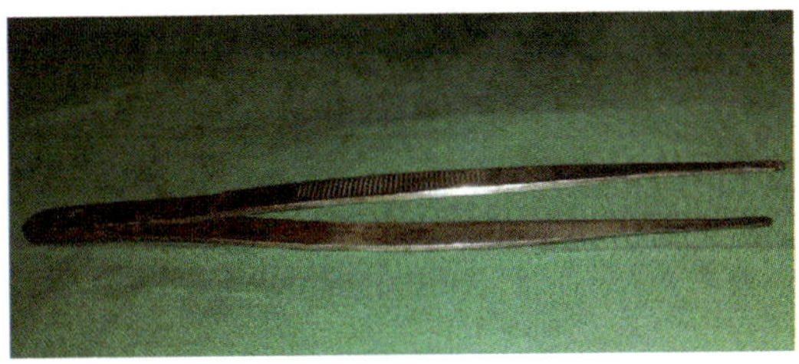

Figure 28.15 DeBakey nontoothed forceps.

DeBakey atraumatic tissue forceps are thumb forceps used in numerous surgical procedures. The narrow tips and atraumatic teeth cause little to no damage to the tissues. It is available in multiple lengths, straight or angled, and with a variety of tip dimensions. It is commonly used for grasping fine tissue and blood vessels and for tissue dissection.

Uses

- To hold delicate structures such as peritoneum, blood vessels, bladder wall, and bowel
- To secure hemostasis with electrocautery

TOOTHED TISSUE FORCEPS (FIGURE 28.16)

Description

Toothed forceps have a toothed end that helps to hold tough tissues.

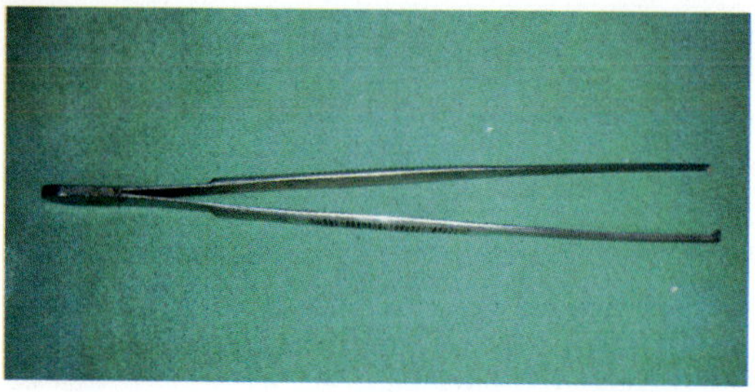

Figure 28.16 Toothed tissue forceps.

Uses

- To hold tough structures such as fascia, skin, and rectus sheath
- Can be used to secure hemostasis

DOYEN'S RETRACTOR (FIGURE 28.17)

Description

- Doyen's retractor is a non–self-retaining, heavy abdominal retractor having a large curved blade with an inward-turning margin.
- It is used to retract the abdominal wall and bladder during abdominal surgeries.

Uses

Obstetrics

- Cesarean section
- Cesarean hysterectomy
- Laparotomy for ruptured ectopic pregnancy

Gynecology

- Abdominal hysterectomy
- Myomectomy
- Exploratory laparotomy
- Sling surgeries

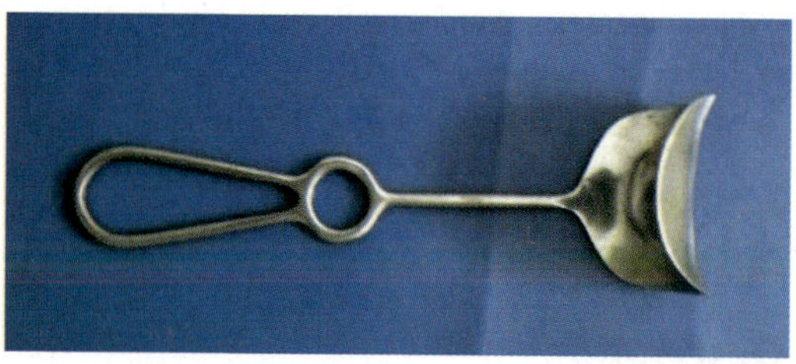

Figure 28.17 Doyen's retractor.

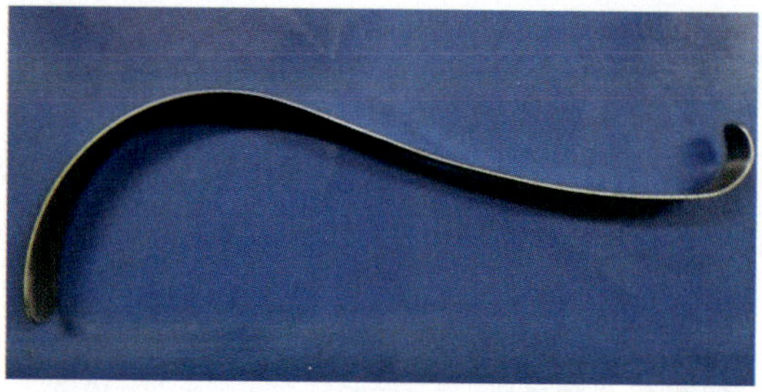

Figure 28.18 Deaver's retractor.

DEAVER'S RETRACTOR (FIGURE 28.18)

- Deaver's retractor is a non–self-retaining, abdominal retractor having a large curved blade.
- It is available in different sizes.
- It is used to retract the abdominal walls and bladder during abdominal surgeries.

Uses

Obstetrics

- Cesarean section
- Cesarean hysterectomy
- Laparotomy for ruptured ectopic pregnancy

Gynecology

- Abdominal hysterectomy
- Myomectomy
- Exploratory laparotomy
- Sling surgeries

SELF-RETAINING ABDOMINAL WALL RETRACTOR (FIGURE 28.19)

Description

- This retractor has movable blades that can be fixed by screws.
- It is self-retaining; hence, an assistant is not required to hold the retractor in place.
- It helps to retract the abdominal wall in more than one direction.

Use

To retract abdominal wall during abdominal surgeries

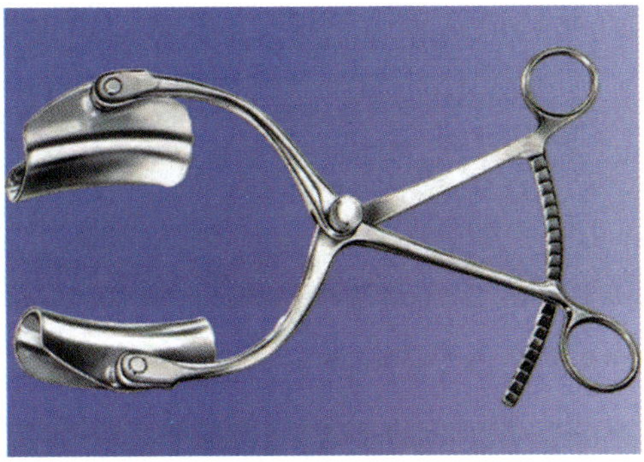

Figure 28.19 Self-retaining abdominal wall retractor.

Disadvantages

- If used for prolonged duration, it can cause bruising of tissues, nerve compression, necrosis of rectus muscles, etc.
- It is space occupying.

DOYEN'S MYOMA SCREW (FIGURE 28.20)

Description

This instrument has a spiral corkscrew with a pointed tip and a ring-shaped handle for gripping.

Uses

- To perform myomectomy
- Can be screwed into the uterine fundus to steady the uterus during abdominal hysterectomy

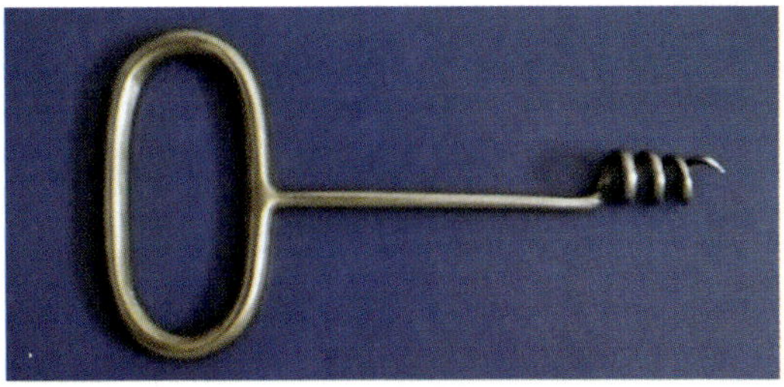

Figure 28.20 Doyen's myoma screw.

VULSELLUM (FIGURE 28.21)

Description

- This is a long instrument with a gentle curve and the tips of the blades have three to four teeth.
- The gentle curve prevents obstruction of the line of vision when introduced into vagina. It should be held with the tip facing upwards.
- It is used to hold and steady the cervix during vaginal procedures.
- It is not preferable to grasp the cervix during pregnancy, as it can cause cervical tears and lacerations. A sponge holding forceps can be used to grasp the cervix during pregnancy.

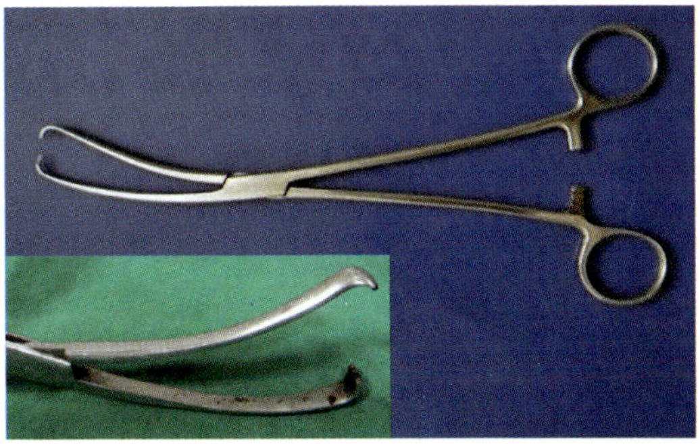

Figure 28.21 Vulsellum (inset: close up).

Uses

- To hold the anterior lip of cervix during:
  - Endometrial biopsy
  - IUCD insertion
  - IUI
  - Vaginal hysterectomy
  - Cervical biopsy
- To hold the posterior lip of cervix during
  - Culdocentesis in suspected ruptured ectopic pregnancy
  - Culdoscopy

SINGLE-TOOTHED TENACULUM (FIGURE 28.22)

Description

The instrument has a single pointed hook at one end to hold the cervix. It is not preferred to grasp the cervix during pregnancy, as it can cause cervical tears and lacerations.

Uses

- Similar to those of vulsellum

Part 3

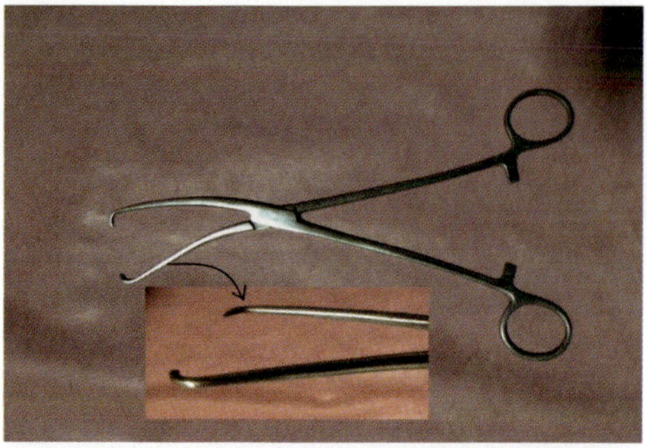

Figure 28.22 Single-tooth tenaculum (inset: close up).

MAYO'S SCISSORS (FIGURE 28.23)

Description

- Mayo's scissors are sturdy scissors used for tough dissection.
- This scissors is curved at an angle along its long axis in the horizontal plane.
- It is used for cutting obliquely directed tissues and pedicles during surgery.

Use

Used for tough tissue dissection such as to cut rectus sheath, uterosacrals and Mackenrodt's ligaments, and vaginal flaps.

METZENBAUM SCISSORS (FIGURE 28.24)

Description

- This scissors is more delicate than Mayo's scissors and is used for cutting thin tissues.
- It is also curved at an angle along its long axis in the horizontal plane.
- It is used for cutting obliquely directed tissues and pedicles during surgery.

Uses

- Used for fine dissection
- To cut delicate tissues such as peritoneum and uterovesical (UV) fold
- Used for retroperitoneal dissection and for releasing adhesions

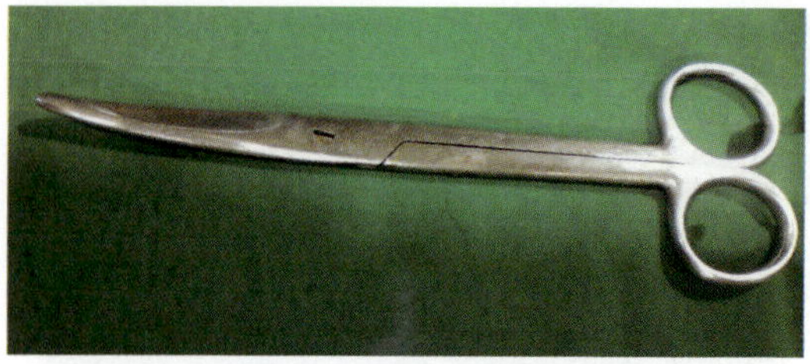

Figure 28.23 Mayo's scissors.

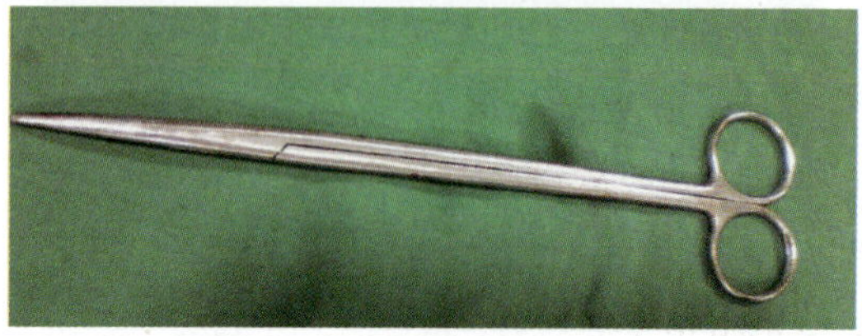

Figure 28.24 Metzenbaum scissors.

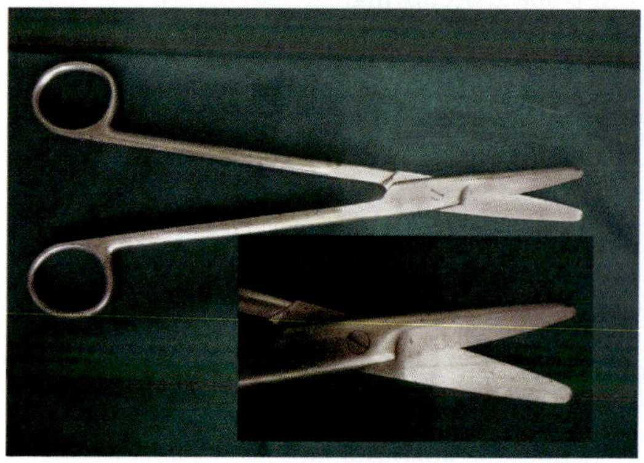

Figure 28.25 Straight scissors.

STRAIGHT SCISSORS (FIGURE 28.25)

Description

This is a straight scissors used for cutting suture material during surgical procedures.

BARD-PARKER SCALPEL WITH BLADE (FIGURE 28.26)

Description

- The instrument has a handle with a notch to fit the blade.
- Scalpel is usually held by pencil grip and its movement is directed by thumb and index finger.
- Blades are available in different sizes.

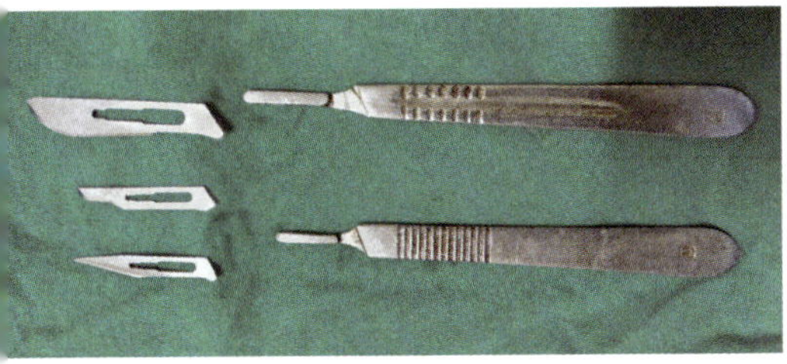

Figure 28.26 Bard-Parker scalpel with blades of different sizes.

Uses

- It is used to incise the skin and subcutaneous tissue.
- It is used to cut the clamped pedicles.
- It is used to perform sharp dissection.
- No. 20 blade offers a long edge, which is ideal for quickly covering distance during initial skin incisions. The small no. 15 blade is selected for finer incisions. No. 11 blade has an acute angle that is used for giving stab incisions, for insertion of drains, and drainage of abscesses.

TOWEL CLIP (FIGURE 28.27)

Description

Instruments used for holding and retracting surgical drapes during surgery

Use in obstetrics and gynecology

- For draping during abdominal and vaginal surgeries
- Used for fixing diathermy, cables, and suction tubes during surgery

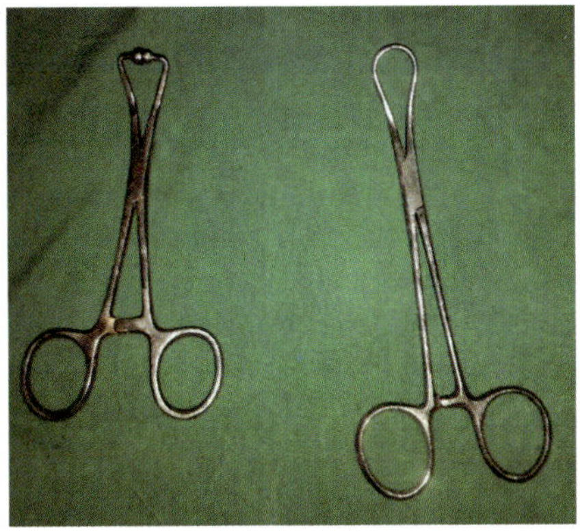

a.

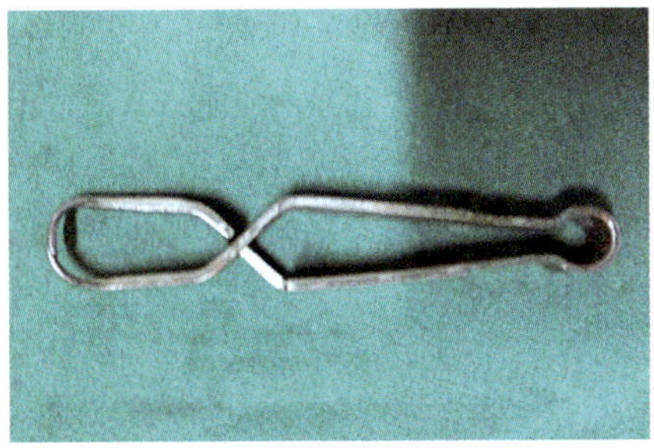

b.

Figure 28.27 Towel clips. a. Peers-Bertman nonperforated towel clip and Mayo's towel clip. b. Doyen's cross action towel clip.

SIMPSON'S GRADUATED METALLIC UTERINE SOUND (FIGURE 28.28)

Description

- It is a long angulated instrument about 30 cm long with a blunt tip.
- It has graduations marked in inches or centimeters.
- About 7 cm from the tip, it is bent at an angle of 30°, which helps to negotiate the curvature of uterus (anteversion or retroversion).

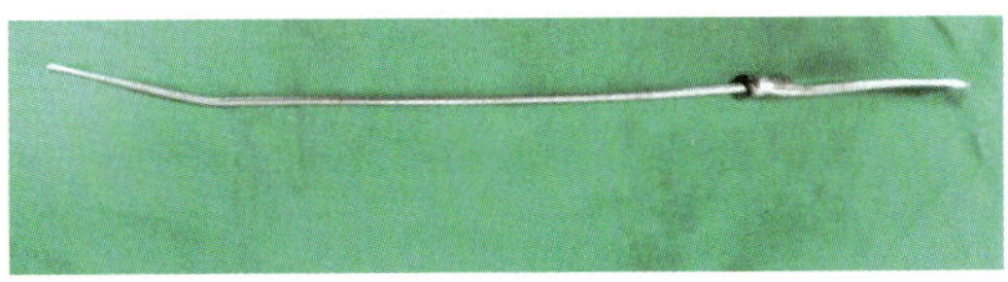

Figure 28.28 Simpson's graduated metallic uterine sound.

- The tip is blunt to avoid injury and perforation when introduced into the uterine cavity.

Uses

- To measure uterocervical length during procedures such as D&E, endometrial sampling, and Manchester repair
- Serves as the first dilator during procedures such as D&E and suction evacuation
- To probe for any pathology inside the uterine cavity
- To diagnose cervical stenosis
- To break adhesions in Asherman syndrome

- To differentiate between chronic uterine inversion and fibroid polyp (uterine sound cannot be inserted in case of uterine inversion)
- To probe for misplaced IUCD
- Can determine the location of IUCD in cases of misplaced IUCD by taking anteroposterior (AP) and lateral pelvic X-rays, by comparing the position of IUCD in relation to the uterine sound in situ

Other uses

- To differentiate cystocele from anterior vaginal wall cyst
- To confirm suspected bladder injury during vaginal hysterectomy
- To sound a calculus or foreign body in the bladder
- To determine length and direction of VVF

Note *Bladder sound is a long instrument having a gentle curve (unlike the uterine sound, which is angled). The instrument has no markings on it and is shorter in length compared with uterine sound.*

Disadvantages

- It can cause uterine perforation, if the direction or size of the uterus is misjudged.
- Uterine sound can cause false passage or perforation in a pregnant uterus where the uterus is very soft.

UTERINE CURETTE (FIGURE 28.29)

Description

- It is a long metallic instrument with an oval fenestrated end and a shaft.
- It is available as blunt curette (edges are blunt) and sharp curette (edges are sharp).
- It is also available as double-ended curette with sharp curette at one end and blunt curette at the other end. The blunt and the sharp curette are in opposite directions.
- It is used for scraping the endometrial cavity. The sharp curette is used for gynecological indications and the blunt curette is used in pregnant uterus.

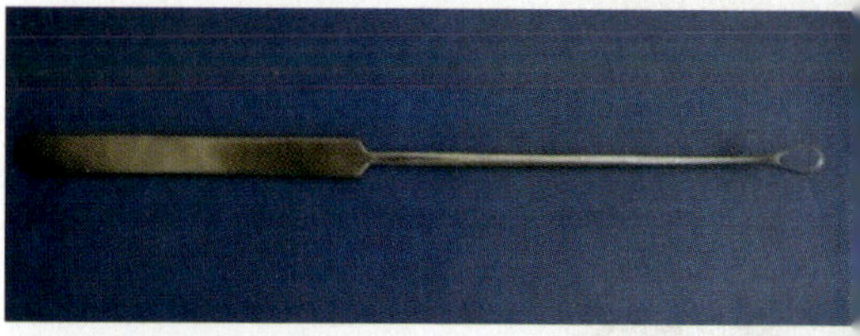

a.

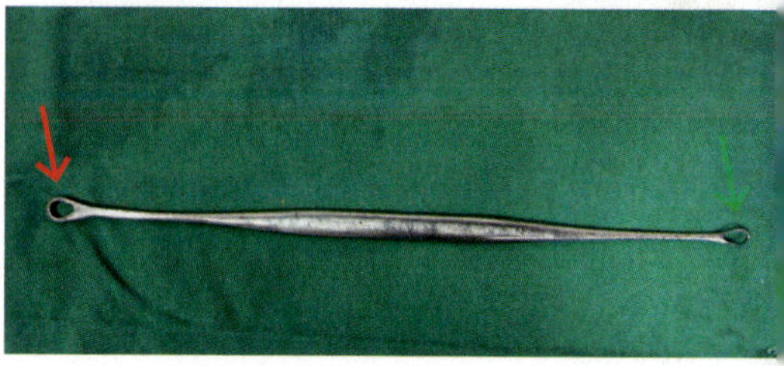

b.

Figure 28.29 Uterine curette. **a.** Sharp uterine curette. **b.** Double-ended curette with sharp curette at one end (green arrow) and blunt curette at the other end (red arrow).

Uses

Obstetrics

To do curettage following surgical abortion

Gynecology

- To perform endometrial sampling in the following:
  - Abnormal uterine bleeding (AUB)
  - Tuberculous endometritis
  - Secondary amenorrhea
  - Postmenopausal bleeding
  - Primary or secondary infertility
- Asherman syndrome—to release adhesions
- To remove embedded intrauterine device

OVUM FORCEPS (FIGURE 28.30)

Description

- It is a long metallic instrument with spoon-shaped fenestrated blades.
- The handle does not have a lock in order to prevent crushing of tissues.

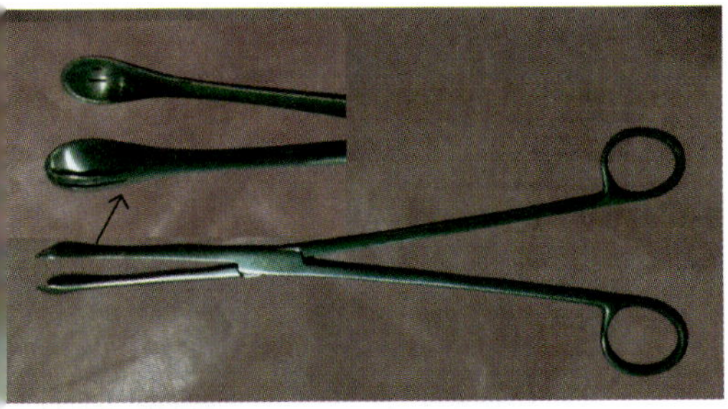

Figure 28.30 Ovum forceps (inset: close up).

Use

It is used to remove products of conception from the uterine cavity during surgical abortion. As it does not have a lock, inadvertent crushing of uterine wall or intra-abdominal structures is minimal, if uterine perforation occurs during the procedure.

Viva corner

Q1 How is an ovum forceps differentiated from a sponge holding forceps?

Ovum forceps:

- Does not have a catch lock
- Does not have transverse serrations

Sponge holding forceps has a catch lock and transverse serrations.

HEGAR'S DILATORS (FIGURE 28.31)

- Hegar's dilators are curved, double-ended dilators with conical tips used for rapid dilatation of cervix. Width of one end is smaller than that of the other.
- These are available in sets, with a minimum size of 1/2 and maximum size of 11/12. The number represents the diameter in millimeter. Both the ends are used, with the lower number side introduced first into the cervical canal.
- The presence of a slight angulation at the ends makes the instrument less traumatic.

Uses

Obstetrics

- For rapid dilatation of cervix during suction evacuation procedure and in molar pregnancy
- Diagnosis of cervical incompetence

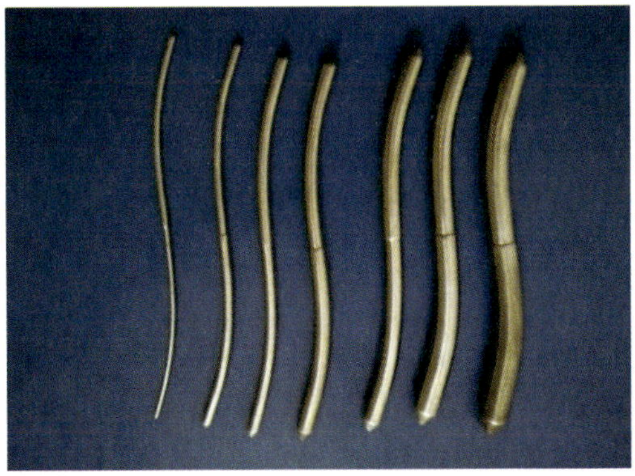

Figure 28.31 Hegar's dilators available in various sizes.

Gynecology

Hegar's dilators are used for dilatation of cervix in the following:

- Endometrial curettage
- Hysteroscopy
- Amputation of cervix and cervical cone biopsy
- Cervical stenosis
- Primary dysmenorrhea

Disadvantage

Risk of uterine perforation, especially in a pregnant uterus

KARMAN'S SUCTION CANNULA (FIGURE 28.32)

Description

- Karman's cannula is a long tubular structure made of plastic or metal.

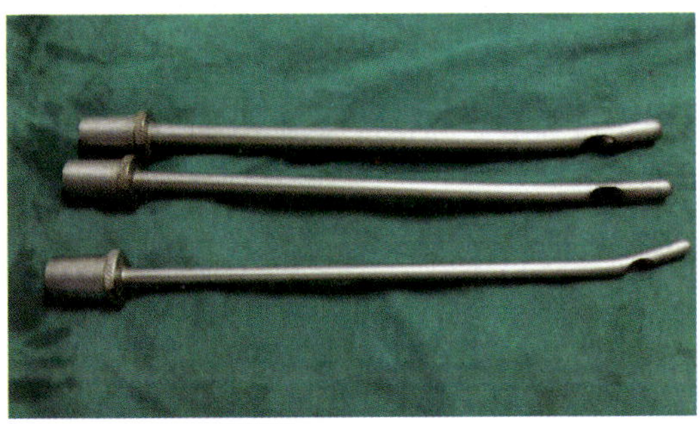

Figure 28.32 Karman's metal suction cannula available in different sizes.

Part 3

Extra edge

Q1 What is a Mathew Duncan's dilator?

Description

- It is a single-ended, metallic cervical dilator.
- The handle is disc shaped and the width of the dilator gradually decreases toward the tip.
- It is available in sets of variable sizes; the smallest is 3/6 and the largest is 18/21. The markings indicate the circumference in millimeter.

Uses

Same as those of Hegar's dilators

- Depending on the constituent material, the cannula can be rigid or flexible.
- A plastic cannula is preferred as it is less traumatic, transparent, and disposable.
- It is available in sizes varying from 4 to 12 mm diameter. The approximate size to be used corresponds to the weeks of pregnancy to be terminated. For example, 10-mm cannula is used for a 10-week pregnant uterus.
- The distal end of cannula is fixed to the suction tubing or apparatus. The proximal end, which is introduced into the uterine cavity, has two side openings to collect the contents.

Uses

- Used for suction evacuation during surgical abortion
- Used for suction evacuation of molar pregnancy

CHEATLE FORCEPS (FIGURE 28.33)

Description

- It is a heavy, metallic, curved forceps having serrations for a better grip.
- It has no lock.
- It is kept sterile by keeping it dipped in Savlon, Cidex, etc.

Use

To pick and transfer sterile linen or instruments from one tray to other

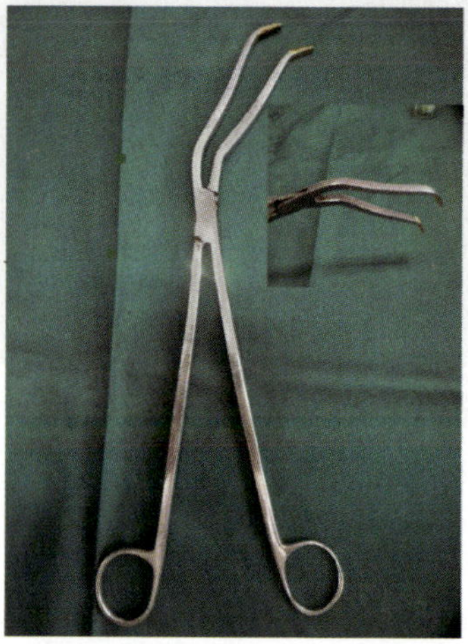

a.

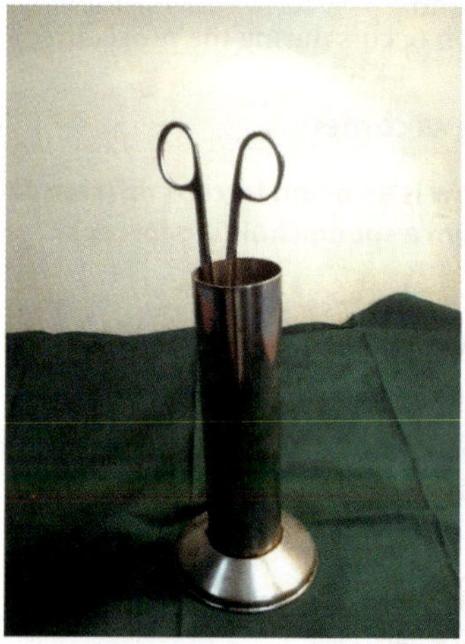

b.

Figure 28.33 Cheatle forceps. **a.** Cheatle forceps with its close-up view. **b.** Cheatle forceps kept inside its container containing antiseptic solution such as Savlon.

EPISIOTOMY SCISSORS (FIGURE 28.34)

Description

This scissors has angulated blades and one of the blades has a blunt tip.

Use

Used for giving episiotomy during vaginal delivery

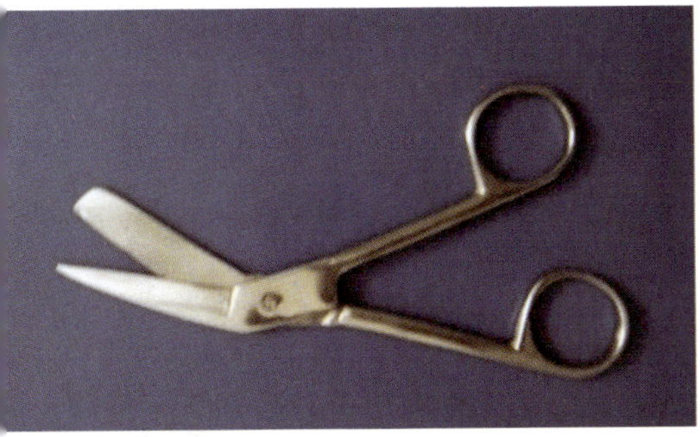

Figure 28.34 Episiotomy scissors.

Advantages

- Angulation of blades helps in better visualization during episiotomy.
- Blunt end is introduced into the vagina to avoid damage to fetal parts.

UMBILICAL CORD-CUTTING SCISSORS (FIGURE 28.35)

Description

It is a short scissors with curved blades.

Use

To cut the umbilical cord following delivery

SUTURE-CUTTING SCISSORS (FIGURE 28.36)

Description

This is a fine scissors especially used for removal of skin sutures.

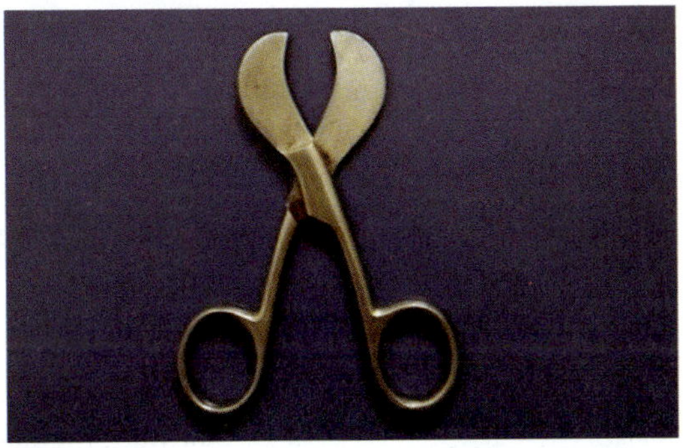

Figure 28.35 Umbilical cord-cutting scissors.

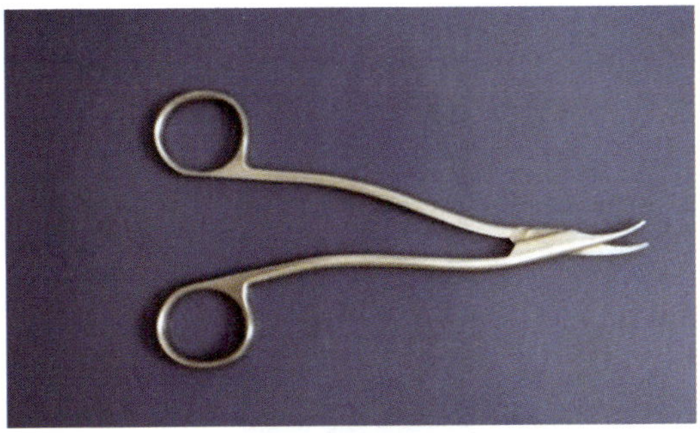

Figure 28.36 Suture-cutting scissors.

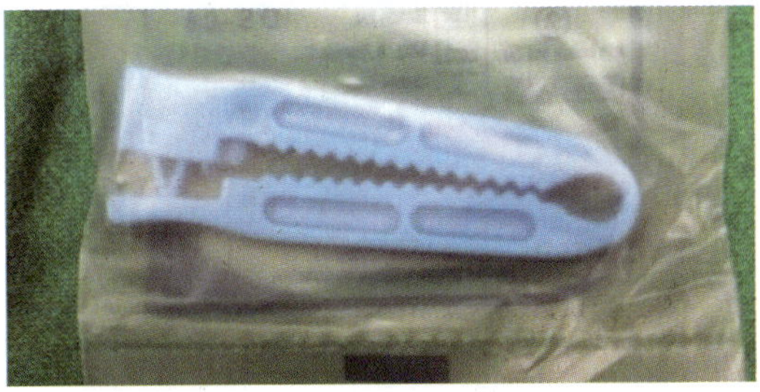

Figure 28.37 Disposable cord clamp.

DISPOSABLE CORD CLAMP (FIGURE 28.37)

Description

- It is made of plastic and is supplied in a sterile pack.
- It has a serrated inner surface and a lock that make its grip firm.

Use

Disposable cord clamp is used to clamp the umbilical cord following delivery. The cord clamp is kept in place, until it falls off with the detached umbilical cord stump.

AYRE'S WOODEN SPATULA (FIGURE 28.38)

Description

- It is a wooden spatula, 15–20 cm in length; one end has a smooth bifurcated edge that fits into the ectocervix and the other end is broad.

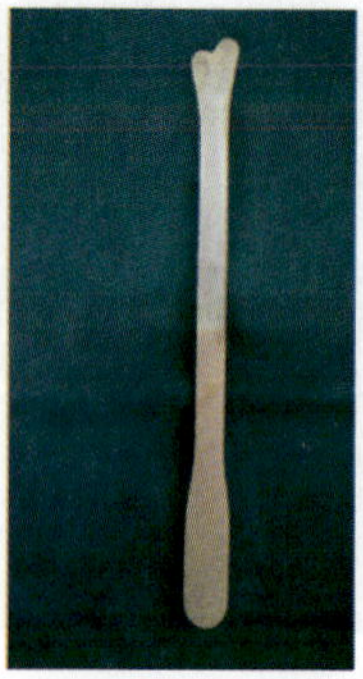

a.

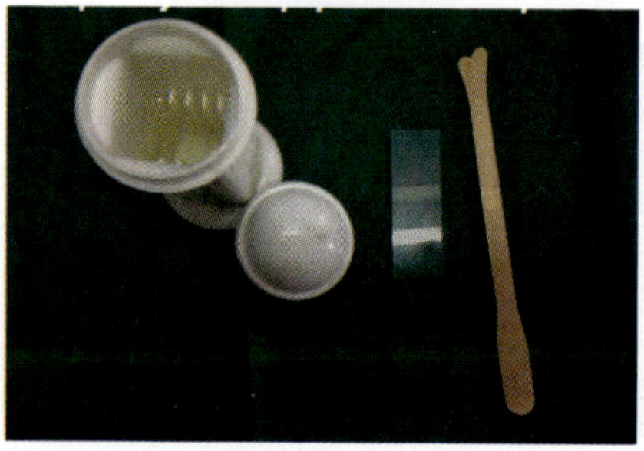

b.

Figure 28.38 Ayre's wooden spatula and the items required for taking a Pap smear. **a.** Ayre's spatula. **b.** Koplin jar containing the fixative, a numbered glass slide, and the Ayre's spatula.

- It is made up of wood so that the cells can adhere to its porous surface.

Uses

- To take Pap smear
- To take surface biopsy in carcinoma cervix
- To collect vaginal secretions from lateral fornix for hormonal cytology
- To take buccal smear

Viva corner

Q1 How is a Pap smear taken?

- The long bifurcated end of Ayre's spatula is introduced into cervical canal and rotated 360°.
- The exfoliated cells are smeared on a glass slide and the slide is placed in Koplin jar containing the fixative (ether and alcohol in equal amount).
- The broad end is used for taking buccal smear, and smear from lateral vaginal wall for hormonal cytology.

CERVICAL BROOM SAMPLING DEVICE (FIGURE 28.39)

Description

Cervical broom is a plastic stick-like structure having a broom-like head.

Uses

- A cervical broom is recommended for taking specimens for liquid-based cytology. The device is rotated around the cervical os in a clockwise direction.
- Sample is rinsed in a vial containing liquid-based medium—80–90% of cells are transferred to liquid medium and transported to the laboratory.

UTERUS HOLDING FORCEPS (FIGURE 28.40)

Description

This instrument has blades with curved transverse bars, with a gap between the bars when locked. The gap between the transverse bars makes it atraumatic.

Use

To lift, hold, and steady the uterus during procedures such as sling surgeries and tubal surgeries

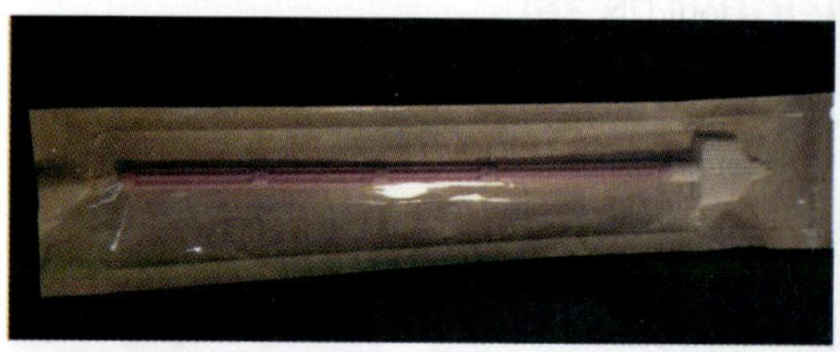

Figure 28.39 Cervical broom.

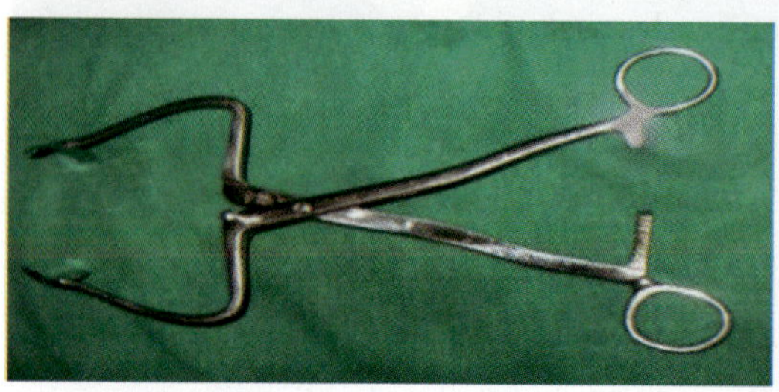

Figure 28.40 Uterus holding forceps.

RING PESSARY (FIGURE 28.41)

Description

- It is a ring-shaped plastic device used in conservative management of uterovaginal prolapse.
- A ring pessary supports the uterus by resting on the levators that act as shelves.

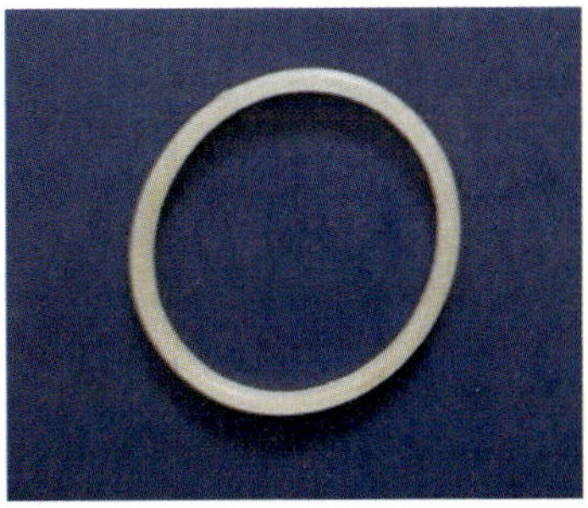

Figure 28.41 Ring pessary.

Uses

Indications for pessary in prolapse

- Pregnancy up to 12–14 weeks
- During lactation
- If surgery is contraindicated
- If the patient refuses surgery
- To promote healing of decubitus ulcer
- As a therapeutic test to confirm whether the symptom of low backache is due to prolapse or orthopedic problem

PINARD'S STETHOSCOPE (FIGURE 28.42)

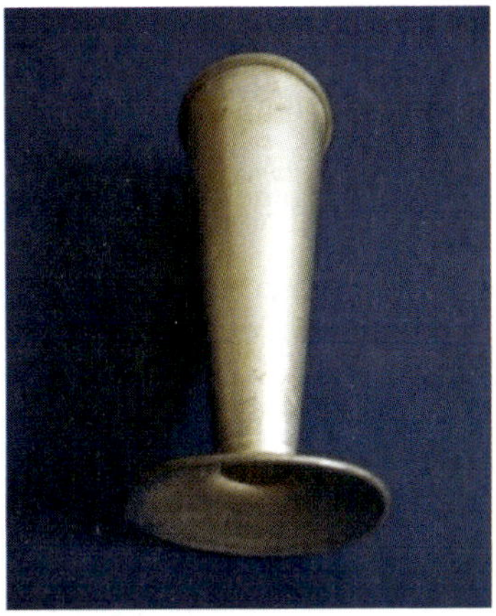

Figure 28.42 Pinard's stethoscope.

Description

- It is a hollow metal tool used for fetal heart rate auscultation. It functions similar to the trumpet by amplifying the sound.
- The wider side is pressed upon the maternal abdomen and the clinician's ear is applied to the tapering rim of the device.
- It should be held firmly at right angle to the point on the abdominal wall.
- It should not be touched by hand while listening to fetal heart sound.

Use

It is used for auscultation of the fetal heart rate. This instrument is currently not used in clinical settings, due to the availability of stethoscope and other advanced devices.

CERVICAL PUNCH BIOPSY FORCEPS (FIGURE 28.43)

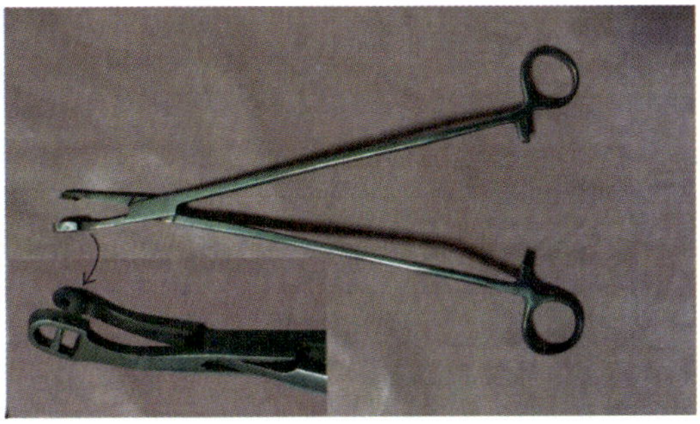

Figure 28.43 Cervical punch biopsy forceps.

Description

This instrument has a smaller blade with a sharp cutting edge that fits into a larger blade and can punch out the tissues when approximated.

Use

To take punch biopsy from cervix or any growth

> **Extra edge**
>
> Bleeding following biopsy procedure can be controlled by applying local pressure or by applying chemical cautery agent such as ferric subsulfate solution (Monsel's solution).

NOVAK'S ENDOMETRIAL BIOPSY CURETTE (FIGURE 28.44)

Description

- It is a long hollow instrument with a blunt tip and a subterminal opening, having serrated cutting edges.
- The instrument is angulated for introduction into the uterine cavity.
- It is provided with a stylet to collect the tissue sample and to clean the instrument.
- It is used for endometrial sampling.

Uses

It is used for endometrial sampling for the following indications:
- Dysfunctional uterine bleeding (DUB)
- Corpus luteal insufficiency—biopsy taken on days 21–24
- Diagnosis of anovulation (premenstrual biopsy is taken)
- Diagnosis of genital tuberculosis (endometrial sampling is taken on day 1 of menses because tubercles come to the superficial endometrial surface only during this time)

LEECH-WILKINSON CANNULA (FIGURE 28.45)

Description

- This is a metal cannula with a conical tip having screw-like serrations that help to screw the cannula into the cervical canal.
- The cannula fits snugly into the cervical canal and is used for instilling dye into the uterine cavity.

Uses

- Hysterosalpingogram—to determine the patency of fallopian tubes and to check for uterine anomalies (oil- or liquid-based solution is instilled into uterine cavity and studied under fluoroscopic guidance)
- Laparoscopic chromopertubation to determine patency of the fallopian tubes during laparoscopy (methylene blue dye is used)

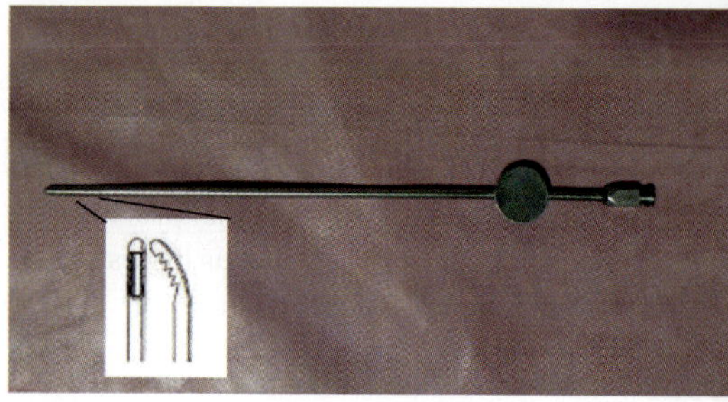

Figure 28.44 Novak's endometrial biopsy curette.

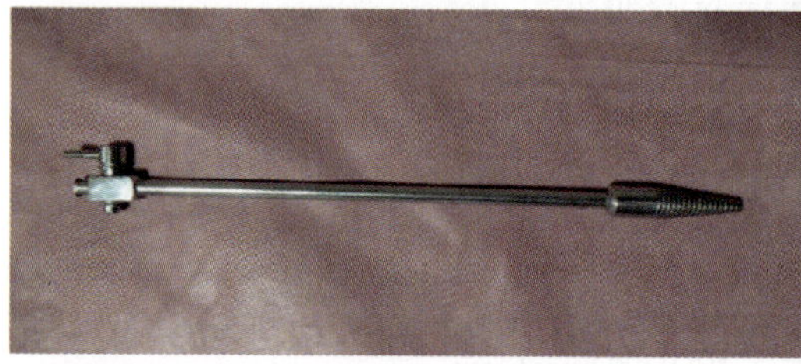

Figure 28.45 Leech-Wilkinson cannula.

MALECOT'S CATHETER (FIGURE 28.46)

Description

It is a red rubber catheter with a flower tip that provides enhanced drainage and catheter retention.

Uses

- Used to provide drainage following open renal and bladder surgeries
- In gynecology, can be used for draining collection from peritoneal cavity following surgery
- In pyoperitoneum for drainage of fluid

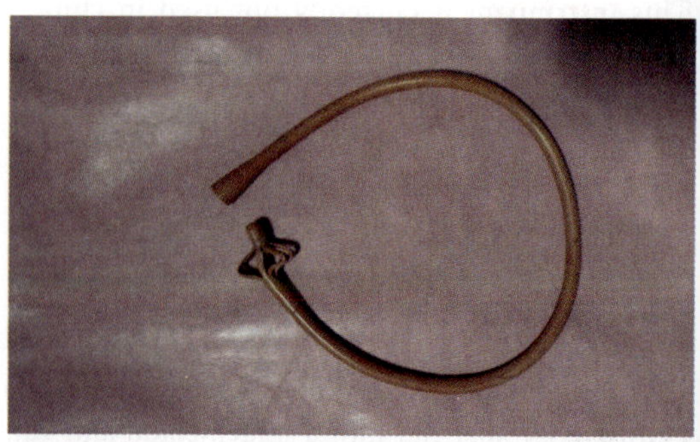

Figure 28.46 Malecot's catheter.

VAGINAL TAMPON (FIGURE 28.47)

Description

It is made of cotton wrapped in gauze piece for insertion into vagina.

Use

It is used for vaginal packing in uterovaginal prolapse. It is soaked in acriflavine and glycerin prior to insertion. It helps in healing of decubitus ulcer by reducing congestion and edema.

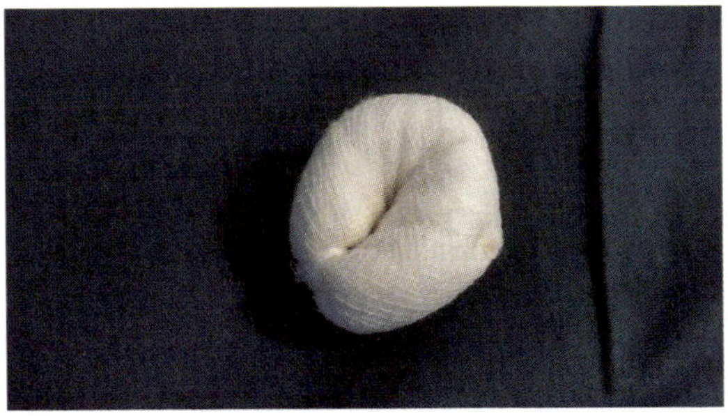

Figure 28.47 Vaginal tampon.

KIDNEY TRAY (FIGURE 28.48)

Description

- Kidney tray is a shallow basin having a kidney-shaped base and sloping walls. It is commonly used in the wards for receiving soiled dressings and other medical waste.
- Reusable kidney trays are made up of metal, while the disposable ones are made up of plastic.

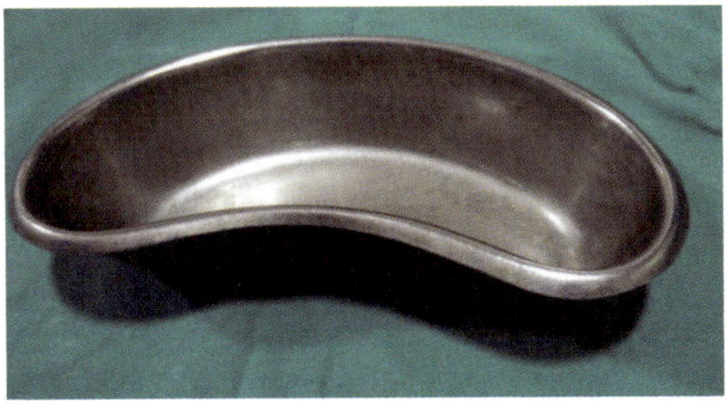

Figure 28.48 Kidney tray.

Uses

- To collect and hold urine during vaginal surgeries such as vaginal hysterectomy and cystocele repair
- To hold swabs for antiseptic painting before any operation
- To collect placenta after delivery of the baby
- To collect blood clots during cesarean section and ruptured ectopic pregnancy
- To collect vomitus

LANE'S TISSUE HOLDING FORCEPS (FIGURE 28.49)

Description

It is an instrument with sharp, fenestrated, curved blades at one end and a handle with a lock at the other end.

Uses

- It is used to hold tough/bulky tissue.
- It is used to hold tissues being excised, such as uterus in vaginal hysterectomy.
- It can be used to hold or grasp dressing and surgical materials.

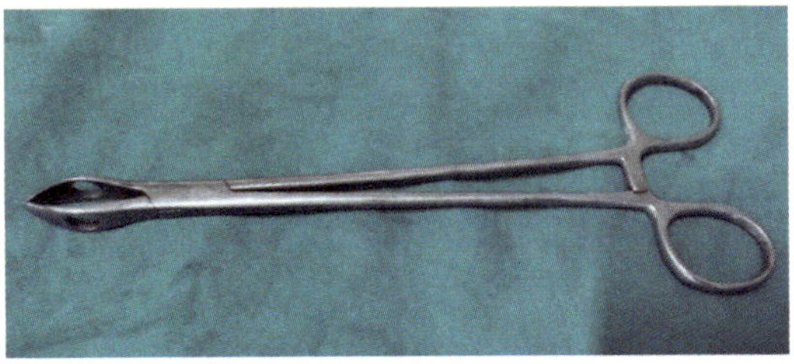

Figure 28.49 Lane's tissue holding forceps.

LANDON'S RETRACTOR (FIGURE 28.50)

Description

- It is an L-shaped instrument with a flat blade at right angles to the handle. The handle has a fenestration for better grip.

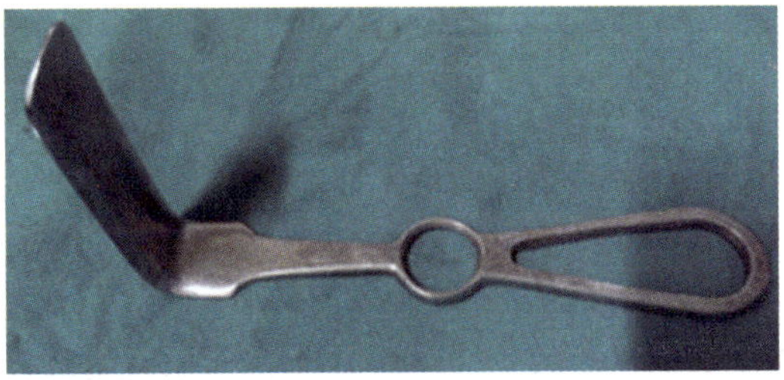

Figure 28.50 Landon's retractor.

Part 3

- It is a non–self-retaining retractor mainly used in vaginal surgeries.

Uses

- To retract the bladder during vaginal hysterectomy (it is introduced into the anterior pouch after the UV fold of peritoneum has been opened)
- To retract the vaginal walls during vaginal procedures

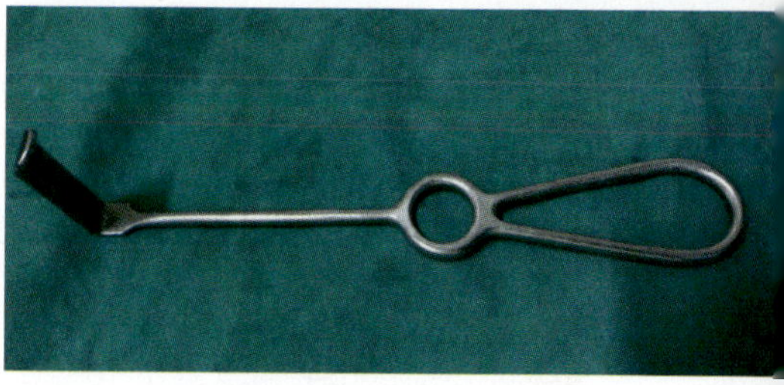

Figure 28.51 Langenbeck's retractor.

LANGENBECK'S RETRACTOR (FIGURE 28.51)

Description

- It is a single-bladed right-angled retractor.
- There is a fenestration between the blade and the handle for gripping the instrument.

Uses

- For retraction of abdominal wall or abdominal organs during abdominal surgeries (adequate retraction ensures that no damage is caused to the underlying organs and tissues during dissection)
- To retract the abdominal wall during tubal ligation
- To retract bladder and vaginal walls during vaginal hysterectomy
- For superficial retraction of skin and subcutaneous tissue

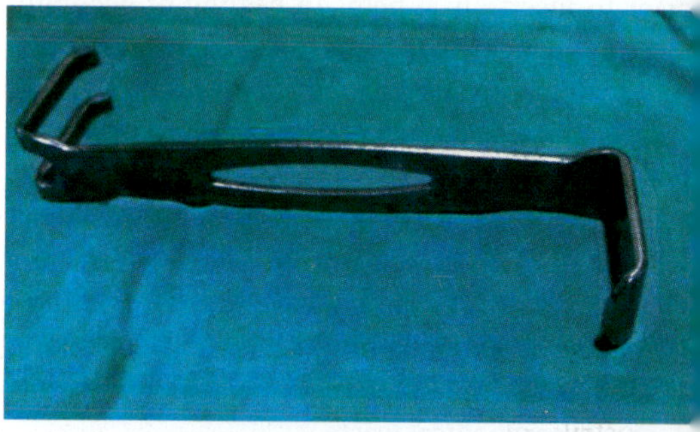

Figure 28.52 Czerny's retractor.

CZERNY'S RETRACTOR (FIGURE 28.52)

Description

Retractor with two spikes on one end and a broad surface on the other

Uses

- Typically used to retract the skin for placing sutures at the angles of rectus sheath during closure of laparotomy incision
- Used to retract the subcutaneous tissue during rectus closure

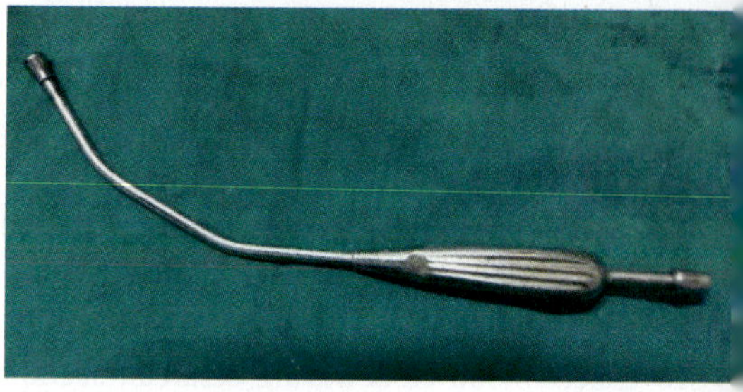

Figure 28.53 Suction cannula.

SUCTION CANNULA (FIGURE 28.53)

Description

It is a cannula that is connected to a suction apparatus by rubber tubing.

Uses

- Used for suction of blood and to clear the field of surgery during abdominal and vaginal surgeries
- Used for suctioning of liquor during LSCS

BULB SYRINGE/SUCTION BULB (FIGURE 28.54)

Description

It is a rubber object with a long tip at the end of a bulb. It is used to remove excess mucus from the mouth and nose.

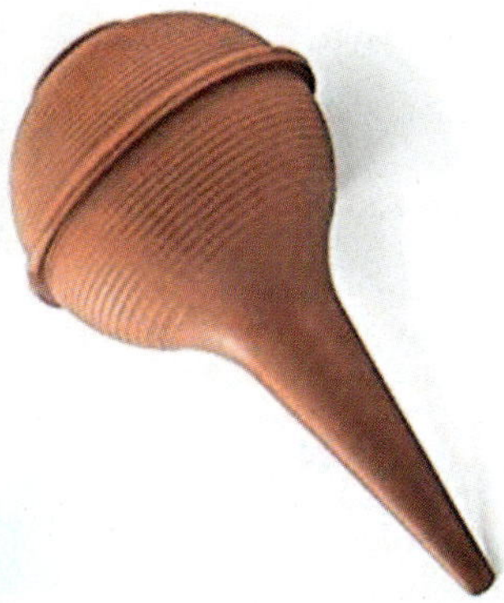

Figure 28.54 Bulb syringe or bulb sucker.

Uses

- To remove excess mucus from the mouth and nostrils of the baby following delivery. The mouth is suctioned first followed by the nostrils to prevent aspiration.
- The air out of the bulb is squeezed out to create a vacuum. The rubber tip is then gently inserted into the mouth or nostril of the baby. The bulb is released slowly to suck out the mucus. The bulb syringe is then removed and the bulb is squeezed forcefully to expel the mucus into a tissue/container.

MICROSURGICAL INSTRUMENTS (FIGURE 28.55)

Uses

- Microsurgical instruments are used during tubal recanalization procedure where tubal reanastomosis is done.
- They are also used in other tubal reconstructive surgeries for treatment of tubal causes of infertility.
- Microsurgical techniques used to minimize postoperative adhesions
  - Use of suction, irrigation, and floatation techniques
  - Use of fine instruments and sutures
  - Use of adhesive barriers.

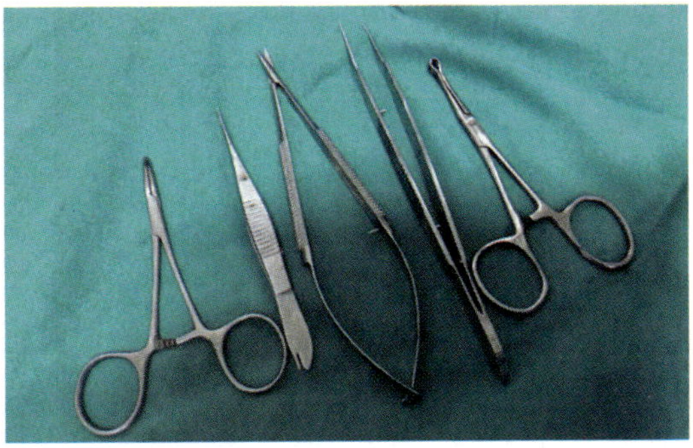

Figure 28.55 Microsurgical instruments used in tubal reconstructive surgeries.

LAPAROSCOPY INSTRUMENTS (FIGURE 28.56)

Veress needle

A Veress needle is a spring-loaded needle used to create pneumoperitoneum during laparoscopic surgery.

Trocar and cannula

- Trocar with the cannula is inserted into peritoneal cavity (port site) for laparoscopy.
- It has a side opening for connecting it to gas source.
- It has a trumpet valve that prevents gas leakage.
- It is available in varying sizes: 10 mm for operative laparoscopy and 5 mm for diagnostic laparoscopy.

Laparoscope

- It is introduced into peritoneal cavity through port site for inspection of cavity and has an inbuilt camera.
- It is connected to the light source cable and monitor cable.
- It is available in two types: 0° and 30° scopes. The 30° scope is mainly used in gynecology.

Accessory instruments

- Grasper, scissors, etc., are used in operative gynecology
- Introduced by creating accessory ports

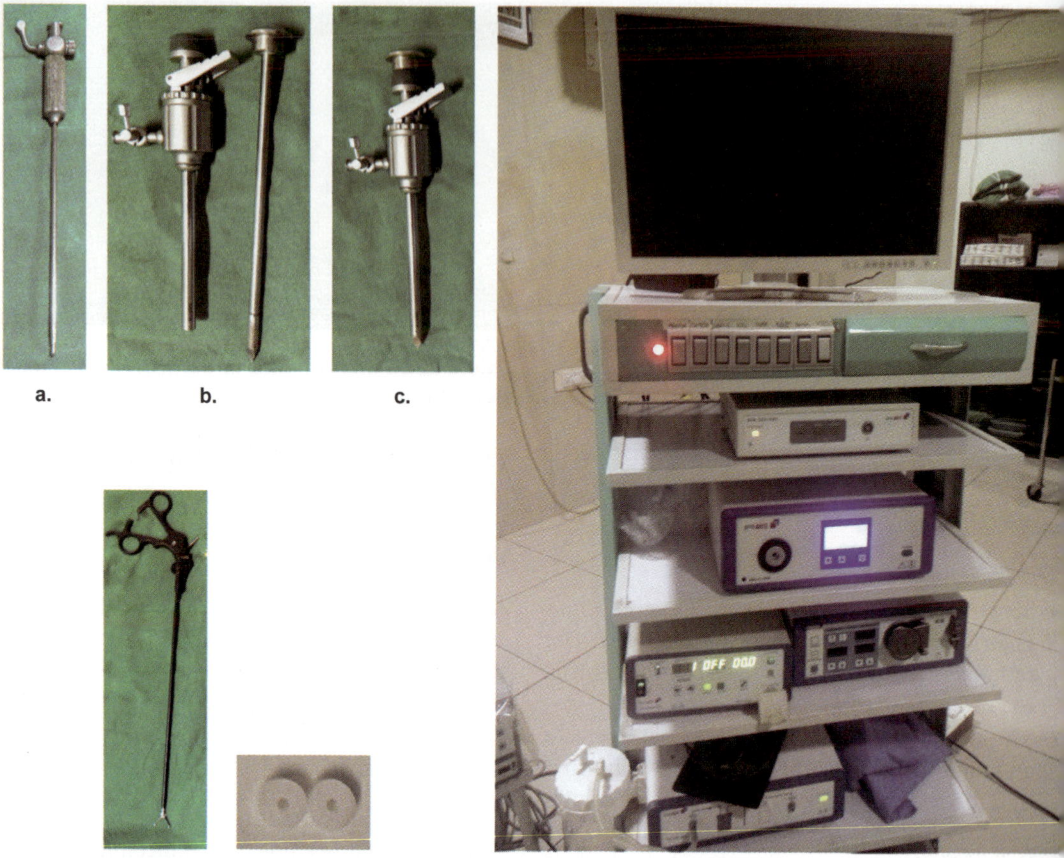

Figure 28.56 Laparoscopy instruments. **a.** Veress needle. **b.** Trochar and cannula. **c.** Trochar placed inside the cannula. **d.** Grasper. **e.** Falope rings. **f.** Display monitor along with other gadgets for laparoscopy.

Note *Vacuum extractor and obstetric forceps used for conducting instrumental vaginal deliveries are described in Part 3, Chapter 37, Common Obstetric Surgical Procedures.*

SURGICAL SUTURES (FIGURE 28.57)

Classification of suture material

- Classification of suture material based on absorbability (Table 28.1)
- Classification of suture material based on material structure (Table 28.2)
- Classification of suture material based on the raw material—natural and synthetic (Table 28.3)
- Classification of suture material based on whether coating is provided or not [specialized coatings may enhance properties such as knotting and easy passage through tissue, and reduce tissue reaction (Table 28.4)]
- Classification based on suture size:
  - Surgical sutures are classified into different sizes based on the diameter of the thread.
  - The United States Pharmacopeia's classification of sutures sizes is widely accepted.
  - No. 1, No. 2, etc., sizes indicate a progressively thicker suture material, and No. 1-0, No. 2-0, etc., sizes indicate a progressively thinner suture material.
- Classification based on usage:
  - Sutures can be classified according to their usage, for example, cardiovascular sutures, ophthalmic sutures, general sutures, and orthopedic sutures.

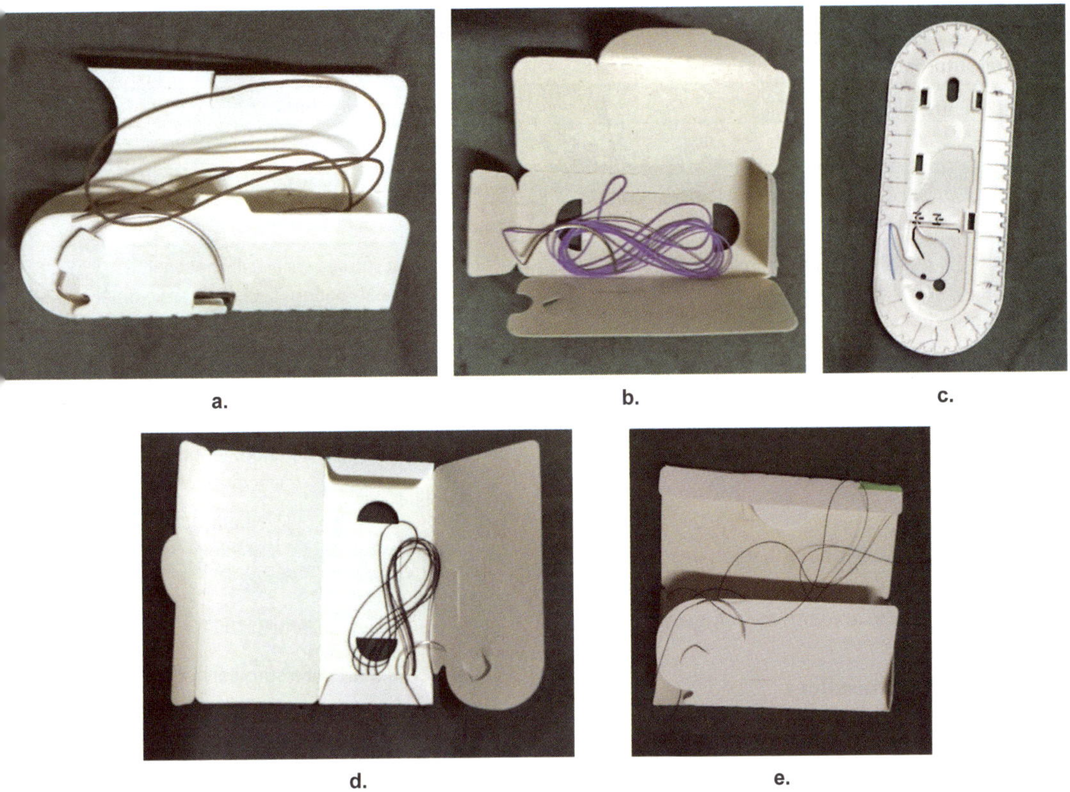

Figure 28.57 Surgical suture. **a.** Chromic catgut suture material. **b.** Vicryl (polyglactin 910) suture material. **c.** Prolene (polypropylene) suture material. **d.** Silk suture material. **e.** Ethilon (nylon) suture material.

Table 28.1 Comparison of absorbable and nonabsorbable suture materials

Absorbable	Nonabsorbable
• Suture material will break down harmlessly in the body over time without intervention • Absorbable sutures are often used internally • *Examples:* – Rapidly absorbable suture materials: catgut, chromic catgut – Delayed absorbable suture material, braided: polyglycolic acid (Dexon), polyglactin 910 (Vicryl) – Delayed absorbable suture material, monofilament: poliglyconate (Maxon), and polydioxanone (PDS)	• Suture material is nonabsorbable unless manually removed • Nonabsorbable sutures are often used externally • For example, polypropylene (Prolene), nylon (Ethilon), silk

Table 28.2 Comparison of monofilament and braided suture materials

Monofilament	Polyfilament or braided
• Monofilament sutures provide better passage through tissues • Monofilament sutures elicit lower tissue reaction compared with braided sutures • For example, polypropylene, catgut, nylon, polyglyconate, and polydioxanone	• Braided sutures provide better knot security than monofilament sutures • Polyfilament sutures are braided and often coated with materials such as silicon, wax, and polycaprolactone • For example, polyglycolic acid, polyglactin 910, silk

Table 28.3 Examples of natural and synthetic suture materials

Natural sutures	Synthetic sutures
Silk and catgut sutures	All other sutures are synthetic in nature

Table 28.4 Comparison of coated and uncoated suture materials

Coated	Uncoated
• Coating is usually applied to braided sutures • Coating materials used are chromium salt, silicon, wax, polycaprolactone, calcium stearate, etc. • For example, polyglycolic acid sutures, chromic catgut, polyglactin 910, silk, and polydioxanone sutures	• Monofilament sutures are usually not coated • Newer functional coatings such as antimicrobial coating are given to both monofilament and multifilament sutures • For example, monofilament polypropylene, monofilament nylon

SURGICAL NEEDLES

Description

Surgical needles are made of steel, are available in different sizes, and can be curved or straight. Parts of a surgical needle are shown in Figure 28.58.

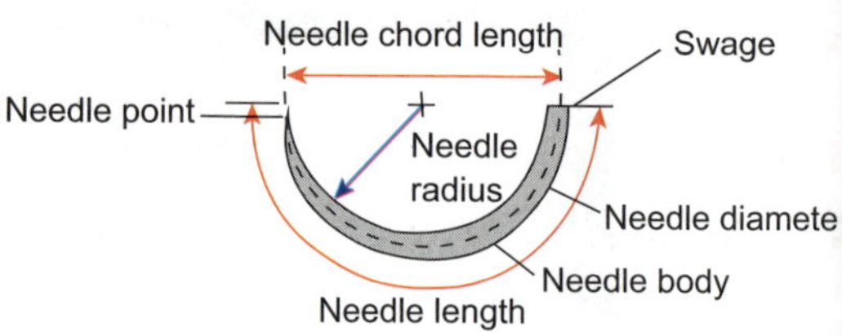

Figure 28.58 Parts of a surgical needle.

Types of surgical needles

Straight needles Straight needles can be used for skin closure. They can be used for suturing without the need of a needle holder.

Curved needles

- Curved surgical needles are used most commonly.
- Curved needles are made in several different configurations: 1/4, 3/8, 1/2, and 5/8 of a circle (Figure 28.59). Types of curved needles are mentioned in Table 28.5 and Figure 28.60.

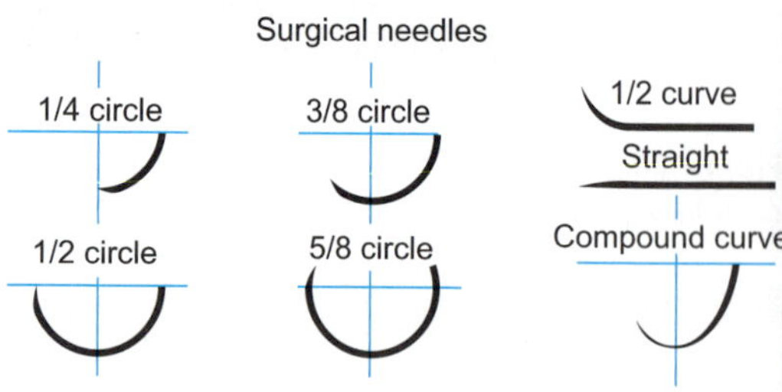

Figure 28.59 Different configurations of curved needles.

Table 28.5 Types of curved needles

Curved needle type	Description	Usage
Taper point needles	Gradually tapers to a point and cross-section is round	Used for tissues that are easy to penetrate—used for structures within peritoneal cavity such as pedicles, bladder, peritoneum, and blood vessels
Cutting needles	Triangular tip with apex forming the cutting surface	Used for tough tissues such as skin
Reverse cutting needle	Similar to cutting needle, but the cutting surface faces down or on the outer side of the needle	Used for tough tissues such as tendon sheath and skin

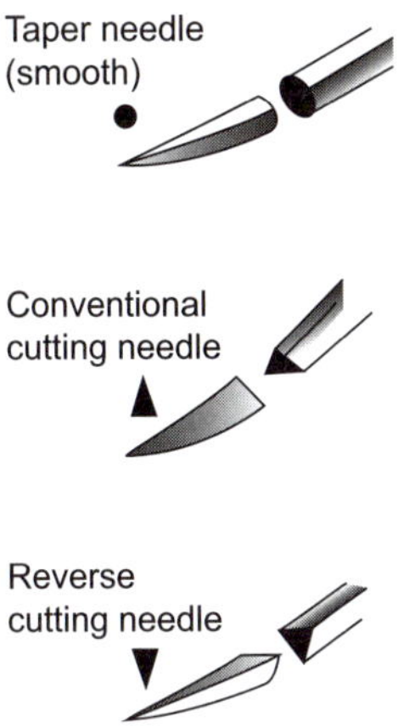

Figure 28.60 Types of curved needles.

SUTURE ATTACHMENT TO NEEDLE

- **Eyeless or swaged needles:** Suture is attached to most surgical needles by a type of connection known as eyeless connection (Figure 28.61).
- **Closed-eye needles:** Suture has to be tied through the eye on the needle, making it more bulky.

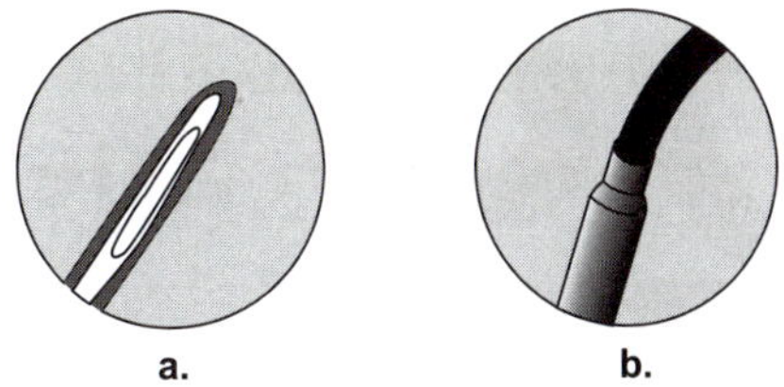

Figure 28.61 Suture attachment to needle. a. Eyed needle. b. Eyeless (swaged) needle.

PROCESSING OF INSTRUMENTS

Instruments can be disinfected by immersing them in the following:

- Boiling water for 20 minutes
- Glutaraldehyde 2% (Cidex) solution for 20 minutes
- 0.5% chlorine solution for 20 minutes [0.5% of chlorine solution is made by adding three teaspoons (15 g) of bleaching powder in 1 L of water]

Sterilization is done by the following:

- Autoclaving
- Immersing in 2% glutaraldehyde (Cidex) solution for 10 hours

29 Specimens

Introduction

It is essential for medical students to be familiar with the pathology of various disease conditions in obstetrics and gynecology, as it forms the basis for understanding of the clinical signs and symptoms and treatment of the disease condition. It is not always possible for the students to be present during all the surgeries and deliveries to see all the pathological lesions. A collection of pathological specimens will serve as an alternative way to study the pathology. This chapter deals with the common pathological specimens that are discussed during practical viva voce examination in obstetrics and gynecology.

The usual pattern for description of a pathological specimen includes a brief description of the gross features of the specimen, followed by the diagnosis or differential diagnosis. Even if the diagnosis is evident on inspection, it is essential to describe the specimen first, in order to justify the diagnosis.

Description of a specimen

It includes the following:

- Identification of the organ
- Description of the pathology as seen on naked eye examination

Note *Orientation of a specimen of uterus:*

1. *The peritoneal reflection on the anterior serosal surface is higher and blunter (from bladder dissection) and posterior serosal surface is lower and comes to a point.*
2. *The attached adnexa (in order of anterior to posterior): round ligament, fallopian tube, ovary and ovarian ligament.*

Gross appearance of the specimen

Do's

- While describing a specimen, the main organ that is visualized must be first described. Other related organs along with the main organ present in the specimen must also be described.
- The gross pathology in the specimen is then described.
- The answer may be concluded by giving a probable diagnosis or differential diagnosis.

Don'ts

When a specimen is given, do not directly jump to the diagnosis, even if the diagnosis is obvious. For example, in a specimen of fibroid uterus, do not start the answer by saying that "this is a specimen of fibroid uterus." Instead, first describe the organ (uterus), then describe the presence of growth in the myometrium, and then describe that it is a specimen of "fibroid uterus."

Cut specimen

In case of a cut section of a specimen, the layers of the specimen organ should be described. For example, in a specimen of cut section of uterus, various layers such as serosa, myometrium, endometrium, and the endometrial cavity are described. The outer surface of the specimen also has to be described in examination along with the cut surface.

Diagnosis

The most probable diagnosis or differential diagnosis must be mentioned. For example, differential diagnosis in case of ovarian cysts and masses.

Surgical procedure by which the specimen has been retrieved must be mentioned, wherever applicable.

Viva corner

Q1 How is the diagnosis of anencephaly confirmed?

- **Ultrasound findings**
  - Absence of cranial vault can be noted as early as 10 weeks of gestation.
  - Biparietal diameter cannot be measured—failure to identify the fetal skull bones and brain tissue above orbits.
- **Maternal serum alpha-fetoprotein (MSAFP)**
  - Increased level of alpha-fetoprotein in amniotic fluid and/or maternal serum at 13–15 weeks of gestation
- **Clinical examination**
  - *Abdominal examination*: There is difficulty in palpation of the fetal head in later half of pregnancy.
  - *Pelvic examination*: Fetal skull bones and sutures are not felt in per vaginal examination in cephalic presentation.

Q2 What complications are associated with anencephaly during pregnancy?

There is an increased risk of poly hydramnios, malpresentations (face and breech presentation), and tendency for postmaturity.

Q3 How should a case of anencephaly be managed?

If diagnosis of anencephaly is made, pregnancy is terminated after counseling the parents, as it is incompatible with extrauterine life.

Q4 What are the common neural tube defects encountered in the clinical practice?

These are anencephaly, meningocele, and spina bifida.

Q5 What are the steps to prevent neural tube defects?

Folic acid supplementation 4 mg daily, started 1 month prior to conception helps in prevention of the occurrence of neural tube defects.

SPECIMENS IN OBSTETRICS

Specimen 1: Anencephaly (Figure 29.1)

Gross appearance

This is a specimen of fetus with the following features:

- Absence of vault of skull and exposed brain tissue with protruding eyeballs
- Chance of presence of associated malformations (the fetal back should be inspected to detect spinal cord anomalies such as spina bifida, meningocele, and myelocele)

Diagnosis

Specimen of fetus with anencephaly

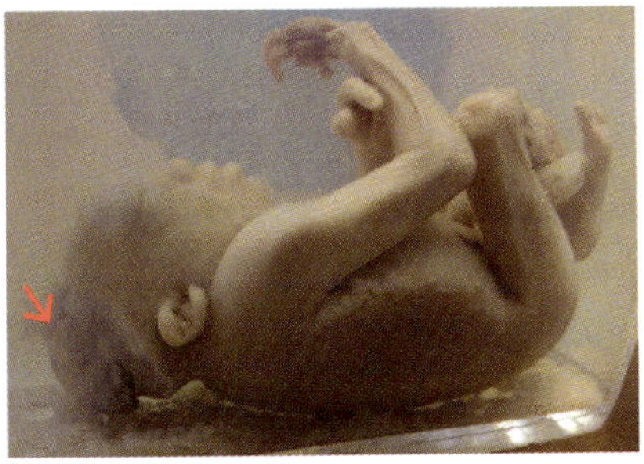

Figure 29.1 Anencephaly.

Specimen 2: Peripartum hysterectomy specimen (Figure 29.2)

Gross appearance

Hysterectomy specimen of a gravid uterus

Diagnosis

Cut section of specimen of gravid uterus, probably removed due to uncontrolled postpartum hemorrhage (PPH) or uterine rupture

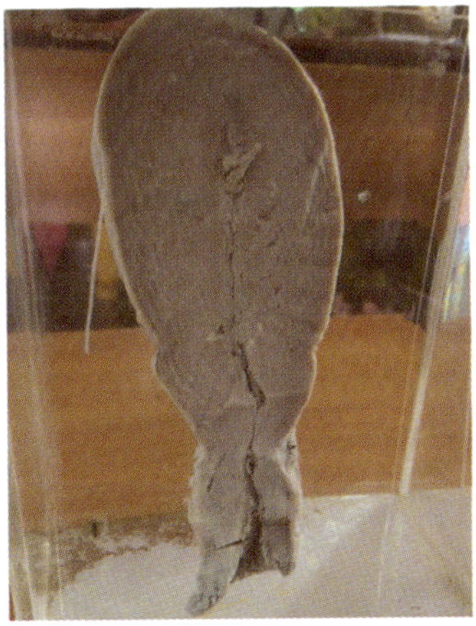

Figure 29.2 Peripartum hysterectomy specimen.

Viva corner

Q1 What are the reasons for performing hysterectomy in a pregnant woman?

- Atonic PPH
- Traumatic PPH
- Ruptured uterus
- Morbidly adherent placenta such as placenta accreta, increta, and percreta

Q2 How do you define PPH?

- **WHO definition:** Amount of blood loss of 500 mL or more following vaginal delivery or blood loss of 1000 mL or more following a cesarean section is defined as PPH.
- **Clinical definition:** Any amount of bleeding from or into the genital tract following birth of the baby up to the end of puerperium, which adversely affects the general condition of the mother, as evidenced by rise in pulse rate or fall in BP is termed PPH.

Q3 What are the important causes of PPH?

(**Acronym:** *Remember "four Ts"*)

- Tone (atonic uterus)
- Trauma (genital tract)
- Tissue (retained products of conception)
- Thrombin (coagulopathy)

The most common cause of PPH is atonic uterus (80%).

Q4 What are the risk factors of PPH?

- Grand multipara
- Uterine overdistension—multiple pregnancy and poly hydramnios
- Anemia
- Antepartum hemorrhage
- Prolonged labor
- Morbidly adherent placenta
- Trauma to genital tract

Q5 What are the medical measures available to control atonic PPH?

Medical management options available for atonic PPH are the following:

- Oxytocin 20 units in 500 mL normal saline started intravenously at the rate of 60 drops/minute
- Injection methergin 0.2 mg IV
- Injection carboprost (PGF2α) 250 μg IM, can be repeated at intervals of >15 minutes, up to maximum of eight doses
- Misoprostol (PGE1) 1000 μg placed per rectally
- Intramyometrial injection carboprost 250 μg

Q6 What are the surgical measures to control PPH?

- Explore the uterus under general anesthesia.
- Repair any genital tract injuries in case of traumatic PPH.
- Uterine tamponade with hydrostatic balloon catheter such as Sengstaken–Blakemore esophageal catheter. Balloon is inflated with 200–500 mL saline and is kept in situ for 4–6 hours to secure hemostasis.
- Hemostatic compression sutures: Hemostatic suture techniques are effective in controlling severe PPH.
  - B-Lynch sutures
  - Modified B-Lynch suture
  - Multiple Cho sutures
- Uterine devascularization procedures
  - Bilateral ligation of uterine vessels and utero-ovarian vessels
  - Bilateral internal iliac artery ligation, which is an effective method to control PPH
  - Uterine artery embolization (it requires the equipment and an interventional radiologist to perform the procedure)
  - Hysterectomy—final step if the patient is not responding to the above-mentioned methods

Q7 What are the components of active management of third stage of labor (AMTSL)?

(CONTD...)

(...CONTD)

Viva corner

AMTSL for prevention of PPH is practiced universally for all deliveries and it has three components:

- Administration of uterotonics, preferably oxytocin (10 units IV/IM), immediately following delivery of the baby
- Controlled cord traction (CCT) to deliver the placenta
- Massage of the uterus

Q8 What are the common causes of ruptured uterus?

- Rupture of uterine scar
- Obstructed labor
- Injudicious use of oxytocin in labor

Q9 How do you manage a case of ruptured uterus?

- Resuscitation and emergency laparotomy are done.
- Repair of the uterus may be done in selected cases. Tubal ligation is recommended along with the procedure.
- If repair is not possible, then hysterectomy is done.

Specimen 3: Ectopic pregnancy (Figure 29.3)

Gross appearance

- The specimen is a tube-like structure, which is identified as fallopian tube by the fimbrial end.
- Adjacent organs (either uterus or ovary) cannot be identified. This implies that salpingectomy was performed for pathology in the fallopian tube.
- The tube appears distended and is ruptured with tissue protruding out (probably gestational sac).

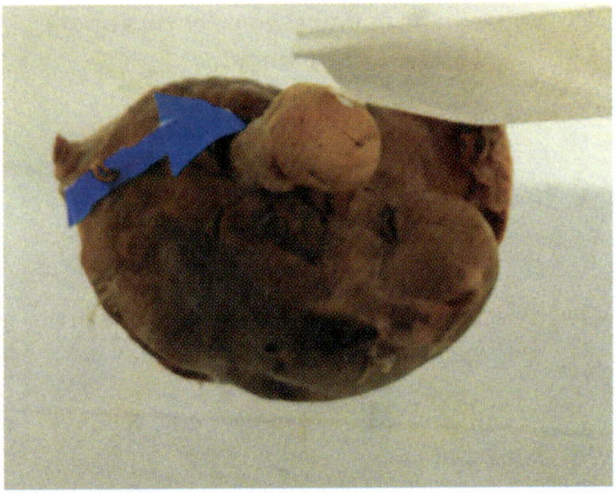

Figure 29.3 Ectopic pregnancy.

Diagnosis

A ruptured ectopic pregnancy for which salpingectomy was performed

Viva corner

Q1 What are the risk factors for ectopic pregnancy?

- History of pelvic inflammatory disease (PID)
- Previous tubal surgeries—history of tubal ligation and tubal reconstructive surgery
- Previous ectopic pregnancy
- Assisted reproductive techniques—especially if tubes are damaged
- Intrauterine contraceptive device (IUCD) usage (if there is failure of IUCD and pregnancy occurs, it is more likely to be an ectopic pregnancy)

Q2 What is the clinical presentation in ectopic pregnancy?

Clinical presentation in ruptured ectopic pregnancy:

- **Symptoms:** Classic triad of amenorrhea, abdominal pain, and vaginal bleeding is present. Positive urine pregnancy test is present.
- **Signs:** Pallor, tachycardia, hypotension, and shock are present.

(CONTD...)

(...CONTD)

Viva corner

- On bimanual examination, uterus appears bulky and forniceal tenderness or cervical motion tenderness may be present.
- Ultrasonography (USG) may show free fluid in pouch of Douglas (suggestive of hemoperitoneum).

Clinical presentation in unruptured ectopic pregnancy:

- Urine pregnancy test is positive.
- An adnexal mass with associated tenderness may be present on bimanual examination.
- Transvaginal sonography (TVS) reveals an adnexal mass with empty uterine cavity.

Q3 What is the management for ruptured tubal ectopic pregnancy?

- Resuscitation and laparotomy are done.
- Total or partial salpingectomy on the side of ruptured ectopic pregnancy is done.
- Blood transfusion is often needed.

Q4 What are the management options for unruptured tubal ectopic pregnancy?

- **Conservative management:** Medical or surgical
- **Definitive management:** Salpingectomy

Conservative medical management The drug commonly used is methotrexate. Other drugs that can be used are potassium chloride, prostaglandin (PGF2α), hyperosmolar glucose, and actinomycin.

- Prerequisites for medical therapy
  - Hemodynamically stable patient
  - Serum beta-human chorionic gonadotropin (hCG) level <5000 IU/L
  - Absent fetal cardiac activity
  - No intra-abdominal hemorrhage
- Single-dose regimen or variable-dose (multiple dose) regimen of methotrexate can be given (D1).
  - *Single-dose regimen*: A single dose of methotrexate 50 mg/m^2 IM injection is given (D1).
    - Monitor with serum beta-hCG on D4 and D7.
      - When decline in beta-hCG between D4 and D7 is >15%, serum beta-hCG is followed up weekly.
      - When decline is <15%, second dose of methotrexate 50 mg/m^2 is given on D7 and followed up.
  - *Variable-dose regimen*: Methotrexate 1 mg/kg IM on D1, 3, 5, and 7 and leucovorin 0.1 mg/kg IM on D2, 4, 6, and 8 are administered. Monitor with serum beta-hCG weekly.

Conservative surgical management

- **Salpingostomy:** Longitudinal incision on the antimesenteric border of fallopian tube over the site of ectopic pregnancy → products of conception are removed → the incision site is kept open that heals by secondary intention.
- **Salpingotomy:** Procedure is the same like that of salpingostomy, but the incision line is closed.

Specimen 4: Hydatidiform mole (Figure 29.4)

Gross appearance

The specimen shows a cluster of translucent vesicles/grape-like structures.

Diagnosis

The diagnosis is probably hydatidiform mole.

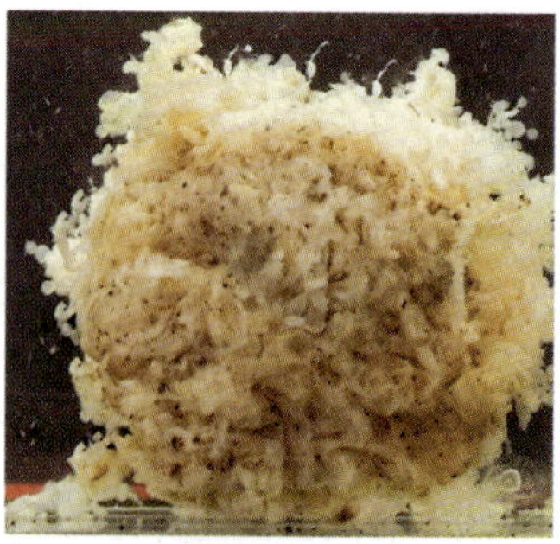

Figure 29.4 Hydatidiform mole.

Viva corner

Q1 What are the types of molar pregnancy?

Molar pregnancy is of two types: partial and complete mole.

On gross inspection:

- **Complete mole:** No fetal/placental tissue is present.
- **Partial mole:** Fetal/placental tissue may be present.

Q2 How is gestational trophoblastic disease (GTD) classified?

Benign GTD (90%)	Malignant GTD (10%)
• Complete hydatidiform mole • Partial hydatidiform mole	• Invasive mole • Choriocarcinoma • Placental site trophoblastic tumor

GTD, gestational trophoblastic disease.

Q3 How will you terminate a molar pregnancy?

A molar pregnancy is terminated by suction evacuation.

Specimen 5: Specimen of fetus with placenta (Figure 29.5a)

Gross appearance

A specimen of fetus is shown with a discoid-shaped structure attached to it. One side of the discoid mass is brown in color, with a rugged look having multiple cotyledons (maternal side; refer to Figure 29.5b). The other side is smooth and covered by thin membranes and a cord-like structure is attached near the center (fetal side; refer to Figure 29.5c).

Diagnosis

Specimen of fetus with placenta

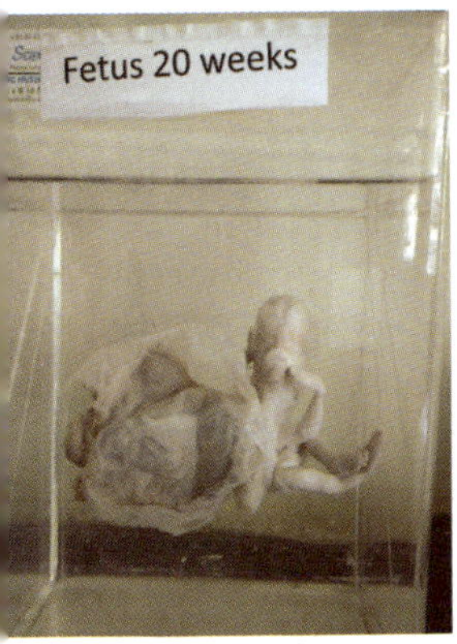

a.

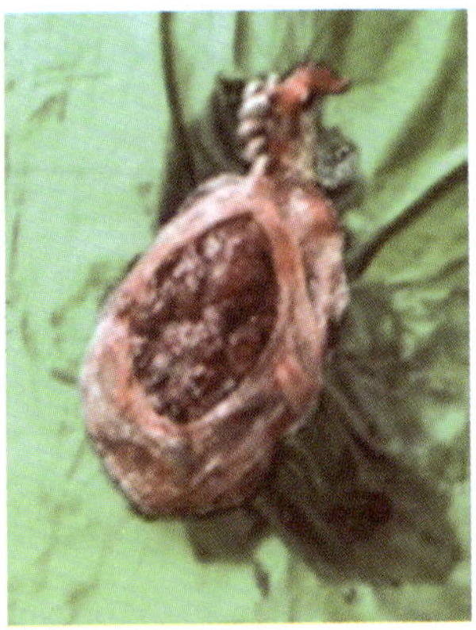

b.

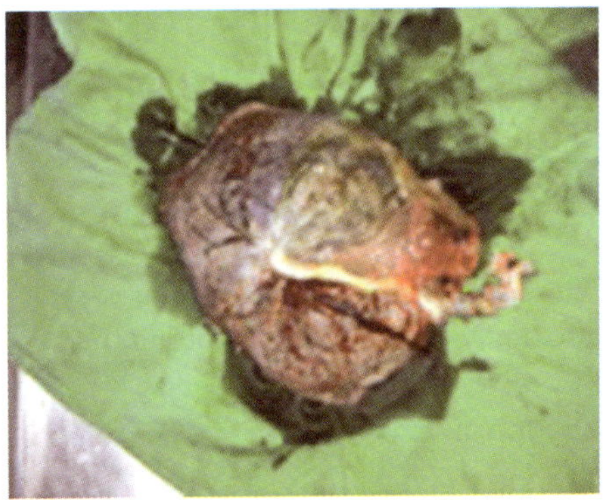

c.

Figure 29.5 Placenta. **a.** Specimen of fetus with placenta. **b.** Maternal surface of placenta. **c.** Fetal surface of placenta.

Viva corner

Q1 What are the functions of the placenta?

- Transfer of nutrients to the fetus and waste products from the fetus across the placenta
- Endocrine function—synthesis of hormones and enzymes necessary to maintain pregnancy
- Barrier function
- Immunological function

Q2 What are the various placental abnormalities?

- **Placenta succenturiata:** One or more small lobes of placenta are placed at varying distances from the main placenta. A leash of vessels traverses through the membranes connecting the main placenta to the small lobe.

(CONTD...)

(...CONTD)

Viva corner

In cases of absence of communicating blood vessels, it is termed placenta spuria.

- *Significance*: If the succenturiate lobe is retained following delivery of the placenta, it can lead to postpartum hemorrhage, subinvolution of uterus, and uterine sepsis.

- **Battledore placenta:** The cord is attached to the margin of the placenta.
- **Circumvallate placenta:** The fetal surface is divided into a central depressed zone surrounded by a thickened white ring situated at varying distance from the margin of placenta. The ring is composed of a double fold of amnion and chorion. Vessels radiate from the site of cord insertion up to the margin of the ring, and then disappear from view.
- **Velamentous placenta:** The cord is attached to the membranes. The branching vessels traverse through the membranes for a varying distance before reaching placenta.
  - *Significance*: If the leash of blood vessels traverses through the membranes overlying the internal os, in front of the presenting part, it is called vasa previa. Rupture of the membranes involving the overlying fetal vessels leads to fetal bleeding, resulting in fetal exsanguination and death. Refer to the figure below for placental abnormalities.

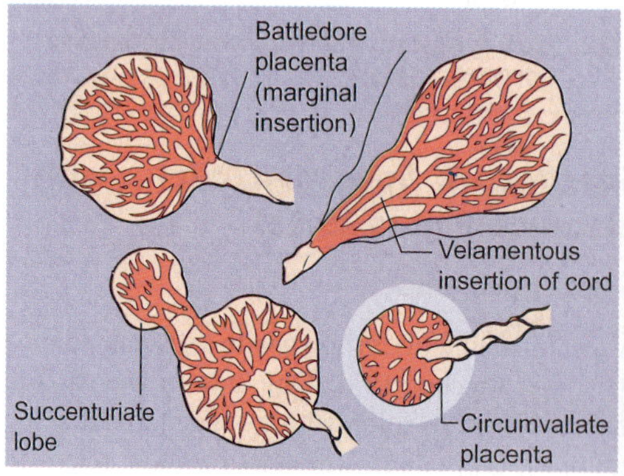

Figure Placental variations.

Part 3

Specimen 6: Conjoint twins (Figure 29.6)

Description

This is a specimen of two fetuses seen in close proximity and attached to one another.

Diagnosis

The most likely diagnosis is conjoint twins.

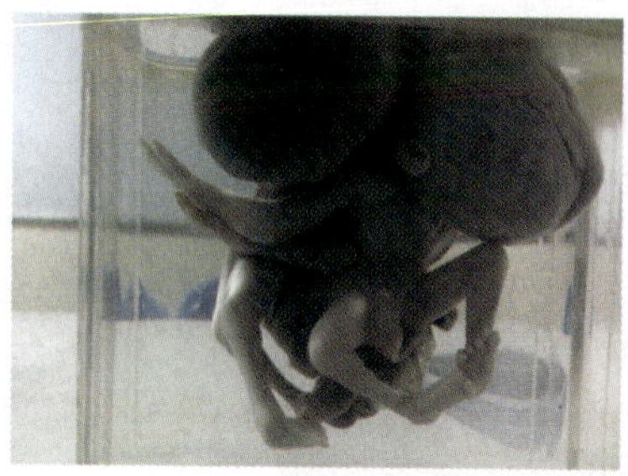

Figure 29.6 Conjoint twins.

Viva corner

Q1 How are conjoint twins formed?

When division of the fertilized ovum occurs after 13 days of fertilization, it is more likely to result in conjoint twins.

Q2 What are the various types of conjoint twins?

Types of conjoint twins are the following:

- **Thoracophagus:** United at chest, commonest
- **Omphalophagus:** Fused at abdomen
- **Pyophagus:** Fused at buttocks
- **Ischiophagus:** Fused at ischium

(CONTD...)

..CONTD)

Viva corner

- **Craniophagus:** Fused at back of the head
- **Cephalophagus:** Fused at head

(**Hint:** *Remember the acronym "TOPIC"*)

Q3 How will you diagnose conjoint twins?

Suspect conjoint twins in USG if the following features are present:

- Inseparable or fused body parts
- No change of relative position of both the fetuses
- Both heads at the same level and plane
- Twins facing each other (thoracophagus, omphalophagus)
- Thorax in close approximation (thoracophagus)

Q4 What will be your plan of management if conjoint twins are diagnosed?

- Termination of pregnancy is offered when the shared organs are vital and single, such as heart and brain.
- Conjoint twins are delivered by cesarean section, as allowing for normal delivery can lead to obstructed labor.
- Feasibility of separation of the twins after birth should be discussed with specialists. Surgical separation may be possible in conjoint twins with no major malformations, such as presence of only fusion of bones

Part 3

SPECIMENS IN GYNECOLOGY

Identification of the organ

Uterus It is identified by the following:

- Pear-shaped structure
- Adnexal attachment
- Cervical os—circular in nulliparous and a transverse slit in parous women

Anterior surface of uterus is identified by the following:

- Attachment of the round ligament
- Loose attachment of uterovesical fold of peritoneum to lower uterine segment

Posterior surface of uterus is identified by the following:

- Attachment of the ovarian ligament with ovary
- Cut margin of posterior peritoneum densely attached to posterior surface and placed at a lower level than the cut margin of anterior peritoneum

Structures attached to the uterine cornu are the following:

- **Round ligament:** A cord-like structure attached anteriorly and running laterally and downwards
- **Fallopian tube:** A tubular structure identified by fimbriae at abdominal ostium
- **Ovarian ligament:** A short cord-like structure (the most posterior structure) attached to the ovary

Ovary Fallopian tube may or may not be attached to the ovarian specimen. There is no other pelvic organ resembling it.

Specimen 7: Fibroid uterus (Figure 29.7)

Gross appearance

- This is a cut section of specimen of uterus. Adnexal structures are not seen.
- The uterus appears enlarged.
- Uterine shape is distorted by a well-circumscribed subserosal growth that has a whorled appearance and is surrounded by a pseudocapsule (describe the site, size, and number, if multiple growths are present).

Diagnosis

Subserosal fibroid is the most likely diagnosis.

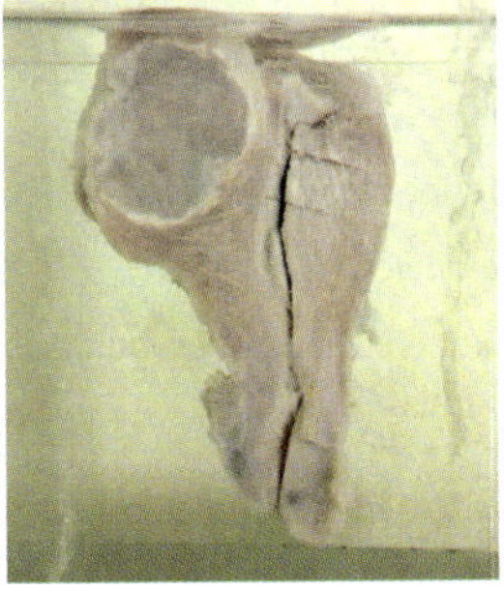

Figure 29.7 Fibroid uterus.

Viva corner

Q1 What are the different types of fibroids?

Depending on the location, different types of fibroids are the following:

- Interstitial or intramural
- Subserous
- Submucous

Q2 What would be the probable age of the woman for whom hysterectomy has been done?

Normal ovaries are usually removed during hysterectomy at ≥50 years. Ovaries are not visualized in the specimen. Oophorectomy had not been done; hence, the probable age of the woman would be <50 years (if the specimen has uterus and ovaries, the probable age is ≥50 years).

Q3 What are the causes of menorrhagia in fibroid?

- Increased surface area of the endometrium
- Increased vascularity and pelvic congestion
- Interference with normal uterine contractility due to interposition of fibroid
- Associated endometrial hyperplasia due to hyperestrogenism
- Altered prostaglandin metabolism

Q4 What are the different treatment options available for fibroids?

- Surgery
  - Myomectomy
  - Hysterectomy
- Medical therapy
- Recent advances
  - Uterine artery embolization
  - Cryomyolysis
  - Magnetic resonance-guided focused ultrasound (MRGFUS)

Q5 What is the role of medical management in fibroid?

The indications for medical management are the following:

- To control menorrhagia
- To correct anemia
- To relieve pain

The various drugs used are the following:

- Prostaglandin synthetase inhibitors
- Progesterone therapy
- Low-dose oral contraceptive pills (OCPs)
- levonorgestrel-releasing intrauterine device (LNG-IUD)
- GnRH analogues—agonists and antagonists
- Anabolic steroids—danazol and gestrinone
- Antiprogesterone (mifepristone)

Q6 What are the secondary changes in a fibroid?

- Degeneration—hyaline, cystic, calcific, and red degeneration
- Infection
- Atrophy
- Necrosis
- Sarcomatous change

Q7 What are the degenerations in fibroid?

- Hyaline degeneration—most common degeneration
- Cystic degeneration—seen in menopause (cystic spaces are seen within the fibroid)
- Fatty degeneration
- Calcific degeneration—"womb stone" appearance
- Red degeneration—seen in pregnancy and puerperium
- Atrophy—usually occurs in menopause
- Necrosis—may occur due to inadequate vascular supply
- Sarcomatous change—can occur in <0.2% of cases

Specimen 8: Submucous fibroid uterus (Figure 29.8)

Gross appearance

This is a specimen of a cut section of uterus, showing a well-circumscribed lesion in the myometrium, protruding into the endometrial cavity, thereby pushing and distorting the endometrial cavity.

Diagnosis

The most probable diagnosis is submucous fibroid.

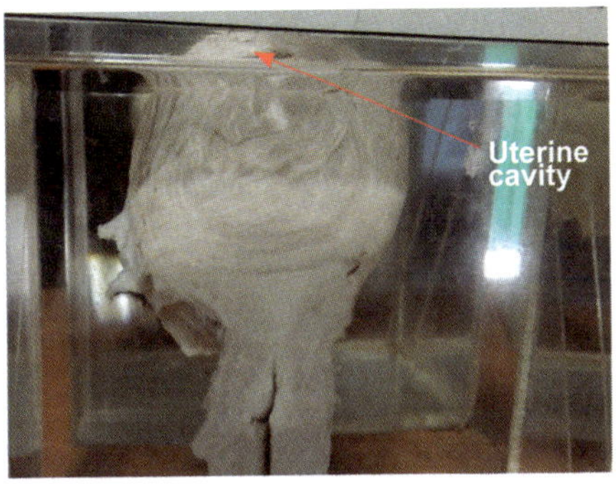

Figure 29.8 Submucous fibroid uterus.

Specimen 9: Cervical fibroid (Figure 29.9)

Gross appearance

- This is a specimen of cut section of uterus with a huge lesion arising from the posterior lip of cervix.
- The uterus sits on the top of the huge mass (lantern on dome of St. Paul's cathedral).
- The uterus is cut open to show the uterine cavity.

Diagnosis

Cervical fibroid is the most probable diagnosis.

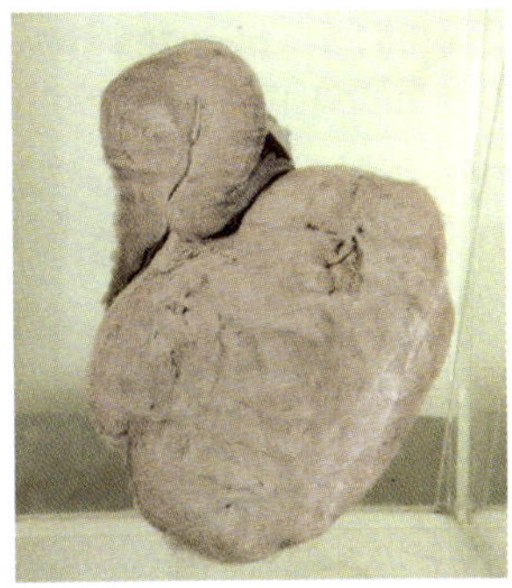

Figure 29.9 Cervical fibroid.

Viva corner

Q1 How is fibroid uterus differentiated from adenomyosis?

See table below

Table Features differentiating a fibroid from adenomyosis

	Fibroid uterus	Adenomyosis
Age	Usually observed in the reproductive age group	Commonly seen in multiparous women older than 40 years
Pathology	It is a benign neoplasia of the smooth muscle of the uterus	It is due to presence of functioning endometrium within the muscle layers of the uterus
Uterus	• Uterus is irregularly enlarged depending on the site, size, and number of myomas • Uterus is firm and nontender on palpation	• Uniformly enlarged uterus due to myohyperplasia • Uterus is soft and tender on palpation
Symptoms	May present with menorrhagia and dysmenorrhea	Menorrhagia—may be present. Dysmenorrhea typically begins a week before and lasts even after menstruation ends
Diagnosis	• Ultrasonography: Homogeneous echogenic area over the fibroid • Cut section: Capsule present, appears smooth and white with a whorled appearance • Histology: Proliferation of smooth muscle and fibrous tissue	• Cystic spaces within the myometrium • Capsule is absent. Diffuse trabeculated appearance, cystic spaces with hemorrhagic spots • Proliferation of endometrial glands and stroma. Phagocytic cells laden with hemosiderin pigment are present

Viva corner

Q1 What are the types of cervical fibroid?

- Anterior cervical fibroid—arises from anterior lip of cervix; may cause urinary retention
- Posterior cervical fibroid—may cause rectal symptoms (constipation)
- Lateral cervical fibroid—compression effect on blood vessels and displacement of the ureter
- Central cervical fibroid

Q2 What would have been the most likely clinical presentation in this woman?

Women with cervical fibroid most likely present with pressure symptoms.

Q3 What are the gynecological pathologies where ureteric injury is more likely to occur during surgery?

- Cervical fibroid
- Broad ligament fibroid
- Pelvic endometriosis
- Gynecological malignancy

(For details related to other clinical questions on fibroid uterus, refer to Part 2, Chapter 20, *Fibroid Uterus.*)

Specimen 10: Submucous fibroid polyp (Figure 29.10)

Gross appearance

This is a cut section of a specimen of uterus showing a pedunculated mass protruding into the uterine cavity near the fundus.

Diagnosis

The probable diagnosis is pedunculated submucous fibroid polyp.

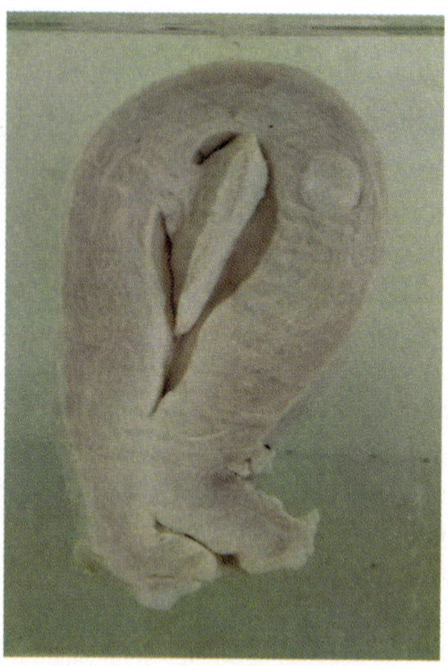

Figure 29.10 Submucous fibroid polyp.

Viva corner

Q1 What would be the clinical presentation in a case of fibroid polyp

- Menstrual abnormalities—menorrhagia, dysmenorrhea, and metrorrhagia
- Pain abdomen

Q2 How will you diagnose the case?

- Speculum examination (the pedunculated polyp can be visualized if it is protruding through the cervical os)
- Ultrasound examination
- Saline infusion sonography
- Hysterosalpingogram—filling defects in the cavity
- Hysteroscopy (direct visualization and removal of the polyp can be done)

Specimen 11: Endometriosis of ovary (Figure 29.11)

Gross appearance

- The mounted specimen shows a cut section of ovary.
- The inner surface contains areas of dark-brown tissue suggestive of clotted blood.
- The outer surface of ovary appears to be thickened.

Viva corner

Q1 What are the common sites of pelvic endometriosis?

- Ovaries
- Pelvic peritoneum
- Pouch of Douglas
- Rectovaginal septum

Q2 What are the treatment options for pelvic endometriosis?

- Expectant management
- Medical therapy
- Surgery
  - Conservative
  - Definitive
- Combined therapy—medical and surgical therapy

Q3 What are the hormones used in the management of endometriosis?

- Combined oral contraceptive pills
- Progestogens (oral, IM, or LNG-IUD)
- Danazol and gestrinone
- GnRH analogues

Q4 What is the management for chocolate cyst (ovarian endometrioma) of the ovary?

- **Small endometrioma <3 cm**: Laparoscopic cystaspiration and destruction of cyst wall epithelium by diathermy or laser can be done.
- **Large endometrioma ≥4 cm:** Ovarian cystectomy with adhesiolysis can be done.

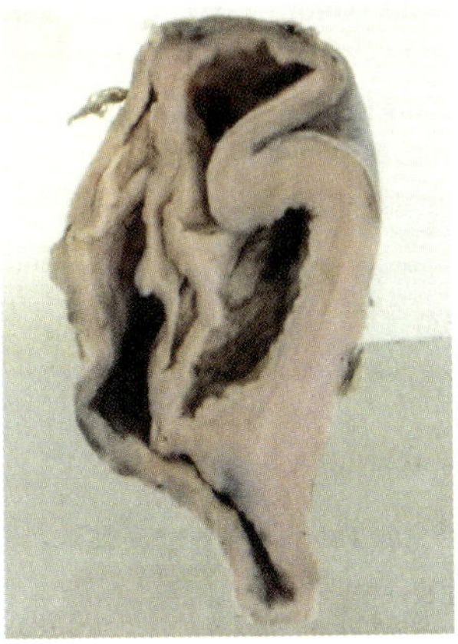

Figure 29.11 Endometriosis of ovary.

Diagnosis

The most probable diagnosis is endometriosis of ovary.

Specimen 12: Endometrial hyperplasia (Figure 29.12)

Gross appearance

- Specimen shows a cut section of uterus with cervix.

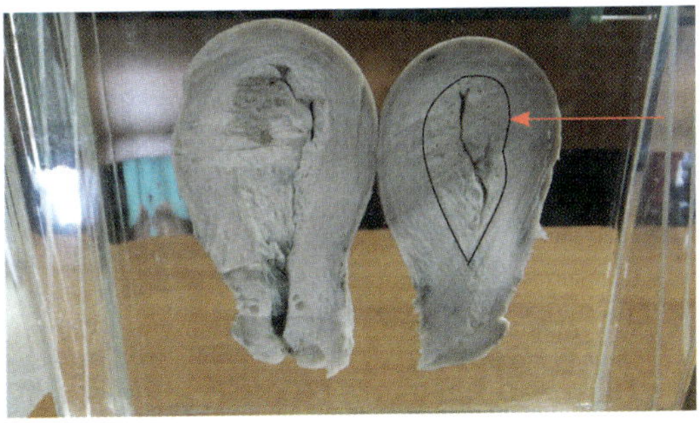

Figure 29.12 Endometrial hyperplasia.

- The endometrium appears irregular and thickened with areas of hemorrhage and necrosis.

Diagnosis

The most likely diagnosis is endometrial hyperplasia or endometrial carcinoma.

Specimen 13: Endometrial carcinoma (Figure 29.13)

Gross appearance

- Specimen shows a cut section of uterus with cervix and B/L adnexae.

Viva corner

Q1 What are the high-risk factors for endometrial carcinoma?

- Nulliparous
- Late menopause
- Persistent unopposed estrogen stimulation of endometrium
- Corpus cancer syndrome (obesity, hypertension, and diabetes)
- Atypical endometrial hyperplasia
- Tamoxifen therapy
- Family history of ovary, breast, or colon cancer

Q2 How will you diagnose a case of endometrial carcinoma?

- History: In all cases of the postmenopausal bleeding and perimenopausal abnormal uterine bleeding (AUB), cervical and endometrial carcinoma are to be ruled out.
- Transvaginal sonography (TVS): Endometrial sampling is recommended if endometrial thickness is ≥4 mm in postmenopausal women.
- Fractional curettage or hysteroscopy-directed biopsy is performed.
- Computed tomography (CT) and magnetic resonance imaging (MRI) are used to identify myometrial invasion and spread of tumor.

Q3 Which is the most common histological type of endometrial carcinoma?

Adenocarcinoma (endometrioid 80%)

Q4 What is the management for endometrial cancer?

- Most patients are identified in early stages; surgery is the first-line therapy.
- Total abdominal hysterectomy (TAH) (extrafascial hysterectomy) + bilateral salpingo-ovariectomy (BSO) + pelvic and para-aortic lymph node sampling is done.
- Clear cell and papillary serous carcinoma: Perform omentectomy and peritoneal biopsy in addition.
- Adjuvant radiotherapy (RT) is given following surgery— for prevention of recurrence.

(For details related to other clinical questions on endometrial cancer, refer to Part 2, Chapter 23, *Carcinoma Endometrium*.)

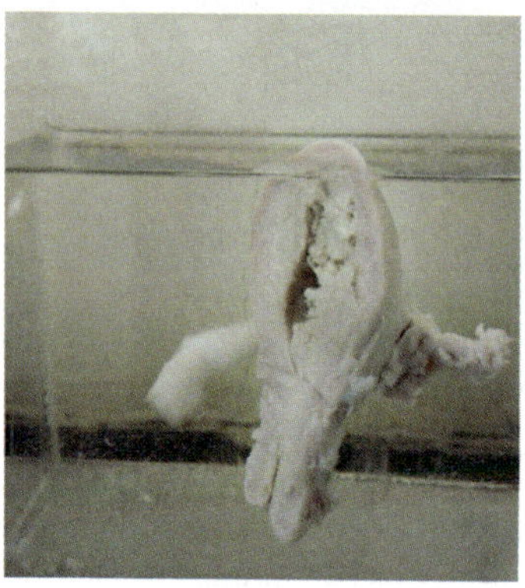

Figure 29.13 Endometrial carcinoma.

- The endometrium appears irregular and thickened with papillary projections and areas of hemorrhage and necrosis.

Diagnosis

The most likely diagnosis is endometrial carcinoma.

Specimen 14: Mucinous cystadenoma (Figure 29.14)

Gross appearance

- Mounted specimen shows a cut section of ovary with a large mass.
- There are multiple septa, which gives it a multiloculated appearance.
- There are no solid areas within the mass.
- Loculi appear to be empty, probably because the contents have been washed out during mounting of the specimen (the specimen prior to mounting may show loculi filled with thick, viscid, mucin-like material).

Diagnosis

The most likely diagnosis is benign ovarian neoplasm, probably a mucinous cystadenoma of the ovary. The diagnosis needs to be confirmed by histopathological examination.

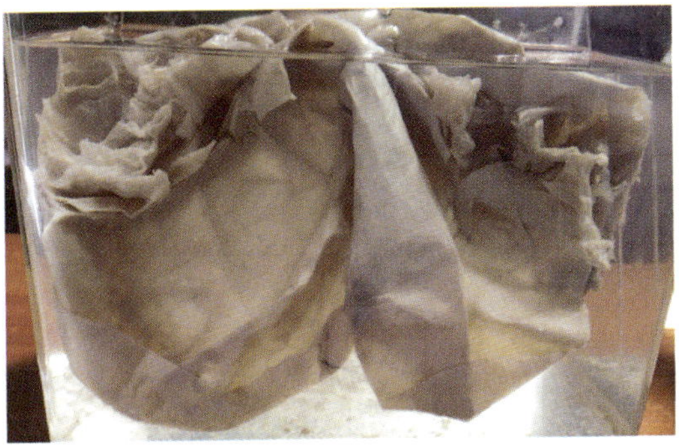

Figure 29.14 Mucinous cystadenoma.

Viva corner

Q1 What are the clinical features of benign ovarian tumors?

- Slow growing
- Unilateral
- Mobile
- Cystic in consistency
- Smooth surface
- No ascites

Differential diagnosis of abdominopelvic mass in reproductive and perimenopausal age groups

- Full bladder
- Pregnancy
- Fibroid uterus
- Adenomyosis
- Chocolate cyst of the ovary
- Tubo-ovarian mass
- Encysted peritonitis (seen in tuberculosis)
- Ascites

(For other details related to benign ovarian neoplasms, refer to Part 2, Chapter 21, *Ovarian Mass*.)

Specimen 15: Serous cystadenoma (Figure 29.15)

Gross appearance

- Specimen shows a cut section of ovary, with a large cystic mass. External surface appears smooth; the capsule appears thin, translucent, and glistening.
- The cut section shows few septations.

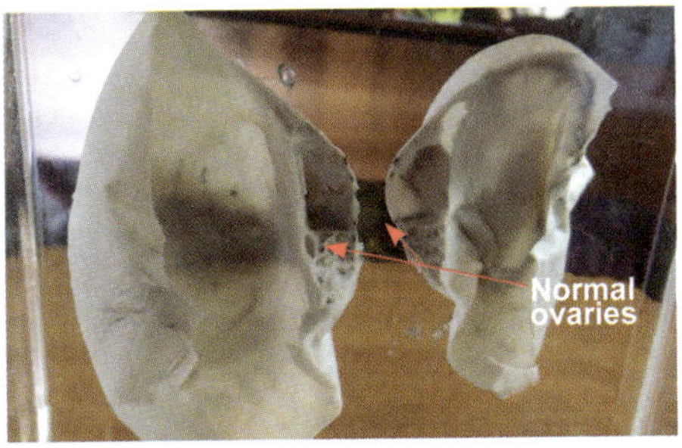

Figure 29.15 Serous cystadenoma.

- There are no solid areas or papillary projections.
- Normal ovarian tissue can be visualized.

Diagnosis

The most likely diagnosis would be a benign ovarian neoplasm, probably a serous cystadenoma of the ovary. A histopathological examination is required to confirm the diagnosis.

Viva corner

Q1 What are the common complications of benign ovarian tumor?

- Torsion
- Intracystic hemorrhage
- Infection
- Rupture
- Pseudomyxoma peritonei
- Malignant change

(For other details related to benign ovarian neoplasms, refer to Part 2, Chapter 21, *Ovarian Mass*.)

Specimen 16: Dermoid cyst (Figure 29.16)

Gross appearance

- Specimen shows a cut section of an ovarian cyst.
- The cut section shows sebaceous material and hair.
- There are no solid areas or areas suggestive of hemorrhage or necrosis.

Diagnosis

The most likely diagnosis is dermoid cyst of the ovary. A histopathological examination is required for confirmation of diagnosis.

Viva corner

Q1 What are dermoid cysts?

The dermoid cysts are mature teratomas with a variety of internal contents such as hair, sebaceous material, teeth, bone, cartilage, thyroid tissues, and bronchial tissues. This leads to anechoic to echogenic appearance in USG.

Dermoid cyst:

- Is the most common germ cell tumor
- Is the most common benign ovarian tumor
- Is the most common benign ovarian tumor in pregnancy
- Contains derivatives of ectoderm, endoderm, and mesoderm (most common element—ectoderm)

Q2 What is the risk of malignant change in dermoid?

The risk of malignancy is 1–2%, usually a squamous cell carcinoma.

Q3 What is the most common complication of dermoid?

Torsion of the dermoid cyst is the most common complication.

(For other details related to benign ovarian neoplasms, refer to Part 2, Chapter 21, *Ovarian Mass*.)

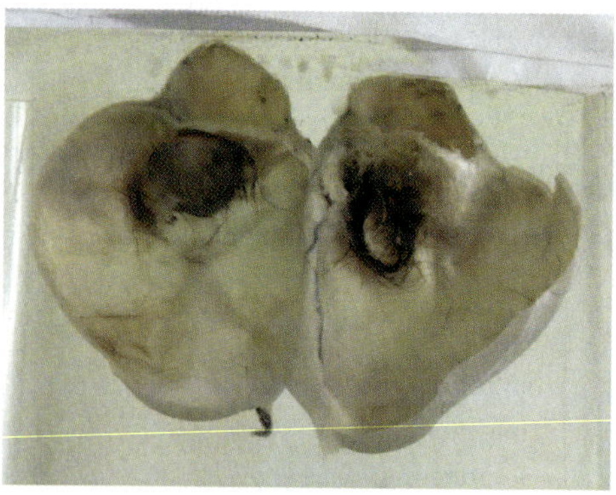

Figure 29.16 Dermoid cyst.

Specimen 17: Malignant ovarian tumor (Figure 29.17)

Gross appearance

- This is a specimen of an irregular-shaped huge mass that appears to arise from the ovary.
- The cut section shows tissues with varied consistency.
- Solid areas are seen within the mass that indicate that the mass is likely to be malignant (in some specimens, areas of hemorrhage, necrosis, and multiple blood vessels can be seen traversing the surface of the ovary).

Viva corner

Q1 What are the common malignant ovarian tumors?

Epithelial ovarian tumors can undergo malignant changes:

- Serous cystadenoma to cystadenocarcinoma —40%
- Mucinous cystadenoma to cystadenocarcinoma —10%
- Malignant endometrioid (rare)

Germ cell tumors are usually malignant. However, dermoid cyst is mostly benign with 1–2% risk of malignancy.

Sex cord stromal tumors may be benign but are potentially malignant.

Q2 What is the primary surgery done for malignant ovarian tumors?

- Exploratory staging laparotomy → total abdominal hysterectomy, bilateral salpingo-oophorectomy, and infracolic omentectomy with pelvic and para-aortic lymph node sampling are done.
- If tumor is not completely resectable, cytoreductive surgery is done that reduces the tumor load. Lesser the residual tumor volume (<1 cm), better is the response to chemotherapy and better is the survival rate.

Q3 How is serum CA 125 measurement helpful?

- Serum CA 125 is a glycoprotein and has got more prognostic value than diagnostic value.

(CONTD...)

(...CONTD)

Viva corner

- It is helpful in the following ways:
  - To assess the prognosis in a known case of ovarian tumor
  - To know the response to treatment
  - For early detection of tumor recurrence

Q4 Name some solid tumors of the ovary.

- **Benign solid tumors:** Fibroma, thecoma, and Brenner tumor
- **Malignant:** Primary epithelial ovarian carcinoma, dysgerminoma, and immature teratoma

Q5 What is Meigs syndrome?

It is a triad of ascites, pleural effusion, and benign ovarian fibroma. The ascites and pleural effusion resolve spontaneously once the ovarian tumor is removed.

If ascites and pleural effusion are seen in association with Brenner tumor or granulosa cell tumor, it is termed pseudo-Meigs syndrome.

Q6 What are the hormone-producing tumors of the ovary?

- **Feminizing tumors:** Granulosa cell and theca cell tumor
- **Masculinizing tumors:** Sertoli–Leydig cell and hilus cell tumor

(For other details related to ovarian cancer, refer to Part 2, Chapter 21, *Ovarian Mass*.)

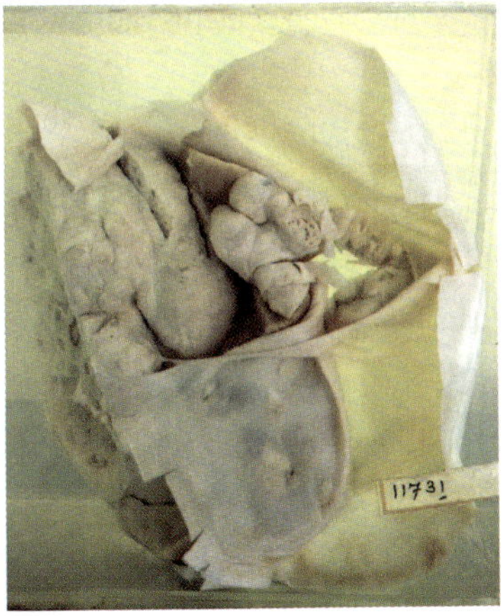

Figure 29.17 Malignant ovarian tumor.

Diagnosis

The most likely diagnosis is a malignant ovarian tumor. However, this needs to be confirmed by histopathological examination.

Specimen 18: Krukenberg tumor (Figure 29.18)

Gross appearance

- This is a specimen of the uterus with tubes and ovaries on both sides.
- The ovaries are enlarged with a lobulated appearance. The shape of the ovary is maintained.
- Uterus and tubes appear normal.

Viva corner

Q1 What is Krukenberg tumor?

- This is a metastatic adenocarcinoma of the ovary.
- Metastasis is from the stomach (most common), breast, colon, or biliary tract.
- The tumor is usually bilateral, lobulated, and solid in appearance with smooth surface, without any adhesions.
- Prognosis is poor with survival rate <1 year.

Q2 What is the mode of spread of tumor to the ovaries?

- Retrograde lymphatics
- Transcelomic spread

Q3 What is the histological picture of the tumor?

The "signet ring" appearance of epithelial cells is characteristic of Krukenberg tumor.

Part 3

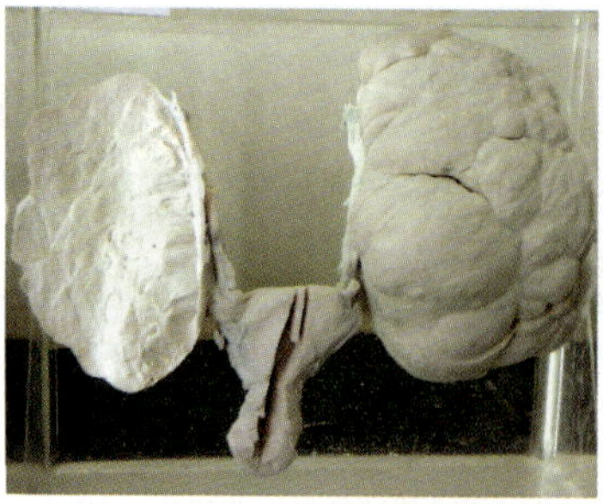

Figure 29.18 Krukenberg tumor.

Diagnosis

The most likely diagnosis is Krukenberg tumor.

Specimen 19: Specimen of uterus with cervix (Figure 29.19)

Gross appearance

- This is a specimen of uterus with cervix. No adnexa is visualized; hence, adnexa has been probably retained during hysterectomy.
- Cervix appears to be elongated. Elongation of the supravaginal part of cervix is commonly associated with uterine prolapse.

Diagnosis

The most likely diagnosis is supravaginal elongation of cervix. The probable cause (prolapse uterus) can be identified if the patient's history is provided.

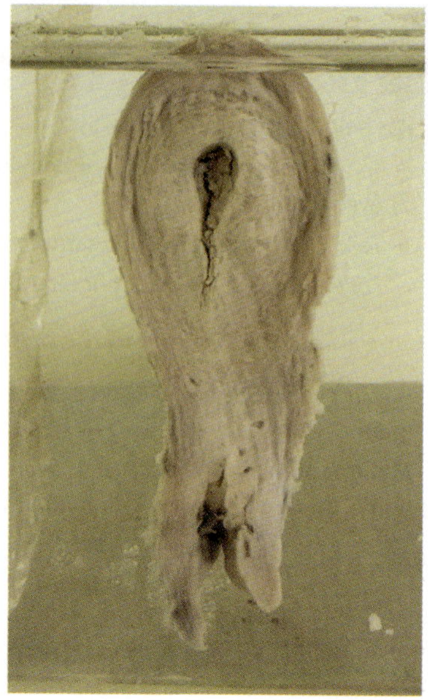

Figure 29.19 Specimen of uterus with cervix.

Viva corner

Q1 Why is supravaginal elongation of cervix present in uterine prolapse?

Elongation of the supravaginal part of cervix is commonly associated with uterine prolapse. The elongation occurs due to pull of the cardinal and uterosacral ligaments on the isthmus of cervix to keep the cervix in position.

30 Imaging Studies: X-Rays, Hysterosalpingogram, and Ultrasound Images

Introduction

Ultrasound is the most common imaging modality in obstetrics and gynecology. The use of radiography in obstetrics and gynecology has decreased considerably with the advent of ultrasonography. This chapter deals with the discussion of radiograph and ultrasound images that are commonly asked during viva voce in obstetrics and gynecology.

X-RAY IMAGES

X-ray—image 1 (Figure 30.1)

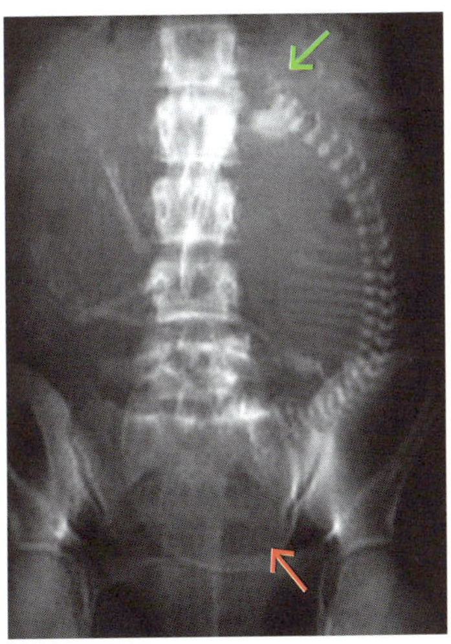

Figure 30.1 X-ray—image 1.

Description

This is a plain X-ray of the maternal abdomen AP view with fetus inside. The fetus is in longitudinal lie with cephalic presentation. The skull bones are seen in the lower pole (red arrow), and the fetal sacrum is seen in the upper pole (green arrow).

Diagnosis

Fetus in longitudinal lie with cephalic presentation.

X-ray—image 2 (Figure 30.2)

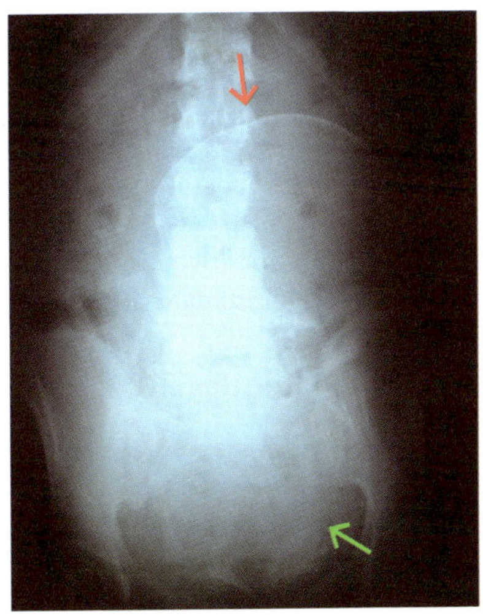

Figure 30.2 X-ray—image 2.

Description

This is a plain X-ray of maternal abdomen anteroposterior (AP) view with the fetus inside. The fetus is in longitudinal lie with breech presentation. The fetal skull bones are seen in the upper pole (red arrow) and fetal sacrum in the lower pole (green arrow).

Diagnosis

Fetus in breech presentation

X-ray—image 3 (Figure 30.3)

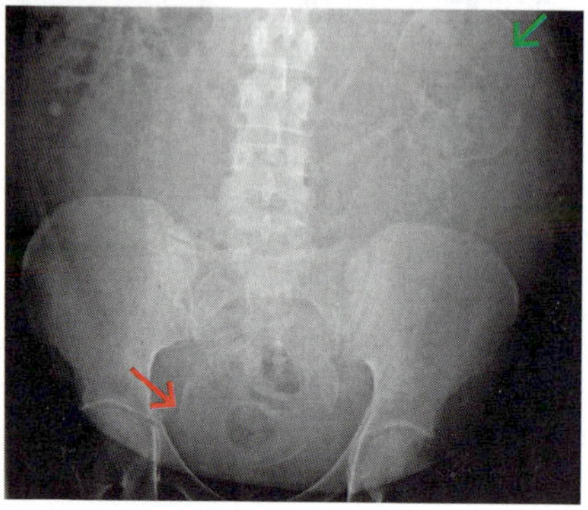

Figure 30.3 X-ray—image 3.

Description

This is a plain X-ray of maternal abdomen AP view with fetus inside. X-ray shows shadows of two fetuses, indicating twin gestation. The first twin is in cephalic presentation (fetal head indicated by red arrow) and the second twin is in breech presentation (fetal head is indicated by green arrow).

Diagnosis

Twin gestation with first twin in cephalic and second twin in breech presentation

X-ray—image 4 (Figure 30.4)

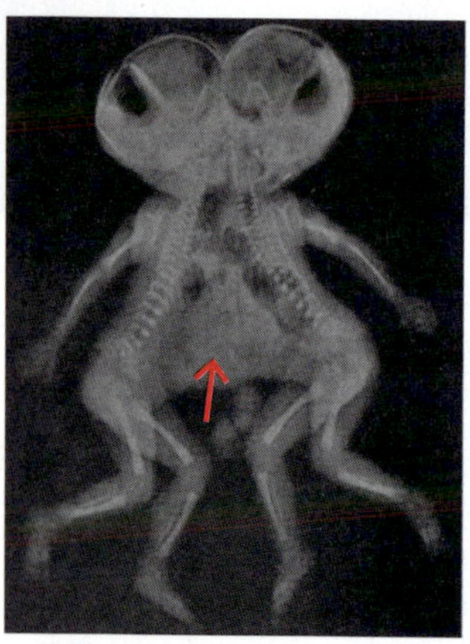

Figure 30.4 X-ray—image 4.

Description

This is a plain X-ray of fetuses after birth, showing two fetuses in close proximity to each other and fused in the region of thorax indicating conjoint twins.

Diagnosis

Conjoint twins—thoracopagus

X-ray—image 5 (Figure 30.5)

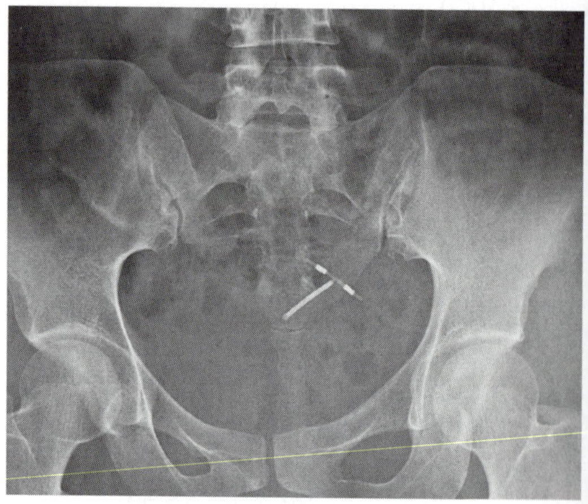

Figure 30.5 X-ray—image 5.

Description

This is a plain X-ray of pelvis AP view showing Cu T. Whether the Cu T is lying within the uterine cavity or outside the uterine cavity following perforation can be made out only if AP and lateral X-ray films are taken with a uterine sound in situ. It is Cu T 380A, as Cu sleeves can be seen in the arms of Cu T (supplied free of cost by the Government of India).

Diagnosis

Pelvic X-ray showing Cu T 380A

HYSTEROSALPINGOGRAM

Hysterosalpingogram (HSG) is a contrast study to assess the uterine cavity and fallopian tubes.
Procedure:

Viva corner

Q1 What is the type of Cu T seen in the image?

- **Cu T 380A:** Copper sleeves in the arms can be seen.

Q2 What are the possible causes of missing threads?

- Threads are coiled inside.
- Threads have torn and are expelled.
- Intrauterine contraceptive device (IUCD) is expelled.
- IUCD has perforated the uterus and has migrated outside into peritoneal cavity.
- In case of pregnancy with IUCD in situ, when the threads can be drawn inside the uterus.

Q3 How is a case with missing threads evaluated?

- Ultrasonography can identify the location of IUCD—within uterine cavity or in abdominal cavity.
- X-ray pelvis is helpful—AP and lateral views with uterine sound in position.
- Hysteroscopy helps in direct visualization of IUCD within the uterine cavity and can be removed at the same sitting.

Q4 What are the complications of IUCD usage?

Immediate complications (during insertion) are the following:

- Syncope
- Cramp-like pain
- Perforation of the uterus

Remote complications (following insertion) are the following:

- Pelvic pain
- Pelvic infections
- Menorrhagia
- Perforation of the uterus
- Expulsion of IUCD
- Failure of contraception—ectopic pregnancy

Q5 What are the advantages of the third-generation IUCD?

- Higher efficacy
- Low expulsion rate
- Longer duration of action
- Reduced risk of ectopic pregnancy
- Reduced risk of PID

Q6 What are the indications for IUCD removal?

- Missing thread
- Persistent pelvic pain
- Persistent menorrhagia
- Woman desirous of pregnancy

- HSG cannula (Leech–Wilkinson's cannula) or no. 8 Foley's catheter is inserted into the cervix, radiopaque dye is instilled slowly through the cannula into the uterine cavity, and the images are studied under fluoroscopic guidance.
- Two radiographic images are generally taken:
  - The first one to show the filling of the uterine cavity
  - The second one after 10–15 minutes to show tubal filling and peritoneal spillage
- Tubal patency is confirmed by peritoneal spillage of the dye.

Indications for HSG

- To assess tubal patency in infertility cases
- To detect the side and site of block, if tubal block is present
- To detect uterine malformations
- For diagnosis of submucous fibroid or polyp
- For diagnosis of uterine synechiae

Time to perform HSG

HSG is done between D4 and D10 of menstrual cycle.

Advantages of HSG

- Noninvasive test
- Relatively simple to perform compared with laparoscopy, which is an invasive procedure

Contraindications of HSG

- Pelvic infections
- Pregnancy
- Vaginal bleeding

Extra edge

Oil-based versus water-based media in HSG

Water-based media: meglumine diatrizoate (Urografin)

- Cause less cramps and discomfort
- Absorbed quickly
- Granuloma formation—rare
- Commonly used

Oil-based media (Lipiodol)

- Give better images (sharp images)
- Higher pregnancy rates
- Slow absorption
- Granuloma formation more with oil-based media
- Risk of lipid embolism in case of extravasation of dye
- Less commonly used

Complications of HSG

- Vasovagal attack
- Pelvic pain
- Flare-up of pelvic infection
- Extravasation of dye into venous or lymphatic channel

HSG—image 1 (Figure 30.6)

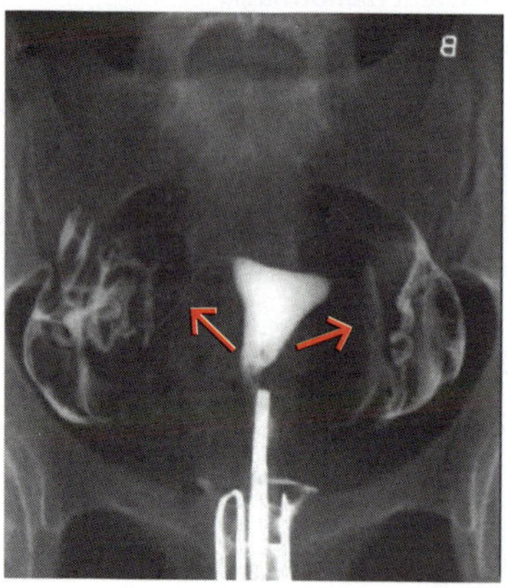

Figure 30.6 HSG—image 1.

Description

It is a HSG image showing radiopaque dye filling the uterine cavity and both the tubes (tubes are indicated by red arrows). There is bilateral spillage of dye into the peritoneal cavity. HSG cannula is in situ.

Diagnosis

Normal uterine cavity with bilateral patent tubes

Viva corner

Q1 What are the tests for tubal patency?

- HSG
- Diagnostic laparoscopy and chromopertubation
- Saline infusion sonography (SIS)

Q2 What is saline infusion sonography?

It involves instillation of saline into the uterine cavity and transvaginal sonography is done simultaneously to study the uterine cavity and tubes. Endometrial polyp and submucous fibroids are better diagnosed by this method.

Q3 What are the methods to detect ovulation?

- Basal body temperature—biphasic pattern
- Cervical mucus study
- Vaginal cytology—progesterone effect
- Serum progesterone estimation
- Endometrial biopsy—secretory changes (D21–D23)
- Serial sonography—detection of dominant follicle and its collapse following ovulation

Q4 Which evaluation is better for evaluation of tubal patency: HSG or laparoscopy?

Advantages of laparoscopy over HSG: Besides testing for tubal patency, it helps in the following:

- Diagnosis of peritubal adhesions and pelvic endometriosis
- Detection of ovarian pathology [polycystic ovarian disease (PCOD) and endometriosis]
- Can perform treatment procedures such as ovarian drilling for PCOD and lysis of peritubal adhesions in the same sitting

Disadvantages of laparoscopy over HSG are the following:

- Laparoscopy cannot evaluate uterocervical factors that can be diagnosed with HSG.
- It is an invasive procedure and needs general anesthesia.
- It is expensive compared with HSG and it needs specialized training.

Hence, HSG and laparoscopy are complementary to each other.

HSG—image 2 (Figure 30.7)

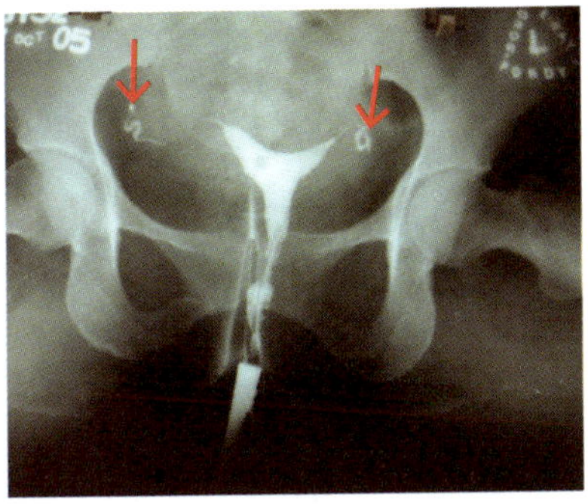

Figure 30.7 HSG—image 2.

Description

HSG shows a radiopaque shadow demarcating the uterine cavity. The radiopaque shadow is visible in both the tubes up to the distal end but there is no peritoneal spillage.

Diagnosis

B/L fimbrial block

Viva corner

Q1 What is the most common cause for bilateral fimbrial block?

Salpingitis is the most common cause.

Q2 What is the most common cause for bilateral cornual block?

Cornual spasm is the most common cause.

HSG—image 3 (Figure 30.8)

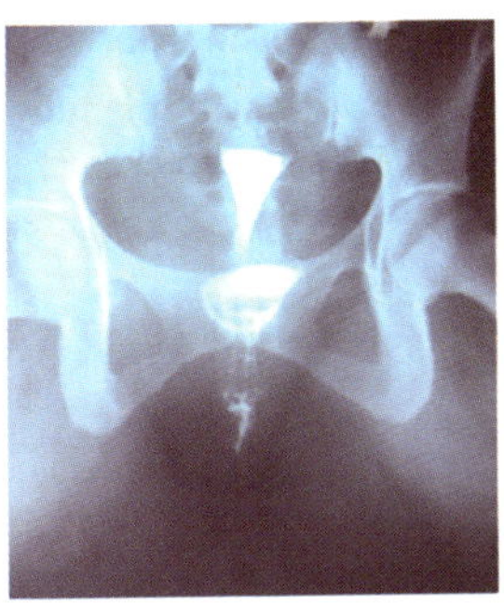

Figure 30.8 HSG—image 3.

Description

HSG shows a radiopaque shadow demarcating the uterine cavity. No radiopaque shadow is visible in either fallopian tube.

Diagnosis

Bilateral cornual block

Viva corner

Q1 What are the causes of tubal block?

- Salpingitis
- Tubal spasm
- Endometriosis
- Tubal surgeries such as sterilization
- Salpingitis isthmica nodosa

Q2 What is the management for tubal block?

Tubal surgery may be considered in young women with mild disease and after tubal sterilization.

- **Proximal tubal block:** It can be overcome by hysteroscopic cannulation.
- **Distal tubal block:** Fimbrioplasty can be done.
- **Midtubal block:** Tubotubal anastomosis can be done.

Assisted reproductive technology (ART) procedures such as in vitro fertilization and embryo transfer (IVF-ET) are considered as the treatment option for any complicated tubal occlusive disease.

Q3 What is the management for infertility if tubes are damaged?

If the tubes are damaged, the couple should be counseled for ART procedures such as IVF-ET.

HSG—image 4 (Figure 30.9)

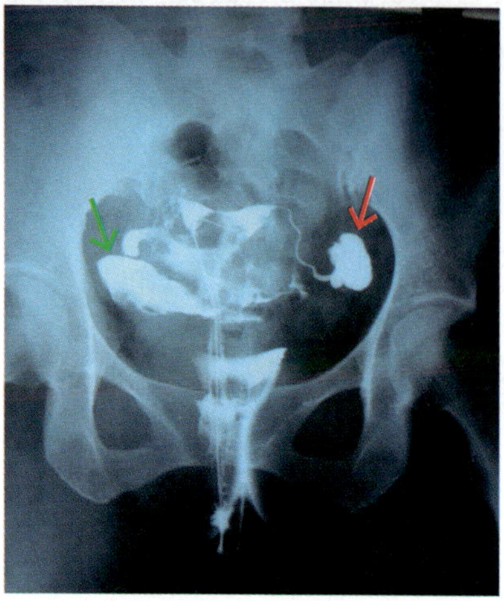

Figure 30.9 HSG—image 4.

Description

HSG shows a radiopaque shadow filling the uterine cavity. Radiopaque dye is seen within both the tubes. The distal end of the left tube is distended with no peritoneal spillage (red arrow) and the right side shows normal peritoneal spillage (green arrow).

Diagnosis

Left-sided hydrosalpinx with fimbrial block and patent tube on the right side

HSG—image 5 (Figure 30.10)

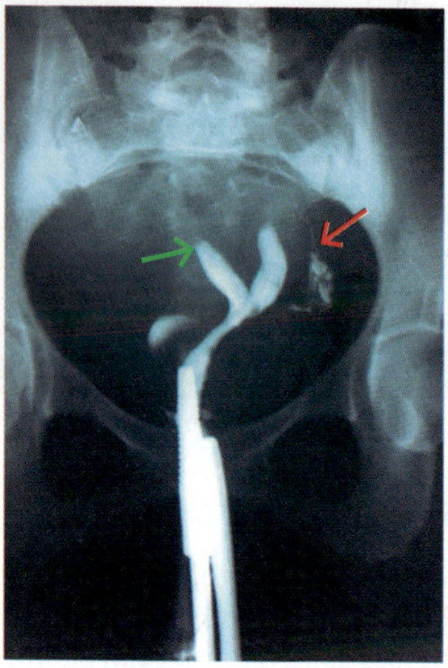

Figure 30.10 HSG—image 5.

Description

HSG shows a radiopaque shadow filling both the horns of the uterus. The radiopaque dye is visible within the left tube (red arrow). The dye has not entered the right-sided tube, indicating cornual block (green arrow). There is no peritoneal spillage on both the sides.

Viva corner

Q1 What are the other methods of diagnosis of hydrosalpinx?

Ultrasonography (USG) and laparoscopy

Q2 What is the danger if HSG is performed in a diagnosed case of hydrosalpinx?

HSG is contraindicated in a case with hydrosalpinx, as there is increased risk of flaring up of pelvic infections.

Q3 Does the presence of hydrosalpinx impair the result of IVF?

Hydrosalpinx reduces the pregnancy rates of IVF by about 50%. Endometrial receptivity is reduced, resulting in implantation failure. Salpingectomy improves the outcome.

Q4 What are the factors related to the success of tuboplasty?

The success of tubal reconstructive surgery depends on the following factors:

- Underlying pathology of the tube (tubercular salpingitis has got poor outcome)
- Presence of adhesions
- Presence of hydrosalpinx
- Length of the reconstructed tube <4 cm—poor outcome

Q5 What is the HSG appearance of the tubes in genital tuberculosis?

- Vascular or lymphatic extravasation of dye
- Rigid tubes (lead pipe appearance)
- Beaded appearance of the tubes

Diagnosis

It is most likely a case of bicornuate uterus or septate uterus with fimbrial block on the left side and cornual block on the right side. Whether it is a septate or bicornuate uterus can be confirmed by doing a hysterolaparoscopy.

Viva corner

Q1 What are the different types of uterine abnormalities?

- Agenesis
- Hypoplasia
- Unicornuate uterus
- Bicornuate uterus
- Didelphys uterus
- Septate uterus
- Arcuate uterus

Q2 What are the different modes of diagnosis of uterine anomalies?

- Hysterosalpingography
- Hysteroscopy
- Laparoscopy
- Ultrasonography
- Magnetic resonance imaging (MRI)

Q3 What are the complications associated with uterine anomalies?

- Infertility
- Recurrent abortions
- Cervical incompetence
- Preterm labor

Q4 How is a bicornuate uterus differentiated from a septate uterus?

- HSG and hysteroscopy may show a similar picture in bicornuate and septate uterus.
- For differentiation, both the internal and the external architecture of the uterus have to be visualized.
- Combined hysterolaparoscopy can differentiate a bicornuate uterus from a septate uterus. The fundus of the uterus appears normal in a septate uterus while there is bifurcation separating the two horns of the uterus in a bicornuate uterus.
- The angle between the two horns is >100° in a bicornuate uterus.

Q5 What is the management of a septate uterus?

Hysteroscopic resection of the uterine septum

Q6 What is the management of a bicornuate uterus?

Metroplasty or unification (Strassman or Tompkins) operation can be done.

HSG—image 6 (Figure 30.11)

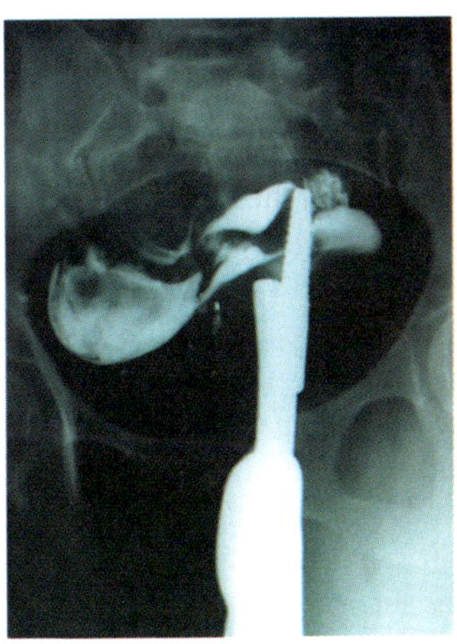

Figure 30.11 HSG—image 6.

Description

HSG shows irregular filling of uterus with extravasation of dye into vascular and lymphatic channels, without any outline of tubes.

Diagnosis

Uterine synechiae (Asherman syndrome)

Viva corner

Q1 What are the common causes of uterine synechiae?

- Following vigorous curettage in abortion and dysfunctional uterine bleeding (DUB)
- Tubercular endometritis

(CONTD...)

Part 3

(...CONTD)

Viva corner

Q2 What are the other methods of diagnosis of uterine synechiae?

Hysteroscopic visualization of the endometrial cavity helps in identifying intrauterine pathology. Adhesiolysis can be done at the same sitting in case of uterine synechiae.

Q3 What is the management of uterine synechiae?

Hysteroscopic adhesiolysis is done. IUCD can be inserted following the procedure to prevent readhesion.

Q4 What are the uterine causes of amenorrhea?

- Primary amenorrhea
  - Mayer–Rokitansky–Küster–Hauser syndrome—Mullerian agenesis
- Secondary amenorrhea
  - Tubercular endometritis
  - Uterine synechiae
  - Surgical removal of uterus (hysterectomy)
  - Postradiation

ULTRASONOGRAPHY

- **Principle in ultrasonography:** High-frequency sound waves are used and they are reflected by the interfaces between tissues of varying density. The reflected sound waves are captured as images.
- Transabdominal (curvilinear, 2- to 5-MHz probe) and transvaginal (curvilinear, 7- to 12-MHz probe) transducers are commonly used (Figure 30.12). Transperineal and transrectal techniques are useful for imaging of the pelvic floor muscles and the anal sphincter.

Obstetric ultrasonography (USG)

Uses of USG in first trimester

- To confirm intrauterine pregnancy
- To confirm viable pregnancy
- To confirm gestational age (dating of pregnancy is most accurate in the first trimester)

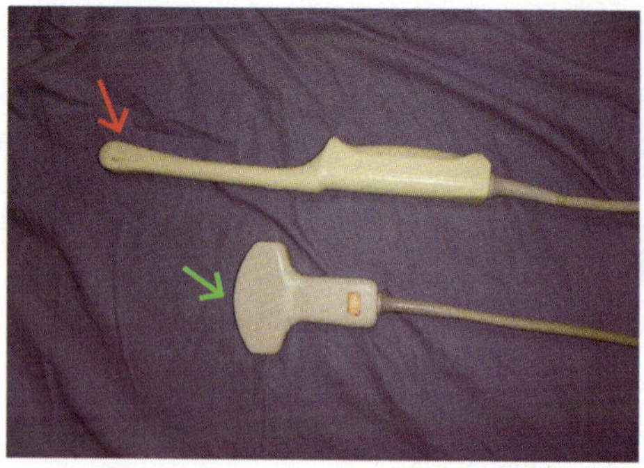

Figure 30.12 Transducers used in ultrasonography. Transabdominal curvilinear probe (green arrow) and transvaginal probe (red arrow).

- To confirm number of fetuses
- To rule out ectopic pregnancy
- To rule out abnormal pregnancies such as molar pregnancy, blighted ovum, and missed abortion
- To measure nuchal translucency at 11–13 weeks
- To assess for any uterine pathology such as fibroid and uterine malformation

Uses of USG in second trimester

- To assess gestational age
- To rule out congenital anomalies (fetal anatomical survey to detect anomalies is usually done between 16 and 24 weeks of gestation)
- For placental localization
- To assess fetal growth (fetal biometry)
- Other uses as in the first trimester such as confirming viability of fetus and detection of multiple pregnancy

Uses of USG in third trimester

- Can obtain all the information of the second-trimester USG in the third-trimester USG
- To assess fetal growth profile by doing fetal biometry
- To do fetal biophysical profile (BPP)
- Estimated fetal weight (EFW) [on the basis of biometric data (biparietal diameter (BPD), head circumference (HC), abdominal circumference (AC), and femoral length (FL)], computer software can calculate estimated fetal weight using formulas such as Hadlock formula]

- Normal fetal weight is between the 10th and 90th percentiles. EFW <10th percentile is considered small for gestational age (SGA) and >90th percentile is considered large for gestational age (LGA).

USG evaluation of early pregnancy

The following events appear in a transvaginal sonography (TVS) in a normal pregnancy (Table 30.1):

- All of the events mentioned in TVS (Table 30.1) appear 1 week later in transabdominal sonography (TAS).
- TVS is most useful in the first trimester, especially in obese women and in case of retroverted uterus.

Table 30.1 Order of appearance of pregnancy events in transvaginal sonography

Event	Time of occurrence in ultrasonography (weeks)
Gestational sac	4.5–5
Yolk sac	5–5.5
Fetal pole	5.5–6
Fetal cardiac activity	6

Fetal biometry

Crown–rump length (CRL) measurement

- It is measured at gestational age 7–13 weeks.
- It gives the most accurate measurement of gestational age (±1 week).
- CRL is the longest length of the fetus excluding the limbs and the yolk sac, measured from the top of the head (crown) to the lowest part of the buttocks (rump).

Biparietal diameter

- BPD is the distance between the two sides of the fetal head.
- The fetal head is imaged in a transverse axial section at the level of falx cerebri, cavum septum pellucidum, and the thalamic nuclei (Figure 30.13).
- BPD is measured from the outer table of the proximal skull to the inner table of the distal skull.
- It is usually measured after 13 weeks of pregnancy for assessing gestational age.

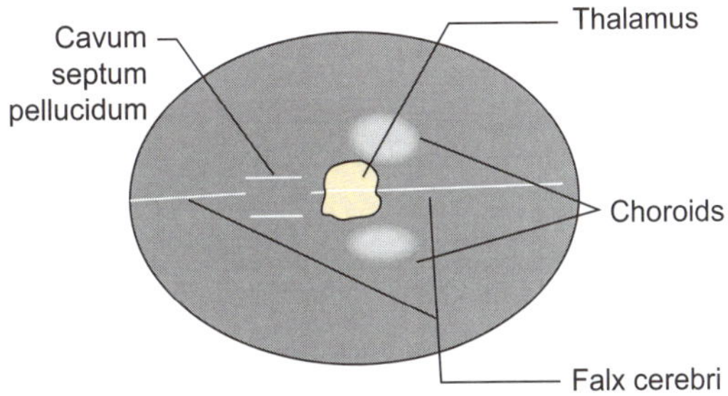

Figure 30.13 Axial plane of measurement of biparietal diameter in ultrasonography.

Abdominal circumference

- AC is a measure of fetal abdominal girth.
- It is measured in an axial plane at the level of the stomach and bifurcation of the portal vein into right and left branches (Figure 30.14).

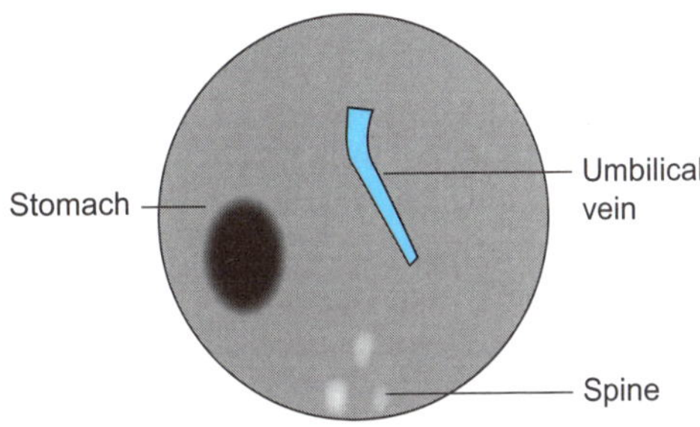

Figure 30.14 Axial plane of measurement of abdominal circumference in ultrasonography.

Fetal femur

- Femur is the longest bone in the body and represents the longitudinal growth of the fetus.
- Femur length is the length of femoral diaphysis.
- It is measured from the origin to the distal end of the shaft—that is, from the greater trochanter to the lateral femoral condyle (Figure 30.15).
- The femoral head and distal femoral epiphysis, which appear after 32 weeks, are not included in the measurements.

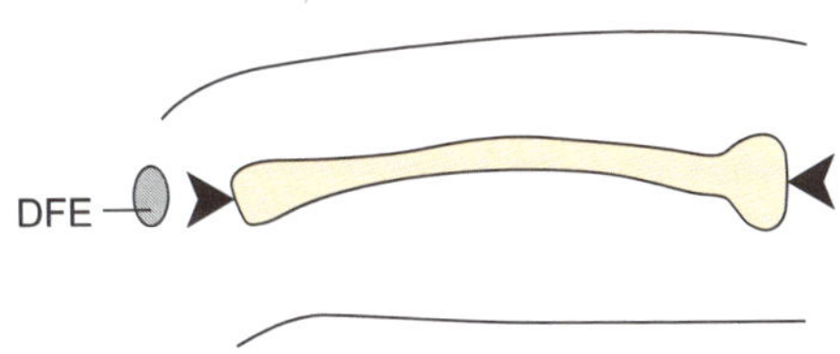

Figure 30.15 Measurement of femur length in ultrasonography. *DFE*, distal femoral epiphysis.

USG—image 1 (Figure 30.16)

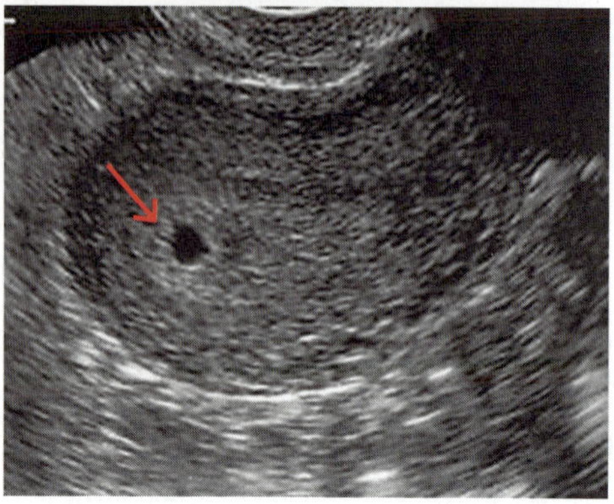

Figure 30.16 USG—image 1.

Description

A well-defined gestational sac (GS) is seen, located eccentrically within the uterine cavity (red arrow). Fetal pole is not seen. The gestational age is around 4–5 weeks.

Diagnosis

Single intrauterine GS

Viva corner

Q1 How is a normal gestational sac (GS) differentiated from a pseudogestational sac in USG?

- A normal GS is regular in shape and is eccentric in position within the uterine activity.
- A pseudo-GS can be seen in ectopic pregnancy. It is irregular in outline and located centrally within the uterine cavity.
- The pseudo-GS gestational remains empty and has no double decidual sac sign (DDSS).

Q2 What is DDSS?

In cases of normal intrauterine pregnancy, hyperechogenic ring of decidua capsularis is surrounded by another hyperechogenic ring (decidua parietalis), giving the double-rimmed appearance around the GS in USG (see figure below).

(CONTD...)

(...CONTD)

Viva corner

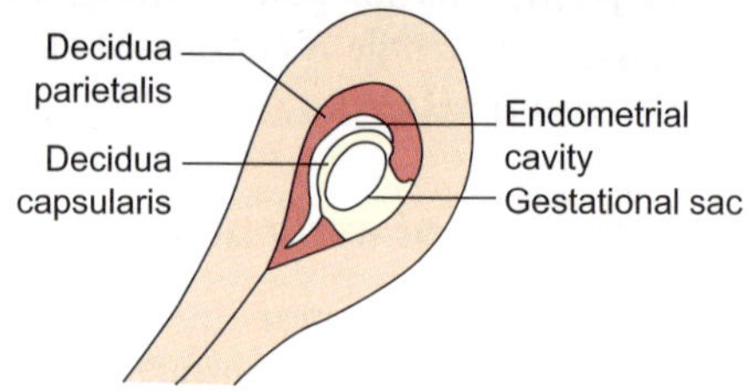

Figure Pictorial representation of double decidual sac sign as seen in ultrasonography.

Q3 What do you mean by discriminatory zone?

It refers to the serum beta-human chorionic gonadotropin (hCG) levels at which GS can be visualized in ultrasonography.

An intrauterine GS should be seen:

- In TVS, when the maternal serum beta-hCG level is 1000–1200 mIU/mL
- In TAS, when the level of maternal serum beta-hCG level is 6000 mIU/mL

GS can be seen in TVS as early as 4.5–5 weeks of gestation.

Q4 What is the significance of visualization of a GS in USG?

- Intrauterine GS is a reliable evidence of intrauterine pregnancy.
- GS outside the uterine cavity suggests ectopic pregnancy.
- Gestational age can be calculated by measuring the mean sac diameter (MSD).

USG—image 2 (Figure 30.17)

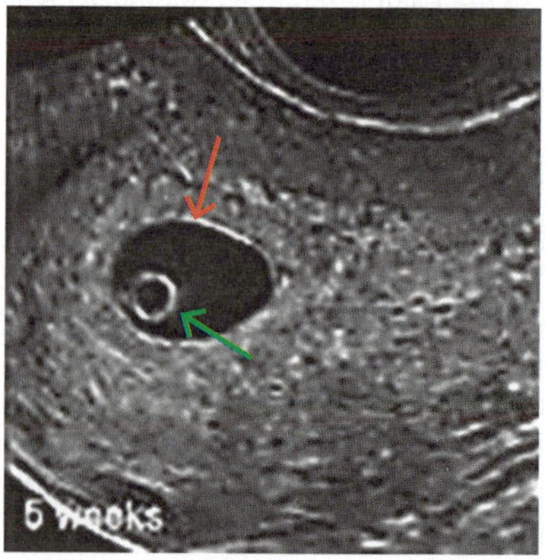

Figure 30.17 USG—image 2.

Description

This is a USG picture showing single intrauterine GS (red arrow). Yolk sac is seen within the GS (green arrow).

Viva corner

Q1 When is a yolk sac visualized in USG?

- Yolk sac is the first structure to be seen within the GS.
- Yolk sac is seen in TVS when the mean sac diameter is 8 mm (5.5 weeks).
- Yolk sac is seen in TAS when the mean sac diameter is 10–15 mm (6 weeks).

Q2 What is the significance of detecting a yolk sac in USG?

- Presence of yolk sac is diagnostic of intrauterine pregnancy.
- Yolk sac differentiates an early intrauterine pregnancy from a pseudosac.
- The number of yolk sacs corresponds to the number of amniotic sacs.

USG—image 3 (Figure 30.18)

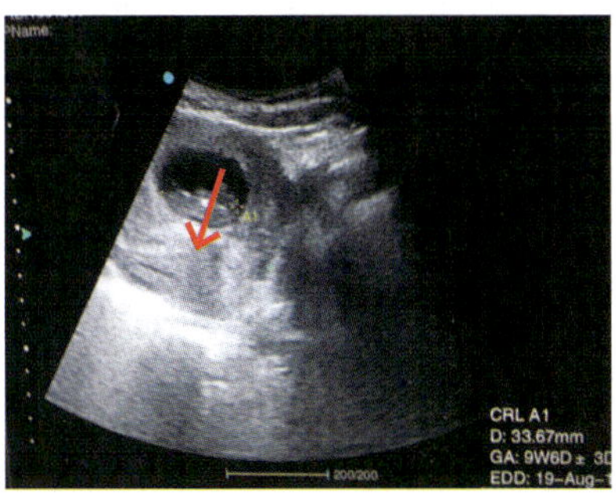

Figure 30.18 USG—image 3.

Description

This is a USG picture showing single intrauterine gestation with fetal pole. CRL measurement has been marked.

Viva corner

Q1 When does embryo appear in USG?

Embryo is first visualized adjacent to the yolk sac at 6 weeks of gestation.

(CONTD...)

(...CONTD)

Viva corner

Q2 What is the significance of CRL measurement?

CRL measurement in the first trimester gives an accurate measurement of the gestational age (±5–7 days).

Q3 When does fetal cardiac activity appear in USG?

Cardiac activity is visualized by 6 weeks in TVS and by 7 weeks in TAS.

Q4 What is the significance of detecting embryonic cardiac activity?

- Presence of cardiac activity indicates a viable embryo.
- Diagnosis of missed abortion is usually made if the fetal pole measures 5 mm or more with no cardiac activity.

Q5 What is the normal fetal heart rate?

Normal fetal heart rate varies between 110 and 160 beats/minute.

USG—image 4 (Figure 30.19)

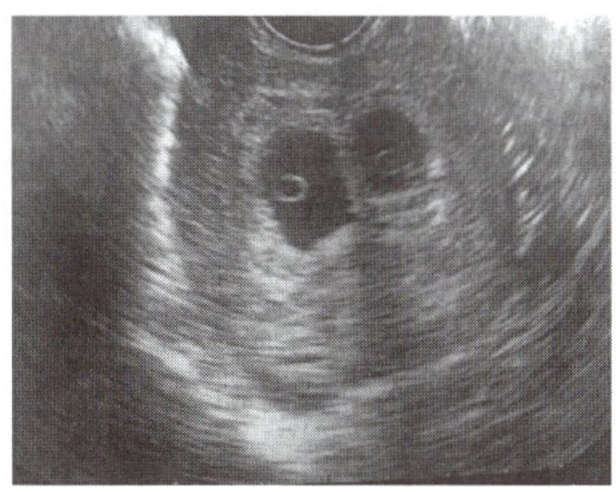

Figure 30.19 USG—image 4.

Description

This is an ultrasound image during early pregnancy showing two GSs. Yolk sac can be visualized within both the GSs.

Viva corner

Q1 What are the uses of USG in multiple pregnancy?

- To assess the following parameters:
  - Gestational age

(CONTD...)

(...CONTD)

Viva corner

- Number of fetuses
- Chorionicity
- Congenital malformations
- Localization of placenta
- Fetal presentation
- Fetal complications such as twin-to-twin transfusion syndrome (acardiac twin) and death of one twin

Diagnosis

Twin gestation

USG—image 5 (Figure 30.20)

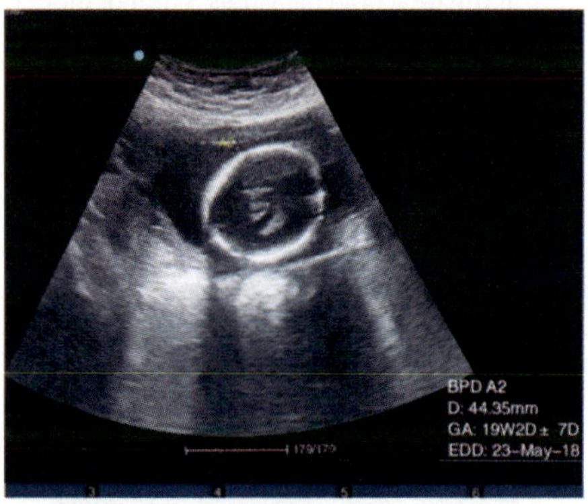

Figure 30.20 USG—image 5.

Description

It is an ultrasound picture showing the fetal head. In this view, the BPD and the HC can be measured as a part of fetal biometry.

Diagnosis

Measurement of BPD of the fetus as part of fetal biometry

Viva corner

Q1 What is the significance of BPD measurement?

- BPD is one of the parameters for the assessment of gestational age in the second and third trimesters.

(CONTD...)

(...CONTD)

Viva corner

- A chart showing serial measurements of BPD is helpful to monitor the fetal growth profile.

Q2 What is the importance of HC?

Head shape—dolichocephaly (flattened) or brachycephaly (rounded)—can be known.

USG—image 6 (Figure 30.21)

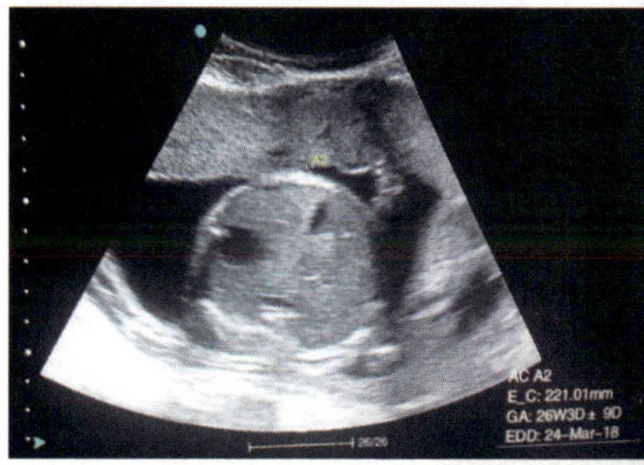

Figure 30.21 USG—image 6.

Description

This is an USG picture showing measurement of AC.

Diagnosis

Measurement of AC of the fetus as part of fetal biometry

Viva corner

Q1 What is the significance of AC?

- AC is one of the parameters for assessment of gestational age in the second and third trimesters.
- A chart showing serial measurements of AC is helpful to monitor the fetal growth profile.
- AC is the first parameter to be affected in intrauterine growth restriction (IUGR).

USG—image 7 (Figure 30.22)

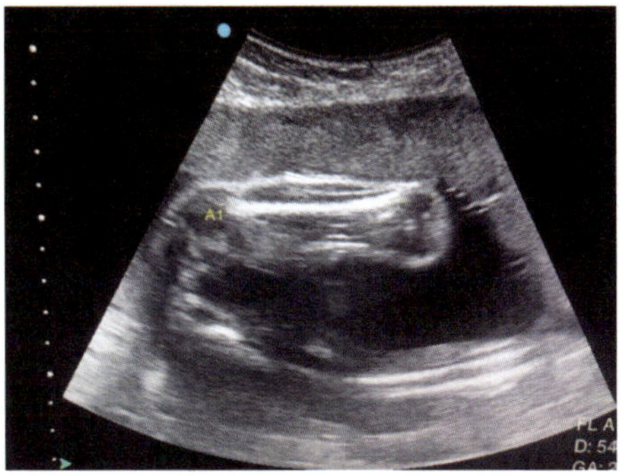

Figure 30.22 USG—image 7.

Description

This is a USG picture showing measurement of femur length of fetus.

Diagnosis

Femur length of fetus

Viva corner

Q1 What are the uses of femur length measurement?

It is used for the assessment of gestational age in the second and third trimesters. It is especially useful when BPD cannot be obtained such as in deeply engaged head, anencephaly, and intrauterine death with collapsed cranial bones.

USG—image 8 (Figure 30.23)

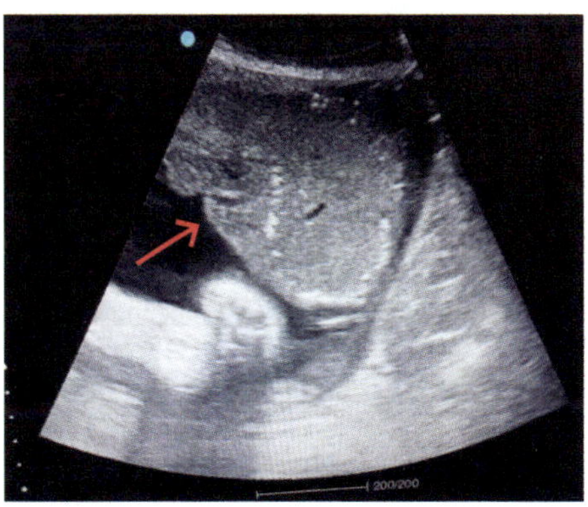

Figure 30.23 USG—image 8.

Description

This is a USG image showing placenta (red arrow). Multiple internal echoes are due to pooling of blood within the cotyledons.

Diagnosis

USG showing normal placenta

Viva corner

Q1 What are the ways in which visualizing the placenta in USG is useful?

- Placental localization: It is normally located in upper segment in the anterior or posterior uterine wall. Placenta previa is diagnosed when the placenta extends into the lower uterine segment. USG helps in placental localization and diagnosis of placenta previa.
- Placental maturity is evaluated as described by Grannum (see table below).

Table Grannum's grading of placental maturity

Grade	Period of gestation (weeks)	Description
Grade 0	<18	• Uniform echogenicity • Smooth chorionic plate
Grade 1	18–29	• Occasional parenchymal calcification/hyperechoic areas • Subtle indentations of chorionic plate
Grade 2	>30	• Occasional basal calcification/hyperechoic areas • Deeper indentations of chorionic plate (does not reach up to basal plate) – Seen as comma-type densities at the chorionic plate
Grade 3	>39	• USG appearance of significant basal plate calcification

- All cases of antepartum hemorrhage should have USG done to rule out placenta previa. Occasionally, a retroplacental clot is seen as

(CONTD...)

(...CONTD)

Viva corner

an echo-free area between the basal plate and the uterine wall.

- Placenta is enlarged (placentomegaly is seen) in Rh isoimmunization and maternal diabetes mellitus.

USG—image 9 (Figure 30.24)

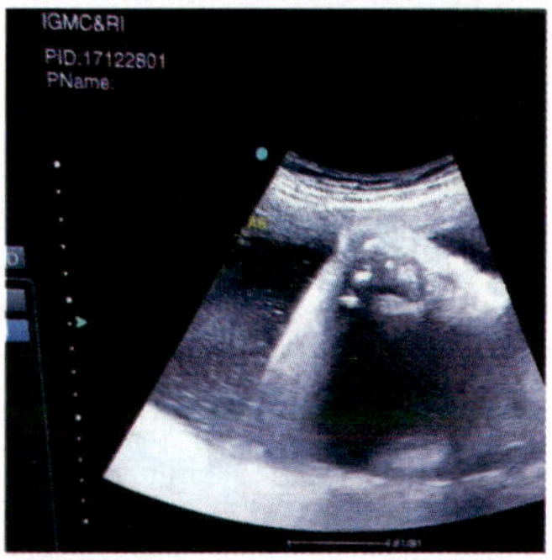

Figure 30.24 USG—image 9.

Description

This is a USG image showing measurement of liquor pocket. Amniotic fluid index (AFI) is calculated by measurement of deepest vertical pocket of liquor in all the four quadrants of abdomen and adding them up. AFI <5 is termed oligohydramnios and AFI >25 is termed polyhydramnios.

Diagnosis

USG showing measurement of liquor pocket in one of the quadrants of abdomen

USG—image 10 (Figure 30.25)

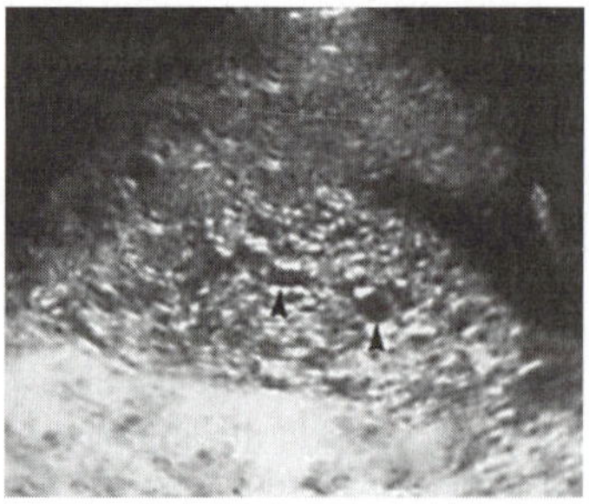

Figure 30.25 USG—image 10.

Description

In the USG image, the uterus is diffusely filled with echoes of moderate strength producing a snow storm appearance.

Diagnosis

USG appearance of molar pregnancy. The differential diagnosis is missed abortion with molar degeneration of placenta.

Viva corner

Q1 What is the clinical presentation of molar pregnancy?

Molar pregnancy presents with amenorrhea and bleeding P/V (typical H/o passing "grape-like vesicles").

Q2 What are the complications of molar pregnancy?

These include hemorrhage, shock, preeclampsia, sepsis, acute pulmonary embolism, and thyrotoxicosis.

Late complications include persistent trophoblastic disease and choriocarcinoma.

Q3 How is a case of hydatidiform mole treated?

- Suction evacuation of the uterus
- Follow-up with beta-hCG

USG—image 11 (Figure 30.26)

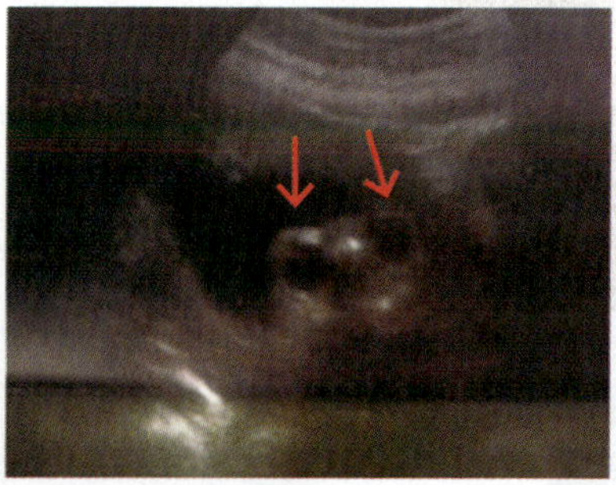

Figure 30.26 USG—image 11.

Description

This is an USG image showing fetal head with absence of circular outline of fetal skull. The fet ves can be seen protruding (red arrows) due to bsence of cranial vault, giving the typical "frog's-eye ppearance" in USG.

iagnosis

nencephaly

SG—image 12 (Figure 30.27)

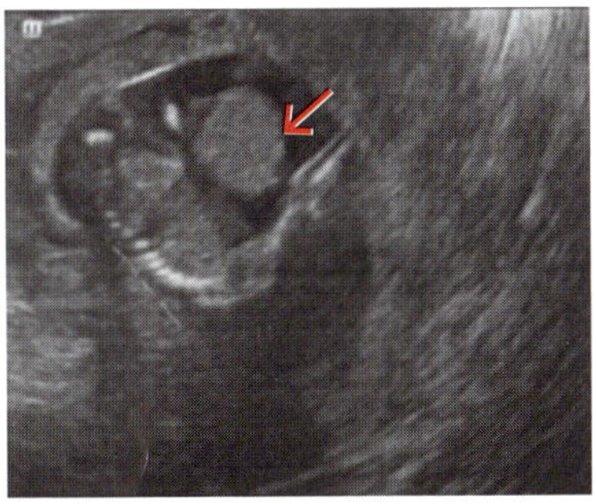

igure 30.27 USG—image 12.

escription

he USG image shows fetus with a large anteior abdominal wall defect and herniation of fetal issue, probably fetal liver through the defect.

iagnosis

mphalocele

JSG—image 13 (Figure 30.28a and b)

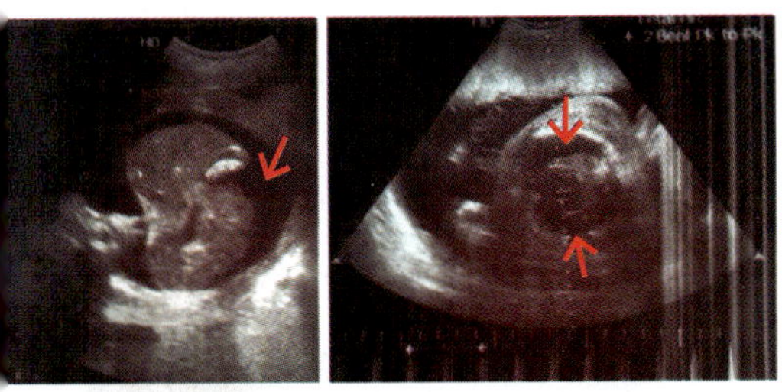

a. b.

igure 30.28 USG—image 13. **a.** Fetal ascites. **b.** Fetal leural effusion.

escription

JSG image in Figure 30.28a shows fetal ascites with he liver floating in fetal ascitic fluid. USG image in igure 30.28b shows fetal pleural effusion.

Diagnosis

- **Fetal hydrops:** It can be a case of immune hydrops due to erythroblastosis fetalis or non-immune hydrops as in TORCH infections, chorioangioma of placenta, etc.

USG—image 14 (Figure 30.29)

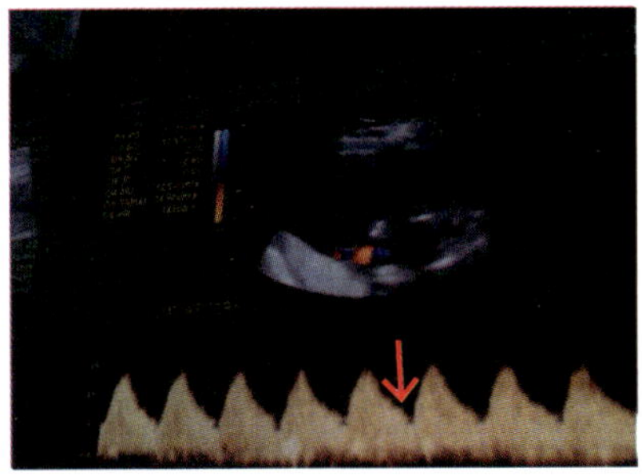

Figure 30.29 USG—image 14.

Description

The image shows Doppler study of fetal umbilical artery. Doppler study of fetal umbilical artery shows normal end-diastolic flow.

Diagnosis

Normal diastolic flow in Doppler study of fetal umbilical artery

USG—image 15 (Figure 30.30)

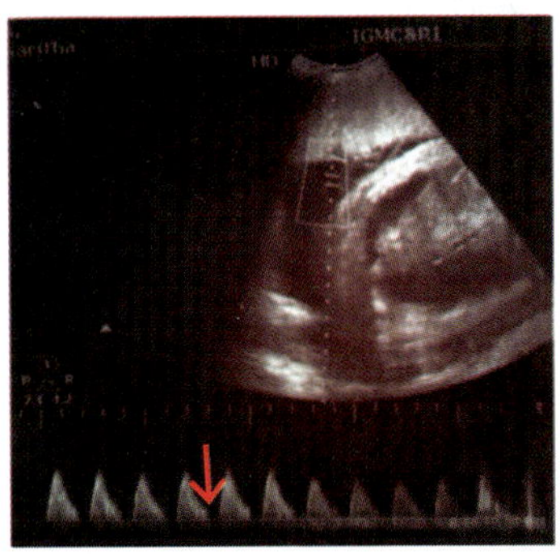

Figure 30.30 USG—image 15.

Description

The image shows Doppler study of fetal umbilical artery. Doppler study of fetal umbilical artery shows absent end-diastolic flow (AEDF). AEDF detected in mid or late pregnancy indicates underlying fetal vascular stress and decompensation, as a result of placental insufficiency. Flow in the umbilical artery should be in the forward direction in normal circumstances. If placental resistance increases, the diastolic flow reduces, later becomes absent, and finally reverses.

Diagnosis

AEDF in Doppler study of fetal umbilical artery

ULTRASONOGRAPHY IN GYNECOLOGY

Uses of ultrasound in gynecology

- To assess uterine shape, size, and contour
- To measure endometrial thickness
- To assess adnexal
- To look for free fluid in pouch of Douglas (POD)
- To look for ascitis
- To look for enlarged lymph nodes in genital malignancy
- To look for the presence of hydronephrosis

Indications for ultrasonography in gynecology

- Postmenopausal bleeding
- Abnormal uterine bleeding
- Pelvic pain
- Dysmenorrhea
- Pelvic infection
- Infertility
- Amenorrhea
- Delayed/precocious puberty
- Congenital anomalies of the genital tract
- Localization of intrauterine contraceptive device (IUCD)
- Abnormal or difficult pelvic examination
- Abnormality noted by other imaging methods
- As a part of screening for genital malignancy in high-risk women
- Urinary incontinence
- Preoperative, for guidance during surgery
- Postoperative pain/bleeding/infection

USG—image 16

Case summary

A 58-year-old woman presents with postmenopausal bleeding. USG was done and the image is shown in Figure 30.31.

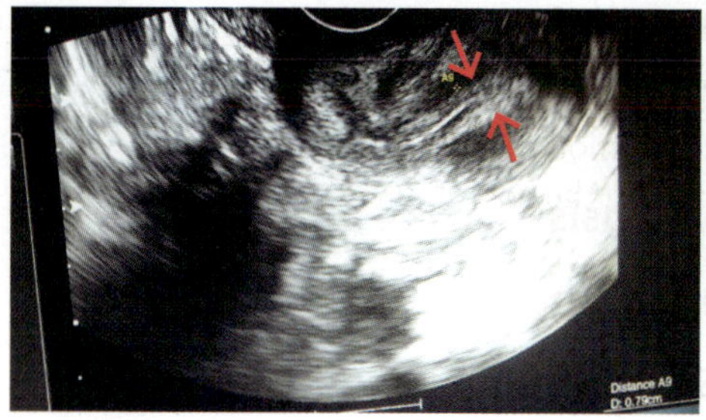

Figure 30.31 USG—image 16.

Description

This is a USG picture showing measurement o endometrial thickness.

Diagnosis

Thickened endometrium in a patient with post menopausal bleeding

Viva corner

Q1 What is the further management in this patient with endometrial thickness of 12 mm?

Women with postmenopausal bleeding with endometrial thickness >4 mm require additional evaluation with investigations such as saline infusion sonography (SIS), hysteroscopy, or endometrial biopsy [American College of Obstetricians and Gynecologists (ACOG) recommendation]. (For further details on postmenopausal bleeding and endometrial carcinoma, refer to Part 2, Chapter 23, *Carcinoma Endometrium*.)

USG—image 17 (Figure 30.32)

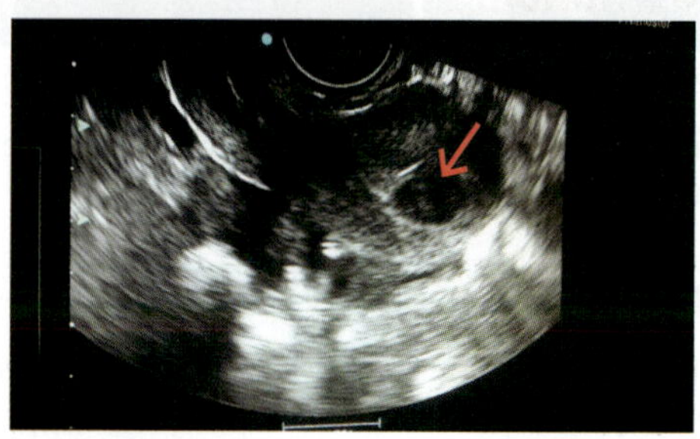

Figure 30.32 USG—image 17.

Description

This is a USG picture showing a well-defined homogenous lesion located within the myometrium in the posterior wall of uterus.

Diagnosis

Intramural fibroid

Viva corner

Q1 What are the uses of USG in fibroid uterus?

- USG is the investigation of choice for diagnosis of fibroid.
- USG helps to assess the size, location, and number of uterine fibroids.
- Preoperative finding on USG can guide the surgeon while performing surgery, hysteroscopy, laparoscopy, etc.

(For further details on fibroid uterus, refer to Part 2, Chapter 20, *Fibroid Uterus*.)

USG—image 18 (Figure 30.33)

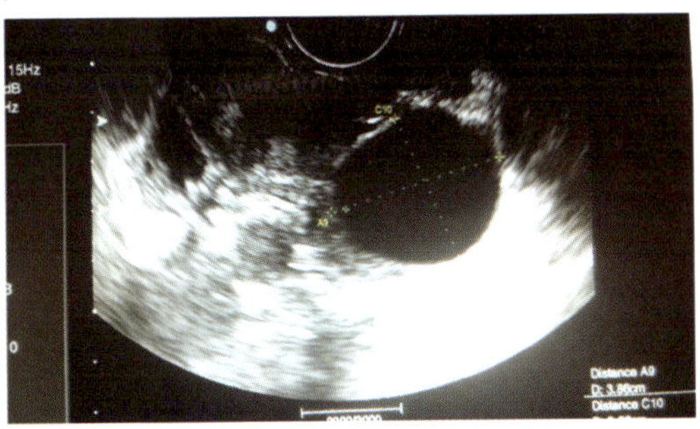

Figure 30.33 USG—image 18.

Description

The USG image shows an anechoic, unilocular cyst in the adnexal region.

Diagnosis

A simple ovarian cyst, probably a follicular cyst

USG—image 19

Case summary

A 50-year-old postmenopausal woman presented with complaints of loss of appetite and loss of weight for 2 months. USG of pelvis was done and image is shown in Figure 30.34.

Description

The USG image shows a mass with cystic and solid areas. There are multiple thick septations within the mass.

Diagnosis

Most likely a case of malignant ovarian tumor

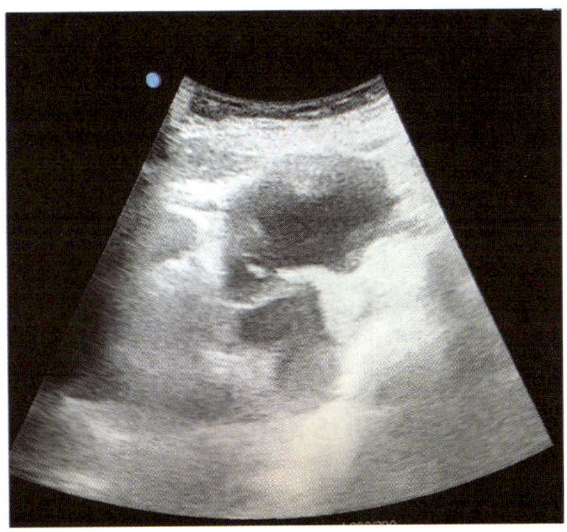

Figure 30.34 USG—image 19.

31 Common Spotters: Drugs and Contraceptives

Introduction

The first part of this chapter deals with the common drugs that are used in obstetrics and gynecology that can be kept as spotters during the viva voce. The drugs are described from a clinician's point of view, giving more emphasis to the indications, contraindications, dosage, side effects, and complications, than to the pharmacokinetics and pharmacodynamics of the drugs.

The second part of this chapter deals with contraceptives. Contraception is an important aspect of undergraduate and postgraduate training program and medical students are often checked for their knowledge in contraception in both theory and practical examinations. During the viva voce, various aspects of contraceptives such as characteristics, mode of action, efficacy, contraindications, advantages, and disadvantages can be discussed.

COMMON DRUGS KEPT AS SPOTTERS IN OBSTETRICS

Oxytocin

- Oxytocin is a polypeptide hormone synthesized in the supraoptic and paraventricular nuclei of hypothalamus and is transported down the axon and stored in the nerve endings within the posterior pituitary and is released during parturition and nipple stimulation.
- The synthetic form of oxytocin (syntocinon or pitocin) is used as a drug.
- Oxytocin ampoule
  - One ampoule of oxytocin contains 5 units in 1 mL (Figure 31.1).
  - The oxytocin ampoules have to be stored in a refrigerator at 2–6°C.

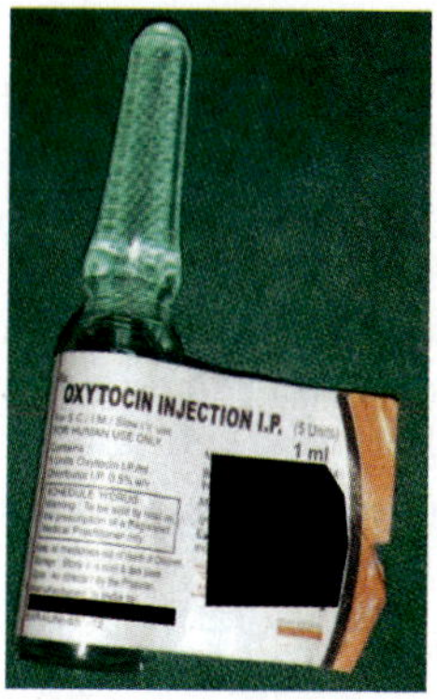

Figure 31.1 Oxytocin ampoule.

Mechanism of action

Uterus Oxytocin has uterotonic action—it causes physiological uterine contractions, that is, contraction of upper uterine segment and relaxation of the lower uterine segment. Uterine sensitivity to oxytocin increases progressively in the third trimester. Oxytocin binds to G-protein-coupled oxytocin receptors in the myometrium, resulting in depolarization of muscle fibers and influx of Ca^{2+} ions.

Breasts Oxytocin contracts the myoepithelial cells of mammary alveoli, resulting in "milk ejection" reflex, which is initiated by suckling of the breast.

Indications

- For induction and augmentation of labor
- For prevention and control of postpartum hemorrhage (PPH)
- To control bleeding following abortion and suction evacuation for molar pregnancy

Routes of administration

- IV route—most common route of administration starts acting immediately

- IM route—starts acting in 2–3 minutes
- Also available as buccal tablets and nasal spray

Note *Oxytocin is not used orally since it is degraded to inactive form when administered orally.*

Dosage

- **Induction/augmentation of labor**
  - Oxytocin is given in titrated doses and the infusion is described in terms of milliunits per minute. Oxytocin is administered as slow IV infusion wherein 2.5 IU of oxytocin is diluted in 500 mL of Ringer's lactate or normal saline solution and infusion is started at a low rate (2.5 mIU/min) and progressively titrated by 2.5 mIU/min every 30 minutes till effective uterine contractions are achieved, that is, uterine contractions of 3 in 10 minutes, each lasting for about 45 seconds.
  - The oxytocin infusion rate can be regulated either manually by counting the number of drops per minute or by using an infusion pump, which automatically controls the infusion rate.
  - Before starting oxytocin infusion, the following prerequisites need to be checked:
    - Confirm cephalic presentation.
    - Cephalopelvic disproportion (CPD) should be ruled out.
    - Placenta previa should be ruled out.
    - There should be no fetal distress.
  - Table 31.1 shows the titration of oxytocin that is widely practiced in labor room and Table 31.2 shows American College of Obstetricians and Gynecologists (ACOG) guidelines for the administration of oxytocin.
- **For prevention of PPH**: Active management of third stage of labor (AMTSL)—prophylactic oxytocin 10 IU is administered IM/IV following delivery of anterior shoulders or immediately following delivery of the baby.
- **For control of PPH:** Oxytocin 10–20 IU in 500 mL of Ringer's lactate is administered by IV infusion at a rate of 125 mL/h (60 drops/min) for an immediate response. Continuous oxytocin infusion is administered for a sustained effect.

Contraindications for oxytocin induction/augmentation

- Grand multipara (risk of uterine rupture)
- If vaginal delivery is contraindicated
- Fetal distress
- Previous uterine scar
- Malpresentations

Adverse effects

See Table 31.3

Table 31.1 Titrated dose of oxytocin

2.5 IU of oxytocin in 500 mL Ringer lactate solution		5 IU of oxytocin in 500 mL Ringer lactate solution	
Drops per minute	Dose (milliunits/min)	Drops per minute	Dose (milliunits/min)
8	2.5	32	20
16	5	40	25
24	7.5	48	30
32	10	56	35
40	12.5	64	40
48	15		
56	17.5		
64	20		

Table 31.2 ACOG guidelines (2011) for administration of oxytocin for induction/augmentation of labor

Regime	Starting dose (mIU/min)	Increase by (mIU/min)	Dosage interval (min)	Maximum dose (mIU/min)
Low dose	0.5–2	1–2	15–40	20
High dose	6	1–6	15–40	42

ACOG, American College of Obstetricians and Gynecologists.

Part 3

Part 3

Viva corner

Q1 What is the difference between low-dose and high-dose oxytocin regimen?

See table below

Table Difference between low-dose and high-dose oxytocin regimen

Low-dose regimen	High-dose regimen
• Lower dose of oxytocin is used • Dose increased less frequently (every 40 minutes) • Lower rates of uterine tachysystole and associated fetal heart rate changes	• Higher dose of oxytocin is used • Dose increased more frequently (every 20–30 minutes) • Increased rates of uterine tachysystole with associated fetal heart rate changes • Associated with shorter duration of labor and lower rates of cesarean section for dystocia

Q2 What is the difference between the actions of oxytocin and methergin?

See table below

Table Difference between the actions of oxytocin and methergin (methyl ergometrine)

	Oxytocin	Methergin
Mechanism of action	Physiological contraction of uterus during labor (law of polarity is maintained, i.e., upper segment contracts and retracts while lower segment relaxes)	Tetanic uterine contraction, i.e., contraction of both the upper and lower segments of uterus
Uses	Used in pregnancy, labor, and postpartum	• Contraindicated in pregnancy and labor with fetus in utero • Mainly used for prevention and control of postpartum hemorrhage

Table 31.3 Adverse effects of oxytocin

Maternal	Fetal
• Uterine hyperstimulation • Rupture of uterus • Water intoxication and antidiuresis at high doses • Hypotension • Formation of constriction ring	Fetal hypoxia and death

Dinoprostone gel

- Dinoprostone is a prostaglandin E2 (PGE2) analogue.
- Dinoprostone gel contains 0.5 mg of PGE2 in 2.5 mL of gel (Figure 31.2).

Indication

For cervical ripening and induction of labor

Route of administration

Dinoprostone is available in the form of gel (Prepidil or Cerviprime) or a vaginal insert (Cervidil).

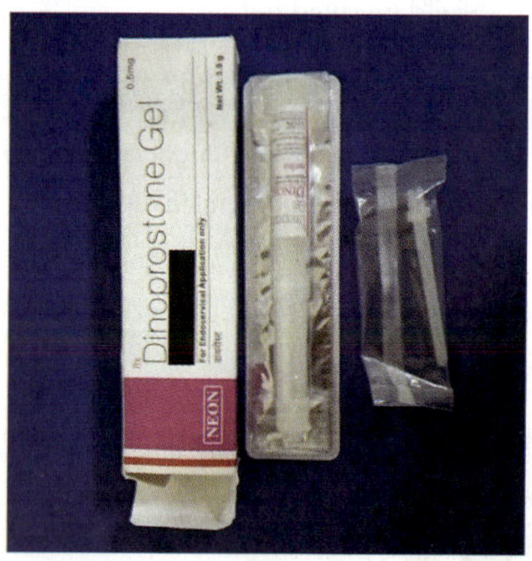

Figure 31.2 Dinoprostone gel.

Dosage

Dinoprostone gel 0.5 mg is given as intracervical application. The preloaded syringe comes with a plastic insertor, which is placed into the cervical canal under direct vision. Reassessment is usually ɔne after 6 hours and, if required, intracervical gel .n be reinstilled for maximum up to three doses a 24-hour period. However, more than two ɔses of PGE2 are usually not used.

Cervidil is a dinoprostone intravaginal insert ɔntaining 10 mg of dinoprostone in a small, white, ɔlymer mesh sac and has an attached tape that ɛlps during removal of the insert from the vagina. is placed high in posterior fornix and is left until :tive labor starts or for 12 hours. The main advan-.ge of vaginal insert is that it can be immediately ·moved in case of hyperstimulation of uterus.

dvantages

- Induces cervical ripening
- Reduces the rate of failed induction
- Reduces the need for oxytocin
- Shortens induction–delivery interval

dverse effects

- Nausea and vomiting
- Hyperstimulation of uterus
- Fetal distress
- Rupture of uterus

lisoprostol

Misoprostol is a synthetic PGE1 analogue (Figure 31.3).

Misoprostol tablets are available in different doses—25-, 50-, 100-, 200-, and 400-µg tablets.

lechanism of action

: acts by stimulating uterine contractions and auses ripening of the cervix.

ndications

- Medical abortion

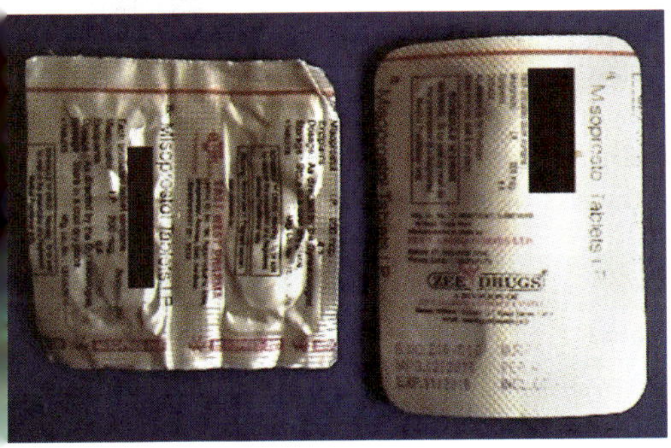

igure 31.3 Misoprostol tablets.

- Cervical priming before surgical abortion
- Induction of labor at term
- Treatment of PPH

Route of administration

Misoprostol can be administered by oral, sublingual, vaginal, and rectal routes.

Dosage

- **First-trimester medical abortion**
  - *Misoprostol as a single agent:* Can use misoprostol 200–800 µg vaginally for first-trimester medical termination of pregnancy (MTP) up to 8–10 weeks of gestation
  - *Misoprostol with mifepristone:* Mifepristone (antiprogesterone) 200 mg oral, followed 36–48 hours later by a single dose of misoprostol 800 µg oral/vaginal.
- **Second-trimester medical abortion:** Misoprostol 400 µg vaginally or orally can be given every 4 hours for four to six doses for termination of pregnancy up to 20 weeks of gestation.
- **Incomplete abortion/missed abortion**: Misoprostol 400 µg vaginally or orally can be given every 4 hours for four to six doses.
- **Cervical priming before surgical abortion:** Misoprostol 400–600 µg is administered vaginally approximately 3–4 hours prior to termination of pregnancy by suction evacuation/dilatation and curettage.
- **Induction of labor at term**
  - Misoprostol 25 µg is administered vaginally (placed in the posterior fornix) every

High-yield points

Advantages of misoprostol over other prostaglandins

- Is cheap
- Has a longer shelf life
- Is stable at room temperature (no need of refrigeration)
- Is easy to administer (can be given via oral, vaginal, sublingual, rectal routes)
- Is ideal for use in low-resource settings
- Is selective for uterus and has no effect on bronchus, hence not contraindicated in bronchial asthma

4–6 hours for cervical ripening and induction of labor.
  - Alternatively, misoprostol 50 μg is administered orally every 4–6 hours for cervical ripening and induction of labor.
- **Medical management of PPH**: Misoprostol 600–1000 μg can be administered sublingually, orally, vaginally, or rectally.

Contraindications

- Previous uterine scar
- Hypersensitivity to the drug
- For treatment of gastric ulcers (misoprostol increases uterine contractions in pregnancy, resulting in abortion)

Adverse effects

- Nausea, vomiting, and diarrhea
- Chills and rigors, and fever
- Uterine hyperstimulation
- Meconium staining of amniotic fluid

Methergin

- Methergin is methylergometrine, a semisynthetic derivative of ergometrine.
- One ampoule of methergin contains 0.2 mg in 1 mL (Figure 31.4). It is also available in tablets of 0.5 and 1 mg.

Mechanism of action

Methergin causes generalized smooth muscle contraction resulting in tetanic contraction of the upper and lower segments of the uterus without any relaxation.

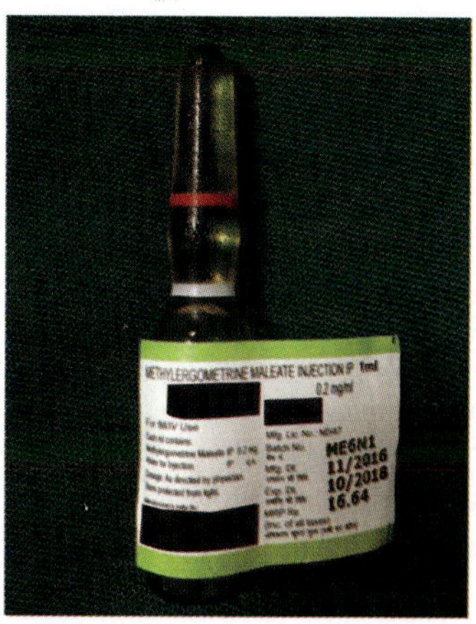

Figure 31.4 Methergin ampoule.

Part 3

Indications

- Early pregnancy—to control bleeding follow-ing abortion and suction evacuation of mola pregnancy
- Prophylaxis and treatment of atonic PPH
- Following cesarean section to facilitate uterin contractions

Note *Methergin causes tetanic uterine contractions unlike oxytocin, hence not used for labor induction or augmentation*

Routes

IV, IM, and oral routes (Table 31.4)

Dosage

- **Prevention of PPH:** Methergine 0.2 mg IV/IM can be administered following delivery of anterior shoulder of baby or immediately following delivery of the baby.
- **Treatment of atonic PPH:** Methergin 0.2 mg IV/IM dose may be repeated as required, at intervals of 2–4 hours.

Viva corner

Q1 What is Syntometrine?

Combined preparation of oxytocin 5 units and ergometrine 0.5 units is called Syntometrine.

Contraindications

- **Severe preeclampsia and eclampsia**: Methergin can result in sudden rise in BP.
- **Heart disease**: Methergin may cause sudden sequestration of the blood from uterine circulation into systemic circulation, causing overloading of the right heart, resulting in pulmonary edema.
- **Following delivery of first twin**: Administration of methergin following the delivery of the first twin can result in entrapment of second twin due to tetanic contractions of the uterus.
- **Rh-negative pregnancy**: Methergin increase the risk of fetomaternal hemorrhage.

Table 31.4 Onset of action of methergin

Route	Onset of action (minutes)
Intravenous	1–1.5
Intramuscular	7
Oral	10

dverse effects

Nausea and vomiting
Increase in BP

arboprost

It is a synthetic prostaglandin F2 alpha (PGF2α). Each ampoule of carboprost contains PGF2α 250 μg/mL (Figure 31.5).

echanism of action

predominantly acts on the myometrium causing terine contractions.

dications

Management of atonic PPH
Medical termination of second-trimester pregnancy

oute of administration

is administered as intramuscular injection.

osage

Atonic PPH: Carboprost 250 μg IM injection can be repeated at 15-minute interval up to a maximum of eight doses. In severe cases of PPH, intramyometrial carboprost can be administered.
- **Second-trimester MTP:** Carboprost 250 μg IM injection, that can be is repeated every 3–4 hours until the patient aborts. A maximum of four injections are usually given.

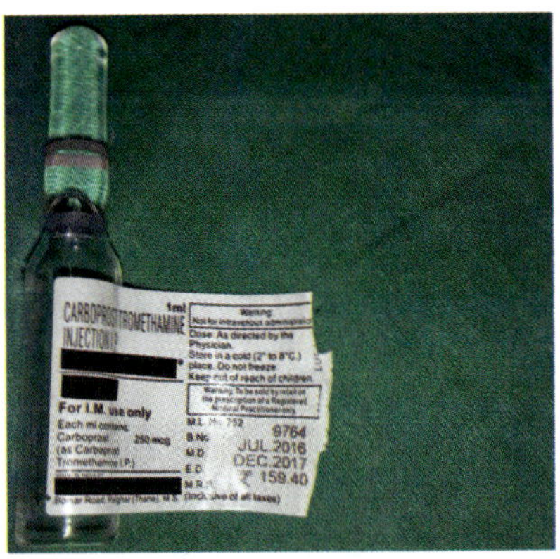

igure 31.5 Carboprost ampoule.

> **Extra edge**
>
> It has been shown that prostaglandins are not preferable over conventional uterotonics such as oxytocin for the active management of third stage of labor and prevention of PPH. However, if PPH occurs, administration of parental prostaglandins serves as an effective form of treatment.

Contraindications

Carboprost should be used with caution in patients with asthma, hypertension, hepatic, or renal diseases.

Adverse effects

- Nausea, vomiting, and diarrhea
- Bronchoconstriction
- Hypertension, headache, flushing, and pyrexia

Mifepristone (RU-486) (Figure 31.6)

- Mifepristone is a progesterone and glucocorticoid antagonist.
- It is available as 200 mg oral tablet.

Mechanism of action

The main action of mifepristone is through its antiprogesterone effect. Mifepristone intake results in the following:
- Prevents implantation of a fertilized ovum
- Prevents further development of an implanted embryo

> **High-yield points**
>
> **Choice of Uterotonics in different clinical situations**

MTP	Mifepristone followed by misoprostol is the preferred drug
Control of bleeding in abortion	• Misoprostol is effective to hasten evacuation and to control bleeding • Methergin is also effective to control bleeding • Oxytocin can also be used to hasten evacuation and to control bleeding

(CONTD...)

(...CONTD)

High-yield points

Induction of labor	• Bishop's score <6 indicates that cervix is unfavorable: Prostaglandins (prostaglandin E2, prostaglandin E1) are the preferred agents • Bishop's score ≥6 indicates that cervix is favorable: Oxytocin and prostaglandins are equally good, oxytocin is preferred
Augmentation of labor	• Oxytocin is the drug of choice
Active management of the third stage of labor (AMTSL) for prevention of PPH	• Oxytocin 10 units IV or IM is recommended
Medical management of atonic PPH	• Oxytocin is the drug of first choice • Methergin (IV or IM) can be given along with oxytocin • Carboprost (prostaglandin F2 alpha) IM injections are effective in severe bleeding • Misoprostol is ideal in low-resource settings

PPH, postpartum hemorrhage.

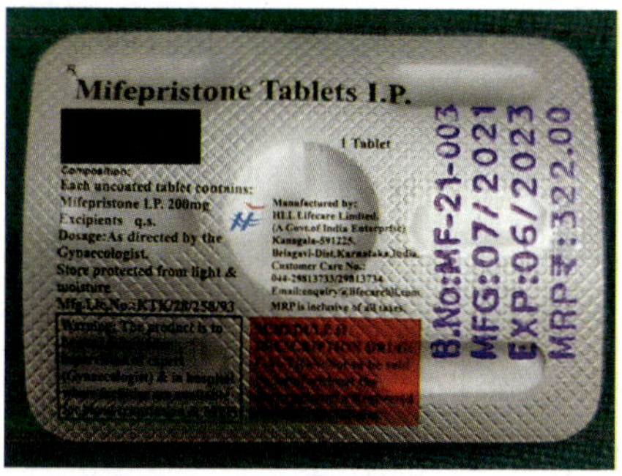

Figure 31.6 Mifepristone tablet.

Indications

- Medical abortion
- Emergency contraception (EC)
- Other uses: Medical management of fibroids and endometriosis

Route of administration

It is administered orally.

Dosage

- **Termination of pregnancy:** Mifepristone 200 mg orally followed up 48 hours later by misoprostol, single oral/vaginal dose of 800 µg, has a success rate of >90% for termination of pregnancy up to 7 weeks of gestation.
- **Emergency contraception:** Mifepristone 10–50 mg administered within 72 hours of unprotected intercourse interferes with implantation and is a highly effective method of EC.

Contraindications

- Ectopic pregnancy
- Bleeding disorders
- Anticoagulant therapy
- Adrenal failure
- Inherited porphyrias
- Long-term corticosteroid therapy

Side effects

- Nausea, vomiting, diarrhea
- Bleeding and lower abdominal cramps

Magnesium sulfate

One ampoule of $MgSO_4$ contains 1 g in 2 ml (Figure 31.7).

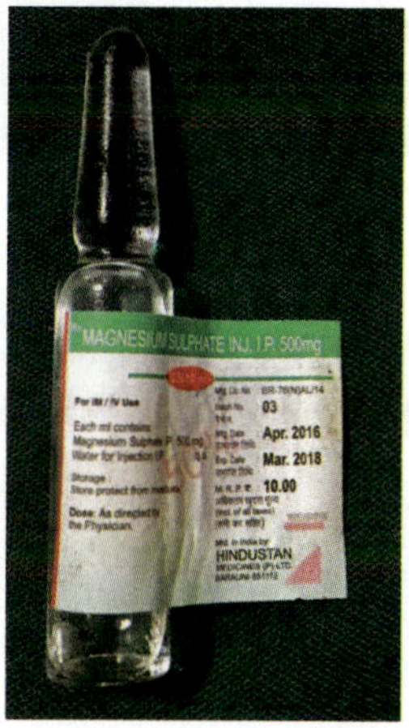

Figure 31.7 Magnesium sulfate ampoule.

Mechanism of action

- Magnesium sulfate is a blocker of *N*-methyl-D-aspartate (NMDA) receptors in the brain.
- It suppresses motor end-plate sensitivity to acetylcholine and the release of acetylcholine from nerve endings.
- It acts as a competitive inhibitor of calcium ion (it acts as a tocolytic by competing with Ca^{2+} ions for entry into myometrium).

Indications

- Anticonvulsant: In eclampsia
- Prophylaxis for prevention of convulsions: in severe preeclampsia and imminent eclampsia
- Tocolytic agent: In preterm labor
- Also has a neuroprotective effect on the fetus

Route of administration

Intramuscular/intravenous route

Dosage

For management and prevention of eclamptic convulsions—Pritchard regimen (Table 31.5) is usually followed.

- Therapeutic level of $MgSO_4$ is 4–7 mEq/L.
- The drug is excreted in urine.
- Excess dose causes loss of patellar reflexes, and respiratory depression.
- The following parameters are monitored before the administration of each dose:
  - Respiratory rate should be >14/min.
  - Patellar reflex should be present.
  - Urine output should be >100 mL/4 hours.
- If convulsions recur after loading dose, additional 2 g of 20% solution IV over 3–5 minutes can be given.
- The dose is the same for prophylaxis and treatment of convulsions.

Table 31.5 **Pritchard regimen for magnesium sulfate therapy**

Dosage	Administration
Loading dose	4 g of 20% solution IV over 5–10 minutes, followed by 10 g of 50% solution given as 5 g in each buttock, deep IM
Maintenance dose	5 g of 50% solution every 4th hourly, on alternate buttocks

- The drug should be discontinued 24 hours after delivery or 24 hours after the last convulsion, whichever occurs later.

For tocolysis—4–6 g IV (20% solution) is given over 20–30 minutes, followed by infusion of 1–2 g/hour, continued up to 12 hours following stoppage of contractions.

Contraindications

- Myasthenia gravis
- Maternal renal disease

Adverse effects

- Respiratory depression
- Muscle weakness
- Reduced fetal heart rate (FHR) variability
- Respiratory and/or neuromuscular depression in the newborn, if the mother has received magnesium sulfate IV therapy, for a prolonged period prior to delivery

Antidote

Calcium gluconate (10 mL of 10% solution given as slow IV)

Labetalol

- Labetalol is currently the first-choice antihypertensive in pregnancy. It can also be used for the control of hypertensive crises in pregnancy.
- Efficacy and safety appear equal to that of methyldopa.
- It is available as 100, 200, 300 mg tablets. Labetalol ampoules contain 5 mg/mL of solution (Figure 31.8).

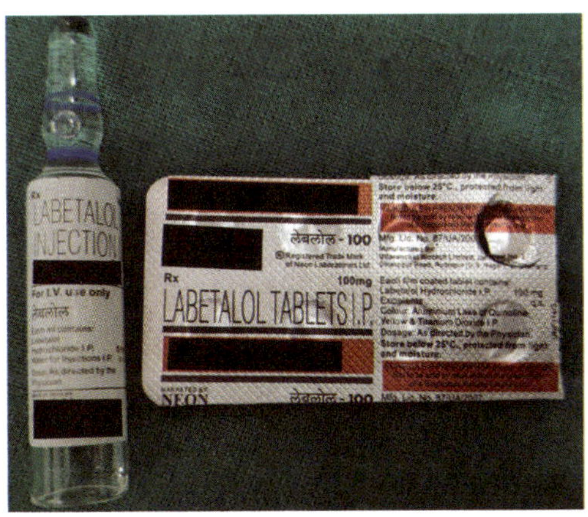

Figure 31.8 Labetalol injectable and oral tablet.

Mechanism of action

Labetalol is a combined alpha- and beta-adrenergic receptor blocker that reduces the peripheral vascular resistance and lowers the BP.

Indications

- Preeclampsia and eclampsia
- Essential hypertension
- Hypertension associated with pheochromocytoma
- Clonidine withdrawal

Route of administration

It can be oral or intravenous.

Dose

- Labetalol 100 mg is given orally every 8 hours, which may be increased up to 800 mg/day.
- Hypertensive crisis: Labetalol 20 mg is given as intravenous bolus over at least 1 minute, followed by 40 mg after 10 minutes. If the first dose is not effective, then 80 mg can be administered every 10 minutes. Maximum total dose of 220 mg can be administered.

Contraindications

- Asthma, airway obstructive disease
- Heart block
- Congestive heart failure
- Cardiogenic shock

Side effects

Tremors, headache, bronchospasm, congestive cardiac failure, and postural hypotension.

Nifedipine

It is a calcium channel blocker

Mechanism of action

Causes direct arteriolar vasodilatation by inhibition of slow inward calcium channels in vascular smooth muscles.

Indications

- Preeclampsia
- Tocolysis in preterm labor

Dose

- **Antihypertensive action**: Dose is 5–10 mg per oral 8 hourly; maximum dose is 60–120 mg/day.
- **Tocolysis**: Dose is 20–30 mg every 6 hours.

Side effects

- Flushing, hypotension, headache, tachycardia, and inhibition of labor.
- Simultaneous use with $MgSO_4$ can be hazardous due to synergistic effect.

Methyldopa

- Methyldopa is an effective antihypertensive during pregnancy. It has been proved to be safe for both the mother and the fetus.
- It is available as 500-mg tablet.

Mechanism of action

It is a central- and peripheral-acting antiadrenergic drug.

Indications

Preeclampsia and eclampsia for control of BP

Route of administration

Oral route.

Dose

Methyl dopa is started at 250 mg, orally two to three times per day, and may be increased to a maximum of 2 g/day in divided doses

Side effects

- **Maternal:** Dry mouth, postural hypotension, sedation, bradycardia, headache, depression, hepatitis, and hemolytic anemia
- **Fetal:** Intestinal ileus

Commonly used antihypertensives in pregnancy

- Andrenergic receptor blocking agents—labetalol
- Calcium channel blockers—nifedipine, nicardipine
- Sympatholytics—methyldopa
- Vasodilators—hydralazine, nitroglycerin, sodium nitroprusside
- ACE inhibitors such as captopril, lisinopril are contraindicated in pregnancy

Isoxsuprine

- Isoxsuprine is a β_2-adrenergic agonist causing smooth muscle relaxation.
- Isoxsuprine hydrochloride (Duvadilan) is available in the form of oral tablets, intramuscular and intravenous ampoules (Figure 31.9).

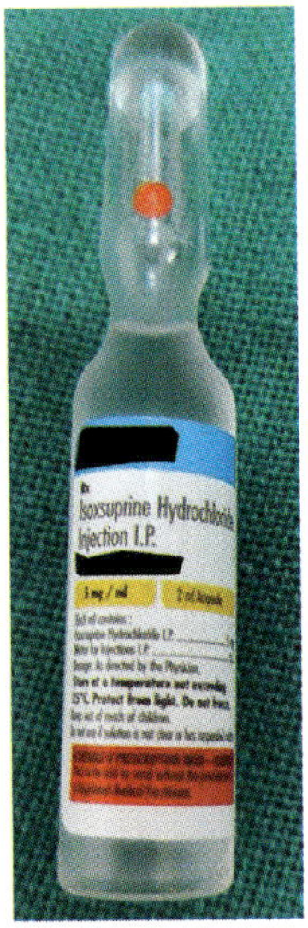

Figure 31.9 Isoxsuprine ampoule.

Mechanism of action

The drug has an antispasmodic and smooth muscle relaxant action on the uterus and blood vessels.

Indications

- Tocolytic agent used for the treatment of preterm labor
- In cases of tetanic uterine contractions—to cause uterine relaxation

Route of administration

Oral/intramuscular/intravenous

Dose

Preterm labor: Isoxsuprine IV infusion is started at the rate of 0.3–0.5 mg/min by adding 40–60 mg in 500 mL of 5% glucose or normal saline. This is followed by 10–20 mg IM 8 hourly for 2 days and then oral isoxsuprine 20 mg 8 hourly for 1–2 weeks.

Side effects

- **Intramuscular/intravenous route**: Flushing, tachycardia, and hypotension
- **Oral route**: Nausea, flushing, giddiness, and headache

Commonly used tocolytic agents

- Beta-mimetics (beta-adrenergic agonists)—isoxsuprine, ritodrine, and terbutaline
- Calcium-channel blockers—nifedipine
- Magnesium sulfate—in addition to tocolytic effect, it has additional neuroprotective effect. Evidence supports magnesium sulphate for women at risk of imminent birth at <32–34 weeks to reduce the likelihood of cerebral palsy in the child
- PG synthetase inhibitors—indomethacin
- Nitric oxide donors—nitroglycerine
- Oxytocin receptor antagonists—atosiban

Drotaverine hydrochloride

It is an antispasmodic agent, commonly used for relieving smooth muscle spasm in various obstetric and gynecological conditions (Figure 31.10).

Mechanism of action

Drotaverine hydrochloride is a phosphodiesterase-4 inhibitor that increases the concentration of cAMP and cGMP, resulting in the smooth muscle relaxation.

Indications

- In active phase of labor—likely to reduce the duration of active phase of labor by hastening cervical dilatation
- Dysmenorrhea
- Uterine cramps following intrauterine contraceptive device (IUCD) insertion
- Nongynecological indications: Treatment of colicky pain such as renal and abdominal colic and in functional bowel disorders

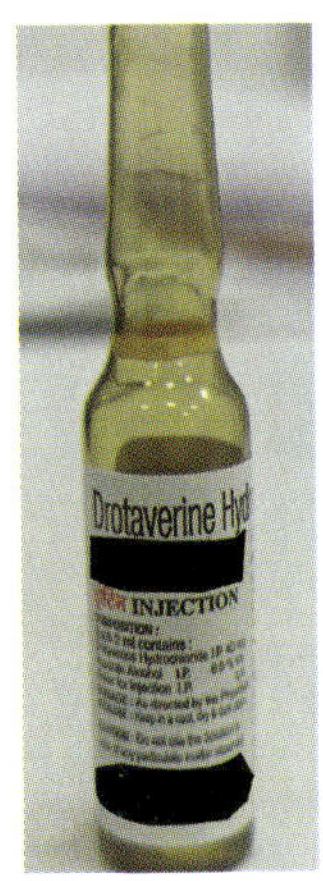

Figure 31.10 Drotaverine ampoule.

Route of administration

Oral/intramuscular/intravenous route

Dosage

- Active phase of labor: Drotaverine 40 mg (one ampoule) is administered IM/IV slowly after dilution. The dose can be repeated every 2–3 hours for a maximum of three doses.
- Dysmenorrhea: Drotaverine 40–80 mg is given orally 8th hourly for 3–5 days.

Side effects

Vertigo, nausea, vomiting, and dry mouth

Dexamethasone and Betamethasone (Antenatal corticosteroids) (Figure 31.11)

- Antenatal corticosteroids accelerate fetal lung maturity and reduce the incidence and severity of respiratory distress syndrome (RDS), thereby reducing neonatal morbidity and mortality.
- Other advantages of steroids: Reduce the incidence of necrotizing enterocolitis, intraventricular hemorrhage (IVH), bronchopulmonary dysplasia, and patent ductus arteriosus

Route of administration

Intramuscular

Dosage

- Inj. Betamethasone 12 mg IM two doses given 24 hours apart or dexamethasone 6 mg IM four doses given 12 hours apart are the standard regimen used.
- Optimal benefit begins 24 hours after therapy and lasts for 7 days.
- Benefit of repeated courses of glucocorticoids is doubtful and not currently recommended.

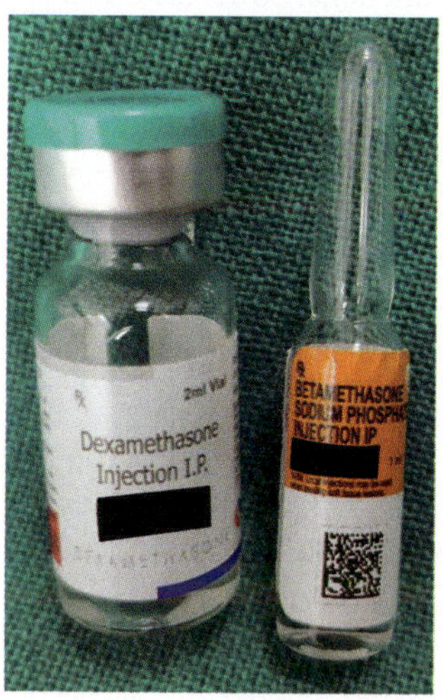

Figure 31.11 Betamethasone and Dexamethasone.

Mechanism of action

- Induce the enzyme system responsible for the synthesis of pulmonary surfactant
- Release the surfactant stored in type II pneumocytes
- Increase lung compliance
- Potentiate the response to postnatal administration of surfactant

Note *In India, the salt Betamethasone acetate + phosphate, which requires only two doses at 12 hourly interval, is not readily available. The available salt in India is Betamethasone phosphate which is short acting and needs more frequent administration as compared to the former. Hence, the dosage schedule of Betamethasone phosphate is similar to that of the Dexamethasone and has no added advantage over it. Further, Betamethasone is more costly and less stable than Dexamethasone at high temperatures. However, where Dexamethasone is not available the service provider may use Betamethasone phosphate to give the advantage of corticosteroids to the newborn.*

RCOG guidelines for use of antenatal corticosteroids

Major Recommendations *(Ref.: Antenatal Corticosteroids to Reduce Neonatal Morbidity RCOG Green-top Guideline No. 74)*

- *Antenatal corticosteroids have no known benefits for the mother.*
- *A single course of antenatal corticosteroids should be administered to women between 24+0 and 34+6 weeks of gestation who are at risk of preterm birth.*
- *The decision to administer corticosteroids at gestations <24+0 weeks should be made taking all clinical aspects into consideration.*
- *Antenatal corticosteroids are most effective in reducing RDS in pregnancies that deliver*

24 hours after and up to 7 days after completion of course of antenatal corticosteroids.

- *Antenatal corticosteroid use reduces neonatal death within the first 24 hours and therefore should still be given even if delivery is expected within this time.*
- *A single course of antenatal corticosteroids does not appear to be associated with any significant short-term maternal or fetal adverse effects.*
- *There is still insufficient evidence on the long-term benefits and risks of multiple courses of antenatal corticosteroids.*
- *Caution should be exercised when giving corticosteroid therapy to women with systemic infection including tuberculosis or sepsis such as chorioamnionitis.*
- *Diabetes mellitus is not a contraindication to antenatal corticosteroid treatment for fetal lung maturation. Women with impaired glucose tolerance or diabetes who are receiving fetal steroids should have additional insulin according to an agreed protocol and be closely monitored.*
- *Antenatal corticosteroids should be given to all women at risk of iatrogenic or spontaneous preterm birth up to 34+6 weeks of gestation.*
- *Antenatal corticosteroids should be given to all women for whom an elective cesarean section is planned prior to 38+6 weeks of gestation.*
- *Clinicians should continue to offer a single course of antenatal corticosteroid treatment to women with multiple pregnancy at risk of iatrogenic or spontaneous preterm delivery between 24+0 and 34+6 weeks of gestation.*
- *Elective lower segment cesarean section should normally be performed at or after 39+0 weeks of gestation to reduce respiratory morbidity.*
- *Pregnancies affected by fetal growth restriction between 24+0 and 35+6 weeks of gestation at risk of delivery should receive a single course of antenatal corticosteroids.*
- *Betamethasone 12 mg given intramuscularly in two doses or dexamethasone 6 mg given intramuscularly in four doses are the steroids of choice to enhance lung maturation.*
- *A single rescue course may be considered with caution in pregnancies where the initial course was given at less than 26+0 weeks of gestation and another obstetric indication arises later in pregnancy.*

ACOG 2017 guidelines recommendations on antenatal corticosteroids

(Ref.: ACOG committee opinion No. 713, 2017):

- *A single course of corticosteroids is recommended for pregnant women between 24 0/7 weeks and 33 6/7 weeks of gestation who are at risk of preterm delivery within 7 days, including for those with ruptured membranes and multiple gestations.*
- *Administration of corticosteroids may be considered in pregnant women between 34 0/7 weeks and 36 6/7 weeks of gestation who are at risk of preterm birth within 7 days, and who have not received a previous course of antenatal corticosteroids.*
- *A single repeat course of antenatal corticosteroids should be considered in women who are less than 34 0/7 weeks of gestation, who are at risk of preterm delivery within 7 days, and whose prior course of antenatal corticosteroids was administered more than 14 days previously.*

Side effects

- Maternal effects: Increased risk of infections and a higher incidence of endometritis and chorionamnionitis in patients with premature rupture of membranes.
- Fetal effects: Reduction of fetal body and breathing movements and a reduction of fetal heart rate variation, without any changes in Doppler waveform patterns of fetoplacental vessels.

Micronized progesterone (Figure 31.12)

Mechanism of action

Progesterone helps in implantation of fertilized ovum in the following ways:

- Stimulates the growth of uterus
- Maintains uterine quiescence by stabilizing lysosomal membranes and inhibiting PG synthesis
- Inhibits myometrial contractions
- Endometrial changes: Induces secretory transformation, increases vascularity of the endometrial lining, stabilizes endometrium
- Immunomodulatory or anti-inflammatory: Progesterone along with HCG and cortisol inhibits tissue rejection and protects the conceptus

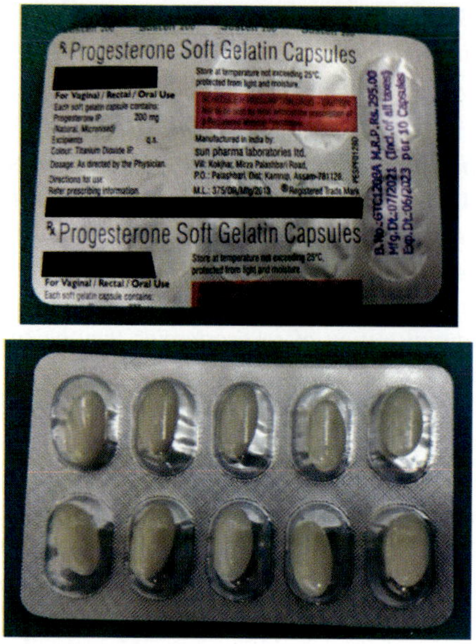

Figure 31.12 Micronized progesterone.

Micronized progesterone (micronization of the natural progesterone)

- It increases the half-life of progesterone.
- Micronization decreases particle size and enhances the dissolution of progesterone.
- Absorption of micronized progesterone is enhanced twofold when taken with food.
- The pharmacologic effects of synthetic progestins (e.g., norethindrone, norgestrel, levonorgestrel, medroxyprogesterone acetate) are slightly different from those of natural progesterone. Androgenic effects of synthetic progestins such as fluid retention, reduction of HDL cholesterol levels, headaches, and mood disturbances are not present with micronized progesterone.

Indications

- **Bad obstetric history (BOH) and luteal phase insufficiency:** In women with spontaneous or recurrent miscarriage, supplementary progesterone provides uterine quiescence by inhibiting uterine contractions. Luteal-phase defect is a progesterone deficient condition and natural progesterone is used to improve luteal function in such cases.
- **Prevention of preterm birth:** Progesterone is used to prevent preterm birth in women with history of spontaneous preterm delivery at less than 37 weeks and in cases with short cervix.
- **Luteal phase support in ART:** Progesterone is used in assisted reproductive techniques (ARTs) as adequate levels of progesterone are essential to support implantation and early pregnancy.

Route of administration

Oral/vaginal

Dosage

Available as 100/200 mg capsules/suppository. Typical doses of progesterone supplementation include 200 mg OD/BD orally or as vaginal suppository.

Side effects

Nausea, bloating, breast tenderness, headache, mood swings, dizziness, or drowsiness

Anti-D immunoglobulin

Anti-D immunoglobulin immunoprophylaxis is given for prevention of Rh isoimmunization. The aim is to prevent antibody formation in the mother (Figure 31.13).

Current recommendations for the prevention of Rh isoimmunization

- Routine antenatal anti-D prophylaxis (RAADP) given at 28 weeks along with postpartum anti-D prophylaxis within 72 hours of delivery.

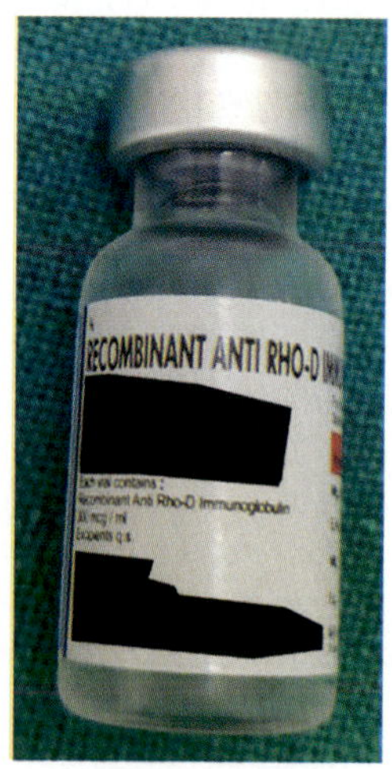

Figure 31.13 Anti-D immunoglobulin.

- Apart from this, anti-D should also be given after potential sensitizing events during pregnancy. *(Refer Part 1, Chapter 10, for further details)*

Iron sucrose

It is a currently used dextran-free parenteral iron preparation available as 5 mL ampoules containing 100 mg iron (Figure 31.14).

(Refer Part 1, Chapter 2, for further details on iron sucrose.)

Ferric carboxymaltose (FCM)

- It is a new dextran-free iron preparation that can be given as a single-dose IV infusion.
- Large dose up to 1000 mg can be administered over 15 minutes. Available as 500 mg/10 mL and 1 g/20 mL vials *(Refer Part 1, Chapter 2, for further details on Ferric carboxymaltose).*

Carbetocin

- Carbetocin is a long-acting synthetic oxytocin analogue.
- Available as 100 µg/mL vial. Stable in room temperature up to 30°C.
- It has a half-life of 40 minutes (around 4–10 times longer than oxytocin) and uterine contractions occur in less than two minutes after intravenous administration of optimal dosage of 100 µg.

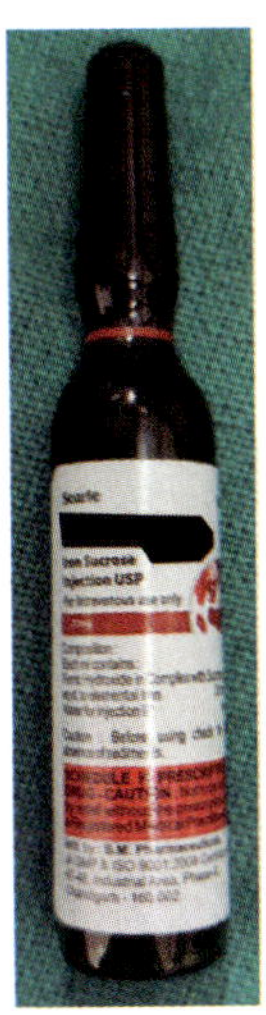

Figure 31.14 Iron sucrose ampoule.

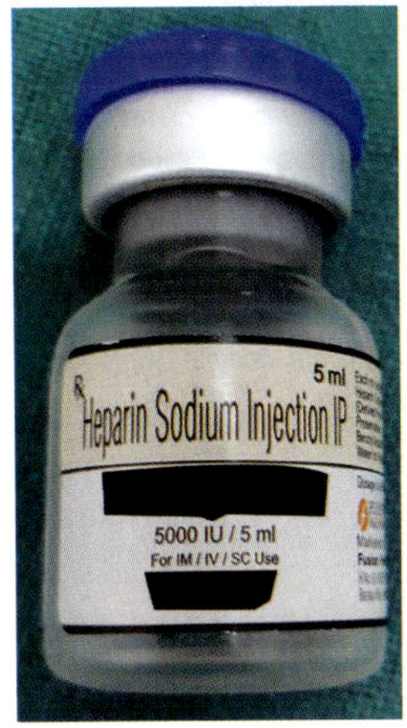

Figure 31.15 Unfractionated heparin.

- Prophylactic administration of carbetocin may be a good alternative to oxytocin to prevent PPH.
- Disadvantage: Highly expensive.

Unfractionated heparin (Figure 31.15)

Mechanism of action

Heparin inhibits the action of thrombin. It enhances the action of antithrombin III and increases factor Xa inhibitor.

Uses in obstetrics

- Treatment of deep vein thrombosis (DVT) and pulmonary embolism
- Prophylaxis against DVT following surgical procedures (cesarean section, cesarean hysterectomy)
- Pregnancy in women who have undergone valve replacement surgery and in atrial fibrillation
- APLA syndrome

Dosage

Heparin prophylaxis is given as 5000–10,000 units SC every 12 hours [monitored with activated partial thromboplastin time (aPTT)].

Side effects

- **Maternal:** Hemorrhage, thrombocytopenia, hyperkalemia, and osteoporosis
- **Fetal:** Does not cross the placenta and is not teratogenic

Extra edge

Advantages of low-molecular-weight heparin (LMWH) over unfractionated heparin

- LMWHs (enoxaparin) are as effective and safe as unfractionated heparin.
- They have a longer duration of action. Hence, they are given as single-daily SC injection.
- Prophylactic regimen of LMWH does not need monitoring.
- Side effects are less compared with those of heparin.

COMMON DRUGS KEPT AS SPOTTERS IN GYNECOLOGY

Tranexamic acid

Tranexamic acid is an antifibrinolytic drug. It is available as 500 mg/5 mL ampoules for IV use and as 250/500 mg oral tablets (Figure 31.16).

Mechanism of action

Tranexamic acid is a competitive inhibitor of tissue plasminogen activator, thereby preventing conversion of plasminogen to active plasmin (activated plasmin binds to the fibrin). It exerts antifibrinolytic effect by preventing the conversion of fibrin to fibrin degradation products (FDP) and hence prevents dissolution of blood clot.

Indications

- Dysfunctional uterine bleeding (DUB)
- Menorrhagia related to uterine fibroid/IUCD insertion, etc.
- Prevention of capillary bleeding after surgical procedures (e.g., cervical conization)
- Obstetric indications—PPH (tranexamic acid is now considered for prevention of PPH)

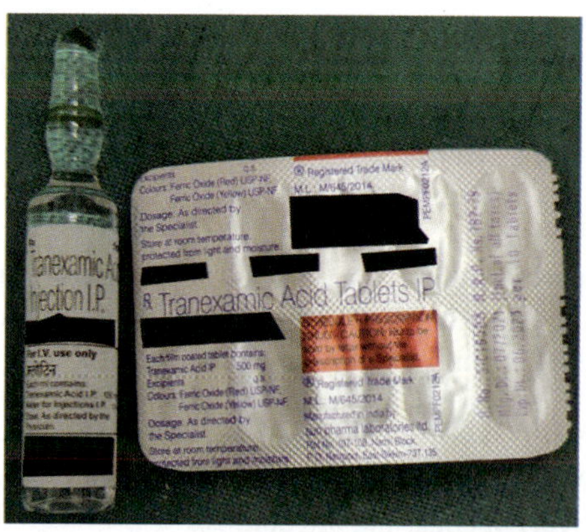

Figure 31.16 Tranexamic acid injectable and oral tablet.

Route of administration

Oral/intravenous route

Dose

- **Treatment of menorrhagia and IUCD-induced bleeding:** Tranexamic acid in dosage of 0.5–1 g, repeated three to four times per day for 4–6 days
- **Prevention of bleeding after surgery:** Tranexamic acid 0.5–1 g intravenously two to three times per day

Contraindications

Severe renal insufficiency, disseminated intravascular coagulation (DIC)

Side effects

Nausea, vomiting, diarrhea, giddiness, hypersensitivity reactions, and potential risk of thrombosis

Metformin

Metformin belongs to biguanide group of oral hypoglycemic drugs (Figure 31.17).

Mechanism of action

Metformin lowers blood glucose by exerting the following actions:

- Metformin suppresses hepatic gluconeogenesis and reduces glucose output from liver.
- It improves peripheral glucose utilization by increasing insulin sensitivity.
- It reduces hyperinsulinemia and hyperandrogenemia.

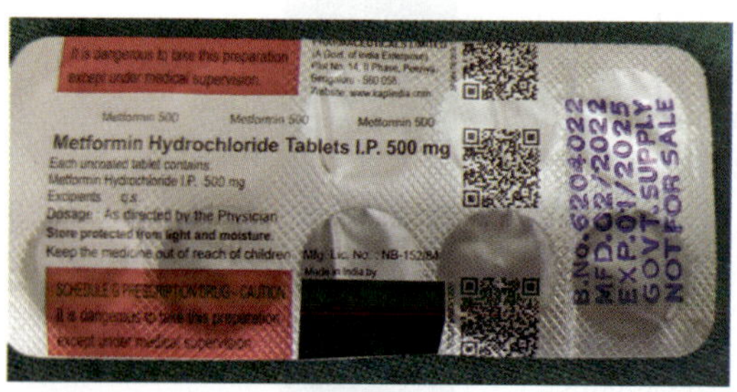

Figure 31.17 Metformin tablet.

Indications in gynecology

In polycystic ovarian disease (PCOD), metformin is used as an insulin sensitizer. In obese women with infertility, metformin may be used along with clomiphene citrate for ovulation induction.

Route of administration

Oral

Dose

In PCOD, metformin is given as 500 mg OD for 7 days, then 500 mg BD for 7 days, and then 500 mg TDS for 3 months. In case ovulation does not occur with metformin as a sole therapy, clomiphene therapy is started along with metformin.

Contraindications

- Hypotension
- Heart failure
- Severe respiratory, hepatic, and renal disease
- Alcoholics (due to an increased risk of lactic acidosis)

Side effects

- Gastrointestinal intolerance, nausea, vomiting, abdominal cramps, anorexia, bloating, metallic taste, diarrhea, and tiredness
- Lactic acidosis, is a rare complication that can be precipitated by alcohol ingestion

Clomiphene citrate

CC is a nonsteroidal drug having both estrogen antagonistic and agonistic effects.

Mechanism of action

CC competes with endogenous estrogen and blocks the estrogen receptors within the hypothalamus, thus alleviating the negative feedback exerted by endogenous estrogen. As a result, release of GnRH, follicle-stimulating hormone (FSH), and luteinizing hormone (LH) gets normalized, thus re-establishing ovulation.

Indications

- Anovulatory infertility
- PCOD
- Unexplained infertility
- Harvesting oocytes before in vitro fertilization (IVF) cycle
- Oligospermia (in males)

Route of administration

Oral

Dosage

Standard protocol

- CC 50 mg OD is given for 5 days, starting on days 3–5 of a spontaneous menstrual cycle or after progesterone-induced bleeding.
- In case there is no response with 50 mg, dose can be increased up to 150 mg/day.
- Follicular monitoring is done with transvaginal sonography (TVS) starting from day 10 of the menstrual cycle.

Combination protocols

- In women who are resistant or refractory to standard treatment with CC, the following combinations can be offered:
  - CC +human chorionic gonadotropin (hCG) (5000–10,000 IU)
  - CC + insulin-sensitizing agents such as metformin (1000–2000 mg/day in divided doses)
  - CC + glucocorticoids (0.5 mg dexamethasone or 5 mg prednisolone daily at night)

Sequential CC with gonadotropins CC 50–100 mg/day is administered on days 5–9 of the cycle, followed by low dose FSH (75 IU/day) on days 9–12 of the cycle.

- **Clomiphene failure:** This is defined as absence of pregnancy, despite the occurrence of ovulation with CC.
- **Clomiphene resistance:** This is defined as absence of ovulation even after treatment with CC in the dosage of 150 mg/day for three cycles.

Contraindications

- Ovarian cysts/tumors
- Ovarian failure
- Hepatic dysfunction
- Pregnancy

Side effects

- Risk of multiple pregnancies
- Thickening of the cervical mucus under the antiestrogenic effect of CC
- Ovarian hyperstimulation

Letrozole

Mechanism of action

- Letrozole is a nonsteroidal highly selective oral aromatase inhibitor which can reversibly bind to the rate-limiting enzyme P450 aromatase in estrogen biosynthesis pathway and inhibit the conversion of testosterone to estradiol and androstenedione to estrone.
- The down-regulated estrogen increases the secretion of pituitary follicle-stimulating hormone (FSH) as feedback to stimulate ovulation.

Indications

- It is approved to be effective for a wide range of breast cancers, which at present is its only registered indication.
- Letrozole is now widely used to induce ovulation in anovulatory infertility patients and to augment follicles for ovulatory women.
- It is used as an adjunct for intrauterine insemination and *in vitro* fertilization (IVF)/intracytoplasmic sperm injection (ICSI) cycles.
- It is also used for fertility preservation in women with estrogen-sensitive cancers.
- Letrozole is more accessible and has fewer adverse side effects and lower cost than injectable gonadotropins.

Route of administration

Oral

Dosage

The most common protocol for ovulation induction is daily dose of 2.5–7.5 mg starting day 3–5 of the cycle for 5 days.

Side effects

Hot flushes, flushed skin, increased sweating, breast tenderness, joint pain, weakness, edema, headache, dizziness

GnRH agonists

Leuprolide and goserelin are the most commonly used GnRH agonists.

Mechanism of action

- The physiological release of GnRH is in pulses, whereas GnRH agonists act continuously. Following the initial episode of pituitary stimulation, GnRH analogues cause downregulation of pituitary secretion of gonadotropins to produce hypogonadotropic hypogonadism.
- Ovulation ceases and estradiol levels fall to the castration levels.

Indications

- Endometriosis
- Adenomyosis
- Uterine fibroids
- Precocious puberty
- Ovarian stimulation protocols (GnRH agonists produce a hypoestrogenic state by causing downregulation of pituitary gonadotropins; FSH is then administered, followed by hCG to trigger ovulation)

Route of administration

Intramuscular/subcutaneous/intranasal

Dosage

- Leuprolide 3.75 mg IM depot injection every month
- Goserelin 3.6 mg SC every month
- Nafarelin administered as a nasal spray 400 µg twice daily

Contraindications

- Pregnancy/lactation
- Hypersensitivity

Side effects

- Hypoestrogenic side effects
  - Loss of trabecular bone density leading to osteoporosis
  - Hot flushes, mood swings, breakthrough bleeding, reduced libido, depression, and vaginal dryness
- Ovarian hyperstimulation (in ovarian stimulation protocols)

Treatment is usually restricted for 6 months due to side effects. Add-back therapy may be helpful in preventing osteoporosis and other hypoestrogenic symptoms associated with the use of GnRH agonists, thereby allowing longer duration of therapy.

Agents used as add-back therapy along with GnRH agonists include the following:

- Hormone replacement therapy (a combination of conjugated estrogen 0.625–1.25 mg with norethisterone 5 mg/day)
- Combined oral contraceptive (COC) pills
- Progesterones (norethisterone 5–10 mg/day)
- Tibolone
- Bisphosphonates

GnRH antagonists

- GnRH antagonists are synthetic peptide molecules having a structure similar to GnRH agonists.
- GnRH antagonists commonly used include cetrorelix, ganirelix, abarelix, and degarelix.

Mechanism of action

These drugs bind to GnRH receptors in pituitary, block the release of LH and FSH, and thereby result in hypoestrogenism. GnRH antagonists block the secretion of pituitary gonadotropins without an initial flare-up effect (unlike GnRH agonists).

The advantages of GnRH antagonists over GnRH agonists are the following:

- GnRH antagonists produce a quick suppression of gonadotropin secretion by competitive antagonism.
- There is a lower risk of ovarian hyperstimulation syndrome in comparison to GnRH agonists.
- They cause more complete suppression of endogenous gonadotropin secretion.

Indications

- Ovarian stimulation protocols
- Endometriosis
- Uterine fibroids

Route of administration

Intramuscular (abarelix) or subcutaneous (cetrorelix, degarelix, and ganirelix) route

Contraindications

- Undiagnosed vaginal bleeding
- Hypersensitivity to the drug
- Pregnancy
- Hepatic/renal insufficiency

Side effects

- Headache, nausea, weight gain, and hot flushes
- Infertility treatment—ovarian hyperstimulation may present with abdominal pain
- Injection site reaction

Danazol

Danazol is an antigonadotropic drug that also has androgenic action.

Mechanism of action

By inhibiting the pituitary gonadotropins, danazol results in a hypoestrogenic state and causes endometrial atrophy.

Indications

- Endometriosis
- DUB
- Medical management of fibroid
- Precocious puberty

Route of administration

Oral

Dosage

- Danazol therapy is started usually on the first day of menses.
- The dose is 800 mg/day orally, given in two divided doses.
- Patients with less severe symptoms may be given 200–400 mg/day.
- Treatment is usually administered for 6 months in endometriosis, but can be extended to 9 months in severe disease.

Contraindications

- Pregnancy and lactation
- Undiagnosed abnormal uterine bleeding
- Porphyrias
- Impaired renal/hepatic/cardiac function

Side effects

- Adverse effects caused by danazol are primarily related to estrogen deficiency and androgenic effects
- Hypoestrogenic effects—flushing, sweating, atrophic vaginitis, and breast atrophy
- Androgenic effects—acne, hirsutism, deepening of voice, and weight gain

Progesterones

Progesterone is a natural hormone (C-21 steroid) produced by the corpus luteum of the ovary and placenta.

Progesterones that are commonly used are the following:

- Natural progesterones
- Synthetic progesterones (progestins)—medroxyprogesterone acetate (MPA), norethisterone, levonorgestrel, and gestodene

Indications

- DUB
- Medical management of fibroid
- Endometriosis
- Endometrial hyperplasia
- Luteal phase support
- Contraception—minipill (progesterone-only pill), combined estrogen + progesterone pills, depot medroxy progesterone acetate (DMPA) injectables, levonorgestrel intrauterine contraceptive device (LNG-IUD), and progesterone-containing implants
- Progesterone challenge test—in cases with secondary amenorrhea, MPA 10 mg/day given orally for 5 days (presence of withdrawal bleeding indicates anovulatory cycles)

Methotrexate

Methotrexate is a folic acid analogue used in the treatment of various malignancies and also for the treatment of several nonmalignant conditions in obstetrics and gynecology.

Mechanism of action

Methotrexate is a folic acid antagonist. It inhibits the enzyme dihydrofolate reductase, thereby blocks the conversion of dihydrofolic acid to tetrahydrofolic acid. Tetrahydrofolic acid is an essential coenzyme required for de novo purine and pyrimidine synthesis. Therefore, methotrexate inhibits the synthesis of DNA, RNA, and proteins.

Indications in gynecology

- Management of persistent gestational trophoblastic tumors
- Choriocarcinoma
- Medical management of unruptured tubal ectopic pregnancy
- Conservative management of placenta accreta and retained placenta
- Medical abortion

Route of administration

IV/IM route. It can also be administered as a direct injection into the ectopic site

Contraindications

- Pregnancy and lactation
- Alcoholism
- Liver diseases
- Hematological disorders
- Hypersensitivity to methotrexate

Side effects

Nausea, vomiting, oral ulceration, stomatitis, alopecia, anemia, and hepatitis

CONTRACEPTIVES

Definition of contraception: Contraception is the planned use of temporary or permanent methods to prevent pregnancy after sexual intercourse.

The agents or methods used for contraception are called contraceptives. Contraceptives prevent pregnancy by one or more of the following methods:

- Prevention of ovulation
- Prevention of fertilization
- Prevention of implantation

Classification of contraceptives

Various options available for contraception are mentioned in Table 31.6.

Efficacy of a contraceptive method Efficacy of a contraceptive method is calculated by Pearl index.

Pearl index is defined as the pregnancy failure rate per 100 women years (HWY) of use. It is calculated by the following formula:

Pregnancy failure rate per HWY (Pearl index) =

$$\frac{\text{No. of accidental pregnancies} \times 1200}{\text{No. of patients observed} \times \text{months of use}}$$

Table 31.6 Classification of contraceptives

Temporary methods			
Natural family planning methods • Calendar or rhythm method • Basal body temperature method • Cervical mucus method or Billings method • Coitus interruptus • Lactational amenorrhea	**Barrier methods** • Male condom • Female condom • Vaginal diaphragm • Cervical cap • Vaginal sponge • Spermicides	**Hormonal contraceptives** • **Oral hormonal contraceptives** – Combined oral contraceptive pills contain both estrogen and progesterone – Progesterone-only pills • **Nonoral hormonal contraceptives** – Injectables – Implants – Hormone-containing intrauterine devices (levonorgestrel intrauterine devices) – Contraceptive dermal patches – Contraceptive vaginal rings	**Intrauterine contraceptive devices** • Copper T devices • Levonorgestrel intrauterine device (LNG-IUD)
Permanent methods			
• Tubectomy • Vasectomy			

The higher the Pearl index, the greater is the chance of failure of contraception and risk of an unintended pregnancy.

CONTRACEPTIVE SPOTTERS

Barrier contraceptives

Male condom

- Male condom is a barrier method of contraception (Figure 31.18).
- It is one of the commonly used methods of contraception.
- A male condom is a thin sheath made of latex or polyurethane. It is closed at one end with a teat and open at the other end.
- The condom is put on an erect penis just before sexual intercourse.
- After sexual intercourse, the condom must be carefully taken off, so that the semen does not leak.
- Each condom is for single usage.

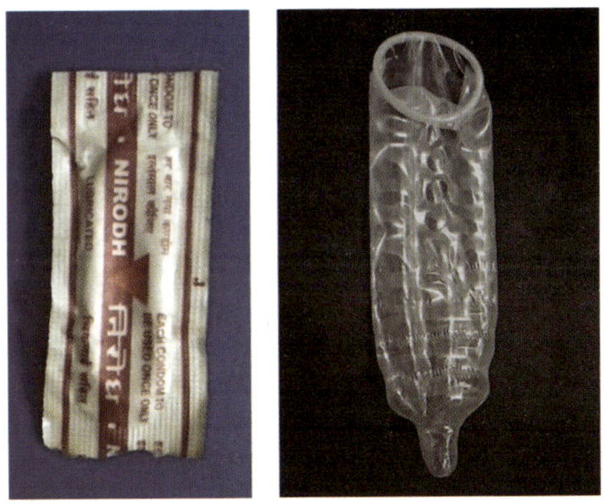

a. b.

Figure 31.18 Male condom. **a.** Foil containing condom. **b.** Male condom.

Advantages

- Not associated with any systemic side effects
- Not expensive
- Easily accessible (supplied free of cost by the Government of India)

Noncontraceptive benefits

- Condoms provide protection against sexually transmitted diseases (STDs), HIV, hepatitis B, and human papillomavirus (HPV) infection.
- Condom is used to cover transvaginal probe during ultrasonography.
- Condom balloon uterine tamponade for management of PPH.

Side effects

- Condoms can cause allergic reactions.
- May tear or leak during coitus.

Disadvantages

- Failure rate is high—14 per HWY of use.
- Concurrent use of spermicides reduces failure rate.

Salient points of other barrier methods of contraception

Female condom

- Female condom is made of transparent polyurethane sheath that is inserted into the vagina before sexual intercourse (Figure 31.19).
- It has two flexible rings, an inner ring and an outer ring. The inner ring is at the closed end, covers the cervix, and holds the condom in place.
- The outer ring at the open end is larger than the inner one. It stays outside the vagina and covers part of the perineum and labia during intercourse.
- In addition to contraception, it also has noncontraceptive benefits like those of male condom—prevention of transmission of STDs, HIV, and hepatitis B infection.
- However, because it is cumbersome to use, the female condom users are very less.
- Failure rate is higher than that of male condom.

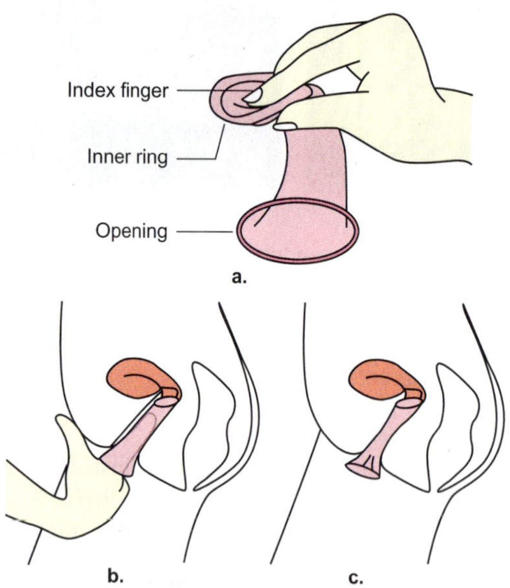

Figure 31.19 Female condom. **a.** Inner ring is compressed to facilitate insertion. **b.** Female condom is inserted into vagina. **c.** Female condom in situ.

Diaphragm

- A diaphragm is a shallow rubber dome with a flexible rim that covers the cervix on insertion (Figure 31.20).
- It is often used in combination with spermicidal jelly.
- It is available in various sizes.
- It can be inserted up to 6 hours before intercourse. It should remain in place for at least 6 hours after the intercourse. However, it must not be left inside the vagina for more than 24 hours.
- Method of insertion: The ring of the diaphragm is lubricated and then folded, so that the two sides of the ring are touching each other and then inserted into the vagina. Following insertion, the anterior rim of the diaphragm rests behind the pubic symphysis and the dome of the diaphragm covers the cervix.
- It can be reused. After usage, it is washed with soap and water, dried, and stored in a case.
- Side effects: It can cause irritation or allergic reaction.
- Failure rate is high.

Cervical cap

- A cervical cap is a soft, rubber cup with a rim that fits snugly over the cervix (Figure 31.20).

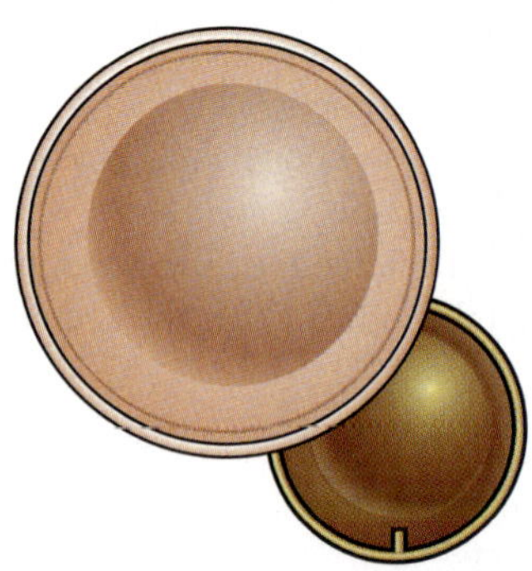

Figure 31.20 The female diaphragm and the cervical cap. The diaphragm is wider compared with the cervical cap.

- It is inserted at least 15 minutes prior to intercourse and should remain in place for a minimum of 6–8 hours.
- It can be reused—after usage, it must be washed with soap and water, dried, and then stored in a case
- Side effects include toxic shock syndrome and discomfort during coitus.
- Failure rate is high.

Contraceptive sponge

- The contraceptive sponge is marketed under the brand name "Today Sponge," which contains a spermicidal agent (nonoxynol-9).
- Spermicide in the sponge causes immobilization of the sperms and prevents sperms from entering the cervix.
- Method of insertion: Prior to insertion, the sponge must be soaked in water, which causes activation of the spermicidal agent. It is then inserted into the vagina so that it covers the cervix.
- It can be inserted up to 24 hours prior to sexual intercourse and should remain in place for about 6 hours following sexual intercourse. However, it should not be worn for more than 24 hours.

Spermicides

- The components of spermicides include the following:
  - Active spermicidal agents such as nonoxynol-9, octoxynol-9, and menfegol
  - Base (carrier) agents such as foams, jellies, creams, foaming tablet, aerosols, soluble films, or vaginal suppositories
- The spermicide is inserted deep into vagina to cover the cervix completely, just before sexual intercourse.
- A second dose of spermicide is required if more than 1 hour passes before sexual intercourse.
- The failure rate is high if spermicides are used alone and hence they are always used in conjunction with other barrier methods.
- Side effects: Spermicides may cause irritation in the vagina or penis, or allergic reaction.

Oral Hormonal Contraceptives

Combined oral contraceptive pills

Composition of COC pills

COC pills contain a combination of ethinylestradiol (EE) and progesterone.

- **Monophasic pills:** Contain the same amount of estrogen and progesterone
- **Phasic pills:** Contain different amounts of estrogen and progesterone over 2 weeks (biphasic pills) or 3 weeks (triphasic pills)

The pills can be classified as standard and low- dose pills based on the dosage of EE in the COC pills.

- Standard dose: 30–35 μg
- Low dose: 20–25 μg (less risk of side effects and thromboembolism)

Mechanism of action

- Inhibits ovulation
- Thickens cervical mucus to prevent sperm penetration
- Makes endometrium nonreceptive to implantation

Note

- *Most COC pills are available in a pack of 21 active pills and 7 placebo pills (Figure 31.21).*
- *Side effects of COC pills are mainly related to the amount of estrogen present in them.*
- *The newer progesterones have higher efficacy and lesser side effects.*
- *The newer COC pills contain low dose of estrogen with third-generation progesterones.*

Government of India has made two types of low-dose COC pills available under the brand name Mala N and Mala D. The pills contain 30 μg of EE plus 150 μg levonorgestrel. Mala D is a pack of 28 pills (21 COCs and 7 Ferrous sulfate 60 mg tablets) and is made available to the consumer through social marketing at a subsidized rate. Mala N is supplied free of cost through PHCs and Government hospitals. Some of the COCs available in market are given in Table 31.7.

Table 31.7 The various combined oral contraceptives available in market

Brand name	Estrogen component	Progesterone component
Mala N (Government of India)	Ethinylestradiol (30 µg)	Levonorgestrel (0.15 mg)
Mala D (Government of India)	Ethinylestradiol (30 µg)	Levonorgestrel (0.15 mg)
Novelon	Ethinylestradiol (30 µg)	Desogestrel (0.15 mg)
Femilon	Ethinylestradiol (20 µg)	Desogestrel (0.15 mg)
Loette	Ethinylestradiol (20 µg)	Desogestrel (0.15 mg)
Yasmin/Dronis 30	Ethinylestradiol (30 µg)	Drospirenone (3 mg)
Krimson 35	Ethinylestradiol (35 µg)	Cyproterone acetate (2 mg)

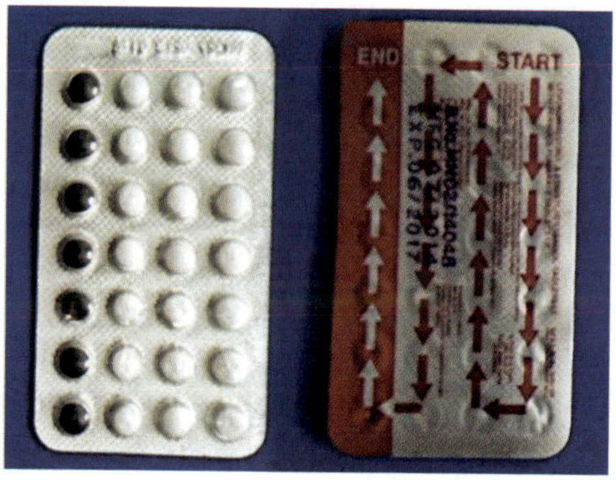

a. b.

Figure 31.21 Combined oral contraceptive (COC) pills. **a.** Foil containing COC pills. **b.** Backside of the foil showing arrow marks for taking the pills.

Advantages

Contraceptive benefits

- COCs are a very effective contraceptive method—failure rate is 0.1 per HWY.
- Usage is not related to sexual intercourse.
- Reversibility rate is prompt.
- COCs have additional noncontraceptive benefits as given below.

Noncontraceptive benefits

- **Treatment of menstrual abnormalities:**
  - Regulation of menstrual cycle
  - Reduction of menorrhagia
  - Reduction of dysmenorrhea
  - Reduction of premenstrual tension syndrome (PMS)
  - Improves anemia
- **Provides protection against the following:**
  - Pelvic inflammatory disease (thick cervical mucus)
  - Ectopic pregnancy
  - Endometriosis
  - Functional ovarian cysts
  - Benign breast diseases
  - Hirsutism and acne
  - Osteoporotic fractures
  - Rheumatoid arthritis
- **Cancer risk reduction**
  - Endometrial cancer
  - Epithelial ovarian cancer
  - Colorectal cancer

Disadvantages

- Do not provide any protection against STDs or HIV infection
- Require education and motivation for usage
- Require initial checkup and periodic supervision
- Inconvenience caused due to daily scheduling

Prescription

When to start a pill for the purpose of contraception?

- New users should start the pill packet on D1 of menstrual cycle, which provides immediate protection.
- The pill should be taken regularly at the same time each day.
- Pills are taken for 21 days followed by 7 days of pill-free interval or placebo. The woman should be cautioned not to exceed the 7-day pill-free interval between packs, and the next pack should be started after 7 days.

Missing the pill

- **One pill is missed:** If one pill is missed, the missed pill should be taken as soon as possible. The next pill is taken as usual.

- **Two pills are missed:**
  - If two pills are missed during the first 2 weeks, two pills should be taken daily for the next 2 days and the pack is completed as usual. A backup method is usually advised for 7 days, though not required.
  - If two pills are missed during the third week, a backup method of contraception must be used for the next 7 days. The next pack is started without a break.
- **More than two pills are missed anytime during the cycle:** A backup method of contraception must be used for 7 days and the next pack is started without a break.

Viva corner

Q1 Indications for backup method of contraception while using COCs

- When the pill-free interval of 7 days is exceeded
- When more than one pill is missed in a cycle
- When broad-spectrum antibiotics such as ampicillin, amoxicillin, and doxycycline are used that impair the absorption of ethinylestradiol
- When enzyme-inducing drugs such as barbiturates, rifampicin, ketoconazole, ritonavir, and nevirapine are used (high-dose preparations containing 50 μg or more of ethinylestradiol are used to counterbalance the increased liver metabolism)

Contraindications

- Valvular or ischemic heart disease
- Uncontrolled hypertension
- Diabetes mellitus with vascular complications
- H/o stroke
- H/o arterial or venous thrombosis
- Migraine with focal neurological symptoms
- Breast cancer (estrogen-dependent neoplasms)
- Liver disease—adenoma and carcinoma
- Smoking at >35 years
- Pregnancy
- Lactation
- Undiagnosed vaginal bleeding
- Major surgery or prolonged immobilization

Side effects

Minor side effects

- Irregular or breakthrough bleeding
- Breast tenderness
- Nausea
- Weight gain
- Mood changes

Major side effects

- Venous thromboembolism
- Myocardial infarction
- Stroke
- Gallbladder disease
- Increased risk of endocervical carcinoma with use of high-dose pills

Progestogen-only pills

Progestogen-only pills (POPs) have lower efficacy than COC pills (pregnancy rate of 2–3 per HWY of use).

Mechanism of action

- Thickens the cervical mucus, thereby reducing sperm viability and penetration
- Makes the endometrium unfavorable for implantation

Prescription

- POPs must be started within 5–7 days of menstruation.
- Unlike the COCs, these pills must be taken on a continuous basis without any break between the packs.
- Strict time schedule should be followed every day (within 3 hours vs. 12 hours for COCs).
- A backup method should be used in the following situations:
  - If there is a delay in taking the pill for more than 3 hours
  - During the first month when the woman starts taking minipills
  - At midcycle every month thereafter (the time when ovulation occurs)

Side effects

- Irregular bleeding, spotting, and breakthrough bleeding
- Depression, headache, and migraine

Part 3

Extra edge

Classification of progestins and their level of androgenic activity

See table below

Table Classification of progestins and their level of androgenic activity

Progestin	Androgenic activity
First generation • Norethindrone acetate • Ethynodiol diacetate • Norethynodrel	Middle
Second generation • Norgestrel • Levonorgestrel	Highest
Third generation • Desogestrel • Gestodene • Norgestimate	Lowest
Unclassified • Drospirenone • Cyproterone acetate	Has mineralocorticoid activity and antiandrogenic properties

Continuous or extended use of COCs

- For extended use of COCs, the woman should take the active pills from the pill pack and immediately start the next pack of active pills without any break. The pills should be continued for 60–80 days, and then a withdrawal bleed is allowed.
- Extended-use COCs are prescribed in women who prefer to bleed at an interval of 60–80 days (three to four times a year) or women with menorrhagia, to give time for correction of anemia or in systemic causes of bleeding such as chronic renal disease)
- Formulations with 84 active pills followed by 7 placebo pills are available under brand name "Seasonale." This results in a "seasonal" withdrawal bleed at an interval of 4 months. Any monophasic pill may be used for this purpose.

- Weight gain
- Ectopic pregnancy
- Breast tenderness
- Mood swings

Advantages

- Failure rate is 0.3 per HWY.
- Unlike the COCs, minipills are not associated with a risk of DVT or cardiac side effects.
- Minipills can be prescribed during lactation as they do not affect milk production.

Extra edge

Progesterone-only contraceptives

Contraceptives containing only progesterone are available in various forms:

- Progesterone-only pill (POP) or minipill (the POPs may contain 350 μg of norethindrone, 75 μg of norgestrel, 30 μg of levonorgestrel, or 75 μg of desogestrel)
- Subdermal implants (Norplant I, II, and Implanon)
- Progesterone-only injectables (POIs), for example, DMPA
- Intrauterine system (Mirena and Progestasert)
- Injectable contraceptives

Nonoral hormonal contraceptives

Hormonal injectables

- Hormones are delivered through deep intramuscular injections in the arms or buttocks.
- Hormonal injectables provide protection starting 1 week after the first injection.
- Two types of injectable contraceptives are available: progesterone-only formulations and combined formulations.
  - *Progestogen-only injectables:* These contain only progesterone, for example, DMPA and norethindrone enanthate (NET-EN). DMPA 150 mg IM is given every 3 months (Figure 31.22); NET-EN 200 mg IM is given at 2-month intervals.
  - *Combined contraceptive injectables:* These contain both estrogen and progesterone, for example, Mesigyna and Cyclofem.

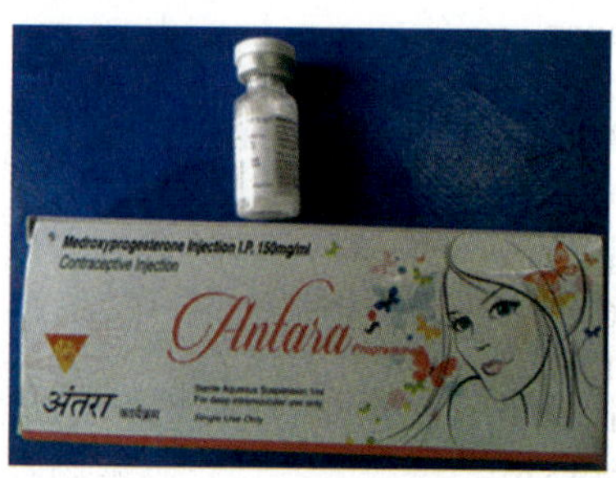

Figure 31.22 Medroxyprogesterone acetate injectable.

Mechanism of action

- Thickening of cervical mucus, thereby reducing sperm viability and penetration
- Make the endometrium unfavorable for implantation

Side effects

- Menstrual irregularities such as amenorrhea, intermenstrual spotting, and heavy or prolonged bleeding
- Weight gain, headache, and dizziness

Advantages

- Hormonal injectables are highly effective and reversible with failure rate of 0.1–0.4%.
- They overcome the inconvenience of daily dosing required with POPs or COCs.
- Progesterone injectables are suitable in women with contraindications for estrogen.
- They can be used during lactation starting at 6 weeks postpartum.
- Fertility is not impaired after discontinuation, although return of ovulation may be delayed.

Disadvantage

Hormonal injectables do not provide protection against HIV and STDs.

Subdermal implants

Contraceptive implant is a device inserted subdermally under the skin that causes sustained release of progesterone.

Mechanism of action

- Thickening of cervical mucus, making it difficult for sperm to pass through
- Inhibition of ovulation

Available subdermal implants

- Norplant I and Norplant II (Jadelle)
- Implanon

Norplant I (Figure 31.23a)

- This contains six silastic capsules made up of siloxane of size 34 mm × 2.4 mm, each containing 36 mg of levonorgestrel.
- The implants release 85 μg of levonorgestrel per day in the first 3 months, which then gradually decreases to 50 μg/day and finally to 30 mg/day.
- Its effect lasts for 5 years.

Norplant II

- This contains two rods of size 2.5 mm × 4.3 cm, each containing 75 mg of levonorgestrel.
- The hormone is released at 80 μg/day in the first month, and then gradually decreases to 50 μg/day and finally to 25–30 μg/day.
- Norplant II provides protection for 3–5 years.

Implanon (Figure 31.23b)

- Implanon is a single rod of size 4 cm × 2 mm, containing 68 mg of a progesterone named etonogestrel (3-keto derivative of desogestrel).
- It usually remains effective for a period of 3 years.
- It releases approximately 30 μg/day of the hormone.

Insertion of implants

- Implants are inserted on the first day of the menstrual cycle.
- Under local anesthesia, a needle-like applicator is used to insert the implant subdermally under the skin, on the medial aspect of upper arm.

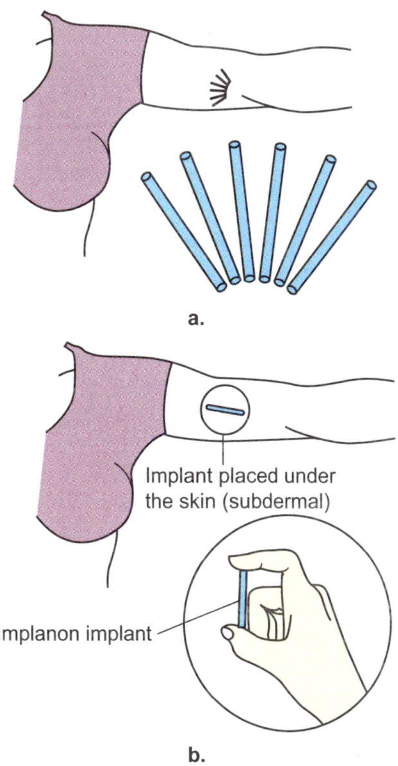

Figure 31.23 Subdermal implants. **a.** Norplant implant. **b.** Implanon implant.

- The capsules are nonbiodegradable and hence need removal at the end of use.
- Removal of an implant requires local anesthesia and a small incision.

Side effects

Side effects are similar to those of progesterone injectables described previously.

Advantages

- Implants are highly effective with a failure rate of 0.2–1.3 per HWY.
- They can be used by lactating mothers starting 6 weeks after childbirth.
- Return of fertility is almost immediate following removal of the implant.

Disadvantages

- Do not provide protection against STDs
- Trained practitioner required for insertion and removal
- Removal sometimes is painful and often more difficult than insertion
- Expensive

Transdermal contraceptive patch

- The patch is of 20 cm^2 that has an outer waterproof layer, an active medicated layer, and adhesive.
- The patch is most commonly applied on the upper arm, hip, thigh, buttock, or lower abdomen.
- Each patch contains a 1-week supply of norelgestromin (150 mg) and EE (20 mg). A sustained low dose of hormones is released daily, equivalent to the COC pills.

Mechanism of action

- The mechanism of action is the same as that of COC pills.

Method of usage

- The patch is initiated on the first day of a month or first Sunday of a month, or as a quick start.
- The patch is changed once a week for 3 weeks (21 total days), followed by 1 week that is patch free.
- It should always be changed/applied on the same day of the week.

Contraceptive vaginal ring

- The contraceptive vaginal ring is a latex-free flexible device measuring 54 mm in diameter and 4 mm in cross-section.
- The ring is composed of EE and etonogestrel.
- The ring is left in place for 3 weeks and then removed for a single ring-free week.
- The dose of hormones released each day is 15 mg of EE and 120 mg of etonogestrel.

Hormone-containing intrauterine contraceptive devices

Levonorgestrel intrauterine device (LNG IUD): Mirena (explained under the subsection "intrauterine contraceptive device" in this chapter

Intrauterine contraceptive devices

- IUCDs are flexible plastic devices made up of polyethylene inserted into the uterine cavity for the purpose of contraception.
- Each device has a nylon thread that protrudes out through the cervical canal into the vagina which can be felt by the patient.
- The efficacy of IUDs varies from 3 to 10 years (depending on the type of IUCD inserted).
- IUCD is commonly used in parous women for spacing of pregnancy.

Types of intrauterine contraceptive devices

- **Inert devices:** Lippes loop and Saf-T-Coil
- **Copper-containing devices:** Cu T 200, Cu 7 multiload Cu T 250, Cu T 380A, Cu T 220, and Nova T (Figure 31.24a and b)
- **LNG-IUS:** Mirena (Figure 31.24c and d)
  - Mirena: It contains 52 mg of levonorgestrel released at the rate of 20 µg/day.
  - Efficacy of Mirena is up to 5 years.

Mechanism of action

- IUCDs cause nonspecific inflammatory and biochemical changes in the endometrium Endometrial inflammatory response prevents transport of sperms.
- Copper is spermatotoxic and gametotoxic.
- Ionized copper prevents implantation by enzymatic interference.

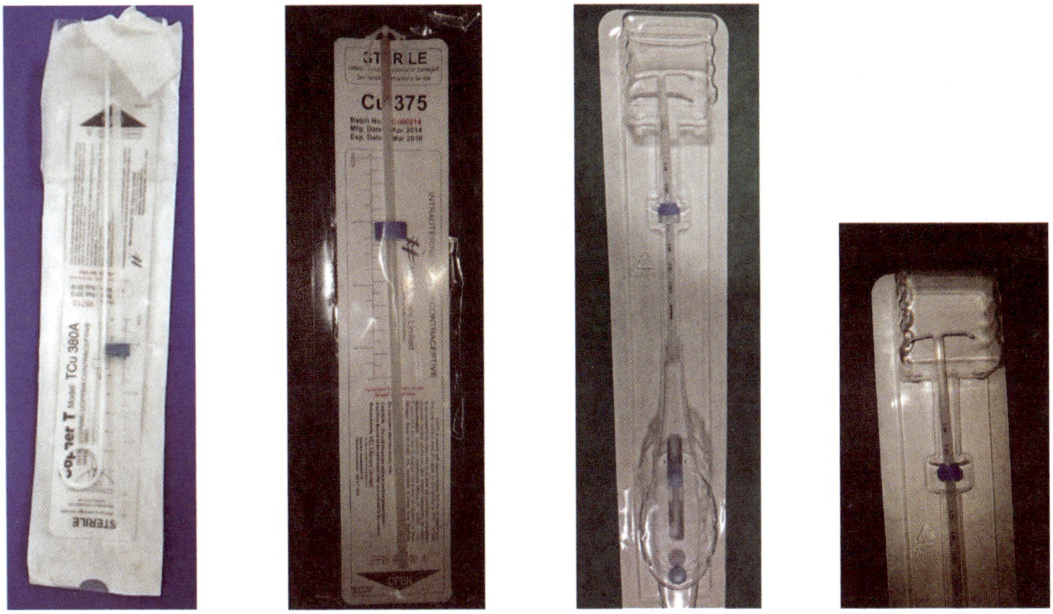

a. b. c. d.

Figure 31.24 Intrauterine contraceptive devices. **a.** Cu T-380A. **b.** Multiload Cu T. **c.** Mirena. **d.** Close-up view of Mirena.

- Lysosomal disintegration from macrophages releases prostaglandins, which are toxic to sperms.
- LNG-IUD (Mirena) induces uniform suppression of endometrium and makes the cervical mucus scanty.

Contraindications

- Suspected pregnancy
- Undiagnosed vaginal bleeding
- Pelvic inflammatory disease or STDs within 3 months

> **High-yield points**
>
> **Cu T 380A**
>
> - Cu T 380 A is supplied free of cost by the Government of India.
> - "380" refers to the total surface area of copper wire wound around the stem (314 mm^2) plus the copper sleeve on the horizontal arms (33 mm^2).
> - "A" refers to the Cu sleeve on the arms.
> - The frame contains barium sulfate, which makes it radiopaque.
> - It has to be replaced every 10 years.

- Severe anemia
- Past history of ectopic pregnancy
- Uncontrolled diabetes (increased risk of pelvic infections)
- Heart disease (increased risk of infections)
- Distorted uterine cavity like in fibroid and congenital uterine malformations (septate uterus/bicornuate uterus)

Complications

- **During insertion:** Difficulty in insertion, vasovagal attack, uterine cramps, and uterine perforation can occur.
- **Abnormal uterine bleeding:** Irregular bleeding, menorrhagia, etc., are common side effects in the first few months after insertion.
- **Dysmenorrhea:** May be present in the initial few cycles following insertion. LNG-IUD is associated with reduced menstrual pain.
- **Pelvic inflammatory disease (PID):** Risk is more in the first few weeks. Infections with *Chlamydia* and *Actinomyces* are common.
- **Spontaneous expulsion:** It is common in the initial few months of insertion (2–10% of users). It is more common following postabortal or puerperal insertion.

Part 3

Viva corner

Q1 What are the causes of missing IUCD?

- Threads coiled inside
- Threads torn and expelled
- IUCD expelled out unnoticed
- IUCD perforated the uterus and migrated into the peritoneal cavity
- IUCD pulled up due to uterine enlargement in pregnancy

Q2 What should be done in case of misplaced IUCD?

- Exclude pregnancy.
- If the IUCD threads are not visible through the external os:
  - An ultrasound can be performed to identify its location within the uterus or in the pelvis.
  - If the IUCD is not identified inside the uterine cavity in ultrasonography (USG), plain X-ray [both anteroposterior (AP) and lateral views] of the abdomen and pelvis are taken, after introducing a radiopaque probe into the uterine cavity to determine the location of the IUCD.
- If the IUCD is inside the cavity in USG, uterine sound can be introduced into the uterine cavity to probe for the IUCD and can be removed with artery forceps.
- If the IUCD is embedded in myometrium, it can be removed under hysteroscopic guidance.
- If the IUCD has perforated the uterus and is in the abdominal cavity, management depends on the type of IUCD inserted:
  - *Lippes loop:* As Lippes loop is made of an inert material, there is no harm if it is left in the peritoneal cavity. Adhesions and intestinal injury are unlikely. But for psychological reason, it is better to remove the Lippes loop by laparoscopy or by laparotomy.
  - *Copper containing device:* A copper-bearing device induces an intense local inflammatory reaction and adhesions. Thus, as soon as the diagnosis is made, it should be removed by laparoscopy or laparotomy.

Q3 What should be done in case of pregnancy following IUCD insertion?

- If threads are visible through the cervix, it is better to remove the device. This will minimize complications such as abortion, preterm labor, sepsis, and low birth weight.
- If threads are not visible, and if the patient wants to continue the pregnancy, it is better to leave the IUCD, after counseling the patient about the risks involved in continuing the pregnancy. The device is expected to be expelled spontaneously with the delivery of the placenta. There is no conclusive evidence of risk of fetal anomalies with IUCD.

- **Uterine perforation:** Uterine perforation is a rare, but serious complication of IUCD insertion. Perforation can occur at the time of insertion or later, following embedment of IUCD in the myometrium and subsequent migration into the abdominal cavity.
- **Ectopic pregnancy:** The failure rate of IUCD in situ is 0.1–2 per HWY. If pregnancy occurs with IUCD in situ, there is a risk of ectopic pregnancy. The risk of ectopic pregnancy is less with LNG-IUD.

Insertion of intrauterine contraceptive device

Prior to insertion

- Informed consent is obtained after explaining the potential benefits, side effects, and alternative methods of contraception.
- A speculum and bimanual examination is performed.

Insertion of IUCD (Figure 31.25)

- Under aseptic precautions, the posterior vaginal wall is retracted with Sims' speculum and the anterior lip of cervix is grasped with vulsellum
- Length of the uterine cavity is determined with a uterine sound.
- The IUCD is available in presterilized packs containing the IUCD, insertion tube, and plunger. It is mounted into the insertion tube and the flange on the insertion tube is adjusted according to the length of the uterine cavity as measured by uterine sound (Figure 31.25a and b).
- The Cu T–loaded insertion tube is then passed into the uterine cavity through the cervix till the flange touches the cervix (Figure 31.25c).

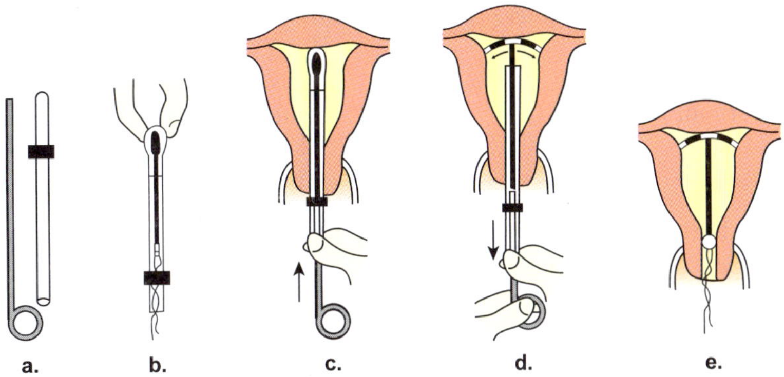

Figure 31.25 Images depicting an intrauterine contraceptive device insertion (withdrawal technique). **a.** Plunger and insertion tube. **b.** Cu-T mounted on the insertion tube and the flange on the insertion tube adjusted according to the length of the uterine cavity. **c.** The loaded Cu-T is inserted through the cervix into the uterine cavity along with the plunger. **d.** Insertion tube is withdrawn over the plunger (withdrawal technique of insertion). **e.** Cu-T in situ inside the uterine cavity.

- The insertion tube is withdrawn over the plunger that makes the IUCD to recoil open within the uterine cavity—withdrawal technique of insertion of IUCD (Figure 31.25d).
- The plunger and the insertion tube are then removed and the nylon threads are cut, up to the required length (Figure 31.25e).
- The speculum and the vulsellum are then removed.

Postinsertion

- The woman is instructed to feel for the threads every week.
- A follow-up visit is scheduled 6 weeks postinsertion to assess the following:
  - Any abnormal bleeding or side effects
  - Exclude presence of any infection
- The woman is instructed to contact her healthcare provider in case of the following:
  - IUCD threads cannot be felt.
  - She experiences persistent abdominal pain, excessive bleeding, fever, dyspareunia, abnormal vaginal discharge, etc.

Advantages

- Most cost-effective of all methods of contraception [failure rate is 0.1–2 (HWY)]
- Prolonged contraceptive protection after insertion (5–10 years)
- No systemic side effects—suitable for breastfeeding women

Viva corner

Q1 What is "no-touch" technique of insertion?

"No-touch" technique of insertion includes the following:

- The IUCD is loaded into the inserter without opening the sterile package.
- The loaded inserter is taken out of the package without touching the loaded end.
- While introducing the loaded IUCD through the cervix, care is taken not to touch the vaginal wall and speculum.

- Reversibility to fertility prompt after removal of the device

Disadvantages

- Requires motivation for insertion
- Has side effects such as menstrual abnormalities, PID, pelvic pain, and risk of ectopic pregnancy
- No protection against STDs and HIV infections

Various time periods for IUCD insertion

- **Postpartum IUCD (PPIUCD) insertion** is the most convenient time period and it can be inserted immediately following delivery or within 48 hours after delivery.

- **Interval IUCD** insertion is done after 6 weeks of delivery.
- **Postabortion IUCD (PAIUCD)** insertion is done after an abortion.

PPIUCD insertion

- The technique for PPIUCD insertion is different from the technique of inserting interval IUCD. This is due to the changes in the cervix and uterus after delivery.
- For the first 48 hours following delivery, the length of the uterus is almost 30 cm. This makes the fundal placement of the IUCD with a typical interval IUCD inserter difficult, as the length of the inserter is not sufficient. Instead, a long PPIUCD insertion forceps with a fenestrated end is used for insertion of the PPIUCD to ensure the placement of IUCD at the fundus.
- Following insertion, the IUCD strings should not be visible at the cervical os. If the strings are visible or appear to be very long, then it implies that the IUCD has not been adequately placed at the fundus and the chance of spontaneous expulsion is high. Removal and reinsertion is needed.
- After 6 weeks of childbirth, the technique of insertion is the same as for regular IUCD insertion. Interval insertion using no-touch technique and the traditional inserter tube assembly is recommended for IUCD insertions starting at 6 weeks after birth when the uterus has returned to its pre-pregnant state.

Types of PPIUCD insertion

- *Postplacental (Figure 31.26).*
  - Postplacental IUCD insertion is done immediately following delivery of the placenta, typically within 10 minutes. The insertion takes place immediately following active management of third stage labor and the delivery of the placenta.
  - Postplacental insertion can be done by using PPIUCD insertion forceps—the IUCD is held in a suitably long forceps without a lock. The instrument is inserted up to the fundus of the uterus and the IUCD is released.
  - Insertion of an IUCD postpartum should not interfere with the routine intrapartum and postpartum management protocols.
- *During cesarean (Figure 31.27).*
  - IUCD is introduced through the uterine incision during a cesaren section and placed at the uterine fundus following removal of placenta.
  - This is performed manually or using a regular sponge holding forceps, as it is not necessary to use a long instrument to reach the fundus. This is followed by uterine closure.
  - It is important not to attempt to pass the strings of the IUCD through the cervical os before closure of the uterus as this will displace the IUCD and leave it lower down in the uterine cavity.
  - There is no need to fix the IUCD with a ligature.
- *Postpartum within 48 hours:*
  - IUCD is inserted within 48 hours following delivery.
  - The IUCD insertion is done in a procedure or examination room in the postpartum ward using PPIUCD insertion forceps.
- *Extended postpartum/interval IUCD:*
  - Women who return for postpartum care at 6 weeks or later can receive the IUCD.
  - The technique of insertion and the related precautions are the same as for regular IUCD insertion.

Post-insertion care

- The client should be advised to report any undue vaginal bleeding or uterine cramps. Hemorrhage related to uterine atony should be managed as per standard procedure with uterine massage and uterotonics as necessary. *(Note: PPIUCD does not increase the risk of uterine atony.)*
- If severe uterine cramping occurs after PPIUCD insertion, a speculum exam should be performed to check for partial or complete expulsion.

Post-insertion instructions to the client

- There may be vaginal bleeding or spotting or cramping for initial few days/weeks after insertion. These symptoms are normally experienced in the postpartum period. Advise ibuprofen, paracetamol, or other pain reliever as needed.
- Spontaneous expulsion can happen in some cases, and is most likely to occur during the first

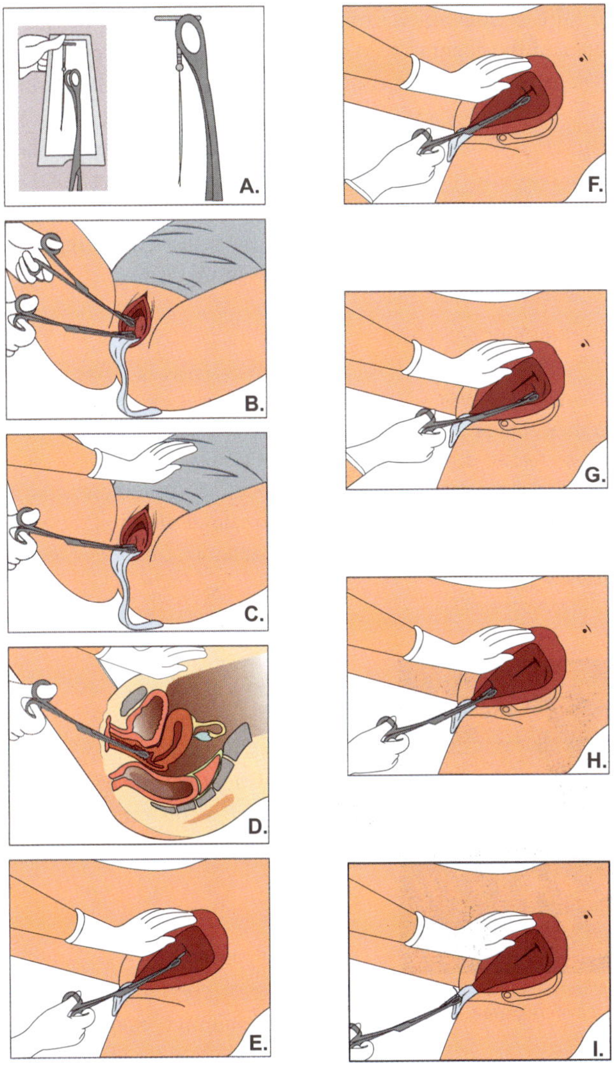

Figure 31.26 Steps of PPIUCD insertion (A-I).

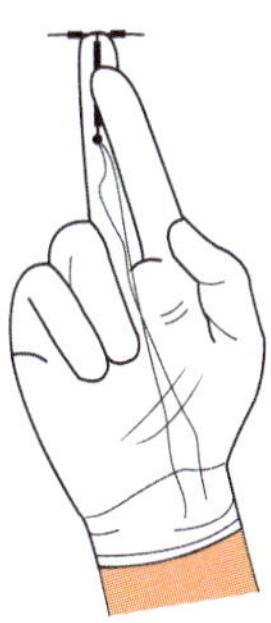

Figure 31.27 Copper T held with 2 fingers for cesarean insertion.

three months postpartum. If the IUCD has been expelled, she should be asked to visit the health facility for reinsertion or another contraceptive.

- At 6 weeks postpartum, the IUCD strings can be felt by some women. The client should be encouraged to visit the health facility if there is any concern about the strings.
- IUCD does not protect against STIs and HIV.
- She can resume intercourse when she feels ready.
- To return for removal of the IUCD at any time she wants a pregnancy and there is immediate return of fertility following removal.

Prior to discharge, the following warning signs should be informed, and the client should be encouraged to come to the health facility immediately for assessment:

- Heavy vaginal bleeding
- Severe lower abdominal discomfort
- Fever

Extra edge

New contraceptive programs launched by the Ministry of Health and Family Welfare

The Ministry of Health and Family Welfare, India, has launched two new contraceptives, an injectable contraceptive medroxyprogesterone acetate (MPA) under the "Antara" program and a contraceptive pill, "Chhaya," containing centchroman (Figure 31.28) to expand the contraceptive choices offered to couples. The contraceptives are available for free in medical colleges and district hospitals at present.

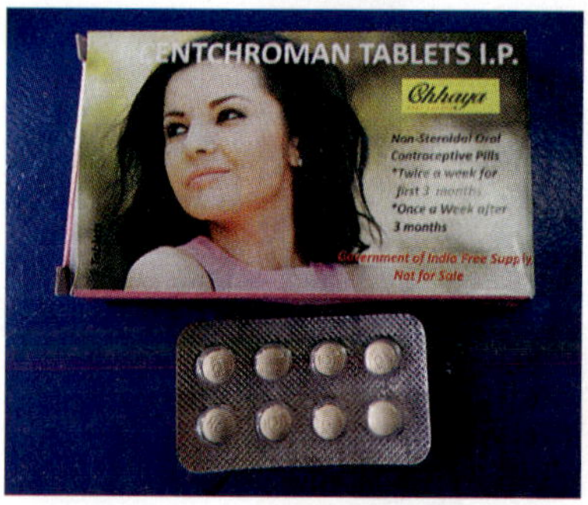

Figure 31.28 Chhaya—centchroman.

The contraceptives are safe and highly effective—"Antara" injectable is effective for 3 months and the "Chhaya" pill for 1 week.

Family Planning Logistics Management Information System (FP-LMIS): To improve the supply and distribution of contraceptives, the Ministry has launched a new software (FP-LIMS) to provide information on the demand and distribution of contraceptives to health facilities and Accredited social health activists (ASHAs).

Mission Parivar Vikas: It is a central family planning initiative launched by the Ministry, to focus on improving access to contraceptives by delivering assured services, ensuring commodity security, and providing access to high-quality family planning services.

- Unusual vaginal discharge
- Expulsion: Can either feel IUCD in the vagina or has seen it expelled from the vagina

A card is given to the client with the following details: Type of IUCD inserted; date of IUCD insertion; month and year when IUCD need to be removed or replaced; date of postpartum follow-up visit.

PERMANENT METHODS OF CONTRACEPTION

Permanent methods of sterilization include tubectomy in females and vasectomy in males. (Female sterilization procedure is described in Part 3, Chapter 37, *Common Obstetric Surgical Procedures.*)

EMERGENCY CONTRACEPTIVES

- EC, also known as "postcoital contraception" or "morning-after pill," is a method of contraception used after sexual intercourse, prior to the potential time of implantation.
- It prevents pregnancy but does not interrupt an already established pregnancy.

Indications

- Failure to use a contraceptive method (unprotected sexual intercourse)
- Condom breakage, slippage, or leakage
- Dislodgment of a diaphragm or cervical cap
- Two or more missed oral contraceptive pills
- Injection Depo-Provera delayed by more than 1 week
- Rape victims

Note

- *EC prevents pregnancy following unprotected sexual intercourse or potential contraceptive failure.*
- *It is a backup method for occasional use and should not be used as a regular method of contraception.*

The various emergency contraceptives available are mentioned in Table 31.8 and described in the subsequent text.

Table 31.8 Various regimens used for emergency contraception

Drug	Dosage	Time period within which the drug has to be taken
Levonorgestrel	0.75 mg given twice, 12 hours apart, or given as a single dose of 1.5 mg	Up to 72 hours following unprotected intercourse
Yuzpe regimen	100 µg of ethinylestradiol + 500 µg levonorgestrel given twice, 12 hours apart	Up to 72 hours following unprotected intercourse
Mifepristone	10 mg single oral dose	Up to 72 hours following unprotected intercourse
Ulipristal	Single oral dosage of 30 mg	Up to 120 hours following unprotected intercourse
Copper intrauterine contraceptive device		Up to 5 days following unprotected sexual intercourse

Part 3

Hormonal methods

- **Levonorgestrel**
  - Two doses of levonorgestrel 750 µg are taken orally 12 hours apart or a single oral dose of levonorgestrel 1500 µg is taken.
  - Single dose of levonorgestrel is as effective as the two-dose levonorgestrel regimen.
  - The regimen should be given within 72 hours of unprotected sexual intercourse.
  - The levonorgestrel EC regimen is more effective and causes fewer side effects than the Yuzpe regimen (see the subsequent text).
- **Combination of EE and levonorgestrel (Yuzpe method)**
  - Two doses of 100 µg EE plus 500 µg levonorgestrel taken orally 12 hours apart.
  - The regimen should be given within 72 hours of unprotected sexual intercourse.

Side effects

- Nausea, vomiting, dizziness, and fatigue are the common side effects.
- Other side effects include headache, bloating, abdominal cramps, and spotting or bleeding P/V.

Postcoital insertion of a copper-containing IUCD

- Highly effective method, which can be used up to 5 days following unprotected intercourse
- Provides continuing contraception after the initial event

Side effects

Pelvic pain, abnormal bleeding, pelvic infection, perforation, and expulsion

Antiprogestins

- Ulipristal acetate (a selective progesterone receptor modulator) and mifepristone are antiprogestins and are highly effective for use as EC.
- They are more effective than progestins as they delay ovulation as well as inhibit implantation.

Disadvantages of ECs

- ECs do not provide long-term or continuing contraception except IUCDs.
- They do not protect against STDs.

32 Maternal Pelvis and Fetal Skull

Introduction

This chapter deals with the description of maternal bony pelvis and the fetal skull, which is one of the viva-voce stations in obstetrics and gynecology.

Importance of study of the maternal bony pelvis

- To understand the mechanism of labor
- To assess adequacy of pelvis for vaginal delivery
- To appropriately manage normal labor and abnormal labor

Articulated pelvis is composed of four bones (Figure 32.1):

- Two innominate or hip bones (each formed by fusion of ilium, ischium, and pubis)
- Sacrum
- Coccyx

The four bones are united by four joints:

- Two sacroiliac joints (between sacrum and ilium)
- Symphysis pubis (between two pubic bones)
- Sacrococcygeal joint (between sacrum and coccyx)

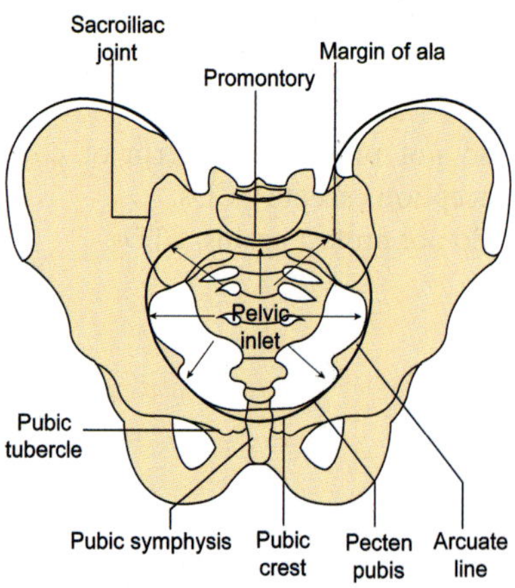

Figure 32.1 Female pelvis—bones and joints of the bony pelvis and the pelvic brim.

Anatomically, the pelvis is divided by the pelvic brim into true and false pelvis:

- **False pelvis:** The part that lies above the pelvic brim
- **True pelvis:** The part that lies below the brim

Pelvic brim (pelvic inlet) The important landmarks on the brim of the pelvis from anterior to posterior are as follows:

- Upper border of the symphysis pubis
- Pubic crest
- Pubic tubercle
- Pectineal line
- Iliopectineal eminence
- Iliopectineal line
- Sacroiliac joint
- Ala of the sacrum
- Sacral promontory
  - To be continued with similar borders on the opposite side

True pelvis is divided into: (a) inlet, (b) cavity, and (c) outlet.

PELVIC INLET

Pelvic inlet is formed by the borders of the pelvic brim and is almost round in shape. It is narrowest in anteroposterior (AP) diameter and widest in transverse diameter.

Angle of inclination

The plane of the pelvic inlet (superior strait) is not horizontal, but is tilted forwards, making an angle of 55° with the horizontal, termed angle of inclination (Figure 32.2).

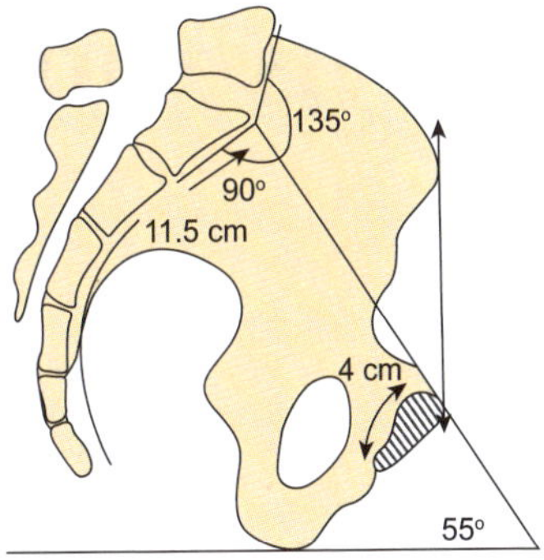

Figure 32.2 Angle of inclination.

Significance of angle of inclination

Increase in the angle of inclination (high inclination):

- May delay engagement and descent of the fetal head
- Favors occipitoposterior position

Reduction in the angle of inclination (low inclination) does not have obstetric significance.

Axis of the pelvic inlet

It is a line drawn perpendicular to the plane of inlet in the midline and is directed downwards and backwards.

Diameters of pelvic inlet

Anteroposterior diameters (Figure 32.3)

- **True conjugate or anatomical conjugate (11 cm):** It is measured from the midpoint of sacral promontory to the upper border of pubic symphysis.
- **Obstetric conjugate (10.5 cm):** It is measured from the midpoint of sacral promontory to the most prominent point on the back of pubic symphysis. This is the shortest AP diameter of the pelvic inlet.
- **Diagonal conjugate (12 cm):** It is measured from the midpoint of sacral promontory to the lower border of pubic symphysis.

Note
- *Only diagonal conjugate can be assessed clinically.*
- *Obstetric conjugate can be calculated by subtracting 1.5 cm from the diagonal conjugate.*
- *True conjugate can be calculated by subtracting 1 cm from the diagonal conjugate.*

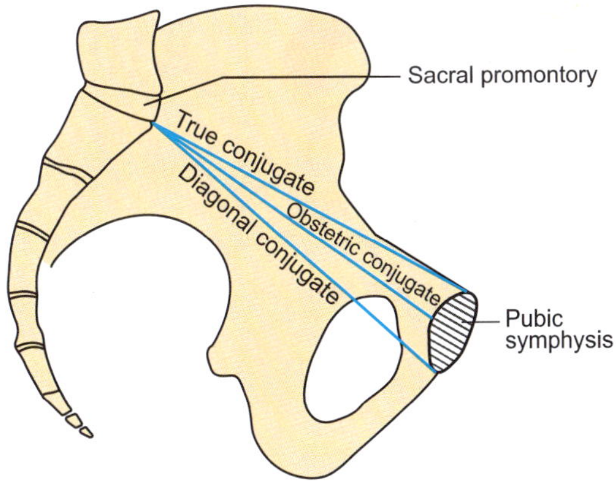

Figure 32.3 Anteroposterior diameters of the plane of pelvic inlet. The three anteroposterior diameters extend from sacral promontory to three different points on the pubis.

Measurement of the diagonal conjugate (Figure 32.4)

- The patient is put in dorsal position with thighs flexed.
- Under aseptic precautions, two fingers are introduced into vagina and the sacral curvature is felt.
- The elbow and the wrist are depressed and the fingers are directed upwards, in order to reach the sacral promontory. The point at which the bone recedes from the finger is the sacral promontory. Normally, it is difficult to feel the sacral promontory.
- A mark is placed over the gloved index finger at the site where it impinges under the pubic symphysis, by the index finger of the other hand.
- After removing the fingers from the vagina, the distance between the marking and the tip of the middle finger is measured to obtain the diagonal conjugate.

Note *It is not always possible to measure the diagonal conjugate, as the fingers cannot be reached up to the sacral promontory. Hence, clinically, if the middle finger fails to reach the sacral promontory, the diagonal conjugate can be considered as adequate.*

Transverse diameter of pelvic inlet (13 cm)

It is the distance between the two farthest points on the iliopectineal line of both sides.

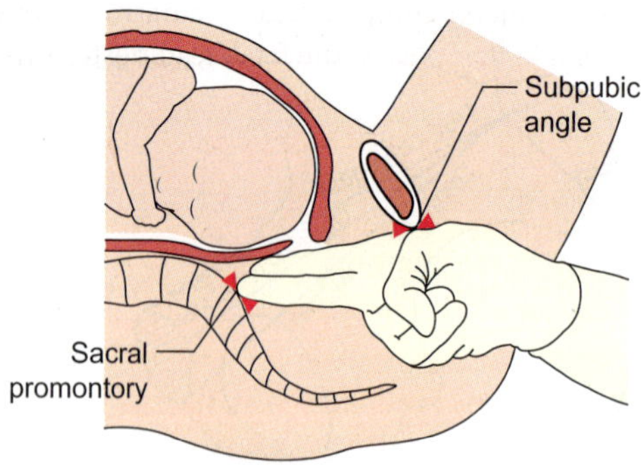

Figure 32.4 Measurement of diagonal conjugate. The diagonal conjugate is the distance between the tip of the middle finger that touches the sacral promontory and the point of contact with the undersurface of pubic symphysis, on the radial border of hand.

Oblique diameters of pelvic inlet (12 cm)

- The right oblique diameter extends from the right sacroiliac joint to the opposite iliopubic eminence.
- The left oblique diameter extends from the left sacroiliac joint to the opposite iliopubic eminence.

PELVIC CAVITY

The pelvic cavity is almost round in shape and is bounded by the following (Figure 32.5):

- **Pelvic brim:** Above
- **Plane of least pelvic dimension:** Below
- **Pubic symphysis:** Anteriorly
- **Sacrum:** Posteriorly

Plane of cavity or plane of greatest pelvic dimension (PGD): This plane passes from the midpoint on the posterior surface of pubic symphysis to the junction between second and third sacral vertebra. It is the roomiest plane of pelvis, hence known as the PGD. It measures 12 cm in all directions and has no obstetric significance.

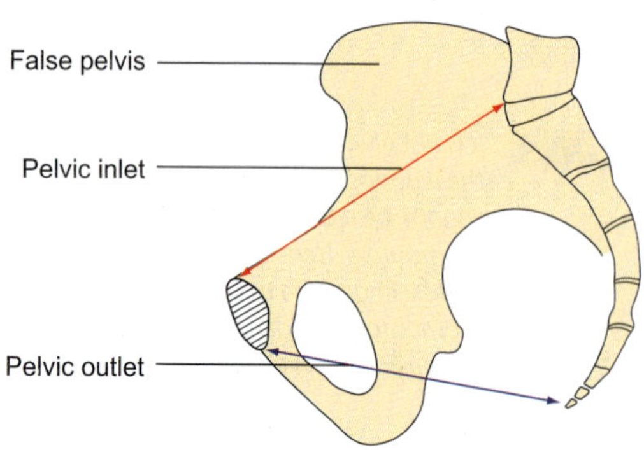

Figure 32.5 Pelvic cavity.

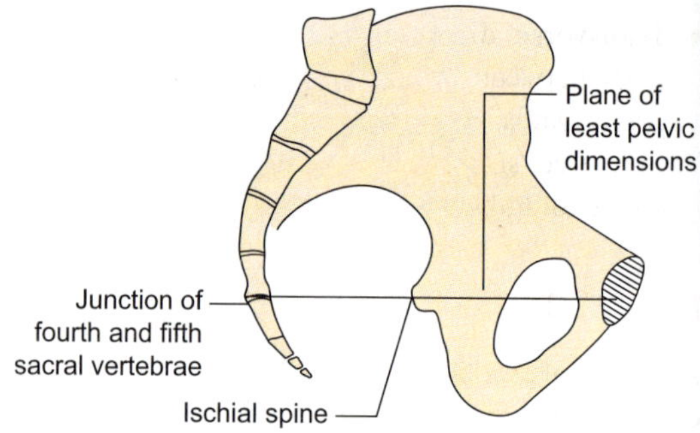

Figure 32.6 Plane of least pelvic dimension.

Plane of least pelvic dimension: This passes from the lower border of pubic symphysis through the tip of ischial spines laterally to the tip of fifth sacral vertebra posteriorly (Figure 32.6).

High-yield points

Significance of plane of least pelvic dimension

- It is the narrowest plane in the pelvis.
- This plane corresponds to the origin of levator ani muscle, also known as the pelvic floor.
- Internal rotation of fetal head takes place in this plane.
- It marks the beginning of the forward curve of the pelvic axis.
- It is a landmark used for pudendal nerve block analgesia. Pudendal nerve hooks around the ischial spine and enters the perineal pouch.
- The bispinous diameter (10.5 cm), which is the distance between the tips of two ischial spines, is in this plane.
- Station of the presenting part is expressed as "–5 to 0 to +5," in relation to this plane.

Diameters of pelvic cavity

- **AP diameter (12 cm):** It is measured from the midpoint on the posterior surface of pubis symphysis to the junction of second and third sacral vertebrae.

- **Transverse diameter (12 cm):** It is the distance between two farthest points on the lateral pelvic walls. The diameter cannot be exactly measured since there are no bony landmarks and is roughly estimated as 12 cm.

PELVIC OUTLET

Anatomical outlet and obstetric outlet are described next.

Anatomical outlet (Figure 32.7)

It is formed by two triangles in different planes with common base formed by a line drawn between the two ischial tuberosities. It is bounded by symphysis pubis and pubic arch anteriorly, ischial tuberosities laterally, sacrotuberous ligaments, sacrospinous ligaments, and the tip of coccyx posteriorly.

- **Plane of anatomical outlet:** It passes along the boundaries of the anatomical outlet.

Diameters of the anatomical outlet

- **Anatomical AP diameter (11 cm):** It extends from the lower border of pubic symphysis to the tip of coccyx.
- **Transverse or the intertuberous diameter of the anatomical outlet (11 cm):** It extends between the inner aspects of ischial tuberosities. If the pelvis is adequate, the intertuberous diameter allows four knuckles of a closed fist.
- **Posterior sagittal diameter (7.5 cm):** It is the part of the AP diameter that lies posterior to the line joining the ischial tuberosities. This diameter compensates for a narrow subpubic angle that pushes the fetal head posteriorly.

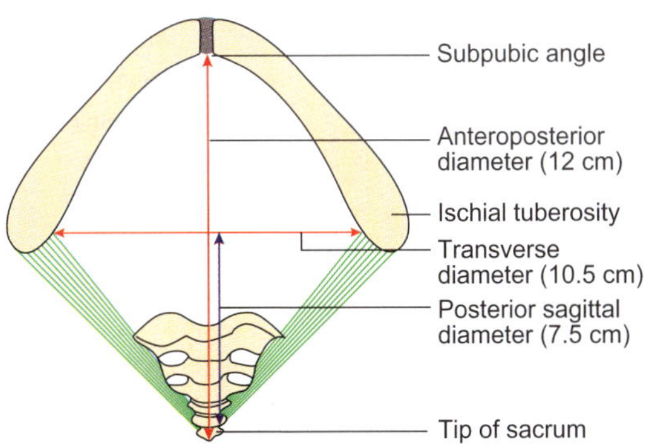

Figure 32.7 Anatomical outlet. Anteroposterior diameter, transverse or the intertuberous diameter, and the posterior sagittal diameters are marked.

Obstetric outlet (Figure 32.8)

It is the segment of pelvis between the plane of least pelvic dimension above and the anatomical outlet below. Obstetric outlet is bounded by the following:

- Anteriorly by the lower border of pubic symphysis
- Posteriorly by the coccyx
- Laterally by the ischial spines
- Superiorly by the plane of least pelvic dimensions
- Inferiorly by the anatomical outlet

Diameters of the obstetric outlet

- **Obstetric AP diameter (13 cm):** It extends from the lower border of pubic symphysis to the tip of coccyx that has moved backwards during the second stage of labor.
- **Transverse diameter of the obstetric outlet or the interspinous diameter (10.5 cm):** It extends between the tips of ischial spines.

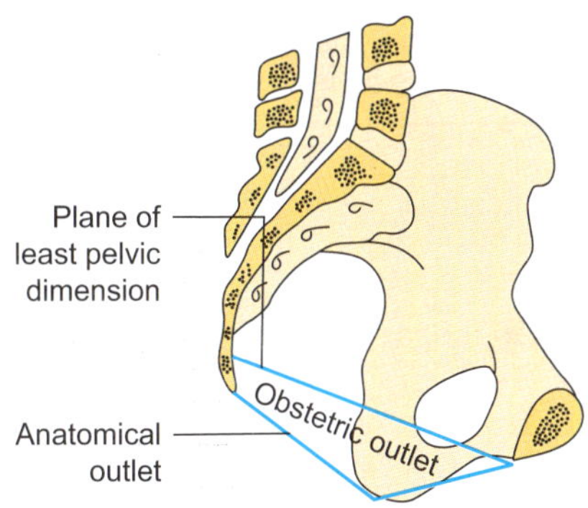

Figure 32.8 Obstetric outlet.

Composite measurements of the diameters of the inlet, cavity, and outlet in centimeters are given in Table 32.1.

Table 32.1 Composite measurements of the diameters of the inlet, cavity, and outlet

Diameter	Pelvic brim (cm)	Pelvic cavity (cm)	Pelvic outlet (cm)
Anteroposterior	11	12	13
Oblique	12	12	—
Transverse	13	12	11

PELVIC AXIS (FIGURE 32.9)

Anatomical axis (curve of Carus)

- This is an imaginary line passing through the central points of the planes of inlet, cavity, and outlet of pelvis.
- This axis is C-shaped with concavity directed forwards.

Obstetric axis

- It is an imaginary line that represents the direction in which the fetal head passes during the labor.
- It is J-shaped and passes downwards and backwards along the axis of the inlet till the ischial spines, and then it passes downwards and forwards along the axis of pelvic outlet.

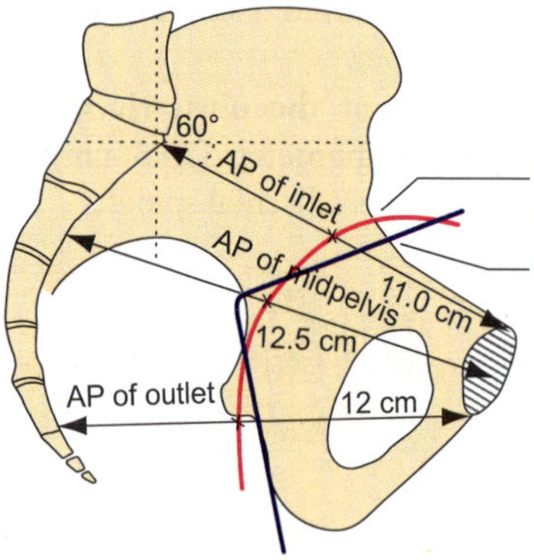

Figure 32.9 The anatomical and obstetric axes of the pelvis.

MIDPELVIS

This is the part of pelvis that is bounded by the following:

- Above by the plane of greatest pelvic dimension
- Below by the midpelvic plane (midpelvic plane extends from the lower margin of pubic symphysis through the ischial spines to the junction of S4 and S5 or the tip of S5, depending on the anatomy of the sacrum)

If the midpelvic plane meets the tip of the S5 sacral vertebra, then it becomes the same as the plane of least pelvic dimension; otherwise, it forms a wedge posteriorly (Figure 32.10).

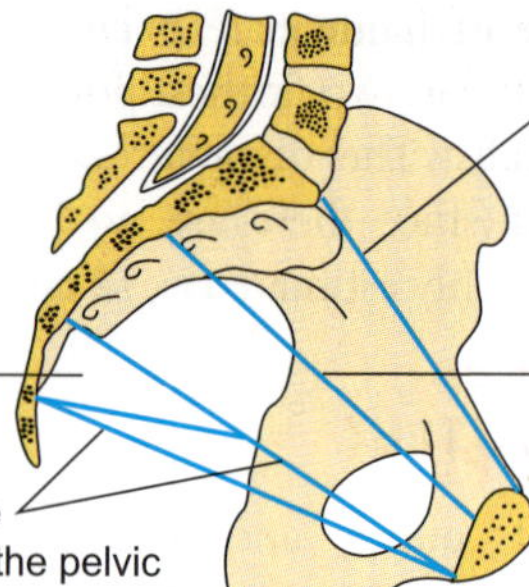

Figure 32.10 Midpelvic plane.

Diameters of midpelvis

- **AP diameter (11.5 cm):** It extends from the lower border of the pubic symphysis to the junction of S4 and S5 or the tip of S5, depending on the anatomy of sacrum.
- **Interspinous diameter or the transverse diameter (10.5 cm):** It is the distance between two ischial spines.

SUBPUBIC ANGLE

It is the angle between the two pubic rami and measures 85° ± 5°.

Waste space of Morris

Normally, a round disk of 9.5 cm (diameter of a well-flexed head) can pass through the pubic arch, at a distance of 1 cm from the inferior border of the symphysis pubis. This distance is known as the "waste space of Morris" (Figure 32.11).

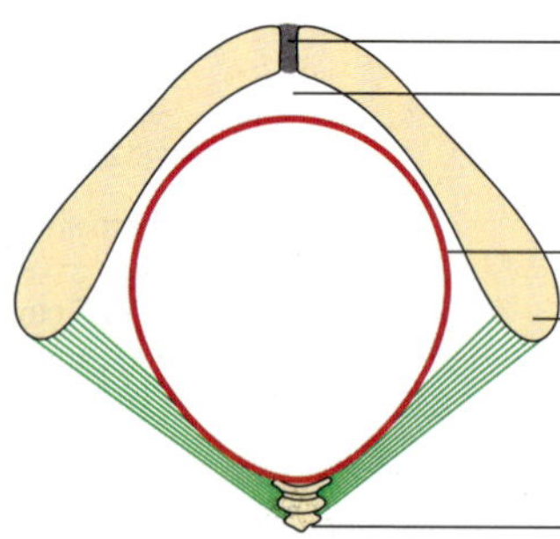

Figure 32.11 Waste space of Morris. This is the space between the fetal head and the subpubic angle.

In case of inadequate pelvis with a narrow pubic arch, the waste space of Morris increases and the fetal head will be pushed backwards, thereby increasing the risk of perineal injuries.

PARAMETERS ASSESSED DURING CLINICAL PELVIC ASSESSMENT

Refer Section 1, Chapter 16, for detailed description of pelvic assessment.

Assessment of pelvic inlet

Sacral promontory is palpated.

Assessment of midpelvis

The following are palpated:
- Curvature of sacrum
- Sacrospinous ligaments
- Ischial spines
- Pelvic sidewalls

Assessment of the pelvic outlet

The following are determined:
- Subpubic angle
- Intertuberous diameter
- Mobility of coccyx (refer to Part 1, Chapter 16, *Primigravida with Mobile Head at Term* for details of pelvic assessment)

TYPES OF FEMALE PELVIS (CALDWELL–MOLOY CLASSIFICATION)

The female pelvis is divided into four parent types based on the various characteristics of inlet, cavity, and outlet (Figure 32.12; Table 32.2):
- Gynecoid (50%)
- Anthropoid (25%)
- Android (20%)
- Platypelloid (5%)

However, in majority of cases, mixed features are present. The gynecoid type of pelvis is the most common, with its diameters being most favorable for vaginal delivery.

Part 3

High-yield points

Clinical significance of anatomy of pelvis

- The transverse diameter is more at the pelvic inlet; hence, the fetal head often engages in the transverse diameter.
- The anteroposterior diameter is more at the outlet; hence, the fetal head has to undergo internal rotation through 90° to achieve delivery.
- The interspinous diameter is the smallest; hence, malrotation, nonrotation, and arrest of descent occur at this level.
- The direction of descent of the fetal head is along the pelvis axis. This axis should be followed while conducting instrumental deliveries.
- Relaxation of the pelvic joints increases the pelvic diameters and helps in descent of the fetal head and delivery.

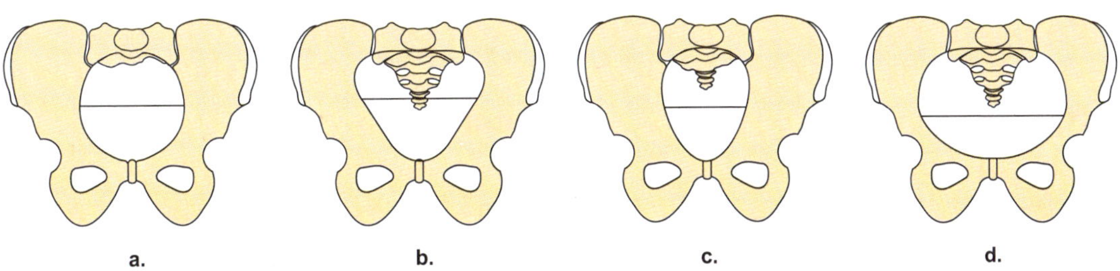

Figure 32.12 Types of pelvis. **a.** Gynecoid. **b.** Android. **c.** Anthropoid. **d.** Platypelloid.

Table 32.2 Types of female pelvis

Pelvis type	Inlet	Cavity	Outlet	Obstetric significance
Gynecoid	Round	• Sidewalls: Straight • Ischial spines: Not prominent	• Subpubic angle—wide (>90°) • TDO 11 cm	• Occipitoanterior position is common • No difficulty in engagement, anterior rotation, and delivery of baby
Anthropoid	Anteroposteriorly oval	• Sidewalls: Straight • Ischial spines: Not prominent	• Subpubic angle—slightly narrow • TDO 11 cm	• Occipitoposterior position is common • No difficulty in engagement except that flexion is delayed • Nonrotation is common • Increased incidence of face-to-pubis delivery
Android	Triangular	• Sidewalls: Convergent • Ischial spines: Prominent	• Subpubic angle—narrow • TDO <11 cm	• Occipitoposterior position is common • Engagement is delayed and difficult • Difficult anterior rotation or nonrotation—deep transverse arrest is common • Difficult delivery with increased chance of perineal injuries • Prolonged labor and obstructed labor are common
Platypelloid	Transversely oval	• Sidewalls: Divergent • Ischial spines: Not prominent	• Very wide (>90°) • TDO 11 cm	• Asynclitism is common • Anterior rotation usually occurs late in labor

TDO, transverse diameter of outlet.

Gynecoid pelvis is an ideal type of pelvis and is characterized by the following features:

- Inlet is round.
- Sacral promontory is not prominent; sacrum is concave and well curved.
- Forepelvis is wide and rounded.
- Sacrosciatic notch is wide and admits two fingers.
- Pelvic sidewalls are straight and parallel.
- Ischial spines are not prominent.
- Subpubic angle is wide and >90°.
- Inter tuberous diameter is adequate and admits four knuckles.

FETAL SKULL

The various landmarks and diameters of fetal skull should be known for the following reasons:

- The sutures and fontanels are used for identification of presentation and position of the fetus.
- The engaging diameter of the fetal head in various degrees of flexion of the fetal head is an important factor determining the progress of labor and vaginal delivery.

Fetal skull is made up of pliable, compressible, flat bones that form the vault, anchored to rigid incompressible bones at the base of the skull (Figure 32.13).

The bones that form the vault of the skull are as follows:

- Two frontal bones
- Two parietal bones
- Two temporal bones
- One occipital bone

Sutures

The flat bones of the vault are not united rigidly, but are separated by membranous spaces termed sutures. The fetal skull has four main sutures:

- **Sagittal suture:** This suture lies longitudinally between the two parietal bones.

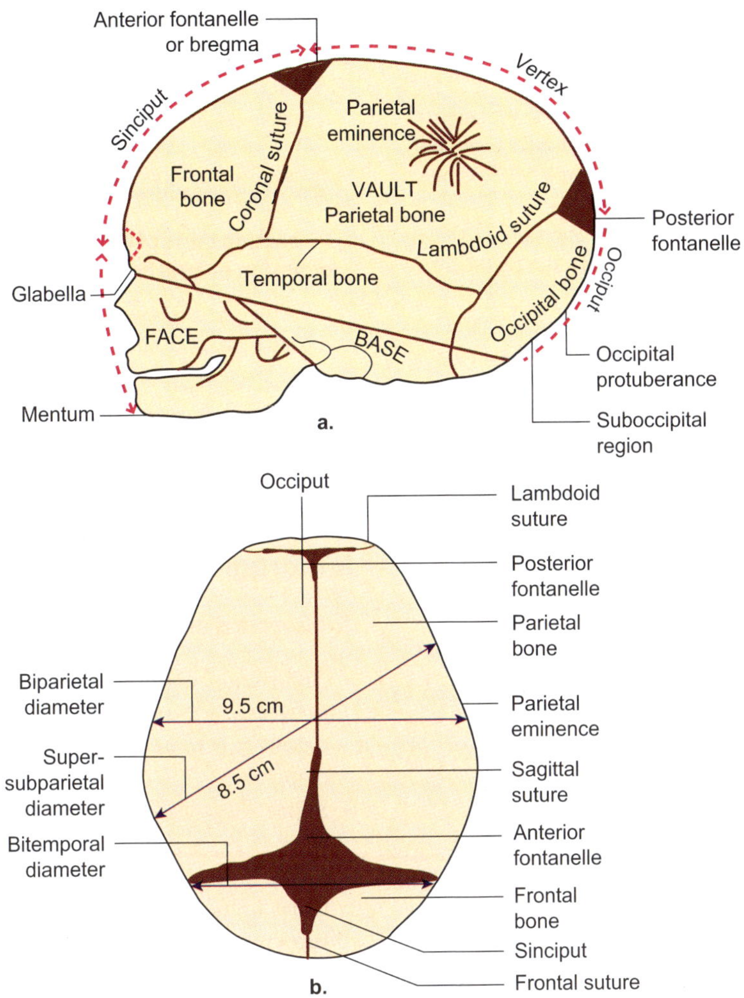

Figure 32.13 Fetal skull. **a.** Fetal skull showing various landmarks of obstetric significance. **b.** Fetal skull showing important sutures, fontanelles, and diameters of obstetric significance.

- **Coronal suture:** This suture lies transversely between the parietal and frontal bones.
- **Lambdoid suture:** This suture lies transversely separating the occipital bone from the two parietal bones.

> **High-yield points**
>
> **Obstetric significance of sagittal suture**
>
> - Allows gliding movement of the skull bones over one another, thereby permitting molding of fetal head
> - Palpating the sagittal suture gives an idea about the degree of asynclitism of fetal head, degree of internal rotation and molding of fetal head

- **Frontal suture:** This suture is present between the two halves of the frontal bone in infants and children, and usually disappears by the age of 6 years.

Fontanel

Where several sutures meet, an irregular space is formed, which is enclosed by membranes and is termed fontanel.

- The anterior fontanel (bregma) is a diamond-shaped quadrangular space situated at the intersection of the sagittal and coronal sutures.
- The posterior fontanel (lambda) is a small triangular space at the intersection of the sagittal and lambdoid sutures.

High-yield points

Obstetric significance of fontanels

- Palpation of fontanels indicates the degree of flexion of fetal head. In a well-flexed head, only posterior fontanel is felt, while in a deflexed head, anterior fontanel is also felt easily.
- It facilitates molding of fetal head—allows sliding of bones under each other, thus reducing the diameter of the fetal skull.
- The membranous nature of anterior fontanel helps in accommodating the growing brain during neonatal period.
- Floor of the anterior fontanel reflects the intracranial status after birth. Depressed anterior fontanel is seen in dehydration, and bulging anterior fontanel is seen in hydrocephalus or conditions with raised intracranial tension.

Areas of skull of obstetrical importance

- **Vertex:** It is a quadrangular area bounded by the following (Figure 32.14):
  - Anteriorly by the bregma
  - Posteriorly by the lambda
  - Laterally by parietal eminences
- **Brow:** This is an area of forehead extending from the root of nose and supraorbital ridges to the bregma and coronal sutures (Figure 32.13a).
- **Face:** This is an area bound above by the root of the nose along with the supraorbital ridges and below by the junction of the chin with the neck (Figure 32.13a).
- **Sinciput:** This is an area lying in front of the anterior fontanel and corresponds to the forehead.
- **Occiput:** Area limited to the occipital bone.
- **Mentum:** It corresponds to the chin of fetus.
- **Parietal eminences:** These are the prominent eminences on each of the parietal bones.

High-yield points

Presenting parts of fetal skull and the degree of flexion of fetal head

- **Vertex:** When vertex is the presenting part, fetal head is in complete flexion.
- **Face:** When face is the presenting part, fetal head is in complete extension.
- **Brow:** When brow is the presenting part, fetal head is in incomplete extension.

Important diameters of fetal skull

Transverse diameters

- **Biparietal diameter (9.5 cm):** It extends between the two parietal eminences. This diameter is most often the engaging transverse diameter.
- **Super-subparietal diameter (8.5 cm):** It extends from a point below one parietal eminence to a point above the other parietal eminence of the opposite side.
- **Bitemporal diameter (8 cm):** It is the distance between the anteroinferior ends of the coronal sutures.
- **Bimastoid diameter (7.5 cm):** It is the distance between the tips of the mastoid process. This diameter is nearly incompressible.

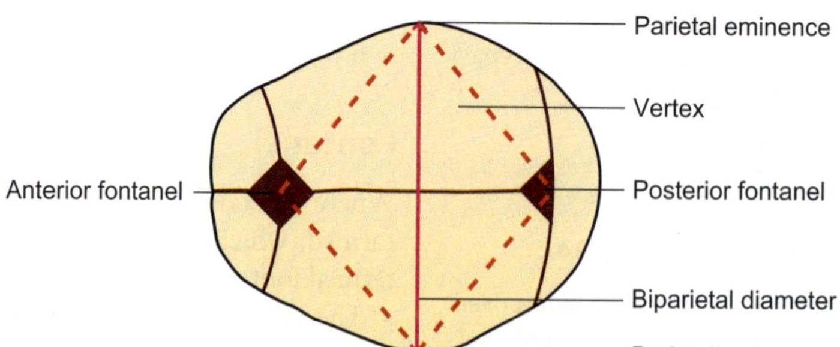

Figure 32.14 Vertex—a quadrangular area bounded anteriorly by bregma, posteriorly by lambda, and laterally by parietal eminences.

Anteroposterior diameters (Figure 32.15; Table 32.3)

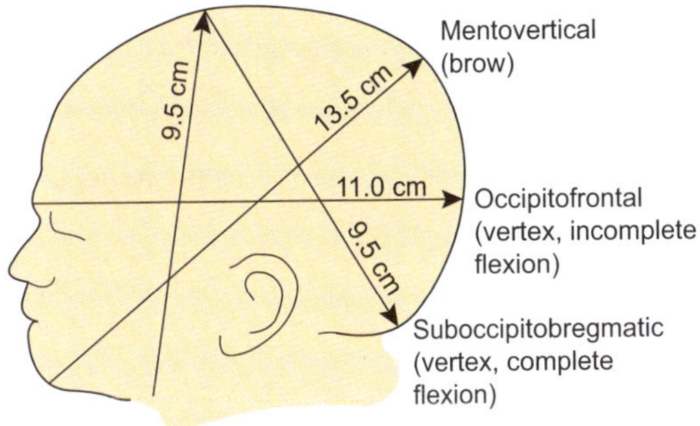

Figure 32.15 Anteroposterior diameters of fetal skull.

Note

- *The engaging AP diameters of fetal skull in vertex and face presentations are suboccipitobregmatic and submentobregmatic, respectively, which are 9.5 cm. Hence, a normal pelvis permits engagement of the fetal skull in vertex and face presentations.*
- *In brow presentation, the engaging AP diameter of fetal skull is mentovertical (14 cm). Hence, engagement does not occur and arrest of labor occurs.*

Table 32.3 Anteroposterior diameters of fetal skull

Diameter	Extent	Length (cm)	Attitude of head	Presenting part
Suboccipitobregmatic	Extends from the nape of the neck to the center of bregma	9.5	Complete flexion	Vertex
Suboccipitofrontal	Extends from the nape of the neck to the center of sinciput	10	Incomplete flexion	Vertex
Occipitofrontal	Extends from the occipital eminence to the root of nose (glabella)	11.5	Marked deflexion	Vertex
Mentovertical	Extends from the chin to the highest point on sagittal suture	14	Partial extension	Brow
Submentobregmatic	Extends from the junction of the floor of the mouth and neck to the center of bregma	9.5	Complete extension	Face

Viva corner

Q1 What are the diameters of obstetric significance that are 9.5 cm?

Diameters of fetal skull (9.5 cm) are as follows:

- Biparietal diameter
- Suboccipitobregmatic diameter
- Submentobregmatic diameter

Diameter of maternal pelvis (9.5 cm) is as follows:

- **Sacrocotyloid diameter:** It is the distance from the midpoint of the sacral promontory to the iliopubic eminence. It represents the space occupied by the biparietal diameter of the head, while negotiating the brim in a flat pelvis.

33 Mechanism of Normal Labor

Introduction

The medical students are expected to know the various fetal presentations and positions, normal and abnormal labor mechanisms, and obstetric maneuvers and may be asked to demonstrate cardinal movements during labor using a dummy fetus and articulated maternal pelvis. A dummy fetus is a soft doll that resembles a term fetus. This chapter deals with the mechanism of normal labor.

Terminologies

Labor

Labor consists of a series of events that take place in the maternal genital organs, which help to expel the fetus and other products of conception from the uterine cavity into the outer world.

Delivery

It is the process of expulsion or extraction of a viable fetus out of the uterus. Delivery can be vaginal or abdominal (cesarean section).

Fetal lie

It refers to the relationship of the long axis (spinal column) of the fetus to the long axis of the uterus or the maternal spine. The fetal lie can be:

- **Longitudinal lie**: The maternal and fetal long axes are parallel to each other (Figure 33.1a and b).
- **Transverse lie:** The maternal and fetal long axes are perpendicular to each other (Figure 33.1c).
- **Oblique lie:** The maternal and fetal long axes cross each other obliquely or at an angle of 45°. The oblique lie is usually unstable and may become longitudinal or transverse during the course of labor (Figure 33.1d).

Fetal presentation

It is described as the fetal part that occupies the lower pole of the uterus and is thereby the first part to enter the pelvic passage. Fetal presentation can be cephalic (head), podalic (breech), or shoulder presentation (Table 33.1).

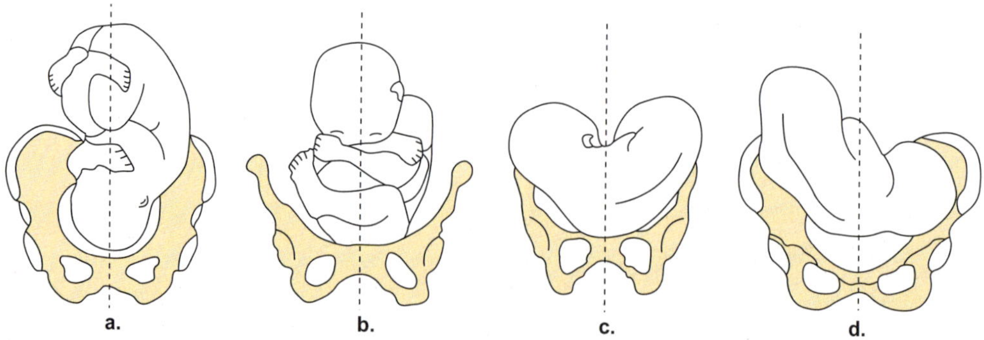

Figure 33.1 Fetal lie and presentation. **a.** Longitudinal lie, cephalic presentation. **b.** Longitudinal lie, breech presentation. **c.** Transverse lie, shoulder presentation. **d.** Oblique lie.

Table 33.1 Various fetal presentations	
Presentation	**Fetal lie**
Cephalic or the head presentation—most common (Figure 33.1a)	Longitudinal
Podalic or breech presentation (Figure 33.1b)	Longitudinal
Shoulder presentation (Figure 33.1c)	Transverse

Note *Breech and shoulder presentations pose difficulty for normal vaginal delivery and are termed malpresentations.*

Presenting part

It is defined as that part of the fetal presentation that overlies the internal os and is first felt by the examining fingers of the clinician.

In cephalic presentation, fetal presenting part varies, depending on the degree of flexion of the fetal head (Table 33.2). Brow and face presentation pose difficulty for vaginal delivery and are termed abnormal cephalic presentation or malpresentations.

Table 33.2 Various presenting parts in cephalic presentation	
Degree of flexion of fetal head	**Presenting part**
Completely flexed fetal head	Vertex (Figure 33.2a)
Partially extended fetal head	Brow (Figure 33.2b)
Completely extended fetal head	Face (Figure 33.2c)

In breech presentation, fetal presenting part varies depending on the degree of flexion at fetal hip and knee joints (Table 33.3).

Table 33.3 Various presenting parts in breech presentation	
Degree of flexion of breech	**Presenting part**
Flexed breech (complete flexion at hip and knee joints)	Buttocks, feet, external genitalia (Figure 33.3a)
Frank breech (flexed at hip joint and extended at knee joint)	Buttocks, external genitalia (Figure 33.3b)
Footling breech (extended at hip and knee joints)	Feet (Figure 33.3c)

Part 3

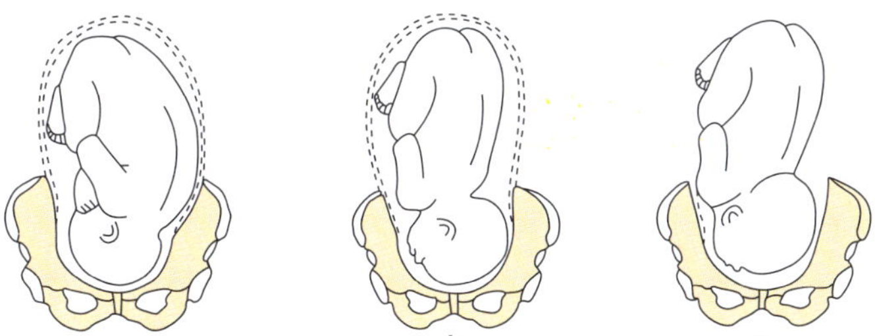

Figure 33.2 Fetal presenting parts in cephalic presentation. **a.** Vertex. **b.** Brow. **c.** Face.

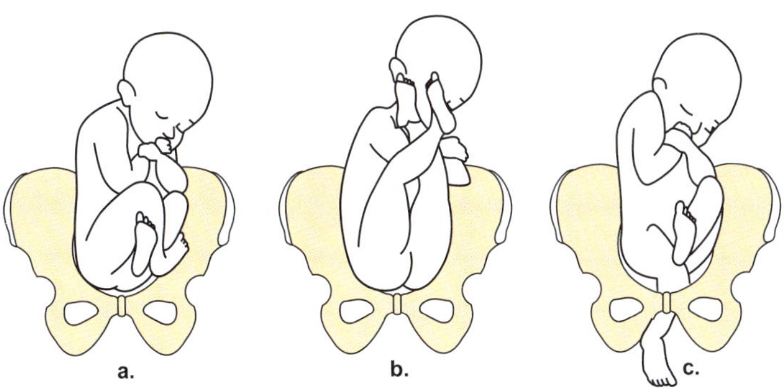

Figure 33.3 Fetal presenting parts in breech presentation. **a.** Complete breech. **b.** Frank breech. **c.** Footling breech.

Fetal attitude

It refers to the relationship of the fetal parts to each other.

- The most common fetal attitude is universal flexion in which the fetal head is flexed over the fetal neck, fetal arms are flexed upon the chest, and fetal legs are flexed over the abdomen.
- Depending on the attitude of the fetal head (degree of flexion), the fetal presenting part varies (Table 33.4).

Table 33.4 Various attitudes of fetal head

Attitude of fetal head	Presenting part
Complete flexion	Vertex (Figure 33.4a)
Marked deflexion	Vertex (Figure 33.4b)
Partial extension	Brow (Figure 33.4c)
Complete extension	Face (Figure 33.4d)

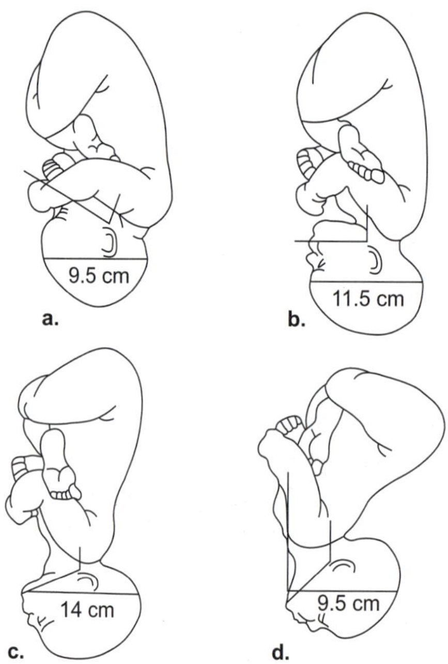

Figure 33.4 Various attitudes of the fetal head and the corresponding engaging diameters, depending on the degree of flexion of head. **a.** Complete flexion (vertex). **b.** Marked deflexion (vertex). **c.** Partial extension (brow). **d.** Complete extension (face).

Denominator

It is described as an arbitrary fixed bony point on the fetal presenting part, which is described in relation to the various quadrants of maternal pelvis (Table 33.5).

Table 33.5 Denominators in various presenting parts

Fetal presenting part	Denominator
Vertex	Occiput
Face	Mentum
Brow	Frontal eminence
Breech	Sacrum
Shoulder	Acromion

Fetal position

It is the description of the denominator of the fetus in relation to the different quadrants of the maternal pelvis (Figure 33.5).

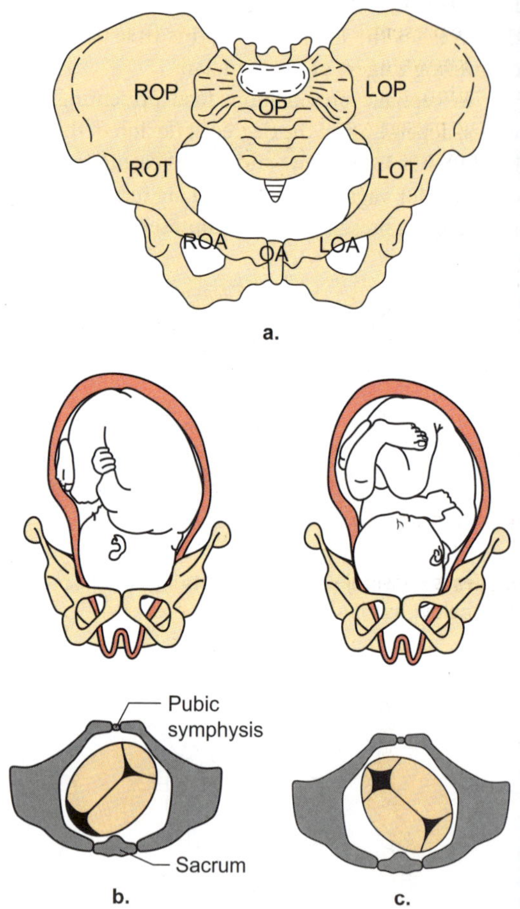

Figure 33.5 Various positions of occiput in vertex presentation. **a.** Various positions of occiput described in relation to quadrants of maternal pelvis. **b.** Left occipitoanterior (LOA) position. **c.** Left occipitoposterior (LOP) position.

In vertex presentation, occiput is the denominator and the various positions described are as follows:

- Left occipitoanterior (LOA)
- Right occipitoanterior (ROA)
- Left occipitotransverse (LOT)
- Right occipitotransverse (ROT)
- Left occipitoposterior (LOP)
- Right occipitoposterior (ROP)
- Direct occipitoanterior (DOA)
- Direct occipitoposterior (DOP)

Station

It is the description of the level of the presenting part in relation to the ischial spines (Figure 33.6).

- When the presenting part is at the level of ischial spines, it is known as station zero.
- The presenting part at levels above ischial spines is known as minus (−1, −2, −3, −4, and −5 cm) station.
- The presenting part at levels below ischial spines is known as plus (+1, +2, +3, +4, and +5 cm) station.

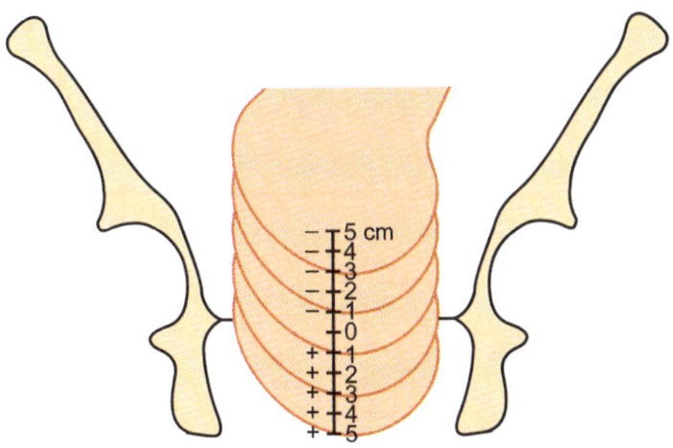

Figure 33.6 Station of the presenting part as determined by vaginal examination. The level of the ischial spines is considered as "0." There are five levels above and below, as minus (–) 1 to 5 and plus (+) 1 to 5.

Asynclitism

Synclitism is when saggital suture lies exactly in the middle of pelvis. When the fetal head descends through the available transverse diameter of the pelvic inlet, the sagittal suture may be deflected either anteriorly toward the symphysis pubis or posteriorly toward the sacral promontory. Such deflection of the head in relation to the pelvis is called asynclitism (Figure 33.7).

Importance

- Mild degree of asynclitism is common.
- Severe degree of asynclitism indicates cephalopelvic disproportion.

Anterior asynclitism or anterior parietal presentation

- When the sagittal suture is deflected posteriorly, the anterior parietal bone becomes the leading presenting part, termed anterior asynclitism or anterior parietal presentation.
- It is common in multipara.

Posterior asynclitism or posterior parietal presentation

- When the sagittal suture is deflected anteriorly, the posterior parietal bone becomes the leading presenting part, termed posterior asynclitism or posterior parietal presentation.
- It is common in primigravida.

Engagement

When the biparietal diameter of the fetal head (maximum transverse diameter of the fetal presentation) enters the pelvic brim, the head is said to be engaged.

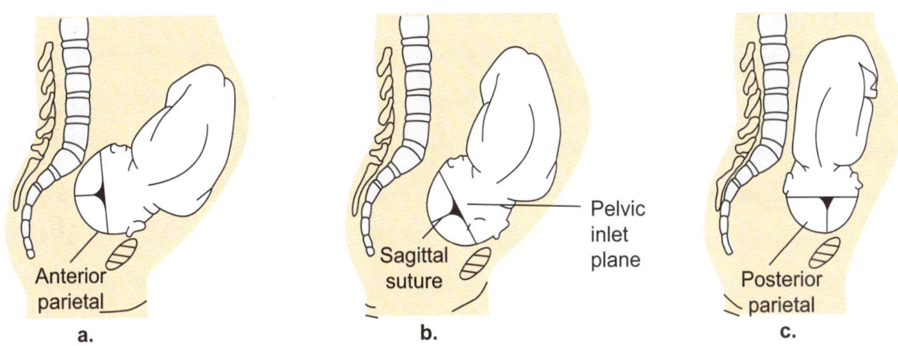

Figure 33.7 Asynclitism. **a.** Anterior asynclitism. **b.** Normal (without asynclitism). **c.** Posterior asynclitism.

Engaging diameter

When the head enters the pelvis, there is girdle of contact of the fetal head with the maternal pelvis at diametrically opposite points that is termed engaging diameter. The engaging diameter varies with the attitude of the fetal head.

Diameter of engagement

It refers to the diameter of the maternal pelvis through which the engaging diameter of the fetus enters the pelvis.

Stages of labor (Figures 33.8 and 33.9)

See Table 33.6

MECHANISM OF LABOR

Mechanism of labor refers to the series of movements that occur in the fetus, as it passes through the maternal pelvis during vaginal delivery.

- In normal labor, the fetal head enters the pelvic brim most often through the available transverse diameter of the pelvic inlet, as the most common fetal position is occipitotransverse position. In some cases, the fetal head may enter the pelvis through one of the oblique diameters of the pelvis (LOA or ROA position).

Note *Right oblique diameter of pelvis extends from right sacroiliac joint to the opposite iliopectineal eminence and left oblique diameter of pelvis extends from left sacroiliac joint to the opposite iliopectineal eminence.*

- The fetal head in LOA position engages in the right oblique diameter, and the fetal head in ROA position engages in the left oblique diameter of pelvic brim.
- LOA position is more common than ROA position because the left oblique diameter is occupied by the sigmoid colon.
- Occipitotransverse and occipitoanterior positions are common in normal labor and hence the mechanism of labor in occipitotransverse and occipitoanterior positions is described.

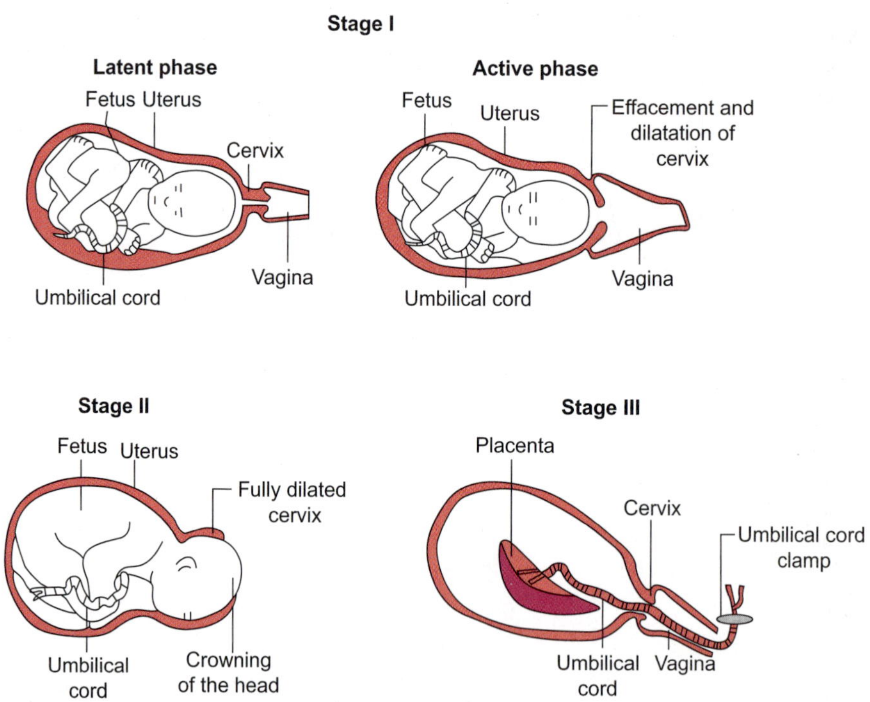

Figure 33.8 Stages of labor. Stage I: Onset of dilatation to full dilatation of cervix; Stage II: Full dilatation of cervix to delivery of the fetus; Stage III: Delivery of the fetus to delivery of the placenta.

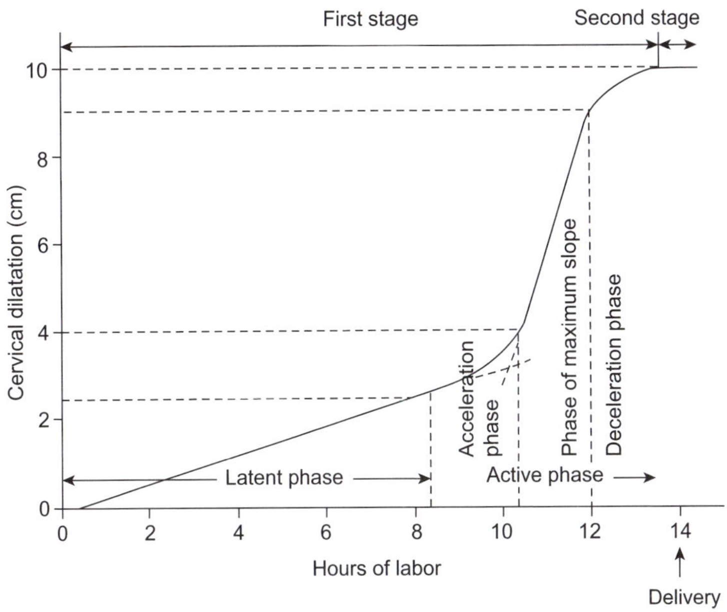

Figure 33.9 Graph showing cervical dilatation during labor.

Table 33.6 Stages of labor

Stages of labor	Description	Characteristics	Duration in primigravida	Duration in multigravida
Stage I	Starts from the onset of true labor pain and ends with full dilatation of cervix	Divided into two phases: • Latent phase: It is of variable duration when slow and gradual cervical effacement and dilatation occurs up to 3–4 cm • Active phase: Active cervical dilatation begins from 3–4 cm dilatation up to 10 cm (full dilatation). In the active phase, cervix dilates at the rate of 1 cm/h in primigravida and 1.5 cm/h in multigravida It consists of the following (Figure 33.9): • Acceleration phase (3–4 cm) • Phase of maximum slope (4–9 cm) • Deceleration phase (9–10 cm)	• 8–20 hours • 6–12 hours	• 6–14 hours • 3–6 hours
Stage II	Starts from full dilatation of cervix and ends with expulsion of the fetus from birth canal		1–2 hours	30 minutes to 1 hour
Stage III	Starts from expulsion of the fetus and ends with expulsion of placenta and membranes		15 minutes	15 minutes
Stage IV	Stage of observation: Starts from expulsion of placenta up to 1 hour after expulsion of placenta		60 minutes	60 minutes

Cardinal movements of labor These are described in Table 33.7. (**Hint**: *"Acronym ED FIERE"*)

Table 33.7 Cardinal movements of labor

Cardinal movement	Explanation
Engagement	Engaging diameter crosses the pelvic brim
Descent	Downward movement of fetus
Flexion	Brings the smallest diameter of the fetal head (suboccipito-bregmatic) in the pelvis
Internal rotation	Internal rotation of the head occurs so that the occiput comes under the pubic symphysis
Extension	Delivery of the fetal head by extension
Restitution	Visible passive movement of the head due to untwisting of the neck sustained during internal rotation
External rotation	Visible external rotation of the head due to internal rotation of the shoulders
Expulsion	Delivery of shoulders and rest of the fetal parts

AP, anteroposterior.

The favorable factors for vaginal delivery are as follows:
- Adequate pelvis
- Average size of the fetus
- Good uterine contractions
- Good flexion of the fetal head
- Elastic recoil of the levator ani muscles

Vertex presentation (LOA position)

Left occipitoanterior is more common than right occipitoanterior, seen in two thirds of anterior positions. Salient parameters in vertex presentation are mentioned in Table 33.8.

Table 33.8 Salient parameters in vertex presentation

Lie	Longitudinal
Presentation	Cephalic
Presenting part	Vertex
Attitude	Well-flexed head
Denominator	Occiput
Position	Left occipitoanterior (most common anterior position)
Engaging diameter	Suboccipitobregmatic (9.5 cm)
Diameter of engagement	Right oblique (in left occipitoanterior position)

Mechanism of labor in occipitoanterior position

- **Engagement:** Fetal head is said to be engaged when the biparietal diameter passes through the pelvic brim. In a primigravida, engagement usually occurs before the onset of labor, while in a multigravida engagement occurs during the course of labor (Figure 33.10). In LOA, head engages in the right oblique diameter of pelvis.
- **Descent:** It is a continuous process that occurs throughout the course of labor. Descent is caused by uterine contractions and in second stage aided by bearing down efforts of the mother.
- **Flexion:** Flexion is achieved when the head meets the resistance of the pelvic floor muscles during descent. It brings the smallest diameter of the fetal head in the pelvis. Flexion causes change in presenting diameter from larger occipitofrontal to smaller suboccipitobregmatic, with a reduction of 1.5 cm in the presenting diameter.

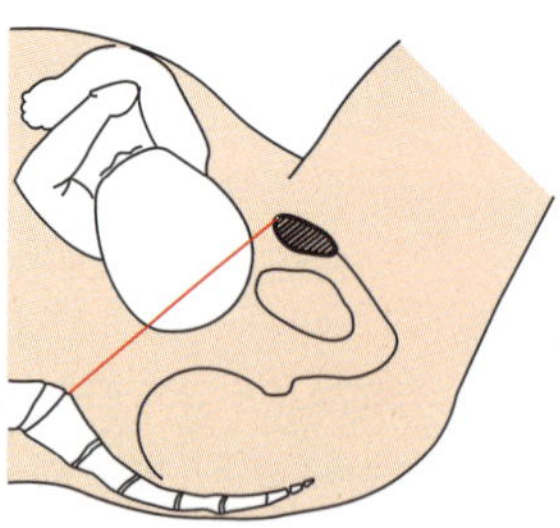

a.

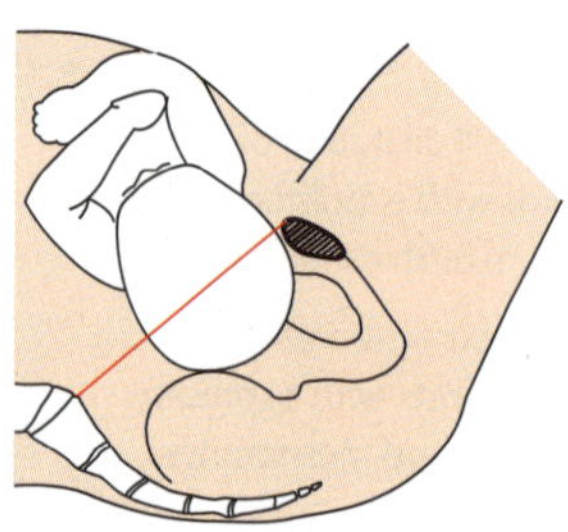

b.

Figure 33.10 Engagement of fetal head. **a.** Biparietal diameter has not crossed the pelvic brim. **b.** Biparietal diameter has crossed the pelvic brim (head is engaged).

- **Internal rotation:** Internal rotation of the head occurs by one-eighth of a circle (45 degrees) in occipitoanterior position so that the occiput comes under the pubic symphysis *and the sagittal suture lies in the anteroposterior diameter of the pelvis.* As a result of the internal rotation of the head, the neck sustains a torsion of one-eighth of a circle. Internal rotation occurs mainly due to the gutter-shaped arrangement of the fibers of levator ani muscle (Figure 33.11).

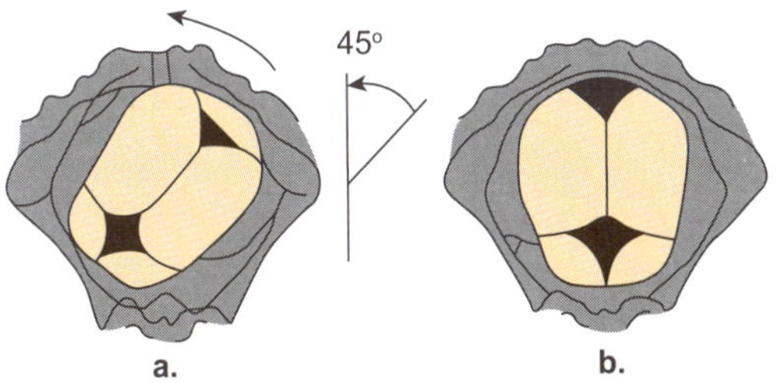

Figure 33.11 Internal rotation of fetal head. **a.** Left occipitoanterior (LOA) position **b.** Anterior rotation of LOA by 45° to direct occipitoanterior (DOA) position.

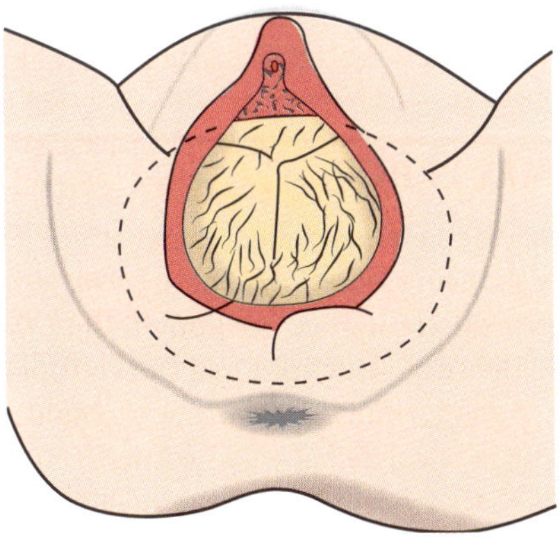

Figure 33.12 Crowning of fetal head.

Note *Prerequisites for internal rotation of the head are as follows: Well-flexed head, efficient uterine contraction, favorable shape of pelvis, and good tone of levator ani muscles.*

- **Crowning:** Following internal rotation of the head, further descent occurs until the subocciput comes underneath the pubic arch. When the biparietal diameter stretches the vulval outlet and does not recede back in between contractions, it is termed crowning of fetal head (Figure 33.12).
- **Extension:** Delivery of the head occurs by extension. The successive parts of the fetal head delivered are vertex, brow, and face. Immediately following the release of the chin, the head drops down, bringing the chin in close proximity to the maternal anus (Figure 33.13a and b).
- **Restitution:** It is the visible passive movement of the head due to untwisting of the neck sustained during internal rotation. During restitution, the head rotates through one-eighth of a circle (45 degrees) in the direction opposite to that of internal rotation. Following restitution, the head *returns to left occipitoanterior from direct occipitoanterior* and aligns along the long axis of the fetus (Figure 33.13c).
- **External rotation:** It is the visible external rotation of the head that occurs due to internal rotation of the shoulders. The anterior shoulder rotates through one-eighth of a circle toward the pubis symphysis and the shoulders engage in anteroposterior diameter of pelvis. This results in visible external rotation of the fetal head by one-eighth of a circle in the same direction as restitution, i.e., *the head rotates from left occipitoanterior by another 45 degrees to left occipitotransverse.* (Figure 33.13d).

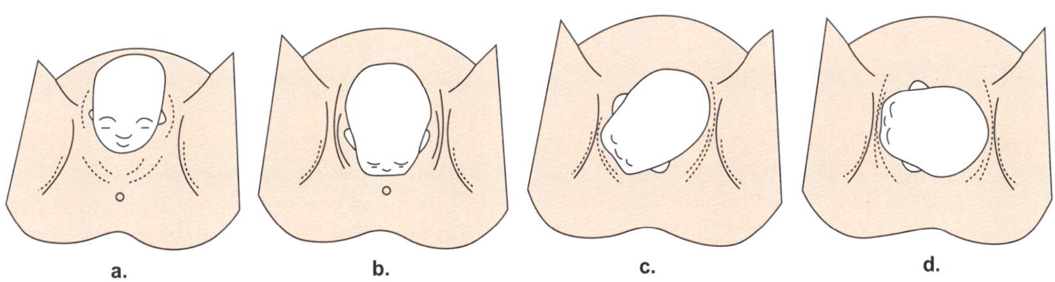

Figure 33.13 Mechanism of labor. **a.** Delivery of the head by extension. **b.** Head drops down to face maternal anus. **c.** Restitution of fetal head. **d.** External rotation of fetal head.

Part 3

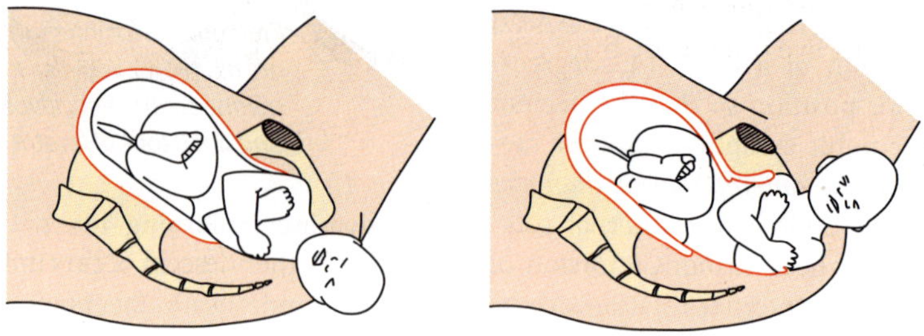

Figure 33.14 Delivery of the shoulders. **a.** Delivery of anterior shoulder. **b.** Delivery of the posterior shoulder.

- **Delivery of the shoulders:** The anterior shoulder delivers first followed by the posterior shoulder (Figure 33.14a and b).
- **Delivery of trunk:** Rest of the baby delivers by lateral flexion of trunk.

Mechanism of labor in occipitotransverse position

- Engagement
- Descent
- Flexion
- Internal rotation [in occipitotransverse position, internal rotation of head occurs by two-eighth of a circle to place the occiput behind the pubic symphysis; the neck fails to withstand such major degree of torsion of two-eighth of a circle as a result of this anterior rotation of the occiput; there will be simultaneous rotation of the shoulders in the same direction to the extent of one-eighth of a circle, and the shoulders will be placed in the oblique diameter with only one-eighth of torsion of neck still remaining (Figure 33.15)]
- Extension
- Restitution
- External rotation
- Expulsion of the shoulders and trunk

Note *Only difference in the mechanism of labor in occipitotransverse position when compared with occipitoanterior position is the degree of internal rotation. Rest of the mechanism of labor is same as in occipitoanterior position.*

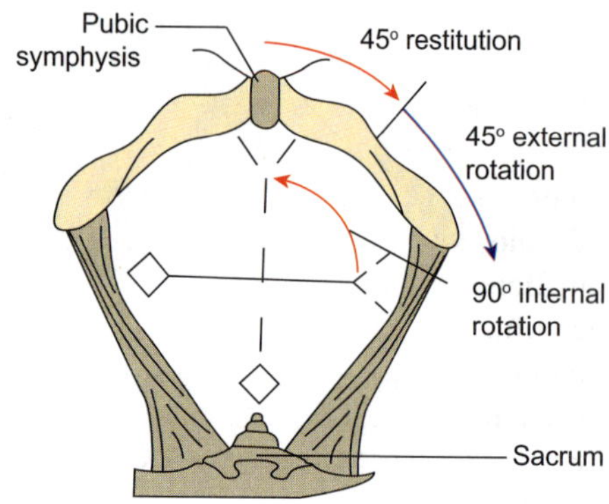

Figure 33.15 Degree of internal rotation, restitution, and external rotation of fetal head in left occipitotransverse position.

NORMAL LABOR

Criteria for normal labor include the following: Spontaneous onset of labor at term, in a fetus with vertex presentation, resulting in spontaneous vaginal delivery with minimal aid, without any undue prolongation of labor or complications, resulting in a healthy baby and mother.

True labor begins when the uterine contractions are of sufficient frequency, intensity, and duration to cause progressive effacement and dilatation of the cervix.

Characteristics of true labor pains

- Painful uterine contractions occur at regular intervals.
- Contractions increase in intensity, frequency and duration as time progresses.
- Contractions are associated with progressive effacement and dilatation of cervix.
- Contractions are associated with "show" (vaginal discharge of "mucus mixed with blood") and formation of "bag of waters."

Effective uterine contractions Uterine contractions are said to be effective if there are three contractions in 10 minutes, each lasting for at least 45 seconds. Clinically, intensity of contractions is considered to be good if uterine wall cannot be indented by the fingers.

Conduct of normal labor

On admission to labor room, detailed history is taken, antenatal records are reviewed, and clinical examination of the woman is performed.

Clinical examination includes the following:

- General physical examination
  - Look for pallor and edema.
  - Assess the patient's vitals—temperature, pulse rate, BP, and respiratory rate.
  - Cardiovascular and respiratory system examinations are done.
- Abdominal examination—assess the following:
  - Fundal height
  - Fetal lie—longitudinal, transverse, or oblique
  - Fetal presentation—cephalic, podalic (breech), or shoulder
  - Whether presenting part is engaged or not (Crichton's fifth formula)
  - Uterine contractions—frequency, intensity, and duration
  - Fetal weight
  - Amount of liquor
  - Fetal heart rate (FHR)
- Per speculum examination—assess the following:
  - Leaking P/V
  - Bleeding P/V
  - Any abnormal discharge P/V
- Per vaginal examination—assess the following:
  - Bishop's score is assessed that includes the following:
  - Cervical dilatation, effacement, consistency, position, and station of fetal head (Table 33.9)
  - Status of fetal membranes—present or absent
  - Color of liquor (if membranes are absent)

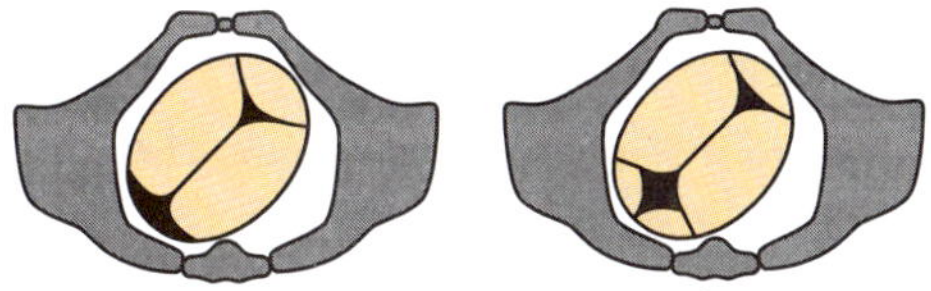

Figure 33.16 Flexion of the fetal head as determined by vaginal examination. **a.** When head is well flexed (vertex presentation), the posterior fontanel is well felt and anterior fontanel is felt with difficulty. **b.** When head is deflexed, anterior and posterior fontanels are felt with equal ease.

  - Fetal presentation and position, degree of flexion of the head (Figure 33.16)
  - Molding of fetal skull bones
  - Pelvic assessment
- Blood grouping and Rh typing, cross matching and reservation are done
- Xylocaine test dose is administered

Conduct of first stage of labor

Important events in first stage of labor

- Dilatation and effacement of cervix
- Formation of the lower uterine segment

Management of first stage of labor

- **Asepsis:** Aseptic precautions should be taken during vaginal examination and during conduct of delivery. The pubic hairs are clipped. The vulva and the perineum are washed with soap and water, and then cleaned with an antiseptic solution such as chlorhexidine. Vaginal examination should be done with sterile gloves after cleaning the vulva with antiseptic swab.
- **Ambulation:** Ambulation in I stage of labor improves maternal comfort and can reduce the duration of labor and the need for analgesia. The woman is confined to bed if she is a high-risk case, if continuous electronic FHR monitoring is required, or if epidural analgesia is given.

Table 33.9 Bishop's score

Score	Dilatation (cm)	Effacement (%)	Station	Cervical consistency	Position of cervix
0	Closed	0–30	–3	Firm	Posterior
1	1–2	40–50	–2	Medium	Midposition
2	3–4	60–70	–1, 0	Soft	Anterior
3	5+	80+	1+, 2+		

Part 3

High-yield points

Assessment of descent by abdominal fifth method—Crichton's score

- In this method, the fetal head felt above the pelvic brim is assessed in fingerbreadths, by placing fingers above the pubis symphysis (see figure below).
- The width of the five fingers of the left hand is taken as a guide to express the fifths of the head present above pelvic brim.
- A freely mobile head will accommodate the full width of five fingers.
- As the head descends, the portion of the head remaining above the brim will be represented by four-fifth, three-fifth, etc.
- When two-fifth or less is palpable above pelvic brim, the head is said to be engaged.

Advantages of "abdominal fifth method" over "station of the head" in assessing descent of fetal head

- It excludes the variability in assessment of descent of head, due to caput and molding and due to different depths in pelvis.
- Repeated vaginal examinations to assess the descent of head can be avoided.
- The assessment is quantitative and can be easily reproduced.

Indications for vaginal examination during labor

- At the onset of labor—to detect cervical changes and to assess pelvis, especially in primigravida
- To assess the progress of labor by noting cervical dilatation, effacement, and station of fetal head
- Following rupture of membranes—to exclude cord prolapse
- To confirm the second stage of labor when the patient starts bearing down

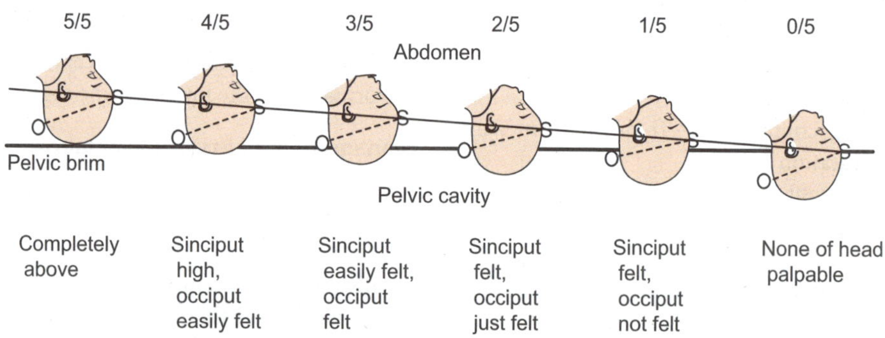

Figure Crichton's score—assessment of descent by abdominal fifth method.

- **Enema:** Soap water enema may be given in early labor to avoid soiling during delivery. However, enema to reduce the use of labor augmentation is not recommended.
- **Bladder care:** The patient is encouraged to pass urine frequently, as full bladder inhibits uterine contractions and may lead to infection.
- **Diet:** Food is withheld during active labor to prevent risk of aspiration of gastric contents, in case general anesthesia is required. Clear fluids such as water or fruit juices may be allowed in early labor.
- **Pain relief:** Analgesics are given in the active phase of labor and can be repeated after 4–6 hours.
- **Monitoring maternal and fetal condition and progress of labor:** Frequent monitoring of maternal pulse, BP, temperature, uterine contractions, and FHR is done and vaginal examination is performed at regular intervals to monitor the cervical changes and descent of head.
- **Partogram:** It is maintained to monitor the maternal and fetal well-being and progress of labor.

High-yield points

- **FHR monitoring:** If facilities are available, continuous electronic FHR monitoring can be done. Otherwise, intermittent auscultation of FHR with stethoscope is done (see table below).

(CONTD...)

(...CONTD)

High-yield points

Table FHR auscultation during labor

Intermittent auscultation of FHR	First stage	Second stage
High-risk patient	Every 15 minutes	Every 5 minutes
Low-risk patient	Every 30 minutes	Every 15 minutes

FHR, fetal heart rate.

Conduct of second stage of labor

Important events in second stage of labor

- Bearing-down efforts by the mother to expel the fetus
- Propulsion and expulsion of fetus

Viva corner

Q1 What are the clinical features indicating onset of second stage of labor?

- Increase in intensity and duration of uterine contractions
- Appearance of maternal bearing-down efforts (pushing efforts)
- Urge to defecate with descent of the presenting part

Vaginal examination is done to confirm the diagnosis (cervical rim cannot be palpated around fetal head—indicates full dilatation of cervix).

Management of second stage of labor

Conducting normal vaginal delivery

- The patient is put in dorsal position with thighs flexed.
- The external genitalia and perineum are cleaned with an antiseptic solution and then draped.
- The patient is encouraged to bear down with uterine contractions.
- FHR is auscultated every 15 minutes in low-risk cases and every 5 minutes in high-risk cases.
- Bladder is emptied.
- The perineum bulges and thins out with descent of the fetal head. When the fetal head distends the vulval outlet and does not recede back in between contractions, it is termed crowning.
- Mediolateral episiotomy may be given at crowning, after infiltrating the perineum with 1% Lignocaine local anesthesia. Episiotomy is given only in indicated cases, to widen the introitus.

Note *Episiotomy is no longer recommended as a routine procedure for conducting vaginal delivery and is performed only in indicated cases.*

- Controlled delivery of the head is facilitated by placing fingers of one hand below the pubic symphysis, against the baby's head to keep it flexed, and perineal support is given with the other hand to prevent perineal injuries (Ritgen maneuver—controlled delivery of the head in between uterine contractions).
- The baby's head delivers by extension and the baby's mouth and nose are suctioned. Check for the presence of any cord around the neck. If a loose cord is present, it should be slipped over the baby's head and if the cord is tight, it is double clamped and cut.
- Following delivery of the fetal head, the fetal head drops down and the baby's face points toward the maternal anus.
- Restitution and external rotation of the fetal head occurs and the occiput turns toward one of the maternal thighs.
- Anterior shoulder appears at the vaginal introitus and is delivered first followed by the delivery of posterior shoulder.
- The rest of the trunk slides out of the introitus and is supported with the clinician's hands.
- The umbilical cord is then clamped and cut, and the baby is handed over to the pediatrician.
- The baby's body is dried and eyes are wiped; the baby is then covered with a dry cloth and placed under a warmer.

Conduct of third stage of labor

Important events in the third stage of labor

Separation and expulsion of the placenta

Management of third stage of labor

Third stage of labor is significant because postpartum hemorrhage (PPH) can occur in this stage, which is an important cause of maternal mortality and morbidity.

Active management of the third stage of labor (AMTSL) is practiced for prevention of PPH. It includes the following:

- Administration of uterotonic agent, oxytocin 5–10 IU (IV/IM) immediately following delivery of the baby
- Delayed cord clamping
- Checking for uterine tone and uterine massage if uterine tone is decreased
- Delivery of the placenta by controlled cord traction (Brandt-Andrews method)

Signs of placental separation

- Appearance of suprapubic bulge due to hardening and contraction of uterus
- Sudden gush of blood
- Apparent lengthening of cord as the placenta passes into the lower uterine segment

Brandt-Andrews method of controlled cord traction (Figure 33.17)

- Slight traction is applied on the cord in downwards and backwards direction and simultaneous counterpressure is applied with the other hand in the suprapubic region on the uterus in upwards and backwards direction.
- The placenta delivers out and as it delivers it is gently twisted until the membranes are stripped off from the uterine wall and removed completely.
- The placenta is examined for any missing cotyledon, to ensure completeness of expulsion.
- Bimanual uterine massaging is done to contract the myometrial muscles.
- Episiotomy and any perineal tears are repaired at this stage.

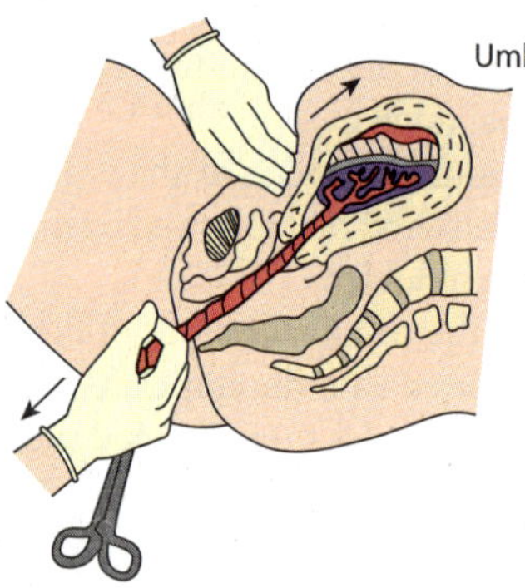

Figure 33.17 Brandt-Andrews method of controlled cord traction.

Extra edge

Indications for early cord clamping

- Rh incompatibility
- Birth asphyxia
- Preterm baby
- Baby of a diabetic mother

Conduct of fourth stage of labor

Events in fourth stage of labor

There are no specific events in this stage of labor. This stage has been included along with the stages of labor due to risk of PPH following delivery. The patient is observed and monitored in labor room for 1 hour following delivery and breast feeding should be initiated.

Management of fourth stage of labor

- **Maternal monitoring is done:** Note the pulse rate, blood pressure, uterine tone, presence of any undue vaginal bleeding, etc.

The patient can be shifted to postnatal ward after 1 hour following delivery, if vitals are stable, uterus is well contracted, and there is no undue vaginal bleeding.

Extra edge

Recommendations on intrapartum care for positive childbirth experience

Adapted from *WHO recommendations: intrapartum care for a positive childbirth experience. Geneva: World Health Organization; 2018.*

- Pregnant women should be treated with dignity, privacy, and confidentiality—respectful maternity care.
- Presence of a companion throughout labor should be allowed.
- The latent first stage in both primigravida and multigravida is characterized by painful uterine contractions, variable effacement of cervix, and slower progression of the cervical dilatation up to 5 cm. The duration of latent phase is variable.
- The active first stage in both primigravida and multigravida is characterized by regular painful uterine contractions, progressive effacement, and rapid cervical dilatation from 5 cm until full dilatation. The duration of active first stage usually does not extend beyond 12 and 10 hours in primigravida and multigravida, respectively.
- Cervical dilatation <1 cm/hour alone (as depicted by the partograph alert line) should not be an indication for obstetric intervention, as labor may not naturally accelerate until 5 cm dilatation. Therefore, oxytocin augmentation/LSCS prior to the threshold of 5-cm cervical dilatation is not recommended, provided fetal and maternal conditions are reassuring.
- Routine clinical pelvimetry and cardiotocography on admission in labor for low risk in spontaneous labor is not recommended.
- Oral fluid and food intake during labor for low-risk women is recommended.
- Encouraging ambulation during labor in women at low risk is recommended.
- Routine perineal shaving and enema prior to vaginal delivery is not recommended.
- Routine vaginal cleansing with antiseptic solution during labor for the purpose of preventing infectious morbidities is not recommended.
- Relaxation techniques such as deep breathing, progressive muscle relaxation, music, and manual techniques, such as application of warm packs or massage are recommended for pain relief during labor.
- Epidural analgesia for women requesting pain relief during labor is recommended.
- Parenteral opioids such as fentanyl, pethidine, and diamorphine for pain relief during labor are recommended.
- Pain relief for preventing delay and reducing the use of augmentation in labor is not recommended.
- Vaginal examination at 4-hour interval for assessment of active labor in low-risk women is recommended.
- Intermittent auscultation of FHR with Doppler device or Pinard fetal stethoscope is recommended rather than continuous CTG for assessment of fetal well-being in cases with spontaneous labor.
- Amniotomy alone/early amniotomy with oxytocin augmentation for prevention of delay in labor is not recommended.
- Routine use of oxytocin for prevention of delay in labor in women who receive epidural analgesia is not recommended.
- Routine use of intravenous fluids and antispasmodic agents with the aim of shortening the duration of labor is not recommended.
- The second stage is the period from full cervical dilatation to the birth of the baby, during which an involuntary urge to bear down is experienced by the woman due to expulsive uterine contractions.
- Delivery is usually completed within 3 hours and 2 hours in primigravida and multigravida, respectively.
- The adoption of a birthing position of their choice for women with/without epidural analgesia should be encouraged.
- Women should be encouraged to bear down in second stage.
- For women with epidural analgesia, delaying pushing for 1–2 hours after full dilatation or until the woman regains the sensory urge to bear down, where resources are available to assess and manage perinatal hypoxia, is recommended.
- Techniques to reduce perineal injury and facilitate spontaneous birth such as perineal massage, warm compresses, and hands on guarding of the perineum are recommended.
- Routine or liberal use of episiotomy is not recommended.
- Manual fundal pressure to facilitate childbirth during second stage is not recommended.
- Oxytocin (10 IU, IM/IV) is recommended as the uterotonic agent of choice for prevention of PPH. If oxytocin is not available, injectable uterotonics such as

(CONTD...)

(...CONTD)

Extra edge

methylergometrine/oxytocin plus ergometrine fixed-dose combination/oral misoprostol is recommended.
- Delayed umbilical cord clamping for improved infant health and nutrition outcomes is recommended.
- Sustained uterine massage as an intervention to prevent postpartum hemorrhage (PPH) in women who have received prophylactic oxytocin is not recommended.
- Controlled cord traction (CCT) for delivery of the placenta is recommended.
- Routine suctioning of the mouth and nose in a neonate born through clear amniotic fluid who start breathing on their own after birth is not recommended.
- Newborn without complications should be kept in skin-to-skin contact with the mother during the first hour after birth to prevent hypothermia and promote breastfeeding.
- All newborns, including low-birth-weight babies who are able to breastfeed, should be put to the breast as soon as possible after birth when the mother and baby are ready.
- All newborns should be given 1 mg of vitamin K IM injection after birth.
- The mother and baby should not be separated and rooming-in should be encouraged.
- Bathing of the newborn should be delayed until 24 hours after birth.

34 Abnormal Labor: Malpositions and Malpresentations

Introduction

Malpositions and malpresentations are common causes of abnormal labor and are associated with increased risk maternal and fetal complications during labor. Students may be asked to demonstrate the mechanism of labor in malpositions such as occipitoposterior (OP) position, and malpresentations such as breech and face presentations.

MALPOSITION

Any position of the vertex other than the flexed occipitoanterior or occipitotransverse position is called malposition. In a vertex presentation, when the occiput is placed posteriorly over the sacroiliac joint or over the sacrum, it is termed OP position.

MALPRESENTATION

Any presentation of the fetus other than the vertex presentation is termed malpresentation. Brow, face, breech presentations, and transverse lie are included under malpresentations.

Viva corner

Q1 Although OP position is a vertex presentation, why is OP described as a malposition?

In 90% of cases of OP position, long anterior rotation of the occiput occurs and the course of labor follows like that of an occipitoanterior position. However, OP position may occasionally cause dystocia during labor due to short anterior rotation, malrotation, or nonrotation and hence is described as a malposition.

OCCIPITOPOSTERIOR POSITION

The salient parameters in OP position are mentioned in Table 34.1.

The factors that favor vaginal delivery in OP position are as follows:

- Adequate pelvis
- Good uterine contractions
- Good flexion of the fetal head
- Average size of the fetus

Outcome of labor in occipitoposterior position

In the presence of all the favorable factors such as adequate pelvis, good uterine contractions, good flexion of the fetal head, and average size of the fetus, there is 90% chance of successful vaginal delivery.

Table 34.1 Salient parameters in occipitoposterior position

Parameter	Finding in occipitoposterior position
Lie	Longitudinal
Presentation	Cephalic
Presenting part	Vertex
Attitude of the head	Deflexed head
Denominator	Occiput
Position	OP: ROP is the most common OP position (Figure 34.1)
Engaging diameter	Occipitofrontal (11.5 cm) or suboccipitofrontal (10.5 cm)
Diameter of engagement	Right oblique in ROP

OP, occipitoposterior; *ROP*, right occipitoposterior.

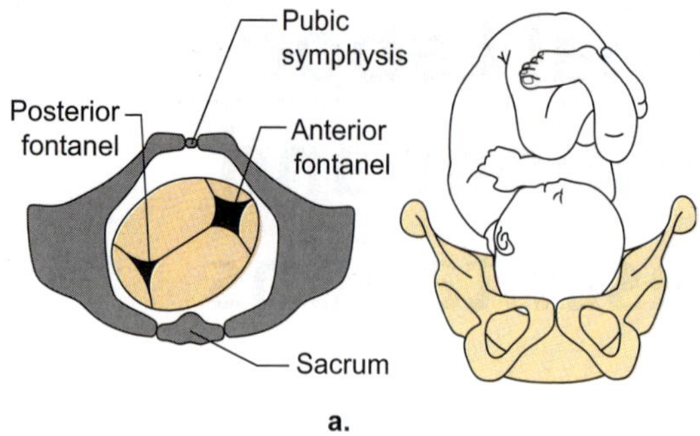

Figure 34.1 Right occipitoposterior position.

- Fetal head undergoes long anterior rotation by three-eighth of a circle, so that the occiput comes under pubic symphysis.
- Shoulders simultaneously rotate by two-eighth of a circle to reduce the torsion on the neck. Torsion of one-eighth of a circle is still present between head and neck, which gets relieved only after delivery of head (by restitution of head).
- Rest of the delivery is similar to that of occipito-anterior position.

Under unfavorable circumstances, the chance of vaginal delivery is less (10%).

Depending on the degree of flexion of the fetal head, uterine contractions, pelvic adequacy, and fetal size, the occiput may fail to undergo complete anterior rotation, resulting in the following outcomes (Figure 34.2):

- In case of mild deflexion of the head → occiput undergoes short anterior rotation through one-eighth of a circle → results in incomplete anterior rotation → results in deep transverse arrest.
- In case of moderate deflexion of the head (sinciput and occiput are at the same level) – nonrotation of head → results in persistent occipitoposterior position → may result in arrest.
- In case of severe deflexion (sinciput is at a lower level than occiput) → malrotation occurs → sinciput, which is at a lower level, rotates anteriorly to come under pubic symphysis → results in direct OP position or occipitosacral position → vaginal delivery is possible as face-to-pubis delivery (Figure 34.3), in the presence of good uterine

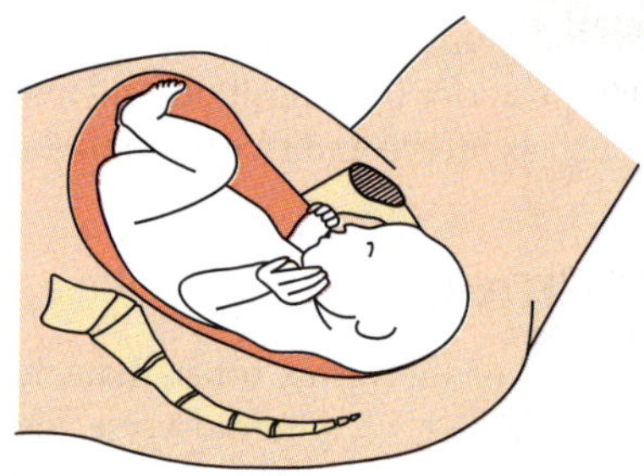

Figure 34.3 Face-to-pubis delivery. When the occiput rotates posteriorly, the fetus is delivered as face to pubis.

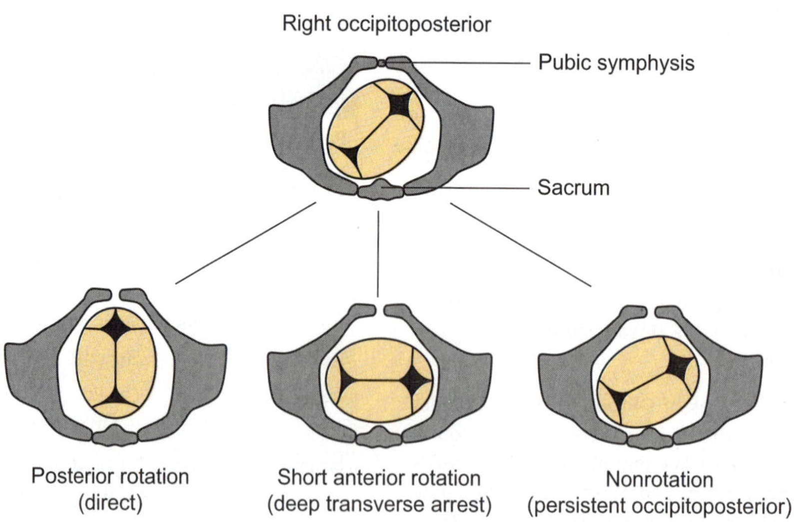

Figure 34.2 Abnormal mechanisms of labor in occipitoposterior position. The occiput, from right occipitoposterior position, can undergo posterior rotation or short anterior rotation, or remain as persistent occipitoposterior by nonrotation.

contractions, adequate pelvis, and average-sized baby. Otherwise, labor may get arrested as occipitosacral arrest.

High-yield points

In face-to-pubis delivery, delivery of the head is by initial flexion to deliver the vertex and occiput, followed by extension of the head to deliver the face of the baby.

BREECH PRESENTATION

Salient parameters in breech presentation are mentioned in Table 34.2.

Table 34.2 Salient parameters in breech presentation

Parameter	Finding in breech presentation
Lie	Longitudinal
Presentation	Breech (podalic pole)
Presenting part	• Buttock, external genitalia, and feet: *In flexed breech* • Buttock and external genitalia: *In extended breech* (Figure 34.4a) • Feet: *In footling breech*
Attitude of the breech	• Complete flexion: *Flexed breech* • Incomplete flexion: *Extended or frank breech*
Denominator	Sacrum
Position (Figure 34.4b)	LSA (most common position)
Engaging diameter*	• Bitrochanteric (10 cm) • Bisacromial (12 cm) • Suboccipitofrontal (10.5 cm)
Diameter of engagement	Left oblique (in LSA)

* In the mechanism of vaginal breech delivery, the cardinal movements occur at three sites: buttocks, shoulders, and the head. Each of the three components undergoes cardinal movements during labor and hence the engaging diameter is mentioned for the three levels.

LSA, left sacroanterior.

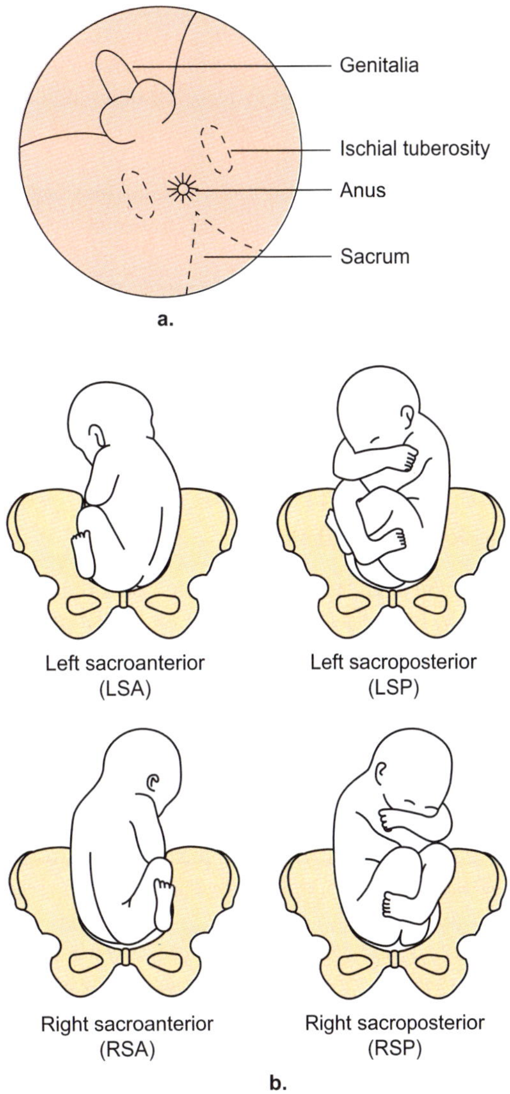

Figure 34.4 Breech presentation. **a.** Vaginal examination findings in frank breech presentation. **b.** Fetal positions in breech presentation. Left and right sacroanterior and sacroposterior positions.

Mechanism of labor in breech presentation

Note *The first two successive parts to be born are compressible (buttocks and shoulders), while difficulty is usually encountered during delivery of the after-coming head because of nonmolding of fetal skull bones.*

Delivery of buttock

- Engagement of the presenting part occurs in one of the oblique diameters [left oblique in left sacroanterior (LSA) position].
- Descent of presenting part occurs.
- Internal rotation of buttocks through one-eighth of a circle to occupy the anteroposterior (AP) diameter of pelvic outlet.
- Anterior buttock hinges under the pubic symphysis and is released first followed by the posterior buttock.
- Lower limbs are then delivered.
- Trunk delivers by lateral flexion.
- When the angle of scapula is seen, hands are delivered from ventral aspect of body.

Delivery of shoulders

- Shoulders engage in the same oblique diameter as the buttocks (left oblique in LSA position).
- Descent and internal rotation of shoulders occur to occupy the AP diameter of the pelvic outlet.
- Delivery of the shoulders occurs.

Delivery of the after-coming head

- Engagement of head occurs in the opposite oblique diameter (right oblique in LSA position).
- Descent of head and increasing flexion of head occurs.
- Internal rotation of the occiput toward pubic symphysis occurs and the occiput impinges against pubic symphysis.
- After-coming head of breech is born by flexion.

High-yield points

Principles of conducting a vaginal breech delivery

- Do not be in a rush to deliver.
- Do not pull from below; instead, push from above.
- Always keep the back of the fetus anterior.

Methods to deliver the after-coming head in assisted vaginal breech delivery

- Malar flexion and shoulder traction (modified Mauriceau–Smellie–Veit technique)
- Burns-Marshall method
- Forceps delivery

FACE PRESENTATION

Salient parameters in face presentation are mentioned in Table 34.3.

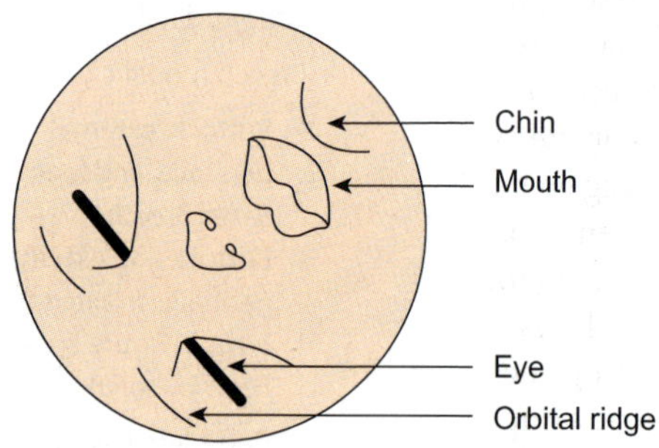

Figure 34.5 Vaginal examination findings in face presentation.

Table 34.3 Salient parameters in face presentation

Parameter	Finding in face presentation
Lie	Longitudinal
Presentation	Cephalic
Presenting part	Face (mentum to nasion; Figure 34.5)
Attitude of the head	Complete extension
Denominator	Mentum
Position (Figure 34.6)	Two-third of cases , mentoanterior position (left mentoanterior position is most common); one-third of cases, mentoposterior position
Engaging diameter	Submentobregmatic (9.5 cm)
Diameter of engagement	Right oblique in left mentoanterior position

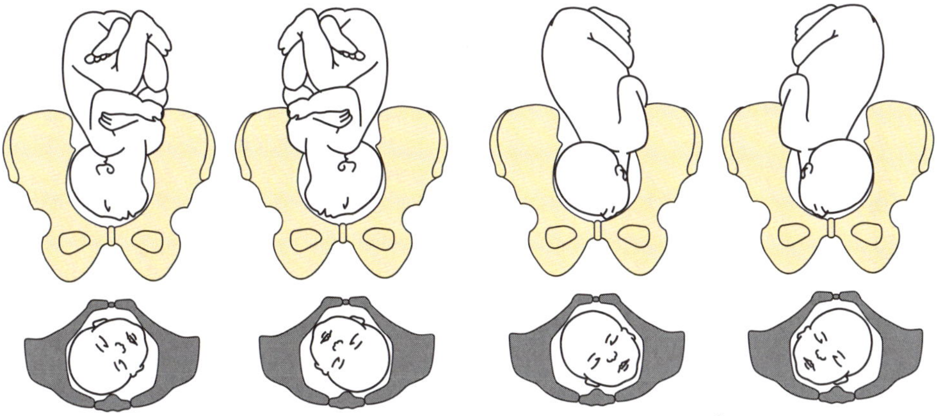

Figure 34.6 Face presentation. **a.** Left mentoanterior and right mentoanterior positions. **b.** Left mentoposterior and right mentoposterior positions.

Mechanism of labor in mentoanterior face presentation

If pelvis is adequate and good uterine contractions are present, the cardinal movements of labor that take place are the following:

- Descent of the presenting part
- Complete extension of head
- Engagement (engagement is delayed in face presentation)
- Internal rotation of mentum toward pubic symphysis
- Impingement of chin of the fetus under the pubic symphysis
- Head born by flexion
- Restitution of the head
- External rotation of head (due to internal rotation of shoulders)
- Trunk born by lateral flexion

Mentoposterior face presentation

- Thirty percent of mentoposterior cases undergo spontaneous rotation to mentoanterior position and can be delivered as mentioned earlier.
- Seventy percent of cases remain as persistent mentoposterior face position.
  - There is no mechanism of labor for persistent mentoposterior presentation because the relatively short neck cannot clear off the total length of the sacrum (12 cm). The thorax is thrust into the pelvis and the sternobregmatic diameter (18 cm) becomes the engaging diameter (Figure 34.7). Vaginal delivery is not possible and results in obstructed labor.
  - Persistent mentoposterior face presentation has to be delivered by cesarean section.

Viva corner

Q1 The clinical course in face presentation is adversely affected in spite of the fact that the engaging diameter of the head in vertex and face presentations is the same, 9.5 cm. Why?

- Ill-fitting presenting part (face) results in early rupture of membranes
- Delay of labor is common due to the following reasons:
  - There is absence of molding of the facial bones.
  - Engagement is delayed because of the long distance between the face and the biparietal plane (7 cm) as compared with distance between vertex and biparietal plane (3 cm).

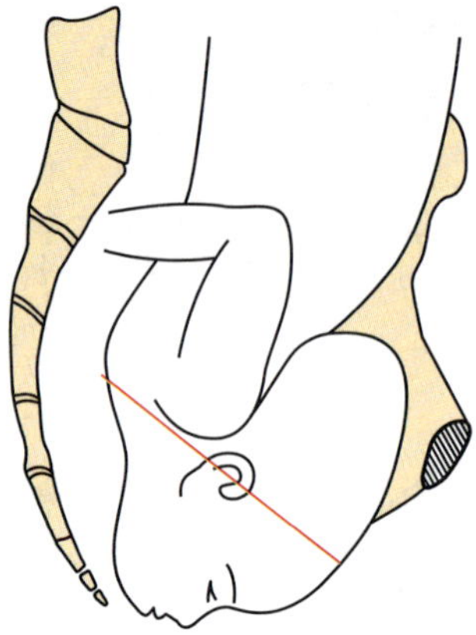

Figure 34.7 The thorax is thrust into the pelvis in persistent mentoposterior face presentation.

BROW PRESENTATION

Salient parameters in brow presentation are mentioned in Table 34.4.

Table 34.4 Salient parameters in brow presentation

Parameter	Finding in brow presentation
Lie	Longitudinal
Presentation	Cephalic
Presenting part	Brow (nasion to anterior fontanelle; Figure 34.8)
Attitude of the head	Partial extension
Denominator	Frontum
Position	Frontoanterior or frontoposterior
Engaging diameter	Mentovertical (14 cm)
Diameter of engagement	–

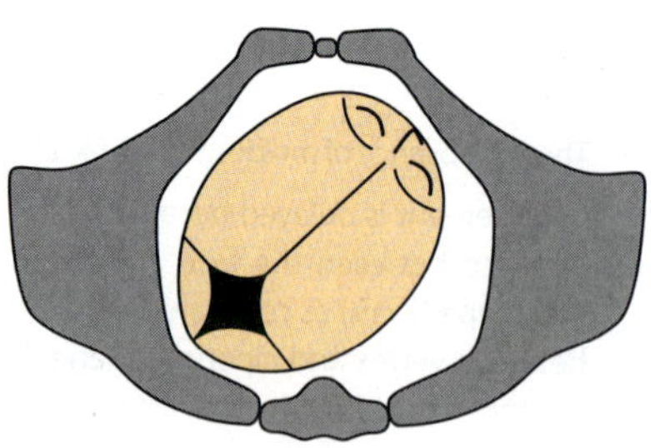

Figure 34.8 Vaginal examination findings in brow presentation.

Mechanism of labor in brow presentation

- There is no mechanism of labor for persistent brow presentation, as the engaging diameter is mentovertical, which is 14 cm. Persistent brow presentation results in obstructed labor, if left unattended.
- Persistent brow presentation in labor has to be delivered by cesarean section.
- In the presence of good uterine contractions and adequate pelvis, spontaneous correction to face or vertex may occur in 30% of cases.
  - Complete extension to face presentation
  - Complete flexion to vertex presentation

TRANSVERSE LIE

Salient parameters in transverse lie are mentioned in Table 34.5.

Table 34.5 Salient parameters in transverse lie

Lie	Transverse lie
Presentation	Shoulder
Presenting part	Shoulder/chest/back/hand (depending on the position of back)
Attitude	Flexion or extension
Denominator	Shoulder/acromion
Position	There are two positions of head (R or L) for each of the four positions of the back: dorsoanterior/posterior/superior/inferior (Figure 34.9)
Engaging diameter	–
Diameter of engagement	–

Mechanism of labor in transverse lie

- There is no mechanism of labor for persistent transverse lie and if left uncorrected leads to obstructed labor. Hence, persistent transverse lie presentation has to be delivered by cesarean section.
- However, under exceptional circumstances, the baby in transverse lie can deliver vaginally by the following mechanisms:

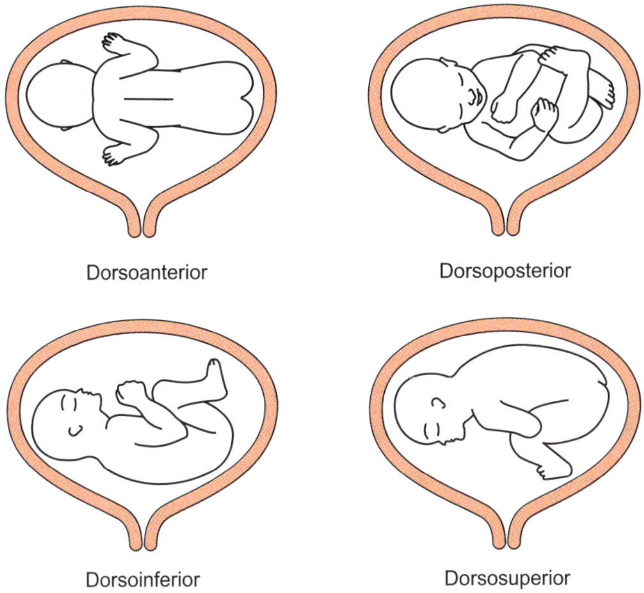

Figure 34.9 Transverse lie. The four positions are: dorsoanterior, dorsoposterior, dorsoinferior, and dorsosuperior.

- Spontaneous correction to vertex or breech.
- Spontaneous evolution can happen in very preterm fetuses: Chest and breech descend simultaneously and baby is born doubled upon itself, termed "corpus con duplicato."

COMPOUND PRESENTATION

When more than one fetal presenting part overlies the internal os, it is termed compound presentation.

Common varieties of compound presentation

- Cephalic with hand or/and foot (Figure 34.10)
- Breech with hand

Mode of delivery

- In uncomplicated cases (vertex with hand): Elevation of the limb with descent of the presenting part usually occurs spontaneously.
- Cesarean section is done for singleton live fetus at term, if associated with complications such as contracted pelvis.

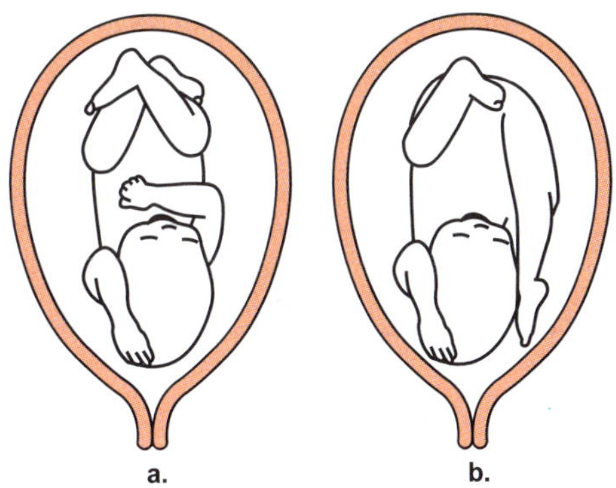

Figure 34.10 Compound presentation. **a.** Hand and head. **b.** Hand, foot, and head.

UNSTABLE LIE

Unstable lie is a condition where the presentation of the fetus keeps constantly changing even beyond the 36th week of pregnancy.

Mode of delivery

- Stabilizing induction of labor: External cephalic version can be done (if not contraindicated) after 37 weeks → oxytocin infusion is started to initiate effective uterine contractions, followed by low rupture of the membranes, anticipating vaginal delivery.

- Cesarean section is done in majority of the cases, especially in the presence of complicating factors such as preeclampsia, placenta previa, and contracted pelvis.

Cord prolapse

There are three types of prolapse of the umbilical cord as mentioned in Table 34.6 (Figure 34.11).

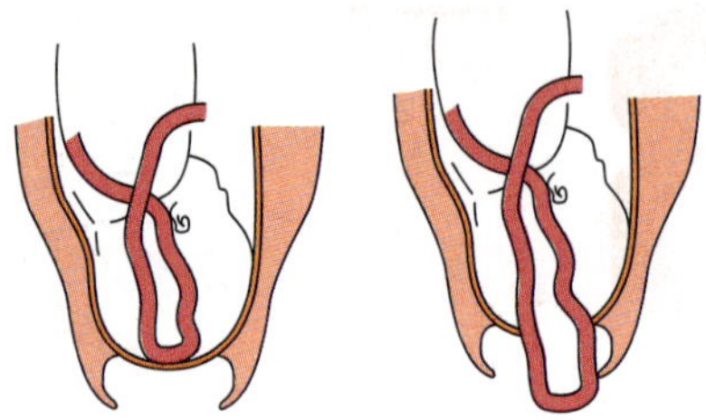

Figure 34.11 Cord presentation and cord prolapse. **a.** Cord presentation with the membranes not ruptured. **b.** Cord prolapse with the membranes ruptured.

Table 34.6 Types of umbilical cord prolapse

Clinical type	Description	Diagnosis	Further management
Occult cord prolapse	The cord is by the side of the presenting part and is not felt by the fingers on internal examination	The possibility should be suspected if there is persistent variable deceleration of fetal heart rate detected on cardiotocography monitoring	Cesarean section is done in case of persistent variable deceleration
Cord presentation	The cord slips down below the presenting part and is felt lying in the intact bag of membranes	Cord pulsations can be felt through the intact membranes	If immediate vaginal delivery is not possible, cesarean section is done
Cord prolapse	The cord lies in the vagina or outside the vulva following rupture of membranes	The cord is palpated directly by the fingers and its pulsation can be felt, if the fetus is alive	• Baby alive: Cesarean section is done • Baby dead: Vaginal delivery is allowed

35 Partogram

Introduction

Partogram is a composite graphical record of the key events of labor on a single sheet of paper.

Medical students should be acquainted with plotting a partogram for a patient in labor and interpretation of any given partogram. This chapter deals with concepts related to a partogram and examples of partogram charts for interpretation.

The evolution of partogram

- **Friedman:** Partogram was first described by Friedman as a record of cervical dilatation versus time.
  - Friedman's cervical dilatation curve is a sigmoid-shaped curve (Figure 35.1).
  - Friedman divided labor into two phases:
    - Latent phase
    - Active phase

  The active phase is further divided into the following:
  - Acceleration phase (cervix dilatation, 3–4 cm)
  - Phase of maximum slope (4–9 cm)
  - Deceleration phase (9–10 cm)
- **Philpott and Castle:** They added the alert line and action line to the cervical graph.
- **Crichton:** Crichton introduced the abdominal examination method of assessing the descent of fetal head by measuring the head palpable above pubic symphysis in fifths.
- **WHO composite partogram**: In addition to cervical dilatation, further details such as the descent of the presenting part, uterine contractions, maternal vitals, oxytocin augmentation, fetal heart rate (FHR), presence of meconium, and molding of the head were added to the original partogram by the WHO in 1990, to make it a composite record of all the important events of labor on a single sheet, known as the "WHO composite partogram." The WHO composite partogram included a latent phase of 8 hours and the alert line began at 3-cm dilatation (beginning of active phase).
- **WHO modified partogram**: Modifications were introduced in the WHO original partogram in the year 2000, to devise the "WHO modified partogram," which is widely used now (Figure 35.2). The modified WHO partograph does not include the latent phase and the alert line (beginning of active phase) starts at 4-cm dilatation.

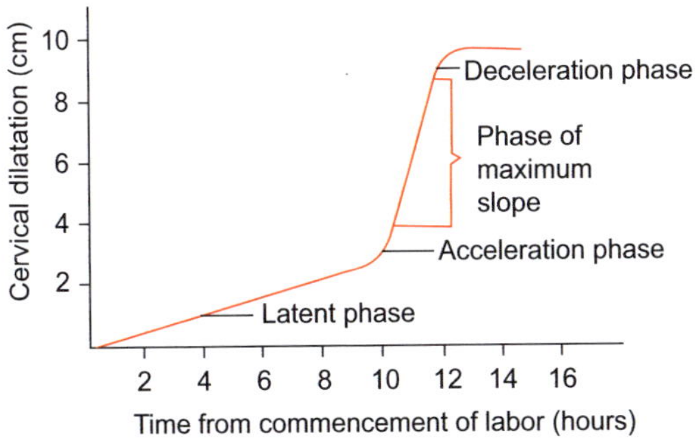

Figure 35.1 Friedman's curve.

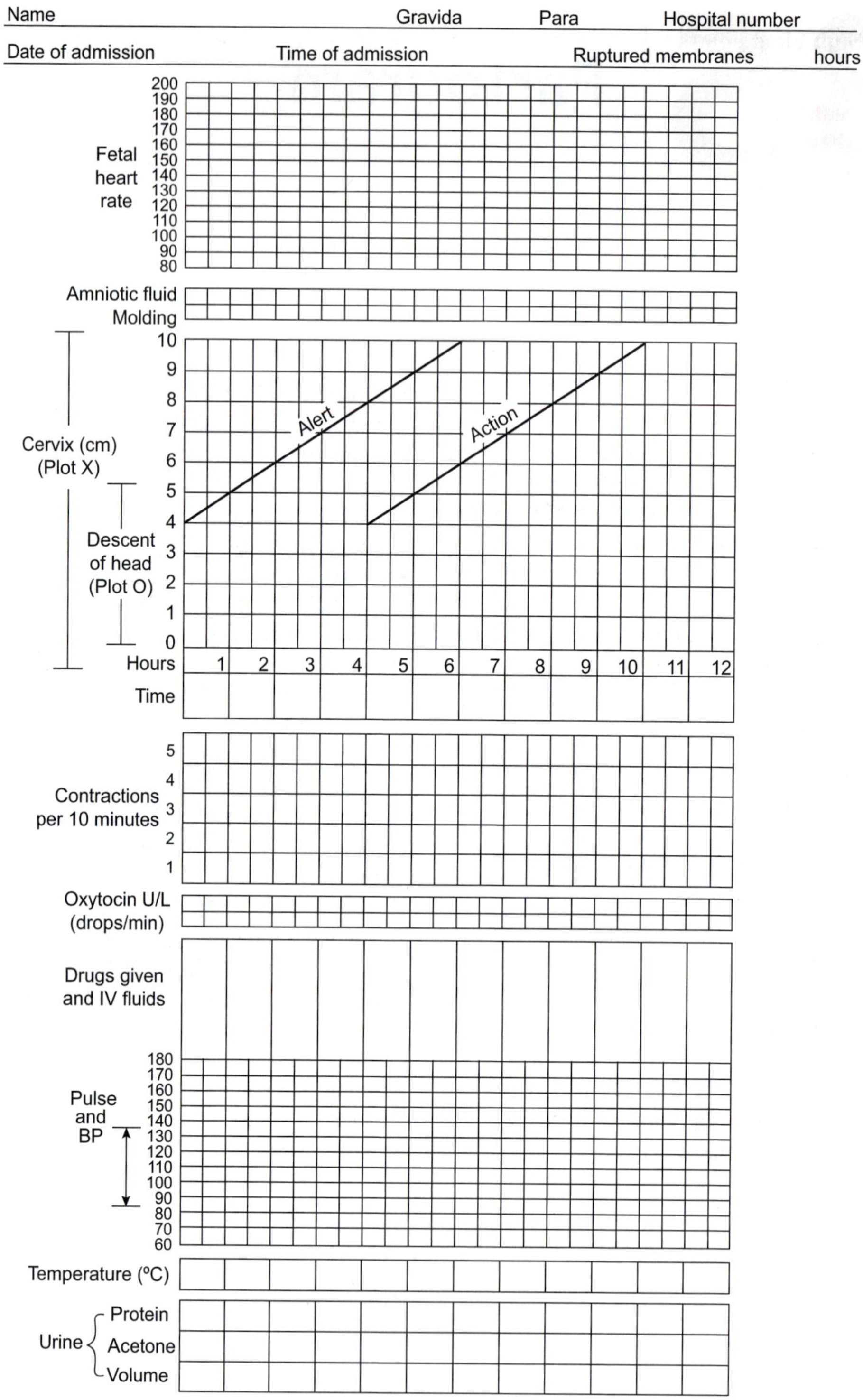

Figure 35.2 WHO modified partogram.

High-yield points

Q1 What are the principle changes in the WHO modified partogram as compared with WHO composite partogram?

- Latent phase has been removed.
- Beginning of the active phase is considered at 4 cm dilatation of cervix instead of at 3 cm.
- There are two squares in 1 hour instead of one square in 1 hour, which means one square is equal to 0.5 hour in the modified partogram. See Figures A and B below comparing WHO composite partogram and WHO modified partogram.

Advantages of WHO modified partogram over the WHO composite partogram

Justification for the changes made in the modified WHO partogram include the following:

- **Removal of latent phase in the graph**
  - Differentiating latent phase from false labor is difficult, as diagnosis is usually made retrospectively.
  - Prolonged latent phase is relatively infrequent and is not associated with poor perinatal outcome. Hence, the usefulness of recording latent phase is questionable.
- **Beginning of active phase at 4 cm instead of 3 cm:** The onset of active phase is clearly understood by making it 4 cm instead of 3 cm.

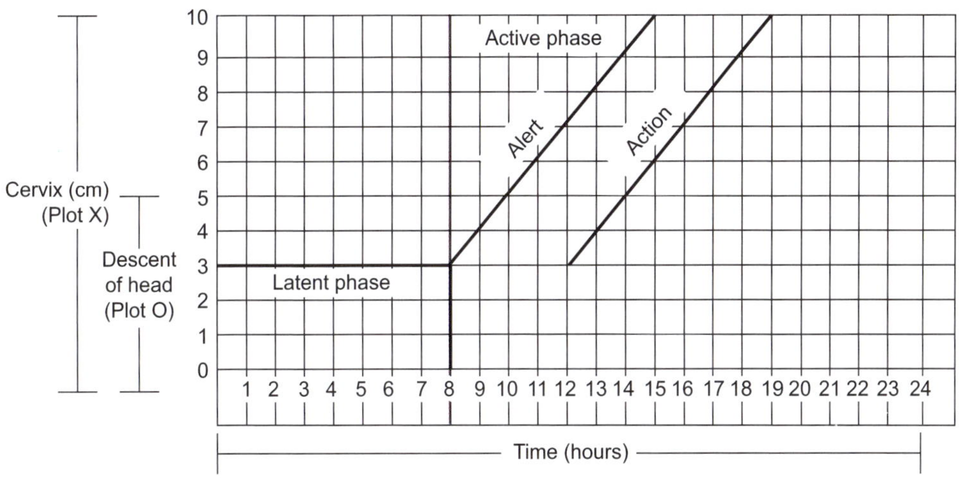

Figure A WHO composite partograph.

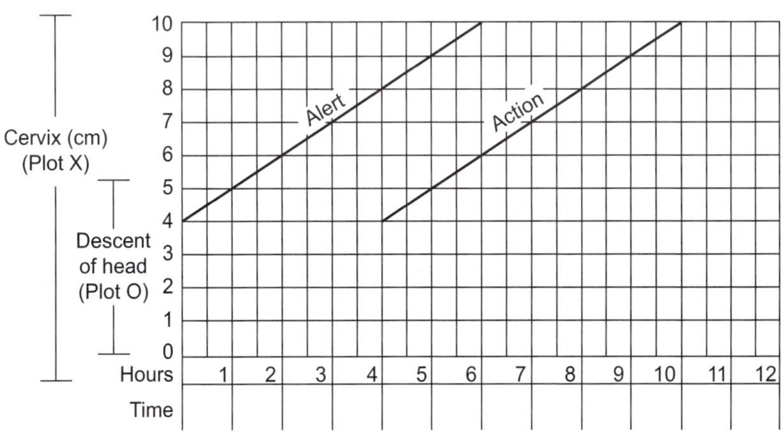

Figure B WHO modified partograph.

COMPONENTS OF WHO MODIFIED PARTOGRAM

The observations recorded are the following (Figure 35.2):

- Patient information: This includes name, age, gravida, parity, hospital number, time of admission, and time of rupture of membranes.
- FHR: It is recorded every 30 minutes in the first stage and 15 minutes in the second stage. Vaginal examination is done every 4 hours to assess cervical dilatation, descent of the fetal head, color of liquor, and molding of skull bones. More frequent examinations are undertaken, if indicated.
- Status of membranes, color of liquor (if membranes are absent), and molding of head are recorded.
- Cervical dilatation, expressed in centimeters, is recorded. Alert and action lines are drawn.
- Descent of fetal head: It is assessed by abdominal examination or by vaginal examination.
- "Hours" is the time elapsed since the onset of active labor.
- "Time" is the actual time of examination.
- Uterine contractions: Frequency, duration, and strength of uterine contractions (assessed by palpation) are recorded every 30 minutes.
- Oxytocin augmentation is recorded in milli-international units per minute (mIU/min), titrated every 30 minutes.
- Drugs and fluids: Drugs are recorded when given.
- Maternal pulse and blood pressure are recorded.
- Maternal temperature is recorded.
- Urine: Urine volume, presence of protein, and ketones are noted.

KEY TO PARTOGRAM (REFER TO FIGURE 35.2)

Fetal heart rate

- It is recorded at the top of the partogram.
- It should be recorded every 30 minutes for a period of 1 minute, immediately after the peak of contraction, preferably with the patient in left lateral position.
- FHR of 110–160 beats/min is considered normal. FHR <110 or >160 beats/min may indicate fetal distress and needs further action.

Status of membranes and amniotic fluid

- **I:** Membranes intact
- **C:** Membranes ruptured, clear liquor
- **M:** Meconium-stained liquor
- **B:** Blood-stained liquor
- **A:** Absent amniotic fluid

Note *Thick meconium or absent liquor warrants more frequent monitoring of FHR as fetal distress is more likely to occur.*

Molding

- **Grade 0:** Bones are separated and sutures can be easily felt.
- **Grade +1:** Bones are just touching each other.
- **Grade +2:** Bones are overlapping but can be reduced.
- **Grade +3:** Bones are severely overlapping and irreducible.

Note *Excess molding is an ominous sign of cephalopelvic disproportion. It is difficult to assess molding in the presence of large caput.*

Cervical dilatation

- The numbers on the *Y*-axis (0–10) represent the cervical dilatation and those on the *X*-axis (0–12) represent the hours.
- Cervical dilatation is plotted with a cross, "X." It is assessed at each vaginal examination and is plotted from 4 cm onwards (i.e., from active labor).

Plotting of cervical dilatation (cervicograph)

- The alert line starts at 4 cm cervical dilatation and ends at 10 cm at the rate of 1 cm/h (cervix dilates at the rate of 1 cm/h in about 90% of primigravidas).
- The action line is drawn 4 hours to the right and parallel to the alert line.
- In normal labor, the cervicograph lies either on the alert line or to the left of it (Zone 1).

Importance of alert and action lines

When the cervicograph crosses the alert line and lies to the right of it (Zone 2), it indicates a delay in labor.

- If the patient is in a peripheral unit, transfer the patient to a referral center.

- If the patient is in hospital, extra vigilance is required.

When the cervicograph crosses the action line and lies to the right of it (Zone 3), the cause for delay has to be critically assessed and specific management decisions must be made.

- Decision has to be made for delivery by cesarean section or augmentation of labor, depending on the abnormality detected.

Extra edge

Q1 Why is there a difference of 4 hours between the alert line and the action line?

A lag time of 4 hours between the slowing of labor and the need for intervention is unlikely to compromise the fetus or the mother and avoids unnecessary intervention.

Descent of the head

- It is assessed by abdominal palpation or vaginal examination and recorded as a circle (O).
- Descent of the head measured abdominally by fifths palpable above the pelvic brim is a more reliable way of measuring the descent than the vaginal examination method of assessment of descent, because it gives a true measure of descent and rules out the false impression due to molding or excessive caput formation noted in a vaginal examination.
- Descent is written on the left-hand side of the graph in partogram, which extends from numbers 0 to 5.

Note *The simplified partograph designed by Rural Health Mission, Govt. of India, has markings for cervical dilatation only, and descent/station is not included.*

Hours

This refers to the time elapsed since the onset of the active phase of labor (1–12 hours).

Time

It is the record of the actual time at 30-minute interval.

Contractions

- Palpate for the number of uterine contractions in 10 minutes and the duration of each contraction in seconds (<20, 20–40, >40 seconds). Contractions are recorded every 30 minutes (Table 35.1).
- "Contractions per 10 minutes" is written on the left-hand side—numbered from 1 to 5. The number of squares filled indicates the number of contractions in 10 minutes.
- The shading shows the strength of contractions (Figure 35.3).

Table 35.1 Depicting the uterine contractions in 10 minutes

Strength of contraction (duration in seconds)	Shading in the graph
<20	Dots
20–40	Crosshatch
>40	Darkened completely

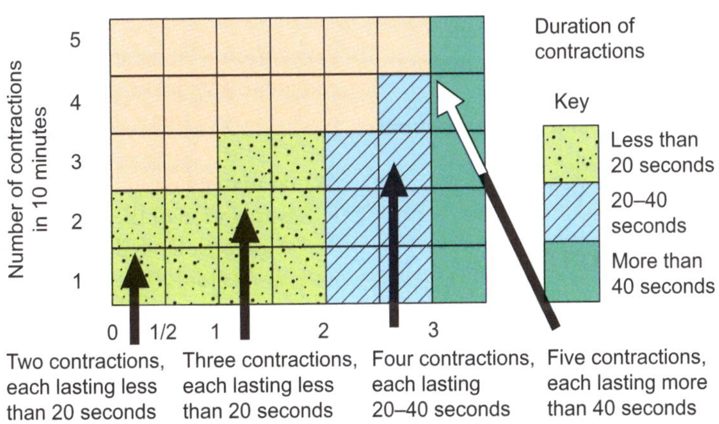

Figure 35.3 Recording of uterine contractions in a partogram.

Oxytocin augmentation

When oxytocin is administered, record the amount of oxytocin in units per volume of IV fluids (mIU/mL) and the number of drops per minute, every 30 minutes.

Drugs given

Any additional drugs given such as analgesics are recorded.

Maternal parameters

Maternal parameters that are recorded are the following:

- Maternal pulse is recorded every 30 minutes and marked with a dot (•).
- Maternal BP is measured every 4 hours and marked with arrows (in patients with hypertensive disorders complicating pregnancy, BP is monitored more frequently).
- Temperature is recorded every 4 hours.
- Urine: Volume, protein, and ketones are recorded every 4 hours. The patient is encouraged to pass urine every 2–4 hours.

Advantages of partogram in management of labor

- Partogram helps in early detection of dysfunctional labor so that appropriate intervention can be done.
- Timely transfer of the mother from peripheral center to higher center can be done on diagnosis of dysfunctional labor.
- Partogram charting reduces the incidence of prolonged labor and cesarean section.
- It helps in early detection of fetal distress.
- A single sheet of paper provides all the necessary information.
- Partogram facilitates the handover procedures among duty teams managing labor room.
- It serves as a document for medicolegal purpose.

ABNORMAL LABOR PATTERNS

A labor pattern that does not follow the usual pattern of normal labor is termed abnormal labor. Abnormal labor patterns are described as follows:

- Protraction disorders: Labor progresses slowly
- Arrest disorders: Labor comes to a stop

Types of dysfunctional labor

- **Primary dysfunctional labor:** Primary dysfunctional labor is when the dysfunctional labor pattern starts after a normal latent phase. This is the commonest abnormal labor pattern.
- **Secondary dysfunctional or arrest of labor:** Secondary dysfunctional labor is when the active phase of labor commences normally, but stops or slows down significantly before full dilatation of the cervix.

Abnormal labor patterns are classified as mentioned in Table 35.2.

OBSTRUCTED LABOR

Definition When the progressive descent of the presenting part is arrested due to some mechanical obstruction, in spite of adequate uterine contractions, it is termed obstructed labor.

Common causes of obstructed labor

- Contracted pelvis and cephalopelvic disproportion (CPD)
- Malpresentations or malpositions—transverse lie, brow presentation, and occipito posterior position
- Fetal malformations—hydrocephalus

Complications in a neglected case of obstructed labor

See Table 35.3

Management of obstructed labor

Prevention Partogram for management of labor can identify dysfunctional labor at the earliest and timely intervention can be provided.

Actual management It includes the following:

- Resuscitation of the patient
  - Correction of dehydration—IV infusion of crystalloids (Ringer's solution)
  - Correction of electrolyte imbalance
  - Control of sepsis (intravenous antibiotics)
  - Blood grouping, typing, and cross-matching and reservation
- Obstetric management

Table 35.2 Abnormal labor patterns

Abnormal labor pattern	Definition	Common causes	Management
Disorders of the first stage of labor			
Prolonged latent phase	Prolonged latent phase is defined as that which lasts for >20 hours in a primigravida and >14 hours in a multigravida		Expectant management is recommended
Protracted disorders • Protracted dilatation • Protracted descent	• Protracted dilatation is when the rate of cervical dilatation is <1.2 cm/h in a primigravida and <1.5 cm/h in a multigravida • Protracted descent is when the rate of descent of fetal head is <1 cm/h in a primigravida and <2 cm/h in a multigravida	Hypotonic uterine dysfunction, malposition, big baby, and CPD	• Abdominal and vaginal examinations are done to assess uterine contractions, to exclude malposition, big baby, and CPD • In the absence of these factors, oxytocin augmentation with ARM achieves vaginal delivery in most of the cases
Arrest disorders • Arrest of dilatation • Arrest of descent (the cutoff limits for arrest disorders are the same for both primigravida and multigravida) • Prolonged deceleration phase	• Arrest of dilation is diagnosed when there is no dilation of the cervix for a period of >2 hours in a woman in active phase of labor, despite adequate uterine contractions • Arrest of descent is diagnosed when there is no descent of the presenting part for a period of >1 hour, despite adequate uterine contractions • Prolonged deceleration phase is that which lasts for >3 hours in primigravida and >1 hour in multigravida	Malposition, big baby, and CPD (in arrest disorders, hypotonic uterine dysfunction may be the result of obstruction; hence, augmentation should be done with caution)	• Abdominal and vaginal examinations are done to exclude malposition, big baby, and CPD • Inadequate uterine contractions: Oxytocin augmentation is successful • Fetal malposition, CPD: Cesarean section is indicated
Disorders of the second stage			
• Protracted descent • Arrest of descent	• Descent of <1 cm/h in a primigravida and <2 cm/h in multigravida • No progress in descent for >2 hours in primigravida and >1 hour in multigravida	Big baby, malposition, CPD, and poor maternal expulsive forces (hypotonic uterine dysfunction may be the result of obstruction)	• Exclude CPD and malposition • If CPD has been ruled out, judicious use of oxytocin and encouraging maternal expulsive efforts may achieve vaginal delivery • Instrumental delivery—if the head is below the level of ischial spines • Cesarean section—if there is CPD or malposition

ARM, artificial rupture of membranes; *CPD*, cephalopelvic disproportion.

Table 35.3 Maternal and fetal complications of obstructed labor

Maternal complications	Fetal complications
• Immediate complications – Dehydration – Metabolic ketoacidosis – Genital tract sepsis – Rupture of the uterus – Postpartum hemorrhage – Maternal death • Late complications – Genital tract fistula: Vesicovaginal fistula, rectovaginal fistula	• Asphyxia • Acidosis • Intracranial hemorrhage • Infection • Increased perinatal morbidity and mortality • Fetal death

High-yield points

I stage of labor

Latent phase

Normal duration: <20 hours in primigravida; <14 hours in multigravida

Active phase

Slope of dilatation

Normal dilatation: 1.2 cm/h in primigravida; 1.5 cm/h in multigravida

Slope of descent

Normal descent: >1 cm/h in primigravida; >2 cm/h in multigravida

II stage of labor

Normal duration: 2 hours if no regional anesthesia is used and 3 hours with regional anesthesia in a primigravida; 1 hour if no regional anesthesia is used and 2 hours with regional anesthesia in a multigravida.

A slope that is below these limits characterizes a labor with protracted dilatation or descent.

– Cesarean section is performed if the baby is alive.
– Vaginal delivery can be done in a dead fetus by performing destructive operations or else cesarean section is performed.

EXAMPLES OF INTERPRETATION OF PARTOGRAM

Partogram 1

Case summary

Mrs. ABC, 26 years of age, G2P1L1 at 39 + 2 weeks, was admitted at 11 pm on February 22nd with labor pains and spontaneous rupture of membranes 1 hour prior to admission. Her first pregnancy was a spontaneous vaginal delivery. On examination, uterine contractions were mild (one to two per 10 minutes) and FHR was 130 bpm and regular. Pelvic examination revealed the following: cervix 50% effaced, os 2 cm dilated, and membranes absent with clear liquor draining. Her partograph is shown in Figure 35.4.

Q1. What was the cervical dilatation at 1 am?
Ans. Cervix was 4 cm dilated.

Q2. How long did the patient take to enter the active phase of labor?
Ans. During admission at 11 pm, cervix was 2 cm dilated, and by 1 am, cervix was 4 cm dilated. The patient entered the active phase of labor by 2 hours since admission.

Q3. What should be the normal rate of cervical dilatation for the patient?
Ans. As the patient is G2P1L1, the cervical dilatation should ideally be 1.5 cm/h.

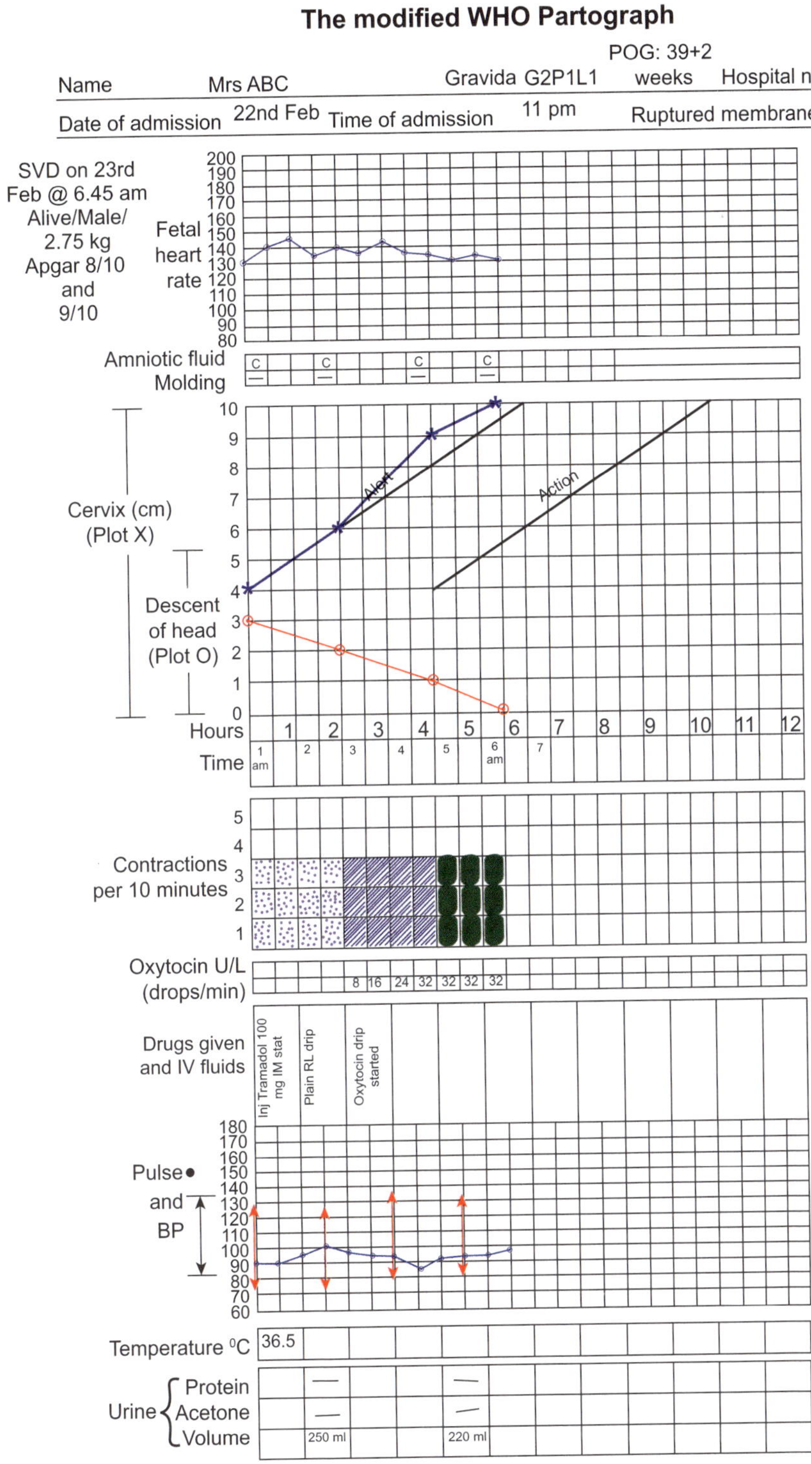

Figure 35.4 Partogram 1.

Q4. When did the patient become fully dilated?
Ans. At 6 am, the patient became fully dilated.

Q5. What was the duration of the active phase of labor?
Ans. It was 5 hours (from 1 to 6 am).

Q6. What was the level of fetal head when the patient was admitted?
Ans. Head was three-fifth palpable above the brim (Crichton method). Head was not engaged at the time of admission.

Q7. How were the uterine contractions during the course of labor?
Ans. During the initial 2 hours of active labor, contractions were mild, each lasting <20 seconds; for the next 2 hours, the frequency of uterine contractions was three per 10 minutes, each lasting for 20–40 second; in the last 1 hour, contractions were strong, each lasting for >40 seconds.

Q8. How was the FHR during the course of labor?
Ans. During the entire course of labor, the FHR varied from 130 to 140 bpm. There was no bradycardia or tachycardia or any FHR irregularity.

Q9. Did the patient require any augmentation of labor?
Ans. Yes. Augmentation of uterine contractions was done with oxytocin drip.

Q10. How was the blood pressure of the patient during the course of labor?
Ans. BP remained between 110/70 and 120/80 mmHg.

Partogram 2

Interpret the partogram given in Figure 35.5.

Q1. What was the cervical dilatation at 11 am?
Ans. Cervix was 4 cm dilated.

Q2. Comment on the rate of cervical dilatation.
Ans. The rate of cervical dilatation expected in a primigravida in the active phase of labor is 1 cm/h. Cervix was 4 cm dilated at 9 am. The patient should have entered the second stage at 3 pm, if the dilatation proceeded at the expected rate, but the patient was only 6 cm dilated at 3 pm and the graph had touched the action line. This patient had a protracted cervical dilatation from 9 am to 3 pm. After starting oxytocin and titration of dose, the patient had effective uterine contractions and cervical dilatation progressed and she was in the second stage at 6 pm.

Q3. What was the duration of the active phase of labor?
Ans. It was 9 hours (9 am to 6 pm).

Q4. What was the level of fetal head during admission?
Ans. Head was three-fifth palpable above the pelvic brim (Crichton method). It was not engaged at the time of admission.

Q5. How were the uterine contractions during the course of labor?
Ans. During the initial 4 hours of active labor, contractions were mild, each lasting <20 seconds; for the next 2 hours, the frequency of uterine contractions was three per 10 minutes, each lasting about 20–40 seconds. In the last 3 hours, contractions were strong, each lasting for >40 seconds.

Q6. How was the FHR during the course of labor?
Ans. During the entire course of labor, the FHR varied from 130 to 140 bpm. There was no bradycardia or tachycardia or any FHR irregularity.

Q7. Did the patient require any augmentation of labor?
Ans. Yes. Augmentation was done with oxytocin drip to achieve effective uterine contractions.

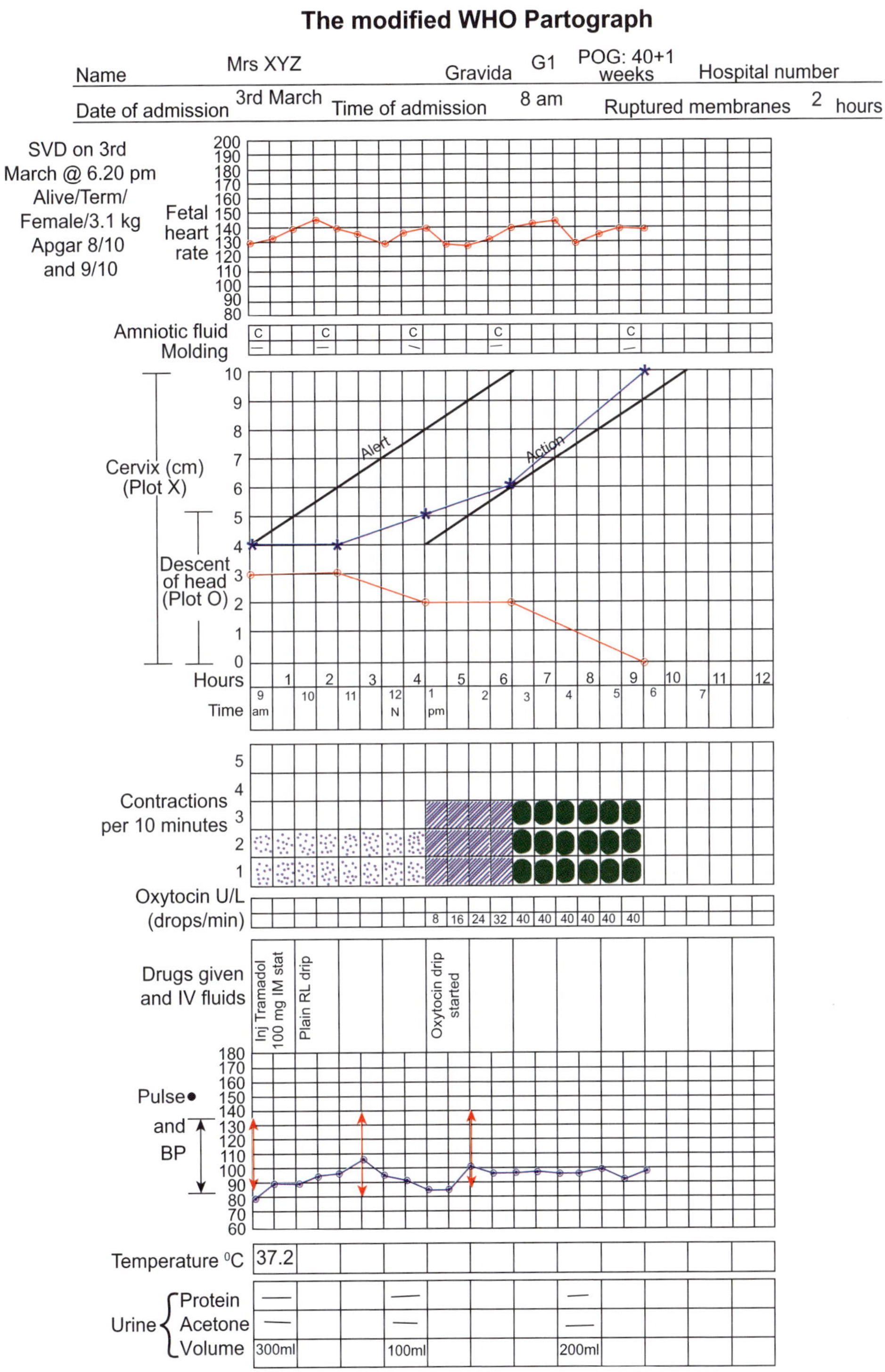

Figure 35.5 Partogram 2.

Partogram 3

Case summary

Mrs. YYY, 30 years of age, a primigravida, was admitted in labor at term pregnancy. Her partograph is shown in Figure 35.6.

Q1. Discuss the partograph observation of the patient during admission at 1 pm.

Ans. The patient had the following: (a) cervical dilatation, 4 cm; (b) fetal head, three-fifth palpable above the brim (not engaged); (c) uterine contractions, mild, each lasting for <20 seconds; (d) FHR, between 120 and 130 bpm, regular; (e) liquor, clear; and (f) blood pressure, 130/70 mmHg. She was in the active phase of labor.

Q2. Discuss the patient's labor progression observed after 4 hours of labor (at 5 pm).

Ans. (a) Cervical dilatation, 6 cm, and has crossed the alert line; (b) fetal head, two-fifth palpable; (c) uterine contractions, three in 10 minutes, each lasting for 20–40 seconds; (d) FHR, 120–130 bpm; (e) liquor, clear; and (f) molding, absent.

Comments Cervical dilatation increased by 2 cm over a period of 4 hours, which was less than expected (normal rate for primigravida is 1 cm/h). Cervicograph is on the right side of the alert line. Uterine contractions were inadequate and hence oxytocin drip started.

Q3. Discuss the partograph as recorded during the course of labor at 10 pm.

Ans. (a) Cervix, fully dilated for 1 hour since 9 pm; (b) fetal head, two-fifth above the brim, no descent at all; (c) uterine contractions, three to four in 10 minutes, each lasting >40 seconds; (d) FHR, bradycardia up to 100 bpm; (e) liquor, clear; and (f) molding, grade 2.

Comments The patient had no further descent of fetal head since the last observation at 5 pm. Fetal bradycardia and molding were observed. Partographic analysis of labor revealed full dilatation of cervix with arrest of descent despite adequate uterine contractions. This indicates that labor is obstructed probably due to CPD. Due to this observation, labor was terminated by emergency cesarean section at 10.15 pm.

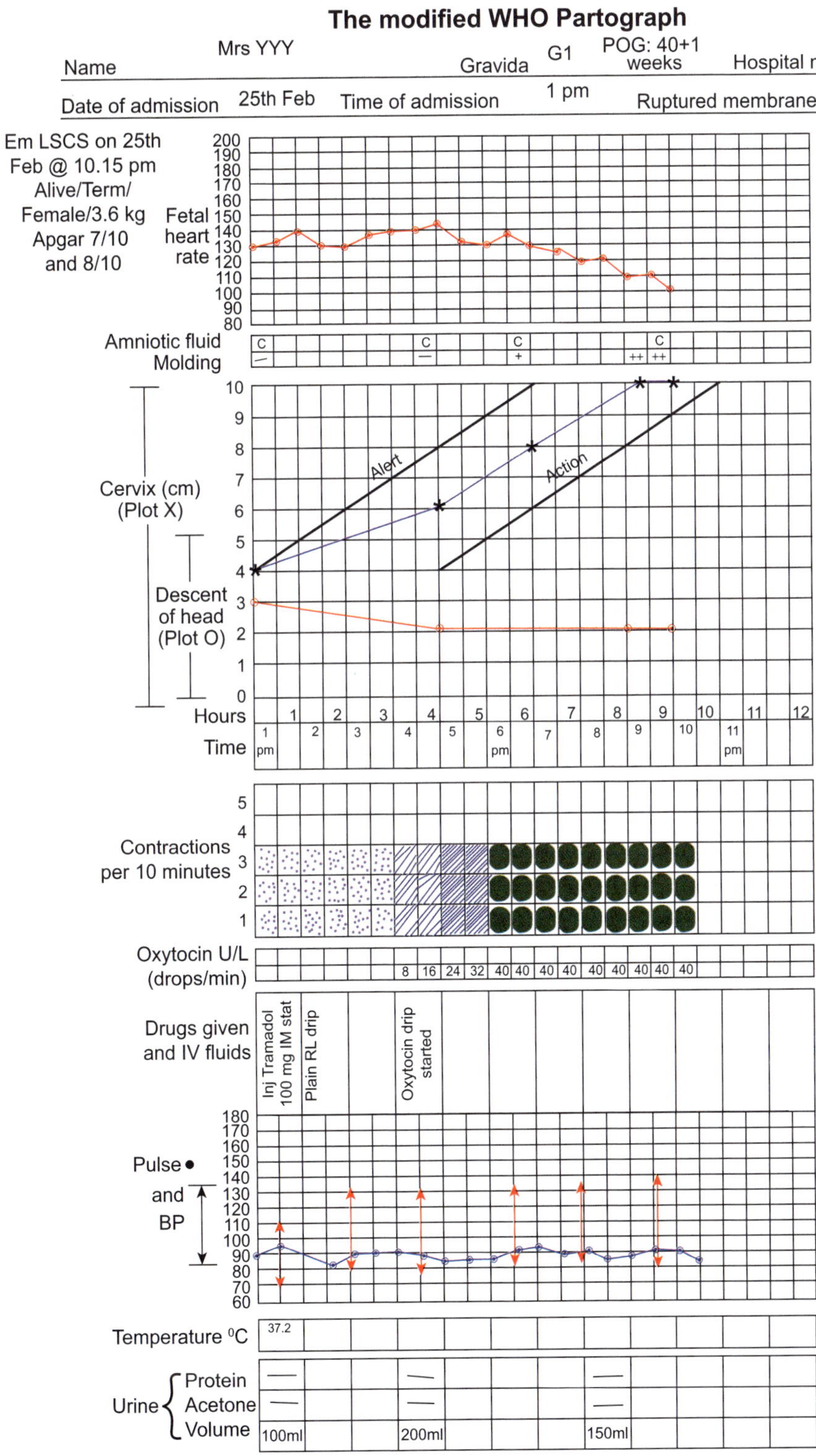

Figure 35.6 Partogram 3.

Partogram 4

Case summary

Mrs. LMN, 28 years of age, a primigravida, was admitted in labor at term pregnancy. Her partograph is shown in Figure 35.7.

Q1. Discuss the partographic observation of the patient during admission at 6 am.

Ans. The patient had the following: (a) cervical dilatation, 4 cm; (b) fetal head, five-fifth palpable above the brim (free floating); (c) uterine contractions, three per 10 minutes, each lasting for 20–40 seconds; (d) FHR, between 120 and 130 bpm, regular; (e) liquor, clear; and (6) blood pressure, 120/70 mmHg. She was in the active phase of labor.

Q2. Discuss the patient's labor progression observed after 4 hours of labor (at 10 am).

Ans. (a) Cervical dilatation, 6 cm, and has crossed the alert line; (b) fetal head, still four-fifth above brim; (c) uterine contractions, three in 10 minutes, each lasting for 20–40 seconds; (d) FHR, 120–130 bpm; (e) liquor, clear; and (f) molding, absent.

Comments Cervical dilatation increased by 2 cm over a period of 4 hours, which was less than expected (normal is 1 cm/h). Cervicograph is on the right side of the alert line. Uterine contractions were inadequate and oxytocin drip was started.

Q3. Discuss the partograph as recorded during the course of labor at 2 pm.

Ans. (a) Cervical dilatation, 6 cm, has crossed the action line; (b) fetal head, three-fifth above the brim, no descent at all; (c) uterine contractions three in 10 minutes, each lasting >40 seconds (d) FHR, significant bradycardia, <110 bpm (e) liquor, meconium stained; and (f) grade 2 molding present.

Comments The patient had slow dilatation of cervix since the beginning of active phase and no further dilatation of the cervix since the last observation at 10 am (4 hours) and there was no descent of the presenting part. Fetal bradycardia, meconium-stained liquor, and molding of head were observed. Partographic analysis of labor revealed arrest of dilatation and descent in the active phase of labor despite adequate uterine contractions. This indicates that labor is obstructed most likely due to CPD. Due to this observation of arrest of dilatation and descent, with the presence of fetal distress, labor was terminated by emergency cesarean section at 2.15 pm.

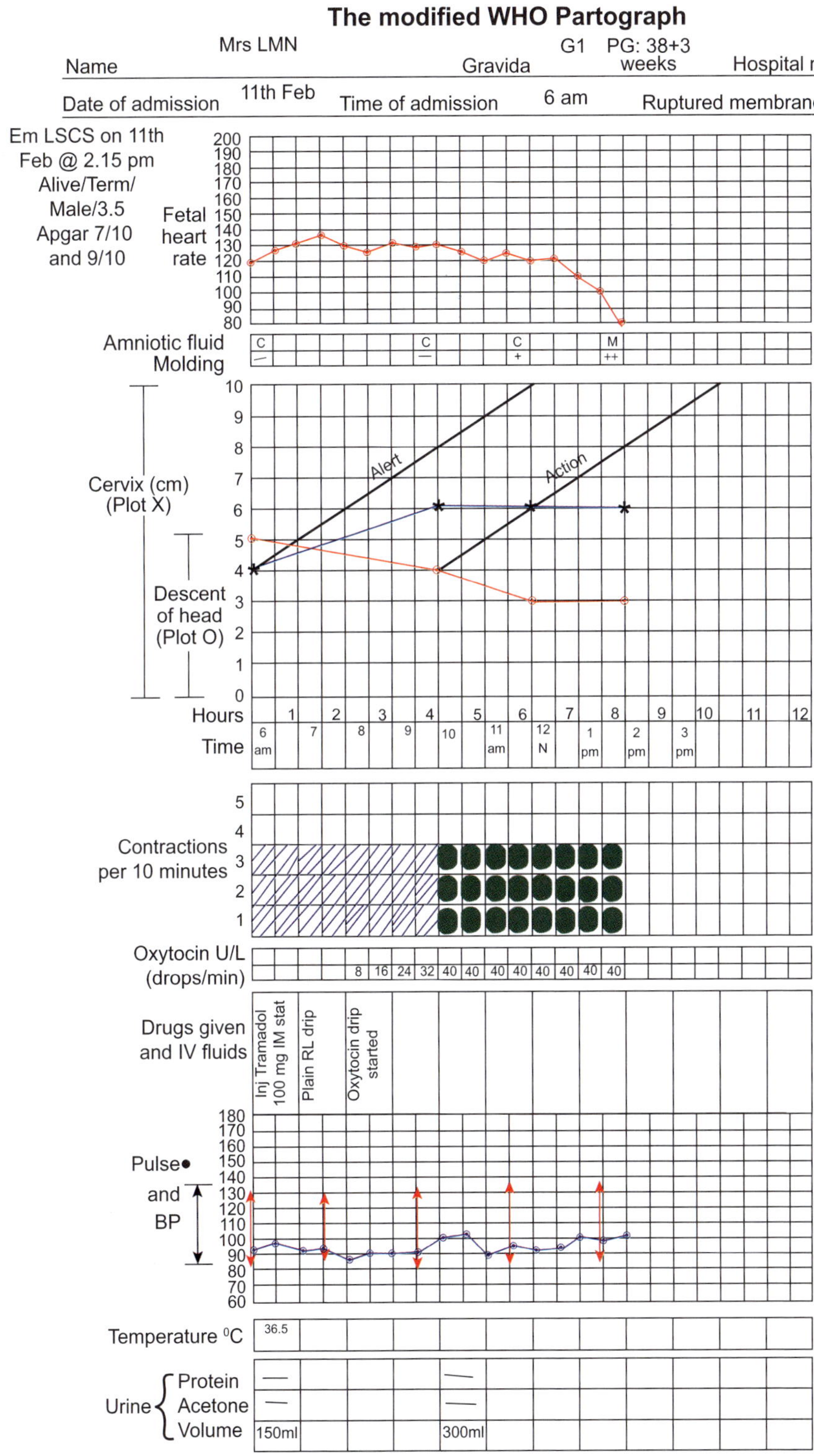

Figure 35.7 Partogram 4.

Partogram 5

Case summary

Mrs. PQY, 24 years of age, a primigravida, was admitted in labor at term pregnancy. Her partograph is shown in Figure 35.8.

Q1. Discuss the partographic observation of the patient during admission at 10 am.

Ans. The patient had the following: (a) cervical dilatation, 4 cm; (b) fetal head, three-fifth palpable above the brim; (c) uterine contractions, three in 10 minutes, each lasting for <20 seconds; (d) FHR, between 120 and 130 bpm, regular; and (e) blood pressure, 120/70 mmHg. She was in the active phase of labor.

Q2. Discuss the patient's labor progression observed after 4 hours of labor (at 2 pm).

Ans. (a) Cervical dilatation, 5 cm dilated, and has crossed the alert line; (b) fetal head, two-fifth above brim; (c) uterine contractions, three in 10 minutes, each lasting for <20 seconds; (d) FHR, 120–130 bpm; (e) liquor, clear; and (f) molding, absent.

Comments Cervical dilatation had increased by only 1 cm over a period of 4 hours, which was less than expected (normal is 1 cm/h). Cervicograph is on the right side of the alert line. Uterine contractions were inadequate and oxytocin drip was started.

Q3. Discuss the patient's labor progress observed at 6 pm.

Ans. (a) Cervical dilatation, 5 cm, and has crossed the action line; (b) fetal head, two-fifth above the brim, no descent at all; (c) uterine contractions, three in 10 minutes, each lasting <20 seconds; (d) FHR, significant bradycardia, up to 90 bpm; and (e) liquor, meconium stained.

Comments The patient had no further dilatation of the cervix since the last observation at 2 pm and there was no descent of the presenting part. Fetal bradycardia and meconium-stained liquor were observed. Uterine contractions were inadequate despite titrating the dose of oxytocin. Partogram revealed arrest of dilatation and descent in the active phase of labor with inefficient uterine contractions. In view of this observation, along with the presence of fetal distress, labor was terminated by emergency cesarean section at 6.20 pm.

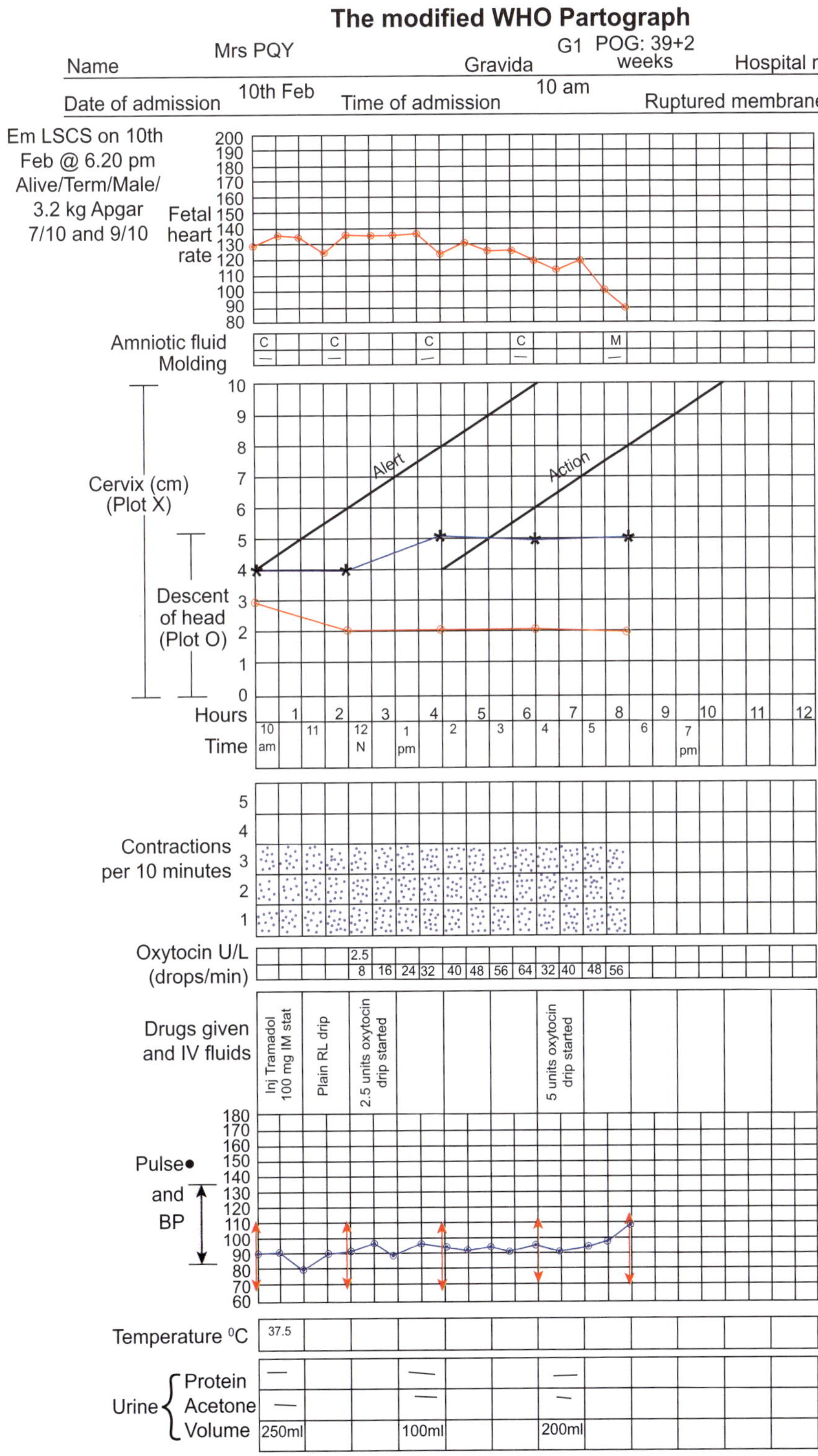

Figure 35.8 Partogram 5.

36 Antepartum and Intrapartum Fetal Surveillance Tests

Introduction

Assessment of fetal well-being is done during the antenatal period and in labor to prevent fetal death and adverse perinatal outcomes. Fetal heart rate (FHR) monitoring is a valuable method of assessment of fetal well-being. The various antepartum and intrapartum fetal surveillance tests are discussed in this chapter. Medical students are expected to be familiar with interpretation of abnormal FHR patterns during pregnancy and labor.

ANTEPARTUM FETAL SURVEILLANCE

Indications

The indications for antepartum fetal surveillance (APFS) include pregnancies with an increased risk for stillbirth such as the following:

- Severe preeclampsia
- Chronic hypertension
- Overt diabetes and gestational diabetes mellitus (GDM)
- Intrauterine growth restriction (IUGR)
- Oligohydramnios/polyhydramnios
- Post-term pregnancy
- Decreased fetal movements
- Multiple pregnancy with discordance in growth
- Previous bad obstetric history such as IUGR and stillbirth
- Maternal vascular diseases
- Advanced maternal age

Antepartum fetal surveillance tests

Fetal well-being during pregnancy can be assessed by several tests. Biochemical tests such as estimation of urinary estriol were used earlier, but have now been replaced by various biophysical tests. The various biophysical tests for fetal well-being include the following:

- Daily fetal movement count (DFMC)
- Nonstress test (NST)
- Vibroacoustic stimulation test
- Contraction stress test (CST)
- Ultrasound assessment of amniotic fluid index (AFI)
- Biophysical profile (BPP)—combination of ultrasonography variables and NST includes the following:
  - Fetal breathing movement
  - Fetal body movement
  - Fetal tone
  - Amniotic fluid volume (AFV)
  - NST
- Doppler ultrasonography of fetal vessels
  - Fetal umbilical artery Doppler
  - Fetal middle cerebral artery (MCA) Doppler
  - Fetal ductus venosus and inferior vena cava (IVC) Doppler

Principle involved in the biophysical tests for antepartum fetal surveillance

- APFS tests are based on fetal biophysical activities that are initiated and regulated through the fetal central nervous system (CNS).
- The fetal CNS is very sensitive to diminished oxygenation. Hypoxia → leads to metabolic acidosis → leads to CNS depression → leads to changes in fetal biophysical activity.
- APFS tests are usually initiated in the third trimester, as the fetus may not respond appropriately in early gestation due to neurophysiological immaturity.

Initiation of antepartum fetal surveillance

- APFS is individualized and initiated depending on the severity of the risk factors associated with the pregnancy.
- There is no specific gestational age cutoff at which it should be initiated.
- APFS tests at 32–34 weeks of gestation are appropriate for most of the high-risk pregnancies such as GDM and preeclampsia.
- When IUGR is diagnosed, a baseline APFS is done and then repeated at regular intervals for follow-up.
- If patient C/o decreased or absent fetal movements in the third trimester, then APFS is initiated immediately.
- If there is H/o of bad obstetric outcome such as stillbirth in the previous pregnancy, then APFS is initiated 2 weeks prior to the gestational age at which the previous adverse event had occurred.
- In a postdated pregnancy, APFS tests such as NST and assessment of AFI are initiated at 40 weeks.
- The frequency of monitoring is usually twice weekly; however, more frequent monitoring may be required in high-risk cases.

The various biophysical tests that are used for APFS are described in the next subsections.

Daily fetal movement count

- It is the simplest method of fetal well-being assessment.
- A pregnant woman usually starts perceiving fetal movements at approximately 18–20 weeks' gestation. Fetus normally has a sleep–wake cycle and a woman usually perceives 80% of fetal movements.

Principle The fetus decreases gross body movements in the presence of fetal hypoxia and placental dysfunction, to conserve oxygen. Decreased fetal movements may precede intrauterine fetal death.

Procedure Women should be taught one of the methods of counting fetal movements as mentioned in Table 36.1 and advised to report decreased fetal movements.

Further management of reduced fetal movements If a patient reports decreased fetal movements, further biophysical tests such as NST and assessment of AFI should be carried out.

Nonstress test

- Continuous recording of the FHR is termed cardiotocography (CTG) and NST is performed using an external CTG. In NST, the FHR is recorded in the absence of contractions and accelerations of the FHR are looked for.
- It is a relatively quick, noninvasive test without discomfort or risk to the mother and fetus.

Principle

The NST is based on the principle that the heart rate of the healthy fetus will temporarily accelerate with fetal movement. The presence of accelerations with fetal movements is called reactivity. A fetus that is acidotic or neurologically depressed will not show accelerations on NST.

Procedure

- The patient should be in lateral recumbent or reclining position in order to avoid supine hypotension in the mother.

Table 36.1 Methods for fetal movement count

Method	Procedure	Interpretation
"Cardiff's fetal kick count to 10" method	The patient is asked to count the fetal movements starting from a particular time of the day up to perception of 10 fetal movements	Lack of perception of 10 movements within a 12-hour time period requires further evaluation
Sadowsky's count	The patient is asked to count the fetal movements for a period of 1 hour after all three meals in a day. The total number of movements is multiplied by 4 to get the fetal movement count over a period of 12 hours	Lack of perception of 10 movements within a 12-hour time period requires further evaluation

- An external transducer is placed on the maternal abdomen, after applying jelly that facilitates better apposition and conduction of signal. The FHR is monitored and the fetal movements perceived by the mother are recorded. The FHR trace is recorded on a graph for at least 20 minutes.

The parameters that are assessed in a NST are mentioned in Table 36.2.

Interpretation of nonstress test

NST is interpreted as reactive or nonreactive as mentioned in Table 36.3.

Evaluation of a nonreactive nonstress test A nonreactive NST may be due to fetal sleep or prematurity but may be indicative of fetal hypoxia, acidosis, or fetal sepsis. Hence, a nonreactive NST needs further evaluation and should be followed by further tests of fetal well-being.

Predictive value of a nonstress test

- NST predicts the fetal status for the next 72 hours; hence, in high-risk pregnancies such as GDM, severe preeclampsia, and post-term pregnancy, NST should be performed twice weekly.
- A reactive NST has a false-negative rate of 0.2–0.8% and hence has high negative predictive value.
- A nonreactive NST has a false-positive rate of 50%. Hence, nonreactive NST should be evaluated further and the management decisions should not be based on the NST alone.
- NST reflects the current fetal status and cannot predict future events or neonatal outcome.
- NST cannot predict sudden events such as placental abruption or cord accidents.

Table 36.2 Parameters assessed in a nonstress test

Parameter	Definition	Normal value
Baseline FHR	• It is the mean level of FHR between the peaks and depressions. It is expressed as beats per minute • Baseline FHR should be determined over a minimum period of 10 minutes	Normal baseline FHR after 30 weeks' gestation is 110–160 bpm
Baseline variability	It is the oscillation of baseline FHR excluding the accelerations and decelerations	Normal variability is 5–25 bpm
Acceleration	• It is the increase in FHR by 15 bpm or more, lasting for at least 15 seconds or more (after 32 weeks' gestation) • It indicates fetal well-being	Two accelerations in 20 minutes
Deceleration	• It is the decrease in FHR below the baseline by 15 bpm or more, lasting for ≥15 seconds in duration • Decelerations may be early, late, or variable in relation to a uterine contraction	No decelerations

FHR, fetal heart rate.

Table 36.3 Interpretation of NST

Interpretation	Criteria
Reactive NST	• NST is considered reactive if it has all the following features (Figure 36.1): – FHR between 110 and 160 bpm – Normal beat-to-beat variability (5–25 bpm) – Two accelerations of at least 15 bpm above baseline, lasting for at least 15 seconds within a 20-minute observation period – No decelerations The duration of the NST should be extended to 40 minutes, if there are no FHR accelerations
Nonreactive NST	A nonreactive NST is defined as one that does not show accelerations over a 40-minute observation period

FHR, fetal heart rate; *NST*, nonstress test.

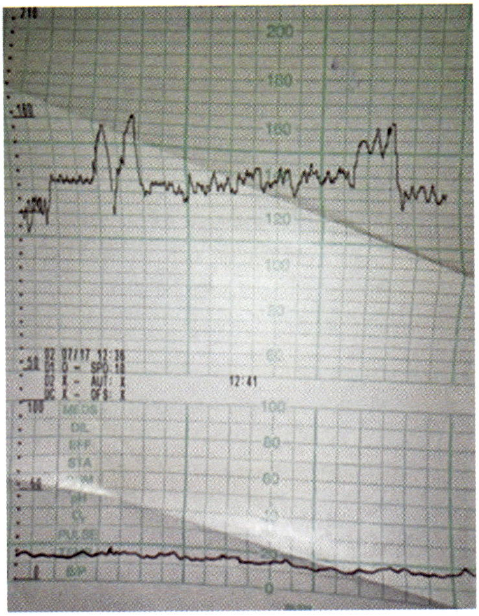

Figure 36.1 An example of a reactive nonstress test.

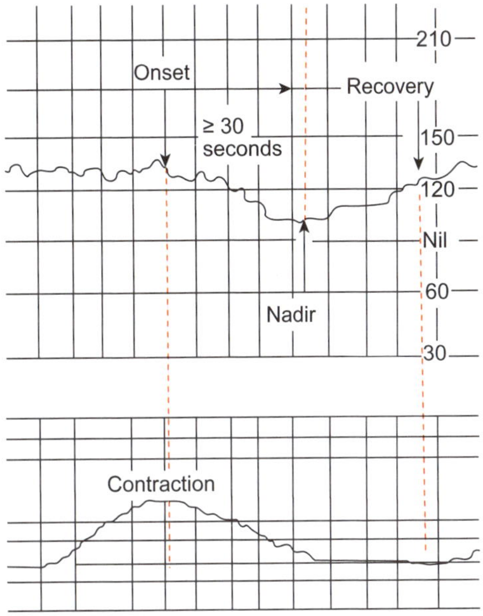

Figure 36.2 Graph showing late decelerations (top) in relation with uterine contractions (bottom).

Vibroacoustic stimulation test

- Auditory stimulus to the fetus can alert a sleeping or inactive fetus resulting in FHR acceleration.
- A short burst of sound is delivered to the fetus for few seconds, through an acoustic stimulator placed on the maternal abdomen.
- This test can be used to reduce the duration of performing a NST.

Contraction stress test

CST is performed using a CTG where the response of the FHR is noted in relation to induced uterine contractions. The FHR is recorded in the presence of induced uterine contractions.

Principle

During uterine contraction, there is a transient decrease in fetal oxygenation. A healthy fetoplacental unit has sufficient reserve to tolerate this short reduction in oxygen supply. If a fetus is already hypoxemic, the intermittent reduction in oxygenation during uterine contraction will result in fetal hypoxia and late decelerations of the FHR.

Late deceleration Under hypoxic conditions, FHR begins to decelerate 15–30 seconds after onset of the contraction, reaches its nadir after the peak of the contraction, and does not return to baseline until after the contraction ends. This FHR pattern is known as a late deceleration (Figure 36.2).

Procedure

- The patient lies in the lateral recumbent position.
- FHR and uterine contractions are simultaneously recorded with an external transducer placed on maternal abdomen.
- Contractions are induced with either nipple stimulation or intravenous administration of dilute oxytocin till there are at least three contractions of 40 seconds' duration within a 10-minute period.
- Any late decelerations associated with uterine contractions are looked for.
- Interpretation of a CST is mentioned in Table 36.4 (Figure 36.3).

Complications

CST-induced contractions can lead to stimulation of regular uterine contraction—risk of preterm labor and premature rupture of membranes (PROM). Hence, CST is currently used less commonly with the availability of other modalities for fetal surveillance.

Table 36.4 Interpretation of contraction stress test (CST)

Interpretation	Criteria
Positive CST	Late decelerations following 50% or more contractions
Negative CST	Absence of late or significant variable decelerations
Suspicious CST	If there are occasional or inconsistent late decelerations
Unsatisfactory CST	If contractions cannot be stimulated or a satisfactory fetal heart rate tracing cannot be obtained
Hyperstimulated CST	If contractions occur more frequently than every 2 minutes or last longer than 90 seconds, the test cannot be interpreted

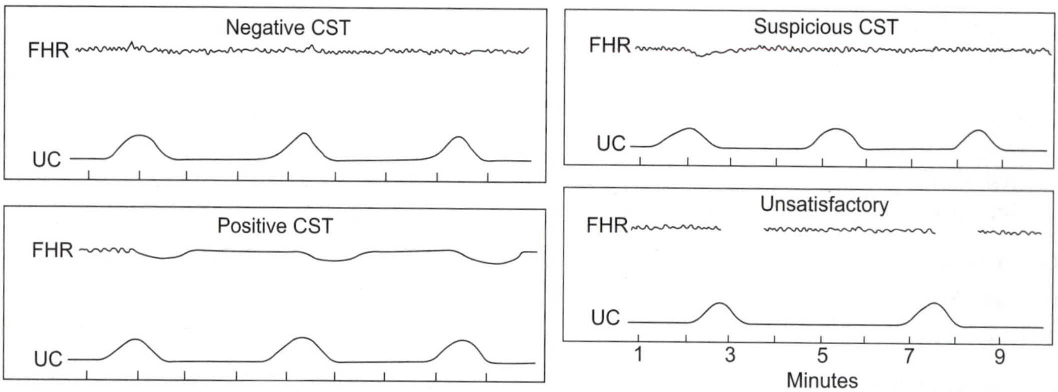

Figure 36.3 Interpretation of contraction stress test. *CST*, contraction stress test; *UC*, uterine contractions.

Contraindications

- Preterm labor or high risk for preterm labor
- Preterm premature rupture of membranes (PPROM)
- Diagnosed case of placenta previa

Predictive value of a contraction stress test

- It has a high negative predictive value. A negative CST is more reassuring than a reactive NST.
- The risk of stillbirth and neonatal mortality is high if a nonreactive NST is followed by a positive CST.
- Cesarean section for persistent late decelerations in labor may be required in one-third of patients with a positive CST.

Biophysical profile (Manning score)

The BPP is a combination of NST along with four biophysical variables measured by ultrasound examination—fetal movements, fetal breathing, fetal tone, and amniotic fluid volume (AFV). BPP is an accurate means for predicting significant fetal hypoxia and acidosis.

Principle

- Fetal biophysical activities such as body movements, breathing, FHR, and tone are regulated and controlled by fetal CNS.
- The presence of these biophysical variables implies normal oxygenation of the CNS.
- Fetal hypoxia and acidosis cause loss of FHR accelerations, decreased body and breathing movements, and hypotonia. These four variables reflect acute hypoxia. Decreased AFV reflects chronic hypoxia.

Procedure

- An ultrasound examination is done, and fetal gross body movements, breathing movements, and tone are noted and AFV is measured.
- A NST is performed using an external CTG.
- Each variable is given a score of 2 (normal) or 0 (abnormal) as mentioned in Table 36.5.

Table 36.5 Scoring of biophysical profile

Parameter	Normal (score = 2)	Abnormal (score = 0)
Nonstress test	Reactive	Nonreactive
Fetal breathing movements	≥1 episode of rhythmic fetal breathing movements within 30 minutes	No fetal breathing movements in 30 minutes
Gross body movements	≥3 discrete body or limb movements within 30 minutes	<3 movements in 30 minutes
Fetal tone	≥1 episode of extension of fetal extremity with return to flexion or opening and closing of a hand in 30 minutes	No movements or slow movements
AFV	Single vertical pocket of AFV >2 cm	No single vertical pocket of AFV is >2 cm

FV, amniotic fluid volume.

nterpretation

- Each assessment is given a score of 0 or 2 points, and then added up to get the total score between 0 and 10. The total score determines the further course of action to be taken.
- A BPP of 8 or 10 is generally considered reassuring.

Recommended management based on the biophysical profile score

See Table 36.6

Predictive value of biophysical profile

- A normal BPP correlates well with good fetal outcome and the false-negative rates are low.
- BPP <4 correlates with fetal asphyxia.
- Nonreactive NST and loss of breathing movements are the earliest manifestations of fetal hypoxia.

Disadvantage

BPP is a time-consuming test

Modified biophysical profile It may take 30–60 minutes to perform the BPP, as the fetus might be in its normal sleep cycle, and it may take time for it to become awake. To make it less time consuming, the modified biophysical profile (mBPP) was introduced. In the mBPP, only two variables are assessed: NST for acute hypoxia and AFI for chronic hypoxia.

Ultrasound assessment of amniotic fluid volume

Assessment of AFV is one of the commonly used APFS tools.

Principle

- With decrease in placental perfusion, there is reduced perfusion of fetal kidneys resulting in decrease in urine production and is reflected as oligohydramnios.

Table 36.6 Recommended management based on the BPP score

BPP score	Interpretation	Recommended management
0–2	Probable fetal asphyxia	Deliver irrespective of POG
4	Strongly suspect asphyxia	• POG >32 weeks: Deliver • POG <32 weeks: Repeat the test in 4–6 hours and deliver if BPP <6
6	Suspect fetal asphyxia	• POG >36 weeks: Deliver • POG <36 weeks: Repeat test in 4–6 hours and: – If BPP ≤6: Deliver – If BPP >6: Follow-up
8, with reduced AFV	Consider chronic hypoxia	• POG < 36 weeks: Repeat BPP at weekly intervals • POG >36 weeks with oligohydramnios: Deliver
8, with normal AFV	Low risk of developing fetal asphyxia	Follow-up
10	Low risk of developing fetal asphyxia	Follow-up

AFV, amniotic fluid volume; *BPP*, biophysical profile; *POG*, period of gestation.

- Assessment of AFV is used to evaluate chronic hypoxia in the fetus.

Procedure

Two methods are described to measure the liquor volume: single deepest pocket (SDP) and AFI.

- **SDP:** It refers to the measurement of vertical dimension of the single largest pocket of amniotic fluid, not containing umbilical cord or fetal extremities in centimeters. This measurement is usually utilized as part of the BPP.
- **AFI:** It is obtained by measuring the maximum vertical pocket of amniotic fluid in each quadrant of the abdomen in centimeters and adding up the values. This measurement is usually utilized as part of the modified BPP.

Interpretation Interpretation of the SDP and AFI measurements are given in Table 36.7.

Table 36.7 Interpretation of SDP and AFI measurements

Interpretation	SDP value (cm)	AFI value (cm)
Normal	≥2 and <8	AFI >5 and <24
Oligohydramnios	<2	≤5
Polyhydramnios	≥8	AFI ≥24

AFI, amniotic fluid index; *SDP*, single deepest pocket.

Recommended management based on amniotic fluid volume

Fetuses with oligohydramnios should be followed up with other APFS tests such as NST, BPP, and Doppler studies.

Doppler ultrasonography of fetal vessels

Doppler ultrasonography of fetal vessels is a noninvasive method to measure the resistance to blood flow in the placenta. It is the main survei lance technique in IUGR fetuses to differentiate compensated healthy fetus from a hypoxemic acidotic fetus, thereby helps in decreasing per natal mortality. The umbilical artery Doppler commonly studied.

Principle

- A healthy fetus will have a good umbilical arter diastolic flow.
- In conditions with abnormal placentatio IUGR sets in, and there may be increase resistance in the placental circulation that reflected as reduced umbilical artery diastoli flow.
- With severe growth restriction, as the placent resistance increases, the diastolic flow can b absent or even reversed, indicating severe fet hypoxia and acidosis.

Procedure

Doppler velocimetry of the umbilical artery measured using Doppler ultrasound. Peak systoli flow and end-diastolic flow in the umbilical arter are measured and various Doppler indices ar calculated such as the following:

- Systolic:diastolic ratio (S/D)
- Resistance index [(S – D)/S]
- Pulsatility index [(S – D)/mean]

Interpretation As the diastolic flow decrease the Doppler indices value increases. Hence, hig Doppler indices indicate increased resistance t blood flow.

Further management based on Dopple studies Further course of action in a case o abnormal umbilical artery Doppler is men tioned in Table 36.8.

Table 36.8 Umbilical artery Doppler interpretation and further management

Doppler indices	Interpretation	Management
Normal indices	Healthy fetus	Continue to observe with weekly Doppler studies, nonstress test, and amniotic fluid index
Absent end-diastolic flow	Ominous finding—increased risk of perinatal mortality	Immediate delivery should be considered, if beyond 34 weeks of gestation
Reversed end-diastolic flow	Preterminal event—associated with poor perinatal outcome	Immediate delivery is warranted

Doppler velocimetry of other fetal vessels

Middle cerebral artery Doppler In the presence of fetal hypoxia, there is preferential blood flow to preserve "vital" organs such as the brain, resulting in increased diastolic flow in the fetal MCA. This is termed the brain-sparing effect and is an early sign of fetal hypoxia.

Ductus venosus and IVC Doppler Abnormal waveform pattern of the fetal ductus venosus and IVC indicate cardiac compromise. It occurs late in fetal hypoxia and indicates imminent fetal demise

Predictive value of Doppler velocimetry

- Doppler studies reduce the perinatal mortality in IUGR fetuses. However, Doppler velocimetry is of little benefit in low-risk fetuses.
- It helps to decide on the time and mode of delivery, in IUGR fetuses and cases with abnormal BPP.

INTRAPARTUM FETAL SURVEILLANCE

Monitoring of the FHR is an integral part of fetus surveillance during labor. Intrapartum fetal surveillance tests are done to detect potential fetal harm due to decrease in fetal oxygenation during labor. Decreased fetal oxygenation may result in brain injury. Timely detection allows prompt intervention, thereby preventing adverse perinatal outcomes

Principle

During the course of labor, uterine contractions cause a temporary reduction in uteroplacental blood flow, thereby decreasing the oxygen delivery to the fetus. A healthy fetus usually tolerates this and shows no adverse effect. In conditions with chronic placental insufficiency such as hypertension, diabetes, and IUGR, the fetus may not tolerate the decrease in oxygenation and may show signs of hypoxia.

Aim Intrapartum fetal surveillance tests aim to identify abnormal fetal heart patterns resulting from fetal hypoxia during labor, so that timely and effective interventions can be initiated to prevent hypoxic brain injury.

Intrapartum fetal surveillance tests The various intrapartum fetal surveillance tests are mentioned in Table 36.9 and are described in the following subsections.

Intermittent auscultation of fetal heart rate

Intermittent auscultation is the recommended fetal surveillance method during labor in the absence of maternal and fetal risk factors.

Procedure

- FHR is auscultated through the maternal abdomen using devices such as Pinard fetoscope, stethoscope, or a handheld Doppler device.
- FHR is usually counted for 1 minute immediately following uterine contraction, when the fetus has been subjected to a temporary decrease in oxygenation.
- FHR has to be compared with the maternal pulse to avoid confusion.

Frequency of auscultation of fetal heart rate in labor

See Table 36.10

Table 36.9 Intrapartum fetal surveillance tests

Noninvasive methods	Invasive methods
• Intermittent auscultation – Pinard fetoscope – Stethoscope – Handheld Doppler device • Cardiotocography or electronic FHR monitoring	• Scalp electrode FHR monitoring • Fetal scalp blood sampling – Scalp pH – Fetal lactate concentration • Fetal electrocardiography • Fetal pulse oximetry

FHR, fetal heart rate.

Table 36.10 Frequency of FHR monitoring during labor by intermittent auscultation

Stage of labor	FHR monitoring in low-risk cases	FHR monitoring in high-risk cases
I stage (active phase)	Every 30 minutes	Every 15 minutes
II stage	Every 15 minutes	Every 5 minutes

FHR, fetal heart rate.

Interpretation

- When FHR remains normal following a contraction, it establishes the ability of the fetus to withstand labor contractions.
- When FHR drops following a contraction, it indicates a decompensated fetus.

Disadvantages

- It may be difficult to auscultate the FHR in obese women and in polyhydramnios cases.
- It is not possible to distinguish the various types of decelerations.
- Baseline FHR variability, which is a marker for the presence or absence of fetal hypoxia, cannot be made out with intermittent auscultation.

Cardiotocography

- Electronic monitoring of FHR is done to observe the response of FHR to uterine contractions during labor.
- CTG is widely being used, although its role in reducing perinatal mortality is not better than that of intermittent auscultation of FHR in low risk cases.

Indications

Continuous electronic monitoring of the fetus is recommended in high-risk cases such as the following:

- IUGR
- Severe preeclampsia/GDM
- Vaginal birth after cesarean (VBAC)
- Previous intrapartum asphyxia/death
- Chorioamnionitis
- Oligohydramnios
- Multiple pregnancy
- Prematurity
- Post-term pregnancy
- Meconium-stained liquor

In low-risk cases, either continuous electronic monitoring or intermittent auscultation of FHR is an acceptable method.

Procedure

FHR is detected with an external transducer and uterine contractions are detected with an external tocodynamometer, both placed on the maternal abdomen with the help of elastic belts. A graphic tracing of the FHR and uterine contractions are obtained and studied.

Advantages and disadvantages of cardiotocography

See Table 36.11

Table 36.11 Advantages and disadvantages of cardiotocography

Advantages	Disadvantages
• Detects fetal hypoxia • Decreases perinatal mortality • Serves as a document for medicolegal purpose	• High false-positive reports result in an increased rate of operative interferences • Expensive • Interpretation of the tracing requires trained personnel

Note

- *CTG is useful in assessing FHR patterns in the presence of meconium-stained liquor or when FHR abnormalities are detected with intermittent auscultation. In these situations, a reassuring FHR tracing allows the obstetrician to continue monitoring the labor without any intervention.*
- *CTG has not shown to improve perinatal outcome in low-risk women.*

High-yield points

Admission test

On admission to labor room, all women are subjected to electronic FHR monitoring for 20 minutes termed the admission test. Based on this trace, a decision is made regarding the need for continuous electronic FHR monitoring in labor.

The fetus is considered to be healthy and capable of withstanding labor if the CTG is reassuring, which is indicated by the following criteria:

- Baseline FHR between 110 and 160 bpm
- Baseline variability >5 bpm
- Two accelerations in 20-minute observation
- No decelerations

Methods to monitor uterine activity

- **Noninvasive method:** A tocodynamometer strapped to the maternal abdomen records the intensity, duration, and number of uterine contractions.
- **Invasive method:** Intrauterine pressure catheter can be inserted following rupture of membranes to directly record the pressure during uterine contraction. It is a very accurate method but not used often due to risk of infections.

Interpretation of cardiotocography

The parameters used for interpretation of CTG include those given in the next subsections.

Baseline fetal heart rate

Normal baseline FHR is between 110 and 160 bpm.

Fetal bradycardia It is defined as FHR <110 bpm. Causes are mentioned in Table 36.12.

Table 36.12 Causes of fetal bradycardia

Fetal causes	Maternal causes
• Fetal hypoxia and acidosis • Sepsis • Fetal heart conduction defects (can occur in maternal systemic lupus erythematosus)	Drugs to mother—pethidine, methyldopa, propranolol, and $MgSO_4$

Fetal tachycardia It is defined as FHR >160 bpm. Causes are mentioned in Table 36.13.

Table 36.13 Causes of fetal tachycardia

Fetal causes	Maternal causes
• Arrhythmias • Infections • Anemia	• Maternal fever • Chorioamnionitis • Hyperthyroidism • Drugs (beta-sympathomimetics used for management of preterm labor—isoxsuprine, ritodrine)

Beat-to-beat variability

FHR of a healthy, awake, term fetus constantly varies from beat to beat by 5–25 bpm. Causes of reduced beat-to-beat variability are mentioned in Table 36.14.

Table 36.14 Causes of beat-to-beat variability

Fetal causes	Maternal causes
• Fetal hypoxia • Fetal sleep • Infections	Medications such as pethidine, propranolol, and $MgSO_4$

Accelerations

Accelerations are transient increase in the basal FHR by >15 bpm, lasting for at least 15 seconds. FHR accelerations are reassuring and rule out fetal hypoxia.

Decelerations

Deceleration of FHR is considered significant if FHR decreases by >15 bpm below baseline, lasting for >15 seconds, and is repetitive. Decelerations are classified into three types based on their relation to uterine contractions (Table 36.15 and Figures 36.4–36.7). Other types of decelerations that can also be observed in CTG trace are mentioned in Table 36.16.

Abnormal cardiotocography patterns

- Baseline FHR: <110 or >160 bpm
- Baseline variability: <5 bpm for >90 minutes or sinusoidal pattern
- Acceleration: None in 40-minute observation
- Deceleration: Late decelerations for >30 minutes or single prolonged deceleration of >3 minutes or atypical variable decelerations
- Sinusoidal pattern

Table 36.15 Types of decelerations in relation to uterine contractions

Type of decelerations	Description	Cause
Early decelerations (type I dips; Figure 36.4)	• Symmetric in shape and closely mirror uterine contractions in time of onset, duration, and ending • The nadir (the lowest point) of the deceleration coincides with the peak of the contraction	Due to fetal head compression
Late decelerations (type II dips; Figure 36.5)	• The onset, nadir, and return to baseline of the deceleration occur after the beginning, peak, and end of the contraction, respectively • The nadir of the deceleration occurs after the peak of the contraction	Due to uteroplacental insufficiency and fetal hypoxia
Variable decelerations (Figure 36.6)	Vary in shape and timing in relation to contractions	• Due to cord compression • Intermittent variable decelerations are often seen even in a normal labor, however, persistent, deep, and recurrent variable decelerations are indicative of fetal acidosis

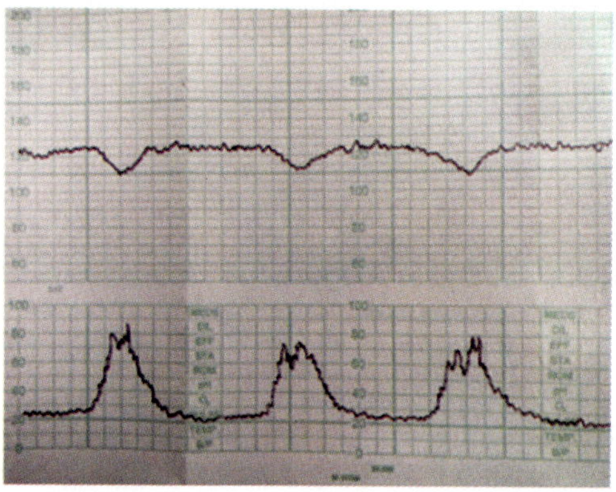

Figure 36.4 Early decelerations.

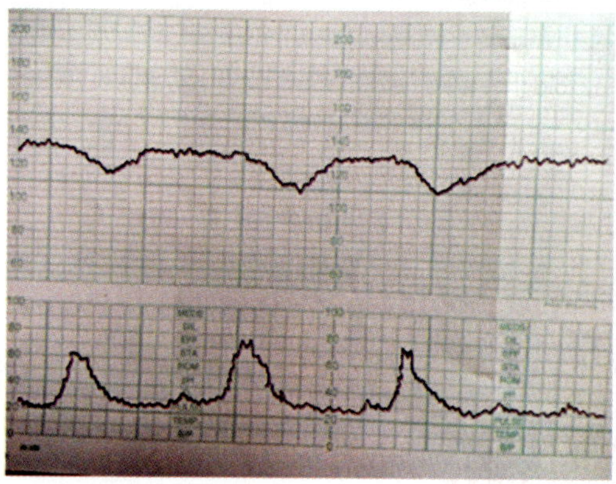

Figure 36.5 Late decelerations.

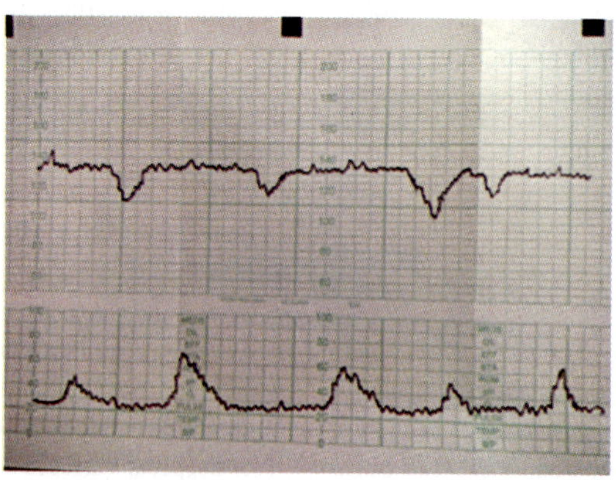

Figure 36.6 Variable decelerations.

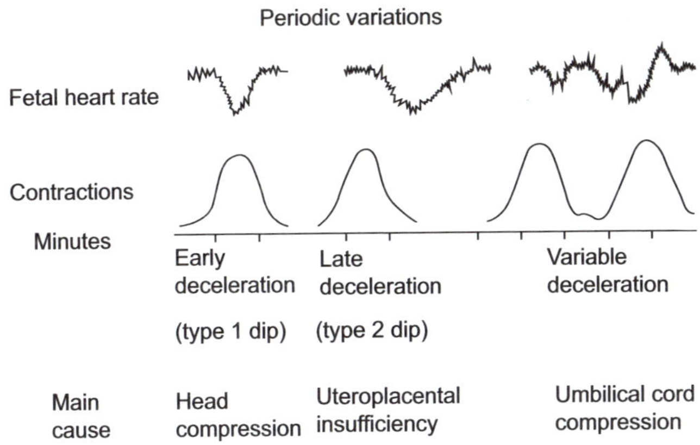

igure 36.7 Types of decelerations.

Table 36.16 Prolonged deceleration and sinusoidal pattern in cardiotocography

Type of decelerations	Description	Causes
Prolonged deceleration	It refers to decelerations that last for >2 minutes but <10 minutes. If deceleration continues for >10 minutes, it is considered as a shift of the baseline FHR (bradycardia)	• Prolonged cord compression • Severe utero placental insufficiency
Sinusoidal pattern	This is a smooth, sine wave–like undulating pattern in the baseline FHR that persists for ≥20 minutes. The characteristic features are as follows: • Baseline FHR is 120–160 bpm • Variability is markedly decreased or absent • Accelerations are absent • Cycle frequency of 3–5/min	• Fetal anemia • Severe hypoxia and acidosis

FHR, fetal heart rate.

NTERPRETATION OF INTRAPARTUM FETAL HEART RATE RECORDINGS—ACOG RECOMMENDATIONS

ee Table 36.17

Cardiotocography patterns in the second stage of labor

Variable decelerations may be associated with contractions in second stage of labor because of fetal head and cord compression. This poses difficulty in interpretation of the FHR tracing.

Patterns suggestive of fetal hypoxia in second stage of labor include the following:

- Decelerations to <70 bpm
- Loss of FHR variability
- Persistent baseline bradycardia/tachycardia

Invasive methods of intrapartum fetal surveillance

Scalp electrode fetal heart rate monitoring

It is the most accurate method for FHR monitoring.

Procedure A small electrode is fixed to the fetal scalp after the membranes are ruptured, to record the fetal electrocardiogram directly. Uterine contractions are monitored by external tocodynamometer. The FHR monitoring is displayed on a fetal monitor and recorded on a graphic paper.

Advantages and disadvantages See Table 36.18

Table 36.17 Intrapartum FHR interpretation recommended by the American College of Obstetricians and Gynecologists

	Criteria	Interpretation	Action required
Category I tracings: Reassuring/ normal	All of the following criteria must be present: • Baseline FHR 110–160 bpm • Baseline FHR variability (5–25 bpm) • Early decelerations may be present or absent • Accelerations may be present or absent • Late or variable decelerations are absent	Tracings that meet these criteria are predictive of normal fetal acid–base balance at the time of observation	Require repeated review
Category II tracing: Indeterminate/ suspicious	FHR tracings that do not meet the criteria for either category I or III are considered indeterminate		Various precipitating factors may be addressed and if unsuccessful, delivery is recommended
Category III tracings: Nonreassuring/ pathological	Include either of the following: • Absent baseline FHR variability with any of the following: – Recurrent late decelerations – Recurrent variable decelerations – Fetal bradycardia • Sinusoidal pattern	Category III tracings are predictive of abnormal fetal acid–base status at the time of observation	Prompt intervention and delivery is indicated

FHR, fetal heart rate.

Table 36.18 Advantages and disadvantages of scalp electrode FHR monitoring

Advantages	Disadvantages
• FHR monitoring is more accurate • It can be used in obese women • It can be used in active labor when use of an external transducer may be difficult due to maternal movements	• Placement of electrode requires rupture of the fetal membranes • There is risk of infection at the electrode site

FHR, fetal heart rate.

Fetal scalp blood sampling

Fetal scalp blood sampling is indicated in cases with FHR abnormality in CTG, to confirm or dismiss the presence of fetal hypoxia and/or acidosis.

Procedure

- Prerequisite: The membranes must be ruptured, cervix must be at least 4–5 cm dilated, and the vertex at –1 station or below.
- Blood sample is obtained from the fetal scalp using a lancet and is checked for pH and lactate concentration.
- The pH values are interpreted as mentioned in Table 36.19.

Disadvantages The test is cumbersome, expensive, and requires special equipment.

Fetal electrocardiography

Fetal electrocardiography can be recorded by internal fetal monitoring and a special equipment called the STAN system processes the fetal ECG. Fetal hypoxia causes ST-segment and T-wave changes in the fetal ECG. This technique is under evaluation.

Table 36.19 Interpretation of scalp pH values

pH value	Interpretation	Further management
>7.25	Normal	Continue monitoring with electronic fetal monitoring
7.25–7.2	Borderline	Repeat test in 20–30 minutes
<7.2	Acidosis	Immediate delivery is indicated

Fetal pulse oximetry

Fetal oxygen saturation (SpO_2) can be measured using a sensor introduced transcervically and positioned against the fetal face. Reduced fetal SpO_2 can be associated with fetal acidosis. As trials failed to show any additional benefit, it is not used currently.

EXAMPLES OF NONSTRESS TEST AND CARDIOTOCOGRAPHY INTERPRETATION

Nonstress test 1

Mrs. H, 24 years of age, a primigravida at 40 + 2 weeks of gestation without any obstetric and medical complications, presented for routine antenatal checkup. Her AFI was 8 and NST was done and is shown in Figure 36.8.

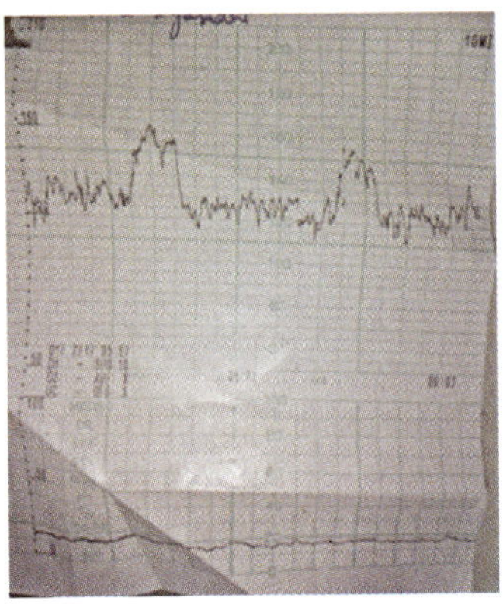

Figure 36.8 Nonstress test 1.

Q1 What is the baseline FHR?
Ans: 130 bpm.

Q2 What is the baseline variability?
Ans: 10–20 bpm.

Q3 How many accelerations are there in the trace?
Ans: Two accelerations are observed.

Q4 Are there any decelerations?
Ans: Nil.

Q5 How do you categorize this NST trace?
Ans: The NST shows a normal baseline, good baseline variability, and presence of accelerations with no decelerations indicating a reactive NST. It is a reactive NST trace indicating a healthy fetus.

Q6 What is your comment on the tocograph in the trace?
Ans: Tocograph showed absence of uterine contractions.

Nonstress test 2

Comment on the NST shown in Figure 36.9.

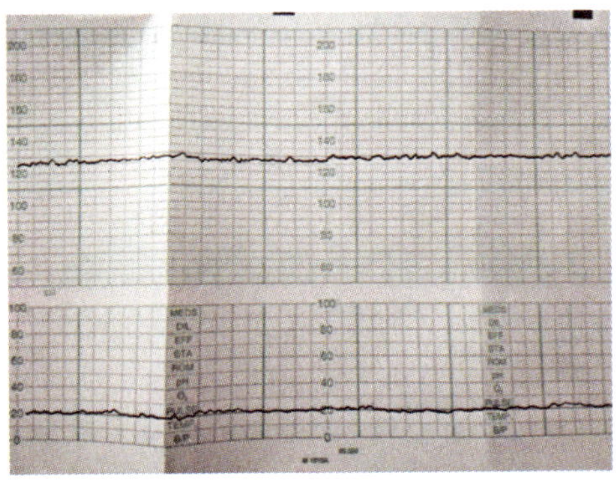

Figure 36.9 Nonstress test 2.

Ans: The NST has the following parameters:
- **Baseline FHR:** 130 bpm
- **Baseline variability:** <5 bpm
- **Accelerations:** Nil
- **Decelerations:** Nil

Interpretation: Nonreactive NST.

Next step in management: NST has to be repeated after some time on the same day. If nonreactive, it has to be followed up with further tests for fetal well-being.

Nonstress test 3

Mrs. S, 28 years of age, G1 at 37 weeks of gestation, presented to OPD with complaints of decreased fetal movements. NST was done and is shown in Figure *36.10.*

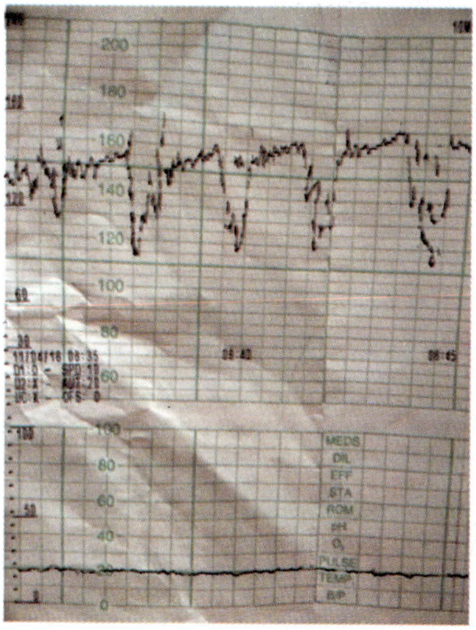

Figure 36.10 Nonstress test 3.

Q1 What abnormalities are shown in the trace?
Ans: The given NST has the following features:

- Baseline FHR is 140 bpm. There are unprovoked repeated decelerations lasting for more than 2 minutes.
- No accelerations are seen.

Q2 What should be the next plan of management?
Ans: This trace is pathological. Immediate delivery should be planned.

Nonstress test 4

Interpret the NST (Figure *36.11) of Mrs. G at 35 weeks of gestation.*

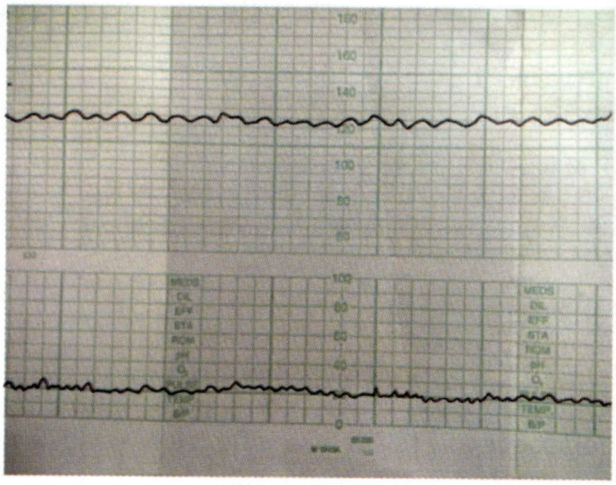

Figure 36.11 Nonstress test 4.

Q1 What abnormalities are seen in the trace?
Ans: The given NST has the following features:

- Baseline FHR is 120 bpm and there is a sine wave-like undulating pattern in the baseline FHR.
- Baseline variability is <5 bpm.
- Acceleration are absent.

Interpretation: Sinusoidal pattern of FHR.

Q2 What should be the next immediate step in management?
Ans: This trace is pathological. Fetus needs to be evaluated further with BPP and Doppler study of fetal vessels.

Q3 What are the probable causes?
Ans: Sinusoidal pattern of CTG trace may suggest fetal acidosis or fetal anemia.

Q4 BPP score is 4. What is the next step in management?
Ans: BPP score of 4 indicates strong suspicion for fetal asphyxia. Patient is already at 35 weeks of gestation and therefore delivery should be planned.

37 Common Obstetric Surgical Procedures

Introduction

Operative procedures form a major part of practical obstetrics and gynecology and hence medical students are expected to have thorough knowledge on this aspect of the subject. The common operative procedures in obstetrics are discussed in this chapter.

COMMON OPERATIVE PROCEDURES IN OBSTETRICS

- Medical termination of pregnancy (MTP)
- Episiotomy
- Operative vaginal delivery that includes obstetric forceps and vacuum application
- Cesarean section
- Female sterilization (tubal ligation)

Medical termination of pregnancy

Definition MTP refers to induced abortion for indications described under the MTP Act.

Indications for MTP

- **Medical causes:** Conditions that can result in risk to the life or grave injury to the physical health of the pregnant woman, for example, cardiac diseases such as New York Heart Association (NYHA) classes III and IV, Eisenmenger syndrome, and primary pulmonary hypertension
- **Social causes:** Conditions that can result in grave injury to the mental health of the pregnant woman
  - Pregnancy resulting from rape
  - Pregnancy resulting from contraceptive failure
- **Eugenic causes:** Conditions that can result in grave injury to the health of the newborn so as to render it seriously handicapped such as:
  - Anencephaly
  - Down syndrome
  - Major congenital malformations

The most common indication for which MTP is performed in current obstetric practice is unplanned pregnancy in a parous woman (presumed grave injury to mental health of the woman).

MTP Act (1971)

- The Medical Termination of Pregnancy (MTP) Act was passed in 1971 by the Government of India.
- The main aim of the act is to improve maternal health by preventing unsafe abortions, legalizing abortion services, and promoting access to safe abortion services for women.

Legal framework

MTP Act:

- Outlines when and where pregnancies can be terminated
- Grants the central government power to make rules and the state government power to frame regulations

MTP Rules outline who can terminate the pregnancy, training requirements, approval process for place, etc.

MTP Regulations specify the forms for opinion, maintenance of records, custody of forms and reporting of cases

MTP: When, where, who?

When can it be performed?

According to the MTP Act 1971, MTP can be done up to 20 weeks of gestation with the clause that *if the period of gestation (POG) ≤12 weeks*, opinion of one medical practitioner is required to take the decision regarding abortion and *if POG >12 weeks*, opinion of two medical practitioners is required to take the decision regarding abortion. This act has been amended in 2021 with key provisions as follows:

Key Provisions of the MTP Amendment Act, 2021 (Table 37.1)

- Increasing the upper gestation limit from 20 to 24 weeks for special categories of women, including survivors of rape, victims of incest, and other vulnerable women such as differently abled women and minors.
- The opinion of one provider needed for the termination of pregnancy up to 20 weeks of gestation. Requirement of the opinion of two providers for the termination of pregnancy at 20–24 weeks of gestation.
- Upper gestation limit does not apply in cases of substantial fetal abnormalities diagnosed by a medical board.
- Confidentiality clause: The name and other particulars of a woman whose pregnancy has been terminated cannot be revealed except under authorization by law.
- Extended MTP services under the failure of contraceptive clause, to unmarried women, in order to provide access to safe abortion irrespective of marital status.

Where can it be performed?

MTP can be done at places established by government or at places approved for the purpose of this Act by a District-level Committee constituted by the government.

Who can perform?

- The eligibility criteria of a registered medical practitioner to perform MTP are the following:
  - A practitioner who has assisted in at least 25 MTP cases of which at least 5 were performed independently in a hospital established or approved for this purpose by the Government (for MTP up to 12 weeks only).
  - A practitioner who has a diploma or postgraduate degree in Obstetrics and Gynecology.
  - A practitioner who has at least 1-year experience in practice of Obstetrics and Gynecology at a hospital which has all facilities.
  - A practitioner who has completed 6 months house job in Obstetrics and Gynecology.

Preprocedure preparations for MTP

- A detailed history is taken and clinical examination is performed.

Table 37.1 Key Provisions of the MTP Amendment Act (2021)

	MTP Act 1971	MTP Act Amendments 2021
Indications (contraceptive failure)	Applies only to married women	Unmarried women are also covered
Gestational age limit	20 weeks for all indications	24 weeks for special categories of women, including survivors of rape, victims of incest, and other vulnerable women (differently abled, minors) Beyond 24 weeks in cases of substantial fetal abnormalities diagnosed by a medical board
Medical practitioner's opinion required before termination	One RMP till 12 weeks Two RMP till 20 weeks	One RMP till 20 weeks Two RMP till 24 weeks Medical board approval after 24 weeks
Breach of women's confidentiality	Fine up to ₹1,000/-	Fine and/or imprisonment of 1 year

MTP, medical termination of pregnancy; *RMP*, registered medical practitioner.

- POG is assessed from last menstrual period (LMP) and clinical examination is performed. Ultrasonography may be performed in doubtful cases.
- The name and identity of the woman seeking MTP should not be revealed and she is alloted a confidential code number.
- Counsel regarding the procedures available for MTP, and regarding complications.
- Counsel for subsequent contraception/sterilization to avoid another unintended pregnancy.
- Investigations that are done include hemoglobin, blood grouping and Rh typing, urine albumin, sugar, and microscopy examination.
- Informed consent: Informed written consent of the pregnant woman is mandatory. Consent of the partner is not essential. If the woman is <18 years, or is mentally ill, consent of parent or legal guardian is obtained.
- Antibiotic prophylaxis is usually not required prior to medical abortion.

Methods of MTP in first trimester

Medical methods

Medical abortion is a nonsurgical abortion method in which medications are used to bring about abortion. The drugs that are commonly used are mifepristone and misoprostol. Medical abortion is usually offered up to 9 weeks (63 days) of gestation.

Protocol for medical abortion See Table 37.2

Mechanism of action (MOA) of the drugs used for medical abortion are as follows:

Table 37.2 Protocol for medical methods of abortion

Visit	Day	Drugs used
First visit	1	• Mifepristone 200 mg administered orally • Anti-D injection given if Rh negative
Second visit	3	• Misoprostol 800 μg administered orally or vaginally • Analgesics may be given The drugs may be administered by the clinician or self-administered by the patient at home
Third visit	14	• To confirm and ensure completion of abortion • Contraceptive advice is given

- **Mifepristone (RU-486)**: Antiprogestin action
  - Binds to progesterone receptors on decidua, resulting in necrosis of decidua and detachment of implanted embryo
  - Softens cervix and increases production of prostaglandins, that cause uterine contractions
  - Sensitizes the uterus to the effect of prostaglandins
- **Misoprostol:** Prostaglandin E1 (PGE1) analogue
  - Causes cervical softening and dilatation
  - Binds to myometrial cells, causing strong uterine contractions resulting in expulsion of conceptus from the uterus

Side effects of the drugs used for medical abortion

- Nausea and vomiting
- Diarrhea
- Fever and chills
- Excessive bleeding and abdominal cramps

Surgical methods

Surgical methods for abortion are the following:

- Dilatation and evacuation (D&E)
  - Rapid method
  - Slow method
- Suction evacuation or vacuum aspiration
  - Electric vacuum aspiration
  - Manual vacuum aspiration (MVA)

Antibiotic prophylaxis Antibiotic prophylaxis is recommended for surgical abortion, as it significantly reduces the frequency of postabortal endometritis. One of the following antibiotics are usually prescribed: Doxycycline 100 mg oral BD, ofloxacin 400 mg oral BD, or ceftriaxone 1 g IV, administered 30 minutes prior to the procedure.

The various surgical methods for abortion are described in the subsequent text.

Dilatation and evacuation

Indications

- Inevitable, incomplete, and missed abortion
- MTP

Steps of rapid method of dilatation and evacuation

- Misoprostol 400 μg is placed vaginally, at least 4 hours before the procedure, that makes the cervix soft and the procedure easier.

- The procedure is done under IV sedation or regional anesthesia or general anesthesia.
- The patient is placed in lithotomy position.
- Parts are cleaned and draped.
- Bladder is drained.
- Per speculum and bimanual examinations are done—to assess cervical dilatation and the size and position of uterus.
- Sims' speculum is introduced, and the anterior lip of cervix is held. (sponge holding forceps is preferred on a pregnant cervix as it is less traumatic, compared to vulsellum that can cause cervical injury and bleeding).
- Dilatation of cervix is done with serial sized Hegar's cervical dilators up to the desired dilatation (rapid dilatation of cervix).
- Ovum forceps is introduced and products of conception are removed completely.
- Blunt uterine curette is introduced and gentle check curettage of uterine cavity is done at the end of the procedure.
- Injection methergin 0.2 mg (IV/IM) is given at the end of the procedure.

Viva corner

Q1 Is there any risk of teratogenicity in case of failure of medical abortion?

Mifepristone is teratogenic. Hence, it is advisable to terminate pregnancy if there is failure of abortion following intake of mifepristone.

Q2 Why is mifepristone termed RU-486?

"RU" stands for the initials of pharmaceutical company "Roussel-Uclaf" that manufactured the drug in 1980, and "486" is a random laboratory serial number.

Q3 When is medical abortion considered to be a failure?

Medical method of abortion is said to be a failure when the clinician has to resort to other methods of abortion for the following reasons:

- Heavy bleeding is present.
- **True drug failure:** True drug failure is the presence of fetal cardiac activity 2 weeks after mifepristone and misoprostol administration, leading to continuing pregnancy; this is to be terminated by surgical methods.
- **Incomplete abortion:** Persistence of gestation sac without cardiac activity 2 weeks after misoprostol administration is termed incomplete abortion. The patient may be prescribed repeat dose of misoprostol or surgical evacuation can be done.
- In some cases, gestation sac is expelled but the woman may have bleeding due to decidual bits in the uterine cavity. This can be managed conservatively, as it will be expelled spontaneously in most of the cases. But if bleeding is profuse, evacuation may have to be done.

Viva corner

Q1 What is slow method of cervical dilatation?

It is a two-step procedure: slow dilatation of cervix is done by laminaria tent followed by rapid dilatation with dilators.

Q2 How will you ensure completeness of surgical abortion procedure?

The following features ensure completeness of surgical abortion:

- Passage of red foam without any tissue
- Significant reduction in amount of bleeding
- Feeling of gritty sensation of uterine wall
- Gripping action of cervix on the instrument inserted
- Well-contracted uterus

Complications of dilatation and evacuation procedure See Table 37.3

Suction evacuation

The products of conception are evacuated by creating a negative pressure with the help of suction cannula.

Table 37.3 Complications of rapid method of dilatation and evacuation

Intraoperative complications	Postoperative complications
• Anesthetic complications • Injury to cervix • Uterine perforation, bowel injury • Hemorrhage	• Infections • Septic abortion • Incomplete evacuation

Indications

- Inevitable, incomplete, and missed abortion
- Molar pregnancy
- MTP

Steps of suction evacuation

- Misoprostol 400 μg is placed vaginally, at least 4 hours before the procedure, that makes the cervix soft and the procedure easier.
- The procedure is done under IV sedation or regional anesthesia or general anesthesia.
- The patient is placed in lithotomy position.
- Parts are cleaned and draped.
- Bladder is drained.
- Per speculum and bimanual examinations are done—to assess cervical dilatation and the size and position of uterus.
- Sims' speculum is introduced and anterior lip of cervix is held.
- Dilatation of cervix is done with serially sized cervical dilators up to the desired dilatation.
- Suction cannula of appropriate size is introduced through the cervical canal and pushed up to midway inside the uterine cavity. The cannula is connected to a suction apparatus by a rubber tubing.
- Negative pressure is created with the suction machine.
- The cannula is moved up and down and rotated in all directions and the products of conception are sucked out till the cavity becomes empty (Figure 37.1).
- Negative pressure is released and cannula is removed.
- Gentle check curettage is done with a blunt curette.
- Injection methergin IV/IM.

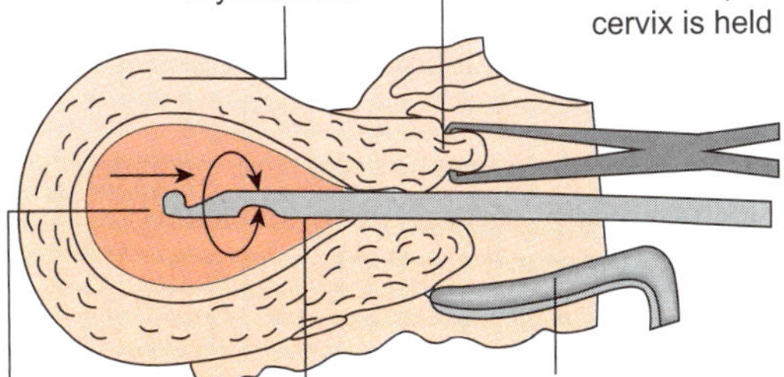

Figure 37.1 Suction evacuation procedure.

Manual vacuum aspiration

- Manual vacuum aspiration (MVA) is a procedure by which a handheld plastic vacuum aspirator is attached with a cannula to suck out the uterine contents.
- It can be used to terminate pregnancy up to 10 weeks.
- Cannula is available in different sizes (4–12 mm) and used according to the gestational age in weeks (e.g., 6-mm cannula for 6 weeks' pregnancy).

Steps

- Misoprostol 400 μg is placed vaginally, at least 4 hours before the procedure, that makes the cervix soft and the procedure easier.
- MVA is an outpatient procedure and can be done under paracervical block.
- The patient is placed in lithotomy position.
- Parts are cleaned and draped.
- Bladder is drained.
- Per speculum and bimanual examinations are done to assess the cervical dilatation and the size and position of uterus.
- Sims' speculum is introduced and anterior lip of cervix is held.
- Cervical canal is dilated with serial dilators.
- Cannula is inserted gently until the tip touches fundus and then it is slightly withdrawn.

Viva corner

Q1 What is menstrual regulation (MR)?

Definition

MR is the induction of uterine bleeding that has been delayed up to 14 days from the date of anticipated menses.

- The most common method of performing a MR is by using a mini vacuum aspiration syringe (MR syringe).
- It is done as an outpatient procedure, without anesthesia.
- It is done without confirming the presence of pregnancy (urine pregnancy test need not be done prior to the procedure).
- It does not require legal approval.
- It is a safe method of inducing uterine bleeding, irrespective of the cause of delay in menses.

- The manual vacuum aspirator is assembled and negative pressure is created. The charged aspirator is attached to the cannula and the valve is released to start suction. Cannula is rotated in all directions and moved up and down till contents are completely aspirated.
- After closing the valve, the cannula and the aspirator are withdrawn.

Complications of suction evacuation or vacuum aspiration

- Cervical injury (during dilatation)
- Vasovagal attack (during dilatation)
- Uterine perforation
- Incomplete evacuation
- Infection
- Hematometra

Complications of suction evacuation/vacuum aspiration are similar to but less than those of D&E (this is the main advantage of suction evacuation/vacuum aspiration over D&E).

Disadvantages of suction evacuation/vacuum aspiration

- It is difficult to perform when fetal parts are well formed, that is, after 10 weeks of gestation.
- The procedure requires a suction apparatus or vacuum aspirator.

Advantages and disadvantages of medical versus surgical methods of MTP

See Table 37.4

Table 37.4 Advantages and disadvantages of medical versus surgical methods of MTP

Parameter	Medical methods	Surgical methods
Hospitalization	Not required	Required
Anesthesia	Not required	Required
Preoperative antibiotics	Not required	Required
Duration of treatment	Days to weeks	Procedure completed at single visit
Number of visits required	Two or more	Single visit
Success rate	95–98%	98–100%
Follow-up	Required to ensure completion	Not routinely required
Cost	Comparatively low	Expensive

Note *In the first trimester, both medical and surgical methods have equal success rates. Since medical abortion does not require admission, anesthesia, and antibiotics, and the cost is comparatively low, it is usually preferred over surgical abortion.*

Methods of MTP in second trimester

- **D&E (as described under first-trimester abortion)**
- **Intra-amniotic hyperosmolar solution instillation:** 20% saline, 40% urea instillation
  - *MOA*: Causes necrosis of the placenta and decidua and release of Prostaglandins, which in turn excites uterine contraction leading to expulsion of fetus
- **Extra-amniotic instillation of ethacridine lactate**
  - *MOA*: Causes separation of membranes with release of Prostaglandins and dilatation of cervix
- **Prostaglandins**
  - Repeated doses of vaginal or oral misoprostol (PGE1)
  - Intracervical dinoprostone (PGE2)
  - Extra-amniotic instillation of PGF2 alpha
- **Oxytocin:** Used as an adjunct to other drugs
- **Hysterotomy:** It is the final option when other methods fail to cause abortion

Contraceptive advice for women undergoing MTP

Contraceptive choices should be discussed with the woman undergoing MTP, prior to the procedure.

- Tubectomy can be performed along with surgical abortion or following medical abortion, in women who have completed family.
- Spacing of pregnancy can be provided with intrauterine contraceptive device (IUCD) or hormonal contraceptives in women who have not completed family. Barrier methods have high failure rates.
- Immediate postabortal insertion of IUCD is safe and is recommended by the World Health Organization (WHO) and American College of Obstetricians and Gynecologists (ACOG).

Episiotomy

Definition

Episiotomy is a planned incision on the perineum during the second stage of labor, to increase the size of introitus, in order to facilitate vaginal delivery.

- It is the most common operative procedure performed in obstetrics.

Indications for episiotomy

Maternal indications

- Primigravida with rigid perineum
- Multigravida with rigid perineum
- To conduct instrumental delivery—forceps or ventouse
- Fetal malpositions and malpresentations allowed for vaginal delivery such as occipitoposterior position, face and breech presentation (to minimize perineal trauma and to perform maneuvers if required)
- Previous H/o complete perineal tear (CPT) repair and pelvic floor repair

Fetal Delivery of preterm fetus—to minimize trauma to the fetal head (to prevent fetal intracranial hemorrhage due to sudden compression and decompression of the fetal head)

Note *Routine use of episiotomy in all cases should be abandoned.*

Advantages of episiotomy

Maternal

- Decreases perineal lacerations and CPT (episiotomy is a planned incision—hence easy to repair and heals well)
- Cuts short the second stage of labor to some extent
- Provides space for application of forceps or vacuum
- Minimizes trauma to pelvic floor, thereby prevents genital prolapse and urinary incontinence (long-term benefit is controversial)

Fetal

- Minimizes trauma to preterm fetal head
- Provides space for manipulation and delivery in vaginal breech delivery

Types of episiotomy (Figure 37.2)

- Mediolateral (most common)
- Median
- Lateral

Advantages and disadvantages of the different types of episiotomy

See Table 37.5

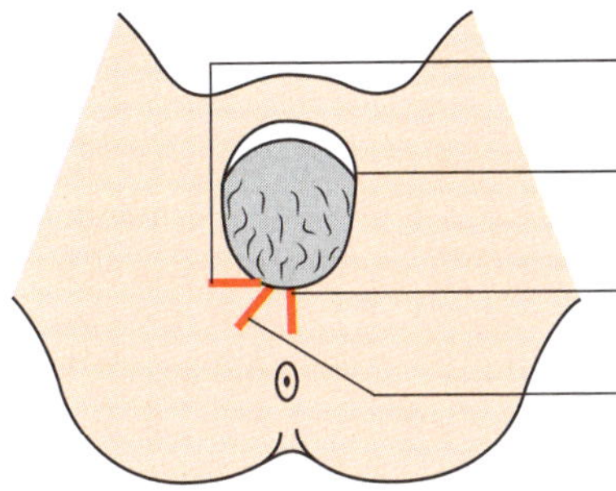

Figure 37.2 Types of episiotomy.

Table 37.5 Advantages and disadvantages of different types of episiotomy

	Advantages	Disadvantages
Mediolateral	Incision can be extended without involvement of rectum	• Blood loss and postoperative discomfort are slightly more compared to that of median episiotomy
Median	• Less bleeding • Perfect anatomical apposition • Postoperative discomfort is less	It can extend downwards to involve the rectum
Lateral	Incision can be extended without involvement of rectum	• Blood loss is more • Poor healing • Injury to Bartholin gland and duct

Viva corner

Q1 What are the structures cut in episiotomy?

- Vaginal mucosa
- Superficial and deep transverse perineal muscles
- Bulbospongiosus
- Few fibers of levator ani
- Subcutaneous tissue
- Skin

Part 3

Principal steps of episiotomy

- The patient is placed in dorsal position with thighs and knees flexed and abducted.
- Parts are cleaned and draped.
- Bladder is drained.
- Per vaginal examination is done.
- Local anesthesia: Perineal infiltration with 10 mL of 1% lignocaine or pudendal block is given.
- Episiotomy is given when head does not recede in between contractions and perineum is thinned out and bulging (at crowning of fetal head).
- Procedure: Two fingers of left hand are inserted into vagina and placed between the fetal presenting part and the posterior vaginal wall. The perineum is cut with episiotomy scissors from midpoint of posterior fourchette extending downwards and laterally on the right or left side (Figure 37.3).
- The baby is delivered out followed by delivery of placenta and membranes.
- Repair of episiotomy is done.
- Repair is done in three layers with absorbable suture material such as 1-0 chromic catgut (Figure 37.4a–d):
  - *Vaginal mucosa*: Continuous sutures
  - *Muscles*: Interrupted sutures
  - *Skin and subcutaneous tissue*: Mattress sutures

Complications

See Table 37.6

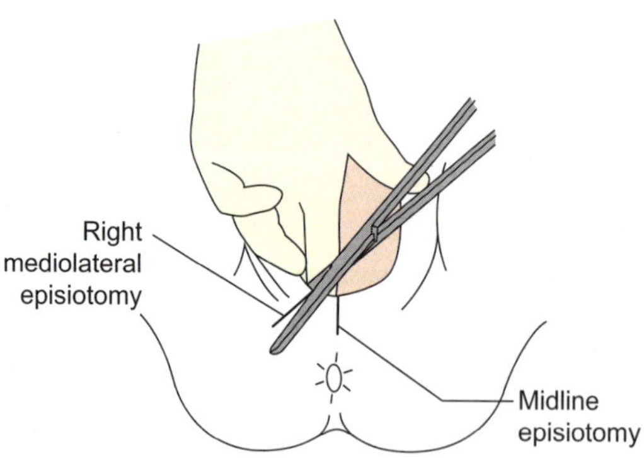

Figure 37.3 Episiotomy procedure.

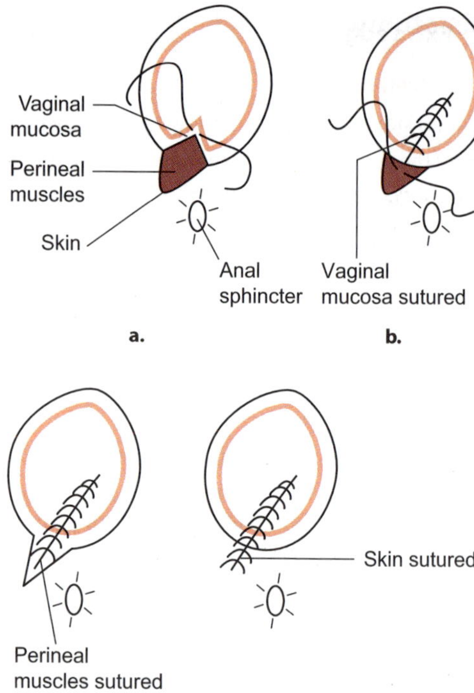

Figure 37.4 Suturing the episiotomy in three layers. **a.** Episiotomy incision. **b.** Suturing the vaginal mucosa. **c.** Suturing the muscle layer. **d.** Suturing the skin.

Table 37.6 Complications of episiotomy

Immediate complications	Delayed complications
• Downward extension of incision causing complete perineal tear • Bleeding • Vulval hematoma • Infection • Wound gaping	• Painful scar • Dyspareunia • Bartholin's cyst, if Bartholin's duct is injured and obstructed • Scar endometriosis

Operative vaginal delivery

Operative vaginal delivery refers to a procedure where the mother is assisted in delivery of the fetal head, by the use of obstetric forceps or ventouse.

A brief description of application of obstetric forceps and ventouse is given in subsequent subsections.

Extra edge

Classification of perineal laceration/tears

Perineal lacerations are classified as mentioned in table below.

Table Classification of perineal lacerations

Degree	Description
First degree	Involves skin and vaginal mucosa
Second degree	Involves skin, vaginal mucosa, and perineal muscles (like an episiotomy)
Third degree	Involves the anal sphincter (complete perineal tear) • 3a: Less than 50% thickness of external anal sphincter is involved. • 3b: More than 50% thickness of external anal sphincter is involved. • 3c: Internal anal sphincter is also involved.
Fourth degree	Involves the rectal mucosa

Principal steps of repair of complete perineal tear

- Repair of rectal mucosa
- Apposition and repair of the torn anal sphincters
- Repair of perineal muscles
- Repair of the vaginal mucosa and skin

Vulvar hematoma

Hematomas are divided into:

Infralevator hematomas (below levator ani)

- Vulvar and perineal hematomas
- Paravaginal hematomas
- Hematoma of the ischiorectal fossa

Supralevator hematoma (above levator ani)

- Spreads to the base of broad ligament or bulge into the wall of upper vagina

Causes

It may occur due to rupture of vulvar varices or more often after perineal repair when a vessel in spasm during repair relaxes and bleeds later.

Clinical features

- Appears as a tender purple swelling on one side of the vulva
- May reach up to 10 cm or more in diameter
- Severe perineal pain and sometimes shock

Treatment

- Swelling >5 cm and rapidly increasing in size: Incision and drainage of clot, ligation of any bleeder if identified
- Swelling <5 cm and not expanding: Managed by observation using ice packs and pressure dressing to limit the expansion

Broad ligament hematoma (Supralevator hematoma)

- These hematomas are the result of upper vaginal, cervical, or uterine laceration extending into the uterine or vaginal arteries.
- Rapid labor, cesarean section, instrumental deliveries, and trauma are predisposing factors in the formation of broad ligament hematoma.
- Clinical features: Persistent postpartum pain together with shock, elevated uterine fundus, and a unilateral fluctuating mass on bimanual examination. Rapid diagnosis is of utmost importance that will determine the treatment options.
- Diagnosis: Even large hematomas can frequently evade adequate assessment by clinical examination alone. Imaging studies such as ultrasound, CT, or MRI are used to diagnose and treat pelvic hematomas.
- Treatment: Based on the patient's hemodynamic situation, treatment differs (conservative management, packing or abdominal hysterectomy).

Obstetric forceps application

Purpose of obstetric forceps

To extract the fetal head during delivery

Types of obstetric forceps

- Long curved obstetric forceps (Simpson's forceps; Figure 37.5a)
- Short curved obstetric forceps (Wrigley's forceps; Figure 37.5b)
- Long straight obstetric forceps (Kielland's forceps)

Parts of obstetric forceps (Figure 37.6)

- It has two halves (right and left blades corresponding to maternal right and left sides, i.e., the maternal side on which it is applied).

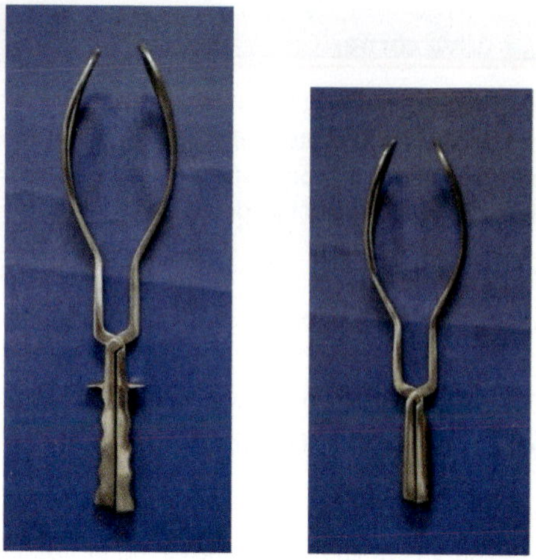

a. b.

Figure 37.5 Obstetric forceps. **a.** Low forceps. **b.** Outlet forceps.

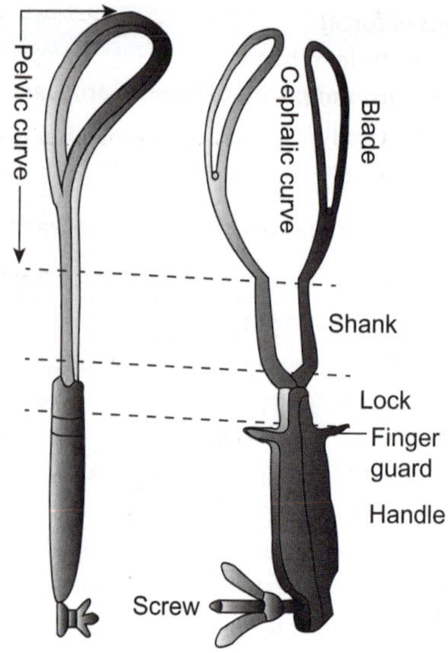

Figure 37.6 Parts of obstetric forceps.

- Each half of the forceps has the following parts:
  - Blade
  - Shank
  - Lock
  - Handle

Blades
- The blades are fenestrated.
- Each blade has two curves:
  - Cephalic curve on the flat or inner surface of the blade (inner surface of the blade which fits with the fetal head during application)
  - Pelvic curve on the edge of the blade (which fits with the curve of sacrum)

Viva corner

Q1 Why are the blades fenestrated?

Fenestrated blades are helpful in the following ways:
- Make the instrument lighter
- Provide a good grip over fetal head
- Provide less compression on fetal head

Shank Shank connects the blade with the handle. Its purpose is for the following:
- Gives length to the instrument
- Facilitates locking
- Makes traction easier

Lock It facilitates articulation of both the blades.
- **Types of lock**
  - *English lock*: Socket system to fit each blade with one another
  - *French lock*: Pivot on left blade that fits with the notch on the right blade

Handle It helps in giving traction.
- It has a finger guard to place the fingers while giving traction.

Note
- *Obstetric forceps may have a fixation screw to keep the blades in position.*
- *Obstetric forceps may have an axis traction device to apply traction in the correct axis of pelvis.*

Viva corner

Q1 What are the features of Wrigley's forceps or outlet forceps?

The features of short curved obstetric forceps or outlet forceps (Wrigley's forceps) are as follows:
- Cephalic curve is marked.
- There is slight or no pelvic curve.
- Shank is short.
- Handle is short.
- Instrument is lighter than long curved forceps.

Functions of forceps

- Traction to fetal head
- Protection—acts as a protective cage to fetal head, especially in preterm fetuses
- Compression—provides good grip on the fetal head
- Rotation of the head—can be done with Kielland's forceps
- Can be used in cesarean section to deliver a floating head or as a vectis to assist delivery of deeply engaged head in cesarean section

Classification of forceps application (American College of Obstetricians and Gynecologists, 2000)

See Table 37.7

Note

- *Station is measured in relation to maternal ischial spines (–5 to 0 and 0 to +5).*
- *Low forceps and outlet forceps are applied in majority of cases.*
- *Cesarean section is preferred over applying midcavity forceps due to increased maternal and fetal morbidity.*

Indications for forceps application

- Prolonged second stage of labor
- Prophylactic cut short of the second stage in maternal conditions such as cardiac disease, severe preeclampsia, eclampsia, and in vaginal birth after cesarean (VBAC)
- Failure of maternal bearing down efforts
- Fetal indications
  - Fetal distress in second stage
  - Cord prolapse in second stage
  - Delivery of after-coming head of breech

Viva corner

Q1 What are the various forceps applications?

- **Long curved obstetric forceps:** For low forceps and midcavity forceps application
- **Short curved obstetric forceps (Wrigley's forceps):** For outlet forceps application
- **Kielland's forceps:** For midcavity forceps application
- **Piper's forceps:** For delivery of after-coming head of breech

Q2 What are the uses of forceps in cesarean section?

- To deliver a floating head
- Can be used as a vectis to assist delivery of deeply engaged fetal head

Prerequisites for forceps application

- Bladder must be emptied.
- Head must be engaged.
- Cervix must be fully dilated.
- Membranes must be ruptured.
- Station must be at +2 or below for low forceps application.
- Presentation and position of presenting part must be known with certainty.
- Cephalopelvic disproportion (CPD) must be ruled out.

Table 37.7 Classification of forceps application (ACOG 2000)

Term	Definition
Outlet forceps	Fetal skull has reached the pelvic floor and head is in the perineum • Fetal head is at the perineum and fetal scalp is visible without separating the labia • Sagittal suture is in the anteroposterior diameter • Rotation is ≤45°
Low forceps	Leading point of the fetal skull is at +2 station or below. Two subdivisions • Rotation of ≤45° • Rotation of >45°
Midcavity forceps	Leading point of the fetal skull is at 0 to +2 stations
High forceps	• Leading point of the fetal skull is above 0 station (head is not engaged) • *Not included in classification and is obsolete in modern obstetrics*

ACOG, American College of Obstetricians and Gynecologists.

- Counseling should be given and informed consent should be obtained.

Contraindications for forceps application

- Head not engaged
- CPD
- Incompletely dilated cervix
- Malpresentations (brow, mentoposterior face)
- Extreme fetal prematurity

Principal steps of low forceps application

- The patient is placed in lithotomy position.
- Parts are cleaned and draped.
- Bladder is drained.
- Examination is done to ascertain whether prerequisites are fulfilled.
- Liberal episiotomy is given after local infiltration with 1% lignocaine or pudendal block.
- Identification of forceps blades is done (blade corresponding to the left side of maternal pelvis is the left blade and blade corresponding to the right side of maternal pelvis is the right blade).
- Left blade is introduced first followed by the right blade, satisfying both cephalic and pelvic applications, and then the blades are locked (Figure 37.7a–d).
- Traction is given along the axis of pelvis during uterine contraction—first downwards and backwards, then forwards, and then forwards and upwards toward maternal abdomen—and head is delivered (Figures 37.7e–f and 37.8).
- Blades are unlocked and removed, and rest of the baby is delivered.
- Placenta and membranes are delivered completely.
- Perineum, cervix, and vaginal walls are examined for any extension of episiotomy, lacerations, etc.

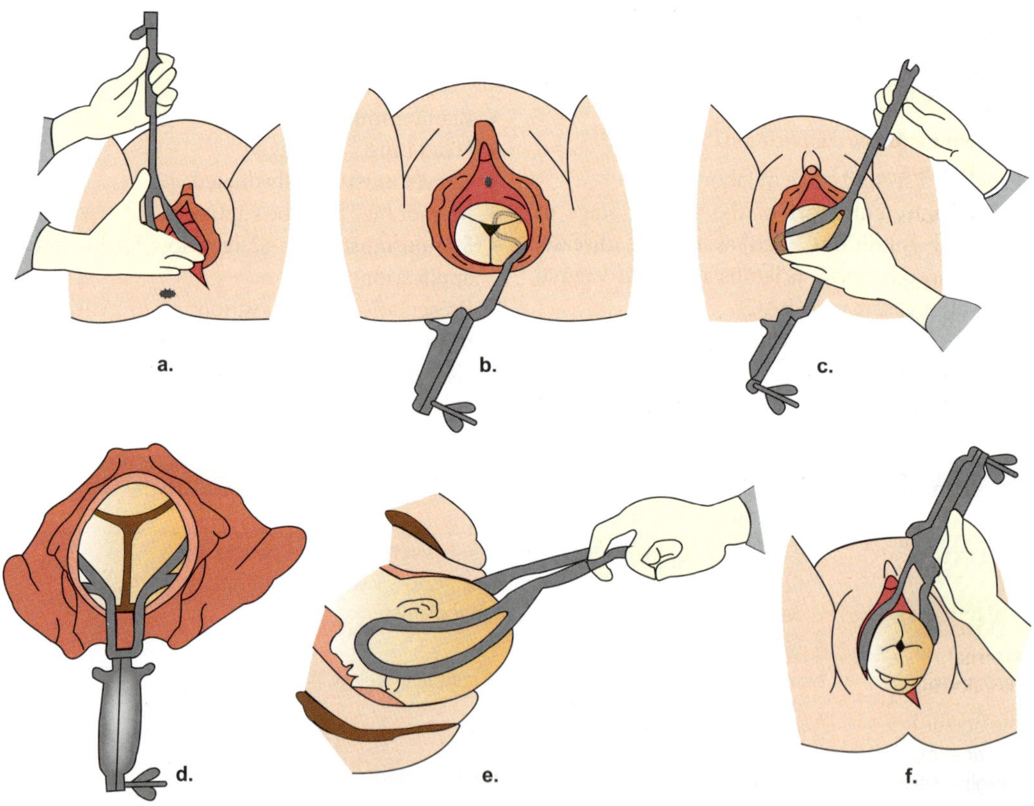

Figure 37.7 Steps of forceps application. **a.** Introduction of the left blade. **b.** Left blade held in position. **c.** Introduction of the right blade. **d.** Apposition and locking of the blades. **e.** Bimalar, biparietal placement of the blades and position of the fingers during traction. **f.** Traction applied to deliver the fetal head.

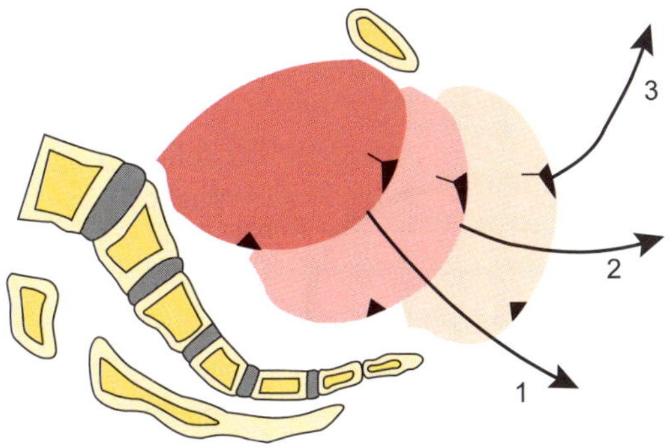

Figure 37.8 Direction of traction of forceps along the axis of birth canal. Initially downwards (1), then forwards (2), and then forwards and upwards (3).

Complications of forceps delivery

See Table 37.8

Ventouse or vacuum extraction

Purpose

Vacuum extractor is a suction–traction device to deliver the fetal head by creating a negative pressure between the vacuum cup and the scalp of the fetus.

> **Viva corner**
>
> **Q1 How is the fetal head delivered by outlet forceps application?**
>
> - Short curved Wrigley's forceps is used.
> - Application is in the same way as that of low forceps application but is easier.
> - Head is already in the perineum during outlet forceps application and it has to be delivered by extension. Traction is given forwards, and then forwards and upwards direction toward maternal abdomen.
>
> **Note** *Downward traction is not required for outlet forceps application as head is already in the perineum.*

Table 37.8 Complications of forceps delivery

Maternal complications	Fetal complications
• Injury to perineum, vagina, cervix • Hemorrhage—traumatic or atonic postpartum hemorrhage • Sepsis	• Fetal scalp injury: Cephalhematoma, skull fracture, abrasion of skin can occur • Intracranial hemorrhage: Due to tears in tentorium cerebelli • Birth asphyxia: Can occur in case of prolonged compression of fetal head

> **Extra edge**
>
> - **Trial forceps:** Trial forceps refers to tentative attempt of forceps delivery if there is doubtful midpelvic contraction, keeping everything ready for cesarean section if there is failure to deliver the head with reasonable traction.
> - **Failed forceps:** Failure to deliver the fetus following an attempt of forceps application is termed failed forceps.

Parts of ventouse (Figure 37.9)

- Suction cup with traction chain and metallic traction bar
  - Suction cup is placed over the fetal scalp for creation of vacuum; traction is given by holding the traction bar attached to the traction chain.
  - Suction cup may be of two types:
    - Metallic cup
    - Soft malleable silastic cup made of silicone rubber
  - Suction cups are available in different sizes (40, 50, 60 mm diameter.)
- Vacuum glass bottle fitted with an airtight rubber cork where vacuum is created
- Rubber tubing that connects the suction cup to the vacuum glass bottle
- Handheld or electric vacuum pump that creates vacuum inside the glass bottle, to build negative pressure between the suction cup and the fetal scalp

Indications for vacuum application

- Prolonged second stage
- Prophylactic cut short of second stage—in maternal conditions such as cardiac disease, severe preeclampsia, eclampsia, and in VBAC

> **Viva corner**
>
> **Q1 What are the advantages of silastic cups?**
>
> - They produce a less marked chignon over the scalp.
> - Negative pressure can be created quickly.
> - Maternal injuries are comparatively less with silastic cups.

Part 3

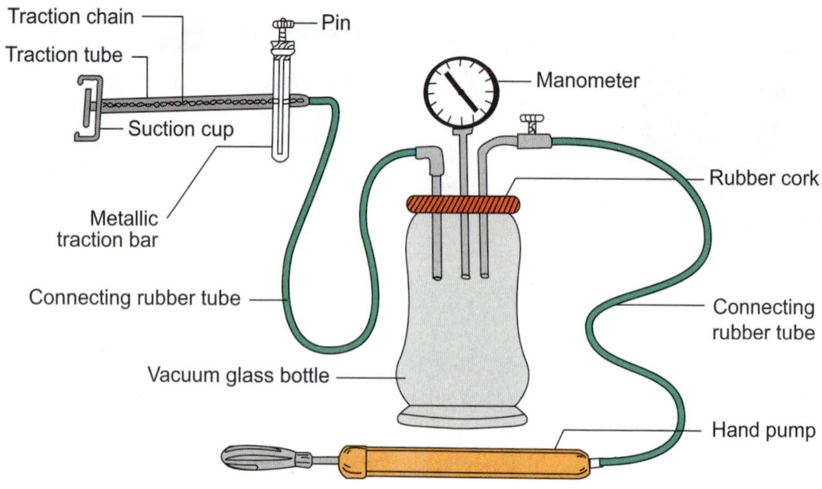

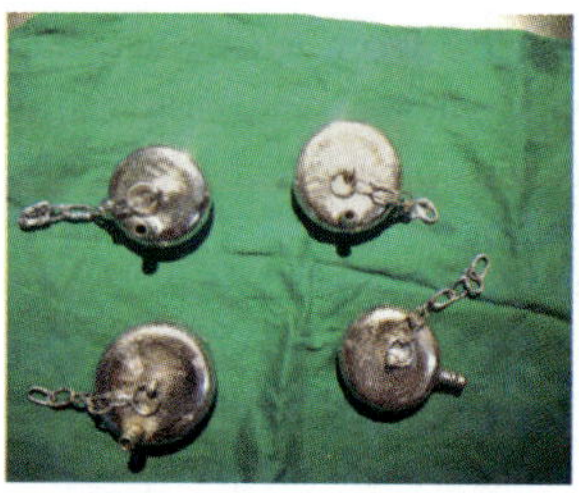

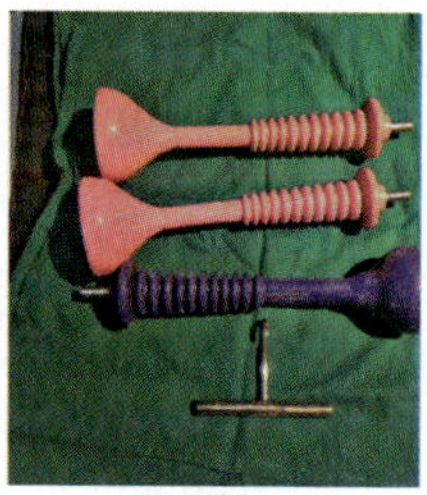

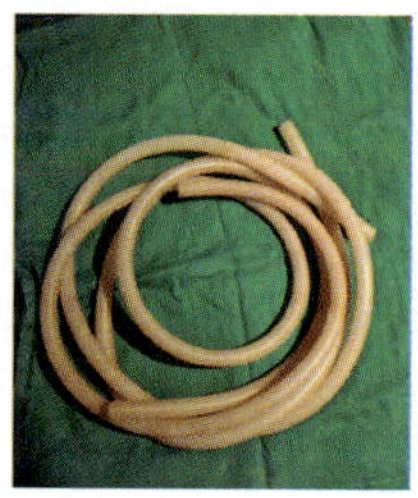

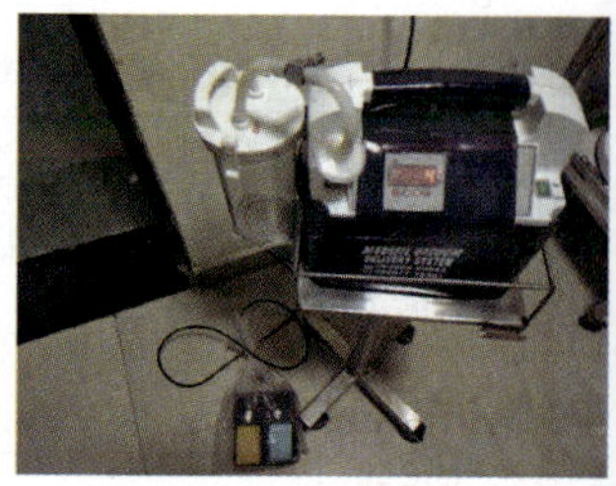

Figure 37.9 Parts of a ventouse. **a.** Pictorial representation of the parts of ventouse. **b.** Metal cups of different sizes. **c.** Silastic cups and metal traction bar. **d.** Rubber tubing that connects the vacuum cup to the suction apparatus. **e.** Electric suction apparatus.

- Failure of maternal efforts
- Fetal indications
  - Fetal distress in second stage of labor

Prerequisites for ventouse application

- Bladder must be emptied.
- Head must be engaged.
- Cervix must be fully dilated preferably (ventouse can be applied even before full dilatation at >6 cm).
- Membranes must be ruptured.
- Station must be at +2 or below (can be applied even at slightly higher station).
- Presentation and position of fetal head must be known with certainty.
- Cephalopelvic disproportion (CPD must be ruled out.
- Counseling should be given and informed consent should be obtained.

Contraindications

- Face presentation
- After-coming head of breech
- Preterm fetus
- Suspected fetal coagulation disorder

Principal steps of ventouse application

- Suction cup is applied to the fetal head more toward the occiput at the "flexion point" that is 3 cm in front of posterior fontanel (facilitates flexion of fetal head during traction).
- Effective negative pressure (vacuum of 0.2 kg/cm^2 is created, which is gradually increased up to a maximum of 0.8 kg/cm^2 over 8–10 minutes) is created between the suction cup and the fetal scalp, which results in the formation of "chignon."
- Traction is given during uterine contraction. Direction of traction is at right angles to the plane of the cup (Figure 37.10a–c).

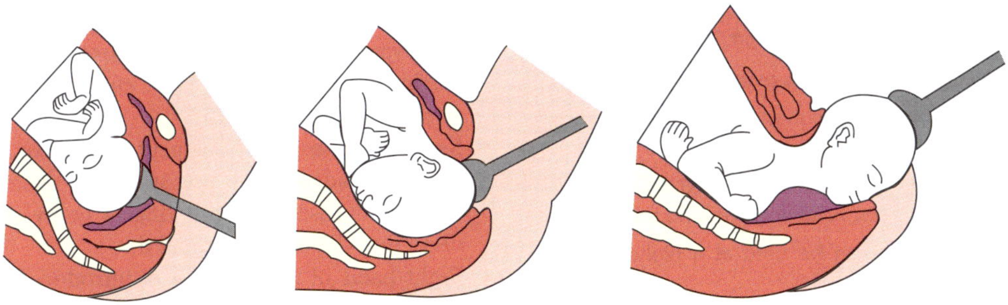

Figure 37.10 Ventouse application. **a.** Vacuum cup applied at flexion point. **b.** Traction given perpendicular to the plane of the cup. **c.** Delivery of the head by extension.

- Head undergoes autorotation and delivers by extension.
- Negative pressure is released, cup is removed, and rest of the baby is delivered.

Complications

See Table 37.9

Viva corner

Q1 What is chignon?

Chignon is artificial caput succedaneum produced during ventouse application that disappears spontaneously within 12–48 hours following delivery (see figure below).

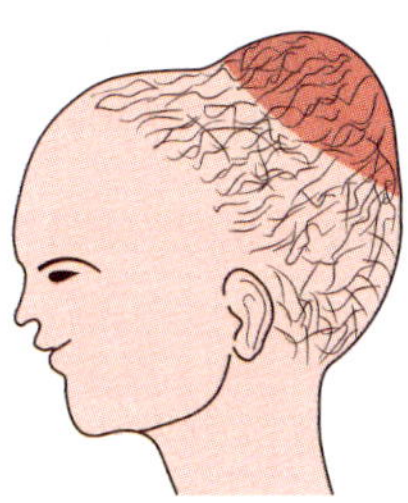

Figure Chignon.

Table 37.9 Complications of ventouse

Maternal complications	Fetal complications
Maternal complications are less. Can occur when tissues are entrapped between suction cup and fetal head	• Cephalhematoma • Abrasion/sloughing of scalp • Intracranial hemorrhage

Lower-segment cesarean section

Definition Cesarean section is defined as delivery of the fetus through an incision on the abdominal wall and another incision on the uterus. It is a common surgical procedure in obstetrics.

Only the steps of lower-segment cesarean section (LSCS) are described in this chapter; for further details, refer to Part 1, Chapter 6, *Postcesarean Pregnancy*.

Preoperative management

- Blood grouping and Rh typing, cross-matching and reservation are done.
- Nil per oral for at least 8 hours is desirable prior to an elective cesarean section (in case of emergency cesarean section, Ryle's tube suctioning can be done and regional anesthesia is preferred).
- Part preparation: Abdominal skin and external genitalia are prepared—cleaned with soap and water and then with antiseptic solution. Hairs that can interfere with the operative site are clipped on the day of surgery.
- Informed written consent is obtained. If the patient is multiparous, then patient is counseled for concurrent sterilization and if the patient is willing, consent is obtained.
- Intravenous injection of ranitidine and antiemetic such as metoclopramide are given before shifting the patient to operation theatre.
- Prophylactic antibiotics decrease the risk of postoperative wound infection and endometritis. A single dose of a first-generation cephalosporin (cefazolin) is usually recommended.

High-yield points

Advantages of ventouse over forceps

- It can be applied even before full dilatation of cervix.
- It can be used in a nonrotated head (autorotation of the head occurs during traction).
- Ventouse can be used at a higher station level.
- Chance of maternal injury is less with vacuum (as it is not a space-occupying device).

Advantages of obstetric forceps over ventouse

- It can be applied in preterm head (acts as a protective cage for fetal head).
- It can be applied in after-coming head of breech.
- It can be applied in face presentation.
- Chance of cephalhematoma is less than in vacuum.
- In suspected midpelvic contraction, when trial of vaginal delivery is attempted, forceps is better than ventouse (chance of failure is more with ventouse).

- Volume preloading with crystalloids is done to reduce the risk of hypotension prior to starting the procedure.

Principal steps of lower-segment cesarean section

- Regional anesthesia (spinal/epidural) is usually given.
- Bladder is catheterized.
- The patient is placed in supine position with 15° left lateral tilt to avoid supine hypotension (alternatively, a wedge may be placed under the right hip).
- Parts are cleaned with povidone–iodine solution and draped.
- Pfannenstiel skin incision (suprapubic transverse incision) is made. It is the most common skin incision for cesarean section (Figure 37.11a).
- The incision is deepened in layers and peritoneal cavity entered (the layers of the abdomen traversed include subcutaneous tissue, rectus sheath, rectus muscle, transversalis fascia, parietal peritoneum).
- Doyen's retractor is introduced.
- Uterovesical fold of peritoneum over the lower uterine segment is incised and bladder is retracted (Figure 37.11b).
- Kerr's incision (lower-segment transverse incision) is made on the uterus and is extended by blunt dissection with fingers or by sharp dissection (Figure 37.11c and d).
- Right hand of the surgeon is introduced into the uterine cavity below the fetal head and the head is delivered out. This is followed by delivery of the rest of the baby. Cord is clamped, cut, and the baby handed over to pediatrician (Figure 37.11e and f).
- Oxytocin infusion 10–20 units in 500 mL Ringer lactate is started and placenta is delivered by controlled cord traction (Figure 37.11g).
- The angles of the uterine incision are held and uterus is closed in double layers; the first layer is continuous/continuous locking sutures and the second layer is continuous sutures, burying the first layer (inverting Lembert's suture). Delayed absorbable suture material such as No. 1 Vicryl is used for uterine closure (Figure 37.11h and i). A single-layer closure technique can be done for women who undergo concurrent tubal sterilization.
- Hemostasis is secured. Mops and instrument counts are checked.
- Abdomen is closed in layers.
  - Parietal peritoneum (optional)
  - Rectus muscle approximated in midline (optional)
  - Rectus sheath closed with continuous or intermittent sutures using a nonabsorbable suture material (No. 1 Prolene) or a delayed absorbable suture material (No. 1 Vicryl). Rectus sheath (it is the most important layer that provides strength to abdominal wall; a properly done rectus sheath closure is essential in preventing incisional hernia later
  - Subcutaneous tissue—optional (if thickness of subcutaneous tissue is more than 2 cm, it is approximated with sutures or a subcutaneous drain is placed)
  - Skin closed with mattress sutures/ subcuticular sutures
- Vaginal toileting is done (to remove the blood collected during surgery, so that any fresh bleeding or postpartum hemorrhage (PPH) can be identified in postoperative ward).

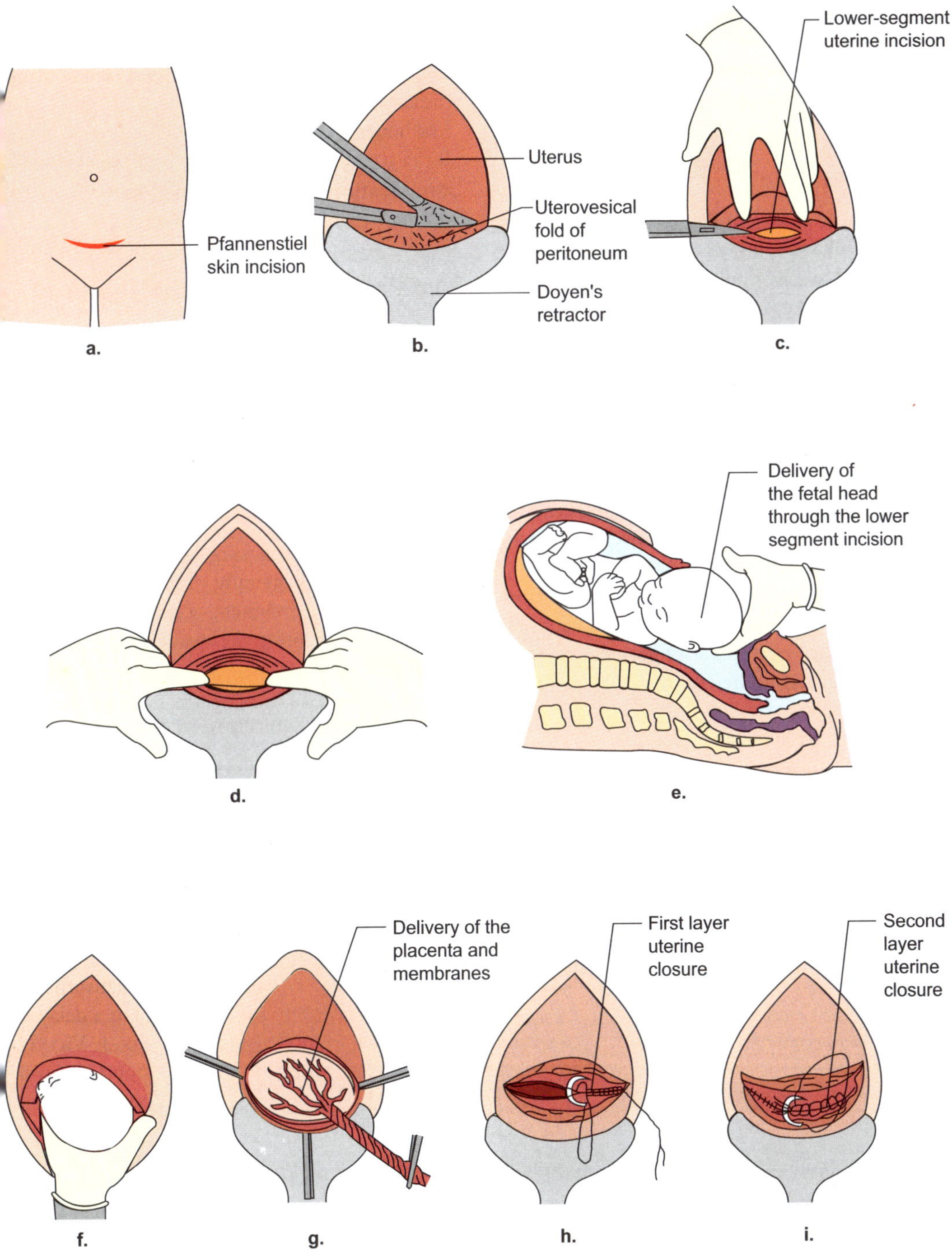

Figure 37.11 Steps of lower-segment cesarean section. **a.** Pfannenstiel incision on the skin and deepened in layers to enter the peritoneal cavity. **b.** The loose uterovesical fold of perineum in the lower uterine segment is incised transversely. **c.** Uterine incision in the lower segment. **d.** Extension of the uterine incision by blunt dissection with fingers. **e.** Introduction of the surgeon's fingers into the uterine cavity. **f.** Delivery of the head. **g.** Delivery of the placenta. **h** and **i.** Closure of uterine incision in two layers.

- Sterile dressing is applied and vaginal pad is kept.
- At the end of the procedure: Check whether urine is clear and vitals are stable.
- The patient is then shifted to the postoperative ward.

Postoperative care

- Temperature, pulse and BP should be monitored.
- Monitor whether uterus is well retracted and watch for excessive vaginal bleeding.
- The patient is kept nil oral for initial 6–8 hours following which clear oral fluids can be started.
- Input/output chart is maintained.
- Intravenous fluids are usually continued for 12–14 hours after cesarean section.
- Pain relief is provided by narcotic analgesics such as pethidine 50–100 mg IM every 6 hours, according to need. Alternatively, analgesics such as Tramadol and Voveran IM injections can be administered every 4–6 hours.
- If prophylactic antibiotics have been administered, then antibiotics are not routinely indicated in the postoperative period.
- Intravenous ranitidine/pantoprazole is given every 12 hours.
- Antiemetics are given as required.
- Urinary catheter may be removed after 12–24 hours.
- Clear oral fluids can be changed to soft diet after 24 hours.
- Oral nonsteroidal anti-inflammatory drugs (NSAIDs) are prescribed for pain relief after 24 hours.

Complications of cesarean section

See Table 37.10

Female sterilization (tubal ligation)

Sterilization is a permanent method of contraception that can be performed in women and men. Female sterilization is called tubectomy and male sterilization is called vasectomy. Female sterilization is one of the most popular methods of permanent sterilization. Women who have completed their family may opt for female sterilization.

Principle It involves surgical occlusion of the fallopian tubes bilaterally. Tubal ligation techniques result in permanent occlusion of the fallopian tubes, preventing the ovum and sperm from meeting each other.

Timing of female sterilization

The various time periods during which tubectomy can be performed are mentioned in Table 37.11.

Table 37.10 Complications of cesarean section

Intraoperative complications	Postoperative complications	
	Immediate	Delayed
• Anesthetic complications – Hypotension – Mendelson syndrome (if general anesthesia is given) • Hemorrhage • Visceral injury—bladder, bowel	• Infections—urinary tract infection, respiratory infections • Paralytic ileus • Deep vein thrombosis	• Incisional hernia • Future obstetric complications such as scar rupture, need for repeat cesarean section

Table 37.11 Timing of female sterilization

Timing of sterilization	Description
Puerperal sterilization	Sterilization following vaginal delivery performed within 7 days of delivery
Interval sterilization	Sterilization performed after 6 weeks following delivery. Ideal time for interval sterilization is the postmenstrual period
Postabortal sterilization	Sterilization performed along with medical termination of pregnancy or following spontaneous abortion
Concurrent sterilization	Sterilization done along with any other procedure such as cesarean section, appendicectomy, and ovarian cystectomy

Table 37.12 Types of surgical approaches for performing female sterilization

Abdominal route (commonly done)	Vaginal route
• Minilaparotomy: The procedure is done through a small skin incision of less than 5 cm, usually 1 inch • Laparoscopic tubal sterilization	• Colpotomy: Tubal sterilization can be done concurrently along with vaginal procedures such as Manchester repair. The tubes are delivered by opening the pouch of Douglas • Hysteroscopy: Hysteroscopic occlusion of the fallopian tube

Types of surgical approaches

The various surgical approaches for performing female sterilization are mentioned in Table 37.12.

Method of sterilization

The sterilization techniques that are commonly performed are the following:
- Modified Pomeroy method
- Parkland method

Other techniques that have been abandoned in modern obstetrics include the following:
- Madlener technique
- Kroener technique
- Irving technique
- Uchida method

Modified Pomeroy method is recommended by Government of India and has been described below.

Modified Pomeroy method of sterilization through minilap route

- Minilap route: It is an abdominal surgical approach to perform puerperal and interval sterilization through a small incision of 2–3 cm.
- The failure rate is 0.5%.

Minilap incision: Two approaches

- Subumbilical approach—to perform postpartum sterilization
- Suprapubic approach—to perform interval sterilization

Preoperative preparation

- History taking and examination are done.
- Investigations—hemoglobin estimation and urine analysis are done.
- Preoperative counseling
  - The patient should be counseled on the following: tubectomy is a permanent procedure, rare possibility of sterilization failure, risk of ectopic pregnancy in case of sterilization failure, and the risk of surgery.
  - Informed written consent is obtained from the patient (consent of the spouse is not mandatory).

Part 3

Principal steps of modified Pomeroy method of tubal sterilization

- The patient must be asked to void before the procedure.
- Anesthesia: Short general anesthesia, spinal, or local anesthesia or intravenous sedation is administered.
- Incision
  - In puerperal sterilization, minilap incision is given approximately two fingerbreadths (1 inch) below the fundus of uterus (uterine fundus is palpable below the umbilicus in the immediate postpartum period).
  - In interval sterilization, minilap incision is given two fingerbreadths above the pubic symphysis.
  - The incision can be transverse or vertical and deepened in layers to enter the peritoneal cavity.
- Delivery of the tubes: The index finger is introduced and is passed along the posterior surface of the uterus to the posterior leaf of the broad ligament and the tube is hooked out.
- The tube is traced laterally and the fimbrial end visualized to differentiate it from the round ligament. The tube is identified by the fimbrial end and the mesosalpinx containing utero-ovarian vessels. In case of interval sterilization, the uterus may be elevated with a uterine manipulator to the level of the incision, to facilitate access of the tubes.
- Tubal ligation is performed by modified Pomeroy technique as follows:
  - A loop of 2–3 cm of tube is picked up with Babcock forceps at the isthmus portion of fallopian tube (2–3 cm from the uterine cornu).

An avascular area on the mesosalpinx is pierced with No. 1–0 chromic catgut suture and the loop is tied (Figure 37.12a and b).
  - A free tie may be placed below the ligature with the same suture material.
  - Segment of the tube about 1–1.5 cm in length distal to the ligature is excised. (The two ends of the cut tube separate after few days; Figure 37.12c and d.)
- Hemostasis is checked.
- The segment of the excised tube is inspected to ensure that the tubal wall has been completely resected.
- The same procedure is repeated on the other side.
- Abdomen is closed in layers.
- Tubal segments are sent for histopathological examination.
- Prophylactic antibiotics are not recommended.
- The patient is usually discharged 24–48 hour after surgery.

Parkland method of sterilization

This is another commonly performed method o sterilization.

- An opening is made in an avascular portion o the mesosalpinx and 1-0 chromic catgut suture i passed through the opening (Figure 37.13a).
- The proximal and distal portions of the tube ar ligated separately. The intervening segment o the tube is excised (Figure 37.13b and c).
- The cut ends separate immediately unlik modified Pomeroy technique where the cut end separate after few days.
- Failure rate is 0.5%.

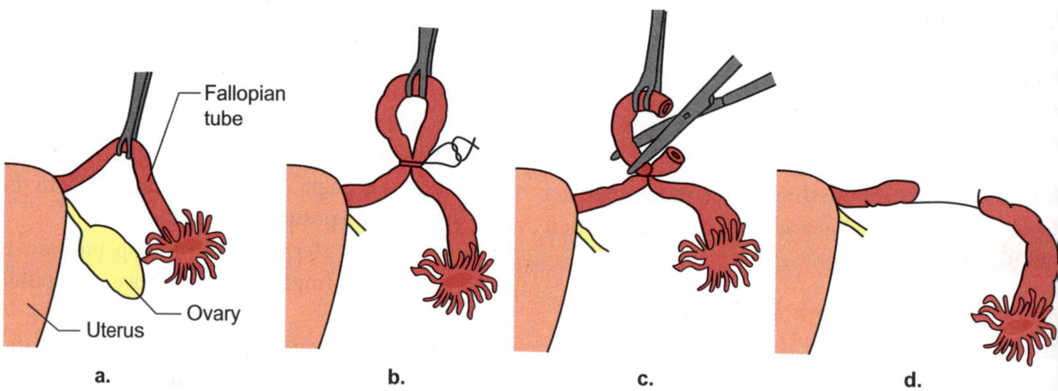

Figure 37.12 Steps of Pomeroy method of tubal sterilization. **a.** The tube is grasped at the isthmic portion **b.** The loop of the tube is then ligated with 1-0 chromic catgut. **c.** The ligated segment of the fallopian tube is excised. **d.** The two ends of the cut tube separate after a few days.

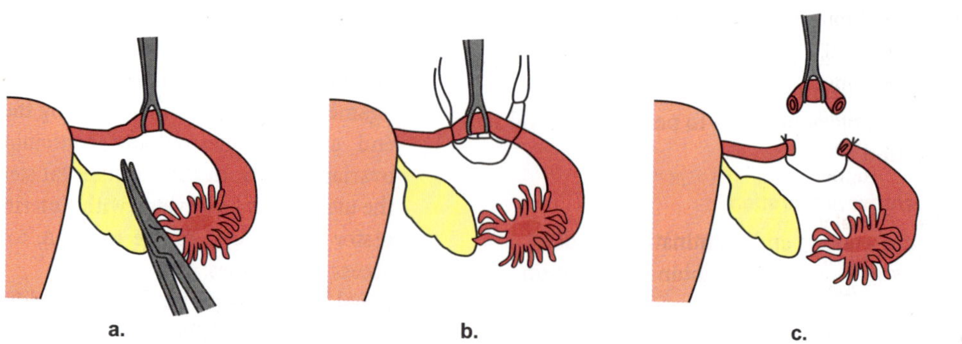

Figure 37.13 Steps of Parkland method of tubal sterilization. **a.** An avascular portion of the mesosalpinx is entered. **b.** A 2-cm segment of the midportion of the tube is ligated proximally and distally with 1-0 chromic catgut. **c.** The intervening segment is then excised.

Extra edge

Absorbable suture material is used for tubal ligation for the following reasons:

- Prompt absorption of the sutures leads to separation of the cut ends of the tube. The cut ends of the tube become sealed off by spontaneous reperitonization and fibrosis and retract from each other .
- If a nonabsorbable suture is used, the ligated tubal segments always remain in close proximity to each other and do not fall apart, thereby increasing the chances of recanalization of tubes and failure of sterilization.

Complications of female sterilization

See Table 37.13

Table 37.13 Complications of female sterilization procedure

Intraoperative	Postoperative	
	Early	Late
• Anesthetic complications • Injury to bowel, bladder, and major vessels, especially in laparoscopic procedure • Broad ligament hematoma	• Pain • Infection	• Failure rate of 0.1–0.5%. Failure of sterilization can result in intrauterine or ectopic pregnancies • Post-tubal ligation syndrome: Constellation of symptoms that include pelvic discomfort, menorrhagia, and ovarian cystic changes. These symptoms are likely due to disruption of utero-ovarian blood supply following sterilization

High-yield points

Methods of laparoscopic sterilization

- Bipolar electrocoagulation is not preferred due to high failure rate.
- Banding—Falope ring is used.
- Clip application—Hulka-Clemens clip and Filshie clip are used.

Advantages of laparoscopic sterilization

- A minimally invasive technique
- Small incision
- Reduced duration of hospital stay
- Rapid recovery
- Provides a chance to inspect the pelvis and upper abdominal organs

No scalpel vasectomy

- No scalpel vasectomy (keyhole vasectomy) is a type of vasectomy procedure, in which a sharp hemostat is used to puncture the scrotum to access the vas deferens, instead of giving an incision as in conventional vasectomy.

Advantages

- Easy to perform hence widely practiced in public health programs.
- It is a day care (outpatient) procedure.
- It can be performed under local anesthesia.
- Procedure can be done in a short time period.
- There is no need for surgical sutures to close the skin.
- Pain, bleeding, and infection are less than conventional vasectomy.
- The individual is able to return to routine activity sooner than conventional vasectomy.

38 Common Gynecological Surgical Procedures

Introduction

The prime objective of this chapter is to make the readers familiar with the basics of operative gynecology. Only the principal steps of the surgical procedures have been described, to help the students remember and recollect the same during exams.

COMMON OPERATIVE PROCEDURES IN GYNECOLOGY

Major procedures

- Abdominal hysterectomy
- Vaginal hysterectomy
- Ward Mayo's surgery
- Manchester repair
- Myomectomy
- Procedures on the ovary

Minor procedures

- Endometrial biopsy/sampling
- Cervical biopsy
- Cervical cone biopsy
- Marsupialization of Bartholin's cyst

PERIOPERATIVE CARE FOR MAJOR GYNECOLOGICAL SURGERIES

It includes the patient care during preoperative, intraoperative, and postoperative periods.

Preoperative preparation

- A complete history is taken and physical examination is done.
- Routine preoperative investigations: These include hemoglobin and complete blood count, blood grouping and typing, urine routine and microscopy, blood glucose and renal function test. ECG, chest X-ray, and serum electrolytes are done in women above 40 years of age for anesthetic fitness. Serology for hepatitis B and HIV are done in high-risk cases.
- Pap smear should be done for all patients prior to surgery.
- Consent: Written informed consent for the surgery must be obtained from the patient.
- Part preparation: Part preparation should be done from inferior rib cage to the midthigh. Routine shaving of the operative site before surgery is not recommended. Hair clipping can be done. The patient is asked to wash the operative area with soap and water.
- Bowel preparation: Enema is administered to the patient in the night before and in the morning of the surgery.

Viva corner

Q1 What is day care surgery?

Day care surgery includes those surgical procedures in which patients are admitted, operated upon, and discharged on the same day.

- **Benefits of day care surgery are the following**: Reduction in hospital stay, inpatient workload, concomitant cost, and least effect on the patient's routine work.
- **Common gynecological day care surgeries**
  - Biopsy procedures
  - Examination under anesthesia
  - Endoscopic procedures such as diagnostic hysteroscopy and laparoscopy
  - Transcervical resection of endometrium

- Injection tetanus toxoid 0.5 mL IM and Xylocaine test dose are administered.
- The patient is kept nil per oral for at least 8 hours prior to the scheduled surgery.
- Night sedation: To ensure good sleep at night prior to the day of surgery, diazepam 5–10 mg or alprazolam 0.5 mg is given orally at bedtime.
- Prophylactic antibiotics: Prophylactic antibiotics are given to maintain adequate tissue levels of antibiotics during the surgery. A broad-spectrum antibiotic, usually a third-generation cephalosporin (ceftriaxone 1 g), is given as slow IV on induction of anesthesia (after test dose). The second dose is repeated after 12 hours.

Intraoperative care

Preparation on OT table

- IV infusion of Ringer lactate solution is started.
- Anesthesia (local, regional, or general) is administered.
- Position of the patient: For abdominal surgeries, the patient is placed in dorsal position, and for vaginal surgeries, the patient is placed in lithotomy position.
- Antiseptic cleaning is done with povidone-iodine or an alcohol based solution.
- Draping is done using sterile linen, towel, and leggings.
- Bladder preparation
  - For minor operative procedures, the patient is asked to void before being taken to the operating room.
  - For major abdominal surgeries, Foley's catheter is inserted for continuous bladder drainage, prior to starting the procedure.
  - For vaginal surgeries, a red rubber or metal catheter is used for intermittent catheterization of bladder prior to and during the procedure, and Foley's catheter is inserted at the end of the operation.

Skin incisions for abdominal surgeries

Transverse incision

Advantages and disadvantages of transverse skin incision are mentioned in Table 38.1.

Table 38.1 Advantages and disadvantages of transverse skin incision

Advantages	Disadvantages
• Good access to pelvic organs • Better postoperative convalescence • Less incidence of postoperative complications • Rapid wound healing • Cosmetically better • Less incidence of wound dehiscence and incisional hernia	Incision is difficult to extend if exploration of the upper abdomen is needed

Vertical (median or paramedian) incision

Advantages and disadvantages of vertical skin incision are mentioned in Table 38.2.

Table 38.2 Advantages and disadvantages of vertical skin incision

Advantages	Disadvantage
• It gives rapid entry into the abdominal cavity • Good access to the whole of abdomen • Excellent exposure • It spares major nerves, vessels, as opposed to transverse incision	It lacks all the advantages of transverse incision

Extra edge

- **Cherney incision**: It is a muscle-splitting incision where the rectus muscle is dissected from its insertion at pubic symphysis.
- **Maylard incision**: It is a transverse muscle-cutting incision. The muscles are approximated during closure.

Surgical procedure

- The required surgical procedure is performed.
- Hemostasis is checked and mop and instrument counts are checked prior to closure of the wound.

Closure of abdominal wound

- Abdominal wound closed in layers
  - Closure of peritoneum—not indicated

- Closure of rectus sheath done
- Closure of subcutaneous tissue—not indicated
- Closure of skin done

Role of intra-abdominal drains

Intra-abdominal drains are used to prevent accumulation of blood, pus, etc. They are less commonly used in gynecological surgeries, when hemostasis is satisfactorily achieved.

Role of closure of peritoneum

Current studies have shown that closure of the pelvic and parietal peritoneum increases adhesions, although it is still done by many surgeons. Peritoneum rapidly spreads across any raw areas left after surgery, and there is no need of peritoneal closure (Royal College of Obstetricians and Gynaecologists, 1998).

Muscle layer

- Muscle does not tolerate suturing well.
- Surgeons prefer to avoid interfering with the blood supply and nerve function of muscle by making a muscle-splitting incision or retracting the muscle toward its nerve supply. During closure, muscles handled in this manner need not be sutured.

Closure of fascia

- Fascial layer (rectus sheath) is a firm connective tissue covering the muscles and provides the main support to the abdominal wall.
- The fascial sutures must hold the wound closed and also help to resist changes in intra-abdominal pressure.
- As the fascial sutures bear the maximum stress of the wound, nonabsorbable or delayed absorbable sutures are used.
- Occasionally, synthetic graft material such as polypropylene mesh may be used when fascia is absent or weak.

Role of closure of subcutaneous fat

- Fat does not tolerate suturing well.
- Some surgeons question the advisability of placing sutures in fatty tissue because it has little tensile strength due to its composition, which is mostly water.
- However, others believe that it is necessary to place at least a few sutures in a thick layer of subcutaneous fat to prevent dead space, especially in obese patients.

Closure of skin

- The skin sutures need only be strong enough to withstand natural skin tension and hold the wound edges in apposition. This is because most of the stress placed upon the healing wound is absorbed by the fascia.
- Closure of skin is usually done by taking interrupted mattress sutures with nonabsorbable monofilament sutures such as Ethilon or Prolene.
- Subcuticular suturing technique of skin can be done by taking continuous short lateral stitches beneath the epithelial layer of skin with absorbable or nonabsorbable sutures.

Postoperative care

Immediate postoperative care

Following the surgical procedure, the patient is shifted to the recovery room adjacent to the operation theater.

Postoperative day (POD)-0: In the first 24 hours

- Monitor vitals: Pulse, respiration, and blood pressure are monitored every half an hour in the initial period. The interval is gradually increased if vitals are stable.
- Watch for soakage of abdominal dressing or vaginal bleeding.
- The patient is kept nil oral for initial 6–12 hours. Orals can be started 6 hours after vaginal hysterectomy, and laparoscopy procedures.
- Fluid replacement: Following major surgeries, fluids are replaced intravenously. Urine output at least 30 mL/h indicates adequate fluid replacement. Fluid requirement during the postoperative period is about 35–40 mL/kg/day, including replacement of insensible loss.
- Analgesics: Adequate pain control ensures deep breathing, adequate oxygenation, early mobilization, prompt wound healing, and lesser duration of hospital stay. Injection tramadol/diclofenac/ketorolac are the common analgesics administered IM in the postoperative period. In some centers, patient controlled analgesia (PCA) is used.

- Antibiotics: Prophylactic antibiotics are usually given during surgery. Alternatively, routine postoperative antibiotics are administered by parenteral route for 24–48 hours followed by oral route for another 3–5 days.
- H2 receptor blocker (Ranitidine) or proton pump inhibitor (Pantoprazole) are administered intravenously in the immediate postoperative period.
- Antiemetics: Nausea and vomiting can be prevented by administration of metoclopramide 10 mg or ondansetron 4 mg IM/IV.
- H2 receptor blockers such as ranitidine or proton pump inhibitors such as pantoprazole are administered IV—decreases the incidence of postoperative emesis, stress ulcers, and aspiration pneumonitis.
- Bladder care: Foley's catheter is kept for 12–24 hours following major gynecological surgeries. It helps to keep the bladder empty, to monitor urine output, and reduces the risk of urinary retention due to pain reflex.

Postoperative day 1

- Vitals are noted.
- Enquire about passage of flatus.
- Check for bowel sounds.
- Vaginal pack (usually kept after vaginal surgeries) is removed.
- Foley's catheter is removed. Catheter is kept for 7–10 days in patients with bladder injury.
- Clear oral fluids are given in small but frequent intervals.
- Early ambulation is advised.
- Deep breathing exercises and leg and arm movements are encouraged.
- Parenteral analgesics and antibiotics are replaced with oral drugs.

Subsequent postoperative days

- Soft diet is started on postoperative day (POD) 2 and then gradually changed to normal diet.
- The abdominal wound dressing can be removed after 48 hours. Sutures may be removed by day 6 for transverse incisions and by day 8 for vertical incisions.
- The patient may be discharged by 5–7 days following major surgeries.

Examination prior to discharge

- Abdominal wound is checked for evidence of infection, hematoma, or dehiscence.
- Vault is checked to assess healing status following hysterectomy.

Advice at discharge

- Avoid lifting heavy weight for 4–6 weeks until the vaginal cuff heals completely.
- Avoid coitus for 6 weeks.
- Follow-up is scheduled after 6 weeks.

Some of the common gynecological surgical procedures are described in the following subsections.

HYSTERECTOMY

Hysterectomy is the procedure of removal of the uterus (with or without removal of ovaries).

Indications for hysterectomy

See Table 38.3

Table 38.3 Indications for hysterectomy

Benign causes	• Dysfunctional uterine bleeding • Fibroid uterus • Adenomyosis • Endometriosis • Endometrial hyperplasia • Uterine prolapse • Tubo-ovarian mass • Benign ovarian tumor in perimenopausal age
Malignant causes	• Carcinoma endometrium • Carcinoma cervix • Carcinoma ovary • Uterine sarcoma • Choriocarcinoma
Traumatic causes	• Uterine perforation • Rupture uterus
Obstetric causes	• Atonic postpartum hemorrhage • Morbidly adherent placenta • Hydatidiform mole at >35 years with completed family • Septic abortion

Routes of performing hysterectomy

- **Abdominal hysterectomy:** Uterus removed abdominally through an abdominal incision
- **Vaginal hysterectomy:** Uterus removed through vaginal route
- **Total laparoscopic hysterectomy (TLH):** It includes laparoscopically detaching the uterine body and cervix from the surrounding supporting structures and suturing the vaginal cuff. It includes bivalving, coring, or morcellating the excised tissues, as required. The uterus is then removed through the vagina or abdomen (uterine vessels are clamped abdominally via the laparoscopic port)
- **Laparoscopically assisted vaginal hysterectomy (LAVH):** It includes laparoscopically detaching the uterine body from the surrounding upper supporting structures. The vaginal portion of the procedure is then performed, uterine vessels are clamped, and the cervix and uterus are detached from the remaining supporting structures. The uterus is then removed through the vagina (uterine vessels are clamped via the vaginal route)

Comparison of advantages of abdominal versus vaginal hysterectomy is mentioned in Table 38.4.

Types of hysterectomy

Depending on the extent of removal of the uterus and adjacent structures, hysterectomy can be of different types as mentioned in Table 38.5.

Piver's classification of hysterectomy

See Table 38.6

Note

- *Hysterectomy Types I–III are commonly performed.*
- *Hysterectomy Types II–V are completed with pelvic lymph node dissection.*

Table 38.4 Comparison of advantages of abdominal with vaginal hysterectomy

Advantages of abdominal hysterectomy over vaginal hysterectomy	Advantages of vaginal hysterectomy over abdominal hysterectomy
• Women with pelvic adhesions or previous history of laparotomy are best managed by abdominal route • Thorough exploration of the abdominopelvic organs can be done • Associated tubo-ovarian pathology (tubo-ovarian mass) or a large uterus (fibroid) is best managed abdominally • Indicated in cases where pelvic and para-aortic lymph nodes are to be sampled	• No abdominal incision and scar • Lesser postoperative pain and need of analgesia • Lesser postoperative morbidity and mortality • Less hospital stay • Preferred in obese patients • Less risk of ureteric injuries when compared to abdominal hysterectomy

Table 38.5 Types of hysterectomy

Type of hysterectomy	Description
Total hysterectomy	Removal of the entire uterus including the cervix
Subtotal hysterectomy	Removal of the body of uterus, leaving behind the cervix
Panhysterectomy (hysterectomy with bilateral salpingo-oophorectomy)	Removal of the uterus along with removal of tubes and ovaries of both sides
Extended hysterectomy	Panhysterectomy along with removal of cuff of vagina
Radical hysterectomy	Removal of uterus, tubes, and ovaries of both sides, upper one-third of vagina, adjacent parametrium, and the pelvic lymph nodes

Table 38.6 Piver's classification of hysterectomy

Classification	Description
Type I (simple hysterectomy)	• It refers to simple extrafascial hysterectomy
Type II (modified radical hysterectomy)	• Paracervical tissues and upper vagina (1–2 cm) are removed • Uterine arteries are ligated at the site of crossing the ureters • Medial half of parametrium is resected
Type III (radical hysterectomy)	• Paracervical and paravaginal tissues with upper one-third of vagina are removed • Uterine vessels are ligated at their origin • Removal of entire parametrium
Type IV (extended radical hysterectomy)	In addition to the structures removed in radical hysterectomy, the other structures that are removed are the following: • Upper three-fourth of vagina • Superior vesical artery • Periureteric tissue
Type V (partial exenteration)	Distal ureter and segment of bladder and rectum are removed

Extra edge

Factors to be considered during hysterectomy

- **Age and parity:** The patient should preferably be in the perimenopausal age group with family completed. However, hysterectomy may have to be done under forced circumstances even in young age group or unmarried or nulliparous women [e.g., atonic postpartum hemorrhage (PPH), torrential hemorrhage during myomectomy ending up in hysterectomy, gynecological malignancies].
- **Total versus subtotal hysterectomy:** The preferred surgery is always a total hysterectomy unless there is sufficient reason to leave behind the cervix.

Indications of subtotal hysterectomy

- Complicated tubo-ovarian mass with obliteration of pouch of Douglas
- Pelvic endometriosis involving the rectovaginal septum
- Emergency hysterectomy (cesarean hysterectomy)

Advantages of subtotal hysterectomy

Controversy exists on the usefulness of subtotal hysterectomy. The potential benefits are as follows:

- Reduced operative and postoperative morbidity
- Reduced rate of vaginal shortening
- Reduced rate of vault prolapse

Risks of leaving behind the cervical stump

- Cervicitis with abnormal vaginal discharge
- Stump carcinoma (1%)

Patients who underwent subtotal hysterectomy should be followed up with Pap smear.

Abdominal hysterectomy

Indications

- Symptomatic fibroid uterus >14 weeks in size
- Chronic pelvic pain due to endometriosis or chronic PID, where dense adhesions are expected and vaginal hysterectomy is not possible
- Hysterectomy required as a part of treatment of malignancies of the genital tract
- Associated tubo-ovarian pathology
- Hysterectomy indicated in a patient with previous pelvic surgeries (adhesions are expected)

Principal steps of abdominal hysterectomy (Figure 38.1)

- Anesthesia: Regional or general anesthesia is given.
- The patient is placed in supine position.
- Bladder is catheterized with Foley's catheter.
- Parts are cleaned with an antiseptic solution and draped.
- Suprapubic transverse skin incision or infraumbilical midline or paramedian incision is made and deepened in layers.
- Intraoperative findings are noted.
- Bilateral (B/L) round ligaments are clamped, cut, and ligated (Figure 38.1a).

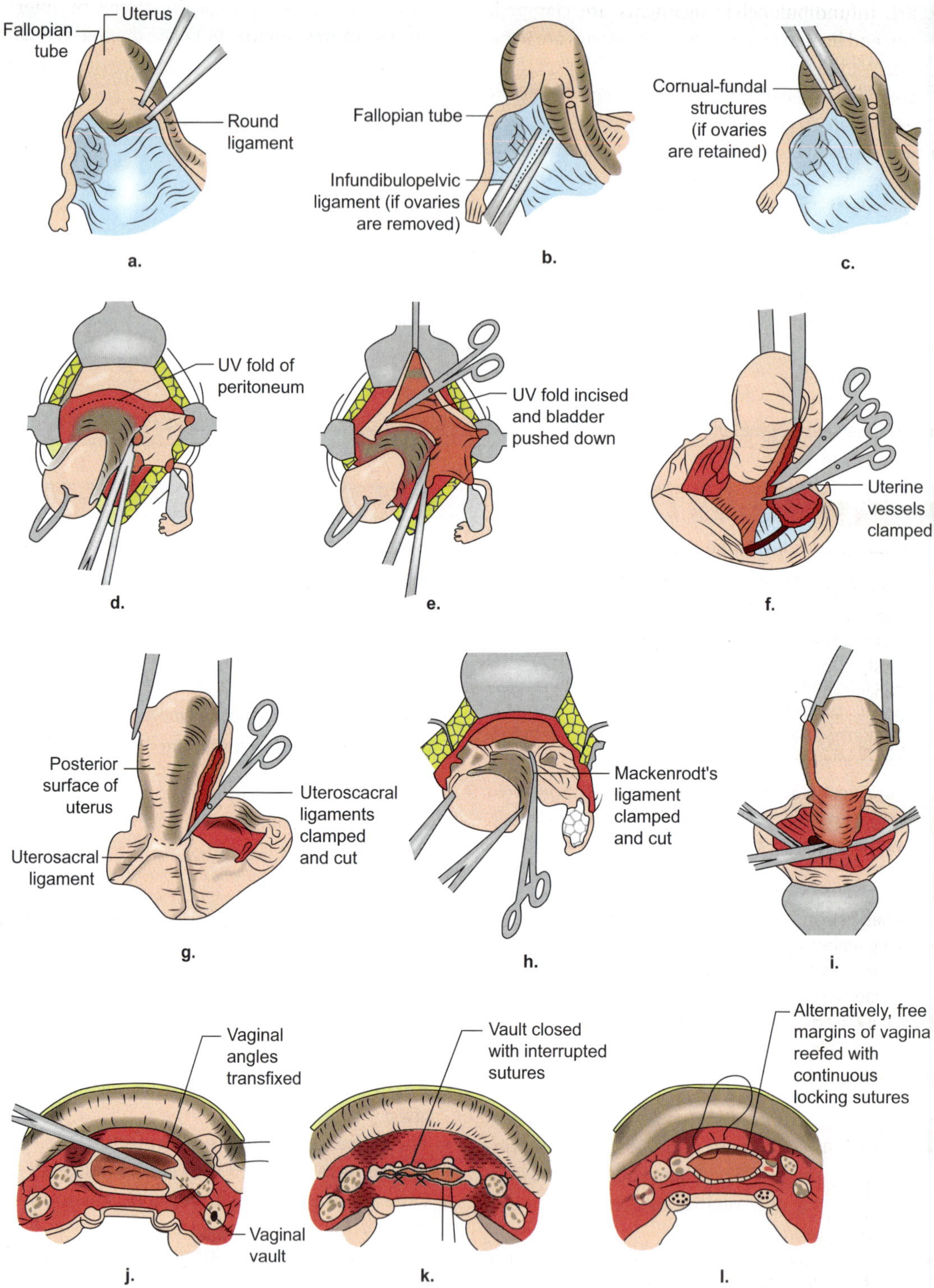

Figure 38.1 Principal steps of abdominal hysterectomy (check the text for description of the procedure).

- B/L infundibulopelvic ligaments are clamped, cut, and ligated (Figure 38.1b) if ovaries are to be removed, *or else*, B/L cornual-fundal structures are clamped, cut, and ligated (Figure 38.1c) if ovaries are to be preserved.
- The loose uterovesical fold of peritoneum is incised and bladder is pushed down (Figure 38.1d and e).
- B/L uterine vessels are clamped, cut, and ligated (Figure 38.1f).
- B/L uterosacrals and Mackenrodt's ligaments are clamped, cut, and ligated (Figure 38.1g and h).
- The vault of vagina is opened, and specimen of uterus with the cervix is delivered out (Figure 38.1i).
- The vaginal angles are transfixed with sutures (Figure 38.1j).
- Vault is closed—vault can be closed by interrupted sutures (Figure 38.1k) or the free vaginal margin can be reefed with a continuous locking suture (Figure 38.1l).
- B/L Mackenrodt's ligament are anchored to the vault.
- Hemostasis and counts are checked.
- Abdomen is closed in layers.

Advantages and disadvantages of abdominal hysterectomy

See Table 38.7

Complications of abdominal hysterectomy

See Table 38.8

Table 38.7 Advantages and disadvantages of abdominal hysterectomy

Advantages	Disadvantages
• Wide exposure of the abdominal and pelvic organs • Tubo-ovarian pathology can be tackled simultaneously • Concurrent surgical procedures such as appendicectomy may be performed, if indicated	• Difficult to perform in very obese patients • More postoperative pain and need for analgesia • Postoperative complications are higher—increased incidence of peritonitis, fever, pulmonary complications • Increased duration of hospital stay • Morbidity and mortality are more when compared to vaginal hysterectomy • Presence of abdominal scar and risk of incisional hernia later

Table 38.8 Complications of abdominal hysterectomy

Intraoperative complications	Postoperative complications	
	Immediate	Late
• Anesthetic complications—lung atelectasis, pulmonary edema, and embolism • Hemorrhage • Injury to adjacent structures such as bladder, bowel, and ureter	• Hemorrhage and shock • Paralytic ileus • Febrile morbidity • Urinary retention—due to pain and spasm • Cystitis • Thrombophlebitis, deep vein thrombosis • Wound infection, dehiscence	• Vault granulation • Vault prolapse • Incisional hernia • Surgical menopause, if ovaries have been removed

Viva corner

Q1 What is the recommendation on preservation versus removal of normal ovaries during hysterectomy?

Recommendation on preservation of ovaries:

- It seems rational to preserve the ovaries in premenopausal and postmenopausal women if ovaries are healthy.
- Refer Part 2, Chapter 20, for further details.

Special considerations for removal of ovaries during hysterectomy:

- If the ovaries are diseased or involved in neoplastic conditions
- Hysterectomy done in a woman who has H/o ovarian or breast cancer in a first-degree relative

(CONTD...)

(...CONTD)

Viva corner

Indications for removal of fallopian tubes:

- International guidelines recommend removal of fallopian tubes (prophylactic bilateral salpingectomy) at the time of hysterectomy to lower the incidence of ovarian cancer.
- Fallopian tubes are removed in most of the instances when ovaries are removed (salpingo-oophorectomy)
- When the fallopian tubes are diseased (salpingectomy)

Benefits and risks of preservation of ovaries during hysterectomy:

See table below

Table Benefits and risks of preservation of ovaries during hysterectomy

Benefits	Risks
• Ovarian function continues till the expected time of menopause • Menopausal symptoms appear late and the severity is less • Decreased incidence of vasomotor symptoms, osteoporosis, and atherosclerotic changes	• Risks of developing ovarian neoplasms (benign or malignant) • Residual ovarian syndrome occurs in 1–3% of cases due to multiple cystic follicles and/or periovarian adhesions • Chronic pelvic pain • Risk of relaparotomy later in life, in 3–5% of cases

Types, causes, and management of hemorrhage during or following surgery

See Table 38.9

Postoperative bowel dysfunction: Paralytic ileus versus obstruction

See Table 38.10

Table 38.9 Types, causes, and management of hemorrhage during or following surgery

Type of hemorrhage	Description	Causes	Management
Primary hemorrhage	Hemorrhage that occurs at the time of surgery	• Incidence is more in cases with adhesions due to endometriosis or pelvic inflammatory disease, in radical hysterectomy, and exenteration procedures • May be due to increased vascularity like in a huge fibroid • Imperfect hemostasis	Managed by hemostatic sutures, compression, internal iliac artery ligation and/or packing
Reactionary hemorrhage	This occurs within 24–48 hours after surgery	• Slippage of ligatures at the pedicles or at the vaginal angles • Dislodgement of clot	The patient usually requires laparotomy to achieve hemostasis
Secondary hemorrhage	This hemorrhage occurs between 7 and 14 days after surgery	It occurs due to sepsis and sloughing away of necrotic material from the uterine vessels or blood vessels at the vault	• In cases of internal hemorrhage, laparotomy has to be done along with resuscitative measures • If hemorrhage is from the vault, hemostasis can be achieved by taking sutures at vault under general anesthesia

Table 38.10 Comparison of paralytic ileus with obstruction in patients with postoperative bowel dysfunction

Feature	Ileus	Obstruction
Distension	Present	Present
Pain	Mild due to distension	Progressively worsens due to cramps
Vomiting	Present	Present
Onset of symptoms	Within 48–72 hours of surgery	Delayed up to 5–7 days postoperative
Bowel sounds	Absent	Peristaltic rushes
X-ray	Bowel loops distended with gas	Distended bowel loops with air–fluid level
Treatment	Conservative—nasogastric suction, IV fluids, correction of electrolyte imbalance, and control of infection	Initially conservative, may need surgical intervention

Viva corner

Q1 What are the causes of fever in the postoperative period?

Postoperative fever is defined as temperature of 38°C or more, after the first 24 hours of surgery, on two occasions at least 4 hours apart. It is the first sign of postoperative sepsis.

Postoperative fever may be due to the following:

- Cystitis
- Abdominal wound infection
- Vault cuff cellulitis
- Peritonitis
- Infected hematoma and abscess formation
- Pulmonary infection and pneumonia
- Thrombophlebitis
- Deep vein thrombosis

Vaginal hysterectomy

Indications

- Uterovaginal prolapse
- In all benign gynecological conditions where uterus is not enlarged more than 14 weeks

Contraindications

Vaginal hysterectomy is difficult to be performed in the following cases:

- Uterus size >14 weeks
- Endometriosis
- Previous abdominal surgeries (adhesions are expected)
- Associated tubo-ovarian pathology
- Gynecological malignancies such as ovarian, cervical, and endometrial carcinoma

Principal steps of vaginal hysterectomy (Figure 38.2)

- Regional or general anesthesia is given. The patient is placed in lithotomy position, and parts cleaned and draped.
- Bladder is drained and vaginal examination is done.
- Circumferential incision is given at cervicovaginal junction, just below the bladder sulcus, and vaginal flaps are raised all around.
- Pubocervical ligaments (bladder pillars) are cut and the bladder is pushed up (Figure 38.2a).
- Uterovesical fold of peritoneum is identified and incised (Figure 38.2b).
- Posteriorly, pouch of Douglas is identified and opened (Figure 38.2c and d).
- B/L Mackenrodt's and uterosacral ligaments are clamped, cut, and ligated (Figure 38.2e).

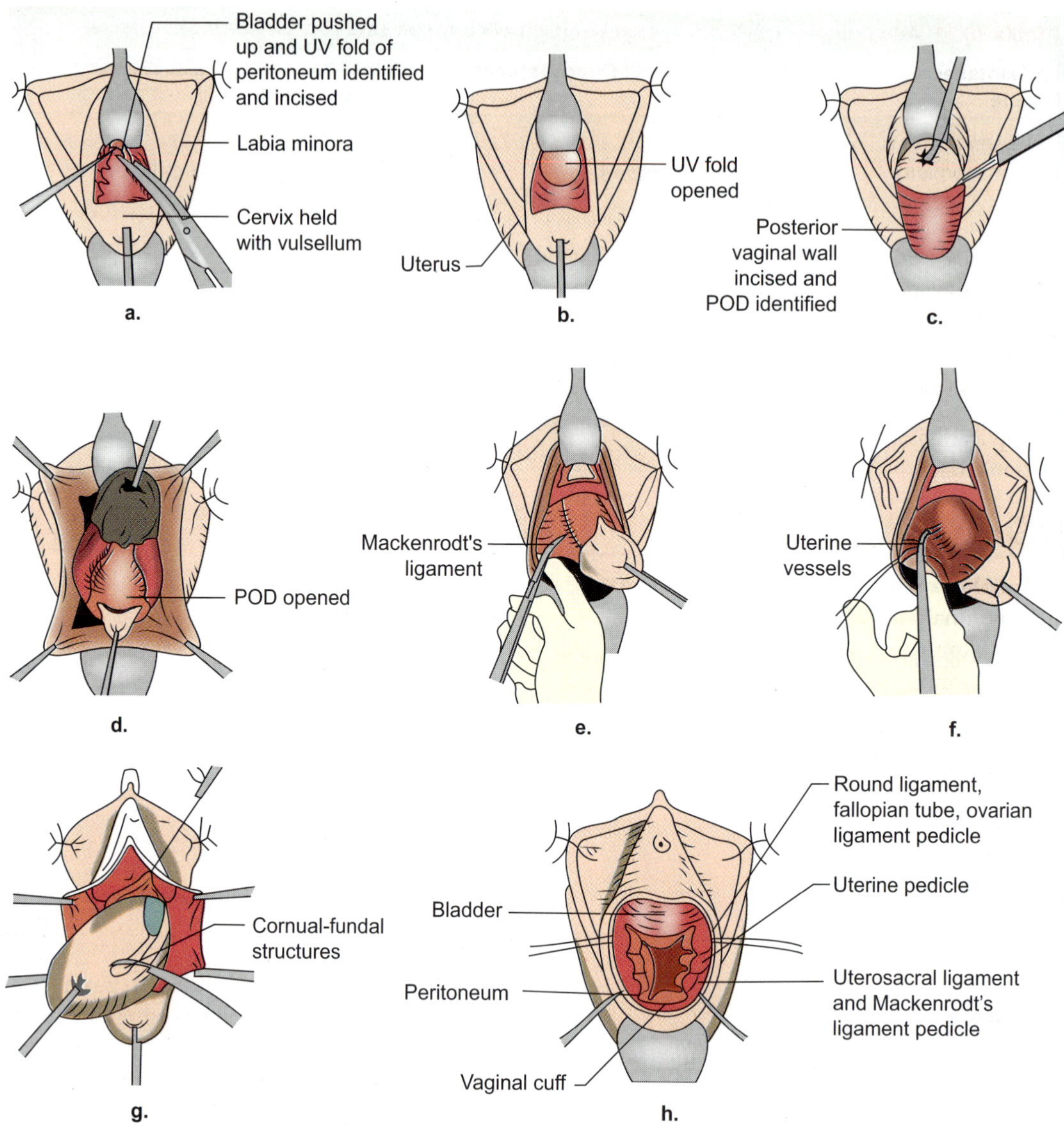

Figure 38.2 Principal steps of vaginal hysterectomy. *POD*, pouch of Douglas; *UV*, uterovesical.

- B/L uterine vessels are clamped, cut, and ligated (Figure 38.2f).
- B/L cornual-fundal structures (round ligament, fallopian tubes, ovarian ligament) are clamped, cut, and ligated if ovaries are to be retained (Figure 38.2g), *or else* infundibulopelvic ligaments are clamped, cut, and ligated if the ovaries are to be removed.
- Uterus specimen is delivered out.
- Hemostasis and counts are checked (Figure 38.2h).
- Vaginal vault is closed with interrupted sutures.
- B/L Mackenrodt's ligament are held to vault.
- Vagina is packed with antiseptic-soaked roller gauze.
- Foley's catheter is inserted for continuous bladder drainage.

Advantages and disadvantages of vaginal hysterectomy

See Table 38.11

Table 38.11 Advantages and disadvantages of vaginal hysterectomy

Advantages	Disadvantages
• Preferred in obese patients • Postoperative complications are less • Less morbidity • Lesser postoperative pain and need of analgesia • Lesser hospital stay • Early resumption of day-to-day activities • No abdominal incision and scar	• Skilled and experienced surgeon required to do the surgery • Exploration of abdominal and pelvic organs cannot be done • Difficult in cases with restricted uterine mobility, limited vaginal space, associated adnexal pathology, uterus >14 weeks size, pelvic adhesions, and previous H/o abdominal surgery

Complications

Complications are similar to those of abdominal hysterectomy.

Ward Mayo's surgery

Ward Mayo's surgery is done for cases with uterovaginal prolapse and refers to vaginal hysterectomy with pelvic floor repair (vaginal hysterectomy with anterior colporrhaphy and posterior colpoperineorrhaphy).

Indications

- Uterovesical prolapse in women aged >40 years (age limit relaxed to 35 years, if there are associated problems such as fibroid or adenomyosis)

Principle steps of Ward Mayo's procedure

Note *Vaginal hysterectomy is performed first followed by correction of the defects. Hence, the initial steps are similar to those mentioned in the section "vaginal hysterectomy."*

- Regional anesthesia is given.
- The patient is placed in lithotomy position, and parts cleaned and draped.
- Bladder is drained and vaginal examination is done.
- Circumferential incision is given at cervicovaginal junction, just below the bladder sulcus.
- Pubocervical ligaments (bladder pillars) are cut and bladder is pushed up.
- Anterior uterovesical fold of peritoneum and posterior pouch of Douglas are identified and opened.
- Hysterectomy is done by serially clamping, cutting, and ligating B/L Mackenrodt's and uterosacral ligaments, B/L uterine vessels, and B/L cornual-fundal structures.
- Uterus specimen is delivered out.
- Hemostasis and counts are checked.
- Vaginal hysterectomy is followed by correction of the defects as mentioned in the subsequent text.

Enterocele repair

Enterocele repair is done by doing a McCall culdoplasty, which includes approximation of the uterosacral ligaments and its fixation to the vault. This procedure, in addition to correction of enterocele, prevents future vault prolapse.

McCall culdoplasty A suture is taken through the vaginal vault from outside in, on the patient's left side, and then through the left uterosacral ligament. This is continued as a series of bites through the peritoneum on the anterior surface of rectum, and then through the right uterosacral ligament, and brought out through the vaginal vault on the right side (Figure 38.3). When the suture is tied, the uterosacrals are approximated and fixed to the vaginal vault.

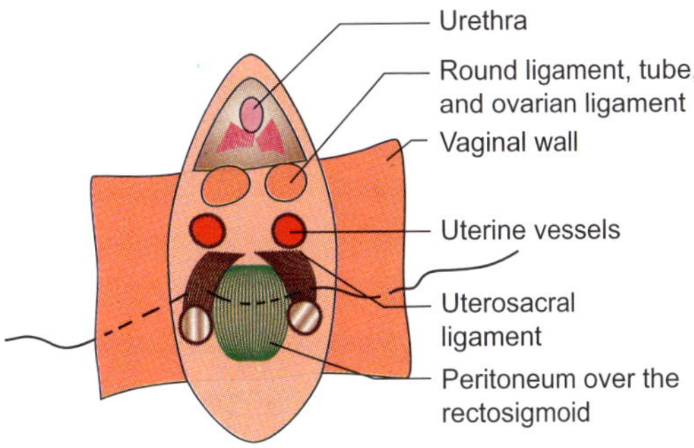

Figure 38.3 McCall culdoplasty.

Cystocele repair (anterior colporrhaphy)

Anterior colporrhaphy is the repair of the defect in the pubovesicocervical fascia by plicating the fascia.

- The circumferential incision that was earlier made at cervicovaginal junction is converted into an inverted "T"-shaped incision by making a vertical incision from the midpoint of the transverse incision up to 1.5 cm below the external urethral meatus on the anterior vaginal wall.
- Triangular vaginal flaps are dissected off from the underlying bladder by sharp and blunt dissection. The lateral dissection should be done up to the pubic rami on both sides (Figure 38.4a).
- Cystocele repair is done by plication of pubovesicocervical fascia with interrupted sutures (Figure 38.4b and c).
- The redundant vaginal mucosa is excised on either side.
- The cut margins of the vagina are closed by interrupted sutures.

Posterior colpoperineorrhaphy

Posterior colpoperineorrhaphy includes repair of rectocele and deficient perineum.

- A horizontal incision is made on the mucocutaneous junction on posterior vaginal wall.
- From the midpoint of this incision, another vertical incision is made up to apex of rectocele.
- Triangular vaginal flaps are dissected off laterally from the rectum (Figure 38.5a).
- The rectocele repair is done by plication of the defect in the rectovaginal fascia (Figure 38.5b).

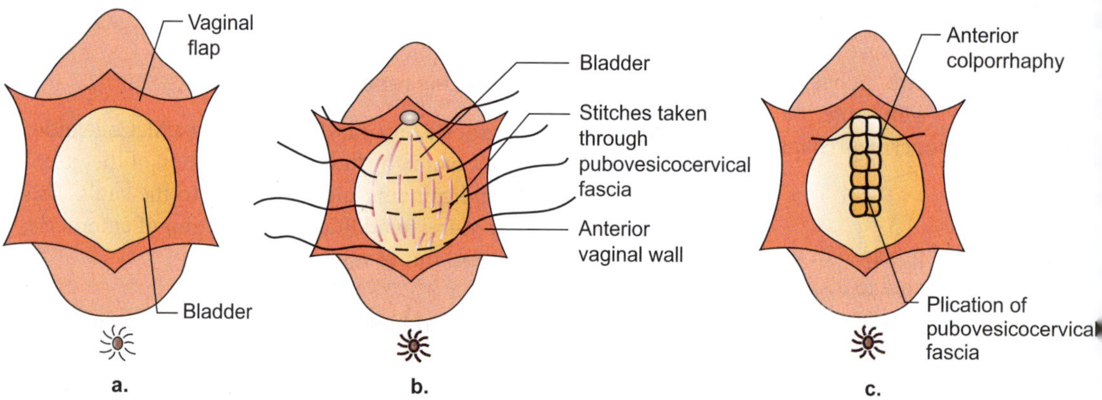

Figure 38.4 Anterior colporrhaphy. **a.** The anterior vaginal wall is dissected away from the bladder. **b.** Interrupted transverse sutures are taken for plication of the pubovesicocervical fascia. **c.** The plication sutures are tied.

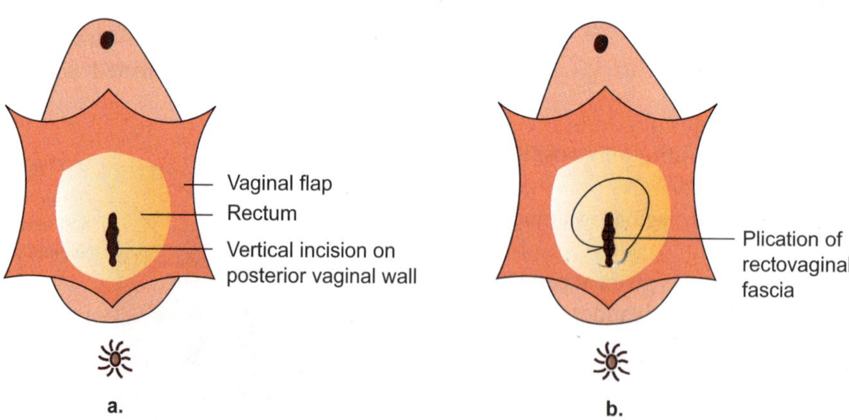

Figure 38.5 Rectocele repair. **a.** The posterior vaginal wall has been dissected away from the rectum. **b.** The defect in the rectovaginal fascia is identified and the fascia is plicated.

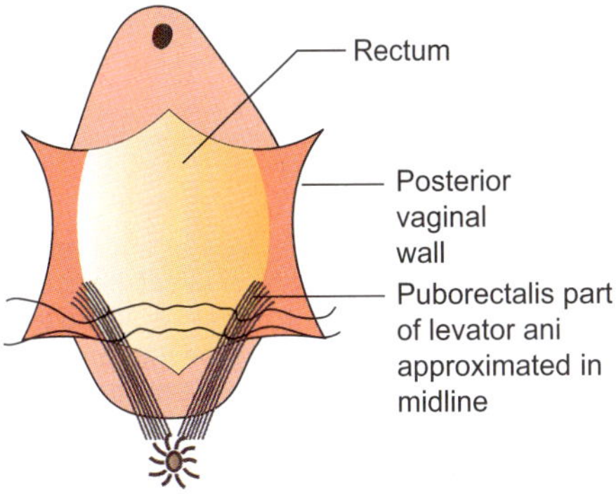

Figure 38.6 Perineorrhaphy. The puborectalis parts of levator ani muscles are brought together in midline and then the muscles of the perineal body are sutured to reconstruct the perineal body.

- The redundant vaginal flaps are excised.
- Puborectalis part of levator ani muscle is identified on both sides and approximated in midline (Figure 38.6).
- The posterior vaginal wall, muscle layer, and skin are approximated (similar to midline episiotomy suturing).
- Vagina is packed with roller gauze soaked with antiseptic solution.

MANCHESTER REPAIR OR FOTHERGILL'S OPERATION

Manchester repair is a conservative surgical procedure done for correction of uterovaginal prolapse.

Indications

- Suitable for women with uterovaginal prolapse, who are <40 years of age and have completed their family, with the intention of preserving menstrual function
- Second- or third-degree uterine prolapse with cystocele/rectocele, with or without supravaginal elongation of cervix

Principal steps of Manchester repair or Fothergill's operation

- Preliminary dilatation and curettage (D&C)
- Amputation of cervix
- Mackenrodt's ligaments shortened and fixed to the front of cervix
- Creation of neocervix
- Anterior colporrhaphy
- Posterior colpoperineorrhaphy

Viva corner

Q1 Why is preliminary dilatation and curettage done in Manchester procedure?

- Uterine sound is introduced to assess the cervical length and uterocervical length.
- Dilatation of the cervix is done for the following reasons:
  - To facilitate the passage of the sutures through the cervix, during creation of neocervix by vaginal flaps.
  - Dilatation ensures uterine drainage in the postoperative period.
  - It prevents cervical stenosis during healing of the neocervix.
- Curettage is done to rule out endometrial pathology as uterus is preserved

Q2 Why is Mackenrodt's ligament plicated in front of the cervix?

It facilitates shortening of Mackenrodt's ligament and takes the cervix up to its normal position.

Steps of Manchester repair/ Fothergill's operation

- Preliminary D & C is done.
- Circumferential incision is given at cervicovaginal junction, just below the bladder sulcus.
- Pubocervical ligaments (bladder pillars) are cut and bladder is pushed up.
- The vaginal walls are dissected off from the cervix by sharp and blunt dissection.
- B/L Mackenrodt's ligaments are clamped, cut, and ligated and sutures are held (Figure 38.7a).
- B/L descending cervical artery are ligated.
- The cervix is now amputated at the desired level to leave behind 2.5 cm of cervix (Figure 38.7b).
- Fothergill's stitch is taken and held. This stitch is taken through the following tissues in a sequence:

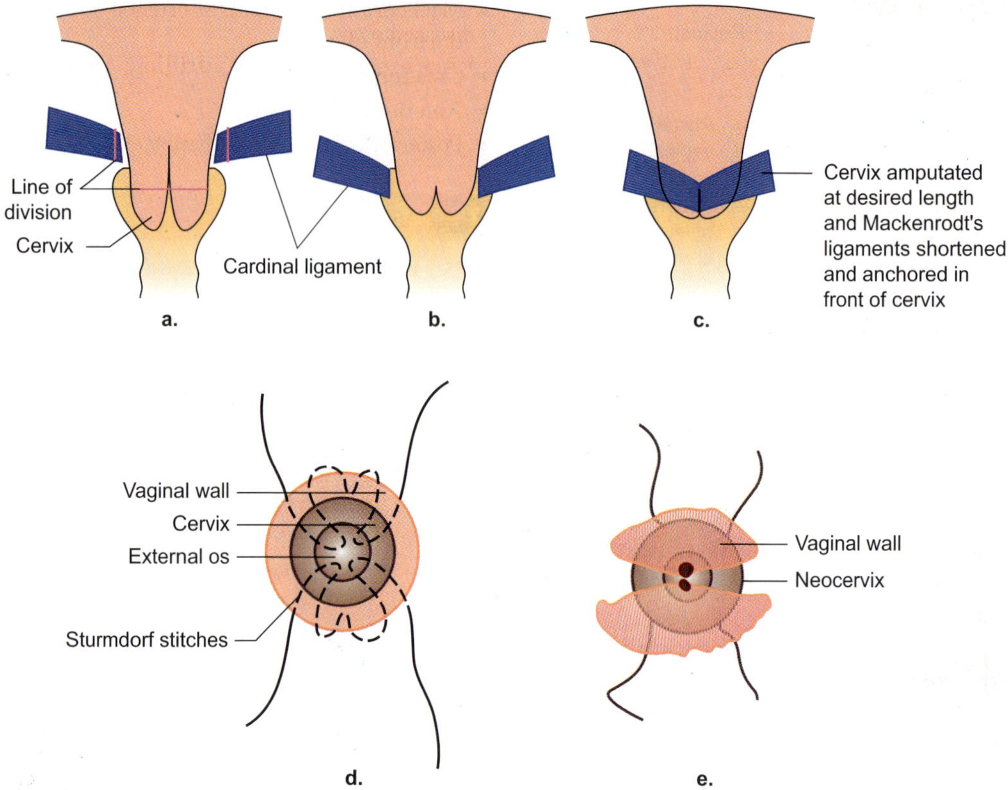

Figure 38.7 Manchester repair. **a.** The cardinal ligaments are cut at the attachment to the cervix. **b.** Amputation of the cervix to the desired length (2.5 cm) is done. **c.** Cardinal ligaments are sutured to the anterior aspect of the cervix. **d.** Sturmdorf sutures are taken with redundant vaginal flaps. **e.** Sturmdorf sutures are tied to form the neocervix with redundant vaginal flaps.

   – Vaginal wall at the level of the Fothergill's lateral point → Mackenrodt's ligament → cervical tissue from outside inwards → cervical tissue from inside outwards → Mackenrodt's ligament of the other side → vaginal wall (Fothergill's lateral point) of the other side. The stitch is held on both sides and tied at the end of the procedure. This stitch helps in anteversion of uterus.
- The shortened Mackenrodt's ligament are anchored to the anterior surface of the cervix (Figure 38.7c).
- Anterior colporrhaphy is done.
- Neocervix is created: The anterior and posterior lips of the amputated cervix are covered by the redundant vaginal flaps by taking Sturmdorf sutures (Figure 38.7d and e).
- Fothergill's stitch is tied anterior to cervix.
- Posterior colpoperineorrhaphy is performed.
- Vaginal pack is placed.
- Self-retaining Foley's catheter is inserted.

Complications of Fothergill's operation

See Table 38.12

Table 38.12 Complications of Fothergill's operation

Intraoperative complications	Postoperative complications	
	Early	Late
• Hemorrhage • Injury to the bladder and rectum	• Urinary retention/ cystitis • Infection	• Infertility • Cervical stenosis • Cervical incompetence

MYOMECTOMY

It refers to surgical removal of the fibroids (myomectomy procedure has been elaborated in Part 2, Chapter 20, *Fibroid Uterus*).

Principal steps of myomectomy procedure

- A single incision is made (preferably) in the midline on the anterior wall of uterus.
- It is deepened through the myometrium till the fibroid is reached.
- The fibroid is grasped with a myoma screw and enucleated from its bed by sharp and blunt dissection.
- The other fibroids are reached through tunneling incision.
- The dead space is obliterated by interrupted mattress or figure-of-eight sutures.

Viva corner

Q1 What are the steps to control hemorrhage during myomectomy?

- Preoperative treatment with GnRH analogues
- Controlled hypotensive analgesia
- Use of vasoactive agents such as vasopressin injection into the myometrium
- Use of Bonney's uterine clamp
- Use of tourniquet to occlude uterine vessels

Complications

Immediate and early postoperative complications are similar to those of abdominal hysterectomy.

Late complications

- Risk of recurrence of fibroid
- Persistence of menorrhagia

SURGICAL PROCEDURES ON THE OVARY

- **Oophorectomy**: Removal of healthy ovaries
- **Ovarian cystectomy**: Removal of ovarian cyst leaving behind healthy ovarian tissue
- **Ovariotomy/ovariectomy**: Removal of the diseased ovary
- **Laparoscopic ovarian drilling:** Done with monopolar/bipolar cautery or laser in polycystic ovarian disease cases
- **Ovarian biopsy:** Indicated in premature ovarian failure and intersex

Principal steps of oophorectomy or ovariotomy (Figure 38.8)

- Paired clamps are placed laterally on the infundibulopelvic ligament and medially over the ovarian ligament and mesovarium.
- Pedicles are cut in between the clamps → ovary is removed → transfixation sutures are placed on the pedicles

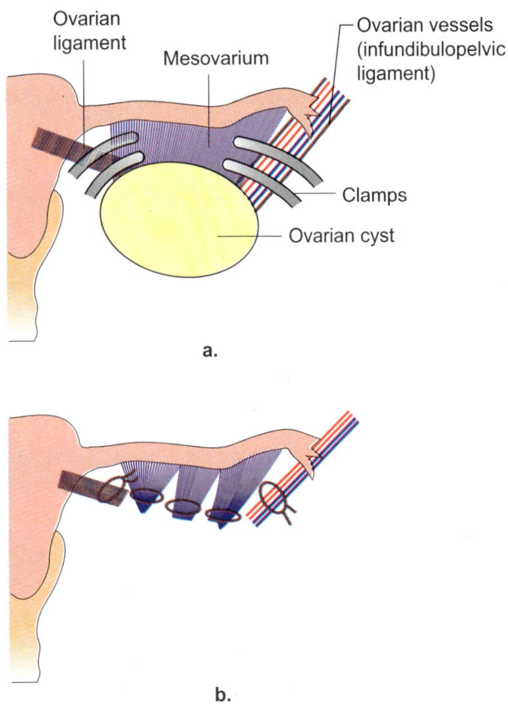

Figure 38.8 Oophorectomy. **a.** The infundibulopelvic ligament, mesovarium, and ovarian ligament are clamped, cut, and ligated. **b.** Stumps or pedicles after removal of ovaries.

LAPAROSCOPY

It is the visualization of peritoneal cavity using a telescope with cold light and fiber optics.

Indications of laparoscopy

Laparoscopy may be done for diagnostic and operative purposes as mentioned in Table 38.13.

Table 38.13 Indications of laparoscopy

Diagnostic purposes	Operative purposes
• Infertility workup (chromopertubation) • Chronic/acute pelvic pain (adhesions and endometrosis) • Evaluation of pelvic mass such as ovarian cyst • Suspected ectopic pregnancy • Suspected uterine abnormalities	• Tubal sterilization • Unruptured ectopic pregnancy • Ovarian cystectomy/biopsy/drilling • Endometriosis • Adhesiolysis • Myomectomy • Hysterectomy (total laparoscopic hysterectomy, laparoscopically assisted vaginal hysterectomy) • Retroperitoneal lymphadenectomy

Principal steps of laparoscopy

- **Patient positioning:** The patient is placed in lithotomy position with head end of the patient slightly lowered (Trendelenburg 15–30°).
- **Creation of pneumoperitoneum:** Veress needle is introduced through subumbilical port and abdominal cavity is distended with gas (CO_2 is commonly used).
- **Introduction of trocar and cannula:** Trocar and cannula are inserted via the subumbilical port.
- **Introduction of laparoscope:** Laparoscope connected to the light source, and camera unit is introduced via the port; the findings are noted and visualized on the monitor.
- **Creation of accessory ports:** Accessory ports may be created for operative procedures.
- **Surgical procedures may be carried out:** Laparoscopic surgical procedures may be performed using basic instruments such as graspers, scissors, aspirator, irrigator, morcellator, uterine

Viva corner

Q1 How will you verify the correct placement of Veress needle inside abdominal cavity?

The correct placement of Veress needle inside abdominal cavity can be verified by the following methods:

- **Hanging drop method**: A small amount of sterile saline is placed on top of the Veress needle. The saline drops into the peritoneal cavity due to negative intraperitoneal pressure.
- **Syringe barrel test**: A 10-mL syringe with normal saline is attached to the Veress needle. Aspiration is done to rule out blood or bowel contents. The saline is then pushed down and aspiration is again done. If the needle placement is correct, the fluid cannot be withdrawn as it goes in the peritoneal cavity.
- Free flow of gas: Intra-abdominal pressure is low (<10 mmHg) on correct placement of the needle and there is free flow of gas.
- Liver dullness is obliterated (on percussion).

Q2 What are the sites of Veress needle insertion?

- Usually a small skin incision is made just below the umbilicus and Veress needle is introduced through this subumbilical incision with 45° angulation into the peritoneal cavity.

Other possible site of insertion:

- Palmer's point: Left subcostal margin (3 cm below in midclavicular line stomach must be decompressed and splenomegaly should be ruled out prior to using this site as port).

Q3 Why is CO_2 gas used for insufflation?

- Creation of a pneumoperitoneum has significant effects on cardiovascular and respiratory physiology. CO_2 is used as the insufflation gas as it is nonflammable, and has a higher blood solubility than air, thus reducing the risk of complications.

Q4 What is Hasson's technique in laparoscopy?

- Hasson introduced the open method of port insertion for laparoscopic procedure to reduce the complications associated with blind insertion of the Veress needle and trocar. However, the closed technique is still more popular than open laparoscopy, as open method is time-consuming and is associated with gas leakage.

manipulator, and electrosurgical energy sources (Figure 38.9).

- **End of the procedure:** After completion of the procedure, the laparoscope is removed, peritoneal gas is deflated, and the ports are closed.

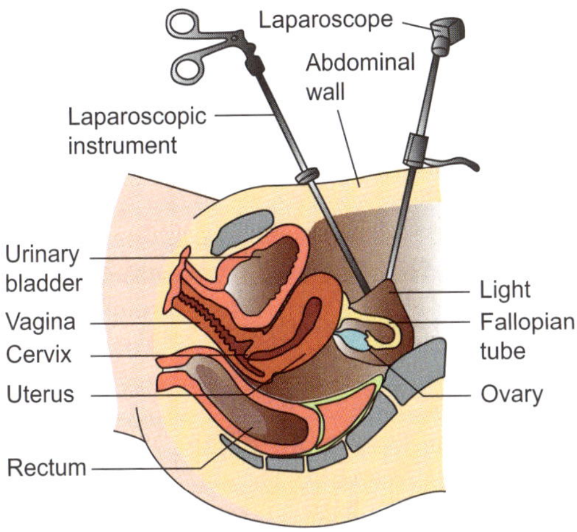

Figure 38.9 Laparoscopy.

Contraindications for laparoscopy

- Severe cardiopulmonary disease
- Patient hemodynamically unstable
- Significant hemoperitoneum
- Generalized peritonitis
- Intestinal obstruction
- Extensive adhesions
- Large pelvic tumor
- Pregnancy >16 weeks

High-yield points

Classic appearance of endometriosis in laparoscopy

Features of endometriosis in laparoscopy include the following:

- Black dots with "powder burn" appearance
- Red flame-shaped lesions
- Yellow brown patches
- White peritoneal areas
- Circular peritoneal defects
- Pelvic adhesions
- Ovarian endometriomas—appear as chocolate cysts of ovary

- Advanced malignancy
- Patient on anticoagulation therapy

Advantages and disadvantages of laparoscopy

See Table 38.14

Table 38.14 Advantages and disadvantages of laparoscopy

Advantages	Disadvantages
• No large abdominal incisions • Less blood loss • Less postoperative pain and lesser need for postoperative analgesia • Rapid postoperative recovery • Shorter hospital stay • Early resumption of day-to-day activity • Increased patient satisfaction • Less adhesion formation • Minimal abdominal scars (cosmetic value) • Reduced risk of incisional hernia	• Operation time—may be longer • Risk of specific iatrogenic complications • Surgeon needs specialized training and expertise • Instruments and equipment are sophisticated

Complications of laparoscopy

- Anesthetic complications—hypercarbia, acidosis, and basal lung atelectasis
- During insertion of Veress needle, trocar, and cannula—injury to bowel, bladder, blood vessels, and surgical emphysema
- During creation of pneumoperitoneum—gas embolism and arrhythmia
- Electrosurgical complications—thermal injury to bowel, etc.
- Other complications like in any surgery—hemorrhage and infection
- Port site hernia

HYSTEROSCOPY

- Hysteroscopy allows direct visualization of uterine cavity by insertion of a rigid or flexible hysteroscope and distension media through the cervix into the uterus.
- Hysteroscopy serves diagnostic as well as therapeutic purposes (Figure 38.10).

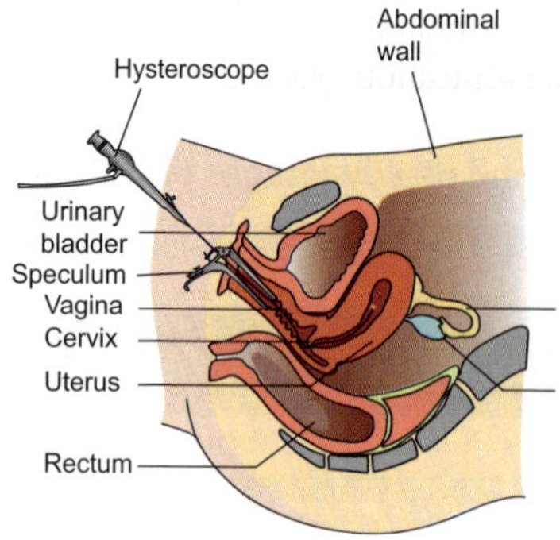

Figure 38.10 Hysteroscopy

Indications of diagnostic hysteroscopy

- Abnormal uterine bleeding
- Infertility
- Müllerian anomalies such as arcuate, subseptate, septate, bicornuate uterus or uterus didelphys can be diagnosed with hysteroscopy. The procedure is combined with laparoscopy for confirmation of diagnosis
- Recurrent miscarriage: Intrauterine pathology such as fibroids, polyps, Asherman's syndrome can be diagnosed and treated
- Misplaced IUD
- Evaluation of chronic pelvic pain

Indications of operative hysteroscopy

- Removal of foreign body or missing IUCD
- Removal of endometrial polyps and submucous myoma
- Endometrial biopsy
- Synechiolysis—lysis of intrauterine adhesions
- Endometrial ablation and resection
- Resection of uterine septum
- Laser coagulation of endometrial hemangioma and AV malformation
- Female sterilization—using Nd:YAG laser or electrocoagulation for destroying the interstitial portion of fallopian tubes or by insertion of Essure

Transcervical resection of endometrium (TCRE) or laser ablation of endometrium (LAE)

- An alternative procedure to hysterectomy in indicated cases of abnormal uterine bleeding.
- Often performed as a day care procedure.
- The principle is to destroy the endometrium up to a depth of 3–5 mm so that the basal layer of endometrium is destroyed and there is no further regeneration of endometrium.
- Preferably performed in women with normal sized uterus in the postmenstrual phase
- It is recommended to treat the patient with danazol, GnRH analogue, or progestogen for 4–6 weeks prior to endometrial ablation to make the endometrium thin, thereby facilitating the procedure.

Contraindications of hysteroscopy

- **Pelvic infection:** Hysteroscopy can cause spread of infection
- **Pregnancy**
- **Cardiopulmonary disorders** put people at higher risk of anesthesia as hysteroscopy carries risk of gas embolism, fluid overload, and pulmonary edema
- **Cervical stenosis:** Can cause cervical trauma. PGE2 gel inserted 2 hours before surgery or PGE1 200–400 microgram placed vaginally 2–4 hours prior to surgery, softens the cervix and help easy dilatation

Complications of Hysteroscopy

Perioperative Complications

- Fluid overload, hyponatremia, pulmonary edema, neurological symptoms, excess glycine absorption leading to ammonia toxicity, and CO_2 embolism due to the distension media used
- Hemorrhage, uterine perforation, injury to surrounding structures, and thermal injury due to electrosurgical energy
- Anesthetic complications
- Infection and procedure failure

Late Complications

- **Abnormal uterine bleeding** due to failure of TCRE
- **Hematometra and pyometra**—may occur due to infection after hysteroscopic surgery with cervical stenosis

MINOR SURGICAL PROCEDURES IN GYNECOLOGY

Preoperative preparations for minor surgical procedures

- Investigations: These include hemoglobin estimation, complete blood count, and urine examination for protein, sugar, and pus cells.
- The patient is advised to be nil per oral for at least 8 hours prior to the procedure.
- Part preparation is done.
- The patient is usually admitted in the morning of surgery.
- The patient is asked to pass urine before entering the operation theater.

Endometrial sampling/biopsy

Indications

See Table 38.15

Different methods for obtaining an endometrial sample

- Dilatation and curettage/fractional curettage
- Pipelle biopsy or other equivalent techniques such as Novak's endometrial biopsy curette and Vabra aspirator
- Hysteroscopy directed biopsy
- Endometrial aspiration cytology

Table 38.15 Indications for Endometrial sampling

Diagnostic indications	Therapeutic indications
• Abnormal uterine bleeding • Postmenopausal bleeding • Detection of endometrial carcinoma/hyperplasia • Follow up of previously diagnosed endometrial hyperplasia • Evaluation of infertility, dating of endometrium • Cancer screening (e.g., heriditary nonpolyposis colorectal cancer) • Abnormal PAP smear with atypical glandular cells favoring endometrial origin • Tuberculosis of endometrium	• Stops bleeding temporarily in abnormal uterine bleeding

Fractional curettage/dilatation and curettage

Principal steps of the procedure (Figure 38.11)

- It is done under IV/IM sedation or general anesthesia.
- The patient is placed in lithotomy position.
- Parts are cleaned and draped.
- Bladder is drained.
- Bimanual examination is done.
- Posterior vaginal wall speculum (Sims') is inserted.
- Anterior lip of the cervix is held with vulsellum.
- Uterine sound is introduced to confirm the uterine position and to measure the uterocervical length.
- Cervix is dilated with graduated dilators (Hegar's dilators).
- After dilatation, uterine curette is introduced and curettage is done. The endometrial tissue

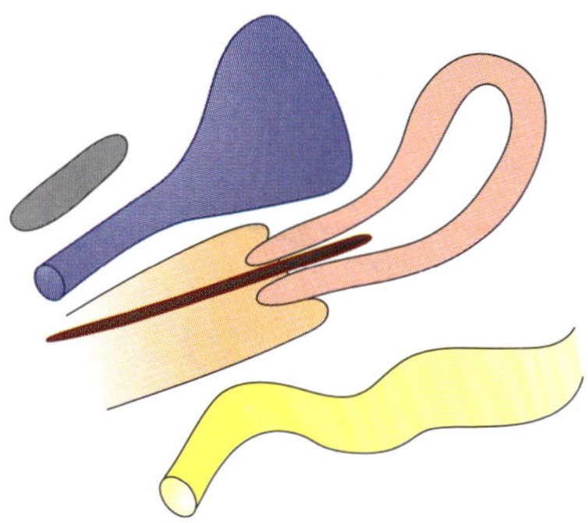

a.

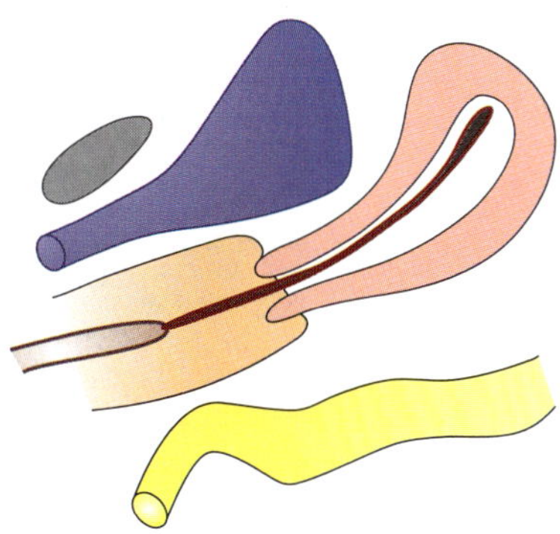

b.

Figure 38.11 Fractional curettage. **a.** Dilatation of cervix. **b.** Uterine curettage.

obtained is preserved in formalin and sent for histopathological examination.

- Vulsellum and speculum are removed at the end of the procedure.

Note
- *A sharp curette is used in gynecology and a blunt curette is used in obstetrics (for removal of products of conception).*
- *In suspected tuberculosis, a portion of the specimen is preserved in normal saline and sent for acid-fast bacillus (AFB) staining, culture, and cartridge based nucleic acid amplification test (CB-NAAT).*
- *D&C procedure may also aid in removal of endometrial polyps and intrauterine contraceptive devices.*

Complications of fractional curettage procedure

See Table 38.16

Table 38.16 Complications of fractional curettage

Immediate complications	Remote complications
• Injury to the cervix • Uterine perforation • Injury to the bladder or bowel (following perforation) • Hemorrhage • Infection	• Cervical incompetence • Uterine synechiae (vigorous curettage can result in removal of basal endometrium and Asherman's syndrome)

Office endometrial biopsy

Endometrial sampling is performed as an outpatient procedure without the need for anesthesia and cervical dilatation using Pipelle endometrial sampler or equivalents such as Novak's endometrial biopsy curette or Vabra aspirator.

Pipelle sampling procedure (Figure 38.12)

- The patient is placed in lithotomy position.
- Parts are cleaned and draped.

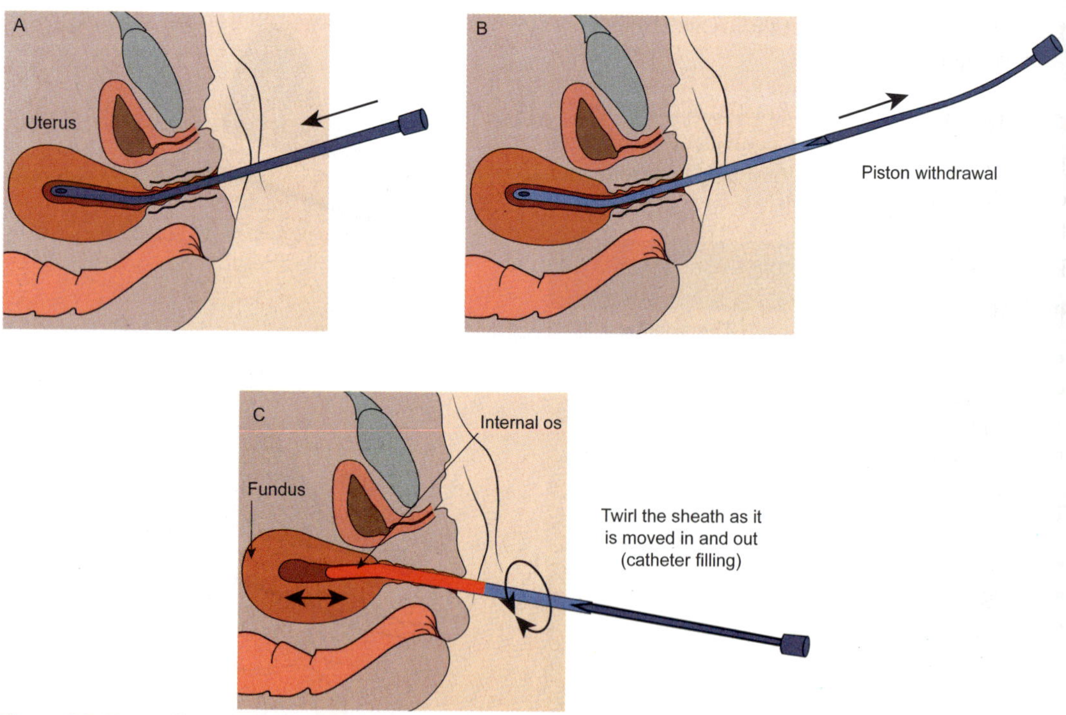

Figure 38.12 Pipelle endometrial sampling procedure

Extra edge

Q1 What are the conditions where only dilatation of cervix is performed?

Indications for performing only dilatation of cervix are as follows:

- Drainage of pyometra or hematometra
- Spasmodic dysmenorrhea
- Prior to hysteroscopy procedure

- Bimanual examination is done.
- Posterior vaginal wall speculum (Sims') is inserted.
- Use of vulsellum to hold the anterior lip of the cervix is optional.
- Pipelle is gently inserted and stopped when resistance is felt (fundus is reached at 6–8 cm).
- Pipelle is held with pincer grasp and piston is pulled out for suction.
- The Pipelle is moved in corkscrew motion along with cephalic–caudal motion to sample the entire endometrial surface.
- The specimen is expelled into a formalin container by syringing.

Cervical biopsy

Removal of a small sample of tissue from the cervix for examination under microscope; used for the diagnosis and treatment of cervical cancer and precancerous conditions.

Indications

- Abnormal Pap smear
- Clinically suspicious cervix (to rule out malignancy)
- Presence of any growth or ulcer on the cervix

Types of cervical biopsy

- Punch biopsy
- Wedge biopsy
- Cone biopsy

Punch Biopsy

- An outpatient procedure without anesthesia.
- Using Cusco's bivalve speculum, biopsy is taken from the suspected area of cervix or a 4-quadrant biopsy is taken using punch biopsy forceps.
- Biopsy is taken with a Punch Biopsy forceps from the edge of ulcer or growth including the healthy tissue for comparative histological study. (the center of the lesion usually contains only necrotic material) (Figure 38.13a).
- Biopsy can be performed after staining with Lugol's iodine or acetic acid or colposcopic directed biopsy (abnormal areas do not take up the iodine stain and appear as acetowhite lesion after 5% acetic acid application).

Wedge Biopsy

With a scalpel, a wedge of tissues is cut from the edge of the lesion including the healthy tissue for comparative histological study.

Cone biopsy (conization of cervix)

Procedure

Removal of cone of the cervix which includes entire squamocolumnar junction, stroma with glands, and endocervical mucous membrane ***(Figure 38.13b)***. Indications for conization of cervix are mentioned in Table 38.17.

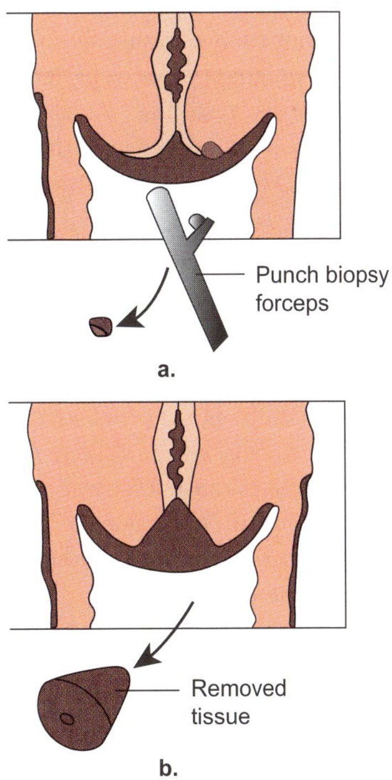

Figure 38.13 Cervical biopsy. **a.** Punch biopsy. **b.** Cone biopsy.

Table 38.17 Indications for cone biopsy conization of cervix

Diagnostic indications	Therapeutic indications
• Unsatisfactory colposcopic findings • Inconsistent findings in cytology, colposcopy, and biopsy • Large lesions and lesion extending into endocervical canal • Positive endocervical curettage • Histological diagnosis of adenocarcinoma in situ • In CIN 2/3 lesions, to exclude microinvasive carcinoma	• Treatment of CIN lesions • Treatment option for carcinoma cervix Stage Ia1 without lymphovascular space invasion (can be done in exceptional cases where childbearing is desired and the patient is strongly motivated for long-term follow-up)

CIN, cervical intraepithelial neoplasia.

Methods

- Cold knife conization–performed with a scalpel
- Loop electrosurgical excision procedure [LEEP], also termed as large loop excision of the transformation zone [LLETZ]) - This procedure is performed using a thin wire loop heated by an electric current that serves as a surgical knife to excise the abnormal cervical tissue for histopathological examination
- CO_2 laser

Complications

- Hemorrhage
- Cervical incompetence resulting in recurrent midtrimester pregnancy loss or preterm labor
- Cervical stenosis resulting in hematometra, infertility and cervical dystocia during labor
- Diminished cervical mucus secretion

Marsupialization of Bartholin's cyst

Bartholin's cyst develops at the junction of anterior two-third and posterior one-third of inner aspect of labia minora.

Marsupialization is a procedure to treat Bartholin's cyst or abscess, in which the cyst is opened and the edges of the cyst wall are sutured to the skin, forming an "open pocket" or "pouch." This technique of suturing keeps the site open, allowing free drainage.

Principal steps of the procedure (Figure 38.14)

- IV/IM sedation is given.
- The patient is placed in lithotomy position.
- Parts are cleaned and draped.

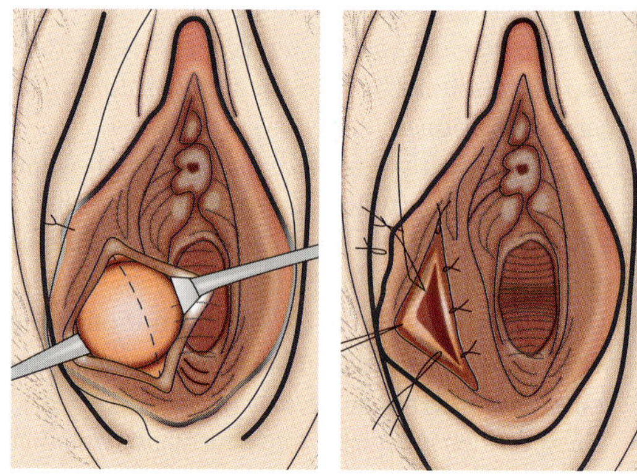

a. b.

Figure 38.14 Marsupialization of Bartholin's cyst. **a.** Incision is made on the inner aspect of labia minora over the cyst and pus is drained out. **b.** Edges of the cyst wall are sutured to the skin, leaving an opening for drainage.

- An elliptical incision is made on the inner side of the labia minora just outside the introitus.
- The pus is drained out. The loculi within the cyst are broken by blunt dissection with fingers.
- The edges of the cyst wall are sutured to the skin by interrupted catgut sutures, thus leaving an opening for drainage.

Advantage of marsupialization over excision of Bartholin's cyst

Gland function (lubrication) is maintained.

Disadvantage of the marsupialization

Risk of recurrence (in case of recurrence following marsupialization, excision of cyst has to be done)

Part 4

Objective Structured Clinical Examination (OSCE)

39 Introduction to OSCE

Competency-based medical education (CBME) curriculum has been introduced in India with the intent to move toward outcome-based education. The emphasis is on the shift from a knowledge-based traditional curriculum to an outcome-based, student-centered approach. Assessment tools suitable for CBME have been suggested to fulfill the essence of the new curriculum.

The objective structured clinical examination (OSCE) is one of the established valid, reliable, and objective tools for assessing clinical skills.

- OSCE is a structured assessment of predetermined competencies including psychomotor, communication, and data interpretation skills.
- An OSCE comprises a circuit of stations in which each candidate is examined on a one-to-one basis with either real/simulated patients or case scenarios. Candidates spend 5–10 minutes in each station, rotate through the stations, and complete all the stations on their circuit.
- OSCE is *Objective* – all candidates are assessed using exactly the same stations with the same marking scheme; *Structured* – stations in OSCEs have a specific task; *Clinical Examination* – the OSCE is designed to apply clinical and theoretical knowledge.

Advantages

- Decreases bias
- Skills/procedures can be assessed without affecting the patient's health
- Broader content coverage

Disadvantages

- Fragmentation of tasks
- Requires preparation time and budget

Skill Assessment

1. CALCULATION OF OBSTETRIC FORMULA, EDD, POG

Skill station

Calculation of Obstetric formula, EDD, POG
(Refer Part 1, Chapter 1 for details)

Situation

You are posted in the Obstetric outpatient department (OPD). Calculate the following, according to the details given by antenatal women who come for their first antenatal visit. Pregnancy has been confirmed by the urine pregnancy test.

a. Client Name: Ms. A, 28 years, gives the following history: First pregnancy – male child delivered at term, alive and healthy at birth but died at 2 years of age due to pneumonia; second pregnancy – male child alive and healthy, 4 years old; this is her third pregnancy at 36 weeks. Calculate her obstetric formula.
b. Client Name: Ms. B, 30 years, with last menstrual period on DD/MM/YYYY. Calculate her period of gestation (POG) and expected date of delivery (EDD).
c. Client Name: Ms. C, 26 years, gives history as: First pregnancy – twins, vaginal delivery, both alive and healthy; second pregnancy – male child delivered at term, alive and healthy. She is 32 weeks in the current pregnancy. Calculate her obstetric formula.
d. Client Name: Mrs. D, 32 years, is not sure of the dates. Ultrasonography done on DD/MM/YYYY shows crown rump length (CRL) of 8 weeks. Calculate her POG.

e. Client Name: Mrs. E, 32 years, is not sure of the dates. Her first-trimester ultrasound EDD is DD/MM/YYYY. Calculate her POG.

2. ELICITING OBSTETRIC HISTORY

Skill station

Eliciting a detailed obstetric history

Skill station setup

Patient/simulated patient

Scenario

You are posted in the Obstetric outpatient department. Elicit a detailed obstetric history of the pregnant woman who has come for an antenatal visit. Example: She is Mrs. P, G2P1L1 at 32 weeks with postcesarean pregnancy, who has come for her routine antenatal checkup.

(Refer Part 1, Chapter 1, History Taking and Examination, for detailed history taking in obstetrics and Chapter 6, Postcesarean Pregnancy, for history taking in postcesarean pregnancy)

- Obstetric history involves asking questions relevant to a patient's current and previous pregnancies.
- Some of the questions are highly personal; hence, good communication skills and a respectful approach are absolutely essential.

Opening the consultation

- Perform hand hygiene
- Introduce yourself to the patient including your name and role
- Confirm the patient's name and age
- Explain that you would like to take the history of the patient
- Gain consent to proceed with history taking

General communication skills

General communication skills are relevant to all patient consultations/encounters. Demonstrating these skills will ensure that your consultation remains patient-centered and not checklist-type. These include:

- Demonstrate empathy in response to patient cues.
- Establish rapport (e.g., calling by her name, asking how she is doing, and offering a seat).
- Listen actively through body language and verbal responses to what the patient has said.
- Maintain eye contact during the consultation.
- Maintain professional body language (uncrossed legs and arms, leaning slightly forward in the chair).
- Use open-ended questions to explore the patient's presenting complaints. Open questions are effective at the start of consultation, allowing the patient to explain the complaints in her own words.
- Closed questions may be asked to explore the symptoms mentioned in a more detailed manner, to gain a better understanding of the presentation. Closed questions can also be asked to identify relevant risk factors and to narrow down the differential diagnosis.
- Provide enough time to the patient to answer and make sure not to interrupt the patient throughout the consultation.
- Explain the patient what has been discussed so far and what you plan to discuss next (sign posting). This will be useful when transitioning between different parts of history taking. Example: "*We have now talked about your present complaints. Next I'd like to ask about your current pregnancy history.*"
- Explore the patient's ideas, concerns, and expectations (ICE) to gain insight into how the patient currently perceives the situation, what are her concerns, and what she expects from the consultation.
- Summarize at regular intervals. This allows to check your understanding of the patient's history and provides an opportunity for the patient to clarify any inaccurate information.

Closing the consultation

- Summarize the key points
- Ask the patient if she has any questions or concerns that have not been addressed
- Thank her for the time
- Perform hand hygiene
- Document the details

3. OBSTETRIC ABDOMINAL EXAMINATION

Skill station I

Obstetric abdominal examination [inspection, fundal height and symphysial fundal height (SFH)]

Skill station setup

Obstetric manikin, measuring tape, cover sheet, stethoscope, gloves, hand sanitizer.

Scenario

Mrs. H, a 23-year-old female, G2P1L1 at 38 weeks of gestation with previous normal vaginal delivery has come for a routine visit. Her antenatal history has been uneventful. Perform obstetric abdominal inspection and demonstrate fundal height and SFH measurement.
(Refer Part 1, Chapter 1 for detailed obstetric examination)

Steps

- Keep the necessary items ready for obstetric abdominal examination (manikin, measuring tape, stethoscope/fetoscope, watch with seconds hand).
- Perform hand hygiene.
- Introduce yourself to the patient including your name and role.
- Confirm the patient's name and age.
- Explain that you would like to examine the patient and explain what you are going to perform.
- Gain consent to proceed with the examination.
- Ensure that the patient has voided.
- Ensure adequate lighting and screen for privacy.
- Stand on the right side of the patient/manikin.
- Ask the patient to be in a dorsal position and expose the parts to be examined. Cover lower limbs with a cover sheet.
- Inspect the abdomen for distension, contour, umbilicus (normal/everted/flushed with skin surface), linea nigra, striae gravidarum, scars if any, cough impulse at hernial orifices.
- For fundal height examination, ask the patient to be in a dorsal position and keep the legs in a flexed and slightly abducted position.
- Correct dextrorotation with the right hand and measure the fundal height using the ulnar border of the left hand to determine the upper border of the uterus (either from below upwards till disappearance of resistance of uterus or from above downwards till the appearance of resistance at the fundus).
- Ask permission of the patient and mark the fundal height on the abdomen.
- For the measurement of the SFH, ask the patient to be in a dorsal position with legs extended.
- Measure SFH with a measuring tape with the inches side facing up from pubic symphysis, across umbilicus, up to the marking of fundal height. Turn the tape to check for the SFH measurement in centimeters.
- Explain the findings to the patient.
- Perform hand hygiene.
- Record the clinical examination findings.

Skill station II

Obstetric abdominal examination (obstetric grips and auscultation of fetal heart rate (FHR))

Skill station setup

Obstetric manikin, measuring tape, cover sheet, stethoscope, watch with second hand, hand sanitizer

Scenario

Mrs. G, a 30-year-old female, primigravida at 38 weeks of gestation has come for a routine antenatal visit. Her antenatal history is uneventful. Perform obstetric abdominal examination to demonstrate the various obstetric grips and FHR auscultation.
(Refer Part 1, Chapter 1 for detailed obstetric examination)

Steps

- Perform hand hygiene.
- Introduce yourself to the patient including your name and role.
- Confirm the patient's name and age.
- Explain that you would like to examine the patient and explain what you are going to perform.
- Gain consent to proceed with the examination.
- Ensure that the patient has voided.
- Ensure adequate light and screen for privacy.
- Stand on the right side of the patient/manikin.
- Ask patient to expose the parts to be examined. Cover lower limbs with cover sheet.
- Ask the patient to be in a dorsal position and to keep the legs in a flexed and slightly abducted position. Palpate the abdomen as follows:
  - Fundal grip (to identify the fetal part in the upper pole of the uterus) – Facing the head end of the patient, palpate the fundus of the uterus with both hands.

- Lateral grip (to assess the side of the fetal back) – Facing the head end of the patient, steady one side of the uterus with the palm of one hand while palpating the other side and then vice versa.
- I Pelvic grip (to assess the fetal head engagement) – Facing the head end of the patient, place the ulnar border of the right hand on the upper border of the pubic symphysis and palpate the fetus between the outstretched thumb and the four fingers of the right hand.
- II Pelvic grip (to confirm the finding of first pelvic grip) – Facing the foot end of the patient, place both hands on either side of the abdomen above and parallel to the inguinal ligament. Palpate simultaneously with both hands, move medially and downward.
- For the auscultation of FHR, place the bell of the stethoscope on the side where the fetal back was felt. Count the FHR for 1 minute using the watch with second hand.

- Explain findings to mother and perform hand hygiene.
- Record the clinical examination findings.

4. PELVIC ASSESSMENT

Skill station

Demonstrate pelvic assessment in the given model

Skill station setup

Maternal pelvis model/manikin, cover sheet, chlorhexidine swabs, lubricant, gloves, hand sanitizer, color-coded waste bins

Scenario

Mrs. J, 30 years of age, at 39 weeks of gestation with uneventful antenatal history is admitted with complaints of labor pains. You have already taken history and have performed the abdominal examination. As part of your examination, demonstrate pelvic assessment in this patient.

(Refer Part 1, Chapter 16 for the detailed description of pelvic assessment)

Steps

- Perform hand hygiene.
- Introduce yourself to the patient including your name and role.
- Confirm the patient's name and age.
- Explain that you would like to examine the patient and explain what you are going to perform.
- Gain consent to proceed with the examination.
- Ensure that the patient has voided.
- Ensure adequate light and screen for privacy.
- Stand on the right side of the patient/manikin.
- Ask the patient to be in a dorsal position and to keep the legs in a flexed and slightly abducted position. Cover lower limbs with a cover sheet.
- Perform hand hygiene and put on a sterile pair of gloves.
- Clean the vulva with wet cotton swabs soaked in antiseptic solution.
- Lubricate the fingers
- Separate the labia and insert fingers (two index and middle fingers) gently into the vagina. Perform pelvic assessment as follows:
  - Attempt/try to reach the sacral promontory, to assess the diagonal conjugate.
  - Follow the curve of sacrum downward along the midline to assess the sacral curvature.
  - After assessing the sacrum, move the fingers laterally, to feel the sacrospinous ligaments.
  - Follow the sacrospinous ligaments laterally, to palpate the ischial spines.
  - Assess the interspinous distance by separating the index and middle fingers wide apart.
  - Next, palpate the retropubic area (forepelvis) by placing two fingers behind the symphysis pubis with the palm of the hand facing forward and then move the fingers laterally to both sides.
- To assess the subpubic angle, turn the examining fingers so that the palm of the hand faces upward and the angle under the pubis is felt.
- Withdraw the fingers from the vaginal introitus and assess the intertuberous diameter with the knuckles of the closed fist of the hand placed between the ischial tuberosities.
- Remove the gloves and dispose in the red bin.
- Perform hand hygiene.
- Explain the findings to the patient and document the findings.

5. MANAGEMENT OF ANTENATAL COMPLICATIONS

Skill station I

Management of antenatal complication

Case scenario

Read the case details and answer the given questions based on the information provided.

Ms. S, 35-year-old G2P1L1, is being seen by you today for a routine antenatal visit at 37 weeks gestation. Her examination findings are as follows: Weight 97 kg; no pallor; BP 140/100 mm of Hg; pedal edema and edema of hands and face present; urine dipstick +3 protein.

Questions

1. What is the most likely diagnosis in the given case?
2. What further questions will you ask Ms. S?
3. What further investigations will you perform for Ms. S?
4. If Ms. S has convulsion when she is in the OPD, what will be your next step of action?
5. What is the loading dose of magnesium sulfate?

(Refer Part 1, Chapter 4 for further details on preeclampsia)

Skill station II

Magnesium sulfate administration for eclampsia

Skill station setup

Manikin, magnesium sulfate injection – 14 ampoules (each ampoule = 2 mL = 1 g), syringes (10, 20 mL syringes and 22 G needle), normal saline, spirit/alcohol swabs, kidney tray, knee hammer, 10% calcium gluconate ampoule, color-coded waste disposal bins

Case scenario

A primigravida at 37 weeks gestation, an admitted case of severe preeclampsia, has one episode of convulsions while in the ward. She is semiconscious. Prepare and administer magnesium sulfate for the patient *(airway, breathing, circulation checked; patient already has an IV line secured).*

(Refer Part 1, Chapter 4 for further details on preeclampsia)

Steps

- Call for help.
- Place woman in left lateral position.
- Take the required number of MgSO4 and check the expiry date.
- Prepare loading dose (IV + IM dose):
  - IV dose is 4 g of 20% magnesium sulfate solution. Take 20 mL syringe, add 4 ampoules $MgSO_4$ (4 g/8 mL) and dilute with 12 mL normal saline which makes 4 g in 20 mL, i.e., 20% solution).
  - IM dose is 10 g of 50% magnesium sulfate solution (take two 10 mL syringes and load each syringe with 5 g $MgSO_4$ (5 g in 10 mL which makes 50% solution).
- Perform hand hygiene and wear gloves.
- Inform woman (if conscious)/patient attender about injection administration.
- Administer IV dose as slow IV over 3–4 minutes.
- For administration of IM injection, clean the injection site with an alcohol swab.
- Administer 5 g (10 mL) by deep IM injection in each buttock (upper outer quadrant).
- Cut the needle with hub cutter.
- Dispose of used syringes as per guidelines.
- Perform hand hygiene and record the details.

Note *Pre-eclampsia, is given as an example. Situation/case scenario may be framed for any other antenatal complication.*

6. VAGINAL EXAMINATION

Skill station

To perform the vaginal examination in labor to assess cervical dilatation and effacement

Skill station setup

Maternal pelvis manikin/cervical dilatation models, cover sheet, sponge holder, chlorhexidine swabs, gloves, lubricant, hand sanitizer, color-coded waste disposal bins

Scenario

Mrs. J, a 30-year-old G2P1L1, with previous normal vaginal delivery with uneventful antenatal history is admitted with complaints of labor pains. You have conducted a quick history and abdominal examination. As part of examination, demonstrate per vaginal examination for assessment of cervix in this patient.

Steps

- Perform hand hygiene.
- Introduce yourself to the patient including your name and role.

- Confirm the patient's name and age.
- Explain that you would like to examine the patient and explain what you are going to perform.
- Gain consent to proceed with the examination.
- Ensure that the patient has voided.
- Ensure adequate light and screen for privacy.
- Stand on the right side of the patient/manikin.
- Ask the patient to be in a dorsal position and to keep the legs in a flexed and slightly abducted position. Cover lower limbs with cover sheet.
- Perform hand hygiene and put a sterile pair of gloves.
- Clean the vulva with wet cotton swabs soaked in an antiseptic solution with a sponge holder and discard the swabs in the yellow bucket.
- Lubricate the fingers.
- Separate the labia and insert fingers (two index and middle fingers) gently into the vagina.
- Rotate the hand 90 degrees so that the palm faces upwards and gently stretch the fingers till the rim of the cervix is felt. Assess the cervical dilatation in centimeters.
- Feel the rim of the cervix with the index and middle fingers. Assess the cervical effacement (in length/%).
- Remove the gloves and dispose of in the red bin.
- Perform hand hygiene.
- Explain the findings to the patient and document the findings.

7. PLOTTING A PARTOGRAM

Skill station I

Read the case details and plot the partogram based on the information provided.

Skill station setup

Blank partogram charts, pen

Case scenario

Ms. K, 24 years of age, primigravida is admitted to the hospital in active labor at **10:00 am.** Examination upon admission reveals the following:

- Vitals: Temperature 37°C; pulse 88/min; BP 110/70 mm Hg
- Obstetric examination: 3/10 min/40"; FHR 142 bpm;
- Vaginal examination: Cervix 4-cm dilated; membranes intact

At 2 pm, she reports a gush of amniotic fluid. On inspection, clear fluid draining per vaginum is noted.

- Vitals: Temperature 37°C; pulse 92/min; BP 120/70 mm Hg
- Obstetric examination: 3/10 min/45"; FHR 150 bpm
- Vaginal examination: Cervix 6–7 cm dilated; membranes ruptured, clear liquor

At 4 pm, she informs of an urge to bear down

- Vitals: Temperature 37°C; pulse 100/min; BP 130/84 mm Hg
- Abdominal examination: 4/10 min/45–50"
- Vaginal examination: Cervix fully dilated; membranes ruptured, clear liquor

She delivers a healthy 3.2-kg female baby by normal vaginal delivery at 5 pm.

Plot the following in the partograph:

1. FHR
2. Membrane status
3. Cervical dilatation
4. Uterine contractions

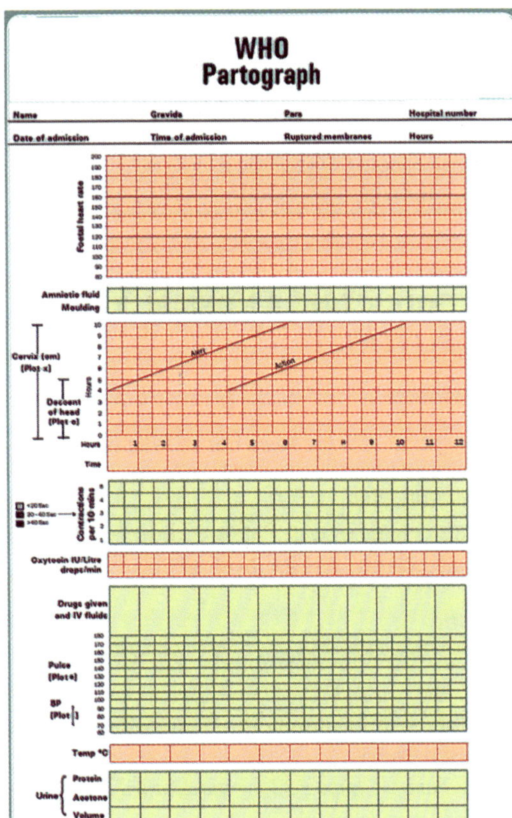

Figure WHO partogram.

Skill station II

Read the given partogram and answer the questions based on the information provided

Skill station setup

Plotted partogram charts

Case study

Ms. L, 24 years of age, primigravida, is admitted in active labor. From the given partogram, please identify the following findings as NORMAL, a cause for ALERT, or immediate ACTION. Put a tick (√) mark in the appropriate column *(plotted partogram chart will be provided).*

Time and condition	Normal	Alert	Action
FHR at __ hours			
Cervical dilation at __ hours			
Cervical dilation at __ hours			
Uterine contractions at __ hours			
Uterine contractions at __ hours			

8. CONDUCTING A NORMAL VAGINAL DELIVERY

Skill station

Demonstrate conducting a normal vaginal delivery

Skill station setup

Manikin, baby towels, gloves, antiseptic swabs, normal delivery set, and disposal bins.

Scenario

You have been monitoring Ms. J, G3P2L2, during labor. She is now fully dilated. She is bearing down and the birth is imminent. Demonstrate normal vaginal delivery.

(Refer Part 3, Chapter 33 for the detailed description of conduct of delivery)

Steps

- All preliminary steps to be followed as mentioned earlier.
- Perform hand hygiene and put on sterile gloves.
- Put on personal protective barriers (goggles, mask, cap, shoe cover, plastic apron).
- Palpate the suprapubic region to ensure that the bladder is not full.
- Clean the perineum with an antiseptic swab and place a clean drape on the abdomen.
- Encourage the woman to take deep breaths and to bear down with contractions.
- Control the delivery of the fetal head with the fingers of the left hand to maintain flexion, and support the perineum with other hand using the clean vulvar pad.
- Once baby's head is delivered, wipe the mucus from the baby's mouth and nostrils. Feel for any cord around baby's neck and loosen it if present.
- Allow the baby's head to undergo restitution and external rotation and with the hands on either side of the baby's head, deliver the anterior shoulder followed by the posterior shoulder.
- Support the rest of the baby's body with one hand as it slides out and place the baby on the mother's abdomen over a clean towel.
- Note the time of birth and sex of the baby. Simultaneously, check for crying/breathing of the baby.
- Perform delayed cord clamping after 1–2 minutes.

9. ACTIVE MANAGEMENT OF THIRD STAGE OF LABOR

Skill station

To perform active management of the third stage of labor (AMTSL)

Skill station setup

Obstetric model with placenta, oxytocin-loaded syringes, gloves, forceps, kidney tray, color-coded waste bins

Scenario

You have conducted vaginal delivery for Mrs. N and the baby Apgar is good. Demonstrate the steps of AMTSL.

(Refer Part 1, Chapter 17 for further details)

Steps

- Rule out the presence of another baby by abdominal examination.
- Administer uterotonic drug – 10 IU oxytocin IM/IV.
- Perform delayed cord clamping.
- Perform controlled cord traction for delivery of the placenta.
- Palpate for uterine tone, to check if contracted well.
- Examine placenta, membranes, and umbilical cord to ensure completeness.
- Put the placenta in the yellow bag.
- Examine the vagina and perineum for any tears.
- Remove gloves and dispose of in the red bin.
- Perform hand hygiene/wash hands.
- Document findings including estimated blood loss.

10. INTRAPARTUM COMPLICATIONS – ABNORMAL LABOR

Skill station

Management of intrapartum complications

Scenario

For each of the following scenarios, state whether NORMAL or ABNORMAL and justify accordingly.

SN	Labor Scenario		
1.	A primi at term presents with c/o labor pains. On examination, cervix is 4 cm dilated and she has 1 uterine contractions in 10 minutes lasting 10 seconds.	NORMAL/ ABNORMAL	Justify
2.	A G2P1L1, 39-weeks POG is admitted in labor at 4 cm dilation. Four hours later she is 5-cm dilated.	NORMAL/ ABNORMAL	Justify
3.	A primi in labor progresses to full dilation. On abdominal examination, both fetal poles are easily palpable.	NORMAL/ ABNORMAL	Justify
4.	A primi is admitted in labor with a cervical dilatation of 4 cm. Five hours later, her cervix is 9 cm dilated.	NORMAL/ ABNORMAL	Justify
5.	A primi at 38 weeks POG presents to the labor room following rupture of membranes for 4 hours. On examination, cervix is 4 cm dilated, the vertex is at -3 station, membranes absent, minimal liquor draining, caput is present, and grade III molding is present.	NORMAL/ ABNORMAL	Justify

11. INITIAL MANAGEMENT OF PPH

Skill station

Demonstrate the initial management of PPH

Skill station setup

Manikin, tourniquet, IV cannula, drip set and drip stand, IV fluids, BP apparatus, stethoscope, oxytocin ampoules, gloves, antiseptic swabs *(Refer Part 1, Chapter 17 for further details)*

Scenario

Following normal delivery of a healthy baby and AMTSL, you note that there is profuse vaginal bleeding. The patient has signs of shock. Demonstrate the initial management of PPH that you will perform

- Call for help and assess the vitals.
- Reassure the woman.
- Insert a wide bore IV cannula and collect blood for cross-matching.
- Start IV fluids with crystalloids.
- Start oxytocin infusion 20 IU in 500 mL of RL at 40–60 drops per minute.
- Wash hands and wear gloves.
- Palpate the uterus to ensure that it is well contracted.
- If atonic, start uterine massage.
- Check for any perineal injuries/tears to rule out traumatic PPH.
- Catheterize the bladder.

- Check for completeness of the placenta and membranes.
- Continue to massage the uterus, if not contracted.

12. ESSENTIAL NEWBORN CARE AND INITIAL STEPS OF NEWBORN RESUSCITATION

Skill station I

Essential newborn care

Skill station setup

Neonatal manikin, gloves, cord clamps, cord-cutting scissors, identification bands, Vit. K ampoules, 2 towels, weighing scale

Scenario

A full-term newborn baby is just born. The baby cried immediately after birth and looks pink. Demonstrate the essential newborn care for the baby.

Steps

- Call out the time of birth and sex and ensure that it is recorded.
- Deliver the baby to a warm, clean towel on the mother's abdomen and assess the baby.
- Perform delayed cord clamping (clamp and cut the umbilical cord after 1 minute).
- Shift the baby under a radiant warmer.
- Dry the baby quickly from head to foot.
- Discard the wet towel and wrap the baby with another clean towel.
- Perform gentle suction - mouth and nose, if secretions are seen.
- Check for any congenital malformation.
- Place an identity band on the baby's hand.
- Record the weight of the baby.
- Give injection vitamin K to the baby.
- Place the baby in between the mother's breast and cover both with a warm sheet.
- Encourage skin-to-skin care and initiation of breastfeeding.
- Document the findings.

Skill station II

Newborn Resuscitation

Skill station setup

Neonatal manikin, gloves, neonatal bag and mask, 2 towels, stethoscope

Scenario

A full-term baby is just born. The baby's heart rate is <100, he is gasping and floppy and unresponsive Demonstrate the initial steps of neonatal resuscitation.

Steps

- Clamp and cut the umbilical cord immediately.
- Place the baby under a radiant warmer.
- Dry and wrap the baby in a pre-warmed towel.
- Do gentle suctioning with bulb syringe or mechanical suction device, if secretions are visible.
- Stimulate the baby by rubbing the back and gently flicking the baby's soles of feet.
- Give supplemental oxygen.
- Assess the breathing and heart rate of the baby. If HR <100 and no spontaneous respiratory efforts, then baby requires positive pressure ventilation (PPV) with bag and mask. Connect and monitor SpO_2.
- Position baby with slight neck extension using a shoulder roll.
- Choose the correct size bag and mask and position it correctly to cover the mouth and nose. Connect to oxygen.
- Give inflation breaths of 2–3 seconds each.
- Reassess the heart rate and breathing.
- Continue bag and mask ventilation at a rate of 40–60 breaths/min.
- Reassess every 30 seconds to check if the heart rate is >100/min and spontaneous breathing is present
  - If HR >100 bpm and adequate respiratory efforts are present, evaluate color, continue oxygen, observe, and monitor.
  - If HR < 100 bpm and respiratory efforts are present, continue PPV till HR > 100 bpm, then ongoing care.
  - If HR < 60 bpm → give CPR (chest compression) with PPV → HR persists at < 60 bpm → IV access, epinephrine, intubation.

13. UNIVERSAL PRECAUTIONS FOR SELF-PROTECTION

Skill station

Personal protective equipment

Skill station setup

Apron, gown, cap, mask, eye cover, shoe covers

Scenario

You are going to conduct a delivery. Wear personal protective equipment prior to the procedure.

Steps

- Ensure that you wear the following:
  - Shoe covers
  - Waterproof apron
  - Eye cover (protective wear)
  - Cap
  - Mask
- Perform hand hygiene/wash hands.
- Then wear the sterile gown followed by sterile gloves.
- Be careful not to touch any unsterile items with gloved hands.
- Keep gloved hands above waist level.

Note *You may be asked about other steps of universal precautions such as testing for HIV, HCV, HBsAg and handling of sharp instruments during rendering patient care services.*

14. SPECULUM EXAMINATION AND PAP SMEAR TEST

Skill station

To demonstrate speculum examination and to perform a PAP smear test

Skill station setup

Gynecology examination manikin, gloves, antiseptic swabs, Cusco's speculum, light source, cover sheet, Ayres spatula, glass slides, Koplin jar with fixative, 0.5% chlorinated solution

Scenario

Ms. D, 45-years of age, presents to Gynecology OPD with the complaint of vaginal discharge. Demonstrate speculum examination and perform a PAP smear with Ayre's spatula on this patient.

Steps

- All preliminary steps to be followed.
  - Introduce yourself to the patient.
  - Confirm the patient's name and age.
  - Explain the procedure to the patient in simple language.
  - Gain consent to proceed with the examination.
  - Ensure adequate lighting and privacy.
- Position the patient in the dorsal position with legs flexed. Cover the patient with the sheet
- Perform hand hygiene.
- Inspect the vulva for abnormalities and for evidence of prolapse. Clean the vulva with antiseptic swab.
- Inform the patient that you are going to insert the speculum.
- **Insertion of speculum:** Use the fingers of your left hand to separate the labia.
- Gently insert the Cusco's speculum sideways with blades closed.
- Once inserted, rotate the speculum back 90° so that the handle is facing upwards.
- Open the speculum blades until an optimal view of the cervix is achieved.
- Tighten the locking screw to fix the position of the blades.
- Inspect the cervix for any abnormality (the cervix is identified by the external os).
- **PAP smear:** Insert an Ayre's spatula through speculum into the cervix, rotate the spatula 360°, in a clockwise direction.
- Remove the spatula and smear it on a labeled glass slide.
- Place the glass slide into a Koplin jar containing the fixative.
- **Removing the speculum:** Loosen the screw on the speculum and close the blades.
- Rotate the speculum 90°, back to its original insertion orientation.
- Gently remove the speculum, inspecting the walls of the vagina during removal.
- Dispose of the used speculum into the container containing antiseptic solution.
- All postprocedure steps to be followed
  - Dispose of gloves and other used material as per guidelines
  - Wash hands
  - Document the findings.

15. ARTIFICIAL RUPTURE OF MEMBRANES

Skill station I

Artificial rupture of membranes in a simulated/supervised environment

Skill station setup

Obstetric manikin, gloves, antiseptic swabs, normal delivery set, 1% lignocaine solution, syringes with needles, disposal bins

Scenario

Ms. Q, a primigravida at term, is in active labor. Demonstrate the steps for performing artificial rupture of membranes (ARM).

Steps

- All preliminary steps to be followed as mentioned in earlier skill stations.
- Check FHR with the stethoscope.
- Ask the woman to be in dorsal position with legs flexed and thighs apart.
- Perform hand hygiene and wear sterile gloves.
- Swab the perineum with antiseptic-soaked swabs.
- Insert 2 fingers of right hand to access the amniotic membranes through the cervix.
- With the left hand, slide the amniohook/Kocher's forceps between the fingers of the first hand which guides the tip to the amniotic sac.
- Make a small nick in the sac as it bulges during a contraction with amniohook or hold and tease the membrane with Kocher's forceps.
- Let the amniotic fluid drain slowly and then opening in the membranes may be widened using the finger.
- Note the color of the amniotic fluid.
- Make sure there is no cord prolapse.
- Check the FHR after the amniotomy procedure.
- All postprocedure steps to be followed as mentioned in earlier skill stations.

16. EPISIOTOMY

Skill station I

Steps of mediolateral episiotomy in a simulated/supervised environment

Skill station setup

Obstetric manikin, gloves, antiseptic swabs, normal delivery set, 1% lignocaine solution, syringes with needles, disposal bins

Scenario

Ms. Q, a primigravida at term, is in labor, the cervix is fully dilated and the head is crowning. Demonstrate the steps for performing a mediolateral episiotomy.

Steps

- All preliminary steps to be followed.
- Perform hand hygiene and put on sterile gloves.
- Clean and drape the perineum.
- Place the patient in a lithotomy position and direct the light source at the perineum.
- Infiltrate the perineum in the line of the proposed skin incision with 10 mL of 1% lignocaine.
- Place 2 fingers in the vagina between the presenting part and the posterior vaginal wall.
- Place episiotomy scissors with the blunt end inside, between the fingers and posterior vaginal wall and the sharp end outside, on the skin.
- Perform episiotomy at the peak of uterine contractions by making a deliberate cut starting from the posterior fourchette extending laterally on either side (left or right).
- Direction should be in a straight line that runs diagonally about 2.5 cm away from the anus.
- Incision should be adequate to serve the purpose.
- Encourage to bear down with contractions.

Skill station II

Suturing of episiotomy

Skill station setup

Episiotomy suturing manikin, gloves, antiseptic swabs, episiotomy suturing set, 1% lignocaine solution, syringes with needles, disposal bins.

Scenario

Ms. N has just had a normal vaginal delivery with a left mediolateral episiotomy. Demonstrate the techniques of episiotomy suturing.

Steps

- All preliminary steps to be followed.
- Perform hand hygiene and put on sterile gloves.
- Clean and drape the perineum.

- Place the patient in lithotomy position and direct light source at the perineum.
- Infiltrate the perineum with 5–10 mL of 1% lignocaine.
- Visualize the apex of the episiotomy in the vaginal mucosa and place a suture (chromic catgut/vicryl rapid No 1–0) 1 cm above the apex. Then place continuous sutures in the vaginal mucosa.
- Place interrupted sutures in the muscles starting at the apex of the wound.
- Place mattress sutures to repair the perineal skin.
- When the suturing is complete, perform per rectal examination to feel if any suture has inadvertently been placed through the rectal mucosa.
- Palpate the uterus for the tone and ensure that it is well contracted.
- All postprocedure steps to be followed.

17. INSERTION AND REMOVAL OF IUCD

Skill station

Insertion and removal of IUCD in a simulated/ supervised environment

Skill station setup

IUCD insertion model, IUCD insertion tray, IUCD, cotton swabs, betadine solution, gloves, bucket with 0.5% chlorine solution, disposal bins

Scenario

Ms. R, P1L1, attends postnatal clinic 6 weeks after delivery. You have discussed the family planning choices and she opts for IUCD. You have provided her counseling on IUCD device. Demonstrate IUCD insertion in this patient.

Steps

- All preliminary steps to be followed.
- Check the IUCD pack for the expiry date and for any tears in the pack.
- Wash hands and wear sterile gloves.
- Provide an overview of the insertion procedure.
- Clean the perineum with antiseptic-soaked swab.
- Perform a bimanual pelvic examination and note the size and position of the uterus.
- Gently insert the Cusco's speculum to visualize the cervix *(steps of speculum insertion to be followed as mentioned in S.No. 14).*
- Clean the cervix and vaginal wall with antiseptic solution.
- Gently hold the anterior lip of the cervix with vulsellum and apply gentle traction.
- Insert the uterine sound using the "no touch" technique and assess the utero-cervical length.
- Load the IUCD in its sterile package.
- Set the blue gauge on the IUCD to the measurement of the uterus.
- Align the blue gauge and folded arms of the Copper T to horizontal position.
- Carefully insert the loaded IUCD into the cervical canal observing a "no-touch technique."
- Advance until the blue gauge comes in contact with the cervix, keeping it in horizontal position.
- While holding the plunger rod, withdraw the insertion tube to release IUCD inside the uterus using the "withdrawal" technique.
- Withdraw the plunger and the insertion tube until the IUCD strings can be seen.
- Use sharp scissors to cut the IUCD strings leaving behind 3–4 cm length in the vagina.
- Gently remove the vulsellum and speculum.
- Examine the cervix for bleeding.
- Show the cut threads to the patient and ask how the client is feeling.
- All postprocedure steps to be followed.
- Provide postinsertion instructions.

18. EMERGENCY MANAGEMENT OF OBSTETRIC HEMORRHAGIC SHOCK

Skill station

Diagnose and provide emergency management of antepartum and postpartum hemorrhage in a simulated/guided environment

Skill station setup

Whole body manikin, resuscitation equipment kit, crash cart, iv fluids

Scenario

A 32-year-old G2P1L1 at 36 weeks of gestation, a diagnosed case of placenta previa, presents with sudden onset painless profuse vaginal bleeding.

Demonstrate the initial steps of resuscitation and supportive management in this case.

(Refer Part 1, Chapters 15 and 17 for further details)

19. URINARY CATHETERIZATION AND REMOVAL

Skill station I

Demonstrate the correct technique of urinary catheterization in a simulated/supervised environment

Skill station setup

Catheterization manikin, red rubber catheter, lubricant, antiseptic cotton swabs, kidney tray, waste disposal bins

Scenario

You are monitoring Ms. V who is in second-stage labor. On suprapubic palpation, the bladder is full. Demonstrate one-time catheterization with a red rubber catheter in this case.

Steps

- All preliminary steps to be followed.
- Perform hand hygiene and put sterile gloves on both hands.
- Uses 2 fingers of one hand to gently separate the labia, clean labia and urethral opening with antiseptic-soaked swabs.
- Place a kidney basin close to the perineum.
- Dip the tip of the catheter in sterile lubricant.
- Uses one hand to separate the labia and gently insert the tip of the catheter into the urethral opening with the other hand.
- Place the other end of the catheter in the kidney basin.
- Slowly move the catheter further into the urethra until the urine starts draining.
- Gently remove the catheter when the bladder is empty.
- All postprocedure steps to be followed.

Skill station II

Foley's catheterization and removal

Skill station setup

Catheterization manikin, Foley's catheter, uro bag, 10-mL syringe, distilled water, antiseptic swabs, sponge holder, kidney tray

Scenario

Demonstrate Foley's urinary catheter insertion and removal.

Steps (for insertion of Foley's catheter)

- All preliminary steps to be followed.
- Ensure adequate lighting and privacy.
- Check the expiry date on the pack (16/18 F Foley's catheter is commonly used for adults).
- Open the outer packing and leave it partially drawn out on the sterile tray.
- Perform hand hygiene and put on sterile pair of gloves.
- Clean the vulva with antiseptic-soaked cotton swabs.
- Open the sterile pack and dip the tip of the catheter in sterile lubricant.
- Separate the labia majora and insert the tip of Foley's catheter into the urinary meatus
- Push the catheter inside gently and connect the other end of the catheter to the urobag.
- Check for the flow of urine.
- Inflate the bulb of the catheter with 10 mL of normal saline.
- Fix the catheter to the medial aspect of the thigh using adhesive tape and secure the catheter bag to side of the bed, below the level of the bladder.
- Dispose of the waste material as per guidelines.
- Perform hand hygiene.

Steps (for removal of Foley's catheter)

- All preliminary steps to be followed.
- Ensure adequate lighting and privacy.
- Perform hand wash and put on sterile gloves.
- Take a 10-mL syringe and attach the barrel of the syringe to the short end of the Foley's catheter.
- Deflate the bulb by withdrawing the normal saline with the help of the syringe.
- Gently pull out the catheter.
- Dispose of the catheter, urobag, and syringe as per the guidelines.
- Performs hand hygiene.

20. ENDOMETRIAL BIOPSY OF UTERUS

Skill station

Demonstrate the correct technique of endometrial biopsy of the uterus in a simulated/supervised environment

Skill station setup

D&C manikin, endometrial biopsy set, antiseptic cotton swabs, waste disposal bins

Scenario

You are managing a case of perimenopausal AUB. Demonstrate the correct technique of endometrial biopsy of the uterus in this case.

(Refer Part 3, Chapter 38 on gynecology procedures for details on steps of endometrial biopsy)

Note *In OSCE procedural stations, the assessment will be done based on various domains such as explaining the procedure and taking informed consent, aseptic precautions, performing the task/procedure correctly, time taken to perform the task without interruption and professional attitude throughout the procedure.*

40 Counseling

GENERAL PRINCIPLES OF COUNSELING

Counseling in medical field is a process of two-way interpersonal communication in which the physician encourages the patient to discuss about his/her health issues to know about the possible medical problems in order to enable the patient to take an informed decision, in a safe and confidential environment.

The counseling process goes through the following stages:

- Opening the conversation and building rapport with the patient
- Exploring the problems/issues
- Facilitating exchange of information
- Closing the counseling process with gratification
- Scheduling the next visit

Skills and attitudes for effective two-way communication:

- Greet the patient and offer a seat
- Smile and make eye contact with the patient
- Reassure privacy and confidentiality
- Listen actively using gestures and nonverbal communication
- Use simple terms and language which she can understand
- Check frequently that she has understood what you have said
- Encourage her to ask questions, express concerns, and seek clarification

Common errors to be avoided during counseling:

- Judging based on her looks, appearance, and complaints
- Interrupting while the patient is talking
- Looking away frequently
- Criticizing cultural and religious values

Ethical principles relevant to counseling:

- Respect for autonomy
- Non-maleficence (do no harm)
- Beneficence (Do good)
- Justice (treat with equality)

Two-way communication during counseling in obstetrics and gynecology helps the woman:

- To know the possible problems and to take appropriate action
- To feel more comfortable to express her concerns and needs
- To make informed decision about the treatment, based on the information provided to her
- Establish a good doctor–patient relationship which indirectly helps to decrease future litigations

COUNSELING DURING PREGNANCY

- Counseling during pregnancy is done for the following reasons:
  - To provide essential information to maintain the health of the mother and fetus during pregnancy and after delivery
  - To advise on health promotion issues such as diet and nutrition
  - To explain the potential risks encountered during pregnancy
- Advantages of involving the husband/partner during antenatal counseling:
  - Makes him more caring and concerned for the pregnant partner

- Helps him to become aware of the danger symptoms that she may encounter during pregnancy
- Alerts the family of the possible expenditure for delivery and emergencies
- Helps the family to get prepared to care for the mother and baby after birth

CHECKLIST BASED ON GENERAL PRINCIPLES OF COUNSELING (ACRONYM 'GATHER')

Greet:
- Welcome the patient
- Discuss in a comfortable and private setup
- Assure confidentiality
- Express care and empathy by words and gestures throughout the session

Ask:
- Ask the reason for the visit
- Ask mostly "open" questions
- Encourage the patient to speak out
- Pay attention to what the patient says
- Express understanding of the problem without criticism or judgment
- Ask about the patient's feelings and preferences

Tell:
- Explain using simple and familiar words to the patient
- Start the discussion focusing on the patient's preference(s)
- Discuss and give information so as to help make her own decisions

Help:
- Help the patient to understand her problems
- Let the patient make an informed decision
- Make sure the patient's choices are based on accurate understanding

Explain:
- Explain the patient of the various available options
- Explain using printed instructions, pictures, and diagrams, if required
- Make her explain in her own words how much she understands

Return:
- Plan the next visit
- Thank the patient

In general, in any counseling station you may be asked to take brief history, explain the nature of the disease, prognosis, reassure the patient, give advice, answer questions, and know the exact management and possible risks to both the mother and the fetus.

An example of a counseling skill station is given below:

Skill Station

Counseling a woman prior to distribution of combined oral contraceptive pills

Case scenario

Ms. N, 32 years of age, P2 L2, has already been counseled on family planning methods. After discussing with her partner, she visits you to get combined oral contraceptives (COCs). Counsel her in detail on COC and distribute the pills.

Opening the session

- Wash your hands
- Introduce yourself to the patient including your name and role
- Confirm the patient's name and age

Data gathering and counseling

- Counsel the woman on the following aspects
  - Family planning method she has chosen: Type—combined oral contraceptive
  - How to take it
  - How it works
  - Effectiveness
  - Advantages and noncontraceptive benefits
  - Disadvantages
  - Common side effects
  - What to do if she misses the pill
- Ask her to repeat the instructions—how to use, side effects, etc.
- Educate the woman about prevention of STIs and HIV. Provide her with condoms if she is at risk/as back up
- Listen attentively and address her questions and concerns

Closing the session

- Summarize the key points
- Ask if she has further questions or concerns that have not been addressed.
- Schedule the follow-up visit.
- You may give the patient information leaflet with further information.
- Encourage the woman to return to the clinic at any time if necessary.
- Record the relevant information and thank her

Note *Contraceptive counseling often features in OSCE stations and it is therefore important to be familiar with the various contraceptive methods.*

41 Informed Consent

DEFINITION OF CONSENT

Consent is defined as an instrument of mutual communication between the doctor and patient with an expression of permission by the patient for the doctor to act in a particular way.

INFORMED CONSENT

- Obtaining consent is an ethical obligation and a legal compulsion.
- Informed consent must be taken after disclosure of adequate, accurate, and relevant information in a language that the patient can understand without any kind of coercion.
- Patient should be given an opportunity to ask questions and clarify all her doubts.
- Consent must be voluntary.
- Consent is mandatory for photographing patients, for participation in clinical trials and research projects.
- Patient should be >18 years to give informed consent. If less than 18 years, consent is obtained from a parent and child accent form is obtained at 12–18 years. In case of incapacitated patients, family members or legal guardian can give consent.

IMPLIED/EXPRESSED CONSENT

- The patient entering a doctor's consultation room and expressing her problem is taken as an implied consent for general physical examination and routine investigations. However, examination, especially in a female, invasive tests, and procedures require specific expressed consent.
- Expressed consent can be oral or written. Written consents are preferable in situations involving long-term follow-up, interventions, procedures, and surgeries.

The information disclosed should include:

- The condition/disease that the patient is suffering from
- Natural course of the condition and possible complications
- Treatment options available
- Consequences of non-treatment
- Potential risks and benefits of treatment options
- Duration and approximate cost of treatment
- Expected outcome
- Follow-up

DOCUMENTATION

It is important to document the process of consent taking.

The consent form should be:

- Prepared in duplicate and a copy handed over to the patient
- Dated and signed by the patient or guardian, the doctor, and a witness

Example of skill station on informed consent that may be kept for OSCE: Administer informed consent to a person wishing to undergo Medical Termination of Pregnancy

Appendices

Appendix 1

Mock Case Presentations

Obstetrics

Case presentation 1 (hypertension in pregnancy)

This is the case of Mrs. J, 27 years of age, W/o Mr. P, residing at Lawspet, Puducherry. She is educated up to 12th standard, works in a textile company, belongs to Class IV socioeconomic status, and her nearest health center is the Primary Health Center, Lawspet, which takes 5 minutes to travel by walk.

- She is a primigravida.
- Her last menstrual period (LMP) was on ___.
- Her expected date of delivery (EDD) is on _____.
- Period of gestation (POG) is 36+2 weeks of gestation; with regular 28 days menstrual cycles.
- She is booked and immunized.

Presenting complaints

She presented to OPD 2 days back with complaints of swelling of feet for the past 2 weeks, when she was found to have raised BP and hence admitted.

H/o presenting complaints

The patient was apparently normal until 2 weeks back when she started developing swelling of feet. The swelling is present throughout the day and does not subside with rest. She also noticed tightening of her toe rings.

- There is no H/o swelling of any other sites.
- There is no H/o headache, blurring of vision, epigastric pain or reduced urine output.
- There is no H/o breathlessness, easy fatigability, or palpitation.
- There is no H/o chest pain or syncope.
- Following admission, she says that her BP is being monitored four times per day, and blood and urine investigations and ultrasound have been done.

H/o present pregnancy

First trimester

- It was a spontaneous conception 10 months after marriage.
- Her pregnancy was confirmed at 45 days of amenorrhea by urine pregnancy test and dating scan was done during the same antenatal visit.
- No H/o hyperemesis gravidarum.
- No H/o bleeding per vaginum.
- No H/o fever with rash.
- No H/o exposure to radiation.
- She was prescribed folic acid tablets. No H/o any other drug intake.
- Blood and urine investigations were done and told to be normal.

Second trimester

- She had two antenatal visits in the second trimester.
- She perceived quickening at around 20 weeks.
- She received two doses of tetanus toxoid immunization at 5th and 6th month of pregnancy.
- She was prescribed iron and calcium supplementation and has been taking the medications regularly.
- There is no H/o bleeding per vaginum.
- There is no history suggestive of preeclampsia such as high BP recordings, excessive weight gain, swelling of feet, decreased urine output, headache, blurring of vision, and epigastric pain.

- Ultrasound was done in the 5th month of pregnancy and was told to be normal. Blood sugars were checked and said to be normal.

Third trimester

- She had two antenatal visits in the third trimester.
- She presented with swelling of feet during the last visit that was 2 days back, when she was found to have raised BP and hence admitted.
- There is no H/o decreased urine output and no H/o imminent symptoms such as headache, blurring of vision, and epigastric pain.
- She has been taking the iron and calcium supplementation regularly.
- She is perceiving normal fetal movements.
- There is no H/o bleeding P/V, leaking P/V, or pain abdomen.

Menstrual history

- She had regular menstrual cycles prior to conception with 4/28 day cycles with moderate blood flow.
- Her LMP was on _____.

Marital history

She is married for the past 1½ years. It is a nonconsanguineous marriage.

Obstetric history

She is a primigravida.

Past history

- No H/o diabetes mellitus (DM) or hypertension (HT).
- No past H/o any surgery or blood transfusion.
- No H/o jaundice, tuberculosis, or any other chronic medical illness.

Personal history

- The patient does not have any addictions such as smoking, alcohol, or tobacco chewing.
- Her sleep and appetite are normal.
- No H/o any drug allergy.

Family history

There is no family H/o DM, HT, multiple pregnancy, congenital anomalies, or tuberculosis.

Dietary history

She takes a mixed diet. Her total calorie intake is 2450 kcal and protein intake is 68 g/day, which is adequate in amount.

Examination

General physical examination

- The patient is comfortable at rest.
- She is averagely built and nourished.
- Her height is 158 cm and weight is 68 kg.
- Her prepregnancy BMI was 22.5.
- Her gait is normal.
- There is no pallor. Bilateral pitting pedal edema is present.
- There is no icterus, cyanosis, clubbing, and lymphadenopathy.

Vitals

- She is afebrile.
- Pulse rate is 80/min, regular in rhythm, normal volume, and character without any radio-femoral delay.
- BP is 150/90 mmHg, measured in right upper limb in sitting position.
- Respiratory rate is 20/min.

Thyroid and breast examinations

Breast and thyroid examinations are normal.

Systemic examination

- Cardiovascular and respiratory system examinations are within normal limits.
- Spine examination is normal.
- Knee jerks are normal.

Obstetric examination

Inspection

- Abdomen is uniformly distended. Umbilicus is everted.
- Linea nigra and striae gravidarum are present.
- Abdominal wall edema is present.
- No scars seen.
- Hernial sites are free of cough impulse.

Palpation

- Fundal height corresponds to 36 weeks.

- Symphysiofundal height is 35 cm.
- On performing the obstetric grips, the following are noted:
  - *Fundal grip:* Broad, soft, irregular mass is felt, suggestive of breech
  - *Lateral grip:* Uniformly curved resistance is felt on right side, suggestive of back; irregular, knobby structures are felt on left side, suggestive of limbs
  - *First pelvic grip:* Smooth, hard, globular, ballotable mass is felt, suggestive of fetal head
  - *Second pelvic grip:* Confirms the finding of first pelvic grip and hands are converging, suggestive that head is not engaged
- Liquor appears average.
- Uterus is relaxed during palpation.

Auscultation Fetal heart rate (FHR) is 140 beats/min, regular, heard on the right spinoumbilical line

Case summary

Example Mrs. J, 27 years of age, a primigravida at 36+2 weeks of gestation, booked and immunized, presents with the complaints of swelling of feet for the past 2 weeks. She was found to have elevated BP and admitted for the past 2 days. There is no H/o imminent symptoms. On examination, there is no pallor; pitting pedal edema is present and her BP is 150/90 mmHg. Her obstetric examination reveals fundal height up to 36 weeks of gestation with a singleton live fetus in cephalic presentation, FHR is 140 beats/min, regular, with adequate amount of liquor, and uterus is relaxed.

Case diagnosis

Example 27 years of age, primigravida at 36+2 weeks of gestation, with pregnancy-induced hypertension (PIH), with a singleton live fetus in cephalic presentation, not in labor, admitted for BP charting and further evaluation and management. Whether it is gestational hypertension (GHT) or preeclampsia (PE) can be made out only after testing for urine proteins. If proteinuria is present, it is PE and if proteinuria is absent, it is GHT.

Case presentation 2 (previous cesarean pregnancy with gestational diabetes mellitus)

This is the case of Mrs. L, 31 years of age, W/o Mr. KL, residing at Mudaliarpet, Puducherry. She is a B. Sc graduate, works as a clerk , belongs to Class III socioeconomic status, and her nearest health center is a Primary Health Center, Mudaliarpet, which takes 10 minutes to travel by walk.

- Her obstetric formula is G2P1L1.
- Her LMP was on ___.
- Her EDD is on _____.
- POG is 35+6 weeks of gestation; with regular 30 days menstrual cycles.
- She is booked and immunized.

Presenting complaints

She is a case of previous cesarean pregnancy, diagnosed with gestational diabetes mellitus (GDM) at 6th month of pregnancy, and is on insulin therapy. She presented to obstetrics OPD for routine antenatal checkup 1 day back and has been admitted for blood sugar profile.

H/o presenting complaints

She has no specific complaints and has been admitted for blood sugar profile. She is perceiving normal fetal movements. She says that after admission, blood sugars have been checked 7 times and other blood and urine tests and ultrasound have been done.

H/o present pregnancy

First trimester

- It was a spontaneous conception 4 years after her first pregnancy.
- Her pregnancy was confirmed 1 week after missed periods by urine pregnancy test.
- No H/o hyperemesis gravidarum.
- No H/o bleeding per vaginum
- No H/o fever with rash.
- No H/o exposure to radiation.
- She has taken folic acid supplementation. There is no H/o any other drug intake.
- Dating scan done, blood and urine investigations were done and told to be normal.

Second trimester

- She had two antenatal visits in the second trimester.
- She perceived quickening at around 20 weeks.
- She received two doses of tetanus toxoid immunization at 5th and 6th month of pregnancy.

- She was prescribed iron and calcium supplementation and has been taking the medications regularly.
- There is no H/o bleeding per vaginum.
- There is no history suggestive of preeclampsia such as high BP recordings, excessive weight gain, swelling of feet, decreased urine output, headache, blurring of vision, and epigastric pain.
- Oral glucose tolerance test done at 6th month of pregnancy was found to be abnormal. She was admitted for blood sugar profile and was started on insulin therapy. She administers the insulin injections by herself and her blood sugars have been monitored once in 2 weeks since then.
- Ultrasound was done in the 5th month of pregnancy and was told to be normal.

Third trimester

- She had three antenatal visits in the third trimester.
- There is no history suggestive of preeclampsia such as high BP recordings, excessive weight gain, swelling of feet, decreased urine output, headache, blurring of vision, and epigastric pain.
- She was admitted earlier at 8th month of pregnancy for blood sugar profile and insulin dose was adjusted.
- She has been taking the iron and calcium supplementation regularly.
- She is perceiving normal fetal movements.
- There is no H/o bleeding P/V, leaking P/V, or pain abdomen.
- She is now admitted for blood sugar profile. Blood and urine tests and ultrasound have been done. Test for fetal well-being probably a nonstress test (NST) has been done.

Menstrual history

- She had regular menstrual cycles prior to conception with 4/30 day cycles with moderate blood flow.
- Her LMP was on ______.

Marital history

She is married for 5 years. It is a nonconsanguineous marriage.

Obstetric history

She is G2P1L1.

First pregnancy

- It was a spontaneous conception 1 year after her marriage.
- Pregnancy was confirmed at 35 days of amenorrhea by urine pregnancy test.
- She was booked and immunized.
- Her antenatal period was uneventful.
- There was no H/o PIH, GDM, or antepartum hemorrhage (APH) during antenatal period.
- She had spontaneous onset of labor at term.
- She had an emergency cesarean section during labor in view of fetal distress.
- Intraoperative details are not available with the patient.
- No H/o fever, foul smelling lochia, wound discharge, wound gaping, or blood transfusion in the postoperative period.
- Urinary catheter was removed on day 1 and skin sutures were removed on day 7.
- It was a male baby, weighing 3.1 kg and the baby cried immediately following birth.
- She breast fed the baby 6 hours after delivery and exclusively breastfeeding was given for 6 months. The child had normal milestones and is doing well at present.
- Barrier method was used for contraception following pregnancy.

Past history

- No H/o DM or HT.
- No past H/o any surgery or blood transfusion.
- No H/o jaundice, tuberculosis, or any other chronic medical illness.

Personal history

- The patient does not have any addictions such as smoking, alcohol, or tobacco chewing.
- Her sleep and appetite are normal.
- No H/o any drug allergy.

Family history

- Her mother is a known diabetic.
- No H/o HT, multiple pregnancy, congenital anomalies, or tuberculosis in the family.

Dietary history

She is on diabetic diet. Her total calorie intake is 2250 kcal and protein intake is 65 g/day, which is adequate in amount.

Examination

General physical examination

- The patient is comfortable at rest.
- She is averagely built and nourished.
- Her height is 155 cm and weight is 72 kg.
- Her prepregnancy BMI was 26.
- Her gait is normal.
- There is no pallor or pedal edema.
- There is no icterus, cyanosis, clubbing, and lymphadenopathy.

Vitals

- She is afebrile.
- Pulse rate is 86/min, regular in rhythm, normal volume, and character without any radio-femoral delay.
- BP is 130/80 mmHg, measured in right upper limb in sitting position.
- Respiratory rate is 18/min.

Thyroid and breast examinations

Breast and thyroid examinations are normal.

Systemic examination

Cardiovascular and respiratory system examinations are within normal limits. Spine is normal.

Obstetric examination

Inspection

- Abdomen is uniformly distended. Umbilicus is everted.
- Linea nigra and striae gravidarum are present.
- Suprapubic transverse scar measuring about 12 cm is present and the scar is healthy. No sinuses.
- Hernial sites are free of cough impulse and no cough impulse at scar site.

Palpation

- Fundal height corresponds to 36 weeks.
- Symphysiofundal height is 37 cm.
- On performing the obstetric grips, the following are noted:
  - *Fundal grip:* Broad, soft, irregular mass is felt, suggestive of breech
  - *Lateral grip:* Uniformly curved resistance is felt on right side, suggestive of back; irregular, knobby structures are felt on left side, suggestive of limbs
  - *First pelvic grip:* Smooth, hard, globular, ballotable mass is felt, suggestive of fetal head
  - *Second pelvic grip:* Confirms the finding of first pelvic grip and hands are converging suggestive that head is not engaged
- Liquor appears average.
- Uterus is relaxed during palpation.
- There is no scar tenderness.

Auscultation FHR is 136 beats/min, regular, heard on the right spinoumbilical line.

Case summary

Example Mrs. L, 31 years of age, G2P1L1 at 35+6 weeks of gestation, booked and immunized, a case of previous cesarean pregnancy diagnosed to have GDM at 6th month of pregnancy and on insulin since then, now admitted during her routine antenatal checkup for blood sugar profile. She is perceiving normal fetal movements. Her first pregnancy was 4 years back. There is no H/o GDM in first pregnancy and she underwent an emergency cesarean section for fetal distress during labor. Her mother is a known diabetic. On examination, there is no pallor or pedal edema and her BP is 130/80 mmHg. Her obstetric examination reveals fundal height up to 36 weeks of gestation with a singleton live fetus in cephalic presentation, with good FHR, and adequate amount of liquor. Uterus is relaxed on palpation and there is no scar tenderness.

Case diagnosis

Example 31 years of age, G2P1L1 at 35+6 weeks of gestation, with previous cesarean pregnancy, with GDM on insulin, with a singleton live fetus in cephalic presentation, not in labor, admitted for blood sugar profile

Case presentation 3 (anemia in pregnancy)

This is the case of Mrs. Z, wife of Mr. D, 27 years of age, resident of Saram, Puducherry. She is educated up to 10th standard, is a housewife, belongs to Class IV socioeconomic class, and her nearest health center is Indira Gandhi Medical College, Kathirkamam, Puducherry, which takes 15 minutes to travel by bus.

Patient details

- She is gravida 3, para 2, with two living children.
- Her LMP was on __ and EDD is on __, with previous regular 28-day cycles.
- Her POG is 32 weeks.
- She is booked and immunized.

Presenting complaints

She presented to antenatal OPD with complaints of the following:
- Weakness and easy fatigability for the past 2 months
- Breathlessness on exertion for the past 2 weeks

H/o presenting complaints

- The patient complains of easy fatigability and weakness for the past 2 months that has gradually worsened over the days, and now she gets tired on doing routine household activities.
- The patient also complains of breathlessness on exertion since the past 2 weeks. It is not associated with palpitations, chest pain, or syncope.
- There is no H/o pedal edema or decreased urine output.
- There is no H/o asthma or chronic cough.
- There is no H/o passage of worms in stool, malena, or hematemesis.
- There is no H/o easy bruising or petechiae.
- There is no H/o fever with chills and rigors.
- During the routine antenatal visit, the patient was found to be anemic and has been admitted for the past 3 days for further evaluation and management.
- Blood and urine investigations and ultrasound have been done and the patient has received two doses of parenteral iron infusions.

H/o present pregnancy

First trimester

- It was a spontaneous conception 2 years following the last pregnancy. Pregnancy was confirmed by urine pregnancy test done at home
- No H/o hyperemesis
- No H/o bleeding per vaginum
- No H/o any drug intake
- No H/o fever with rash
- No H/o exposure to radiation
- No antenatal visits in the first trimester

Second trimester

- The patient had two antenatal visit in the second trimester at fourth month of pregnancy.
- She perceived quickening at around 20 weeks.
- She received one booster dose of tetanus toxoid immunization at fourth month of pregnancy.
- The patient was prescribed iron and calcium supplementation but she did not take the medications (on enquiring as to why she has not taken the medications, she said that as this was her third pregnancy, she was very casual about it).
- There is no H/o bleeding per vaginum.
- There is no history suggestive of preeclampsia such as high BP recordings, excessive weight gain, pedal edema, headache, blurring of vision, or epigastric pain.
- Blood investigations and ultrasound were done and told to be normal.

Third trimester

- The patient had one antenatal visit in the third trimester during which she was found to be anemic and has been admitted.
- She did not take the iron and calcium supplementation regularly.
- There is no history suggestive of preeclampsia such as high BP recordings, excessive weight gain, pedal edema, headache, blurring of vision, or epigastric pain.
- She is perceiving normal fetal movements.
- There is no H/o bleeding P/V, leaking P/V, or pain abdomen.

Menstrual history

- Her menstrual cycles prior to conception were regular 4/28 days cycles with normal blood flow.
- Her LMP was on _____.

Marital history

She is married for the past 4 years. It was a nonconsanguineous marriage.

Obstetric history

She is gravida 3, para 2, with two living children.

First pregnancy

- It was a spontaneous conception 6 months following marriage.
- The patient was booked and immunized.
- Her antenatal period was uneventful.
- It was a full-term normal vaginal delivery at Indira Gandhi Medical College, Puducherry. It was a female child weighing 2.8 kg with good Apgar scores.
- There is no history suggestive of postpartum hemorrhage (PPH). Postnatal period was uneventful.
- The child is at present alive and healthy, 3 years of age, and has been immunized.

Second pregnancy

- It was a spontaneous conception 1 year following the first pregnancy.
- The patient was booked and immunized. Her antenatal period was uneventful.
- It was a full-term normal vaginal delivery at Indira Gandhi Medical College, Puducherry. It was a female child weighing 3 kg with good Apgar scores.
- There is no history suggestive of PPH. Postnatal period was uneventful.
- The child is alive and healthy, 2 years of age, and has been immunized.
- She did not use any contraceptive methods in between pregnancies.

Past history

- There is no H/o DM or HT.
- There is no H/o surgery or blood transfusion in the past.
- There is no H/o jaundice, tuberculosis, or any other chronic illness.

Personal history

- The patient does not have any addictions such as smoking, alcohol, or tobacco chewing.
- Her sleep is normal.
- Her appetite has reduced for the past 2 months.

Family history

There is no family H/o DM, HT, multiple pregnancy, congenital anomalies, or tuberculosis.

Dietary history

She takes a mixed diet. Her total calorie intake is 1550 kcal and protein intake is 24 g/day, which is grossly deficient.

Examination

General physical examination

- The patient is thin built and averagely nourished.
- Her height is 158 cm and weight is 52 kg. Her prepregnancy BMI was 19.
- Her gait is normal.
- Pallor is present. There is no pedal edema.
- There is no icterus, cyanosis, clubbing, and lymphadenopathy.

Vitals

- She is afebrile.
- PR is 80/min, regular, good volume, and normal character without any radiofemoral delay.
- BP is 120/80 mmHg, measured in right upper limb in sitting position.
- Respiratory rate is 20/min.
- JVP is not raised.

Thyroid and breast examinations

Breast and thyroid examinations are normal.

Systemic examination

Cardiovascular system

S1 and S2 are normal. Ejection systolic murmur of grade II is heard over pulmonary area not radiating to any site.

Respiratory system

Air entry is equal on both the sides. There are no added sounds or crepts.

- Spine examination is normal.

Obstetric examination

Inspection

- Abdomen is uniformly distended. Umbilicus is everted.
- Linea nigra and striae gravidarum are present.
- No scars are seen.
- Hernial sites are free of cough impulse.

Palpation Fundal height corresponds to 32 weeks. Symphysiofundal height is 31 cm.

- **Fundal grip:** Broad, soft, irregular mass is felt, suggestive of breech.
- **Lateral grip:** Uniformly curved resistance is felt on right side, suggestive of back; and irregular, knobby structures are felt on left side, suggestive of limbs.
- **First pelvic grip:** Smooth, hard, globular, ballotable mass is felt, suggestive of fetal head. Liquor appears to be average and uterus is relaxed.
- **Second pelvic grip:** Confirms the findings of first pelvic grip.

Auscultation FHR is 140 beats/min, regular, heard on the right spinoumbilical line.

Case summary

Example Mrs. A, 28 years of age, G3P2L2 at 32 weeks of gestation, presents with complaints of tiredness and easy fatigability for the past 2 months and breathlessness on exertion for the past 15 days. She has not taken the iron and calcium prophylaxis regularly during this pregnancy. On examination, pallor is present; there is no pedal edema and the patient's BP is 120/80 mmHg. Her cardiovascular system examination reveals Grade II ejection systolic murmur in pulmonary area and respiratory system examination is normal. Her obstetric examination reveals fundal height up to 32 weeks with single live fetus in cephalic presentation, FHR 140 beats/min, regular, with adequate amount of liquor, and she is not in labor.

Case diagnosis

Example 28 years of age, G3P2L2 at 32 weeks of gestation, with anemia complicating pregnancy with a single live fetus in cephalic presentation, not in failure, not in labor, admitted for further evaluation and management

Gynecology

Case presentation 1 (fibroid uterus)

This is the case of Mrs. C, 41 years of age, W/o Mr. H, residing at Villianur, Puducherry. She is educated till 10th standard, a homemaker, and belongs to class III socioeconomic status.

Presenting complaints

She is a multiparous, sterilized woman presenting with complaints of heavy menstrual bleeding for the past 20 days.

H/o presenting complaints

- The patient presented to gynecology OPD with complaints of heavy menstrual bleeding for the past 10 days. The bleeding is associated with clots and she changes about five pads per day. There is H/o associated dysmenorrhea.
- There is no H/o preceding amenorrhea.
- She gives H/o similar episodes of excessive and prolonged bleeding lasting for 7–10 days during her menstrual cycles for the past 1 year for which she has been receiving symptomatic treated on and off.
- No H/o intermenstrual bleeding or post coital bleeding.
- No H/o pain abdomen, fever, or abnormal discharge P/V.
- No H/o dyspareunia.

Menstrual history

- She attained menarche at 14 years.
- Her previous menstrual cycles until 1 year back were regular 4/30 days cycle with no associated dysmenorrhea.
- Her LMP was 20 days back and is having bleeding since then.

Marital and sexual history

- She got married at the age of 25 and is married for the past 16 years. It was a nonconsanguineous marriage.
- She is sexually active with her partner. There is no H/o dyspareunia.

Obstetric history

- She is a multiparous woman (P2L2A1) with two living children.

- Her first pregnancy was at the age of 26 years and had a spontaneous vaginal delivery at term.
- Her second pregnancy was a spontaneous abortion at 60 days of pregnancy. D&E was not done.
- Her third pregnancy was at the age of 29 years and had a spontaneous vaginal delivery at term.
- There is no H/o obstetric complications.
- Her last child birth was 12 years back.
- She underwent puerperal sterilization following delivery of the second child.

Past medical/surgical history

- No H/o DM or HT.
- No H/o tuberculosis, jaundice, and thyroid disorders.
- No past H/o surgery except for the puerperal sterilization.
- No past H/o blood transfusion.
- No H/o sexually transmitted diseases.
- No H/o drug intake for any chronic medical illness.

Personal history

- No H/o alcohol intake, smoking, tobacco chewing, and drug addictions.
- No H/o drug allergy.
- Her sleep and appetite are normal.

Family history

- There is no H/o HT, DM, and tuberculosis in the family.
- There is no H/o genital malignancy among family members.

Examination

General physical examination

- The patient is comfortable at rest.
- She is averagely built and nourished.
- Her height is 156 cm and weight is 58 kg. Her BMI is 24.1.
- Pallor is present.
- There is no pedal edema, icterus, and lymphadenopathy.

Vitals

She is afebrile, PR is 84/min, BP is 130/80 mmHg, and respiratory rate is 18/min.

Breast and thyroid examinations

Her breast and thyroid examinations are normal.

Abdominal examination

Inspection

- Abdomen is symmetrical in shape and there is no abdominal distension.
- Umbilicus is normal and midline in position.
- Tubectomy scar is present.
- No sinuses or engorged veins are seen.
- There is no cough impulse at hernia orifices and at tubectomy scar site.

Palpation

- There is a mass arising from pelvis palpable up to 20 weeks in size. The mass is firm in consistency, with irregular surface; margins are well defined; upper and lateral borders are clearly made out but lower border is not made out. Side to side mobility is present and the mass is nontender on palpation.
- No hepatosplenomegaly.

Percussion There is a dull note on percussion over the mass.

Genital examination

External genitalia

External genitalia is healthy.

Per speculum examination (expected only from postgraduates)

- Vagina is healthy.
- Cervix is pointing downwards and is healthy.
- Bleeding through os is present.

Bimanual examination There is an irregularly enlarged mass arising from pelvis, palpable up to 20 weeks size. Uterus is not felt separately and movement of the mass is transmitted to the cervix.

Case summary

Example Mrs. C, 41 years of age, multiparous, sterilized woman presenting with complaints of menorrhagia for the past 20 days, and H/o similar complaints for the past 1 year. On examination, pallor is present, and her vitals are normal.

Abdominal examination reveals an irregularly enlarged mass arising from pelvis up to 20 weeks size. Cervix and vagina are healthy on speculum examination and on bimanual examination there is an irregularly enlarged mass arising from the pelvis up to 20 weeks size. Uterus is not separately felt and movement of the mass is transmitted to the cervix.

Case diagnosis

Example 41 years of age, multiparous, sterilized woman, with history and clinical examination findings suggestive of fibroid uterus.

Case presentation 2 (uterovaginal prolapse)

This is the case of Mrs. L, 61 years of age, W/o Mr. R, residing at Thengaithittu, Puducherry. She is educated up to 8th standard, an agricultural worker, and belongs to class IV socioeconomic status.

Presenting complaints

She is a multiparous, postmenopausal woman presenting with complaints of mass descending P/V for the past 6 months.

H/o presenting complaints

- The patient presented to gynecology OPD with complaints of mass descending P/V for the past 6 months. She was apparently healthy 6 months back when she started developing a mass descending per vaginum which kept progressively increasing in size up to the present size. The mass increases in size during coughing, straining at micturition, and defecation and reduces in size on lying down.
- She has inconvenience during walking due to the mass descending P/V.
- She has difficulty in micturition and is able to void only on reducing the mass. There is no H/o stress urinary incontinence.
- She has difficulty in defecation and is able to defecate only on keeping the mass reduced.
- She attained menopause 12 years back.
- No H/o postmenopausal bleeding or abnormal discharge P/V.
- No H/o chronic cough or constipation.

Menstrual history

- She attained menarche at 14 years.
- She used to have regular 4/30 day menstrual cycles.
- She attained menopause 12 years back.

Marital and sexual history

She got married at the age of 20 and is married for the past 21 years. She is currently not sexually active.

Obstetric history

- She is a multiparous woman (P3L3) with 3 living children.
- Her first pregnancy was at the age of 21 years. She delivered at a Government hospital. It was a spontaneous vaginal delivery at term, conducted by staff nurse. There is no H/o undue prolongation of labor and episiotomy was given. The baby was of average size and she exclusively breastfed the baby for 6 months. She resumed her routine activities immediately following the delivery and postnatal exercises were not done.
- Second pregnancy was 1 year after the first pregnancy. She delivered at a Government hospital. It was a spontaneous vaginal delivery at term, conducted by staff nurse. There is no H/o undue prolongation of labor and episiotomy was not given. The baby was of average size and she exclusively breastfed the baby for 6 months. She resumed her routine activities immediately following the delivery and postnatal exercises were not done.
- Third pregnancy was 2 years after the second pregnancy. It was a home delivery conducted by a dai (traditional birth attendant). It was a spontaneous vaginal delivery at term. There is no H/o undue prolongation of labor and episiotomy was not given. The baby was of average size and she exclusively breastfed the baby for 6 months. She resumed her routine activities immediately following the delivery and postnatal exercises were not done.
- There is no H/o obstetric complications in all the three pregnancies.
- Her last child birth was 37 years back.
- She underwent interval sterilization 1 year after delivery of the third child.

Past medical/surgical history

- No H/o DM or HT.
- No H/o tuberculosis, jaundice, and thyroid disorders.

- No H/o chronic cough.
- No past H/o surgery except for the puerperal sterilization.
- No past H/o blood transfusion.
- No H/o sexually transmitted diseases.
- No H/o drug intake for any chronic medical illness.

Personal history

- No H/o alcohol intake, smoking, tobacco chewing, and drug addictions.
- No H/o drug allergy.
- Her sleep and appetite are normal.

Family history

- There is no H/o HT, DM, and tuberculosis in the family.
- There is no H/o genital malignancy among family members.

Examination

General examination

- The patient is comfortable at rest.
- She is averagely built and nourished.
- Her height is 150 cm and weight is 56 Kg. Her BMI is 24.8.
- There is no pallor, pedal edema, and lymphadenopathy.

Vitals

She is afebrile, pulse rate is 88/min, BP is 136/84 mmHg, and respiratory rate is 16/min.

Breast and thyroid examinations

Breast and thyroid examinations are normal.

CVS and RS examinations

CVS and RS examinations are normal.

Abdominal examination

Inspection

- Abdomen is symmetrical in shape and there is no abdominal distension.
- Umbilicus is midline in position.
- Tubectomy scar is present.
- No sinuses or engorged veins are seen.
- There is no cough impulse at hernia orifices and at scar site.

Palpation Abdomen is soft and nontender on palpation.

Pelvic examination

External genitalia

- External genitalia appears atrophic with reduced labial pad of fat and sparse pubic hairs.
- There is no stress urinary incontinence.
- The introitus is gaping and cervix is lying 4 cm outside the introitus.
- Cervix appears congested; the vaginal mucosa is dry with loss of rugosities.
- There is a decubitus ulcer of size 1 × 1 cm in the anterior lip of cervix with healthy granulation tissue at the base of the ulcer.
- There is a visible bulge in the anterior vaginal wall with impulse on coughing suggestive of cystocele.

Palpation

- The mass can be reduced.
- On examination of the posterior vaginal wall after reducing the mass, a bulge is seen in the upper one-third of the posterior vaginal wall, suggestive of enterocele.
- There is a bulge in the lower two-third of the posterior vaginal wall, suggestive of rectocele.

Bimanual examination

- Uterine is retroverted, mobile, and atrophic.
- Fornices are free.

Examination of perineum Perineal body length is 3 cm and tone of the levators is average.

Case summary

Example Mrs. I, 61 years of age, para 4 live 4, presents with complaints of mass descending per vaginum for 2 years. On examination, there is no pallor and vitals are stable. Local examination reveals that cervix is lying 4 cm outside the introitus; cystocele, rectocele, and enterocele are present and the mass is reducible.

Case diagnosis

Example 61 years of age, multiparous, postmenopausal woman with third-degree uterovaginal prolapse with cystocele, rectocele, and enterocele.

Case presentation 3 (ovarian tumor)

This is the case of Mrs. V, 64 years of age, W/o Mr. G, residing at Muthirapalayam, Puducherry. She is educated up to 8th standard, a homemaker, and belongs to class III socioeconomic status.

Presenting complaints

She is P1L1, postmenopausal woman presenting with complaints of abdominal distension and pain abdomen for the past 2 months. She also gives H/o loss of appetite for the past 2 months.

H/o presenting complaints

- The patient was apparently healthy 2 months back, when she started developing abdominal distension that progressively increased over the past 2 months. There is H/o associated diffuse dull aching pain abdomen with no specific aggravating or relieving factors.
- She gives H/o bloating sensation and dyspeptic symptoms for the past 2 months.
- There is H/o decreased appetite for the past 2 months. There is no H/o loss of weight.
- No H/o postmenopausal bleeding.
- No H/o fever or abnormal discharge P/V.
- No H/o bowel or bladder disturbances.

Menstrual history

- She attained menarche at 12 years. She used to have regular 4/30 days menstrual cycles.
- She attained menopause at the age of 50 years.

Marital and sexual history

She got married at the age of 24 and is married for the past 40 years.

Obstetric history

- She is a P1L1 with 1 living child.
- It was a spontaneous conception at the age of 29 years. She had a full term vaginal delivery and postnatal period was uneventful.
- She did not use any contraception following delivery; however, did not have any further pregnancies.

Past medical/surgical history

- No H/o DM. She is a known hypertensive for the past 10 years and is on medications.
- No H/o tuberculosis, jaundice, and thyroid disorders.
- No past H/o surgery or blood transfusion.
- No H/o sexually transmitted diseases.
- No H/o drug intake for any chronic medical illness.

Personal history

- No H/o alcohol intake, smoking, tobacco chewing, and drug addictions.
- No H/o drug allergy.
- Her sleep is normal.
- Appetite is reduced for the past 2 months.

Family history

- There is no H/o HT, DM, and tuberculosis in the family.
- There is no H/o genital malignancy among family members.

Examination

General examination

- The patient is comfortable at rest.
- She is averagely built and nourished.
- Her height is 156 cm and weight is 68 kg.
- Pallor is present.
- There is no pedal edema, icterus, and lymphadenopathy.

Vitals

She is afebrile, pulse rate is 86/min, BP is 140/80 mmHg, and respiratory rate is 20/min.

Breast and thyroid examinations

Breast and thyroid examinations are normal.

Abdominal examination

Inspection

- Abdomen appears distended. The skin over the abdomen is stretched and shiny.

- Umbilicus is everted and midline in position.
- No scars, sinuses, or engorged veins are seen.
- There is no cough impulse at hernia orifices.

Palpation

- There is a mass arising from pelvis enlarged up to 24 weeks size with variegated consistency, irregular surface, restricted mobility, and is nontender on palpation. The margins of the mass are not well defined and the lower border of the mass is not palpable.
- There is no hepatosplenomegaly.
- No fluid thrill is present.

Percussion There is a dull note over the mass. Shifting dullness could not be elicited.

Pelvic examination

External genitalia

External genitalia is healthy.

Per speculum examination (expected only from postgraduates)

Cervix and vagina are healthy.

Bimanual examination

It confirms the palpation findings. There is a mass arising from pelvis, enlarged up to 24 weeks size and the mass is firm in consistency, with irregular surface. The mass is tipped through the right fornix. The mass is felt separately from the uterus and the uterus is normal in size. The movement of the mass is not transmitted to the cervix.

Rectal and rectovaginal examinations

Nodules are felt in pouch of Douglas (POD). Rectal mucosa and parametrium are free.

Case summary

Example Mrs. V, 64 years of age, para 1 live 1, postmenopausal woman, presents with complaints of progressively increasing abdominal distension with diffuse pain abdomen and dyspeptic symptoms for 2 months. Associated loss of appetite is present. On examination, a 24-week-sized, ill-defined, nontender mass with variegated consistency, irregular surface, and restricted mobility is felt arising from the pelvis. Bimanual examination confirms the inspection findings and the mass is tipped through the right fornix. The mass is felt separately from the uterus and the movement of the mass is not transmitted to the cervix. On rectal and rectovaginal examinations, POD nodules are present.

Case diagnosis

64 years of age, para 1 live 1, postmenopausal woman with abdominopelvic mass. Considering her history of rapid progression of symptoms and presentation within a short time span and the examination findings, it is most likely to be a case of ovarian tumor, probably malignant.

Appendix 2

Reference Intervals of Common Laboratory Parameters

This appendix contains tables of reference values for common laboratory tests used in Obstetrics and Gynecology. A variety of factors can influence reference values such as the population studied, duration and means of specimen transport, and the laboratory methods used. The reference ranges given in this appendix may therefore not be appropriate for all laboratories, and these values should only be used as general guidelines. Whenever possible, reference values provided by the laboratory performing the tests should be used in the interpretation of laboratory data.

Table 1 Biochemistry

Parameter	Specimen	Reference interval	Units
Glucose (fasting)	P	75–100	mg/dL
Glycated hemoglobin	B	5.8	%
Liver function tests			
• Alanine aminotransferase (ALT)	S	5–40	IU/L
• Aspartate transaminase (AST)	S	10–40	IU/L
• Alkaline phosphatase	S	35–100	IU/L
• Lactate dehydrogenase (LDH)	S	70–250	IU/L
• Bilirubin (total)	S	0.3–1.3	mg/dL
• Bilirubin (direct)	S	0.1–0.4	mg/dL
• Bilirubin (indirect)	S	0.2–0.9	mg/dL
• Protein (total)	P	6.7–8.6	g/dL
• Albumin	P	3.5–5	g/dL
• Globulin	P	2–3.5	g/dL
Renal function tests			
• Serum creatinine	S	Female (0.5–1) Male (0.6–1.2)	mg/dL mg/dL
• Blood urea	P	15–40	mg/dL
Uric acid	S	2.5–5.6	mg/dL
Serum electrolytes			
• Bicarbonate	S	24–30	mmol/L
• Chloride	S	102–109	mmol/L or meq/L
• Sodium	S	133–145	mmol/L or meq/L
• Potassium	S	3.5–5.0	mmol/L or meq/L
• Magnesium	S	0.6–0.9 or 1.5–2.3	mmol/L mg/dL
• Calcium (ionized)	WB	4.5–5.3	mg/dL
• Calcium (total)	S	8.7–10.2	mg/dL
• Osmolality	P	275–295	mOsmol/kg serum water

(CONTD...)

Table 1 *(CONTD...)*

Parameter	Specimen	Reference interval	Units
Lipid profile	S		
• Cholesterol		150–200	mg/dL
• Triglycerides		80–150	mg/dL
• High-density lipoprotein		35–60	mg/dL
• Low-density lipoprotein		80–150	mg/dL
• Very low-density lipoprotein		10–30	mg/dL
Folate	S	5–18	ng/mL
Red cell folate	B	150–450	ng/mL cells
Ferritin	P	10–150	µg/L
Total iron binding capacity	S	54–75	µmol/L
Transferrin	S	200–400	mg/dL
Vitamin B_{12}	S	280–1000	pg/mL
Follicle-stimulating hormone (FSH)	S, P		
• Menstruating			
– Follicular phase		3–20	mIU/L
– Ovulatory phase		9–26	mIU/L
– Luteal phase		1–12	mIU/L
• Postmenopausal		18–150	mIU/L
Luteinizing hormone (LH)	S, P		
• Menstruating			
– Follicular phase		2–15	mIU/mL
– Ovulatory phase		8–76	mIU/mL
– Luteal phase		0.6–19	mIU/mL
• Postmenopausal		16–64	mIU/mL
Estradiol—female	S, P		
• Menstruating			
– Follicular phase		20–145	pg/mL
– Midcycle peak		112–450	pg/mL
– Luteal phase		20–241	pg/mL
• Postmenopausal		<59	pg/mL
Testosterone, free	S		
• Female		3–20	pg/mL
• Male		90–300	pg/mL
Testosterone, total	S		
• Female		6–86	ng/dL
• Male		270–1070	ng/dL
Thyroid function tests			
• Thyroid-stimulating hormone (TSH)	S	0.5–5.7	mIU/L
• Thyroxine (T4)	S	70–140	nmol/L
• Thyroxine (free T4)	S	9–16	pmol/L
• Tri-iodothyronine (T3)	S	2.5–6.7	nmol/L
Prolactin	S	Female 40–530	mg/L
HCG	S		
• Nonpregnant females		<5	IU/L
• 1–2 weeks post conception		9–130	IU/L

(CONTD...)

Table 1 (*CONTD...*)

Parameter	Specimen	Reference interval	Units
• 3–4 weeks post conception		75–2600	IU/L
• 4–5 weeks post conception		4000–1,00,200	IU/L
• 5–10 weeks post conception		11,500–2,89,000	IU/L
• 10–14 weeks post conception		18,300–1,37,000	IU/L
• Second trimester		1400–53,000	IU/L
• Third trimester		940–60,000	IU/L
CA 125	S	<35	U/mL

Table 2 Urine

Parameter	Specimen	Reference interval	Units
Protein		Negative	
Sugar		Negative	
Microscopy			
• RBC		0–2	Per high power field
• WBC		0–5	Per high power field
24-hour urine protein	U	<150	mg/24 h

Table 3 Hematology

Parameter	Specimen	Reference interval	Units
Total white blood cell (WBC) count	WB	4000–11000	Cells/µL
Differential WBC count	WB		%
• Neutrophils		40–70	
• Lymphocytes		20–50	
• Eosinophils		0–6	
• Basophils		0–2	
• Monocytes		4–8	
Red blood cell (RBC) count	WB	4–5.5	Million cells/cu. mm
Hemoglobin	WB	• Male 13–16 • Female 12–15 g/dL	g/dL g/dL
Hematocrit	WB	36–46	%
Mean corpuscular volume (MCV)	WB	76–96	fL
Mean corpuscular hemoglobin (MCH)	WB	27–32	pg/cell
Mean corpuscular hemoglobin concentration (MCHC)	WB	32–36	g/dL
Platelet count	WB	1.5–4	Lakhs/cubic mm
Reticulocyte count	WB	0.8–2	%
Prothrombin time (PT)	P	12–16	Seconds
Activated partial thromboplastin time (aPTT)	P	26–40	Seconds
Erythrocyte sedimentation rate (ESR)	WB	• Males 0–15 • Females 0–20	mm/h
Fibrinogen degradation product (FDP)	P	0–1	mg/L
Fibrinogen	P	230–500	mg/dL

P, plasma (heparin bottle); *S*, serum (clotted); *WB*, whole blood (EDTA bottle).

Appendix 3

Calorie and Protein Values of Some Common Food Items

Table Calorie and protein values of some common food items

Beverages			
Food item	**Quantity**	**Calories (Cal)**	**Proteins (g)**
Cow's milk	100 mL	70	3.3
Buffalo's milk	100 mL	107	3.7
Skimmed milk	100 mL	30	2.6
Curd	100 mL	60	3.1
Tea (without sugar)	250 mL	86	4.3
Tea (with sugar)	250 mL	102	4.3
Instant coffee	250 mL	136	3.8
Buttermilk	100 mL	30	1
Lemonade	100 mL	16	0.1
Orange juice	100 mL	48	0.7
Breakfast items			
Cornflakes with milk	1 cup	220	5
• White bread • Brown bread	1 slice (22 g)	54 50	1.7 1.8
Boiled egg	1 no	90	6.5
Omelette	1 no	160	6.5
Upma	1 cup	170	4.4
Poha	1 cup	270	5.7
Kichidi	1 cup	200	3.5
Plain chapati	1 no (35 g)	85	2.5
Plain paratha	1 no (50 g)	150	4.5
Puri	1 no (25 g)	80	2
Idli	1 no (40 g)	55	2.2
Dosa (plain)	1 no (40 g)	80	2
Vada (masala vada)	1 no (40 g)	103	2.6
Vada (medu vada)	1 no (65 g)	226	6.8
Pongal	100 g	103	2.6

(CONTD...)

Table *(CONTD...)*

Food item	Quantity	Calories (Cal)	Proteins (g)
Tomato chutney	1 tablespoon	10	0.3
Coconut chutney	1 tablespoon	60	0.5
Instant noodles	100 g	413	9.2
Cheese	100 g	350	24
Butter	100 g	730	0
Main meals			
Boiled rice	100 g	54	1.2
Pulao	100 g	108	3.4
Dal (cooked lentils)	100 g	100	6
Sambar	100 g	55	2
Cooked vegetables	100 g	36	1.2
Beans (boiled)	100 g	20	2
Cabbage (boiled)	100 g	17	1.2
Carrot (boiled)	100 g	20	0.6
Cauliflower (boiled)	100 g	10	1.5
Cucumber (raw)	100 g	10	0.6
Peas (boiled)	100 g	50	5
Potatoes (boiled)	100 g	80	1
Tomato	100 g	20	0.5
Tapioca	100 g	80	0.2
Sweet potato	100 g	100	0.3
Lady finger	100 g	27	0.2
Brinjal	100 g	27	0.4
Pumpkin	100 g	24	0.2
Chicken curry	100 g	110	25
Mutton curry	100 g	200	30
Fish curry	100 g	100	18
Desserts and snacks			
Ice cream (vanilla)	100 g	260	2
Halwa	100 g	200	1.7
Good day biscuit	1 no	40	0.7
Parle-G/marie gold/krackjack	1 no	20	0.5
Samosa	Regular size (100 g)	270	4
Pizza	1 slice (100 g)	370	12
Pav bhaji	1 plate (250 g)	118	8
Sandwiches	2 slices	200	5
Peanuts (roasted)	100 g	570	20

(CONTD...)

Table (*CONTD...*)

Food item	Quantity	Calories (Cal)	Proteins (g)
Fruits			
Banana	100 g	110	1.3
Jackfruit	100 g	90	2
Sapota	100 g	100	0.7
Mango	100 g	80	0.8
Apple	100 g	60	0.2
Cherries	100 g	50	0.6
Grapes	100 g	60	0.6
Oranges	100 g	35	1
Guava	100 g	32	0.3
Nuts			
Almond	100 g	655	21
Cashew nuts	100 g	600	21
Raisins	100 g	300	2
Groundnuts	100 g	570	25
Pista	100 g	630	20
Dates	100 g	300	2.5

Note: This appendix contains calorie and protein values for common food items, so as to help the students calculate dietary intake of calories and proteins during pregnancy while taking a diet history. The values may vary depending on the variety of food item, oil content, etc. The values given in this appendix are only appropriate values and these values should only be used as general guidelines.

Index

Note: Page numbers followed by *t* and *f* indicate table and figure respectively.

H

J

K

L

P